CLINICAL MANUAL OF

ELECTROPHYSIOLOGY

CLINICAL MANUAL OF
ELECTROPHYSIOLOGY

Edited by

IGOR SINGER, M.B.B.S., F.R.A.C.P., F.A.C.P., F.A.C.C.

Associate Professor of Medicine
Chief, Arrhythmia Service
Director of Cardiac Electrophysiology and Pacing
School of Medicine
University of Louisville
Louisville, Kentucky

JOEL KUPERSMITH, M.D., F.A.C.P., F.A.C.C.

Professor and Chairman
Department of Medicine
College of Human Medicine
Michigan State University
East Lansing, Michigan

SANS TACHE
WILLIAMS & WILKINS
BALTIMORE • HONG KONG • LONDON • MUNICH
PHILADELPHIA • SYDNEY • TOKYO

Editor: Jonathan W. Pine, Jr.
Managing Editor: Carol Lindley Eckhart
Copy Editor: Joseph Pomerance
Designer: Karen S. Klinedinst
Illustration Planner: Ray Lowman
Production Coordinator: Barbara J. Felton

Accurate indications, adverse reactions, and dosage schedules for drugs are provided in this book, but it is possible that they may change. The reader is urged to review the package information data of the manufacturers of the medications mentioned.

Printed in the United States of America

Chapter reprints are available from the Publisher.

Library of Congress Cataloging-in-Publication Data

Clinical manual of electrophysiology / edited by Igor Singer. Joel Kupersmith.
p. cm.
Includes index.
ISBN 0-683-07735-X
1. Cardiac pacing. 2. Electrophysiology. I. Singer. Igor. II. Kupersmith, Joel.
[DNLM: 1. Arrhythmia—physiopathology. 2. Arrhythmia—therapy. 3. Electric Countershock.
4. Electrophysiology. WG 330 C6416]
RC684.P3C55 1992
616.1′280645—dc20
DNLM/DLC
for Library of Congress

92-5082
CIP

92 93 94 95 96
1 2 3 4 5 6 7 8 9 10

To my wife, Sylvia, my children, Justin, Jessica, and Christina, and my parents for their untiring support and encouragement.

I owe a great deal to the late Dr. Michel Mirowski, who encouraged me to pursue a career in electrophysiology, and Dr. Myron Weisfeldt, who supported and continues to support my career goals.

I.S.

To my wife, Judy, and my children, David, Rebecca, and Adam, whose support and help have been crucial to this book.

To my teachers and to house staff and students who have been a constant source of inspiration.

J.K.

FOREWORD

Cardiac electrophysiology has a centuries-old research heritage using myriad techniques from counting the pulse to molecular genetics. This work has produced a large body of knowledge about the electrical properties of the heart. With the advent of the body surface electrocardiogram almost 100 years ago, a serious and productive study of human cardiac arrhythmias was launched. Clinical electrophysiology began in the mid 1960s and this relatively new discipline forges a link between basic and applied animal research and clinical arrhythmias as detected by the body surface electrocardiogram (12-lead ECG, intensive care unit monitors, Holter (24-hour continuous) ECG recordings, and transtelephonic ECG). In the 25-year span of clinical electrophysiology, diagnostic methods have produced a deluge of information about the electrophysiologic basis for clinical arrhythmias and conduction defects in human disease. Also, clinical electrophysiologic methods have played a major role in developing treatments for cardiac rhythm disturbances like new drugs, surgical techniques, and devices for treating either brady- or tachyarrhythmias.

More recently, clinical electrophysiology has experienced another breakthrough with the advent of interventional electrophysiology. Now in its early stages of development, interventional electrophysiology has developed and is applying methods for mapping cardiac arrhythmias with catheter electrodes under fluoroscopic guidance and for ablating tissues that are critical components of the abnormal circuits that generate cardiac arrhythmias. The primary targets of these early efforts with catheter ablation are atrioventricular (AV) reentrant tachycardia using accessory AV connections (Wolff-Parkinson-White Syndrome) and AV nodal reentrant tachycardia. Other arrhythmias have been attacked with limited success and many more should soon be amenable to treatment with catheter ablation as future technical advances are made. The technical advances developed for interventional electrophysiology will form a firm platform from which to launch additional research efforts and another flood of information about the electrophysiology of the human heart will inevitably result.

The result of the intense research activity in basic and clinical electrophysiology is a bewildering breadth and depth of knowledge about cardiac electrophysiology and cardiac arrhythmias. At the same time, many pieces of the electrophysiologic puzzle are still missing so that a totally coherent framework is not available to organize all this information. Accordingly, a medical student, medical house officer, or cardiology fellow is confronted with a monumental mass of information when he or she turns to the cardiac electrophysiology literature. There is a need for a collection of fundamental information about the various subspecialty areas of clinical electrophysiology to help physicians deal with the practical issues involved in the diagnosis and treatment of cardiac arrhythmias and conduction defects.

In *Clinical Manual of Electrophysiology*, Singer and Kupersmith attempt to provide a rational view of the information explosion in cardiac electrophysiology to guide physicians to the information they need to understand and treat patients with cardiac arrhythmias or conduction defects. Their book starts with two chapters that explore basic concepts of electrophysiology and mechanisms of cardiac arrhythmias. The introduction continues with chapters on clinical approaches to human cardiac arrhythmias and a discussion of the basic cardiac electrophysiologic study. After providing this general information, the book devotes chapters to the workup of several specific clinical problems: syncope, cardiac arrest, tachycardia with narrow QRS, ventricular tachycardia, the Wolff-Parkinson-White syndrome, and the long QT syndrome. Finally the book devotes one or more chapters to discuss each of the following treatment options for cardiac arrhythmias and conduction defects: antiarrhythmic drugs, implanted electronic pacemakers, external cardioversion and defibrillation, cardiopulmonary resuscitation, implanted cardioverter-defibrillators, antitachycardia pacemakers, operative treatment of supraventricular or ventricular tachycardia and catheter ablation. The book is generously referenced with classic and contemporary literature citations and also provides helpful illustrations to clarify important points.

Clinical Manual of Electrophysiology, will provide a valuable resource for students, house staff, cardiology fellows, internists, and cardiologists. It will provide an excellent introduction to electrophysiologic concepts and practice. The organization of the book will permit physicians faced with specific problems to rapidly find the information they need to manage their patients. Physicians who want more details or to review the original data supporting conclusions and recommendations will find ample literature citations to provide this information.

Because there is nothing quite like *Clinical Manual of Electrophysiology* available today, this book will fill a niche between cardiology textbooks/monographs and journal articles. As a result, the book should prove a useful resource for students and physicians in teaching hospitals and for internists and cardiologists who are in practice.

J. THOMAS BIGGER, JR., M.D.
Professor of Medicine and of Pharmacology
Columbia University
New York, New York

PREFACE

Few fields have had such a vast explosion of knowledge as clinical electrophysiology since its establishment as a discipline more than twenty years ago. These include the advent of highly sophisticated devices such as implantable cardioverter defibrillators, antitachycardia and rate adaptive pacemakers, new methods of mapping and arrhythmia surgery, and vastly expanded knowledge about pharmacotherapy. We have seen the development of techniques, essential now, that were unknown just a few years ago. These advances have made clinical electrophysiology an important part of modern clinical cardiology.

With the increased importance of these disciplines it is essential that the clinician have an understanding of the field. There is also a need to present the massive amounts of material available in a coordinated fashion.

The impetus for writing this book was provided by a perceived need to provide a comprehensive, contemporary view of clinical electrophysiology and to provide a text for fellows, residents, general cardiologists, and associated professionals who have a need for specialized knowledge in electrophysiology. Many excellent texts that are devoted to basic and applied electrophysiology already exist. Some are specialized or focused, some presume knowledge of electrophysiology, some, on the other hand, are too basic.

The objective of this book is to provide an integrated textbook for the novice or generalist but one comprehensive enough for the more advanced student. *Clinical Manual of Electrophysiology* is written with both of them in mind. It has useful information of both practical and conceptual nature. Thus its purpose is to present this discipline to the generalists in an understandable way and to synthesize and organize techniques, concepts, and methods of clinical electrophysiology for the more advanced student of the field.

Clinical Manual of Electrophysiology is divided into five parts. Part I describes the basic field of electrophysiology and mechanisms of arrhythmia. Part II is devoted to the clinical approach to arrhythmias, focusing on the clinical electrophysiologic techniques used to diagnose and manage patients with specific arrhythmias. Part III reviews pacing for bradyarrhythmias and the approach to pacing therapy. Part IV is focused on therapy for tachyarrhythmias, including basic concepts of cardioversion and defibrillation, discussion of cardioverter-defibrillators, and antitachycardia pacemakers. Part V discusses surgical and catheter ablation techniques for supraventricular and ventricular tachycardias. A special section is devoted to resuscitation.

We hope that this book will bridge the gap between the very basic and the specialized texts. Further, we hope that this book will lead to a better understanding of the growing field of clinical electrophysiology and the approaches it offers ultimately benefitting our patients.

ACKNOWLEDGMENTS

I would especially like to acknowledge the help of my secretaries Mary Lou Kapfhammer and Sharon J. McGregor for tireless typing effort, many revisions of the manuscript, and their patience.

I. S.

I would like to acknowledge Nancy Farmer, Donna Robbins, Martha Muth, and Gayle Vietti for their secretarial assistance. I would also like to acknowledge Claudio Maldonado and Dr. Zhen Yuan Li for their valuable collaboration in work cited and support from the Hearst Foundation, National Heart, Lung and Blood Institute, and American Heart Association, New York City and Kentucky affiliates.

J. K.

CONTRIBUTORS

Antonio Asso, M.D.
Fellow, Cardiac Electrophysiology
University of Minnesota Hospital
Minneapolis, Minnesota
5. Evaluation of Syncope

Stanley M. Bach, Jr., B.S.E.E., M.D.
Scientific Advisor
Cardiac Pacemakers, Inc.
St. Paul, Minnesota
19. Electrical Cardioversion and Defibrillation

S. Serge Barold, M.B., B.S., F.R.A.C.P., F.A.C.P., F.A.C.C., F.E.S.C.
Professor of Medicine
Chief of Cardiology
The Genesee Hospital
University of Rochester School of Medicine and Dentistry
Rochester, New York
14. Indications for Permanent Cardiac Pacemakers
15. Single- and Dual-Chamber Pacemakers: Electrophysiology, Pacing Modes, and Multiprogrammability
16. Hemodynamics of Cardiac Pacing and Rate-Adaptive Pacemakers
17. Pacemaker Selection for the Individual Patient
18. Complications and Follow-up of Cardiac Pacemakers

David G. Benditt, M.D., F.A.C.C.
Professor of Medicine, Cardiovascular Division
Director, Cardiac Arrhythmia Service
University of Minnesota Medical School
University of Minnesota Hospital
Minneapolis, Minnesota
5. Evaluation of Syncope

Frank J. Callaghan, M.S., M.S.E.E.
Director of Research and Development
Telectronics Pacing Systems
Miami, Florida
13. Current and Future Lead Technology

Mark S. Christensen, B.A.
Lead Systems Product Development
Telectronics Pacing Systems
Englewood, Colorado
13. Current and Future Lead Technology

Alan D. Guerci, M.D., F.A.C.C.
Executive Vice President for Medical Affairs
Director of Research
St. Francis Hospital
Roslyn, New York
25. Cardiopulmonary Resuscitation

Gerard M. Guiraudon, M.D., F.R.C.S. (C), F.A.C.C.
Professor of Surgery
University of Western Ontario
Cardiovascular and Thoracic Surgeon
University Hospital
London, Ontario
Canada
22. Operative Treatment of Supraventricular Tachycardia
23. Surgical Management of Ventricular Tachycardia

George J. Klein, M.D., F.R.C.P. (C), F.A.C.C.
Professor of Medicine
University of Western Ontario
Director, Arrhythmia Service
University Hospital
London, Ontario
Canada
22. Operative Treatment of Supraventricular Tachycardia
23. Surgical Management of Ventricular Tachycardia
24. Catheter Ablation

Joel Kupersmith, M.D., F.A.C.P., F.A.C.C.
Professor & Chairman
Department of Medicine
College of Human Medicine
Michigan State University
East Lansing, Michigan
1. Basic Concepts
2. Mechanisms of Arrhythmia
3. Clinical Approach to the Patient with Arrhythmia
10. Long QT Syndrome
11. Antiarrhythmic Drugs: General Principles
12. Antiarrhythmic Drugs: Specific Agents

Morton Mower, M.D., F.A.C.P., F.A.C.C., F.C.C.P.
Vice President
Cardiac Pacemakers, Inc.
St. Paul, Minnesota
Visiting Associate Professor
The Johns Hopkins Hospital
Baltimore, Maryland
20. Implantable Cardioverter Defibrillator

Andrea Natale, M.D.
Fellow, Cardiac Electrophysiology
Department of Medicine
University of Western Ontario
University Hospital
London, Ontario
Canada
22. Operative Treatment of Supraventricular Tachycardia
23. Surgical Management of Ventricular Tachycardia
24. Catheter Ablation

Stephen Remole, M.D.
Fellow, Cardiac Electrophysiology
University of Minnesota Hospital
Minneapolis, Minnesota
5. Evaluation of Syncope

Igor Singer, M.B.B.S., F.R.A.C.P., F.A.C.P., F.A.C.C.
Associate Professor of Medicine
Chief, Arrhythmia Service
Director of Cardiac Electrophysiology and Pacing
School of Medicine
University of Louisville
Louisville, Kentucky
3. Clinical Approach to the Patient with Arrhythmia
4. Electrophysiologic Study
6. Evaluation of a Resuscitated Patient with Aborted Sudden Cardiac Death
7. Narrow QRS Complex Tachycardia
8. Ventricular Tachycardia
9. Wolff-Parkinson-White and Other Preexcitation Syndromes
20. Implantable Cardioverter Defibrillator
21. Antitachycardia Pacemakers
26. Approach to Resuscitation in the Electrophysiology Laboratory

David Slater, M.D., F.A.C.C.
Associate Professor of Surgery
University of Louisville
Louisville, Kentucky
20. Implantable Cardioverter Defibrillator

Marcus F. Stoddard, M.D., F.A.C.C.
Assistant Professor of Medicine
Director, Noninvasive Cardiology
University of Louisville
Louisville, Kentucky
3. Clinical Approach to the Patient with Arrhythmia

Tibor S. Szabo, M.D.
Instructor in Medicine
Cardiology Division
Staff Electrophysiologist
V.A. Medical Center
University of Louisville
Louisville, Kentucky
7. Narrow QRS Complex Tachycardia
9. Wolff-Parkinson-White and Other Preexcitation Syndromes

Mark Wathen, M.D.
Assistant Professor
Vanderbilt University
Nashville, Tennessee
24. Catheter Ablation

Raymond Yee, M.D., F.R.C.P. (C), F.A.C.C.
Assistant Professor
Department of Medicine
University of Western Ontario
Director, Arrhythmia Monitoring Unit
University Hospital
London, Ontario
Canada
22. Operative Treatment of Supraventricular Tachycardia
23. Surgical Management of Ventricular Tachycardia
24. Catheter Ablation

CONTENTS

I

BASIC MECHANISMS

BASIC CONCEPTS

Joel Kupersmith, M.D., F.A.C.P., F.A.C.C.

Basic concepts in electrophysiology are crucial in understanding and evaluating the clinical situation. In no other clinical discipline is information gained in the basic laboratory so closely related to clinical endeavor. This chapter will deal with recording techniques, normal and abnormal action potentials, ionic currents and other aspects of basic electrophysiology.

PART I
RECORDING TECHNIQUES

INTRACELLULAR RECORDINGS

The fundamental recording of electrophysiology is the intracellular action potential. The first such recording in the heart was reported by Ling and Gerard in 1949. Subsequently, the technique was elaborated in several important laboratories, including those of Weidmann (1), Hoffman (2), Cranefield (2), Hecht, Trautwein, and Carmeleit.

Intracellular action potentials are recorded by glass microelectrodes filled with highly conductive 3M K^+ and designed to detect voltage deflections. Tip diameter of the microelectrodes is approximately 1 μm so as to enable them to puncture cardiac cells. Apparatus associated with the electrodes includes high-resistance preamplifiers which then transfer the signal to an oscilloscope, a heat or ink paper recorder (not as good for fast transients that occur in the action potential upstroke), or more recently, computer analog to digital converters for data storage and analysis.

Figure 1.1 shows an example of action potentials recorded by this technique in myocardium and sinus node. The action potentials shown are recordings of voltage changes that occur during a cardiac electrical cycle. In a related technique called "voltage clamp," voltage is kept constant and one thus records intracellular current rather than voltage changes. Voltage clamp, which will not be discussed further, has been the primary method of elucidating the various types of ionic currents that occur in the heart.

Although the above-mentioned intracellular techniques predominate, others have recently come into use for sophisticated analysis. Using ion-sensitive resins placed in glass microelectrodes, it is possible to record both intracellular and extracellular ionic changes. These electrodes have been particularly employed for K^+ (4), Na^+, and Ca^{++}.

Fluorescent dyes have also been used, both to detect intracellular ionic change (especially Ca^{++}) (5) and to record cellular potential changes (6). A number of ion and potential sensitive fluorescent dyes exists for this purpose along with the sophisticated spectroscopic apparatus that is necessary to process the signals. Unfortunately, because of the toxicity of the dyes and the technical complexity of applying these techniques, they have not yet come into clinical use.

EXTRACELLULAR RECORDINGS

At present, intracellular recordings are only experimental and not a part of clinical electrophysiology. Clinical testing is involved solely with extracellular recording techniques. Extracellular recordings can be made either endo- or epicardially. Clinical invasive electrophysiologic testing involves recordings made by catheters placed transvenously and/or rarely transarterially. Surgical mapping techniques involve recordings made directly on the heart in the open chest and can be either endo- or epicardial (7). Additionally, implanted pacemakers and defibrillators now have the capacity to make and measure extracellular recordings for long-term device assessment and monitoring purposes.

A recording made directly on the heart is called an electrogram in contrast to the electrocardiogram which is recorded from the body surface (7). Electrograms may be unipolar or bipolar (Figure 1.2). Virtually all clinical electrophysiologic recordings are bipolar. Bipolar electrograms are recordings of electrical potential differences between two electrodes placed on the heart, while unipolar electrograms are recordings of potential differences between an electrode placed on the heart and a distant reference electrode. This reference electrode can be on the body surface or in a Wilson-type central terminal as in a standard electrocardiogram (ECG) machine. In the surface electrocardiogram, standard leads I, II, and III are bipolar (RA-LA, LA-LL,

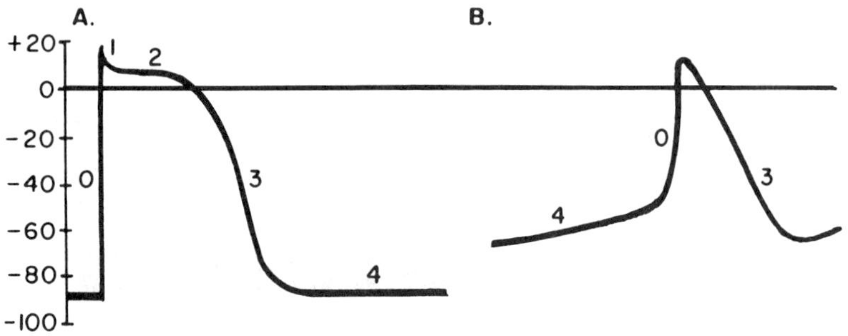

Figure 1.1. Types of action potentials in the heart. **A** "Fast response" which exists in normal myocardial (shown here) and His-Purkinje tissue. **B** "Slow response" which occurs in the sinus (shown here) and AV nodes. The upstroke in these tissues is slower and smaller than in the "fast response" action potentials in **A.** Fast response action potentials are mediated by rapid inward movements of Na^+ while slow response action potentials are mediated mainly by slow inward movement of Ca^{2+}. Note that the sinus node action potential also displays phase 4 depolarization (automaticity). Numbers to the left of vertical bar are mV. Numbers associated with action potentials indicate phases. Reprinted from Kupersmith J: Cellular mechanisms of the antiarrhythmic action of beta blockers. In Deedwania P (ed): Beta Blockers and Cardiac Arrhythmias. Marcel Dekker, New York, 1992, with permission.)

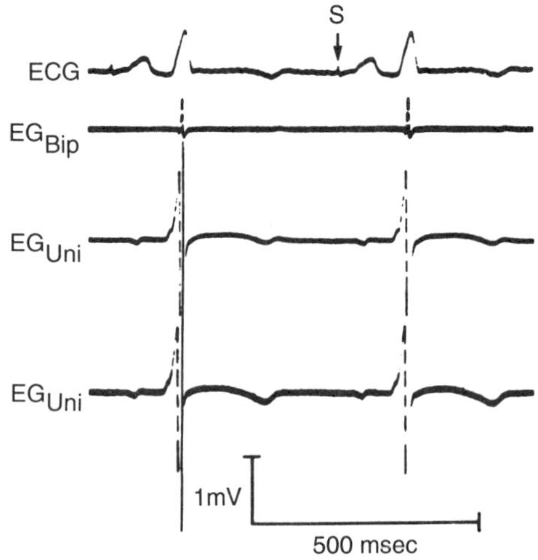

Figure 1.2. Electrocardiogram (ECG) and bipolar (EG_{BIP}) and unipolar (EG_{UNI}) electrograms were recorded from the ventricular epicardium of a dog during atrial stimulation (S = stimulus). The vertical line represents the time of the major deflection in the bipolar electrogram and is thus the time of local activation. The ECG lead and unipolar electrograms were recorded at 0.1–500 Hz, while the electrogram was recorded at 12–500 Hz. Note: it is difficult to determine the precise time of local activation from the unipolar electrograms. Also, the P and the T wave are much more apparent on the unipolar electrograms. The reason for this difference is that the low-frequency components (T wave) are filtered out on a bipolar electrogram, slow components are more difficult to record with closely spaced electrodes, and the contribution of distant electrical events (P wave) is greater on unipolar recordings. Voltage calibrations are for unipolar recordings. (Reprinted from Kupersmith J: Electrophysiologic mapping during open heart surgery. Prog Cardiovasc Dis 1976;19:167–202, with permission.)

etc.) while chest leads V^1–V^6 are unipolar (local chest lead site versus central terminal).

Bipolar recordings are used to time local cardiac activation. In clinical electrophysiology laboratories these recordings are made with catheters. In operating room mapping studies they are made with hand-held probes of various kinds or with arrays of multiple electrodes (e.g., "stockings" that envelop the heart) to enable instantaneous determination of the sequence of activation over the entire heart (see Chapters 22 and 23).

Generally, bipolar electrodes are spaced 1–10 mm apart. The closer the spacing, the more precise the local timing. This is desirable in cardiac mapping studies. On the other hand, more widely spaced electrodes make it easier to find and record special structures such as the His bundle.

Recorded filter frequencies are an important particular for the bipolar electrogram. Cardiac impulses are comprised of signals covering a wide range of electrical cycles (frequencies) from zero (direct current (DC)) to several thousand cycles per second. Generally, faster signals are associated with more rapid conduction. In electrophysiologic studies as well as surgical mapping studies low-frequency signals are eliminated. Generally, low-limit filters are set at 40 Hz with recordings made between 40 and 500 Hz (or 40–200 Hz). Use of low-limit filters enhances recording by increasing baseline stability and accentuating local fast transients. However, it also causes omission of important information recordings from structures that contain predominantly low-frequency components, such as the sinus node and AV node. Recording from these structures requires highly specialized techniques that are not now in common use. Low-limit filters also considerably diminish or eliminate ST segment changes and T waves that have predominantly low-frequency components.

Figure 1.2 shows how one determines local timing in recorded electrograms. Shown are a surface ECG lead recording, along with bipolar and unipolar electrograms recorded from a single site. The major deflection of the locally recorded bipolar electrode, coincident with the vertical line in the first beat of the tracing, is considered the time of local activation. This has been found to correlate well with timing in intracellular recordings (2,7,8).

One point to remember is that the bipolar recording measures potential differences between the two electrodes. Therefore, if activation proceeds in the direction of the electrode sequence, there is a maximum potential difference and therefore, a maximum deflection. However, if the spread of activation is perpendicular to the recording electrodes, there is minimal potential difference and minimal deflection.

Clinical electrophysiologic studies generally consist of bipolar recordings made by endocardial catheter electrodes in atrium, ventricle, His bundle, proximal bundle branches, along with simultaneous surface ECG leads. In cardiac mapping studies, composites of closely spaced bipolar electrodes recorded from multiple sites endocardially or epicardially are constructed to give the cardiac sequence of activation (see Chapters 22 and 23).

Although local timing in mapping studies is generally established by measuring the major deflection of locally recorded electrograms, in certain instances other approaches are used. For example, when determining the interval from His bundle to ventricle (HV interval), the onset of the His and ventricular electrograms is used for timing (see Chapter 4). Here, one wants to determine the time from the earliest His bundle activation to the earliest ventricular activation and not necessarily the time when the activation crosses the midpoint of the electrodes.

Unipolar electrograms (Figure 1.2) are used in clinical electrophysiology and are important in the surface ECG. They record a combination of local and distant events, unlike bipolar electrodes which record predominantly local events. Unipolar recordings are generally not made with a low-limit filter, i.e., they are recorded at 0.1 to 200–500 Hz. They have been used as reference electrodes since the recording from a unipolar electrogram reflects total activation. Unipolar electrograms have also been used to record ST segments and T waves, and for other specialized purposes. They are less useful than bipolar recordings for local timing.

One type of recording that has been recently used clinically is the monophasic potential (Fig. 1.3). Monophasic potentials are essentially local injury potentials recorded with unipolar electrodes at filter frequencies of 0.1 Hz or DC to 500 Hz. The

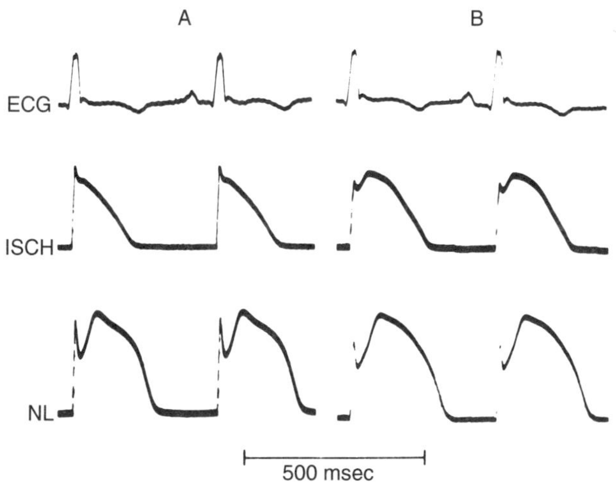

Figure 1.3. Examples of monophasic action potentials recorded from ischemic (ISCH) and normal (NL) zones of a dog heart after ligation of the left anterior descending coronary artery. The upper trace is a surface ECG. **A** At baseline; **B** shows effects of the beta blocker practocol, administered intravenously. Practolol prolonged monophasic action potential duration. This type of recording is useful for determining action potential duration and certain other features of the action potential. It also can detect early afterdepolarizations and triggered activity (see Chapter 2). (Reprinted from Kupersmith J, Shiang HS: Electrophysiologic effects of beta adrenergic blockade with practolol in canine acute myocardial ischemia. J Pharmacol Exp Ther 1979; 207:975–982, with permission.)

recordings closely resemble intracellular action potentials and, when compared to the intracellular recording at the same site, have been found to reliably reflect local action potential duration (10). Local "injury" to enable such recordings has been accomplished by suction. However, recently, an electrode has been devised that uses gently applied pressure (and thus, no lasting injury) to record the local monophasic potentials (11). These recordings may be of use in examining drug effects and certain arrhythmia mechanisms.

SURFACE ECGS

Surface electrocardiographic recordings are either unipolar (chest leads), or bipolar (standard leads) and are recorded at approximately 0.1–200 Hz. The ECG wave form is highly complex and over the years a number of sophisticated techniques have been used to glean more information from it.

Vectorcardiography was a technique in which instantaneous electrical cardiac vectors were recorded over the time of the entire cardiac electrical cycle. These vectors were displayed in three planes—coronal, lateral, and sagittal. Occasionally ECGs using this technique are performed in which X (coronal), Y (lateral), and Z (sagittal) leads are recorded. Body surface mapping techniques of various kinds are another technique to more precisely identify components of cardiac depolarization or repolarization. None of these are now in widespread use.

Signal averaging to improve signal/noise ratio has been an important device to bring out possibly hidden electrical information not detected by the usual surface ECG or mapping procedures. The basic concept is that repetitive recordings of a signal improve the signal/noise ratio. For example, if one records a large number of QRS complexes over and over again and averages them, the electrical activity that represents true signals from the heart is enhanced, while random (or gaussian) noise, which doesn't occur with every beat, is diminished. This improvement of signal/noise ratio then allows one to detect signal information that would not be apparent on standard recorded leads. The rule is that the signal/noise ratio is enhanced by a factor equal to the square root of the number of signals recorded. Thus, if 100 QRS complexes are recorded, signal/noise ratio improves 10-fold. Therefore, if a signal equals 6 mV and noise equals 6 mV, we would not be able to detect it in a usual ECG no matter how high the gain. On the other hand, with averaging of 100 beats, the signal would be 10 times greater than the noise (60 vs. 6 mV) and thus detectable.

Signal averaging has been used in a number of ways in clinical electrophysiology. For example, it has been used to record His bundle electrograms on the body surface. More recently, it has formed the basis of a widely used technique to detect slow waves believed associated with arrhythmias (12,13) and poor long-term prognosis. Related techniques have examined enhanced waveforms in narrow frequency ranges (see Chapter 3 for a more complete discussion of this technique).

BASIC ELECTROPHYSIOLOGY

ACTION POTENTIALS

The action potential is the basic unit of cardiac electrical activity. Atrial and ventricular myocardium, as well as each locus of the specialized conduction system (i.e., sinus and atrioventricular (A-V) nodes and His-Purkinje system) has its own characteristic action potential (2). Virtually all of our knowledge about action potentials is derived from animal studies. However, there is also a body of work in myocardium obtained during open heart surgery showing similarity of humans to other mammalian tissues (14).

Overall, there are two categories of action potential in the heart shown in Figure 1.1. Figure 1.1A is the so-called "fast response." This general type of response occurs in normal atrial and ventricular myocardium and in the His-Purkinje system (although action potentials at each of these loci do have certain individual characteristics). The "fast response" action potential has five phases. Phase 0 is the upstroke in which membrane potential moves from a resting level of about −90 to about +30 mV (on these recordings, membrane potential movement upward is in a positive direction and represents inward current or depolarization, while downward movement is in a negative direction and represents outward current and hyperpolarization or repolarization).

Phase 0 is so called because it was so fast that the earliest devices could not record it. The upstroke of the fast response is mediated by a rapid inward movement of Na^+ ions. Phase 1, which follows it, is a slight movement of membrane potential in an outward current direction towards baseline. During Phase 2, the "plateau phase," membrane potential remains relatively constant. Phase 3 represents repolarization and Phase 4, electrical diastole. In some tissues, there is a slow inward current movement during Phase 4 or "automaticity" (see below).

The other type of action potential in the heart is the so-called "slow response" (Figure 1.1B) which exists in the sinus and A-V nodes and, perhaps, in certain abnormal states. Here, Phase 0 is small, Phase 2 abbreviated, and Phase 3 gradual. Slow response action potentials are mediated by the slow inward movements of ions, mainly Ca^{++}, in the "slow" channel.

Cardiac specialized tissues possess a crucial property, that of self-excitation or automaticity which is responsible for the ability of the heart to initiate its own beats. During Phase 4 of automatic tissue, there is a gradual depolarization which brings the tissue to threshold for another excitation. The action potential in Figure 1.1B displays Phase 4 depolarization. In a normal heart, the sinus node has the fastest automatic rate and therefore is the initiator of cardiac electrical activity. Next in order is the A-V "junction" (i.e., junction of A-V node and His bundle) which assumes the role of initiator when the sinus node fails. The Purkinje system is next in line and takes over when the A-V junction fails or when there is complete heart block. Automaticity in this last site is believed to be responsible for idioventricular rhythms that occur in complete heart block. Atrial and ventricular myocardium are not capable of normal automaticity (however, see also Chapter 2).

Correlation of the various cardiac action potentials with the ECG is as follows (Figure 1.4). Sinus node activation immediately precedes the P wave. Atrial depolarization coincide with and is responsible for the P wave. A-V nodal, His bundle, and bundle branch activation coincide with the P-R segment. Ventricular depolarization coincides with and is responsible for the QRS complex and ventricular repolarization with ST-T segment. Atrial repolarization occurs during the QRS complex and at the earliest part of the ST segment. Purkinje fiber repolarization occurs after the T wave and appears to be responsible for U waves when they are present.

IONIC CURRENTS

A large body of scientific work has dealt with the ionic currents that comprise the various components of the action potential. This work has mainly employed voltage clamp technique (in which voltages are held constant during various electrical and pharmacologic perturbations to study current flows) and the use of a variety of biochemical and pharmacologic probes. Recently, molecular techniques are beginning to define the structure of ionic channels themselves.

An array of inward and outward currents are responsible for cardiac electrical activity. These currents derive from either ionic movement through specific ionic channels or via ionic exchange or pump mechanisms.

Ionic channels exist for Na^+, K^+, Ca^{++} (16), Cl^-, Mg^{2+}, and probably other ions. Current flow through these channels is determined by ionic gradients across the sarcolemmal membrane between the intracellular and extracellular spaces. For example, K^+ exists in higher concentration in the intracellular space and therefore its flow is outward. Na^+ and Ca^{++} are in higher concentration extracellularly and ionic flow through these channels is inward. Channels have thresholds for opening and closing to ion flow. The threshold for opening the inward Na^+ channel is about −60 to −70 mV. That is, at voltage positive to these, the channel opens and Na^+ ions flow inward. The channel closes at about +30 mV.

There are two types of Ca^{++} current—T type which activates at a rather negative membrane potential and probably plays a role in automatic activity, and L type which activates at more positive voltages, is larger, and is responsible for the major Ca^{++} movement during the plateau. (17).

K^+ currents are the main outward ionic currents and a large number have been described. These include an inwardly rectifying instantaneous I_{k1} (18), the delayed (so-called "time dependent") rectifier I_x (a difficult current to study which may be related to K^+ accumulation in intercellular clefts), adenosine triphosphate (ATP)-sensitive K^+ current (interestingly, this channel is blocked by ATP and opens to increase outward current when ATP levels decline).

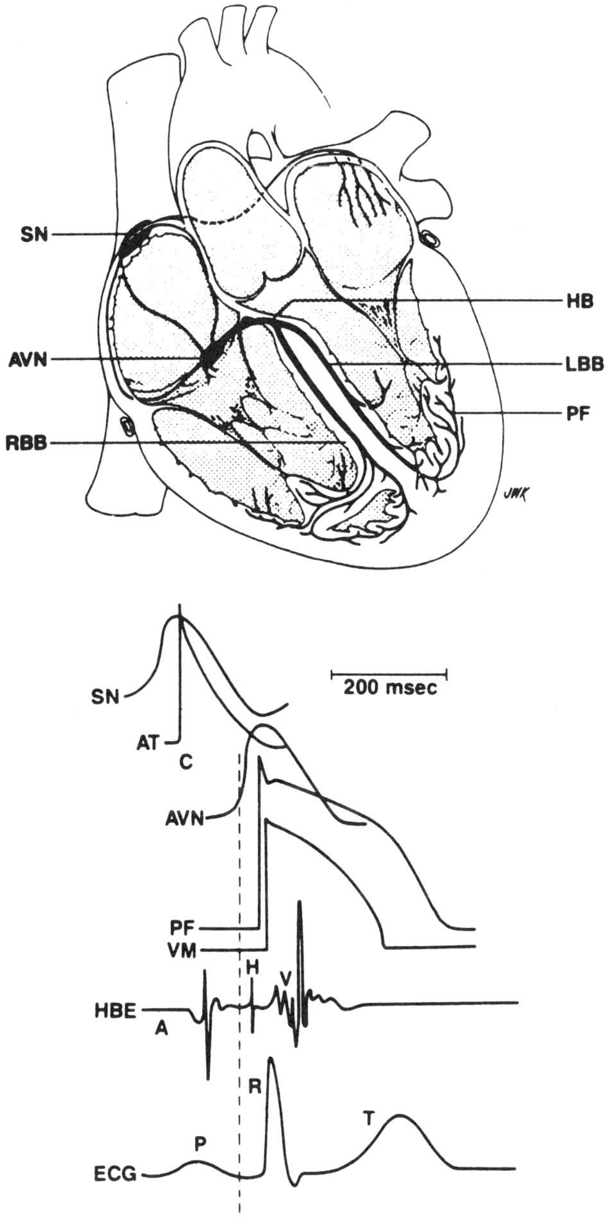

Figure 1.4. Upper drawing shows schematic of the anatomy of the specialized conduction system in the heart. Lower traces show sequence of action potentials, His bundle electrogram (next to **bottom trace**), and ECG (**bottom trace**). In the upper portion, activation begins in the sinus node (SN) then proceeds through the atrium (AT) and specialized tracts to the AV node (AVN) then into the His bundle (HB), right and left bundle branches (RBB and LBB), peripheral Purkinje fibers (PF), and ventricle (VM). **Lower portion** shows characteristic action potentials at each juncture. Note that atrial, Purkinje fiber, and ventricular muscle action potentials have rapid upstrokes, although they are of rather different durations. Sinus nodal and AV nodal action potentials have slower upstrokes and are similar to each other. These are slow responses. The "His bundle electrogram" (HBE) displays an atrial electrogram (A), His bundle electrogram (H), and ventricular electrogram (V) These are coincident with upstrokes of appropriate action potentials. The **bottom trace** shows an electrocardiographic recording (ECG) with P, R, and T waves. Note that the sinus node upstroke begins just prior to the P wave; atrial electrogram is coincident with the P wave, AV nodal upstroke and His bundle electrogram occur in the PR segment; and QRS segment is coincident with ventricular muscle action potential upstroke and ventricular electrogram. (Reprinted from Bigger JT Jr: The electrical activity of the heart. In Hurst JW (ed): The Heart Arteries and Veins. McGraw-Hill, New York, 1990; pp. 77–91, with permission.

Other transmembrane currents derive from ionic exchange pumps. For example, the Na-K pump exchanges three K^+ for two Na^+ ions and thus, results in net outward current, favoring repolarization and/or a more negative resting potential (19). The Na-Ca exchange mechanism which exchanges one Ca^{++} for three or four Na^+ ions adds inward current when removing Ca^{++} outward from the cell (20).

A complex interplay of these ionic mechanisms is responsible for normal and abnormal action potentials. When the threshold for activation of inward current is reached (via intrinsic automatic activity, transmission of current from a neighboring cell or electrical stimulation), an upstroke occurs. In fast-response tissue (atrial and ventricular myocardium and His-Purkinje system), this upstroke is rapid and via Na^+ current (1,21), although there is a component of Ca^{2+} current at its peak (in the 0 to +30 mV range). In slow response tissues (sinus node, AV node and certain abnormal states), the upstroke is predominantly via slow inward Ca^{2+} current (see Figure 1.1).

After the upstroke, a brief outward current, I_{to}, comprised of either outward potassium or inward chloride current, occurs to account for Phase 1 (Fig. 1.1). During Phase 2, both I_{Ca} (22) and a small component of I_{Na} (called "window" sodium current) (23) maintain the plateau. I_{Ca} is also responsible for excitation-contraction coupling.

Repolarization of the action potential (Fig. 1.1) occurs due to a decline in I_{Ca} and window I_{Na} and the occurrence of outward K^+ current. We have also shown that another factor in repolarization is extracellular K^+ accumulation in the tightly spaced intercellular myocardial clefts. This phenomenon increases conductance to I_K to favor outward current (4).

Normal automaticity occurs when gradual depolarization during Phase 4 brings membrane potential to threshold of about −60 mV and it derives from an interaction of several currents. In early Phase 4, there is a decline in outward I_K favoring depolarization, and in later Phase 4 there is activation of both depolarizing Na^+ pacemaker current (called I_f) (24) and T-type I_{Ca}.

A noteworthy phenomenon worthy in regard to automaticity and the basis of certain of the tests of sinus node function is "overdrive suppression." (25) After a rapid beating sequence, there is a suppression of automatic activity, i.e., Phase 4 is moved in an outward current (negative direction) and its slope flattened, leading to slowing of automatic rate. This phenomenon of overdrive suppression is mainly caused by activation of the Na-K pump during rapid beating (via intracellular sodium loading) with a consequent increase in outward current to suppress automaticity (4,19). In brief rapid beating sequences, extracellular K^+ accumulation (causing increased conductance to and, therefore, increased magnitude of outward current) appears to play the important role (4).

ACTION POTENTIAL PARAMETERS

In evaluating antiarrhythmic drugs or the effects of interventions that induce abnormalities, certain action potential parameters are quantitatively analyzed. These include resting potential, action potential amplitude, mean or maximum rate of change of the upstroke (V_{max}), maximum diastolic potential (i.e., membrane potential at the end of the action potential), action potential duration, and effective refractory period.

V_{max} and membrane responsiveness curves (1) are important parts of the analysis. $V_{max,}$ i.e., the maximum rate of change of the action potential upstroke, is a measure in part of inward Na^+ current (though not a perfect one). It also correlates in general with the rate of conduction of an impulse. An intervention that slows V_{max} (e.g., a local anesthetic antiarrhythmic drug) also tends to slow the rate of conduction. Membrane responsiveness curves are a more detailed form of analysis of V_{max}. As membrane potential is reduced, i.e., made more positive, there is partial inactivation of the sodium channel and therefore, a slower rate of rise of the action potential upstroke. One can construct curves (see Chapter 11) plotting membrane potential versus V_{max}, the so-called "membrane responsiveness curves." Interventions that reduce inward Na^+ current shift membrane responsiveness currents so that V_{max} is lower at a given membrane potential. Local anesthetic antiarrhythmic agents do this (see Chapter 11).

Action potential duration is a commonly measured parameter. Generally, one determines the time from the upstroke to 50% (APD_{50}) and/or 90% (APD_{90}) of repolarization.

The most common measure of refractoriness is effective refractory period, the time from the onset of the action potential to the earliest stimulus that elicits a new impulse (usually for this measurement stimulus strength is set at two times diastolic threshold). Effective refractory period is, of course, commonly measured in clinical electrophysiology.

Quantitative analysis of automaticity involves examining the rate of firing of the given tissue, the slope of Phase 4 (more gradual slope equals slower rate), threshold of activation of the upstroke (higher threshold means later firing and slower rate), and maximum diastolic potential at the end of the action potential (more negative maximum diastolic potential at the onset of Phase 4 means that, all other factors being equal, tissue will reach threshold later and rate will be slower) (Fig. 1.5). For example, an intervention that increases maximum diastolic potential and/or depresses the slope of Phase 4, and/or makes threshold more positive, will depress automaticity (Figure 1.5) (2).

Changes in certain action potential parameters can be detected on surface ECGs. For example, decreased V_{max} of the upstroke in ventricular muscle leads to slowing of conduction which, in turn, leads to prolonged QRS duration. Certain antiarrhythmic drugs such as quinidine do this. Prolongation of ventricular muscle action potential duration tends to prolong QT interval on surface ECG (although QT interval is a rather complex parameter, discussed in more detail in Chapter 10).

CABLE PROPERTIES

Cable properties refer to factors pertinent to transmission of electrical activity. Since clinical electrophysiology is involved

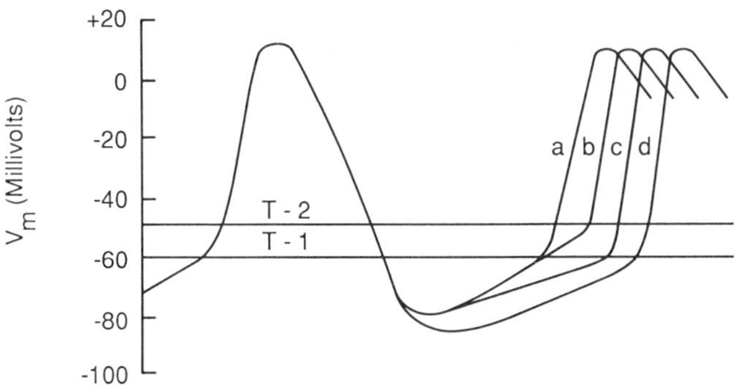

Figure 1.5. Factors influencing automaticity. Shown are a sinus node type action potential which exhibits phase 4 depolarization. T-1 stands for the usual threshold for activation while T-2 is a somewhat more positive threshold. **a** is the action potential which represents baseline sinus rate; **b, c,** and **d** show effects of three changes which slow sinus rate. **b** shows effects of moving threshold in a positive direction; **c** of decreasing the slope of diastolic depolarization; and **d** making the maximum diastolic potential more negative (with same slope as **c**). See text for further discussion.

with stimulation and transmission of impulses, concepts related to cable properties are a part of its information base.

Mathematical analysis of factors affecting transmission of impulses makes the assumption, however imperfect from a geometric as well as a physiologic point of view, that the cardiac conducting tissue acts as a perfect cable for transmission of electricity. We will not review these assumptions or the formulae derived from them (26).

The heart and its specialized tissues have a complex though extremely functional method of transmitting electrical current. Intracellularly, in mammals, a system of transverse tubules (T system) transmits action potentials throughout the individual cell. Intercalated disks are the longitudinal connection between cells. Within these interrelated discs are the gap junctions which are low-resistance highly efficient electrical connections. These longitudinal connections make for more efficient transmission of impulses in this direction than transversely. The junction between the T system and sarcoplasmic reticulum is the connection between the intracellular and extracellular systems. All these systems involving impulses transmission can be compromised by disease states and by drugs.

Much experimental effort has been applied to examining cable properties. For greater understanding of clinical electrophysiology, we will review the concepts and terminology involved.

Electrical current circuits by definition arise at so-called sources of current and are directed at so-called current sinks. *Electrotonic* transmission of current refers to local spread of current between cardiac cells. More electrotonic current and more favorable spread of it, in turn, favor propagation of action potentials and transmission of impulses. If, however, electrotonic current does not ultimately cause cells to reach threshold for a propagated action potential, it will die out.

Space constant refers to the area over which such current theoretically would die out. By definition, the space constant is the distance over which voltage falls to $1/e$ (e = natural log) of its original amplitude (i.e., to about 37%). The higher the space constant, the further the spread of electrotonic current, ultimately resulting in more favorable conditions for transmission of propagated impulses. The space constant is reduced by interventions or disease states that interfere with the intercellular connections described above.

Time constant refers to the time it takes for the electrotonic current to die out. By definition, time constant equals the time it takes for voltage to fall to 84% of its final value in long fibers or 63% in short fibers. The longer the time constant, the more favorable are conditions for transmission of impulses.

Electrotonic current may die out or be sufficient to initiate a new action potential. However, another role is possible. It may, if appropriately timed, influence action potentials in the vicinity. For example, electrotonic impulses from a region of prolonged action potentials may serve to prolong action potentials in neighboring tissues (27), or as we have found, it may enhance automaticity (28) (see Chapter 2).

In the transmission of cardiac impulses the current source can be thought of as already excited tissue and the current sink as the yet unexcited tissue to which the current is directed. When this local current depolarizes a sufficient amount of tissue (in a perfect cable called "liminal length" of the cable) (29), the impulse propagates, i.e., activates another portion of tissue. In electrical terms, this excitable tissue acts as a resistance-capitance (R-C) circuit and formulae to examine quantitatively are based on that assumption (see ref. 26 for further analysis).

The *safety factor* for conduction is the amount of current in excess over that needed to propagate an impulse. Tissues with a high safety factor for conduction easily propagate impulses while tissues with a low safety factor are subject to conduction failure with slightly adverse alterations in the system. In the heart, the His-Purkinje system tends to have a high safety factor, while the A-V node has a lower safety factor. Disease states also influence safety factor.

Threshold refers to the level at which local excitation occurs, and has taken on more than one meaning. In cellular electrophysiology, it may refer to the level of membrane potential at which an excitation occurs, i.e., at which activation of inward Na^{2+} current (or in, slow response tissue, inward Ca^{++}) current occurs. For inward Na^{2+} current, threshold is about -60 to -70 mV. In in situ experimental studies and in clinical electrophysiology (a form of in situ study), threshold refers to the amount of current or voltage required to excite tissue with a given set of electrodes. Threshold measurements are important in performing studies of local refractoriness (which one usually measures at two times diastolic threshold) and in evaluating temporary and permanent pacemakers. (Note: "threshold" may also refer to the amount of current or voltage required to fibrillate ("fibrillation threshold") or defibrillate ("defibrillation threshold") the heart.)

The likelihood and speed of impulse transmission then depends on a number of factors. For example, an electrotonic current will more likely spread over greater distance and excite tissue if local anatomic connections are intact, if thresholds for excitation are low, and if there is an absence of certain ionic changes (e.g., diminished Ca^{2+} and low pH) which may adversely affect cable properties. In this situation, space and time constants will be higher as will the safety factor for conduction. The above factors are, in turn, affected by acute and chronic disease states as well as by drugs and metabolic status.

ACTION POTENTIAL AND CABLE PROPERTY ABNORMALITIES

A number of conditions influence local action potentials and cardiac cable properties to make arrhythmias more likely. In general, acute and chronic injury to cardiac tissue lowers resting membrane potential (i.e., makes it more positive), lowers V_{max}, either shortens (in acute ischemia) or prolongs (in chronic states) action potential duration and alters automaticity in a variety of ways (see Chapter 2 for discussion of abnormal automaticity) (30–32). In ischemia elevated local K^+ plays a role in the lowered membrane potential upstroke velocity and conduction as does acidosis (33).

In addition, disease states alter cable properties by disturbing intracellular and intercellular connections. For example hypoxia (34), ischemia and infarction (35), low pH, Ca^{2+} alteration, certain drugs, and inhibition of metabolic function may disturb these connections. In certain fibrotic states such as chronic infarction or cardiomyopathy, there may be islands of relatively normal cardiac cells between which cable property alterations serve to weaken impulse transmission and promote arrhythmias. Usually, however, an interplay of cellular electrical and intercellular cable property abnormalities (which may be greater in the transverse than in the longitudinal direction) (36,37) combine to interfere with normal cardiac impulse generation and transmission. The consequence of these alterations are bradyarrhythmias and tachyarrhythmias.

References

1. Weidmann S: Effect of current flow on the membrane potential of cardiac muscle. J Physiol (Lond) 1951;115:227–236.
2. Hoffman BF, Cranefield PF: Electrophysiology of the Heart. New York, McGraw-Hill, 1960.
3. Kupersmith J: Cellular mechanisms of the antiarrhythmic action of beta blockers. In Deedwania P (ed): Beta Blockers and Cardiac Arrhythmias. Marcel Dekker, New York 1992.
4. Kline RP, Kupersmith J: Effects of extracellular potassium accumulation and sodium pump activation on automatic canine Purkinje fibers. J Physiol (Lond) 1982;324:517–533.
5. Allen DG, Eisner DA, Orchard CH: Factors influencing free intracellular calcium concentration in quiescent ferret ventricular muscle. J Physiol 1984;350:615–630.
6. Dillon SM, Morad M: A new laser scanning system for measuring action potential propagation in the heart. Science 1981;214:453–456.
7. Kupersmith J: Electrophysiologic mapping during open heart surgery. Prog Cardiovasc Dis 1976;19:167–202.
8. Sano T, Ono M, Shimamoto T: Intrinsic deflections, local excitation and transmembrane action potentials. Circ Res 1956;6:444–449.
9. Kupersmith J, Shiang HS: Electrophysiologic effects of beta adrenergic blockade with practolol in canine acute myocardial ischemia. J Pharmacol Exp Ther 1979;207:975–982.
10. Hoffman BF, Cranefield PF, Lepeschkin E, *et al.*: Comparison of cardiac monophasic action potentials recorded by intracellular and suction electrodes. Am J Physiol 1959;196:1297–1301.
11. Franz MR: Long-term recording of monophasic action potentials from human endocardium. Am J Cardiol 1983;51:1629–1634.
12. Simson MB: Use of signals in the terminal QRS complex to identify patients with ventricular tachycardia after myocardial infarction. Circulation 1981; 64:235–242.
13. Breithardt G, Becker R, Seipel L, *et al.*: Noninvasive detection of late potentials in man—a new marker for ventricular tachycardia. Eur Heart J 1981;2:1–11.
14. Gelband H, Bush H, Rosen M, *et al.*: Electrophysiologic properties of isolated preparations of human atrial myocardium. Circ Res 1972;30:293.
15. Bigger JT Jr.: The electrical activity of the heart. In Hurst JW (ed): The Heart Arteries and Veins. McGraw-Hill, New York, pp. 77–90, 1990.
16. Tsien RW: Calcium channels in excitable cell membranes. Annu Rev Physiol 1983;45:341–358.
17. Hirano Y, Fozzard HA, January CT: Characteristics of L- and T-type Ca^{++} currents in canine cardiac Purkinje cells. Am J Physiol 1989;H1478–H1492.
18. McDonald TF, Trautwein W: The potassium current underlying delayed rectification in cat ventricular muscle. J Physiol (Lond) 1978;274:217–246.
19. Gadsby D, Cranefield PF: Electrogenic sodium extrusion in cardiac Purkinje fibers. J Gen Physiol 1979;73:819–837.
20. Mullins LJ: Ion Transport in Heart. Raven Press, New York, 1981.
21. Brown AM, Lee KS, Powell T: Sodium currents in single rat heart muscles cells. J Physiol (Lond) 1981;318:479–500.
22. Vitek M, Trautwein W: Slow inward current and action potentials in cardiac Purkinje fibers. Pflugers Arch 1971;323:204–218.
23. Attwell D, Cohen I, Eisner D, Ohba M, Ojeda C: The steady-state TTX sensitive ("window") sodium current in cardiac Purkinje fibers. Pflugers Arch 1979;137–142.
24. Brown HF, DiFrancesco D: Voltage-clamp investigations of membrane currents underlying pacemaker activity in rabbit sinoatrial node. J Physiol (Lond) 1980;308:331–351.
25. Vassalle M: An analysis of cardiac pacemaker potential by means of a voltage clamp technique. Am J Physiol 1966;1335–1341.
26. Jack JJB, Noble D, Tsien RW: Electric current flow in excitable cells. Oxford University Press, London, 1975.
27. Kupersmith J, Hoff P: Occurrence and transmission of repolarization abnormalities *in vitro*. J Am Coll Cardiol 1985;6:152–160.
28. Li Z, Noda T, Maldonado C, *et al.*: Junctional zone between segments of varying action potential duration appears to be a site of arrhythmogenesis (Abstr). J Am Coll Cardiol 1990;15:145A.
29. Fozzard HA, Schoenburg M: Strength-duration curves in cardiac Purkinje fibers: effects of liminal length and charge distribution. J Physiol (Lond) 1972;226:593–618.
30. Friedman PL, Stewart JR, Fenoglio JJ Jr, *et al.*: Survival of subendocardial Purkinje fibers after extensive myocardial infarction in dogs: In vitro and in vivo correlation. Circ Res 1973;33:597–611.
31. Lazzara R, El-Sherif N, Scherlag BJ: Electrophysiological properties of canine Purkinje cells in one-day-old myocardial infarction. Circ Res 1973; 33:722–734.
32. Kleber AG: Resting membrane potential, extracellular potassium activity, and intracellular sodium activity during acute global ischemia in isolated perfused guinea pig hearts. Circ Res 1983;52:442–450.
33. Morena H, Janse MJ, Fiolet JWT, *et al.*: Comparison of the effects of regional ischemia, hypoxia, hyperkalemia and acidosis on intracellular and excellu-

lar potentials and metabolism in the isolated porcine heart. Circ Res 1980; 46:634–646.
34. Wojtczak J: Contractures and increase in internal longitudinal resistance of cow ventricular muscle induced by hypoxia. Circ Res 1979;44:88–95.
35. Spear J, Michelson E, Moore EN: Reduced space constant in slowly conducting regions of chronically infarcted canine myocardium. Circ Res 1983;53:176–185.
36. Spach MS, Miller WT Jr, Geselowitz DB, *et al.*: The discontinuous nature of propagation in normal canine cardiac muscle. Evidence for recurrent discontinuities of intracellular resistance that affect the membrane currents. Circ Res 1981;48:39–54.
37. Kadish AH, Spear JF, Levine JH, *et al.*: The effects of procainamide on conduction in anisotropic canine ventricular myocardium. Circulation 1986; 74:616–625.

2

MECHANISMS OF ARRHYTHMIA

Joel Kupersmith, M.D., F.A.C.P., F.A.C.C.

Mechanisms that cause tachyarrhythmias can be placed under three main headings: abnormalities of impulse conduction, abnormalities of impulse generation, and a combination of the two. Reentry is the abnormality of impulse conduction and it is also considered the primary cause of clinical arrhythmias. Much of clinical electrophysiology is grounded in concepts related to reentry. It is therefore important for the clinician to have an in-depth understanding of this important mechanism of arrhythmogenesis and it will be considered first.

ABNORMALITIES OF IMPULSE CONDUCTION—REENTRY

Reentry is a concept that has a long history among cardiac investigators. The first proposal that a reentrant-like abnormality of the conduction was possible has been attributed to McWilliams who suggested it as a mechanism for fibrillation in 1887 (1). McWilliams also found that fibrillation occurred more easily in large rather than in small hearts, a concept that has stood the test of time. Mayer (1906) (2) as well as Mines (1914) (3) and Garrey (1914) (4) validated the concept in a jellyfish preparation with a circus pathway of muscular contraction around its periphery. Interestingly, Mines also postulated that accessory atrioventricular (A-V) connections, then recently described by Kent (1913) (5), could be associated with atrioventricular circus movement as we now know occurs in the Wolff-Parkinson-White syndrome. Mines (1914) (6) further postulated that reentrant arrhythmias can be induced by electrical stimuli. Unfortunately, he tried it on himself and induced a lethal arrhythmia, a tragic ending to a brilliant career.

The noted cardiologist, Lewis (1905) (7), took up the circus movement hypothesis as a cause of atrial flutter and in 1928, Schmitt and Erlanger (8) further elaborated the concept of reentry.

Perhaps the best way to prove a concept of reentry is by abolishing it via transection of the reentrant pathway (9). Mines in 1914 (6) accomplished this in the jellyfish. In the modern era, Burchell *et al.* in 1967 (10) were the first to accomplish it in a human being with Wolff-Parkinson-White syndrome. This case was proof of the valuable concept of reentry in clinical arrhythmias as well as the opening of an era of surgical and ablative therapy for arrhythmias.

Characteristics of Reentry

Figure 2.1 shows a simple model of reentry. Here in the reentrant pathway (R), there is a central zone of anatomic block and a zone of potential one way block. In panel A, an impulse enters the reentrant pathway zone and passes through both limbs around the central zone of anatomic block. In clinical electrophysiology studies the impulse would come from a stimulating (S) site. In panel B, the impulse is unidirectionally blocked in one limb and proceeds around the other limb back through the site of one way block (which by this time has lost its refractoriness) to complete a circuit. Panel C shows the established reentrant circuit. Impulses will then spread out from this established reentrant site or focus to activate the remainder of the heart and result in a new ("echo" or "reciprocal") beat and if repetitive a reentrant tachycardia.

The key features of reentry as displayed in a variety of in vitro models (3,11–16) are one-way or unidirectional block, which is typically due to disparity in refractoriness between the area of block and the rest of the pathway, and slow conduction, slow enough for the impulse to meet continuously excitable (i.e., nonrefractory) tissue. Note also that with reentry, there is of necessity continuous electrical activity. Such activity can and has been recorded during presumed reentrant arrhythmias in in situ experiments (17), during open heart arrhythmia surgery (18), and with surface signal averaging techniques (19).

From the above simple concept derives numerous characteristics which serve to explain a wide variety of arrhythmias.

First, anatomic reentrant pathways (i.e., those with central anatomic obstruction as show in Figure 2.1—other types are described below) have certain components as follows (Figure 2.2): there is a "leading edge" or "head," of the wave of activation. At the "trailing edge" or "tail" there is a zone of relative refractoriness. Between the trailing and leading edges

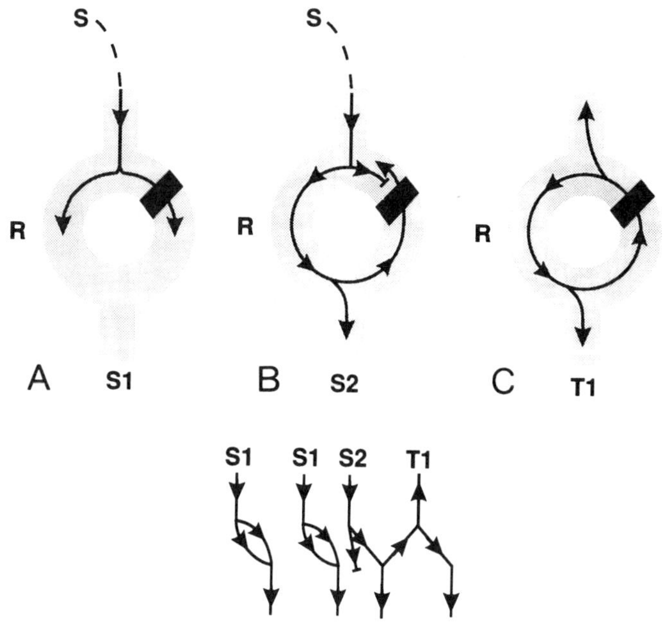

Figure 2.1. Schematic of anatomic reentry. R = site of reentry, S = stimulation site. In R there is a central zone of anatomic block and a zone of slowing of conduction and potential one way block shown on the right limb (darkened area). **A** (S_1) shows a basic stimulated beat in which the impulse passes through both limbs of the circuit. **B** (S_2) shows a premature stimulus. Here, the impulse meets refractory tissue and is blocked in the right limb, darkened area. It continues around the left limb to complete a reentrant cycle. **C** (T_1, i.e., first beat of tachycardia) shows the established reentrant pathway. The lower portion of the figure is a ladder diagram showing two basic beats (S_1), a premature beat (S_2), and the first tachycardia beat (T_1). Note that the S_1–S_2 interval is short and the S_2–T_1 interval is long. See text for further discussion.

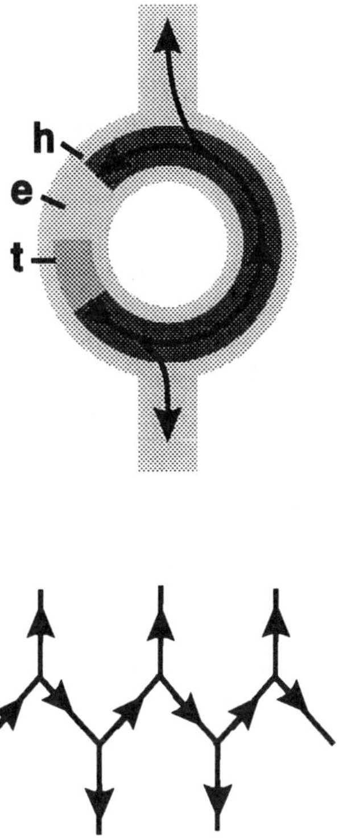

Figure 2.2. Components of reentrant pathway. Shown are an established reentrant pathway and a ladder diagram. In the established reentrant pathway, h = the head, t = the tail, generally a zone of relative refractoriness, and e = the excitable gap. Impulses arriving at the excitable gap reset or abolish the pathway as shown in Figure 2.4.

there may or may not be a zone of excitable tissue called the "excitable gap."

A basic formula can be applied to determine pathway length (or wavelength): the wavelength must equal at least the average conduction velocity times the refractory period.

$$l = CV \times RP \tag{2.1}$$

l = wavelength, CV = conduction velocity,
RP = refractory period

That is, if the average conduction velocity is 1.5 m/sec (as in the human His bundle) (20) and the refractory period is 300 msec (0.3 sec), pathway length would have to be 0.45 meters, an impossibility in the human heart. If on the other hand, the average conduction velocity is 0.03 m/sec (as has been found with certain slow response preparations) (13) the pathway length would have to only be 0.009 m (9 mm) a plausible length for the human heart. If the refractory period shortens to 200 msec, the pathway would only have to be 0.006 M (6 mm). Of course, if there is an excitable gap, the pathway would be somewhat larger. Experimental documentation exists for pathways of circus movement as small as 12–35 min in Purkinje fiber (13).

From this simple equation (Eq. (2.1)) we see that slower conduction and shorter refractoriness make for a greater likelihood of reentry occurring with a given pathway, i.e., these factors make it less likely for the impulse in the pathway to meet refractory tissue and be extinguished.

Induction of Reentry

The centerpiece of the clinical electrophysiologic study is induction of reentrant arrhythmias via programmed stimulation protocols. These protocols are designed to test abilities to induce arrhythmias in patients, and then test ability of interventions such as drugs or pacemakers to prevent or reverse the arrhythmias. It is therefore important for the clinician to have an understanding of the nuances of stimulation protocols designed to examine reentry.

Clinical as well as experimental induction of reentrant arrhythmias depends on applying programmed premature stimuli with varying S_1–S_2 (i.e., basic to premature beat) intervals, at one site to activate a reentrant pathway at a variable distance in space and time from the site of stimulation. Note in Figure 2.1 that there are two components to the reentrant complex, a "stimulation" or "trigger" site (S) and a "substrate" or reentrant pathway (R). The "trigger" is the impulse that activates the pathway. In electrophysiologic studies, the stimulated beat is the trigger. In spontaneously occurring arrhythmias, the trigger may be an atrial or ventricular premature beat. The reentrant pathway is the "substrate," i.e., a potential zone of arrhythmogenesis.

As indicated above, Figure 2.1 shows how an impulse acts in a potential reentrant circuit. Ordinarily, impulses proceed in both directions around the central zone of anatomic block (panel A). However, under certain circumstances one-way block may occur as shown in panel B (21), e.g., if there is a longer refractory period at the site of potential block. This will then result in an unmasking of the potential reentrant circuit. Premature beats tend to expose differences in refractoriness and therefore serve to "stress" the system and induce reentrant arrhythmias (22,23). The critical S_1–S_2 (basic to premature beat interval) time window for initiating a tachycardia is called the "excitable (or vulnerable) window" (21).

The fact that premature beats (whether stimulated or spontaneous) initiate reentry also leads to another of its characteristics. That is, after the reentrant impulse completes one loop around the circuit (Fig. 2.1), some changes in timing may occur. The first reentrant beat is premature with a cycle length shorter than in the baseline rhythm. This would tend to shorten the refractory period and also to influence conduction velocity. In addition, there may be some electrotonic interactions between head and tail of the pathway. These influences tend to further shorten cycle length as the tachycardia gets underway and at times there may be alternans. For this reason, many tachycardias have a warm-up period or irregularity until the cycle length arrives at its final set point.

With these basics in mind we can review specific factors related to inducing reentry in the electrophysiology laboratory. These involve the reentrant pathway site itself, the stimulation protocol, and the pathway from stimulation to reentry site. Stimulation protocols may be via pacing at one or another site in the atrium or ventricle, have shorter or longer S_1–S_1 cycle lengths (where S_1 is the basic stimulus), involve use of from one to three extra stimuli (S_1–S_2; S_1–S_2–S_3; S_1–S_2–S_3–S_4). We will use the example of ventricular tachycardia and discuss two general categories of factors: those related to the reentry site itself and to the stimulation to reentry site pathway.

REENTRY PATHWAY SITE

The following factors related to reentry pathway site influence inducibility of arrhythmias:

1. Basic (S_1–S_1) cycle length—slower rates tend to increase disparity in refractoriness favoring reentry. On the other hand, a more rapid basic cycle length tends to cause slower conduction and shorter refractoriness in the reentrant pathway, both of which favor the ability of echo cycles to occur. Also when ischemia is present, more rapid rates tend to increase the abnormality and occasionally rapid pacing sequences induce ischemia. Probably for a given arrhythmia there is an optimal basic cycle length for induction (13), a reason to use a variety of basic cycle lengths.

2. Use of two or three premature stimuli—Additional premature stimuli will cause cycle length related changes in refractoriness and conduction in the reentrant pathway to facilitate induction of reentry by: (a) further shortening refractory period or slowing conduction in the circuit; (b) increasing the disparity in refractoriness at the site of one-way block if refractoriness of one limb of the circuit is more cycle length sensitive; (c) "peeling back" refractoriness (11). Here the 1st premature stimulus (S_2) moves refractoriness in the reentrant pathway to an earlier place in time. Thus a subsequent stimulus (S_3) is allowed to penetrate the reentrant site at a time when there will be an enabling disparity in refractoriness at the site of potential one-way block.

3. The autonomic nervous system plays a role in both conduction and refractoriness.

4. Atrial versus ventricular pacing—with atrial pacing, the full His-Purkinje system in the ventricle is utilized and therefore, there is the most ordered sequence of activation. Ventricular pacing, on the other hand, is more likely to lead to disparities of conduction and therefore disparities in refractoriness in the reentrant pathway to favor one-way block and reentry (and thus inducibility). This effect may be more exaggerated at one particular ventricular site over another.

5. Effects on conduction rate in the pathway have potentially variable influences. Slowing of conduction by more rapid pacing, for example, might favor one-way block and reentry, but if profound, might cause two-way block. Also conduction may not be uniform within the circuit.

STIMULATION TO REENTRY SITE PATHWAY

Factors related to the pathway between the stimulation and the reentry site are extremely important in clinical electrophysiologic studies (24) and are perhaps not sufficiently discussed.

A crucial point in arrhythmia induction is that an effective trigger will be favored by a short time interval from the S (stimulation) to the R site (Fig. 2.1). This in turn is favored by a short distance from S to R and/or a more rapid (higher) conduction velocity. In addition, timing of refractory periods and excitable windows (intervals when an arrhythmia can be induced) at the S and R sites are also important. Figure 2.3 shows examples of refractory periods and excitable windows at the S and R sites in a number of different situations in which triggering stimuli do and do not initiate reentry (see caption for descriptions).

Some factors related to stimulation site that are pertinent to the clinical electrophysiology study are as follows.

1. Location of the site of stimulation in relation to the reentrant pathway—most important and the closer the better to facilitate induction of reentry (24). In fact, the closer the S site is to the precise site of one-way block in the reentrant circuit, the easier to induce reentry. These aspects emphasize why, in the case of ventricular tachycardia, the use of multiple sites (including at times left ventricular sites when there is a left ventricular origin of arrhythmia) is helpful.

2. Basic cycle length—changing the cycle length may influence refractoriness at S so as to facilitate induction of reentry. For

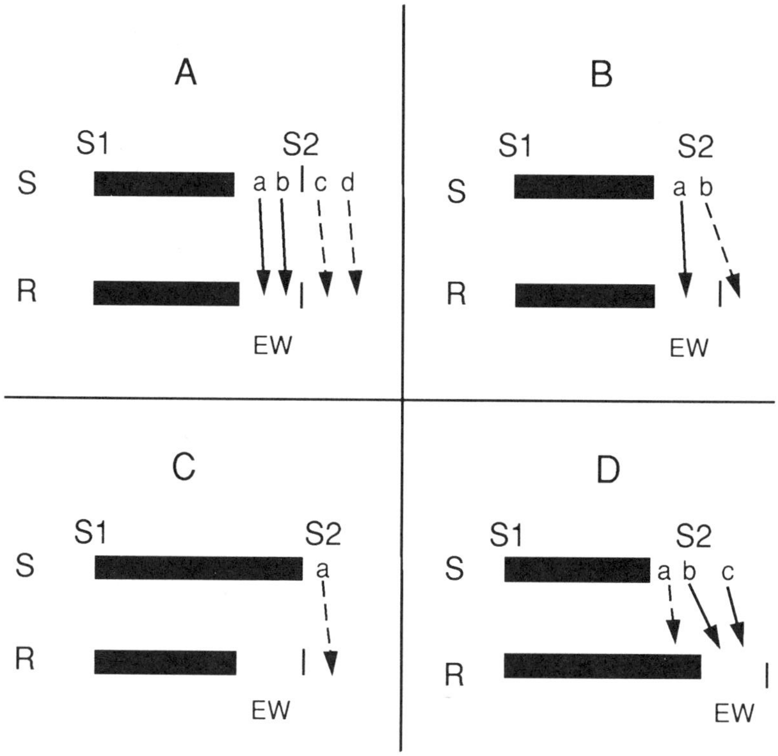

Figure 2.3. Representation of induction of arrhythmia via premature stimulation. Horizontal bars represent refractory periods at stimulation (S) and reentrant pathway sites (R). S_1 is basic cycle and S_2 is premature stimulus. The *arrows* represent conduction from stimulation to reentrant pathway site. Excitable window (EW) indicates time during which a reentrant arrhythmia can be initiated at the R site. It extends from the end of the horizontal bar (refractory period) of (R) to the small vertical bar. (It is assumed that the EW at R begins coincident with the end of the refractory period.) *Solid arrows* are stimuli that induce impulses which arrive at R during the excitable window and therefore induce an arrhythmia. Dashed arrows arrive outside the excitable window and do not induce an arrhythmia. In **A,** the excitable window at S is the same as that at R. S2's at **a** and **b** initiate an arrhythmia and those at **c** and **d** do not. In **B, a** conducts relatively rapidly and arrives within the excitable window in R to initiate an arrhythmia while **b**, which is initiated at almost the same time, conducts slowly and arrives at R after the end of the excitable window. In **C,** refractory period at S is longer than at R and extends beyond the excitable window. It is therefore impossible for impulses initiated at S to induce tachycardias. In **D,** the refractory period of S is much shorter than at R. **a** which is initiated very early, arrives at R before the end of its refractory period and thus before the excitable window begins. **b** and **c,** however, arrive within the excitable window and induce a tachycardia.

example, in Figure 2.3C, where induction of arrhythmias is impossible because of the longer refractory period at S than R, a shorter cycle length might shorten this refractory period relative to that of R sufficiently to make induction possible. On the other hand, a shorter cycle length might also slow conduction from S to R sufficiently to make induction possible. There may be optimal cycle lengths for induction of arrhythmias related to stimulation versus reentry site.

3. The use of two or three premature stimuli. This may have a variety of effects on conduction and refractoriness at S versus R or on S to R conduction intervals to facilitate reentry.

4. Autonomic nervous system—increased advenegic tone, isoproterenol (25) and at times atropine (in atrium/A-V node), may shorten conduction intervals or shorten refractory periods on the S to R pathway so as to favor induction. This is an important way in which isoproterenol, which is commonly used in electrophysiologic laboratories, facilitates induction of arrhythmias(25).

These factors related to stimulation site are important considerations in electrophysiologic studies. They also represent an artificiality in the study, perhaps not related to the spontaneously occurring arrhythmias. However, it is also true that spontaneously occurring arrhythmias may be triggered by spontaneously occurring premature beats arising at a distance from the reentrant site. For example, a ventricular premature beat arising at one site in the heart may initiate a reentrant tachycardia arising elsewhere. In this instance the factors described above that relate to arrhythmias induced by stimulation in the electrophysiologic laboratory also apply to spontaneous arrhythmias induced by premature beats.

Termination of Reentrant Tachycardias Via Stimulation

Reentrant arrhythmias can be terminated or reset by individual stimuli and similar principles apply to termination as to induction of arrhythmias (21). As indicated in Figure 2.2, anatomic reentrant pathways have certain components. When an individual impulse arrives at the anatomic reentrant circuit, its effect depends on where among the components it arrives as follows (Fig. 2.4): (a) If it arrives and meets refractory tissue, it will have no effect, or perhaps a slight effect via electrotonus. (Fig. 2.4A) (b) If it arrives in the excitable gap and finds excitable tissue in both an antegrade and retrograde direction, impulses will collide with the leading edge of the tachycardia and abolish it (Figure 2.4B). (c) If it finds excitable tissue in an anterograde but not a retrograde direction, it will excite the pathway early and reset it (Fig. 2.4C). With repeated pacing, the rhythm can then be entrained and may remain and be faster, but will perhaps be more likely to die out when the pacing is terminated (26,27). (d) Sometimes double stimuli (or more) are required, to intercept the circuit. The first stimulus can alter the refractory period (peel it back) or other factor along the S to R pathway so that the next impulse can have appropriate timing to reach the reentrant circuit.

Aspects related to location of and time interval from stimulation to reentry site are similar when terminating reentrant arrhythmias as when inducing them (closer distance and shorter time are better) (24). It should be noted the considerations of site of stimulation are important for antitachycardia pacemakers (see

Chapter 21), in that one should be careful to assure that sites of testing and implantation correspond.

Clinical Criteria for Reentrant Arrhythmias

Clinically, certain features have been promulgated as minimum requirements to classify a given arrhythmia as reentrant. The criteria in fact date back to the work of Mines in 1914. (6,21,24) and are based on considerations discussed in the above sections. These criteria are as follows:

1. The rhythm must be inducible by single premature beats (as in Fig. 2.1). Generally, but not always, the first return echo beat is delayed (28,29).
2. The rhythm must have the ability to be terminated with a critically timed individual stimulus (Fig. 2.4B). Such a stimulus would penetrate the reentrant pathway and alter conduction and refractoriness so as to abolish the circuit(24,27,30–32).
3. The rhythm must have the ability to be reset by an individual premature stimulus. (24,27,33) (as in Fig. 2.4C).

While these three characteristics have been considered unique for reentry, it has become clear that triggered automatic rhythms due to delayed afterdepolarizations (DADs) may display similar features creating pitfalls in our analysis (see below for further discussion of DADs). One distinguishing feature for reentry is that the first return cycle (T_1) in the case of reentrant arrhythmias is delayed because of slow conduction and relative refractoriness in the reentrant loop (Fig. 2.5) while the return cycle in the case of DAD-induced triggered activity should be early (29,34). (Fig. 2.6). Or, in other words, the premature (S_1–S_2) and echo (S_2–T_1) cycles are inversely related in reentry (Fig. 2.5) and directly related in DAD-induced triggered activity (Fig. 2.6). This distinction is useful but it is not certain as short return cycles occasionally occur in, reentry due to Wolff-Parkinson-White syndrome (29) and probably other reentrant rhythms as well (Fig. 2.7). At times the S_1–S_2/S_2–T_1 relationship pattern is in the same patient at different cycle lengths (Fig. 2.7). (Also see below for a more complete discussion of DAD-induced triggered activity.)

In addition, in contrast to triggered arrhythmias, reentry has been found to be associated with: (a) abrupt rather than with delayed termination of a tachyarrhythmia via a premature beat. Delayed termination is associated with DAD-induced triggered rhythm though either can sometimes occur in reentrant or triggered rhythms (21,29,31) (see below); (b) induction only in certain regions, depending on the characteristics of stimulation to reentry site conduction as described above (24); and (c) a less variable rate response of the induced arrhythmia when basic cycle length during the induction protocol is changed (13,24).

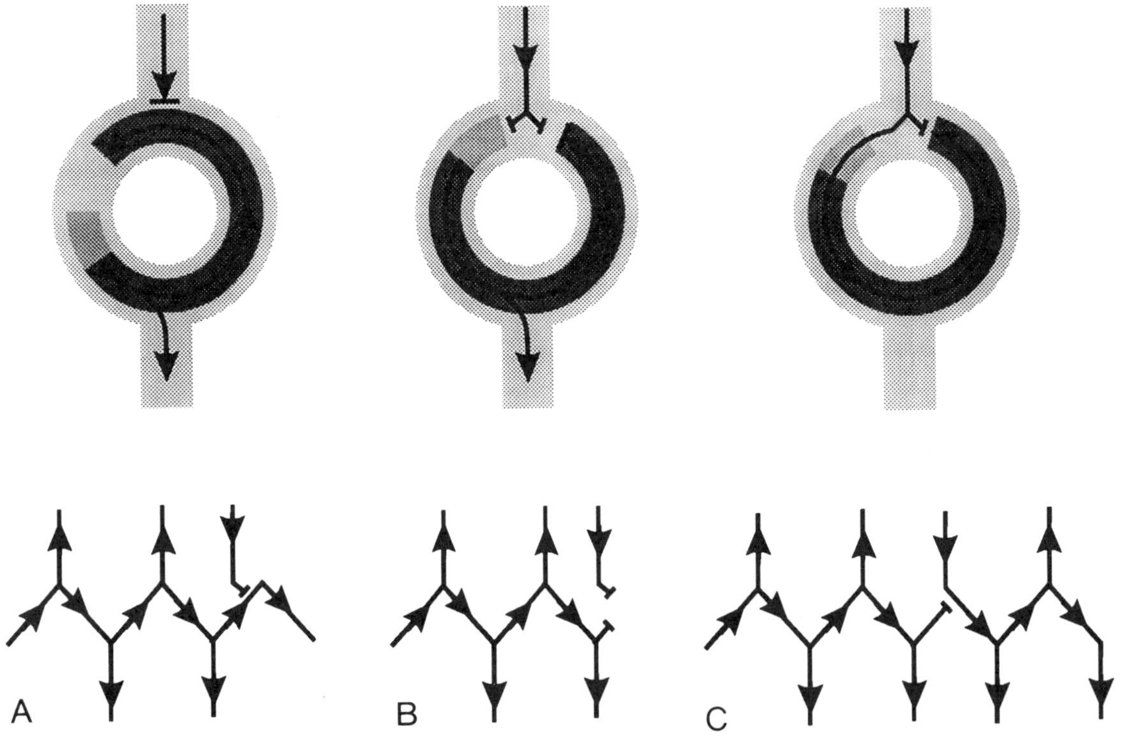

Figure 2.4. Effects of premature stimulation applied to an established reentrant pathway. The upper parts of **A, B,** and **C** show schematic of reentrant pathway and the lower portion is a corresponding ladder diagram. In **A,** stimulus arrives during a time when the pathway is refractory and has no effect. In **B,** stimulus arrives during the excitable window and blocks the head and is in turn blocked at the tail so that the reentrant pathway is abolished. In **C,** stimulus arrives with appropriate timing to be blocked at the head, but it conducts in the other direction to reset the tachycardia.

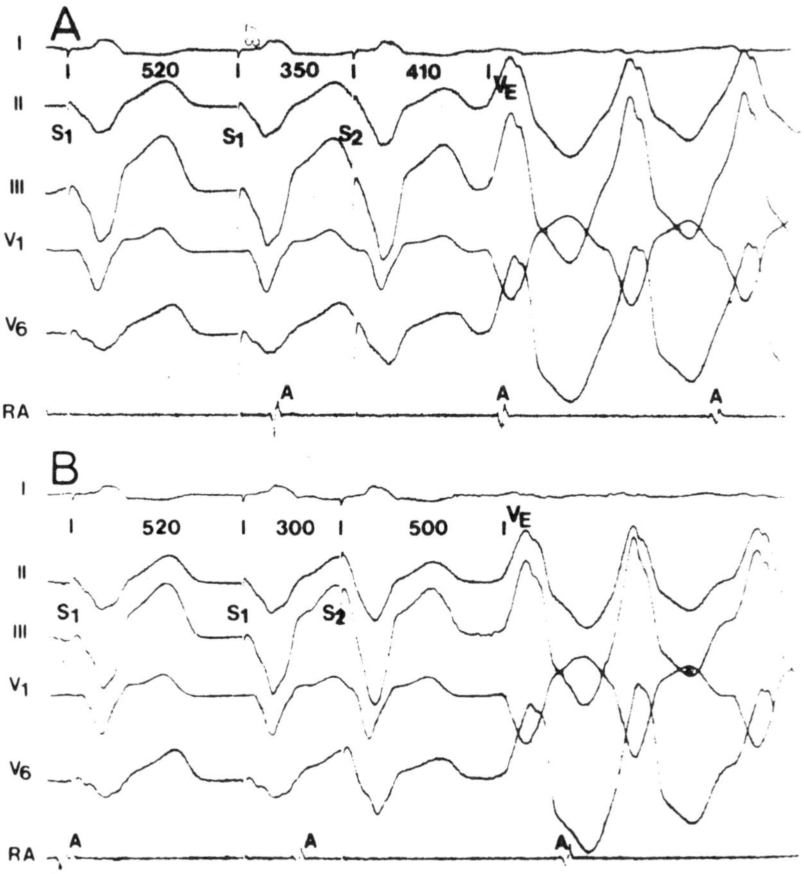

Figure 2.5. Programmed premature stimulation in a patient with ventricular tachycardia. Response to premature stimulation is of the type believed associated with reentrant arrhythmias. Basic recordings from two sequences are shown. Numbers are of cycle lengths are in milliseconds. The basic cycle length is 520 msec. On **A,** first premature S_1–S_2 is 350 msec and this is followed by a return cycle (S_2–T_1) of 410 msec. In **B,** the lower recordings shown in **B,** S_1–S_2 is 300 msec and this is followed by a longer S_2–T_1 (premature stimulus to first tachycardia beat) cycle of 500 msec. Thus, there is an inverse relationship between S_1–S_2 and S_2–T_1, as is believed to occur with reentrant arrhythmias. Leads I, II, III, V_1, and V_6 = ECG leads; RA = right atrium. (From Brugada P, Wellens HJJ: The role of triggered activity in clinical arrhythmias. In Rosenbaum MB, Elizart MV (eds): Frontiers of Cardiac Electrophysiology. The Hague, Martinus Nijhoff, 1983: 195, with permission.)

Rates of triggered activations tend to increase with increase in basic rate of pacing.

None of these distinctions has been proved for in situ arrhythmias, nor have they been subject to any rigorous clinical investigative analysis. In addition, though DAD-induced triggered activity is a hypothetical cause of clinical arrhythmia, clinical evidence for its existence (other than in digitalis toxicity) is still relatively sparse while considerable evidence exists for the occurrence of reentrant arrhythmias.

Effects of Antiarrhythmic Drugs

Antiarrhythmic drugs may influence the reentry circuit and/or the stimulus to reentrant site pathway in various ways to prevent, diminish, or at times enhance the likelihood of inducing reentry. They may do the following:

1. Alter or prolong refractoriness within the reentrant circuit so as to make induction of reentry impossible or unlikely (35). On the other hand, a drug might increase disparity in refractoriness in the circuit to facilitate reentry (22), or change refractoriness within the circuit once reentry has begun to make continuance of reentry more or less likely via Eq. (2.1) above.
2. Slow conduction to the point of block in the circuit to make completion of the loop impossible or to convert one-way to two-way block (35). On the other hand and in other situations, a drug may slow conduction so as to facilitate reentry via Eq. (2.1).
3. Influence cycle length–related changes in conduction or refractoriness to alter the excitable window, the necessity of one versus two or three premature stimuli, optimal basic cycle length, etc. for reentry to occur.
4. Enhance conduction to make maintenance of the reentrant circuit impossible (Eq. (2.1)). This may occur via hypopolarization of membrane potential (through at other sites hypopolarization may make inexcitable tissue excitable opening up another site of slow conduction and one-way block.)
5. Have a primary influence on the S to R pathway. A drug might prolong refractoriness more at S, slow S to R conduction (Fig. 2.3) or have other primary effects on the S to R pathway to prevent induction of reentrant arrhythmia without actually influencing the reentrant circuit (24). In this instance, there might still be spontaneously occurring arrhythmias in the absence of inducibility in the electrophysiologic laboratory. Use of multiple S sites, catecheolamines, or other interventions to shorten refractoriness in the S to R pathway, as well as use of complete stimulation protocols help minimize this potential problem in interpretation of electrophysiologic studies.

From these factors, it is easily seen why an antiarrhythmic drug may also at times be "proarrhythmic." Any factor that can help to prevent induction of tachycardia can, if slightly altered or active in another site, also help enhance tachycardia induction. Also, as indicated above, one should also keep in mind the distinction between trigger and substrate. In this instance "trig-

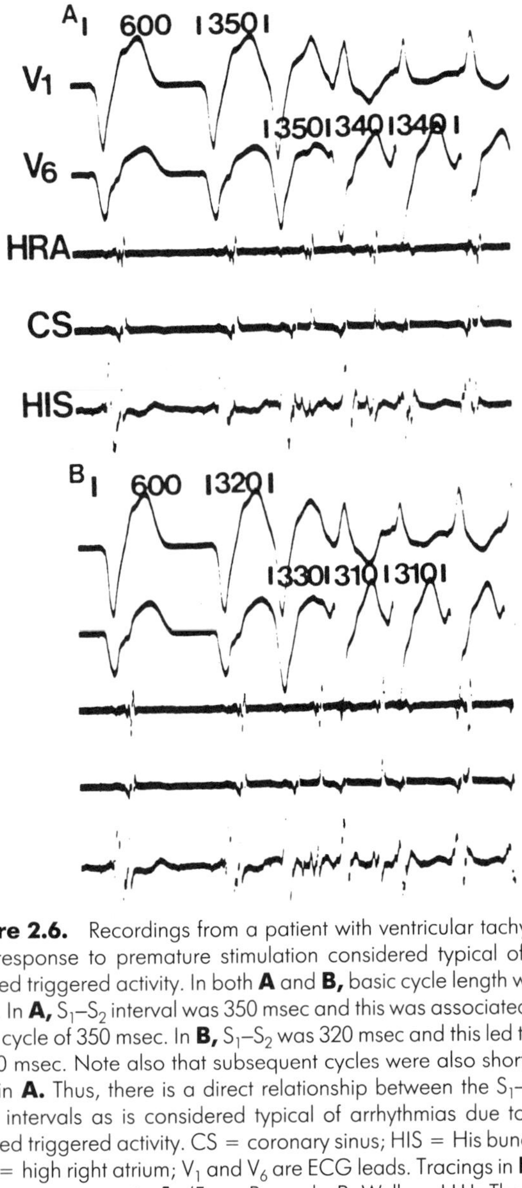

Figure 2.6. Recordings from a patient with ventricular tachycardia with response to premature stimulation considered typical of DAD-induced triggered activity. In both **A** and **B,** basic cycle length was 600 msec. In **A,** S_1–S_2 interval was 350 msec and this was associated with a S_2–T_1 cycle of 350 msec. In **B,** S_1–S_2 was 320 msec and this led to S_2–T_1 of 330 msec. Note also that subsequent cycles were also shorter in **B** than in **A.** Thus, there is a direct relationship between the S_1–S_2 and S_2–T_1 intervals as is considered typical of arrhythmias due to DAD-induced triggered activity. CS = coronary sinus; HIS = His bundle site, HRA = high right atrium; V_1 and V_6 are ECG leads. Tracings in **B** are in same sequence as in **A**. (From Brugada P, Wellens HJJ: The role of triggered activity in clinical arrhythmias. In Rosenbaum MB, Elizart MV (eds): Frontiers of Cardiac Electrophysiology. The Hague, Martinus Nijhoff, 1983; 195, with permission.)

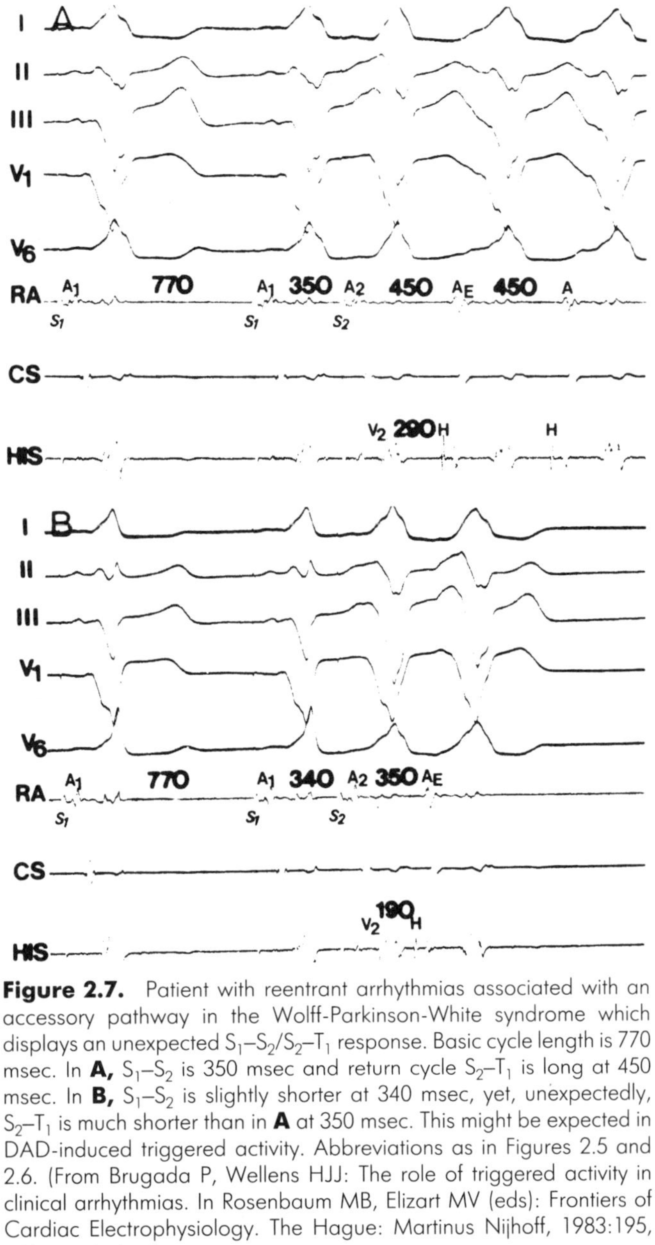

Figure 2.7. Patient with reentrant arrhythmias associated with an accessory pathway in the Wolff-Parkinson-White syndrome which displays an unexpected S_1–S_2/S_2–T_1 response. Basic cycle length is 770 msec. In **A,** S_1–S_2 is 350 msec and return cycle S_2–T_1 is long at 450 msec. In **B,** S_1–S_2 is slightly shorter at 340 msec, yet, unexpectedly, S_2–T_1 is much shorter than in **A** at 350 msec. This might be expected in DAD-induced triggered activity. Abbreviations as in Figures 2.5 and 2.6. (From Brugada P, Wellens HJJ: The role of triggered activity in clinical arrhythmias. In Rosenbaum MB, Elizart MV (eds): Frontiers of Cardiac Electrophysiology. The Hague: Martinus Nijhoff, 1983:195, with permission.)

ger" refers to a spontaneously occurring premature beat (of any type or mechanism) which initiates a reentrant tachycardia. Antiarrhythmic drugs may affect the trigger (i.e., suppress spontaneously occurring premature beats), the substrate (reentrant pathway), or the pathway from trigger to substrate.

Forms of Reentry

Many of the factors involved in reentry described above, for the most part, assume an anatomic site of block around which the reentrant circuit occurs. However, research particularly over the last 20 yr has brought to light a number of possible variations that reentry might take. These forms have been examined in in vitro, in situ, as well as in clinical situations.

ANATOMIC VERSUS FUNCTIONALLY DEFINED REENTRY

The important concept of "functionally defined" pathways, also referred to as the "leading circle hypothesis" was forwarded by a Allessie and others in the 1970s (36,37). In this type of reentry there is no fixed anatomic obstruction. Rather, reentry depends on a certain electrophysiologic pattern of conduction and refractoriness being present at a particular site. That is, if there is an appropriate pattern of conduction and refractoriness a triggering impulse can "functionally" define for itself a pathway of reentry with no anatomic obstacle (36,37). A typical established functionally defined pathway is shown in Figure 2.8. As proven by extensive activation maps, when this type of reentrant pathway is formed, impulses proceed around a vortex which consists of tissue that is functionally refractory but not anatomically blocked (36,37) (Fig. 2.8). For this to occur requires an initiating impulse to meet a precise arrangement of refractory tissue in the center (or vortex) and some sort of available excitable pathway more peripherally. It is a tight fit, with the advancing wavelength of necessity meeting refractory tissue with no excitable gap, and centripetal wavelets arising at the periphery and constantly trying to penetrate the center but not able to because they meet refractory tissue (Fig. 2.8). For various reasons (e.g., shortening of refractoriness at the vortex due to increase in rate or drugs), these impulse wavelets may in fact succeed in penetrating the vortex to abolish the pathway.

Anatomically and functionally defined reentrant pathways each have their own characteristic features (Fig. 2.9). In anatomically defined reentry, the length of the pathway is determined by the parameter of the anatomic obstacle while in functional reentry it is determined by electrophysiologic factors such as refractory period, conduction velocity, etc. Anatomically defined reentry has a fixed circuit length, an excitable gap between head and tail of pathway, and a revolution time (therefore cycle length) that is inversely related to conduction velocity more than to refractory period (because of the presence of the excitable gap). In functionally defined reentry, there is no excitable gap, revolution time is proportional to refractory period more than conduction velocity (since there is no excitable gap), and shortcut of the circuit is possible (36,37) (Fig. 2.9).

Because of the lack of an excitable gap and other factors, functional reentrant pathways are inherently less stable than anatomic pathways and termination occurs in somewhat different ways than shown in Fig. 2.4. For example, functionally defined pathways may change their configuration due to cycle length and other factors. Electronic influences due, for example, to impulses that arrive in the region of the pathway but do not penetrate it because of the lack of an excitable gap, may alter the precise arrangement of refractoriness and conduction in the pathway and abolish it. Entrainment also seems less likely than in anatomic reentry.

To what extent anatomically versus functionally defined circuits or a combination of the two play a role in specific arrhythmias is not clear. There has been perhaps the most interest in

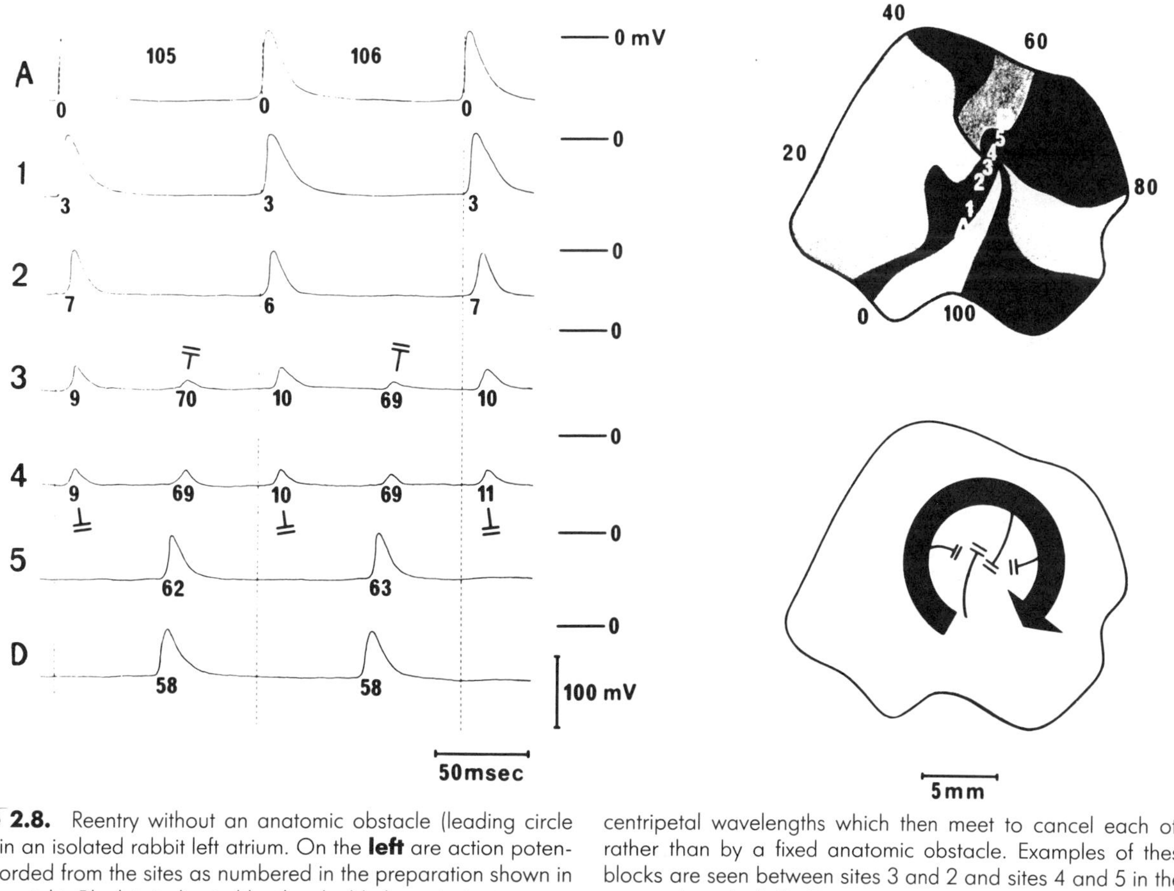

Figure 2.8. Reentry without an anatomic obstacle (leading circle model) in an isolated rabbit left atrium. On the **left** are action potentials recorded from the sites as numbered in the preparation shown in the upper right. Block is indicated by the *double bars.* Activation proceeds around a central vortex, as shown in the upper and more schematically in the **lower right.** The vortex is maintained by converging centripetal wavelengths which then meet to cancel each other out rather than by a fixed anatomic obstacle. Examples of these local blocks are seen between sites 3 and 2 and sites 4 and 5 in the action potentials on the **left.** (From Janse MJ: Reentry rhythms. In Fozzard HA, Haber E, Jennings RB, *et al.* (eds): The Heart and Cardiovascular System. Raven Press, New York, 1986:1203–1238, with permission.)

functionally defined pathways as causes of atrial and ventricular fibrillatory rhythms (see below) but they probably play a role in others as well.

ANISOTROPIC REENTRY

Recently, there has been interest in a form of reentry that may be particularly likely to occur in infarcted tissue—anisotropic reentry (38,40) (Fig. 2.10 and 2.11). This mechanism involves essentially an exaggeration of the natural tendency of the heart to conduct impulses differently in a longitudinal than in a transverse direction (41–43).

In the normal heart, impulses conduct more rapidly parallel to long axis of fibers than transverse (43). In myocardial infarction and perhaps other states this tendency is exaggerated at least in certain regions, due to edema, inflammation, and connective tissue encroaching on intracellular spaces transversely causing separation of fiber bundles, etc. Such an effect sets up the possibility of a reentrant pathway with pivot points occurring as the impulse moves from a transverse into a longitudinal direction (Fig. 2.10 and 2.11). In one study, longitudinal conduction velocity conduction was found to be 0.25–0.5 m/sec while it was less than 0.005 m/sec transversely (39).

Anisotropy seems to be a mixture of functional and anatomic reentry. There is no clear-cut anatomic boundary, though there are some anatomic abnormalities. Block of impulses to establish reentry will not occur unless there is a precise set of pacing, conducting, and milieu influences occurring as in functional reentry. However, there is one interesting difference. In anisotropic reentry, there appears to be an excitable gap. This is evidenced by the fact that single properly timed impulses can interrupt the circuit. The excitable gap appears to occur at pivot

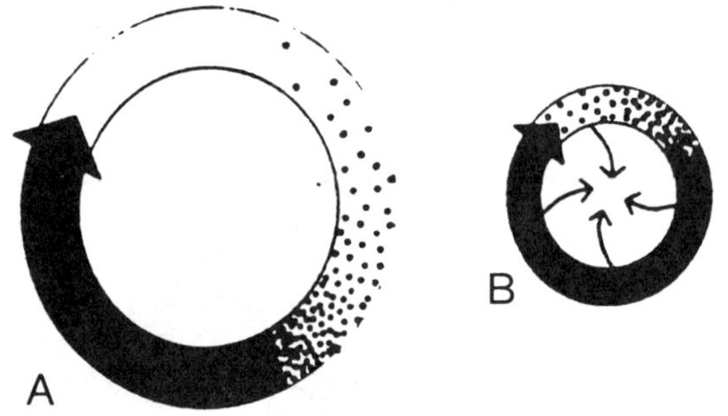

Figure 2.9. Comparison of the properties of circus movement with (**A**) and without (**B**) a central anatomic obstacle. (From Allessie MA, Bonke FIM, Schopman FJG: Circus movement in rabbit atrial muscle as a mechanism of tachycardia. III. The "leading circle" concept: A new model of circus movement in cardiac tissue without the involvement of an anatomical obstacle. Circ Res 1977;41:9–18, by permission of the American Heart Association.)

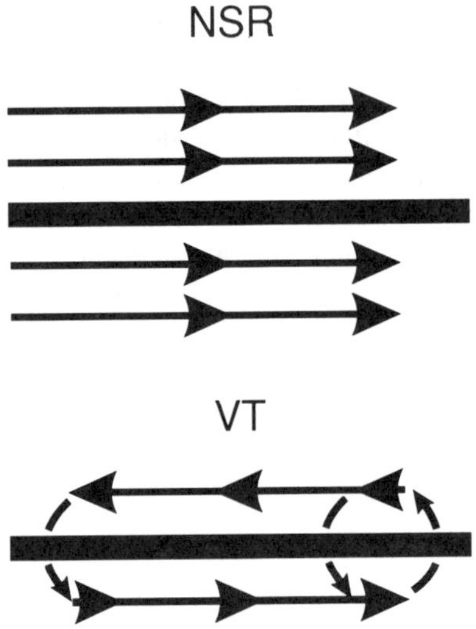

Figure 2.10. Representation of anisotropic reentry. The **upper panel** (NSR) shows conduction proceeding in a longitudinal direction normally. The *black bar* represents an area of potentially slow conduction in a transverse direction. The **lower panel** (VT) shows established anisotropic reentrant circuit with **dashed areas** representing slow conduction in a transverse direction. In these pathways there may be either long or short pathways as indicated.

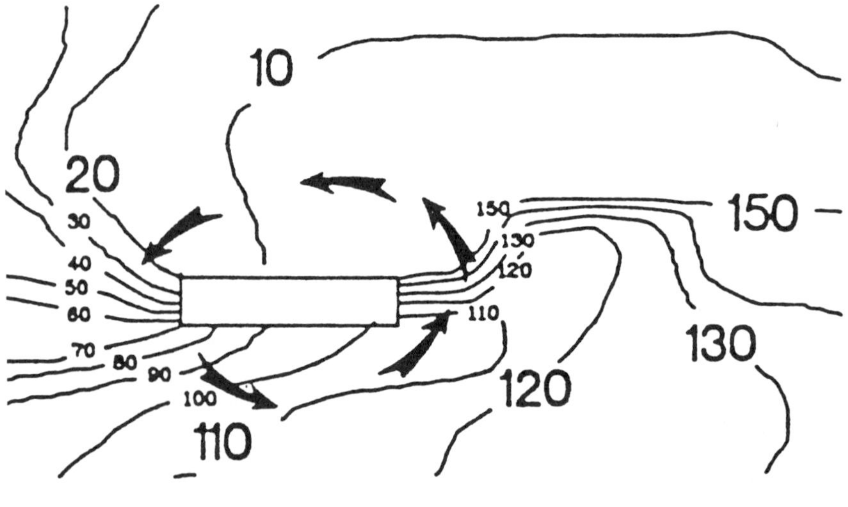

Figure 2.11. Anisotropic reentry in an infarcted preparation. Figure shows isochrone lines from an anisotropic reentry circuit. The widely spaced isochrones are in a longitudinal direction indicating more rapid conduction and are parallel to the muscle bundles (horizontal in this figure) and the closely spaced isochrones indicating slow conduction are in a direction transverse to muscle bundles (vertical in the figure). Anisotropic reentry is associated with rapid conduction longitudinally along muscle fiber bundles and slow conduction transversely. (From Dillon S, Allessie MA, Ursell PC, *et al.*: Influences of anisotropic tissue structure on reentrant circuits in the epicardial border zone of subacute canine infarcts. Circ Res 1988;63:182–206, by permission of the American Heart Association, Inc.)

points of the circuit where impulses conducting transversely turn to a longitudinal direction. Also, anisotropic circuits tend to be very stable, perhaps in part because of the presence of this excitable gap. These features are more characteristic of anatomic rather than functional reentry.

Undoubtedly, anisotropic reentry is important in arrhythmias due to myocardial infarction. Future work is expected to further elucidate and clarify this interesting mechanism of arrhythmia.

REFLECTION

In reflected reentry, impulses proceed to a point of block and then turn backward along the same pathway. One mechanism for this involves electrotonic transmission back from zones of block to cause reexcitation with markedly delayed return loops (16,44). The concept of reflected reentry is most interesting, though it still awaits a proven clinical situation.

MACROREENTRY VERSUS MICRO REENTRY

Macroreentry involves large anatomic pathways (12,21,45–47). A good example is the Wolff-Parkinson-White syndrome where the basic reentrant pathway is atrium–A-V node–ventricle–accessory pathway–atrium, etc. Other types of reentrant pathways may also utilize large cardiac anatomic structures such as bundle branches (46,48).

Macroreentrant pathways may also be the result of atrioventricular pacemakers (see Chapter 20). The circuit here includes paced atrium–paced ventricle–retrograde ventriculoatrial (V-A) conduction using His-Purkinje system and A-V node–atrium (63). Pacemaker modification to alter atrial refractory period and the paced A-V interval prevent these arrhythmias; drugs have been used as well.

Microreentry, as implied, involves small pathways. As indicated earlier, pathways as small as 12–35 mm (13) in vitro have sustained reentrant loops and probably smaller pathways are possible in anatomically disrupted (e.g., chronically infarcted) tissue.

The microreentry concept has been the basis of endocardial resections and other surgery for ventricular arrhythmia and is also the basis for certain types of arrhythmia ablation (18,49). That is, one can eliminate a relatively small reentrant circuit without substantial damage to the heart. Clinical features of microentry include the possibility of capture of the ventricle via sinus, ventricular, or paced beats without terminating the rhythm (i.e., the impulses do not reach the circuit) whereas this is less likely or impossible for macroreentry (18,49).

BOUNDARY OR INJURY CURRENT

It has been postulated that zones with prolonged action potentials or depolarized resting potentials (especially in ischemia) might act as a source of current to cause reentry by exciting contiguous tissue (50–52). One possibility is that electrotonic current arising from zones with prolonged action potentials will reduce membrane potentials and cause slowed conduction in contiguous tissues (53). This slowed conduction could promote reentry. However, while these concepts are attractive, there is little or no substantive evidence for reentry on the basis of injury current. As will be seen below (see Border Zone Automaticity Due to Injury Currents, below) we have recently provided evidence for another possibility—automatic arrhythmias on this basis (54).

FIGURE-OF-EIGHT REENTRY

An interesting phenomenon may occur in infarction whereby circulating wave fronts conduct around two separate areas of block forming a "figure-of-eight" through an isthmus of normal tissue (55,56).

LONGITUDINAL DISSOCIATION

Longitudinal dissociation refers to those forms of reentry in a linear bundle, one side of which has a zone of depressed tissue. Functional longitudinal dissociation is the functional counterpart of this in which critically timed beats arrive at refractory segments in a linear bundle (11,57).

FIBRILLATION—MULTIPLE WAVELET HYPOTHESIS

Fibrillation is, of course, a highly disorganized rhythm which has, in turn, led to postulations of highly disorganized reentrant mechanisms as its basis. In the multiple wavelet hypothesis, wave fronts fractionate, split, coalesce, summate, and collide in a variety of functionally derived circuits. These circuits are, in turn, constantly changing in size and rate of conduction and in site of block depending on changing excitability and refractoriness (in part cycle length related) of tissue it encounters. Figures 2.12 and 2.13 show examples from an ischemia model (21,58). Figure 2.12 shows a reasonably ordered reentrant cycle occurring during ventricular tachycardia while Figure 2.13 shows multiple wavelets developing as the rhythm changed to ventricular fibrillation. In some instances, there may be both anatomically as well as functionally defined circuits.

While the multiple wavelet hypothesis has long been accepted as a mechanism for fibrillation (58,59), mechanisms involving multiple sites of automaticity, perhaps coexistng with reentrant circuits, cannot at this point be excluded.

It should also be noted that, as the mechanism of fibrillation is unclear so is the precise mechanism of electrical defibrillation. According to the currently held postulate, during fibrillation, myocardial cells will be in all different phases of the action potential. The defibrillating shock may uniformly depolarize all cells and prolong the duration of cells that are in the plateau phase so as to create uniformity and an ordered sequence of activation. See Chapter 19 for a more complete discussion of mechanism of defibrillation.

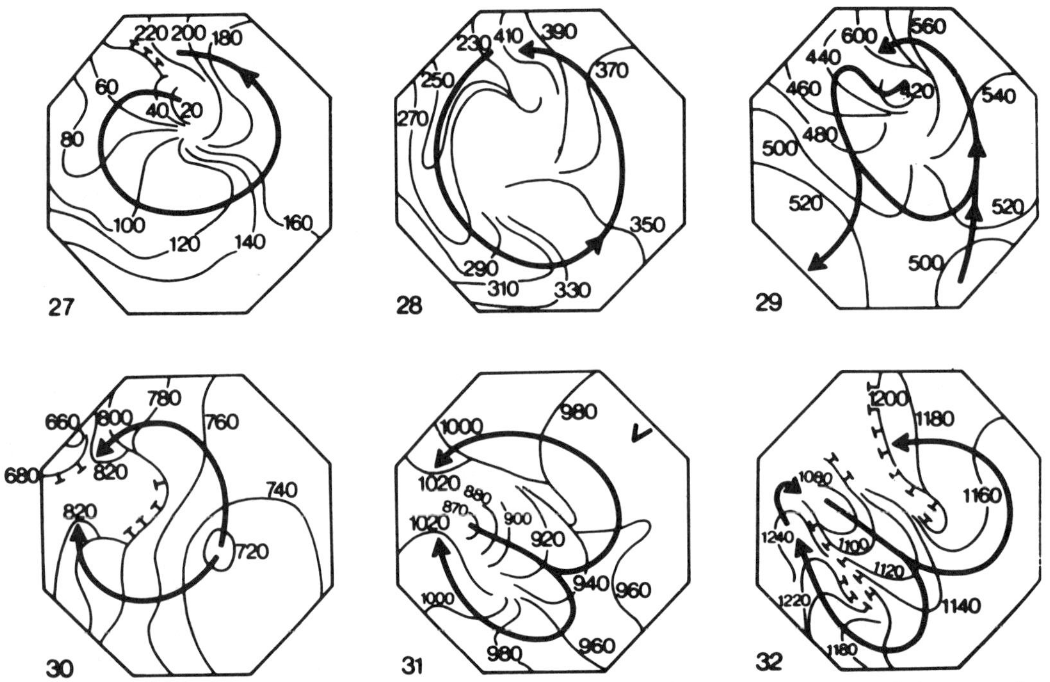

Figure 2.12. Isochrone activation patterns of six consecutive beats during ventricular tachycardia occurring after occlusion of the left anterior descending coronary artery in an isolated perfused pig heart. Recordings were made at 60 sites in the left ventricle. Numbers in isochrones are milliseconds with time zero arbitrarily chosen. *Arrows* indicate general direction of spread of activation. Note that the reentrant circuit changes its position and dimension from beat to beat. Reentry is due to a single circulating wave front. (From Janse MJ: Reentry rhythms. In Fozzard HA, Haber E, Jennings RB, *et al.* (eds): The Heart and Cardiovascular System. Raven Press, New York, 1986;1203–1238, with permission.)

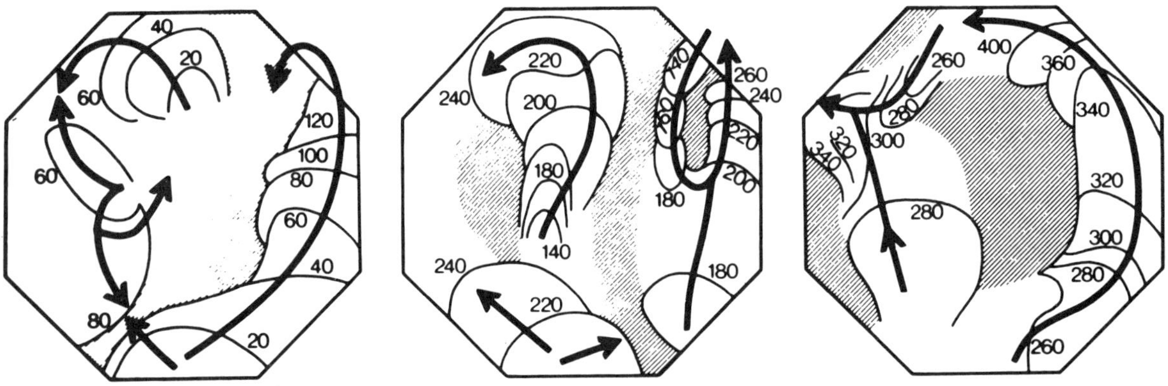

Figure 2.13. Isochrone activation patterns during ventricular fibrillation in an isolated perfused pig heart, after occlusion of left anterior descending coronary artery. This figure is from the same series of experiments as in Figure 2.12. During three successive beats, there is disorganization of electrical activity with collision of wave fronts and occasional complete circus movements. (From Janse MJ: Reentry rhythms. In Fozzard HA, Haber E, Jennings RB, *et al.* (eds): The Heart and Cardiovascular System. Raven Press, New York, 1986;1203–1238, with permission.)

REENTRY AT SPECIFIC ANATOMIC SITES

Specific reentrant arrhythmias are discussed in more detail in Chapters 7–9. However, a few points are worth noting in the context of mechanisms. Paroxysmal atrial tachycardia is most commonly caused by reentry within the AV node via longitudinal dissociation (possibly functional) (11,33,60,61). An α and β pathway have been hypothesized, the α being the slower pathway with the longer absolute refractory period (and more sensitive to drugs influencing slow channels) and the β pathway faster with a usually longer refractory period (and more sensitive to fast channel blocking local anesthetic drugs) (11,60,61). Reentry involving accessory pathways is most interesting and is discussed in Chapter 9. Atrial flutter has been the subject of long-term investigation and appears to involve reentry around anatomic obstacles in the atrium (15,24,27,32,62).

AUTOMATIC ARRHYTHMIAS

Automatic arrhythmias are generally considered to occur less commonly than those due to reentry. However, our methodology for making this distinction clinically is far from perfect. Two general categories of automatic arrhythmia have been promulgated—those associated with and those without triggered activity. Causes of automatic arrhythmias not based on triggered activity have been further subdivided into normal and abnormal automaticity (44). Arrhythmias based on triggered activity are further subdivided into those associated with delayed (DADs) or early (EADs) afterdepolarizations (44,64,65).

Normal and Abnormal Automaticity

NORMAL AUTOMATICITY

Enhanced normal automaticity is probably not a common mechanism for tachyarrhythmias. It is possible that under certain influences, most notably catecholamines (66,67), the normal automatic mechanisms in, e.g., peripheral Purkinje or A-V junction tissue may greatly accelerate. Atrial or ventricular arrhythmias occurring during catecholamine storms such as pheochromocytoma, cocaine abuse, or extreme emotional upset may be based on these mechanisms. Such arrhythmias tend not to be induced by the usual stimulation protocols and tend to display overdrive suppression.

ABNORMAL AUTOMATICITY

A postulated mechanism for certain arrhythmias based on automatic activity associated with cellular depolarization. Both specialized and myocardial tissue (which is not automatic at the usual resting membrane potentials) display automatic activity when depolarized—so-called "depolarization-induced automaticity (68–71). (This phenomenon is also associated with EAD-induced triggered activity—see below.) Abnormal automaticity has been elicited in a variety of preparations which may have clinical relevance, e.g., myocardial infarction (72,73), hypoxia, acidosis, and exposure to lysophospholipids (these are accumulation products of ischemia). Such abnormal automatic rhythms tend to be incessant and do not display overdrive suppression (74). It is not unlikely that some ventricular arrhythmias occurring during the course of myocardial infarction are based on abnormal automaticity. These arrhythmias are probably highly resistant to treatment as pharmacologic agents and are not effective in suppressing this abnormality (74,75).

Triggered Activity

Triggered activity is defined as the occurrence of nondriven action potentials that arise from afterdepolarizations that follow and are caused by previous action potentials (64). It is associated with two types of afterdepolarizations. These are shown in Figure 2.14. An EAD is a persistent depolarization that occurs during or delays repolarization (64) (Fig. 2.14A). A DAD (Fig. 2.14B) is a low-amplitude oscillation occurring in diastole after repolarization of an action potential (64).

An EAD or DAD may or may not lead to a triggered activation. When present, the triggered activation occurs on top of the EAD or DAD (Fig. 2.14). It is "nondriven" in that it depends on the initial "driven" (or triggering) action potential to occur and lead to the afterdepolarization which then leads to the triggered activation.

DELAYED AFTERDEPOLARIZATIONS

Causes of DADs

DADs occur in a number of experimental conditions, many with clinical relevance. The classic DAD model is glycoside toxicity (76–78). However, a body of literature also exists describing DADs in catecholamine excess (79,80) (which is, incidentally, involved in every type of automatic and triggered arrhythmia), low pH (81), histamine (H_2) receptor stimulation (82), lysophospholipids (83), hypertrophied myocardium (84), and infarcted (85,86) and chronically diseased human tissue (70). Also increased intracellular Na^+ (87), decreased extracellular K^+ (87,88), and increased extracellular Ca^{2+} (79,89) may be associated with DADs. The common feature in all of these causes is an increase in intracellular Ca^{2+} in myoplasm and/or sarcoplasmic reticulum.

The ionic current responsible for the DAD has been much studied and labeled "transient inward current" (90). It is believed related to electrogenic Na-Ca exchange. The prevailing

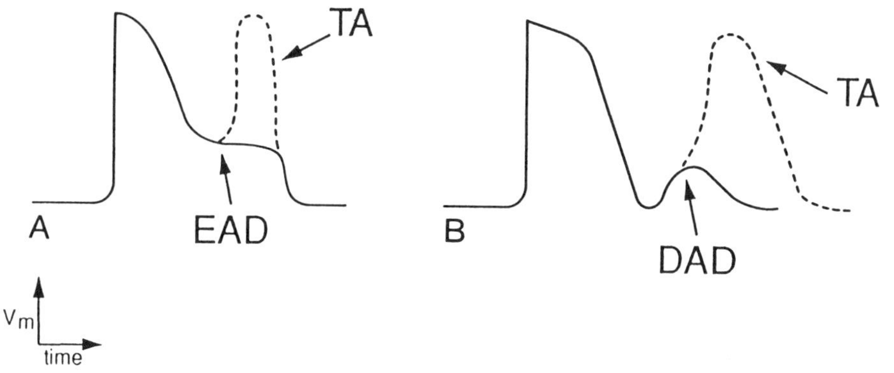

Figure 2.14. Schematic of early (EAD) and delayed (DAD) afterdepolarizations and corresponding triggered activations (TA). **A** shows EAD while **B** shows DAD.

hypothesis is that there is intracellular Ca^{2+} overload and a consequent oscillating, rhythmic movement of Ca^{2+} from the free intracellular space into and out of the sarcoplasmic reticulum. During any increase in free intracellular Ca^{2+}, an important mechanism for cellular calcium extrusion is Na-Ca exchange. Since three or four Na^+ ions enter the cell for each Ca^{2+} ion (91), there is net inward current and an afterdepolarization (92) (another theory holds that increased intracellular Ca^{2+} enhances conductance to gated inward currents such as Na^+) (93).

Characteristics of DADs and DAD-Induced Triggered Activity

The most characteristic feature of the DAD is its response to rapid pacing. As indicated above, the DAD is a low-amplitude oscillation that follows repolarization of an action potential. Under certain circumstances it enlarges and reaches a threshold for an activation to occur. The main circumstance for this sequence of events is rapid pacing, i.e., DAD-induced triggered activity is markedly enhanced with shortened cycle length (84,85,94–96). With a run of rapid pacing or a premature beat, DADs enlarge, reach threshold, and triggered activations occur (Fig. 2.15 and 2.16). When triggered activity is already underway, rapid pacing tends to make it faster.

This phenomenon, also called "overdrive excitation," is considered the essential feature of DAD-induced triggered activity. However, the response of tissue exhibiting DADs is more complex. With rapid pacing or prematurity, the following occur: (a) increased intracellular Ca^{2+} and increased intracellular Na^+ ions which tend to promote DADs; (b) increased extracellular K^+ ions and increased activity of the Na-K pump, both of which tend to promote outward currents and diminish DADs and triggered activity secondary to DADs. These underlying influences interact as follows: with short runs of pacing or single premature beats, the Ca^{2+} loading influence predominates and triggered activity is enhanced causing overdrive excitation. With longer runs of pacing, increased extracellular K^+ and ionic pump currents tend to predominate and the triggered activations are suppressed. In this instance, with long and very rapid pacing, overdrive suppression rather than excitation may occur. One more point: triggered activity due to DADs tends to be self-limited. Why? When the rhythm is initiated, increased intracellular Ca^{2+} loading which occurs with rapid beating tends to perpetuate it. However, as the tachycardia proceeds, outward Na-K pump and potassium currents tend to suppress and terminate it. (The role of Na-K pump mechanisms is much less prominent with DADs induced by glycosides which inhibit Na-K pump activity.) Because of the above influences, DAD-induced

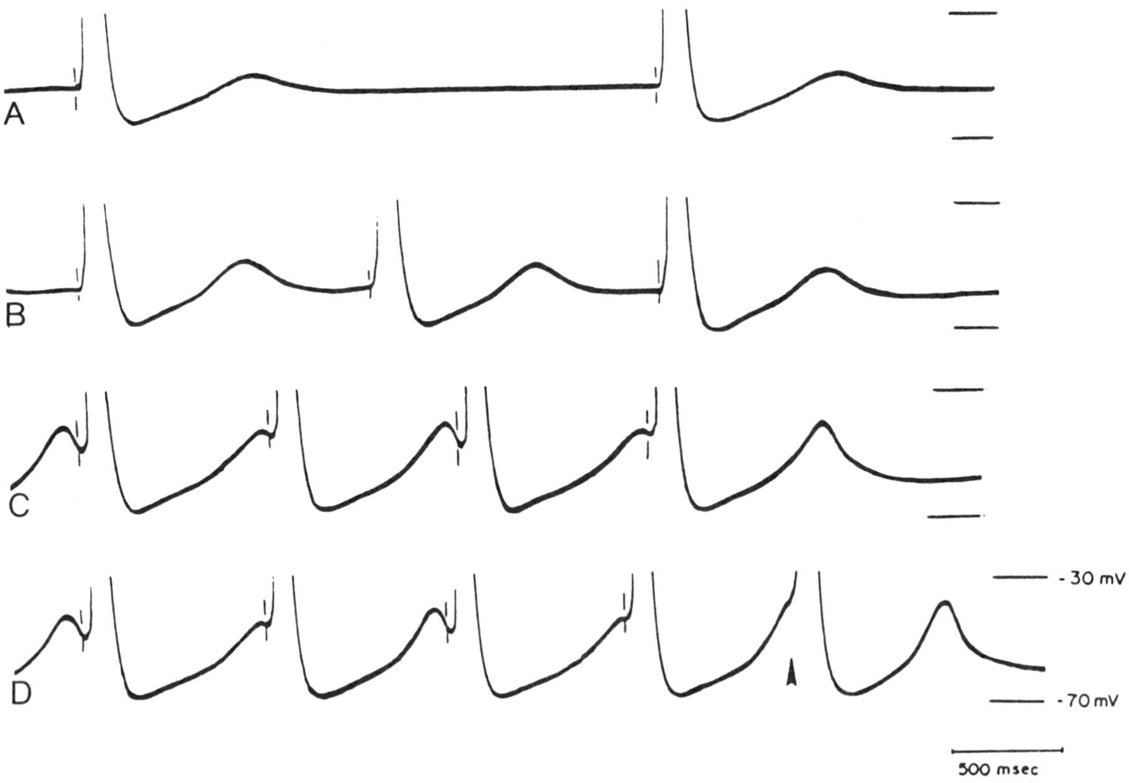

Figure 2.15. Effect of decreasing cycle length on amplitude of delayed afterdepolarizations. From **A** to **C,** driving rate is increased and DADs consequently become larger. In **D,** a further increase results in the DAD reaching threshold to initiate a triggered activation (*arrow*) followed by a DAD. These recordings were from a mitral valve preparation. (From Wit AL, Cranefield PF; Triggered activity in cardiac muscle fibers of the simian mitral valve. Circ Res 1973; 38;85–98, by permission of the American Heart Association, Inc.)

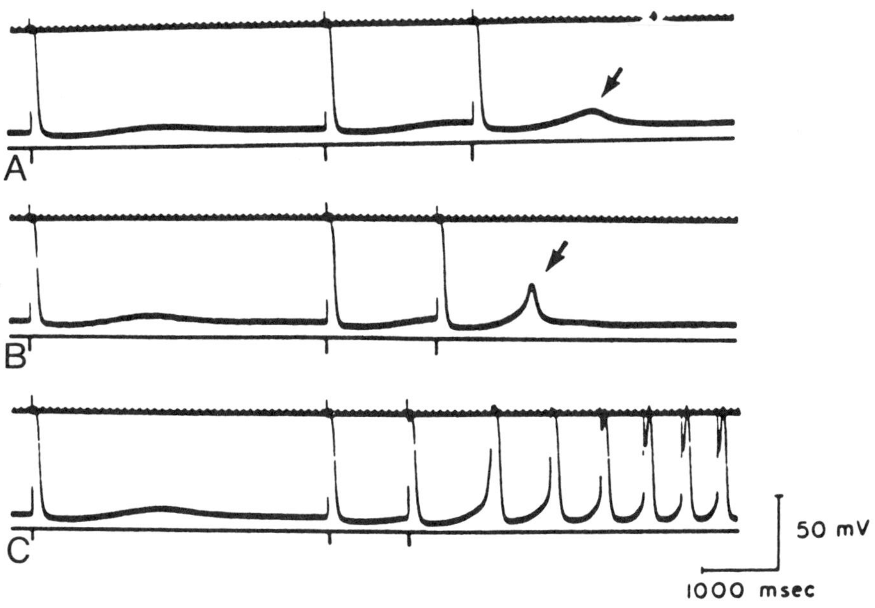

Figure 2.16. Induction of DAD-induced triggered activity via programmed premature stimulation. **A, B,** and **C** show premature beats at progressively earlier intervals. Note that in **B,** premature stimulus is somewhat earlier and the DAD (*arrow*) is somewhat larger. In **C,** an even earlier stimulus causes DAD to reach threshold and initiate a run of triggered activity. This response to programmed premature stimulation can mimic that of reentry. (From Wit AL, Cranefield PF: Triggered automatic activity in the canine coronary sinus. Circ Res 1977;41:435–445, by permission of the American Heart Association, Inc.)

triggered activity tends to have a "warm-up" and "wind-down" period and tends to be self-limited.

Clinical Criteria to Diagnose DAD-Induced Triggered Activity

Certain features elucidated in vitro and in some in situ models of DADs may be helpful in distinguishing clinical arrhythmias related to this mechanism. The most studied model has been digitalis toxicity but it is worthwhile to remember that a number of other models exist and that each model differs somewhat in certain key characteristics. It is also worthwhile to remember that clinical examples with good circumstantial evidence for triggered activity are uncommon and the bulk of clinical arrhythmias appear to be reentrant. Or, to put it another way to physicians evaluating these tests based on current state of knowledge, the pretest probability for given arrhythmia being reentrant rather than triggered is high. It is generally considered that the burden of proof rests on one who postulates that a given arrhythmia is triggered.

The following have been considered in situ and in clinical guidelines (29,34,94,95,97,98) to detect arrhythmia due to DAD-induced triggered activity:

1. Triggered activations can be induced by premature beats and short bursts of rapid pacing (Fig. 2.15 and 2.16). However, unlike reentry, triggered activations often cannot be reproducibly induced by the same stimulation protocol and are more likely, in any case, to be induced by burst pacing rather than single premature beats (34,94,98).

2. Triggered activations are more likely induced when the preceding basic cycle length is short (500–700 msec) (98) whereas reentry is more likely induced with longer basic cycle lengths.

3. Premature beats initiating tachycardia due to DADs tend to occur late in the cycle (97,98) while those initiating reentry tend to occur early.

4. With triggered activity, there tends to be a direct relationship between coupling interval of the initiating premature beat and the interval to the first beat of the tachycardia (T_1) (i.e., with shorter S_1–S_2, there is also a shorter S_2–T_1 interval.) (34,99) (Fig. 2.6). With reentry, on the other hand, this relationship is reversed (shorter coupling interval of S_1–S_2 leads to longer S_2–T_1 interval) (Fig. 2.5). Many consider this an important distinction, although reentrant arrhythmias (e.g., due to the Wolff-Parkinson-White syndrome) may at times display the coupling interval relationship expected for DAD-induced triggered activity (29) (Fig. 2.7). As also seen in Figure 2.7, change in basic cycle length can lead to a change in S_1–S_2/S_2–T_1 ratio from that suggestive of reentry to that suggestive of DAD-induced triggered activity.

5. With a faster basic cycle length the induced tachycardia related to DAD-induced triggered activations should also be faster (97) (though exceptions occur). This should not occur in reentry, though transient acceleration of reentrant arrhythmias can occur during rapid pacing (27), i.e., "entrainment."

6. Overdrive pacing tends to enhance triggered activations while it abolishes reentry. However, as noted above, rapid pacing has a complex relationship with triggered activity, with longer and faster pacing suppressing it.

7. Triggered activations can be terminated by a single premature beat (77,95,100) (Fig. 2.17). However, this is far less likely than with reentry. When triggered activations are terminated in this manner, there are usually but not always additional beats before termination, so-called "delayed termination." In the case of reentry, the rhythm terminates immediately.

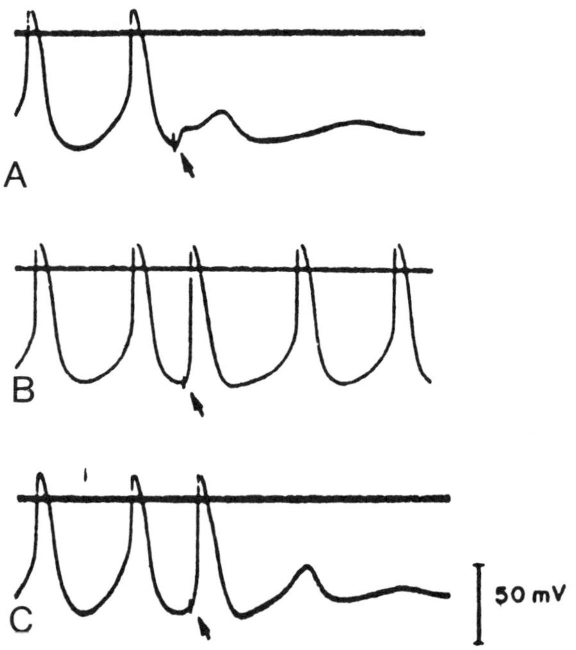

Figure 2.17. Effects of premature stimulation at somewhat different coupling intervals applied during a run of triggered activity due to DADs. **A** shows a premature stimulus terminating the tachycardia without initiating an activation. **B** shows a premature stimulus initiating an activation but not terminating the tachycardia. **C** shows a premature stimulus which results in an activation which is then followed by termination of the triggered activity. Preparation is a simian mitral valve. (From With AL, Cranefield PF: Triggered activity in cardiac muscle fibers of the simian mitral valve. Circ Res 1976;38:85–98, by permission of the American Heart Association, Inc.)

8. As explained above, runs of triggered activations tend to exhibit a "warm-up" and "wind-down", i.e., gradually increase in rate and tend to end spontaneously. However, reentrant arrhythmias may also display both of these peculiarities.

9. Premature beats should be able to reset runs of triggered activity as they do reentrant arrhythmias (34).

It is apparent from the above that, while there are distinguishing features, reentry and DAD-induced triggered activity can mimic each other well in situ.

Clinical Arrhythmias Associated with DADs

Brugada and Wellens (99) examined a large number of arrhythmias induced in electrophysiologic studies using roughly the above guidelines. They found that only a small percent appeared due to triggered activation. In their view, about 10% of ventricular tachycardias or atrial arrhythmias associated with mitral valve prolapse were based on triggered activity.

On the other hand, certain specific clinical arrhythmias have been thought to be based on triggered activity due to DADs (101–104). Accelerated junctional rhythms obey many of the guidelines considered characteristic for triggered activations, especially a tendency to increase in rate over several cycles and then terminate spontaneously (98). Many nonsustained ventricular tachycardias also seem to have these characteristics.

Exercise-induced ventricular tachycardia is another rhythm with many characteristic features of DAD-induced triggered activity. It is initiated by exercise (i.e., with rapid rates) as well as often by rapid pacing (to a certain rate as expected) (105,106). The first beat of the tachycardia tends to occur late in the cycle and the cycle length of the first or second beat is short. This type of ventricular arrhythmia responds to verapamil (107) and adenosine (108). (Interestingly, triggered activations responsive to adenosine have been thought to be mediated by cyclic adenosine monophosphate (cAMP)).

Pharmacology of DAD-Induced Triggered Activity

β-agonists enhance DAD-induced triggered activity. Beta blockers, some local anesthetic agents (74,109), calcium channel blockers (80,95,110,111), and adenosine (108,112) suppress such activity.

EAD & EARLY AFTERDEPOLARIZATIONS

As noted above, EADs are afterdepolarizations that occur during or delay repolarization and they, like DADs, are associated with triggered activations (Fig. 2.14). (Unfortunately, there is no distinction in the term "triggered activation" between the different types of triggered activations associated with DADs and EADs). An action potential displaying EADs may be unique appearing, especially if it also has triggered activations (113–117) (Fig. 2.18). Such an action potential could lead to tachycardia secondary to the triggered activations (Fig. 2.18C). In addition, the phenomenon could lead to marked prolongation of action potential duration without triggered activations (Fig. 2.18A and B). As will be discussed below and in Chapter 10, certain clinical tachycardias have been ascribed to EAD-induced triggered activations.

EADs and resulting triggered activity can occur at various levels of membrane potential. Damiano and Rose (116) have suggested that EADs be classified as high (i.e., more negative) and low (more positive) membrane potential (Fig. 2.19). It has also been suggested that EADs arising at takeoff potentials above (positive to) -30 mV be considered "Phase 2 EADs" and those arising negative to -30 mV, "Phase 3 EADs."

Correlations of EADs and EAD-induced triggered activity with surface ECG recordings have been made. EADs appear to be associated with U waves in the ECG and triggered activations with polymorphic ventricular tachycardia or torsade de pointe.

EADs are more likely to occur in Purkinje fiber than ventricular muscle (119,120). We have also found that transmission of triggered activations occurs from localized abnormal to normal zones (leading to generalized arrhythmias), and that conduction depends on amplitude and upstroke velocity of the individual triggered activation (119,120).

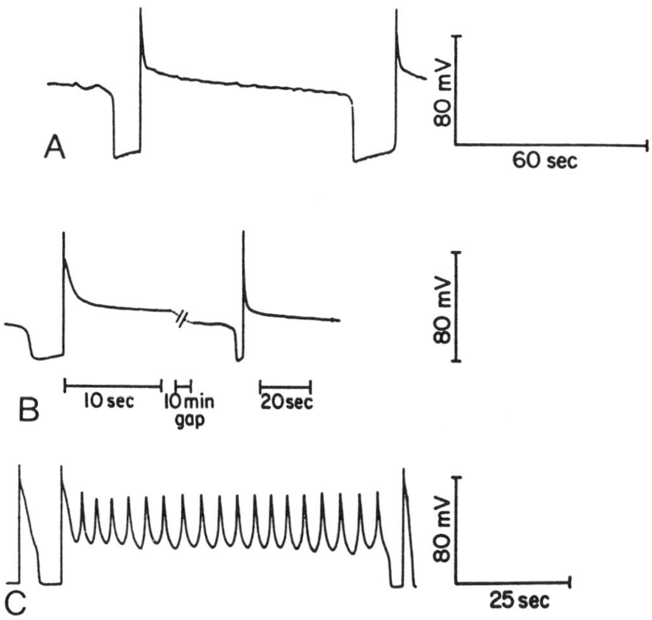

Figure 2.18. Abnormally prolonged action potentials and EADs recorded in three separate experiments utilizing nickel (2FmMol) and moderate hypothermia in Purkinje fiber. **A** and **B** show prolonged action potentials. Note that in **B,** action potential is greater than 10 min long. **C** shows first a normal action potential, then a prolonged action potential, EADs, and triggered activations. (Note: there may be some variance in terminology concerning triggered activations. One might consider that this is one long action potential with multiple triggered activations before a final repolarization. Others consider that each triggered activation in such a situation should be considered a new action potential.) This is followed by another normal action potential. (From Kupersmith J, Hoff P, Guo S: In vitro characteristics of repolarization abnormality—a possible cause of arrhythmias. J Electrocardiol 1986;19:361–370, with permission.)

Causes of EADs

A key point about the EAD phenomenon is movement of membrane potential to and from plateau level. The usual basis of the abnormality in that membrane potential tends to stay at or toward plateau levels for prolonged intervals, i.e., complete repolarization is delayed. Maintenance of membrane potential at depolarized levels leads to "depolarization induced automaticity" a well-described form of automatic activity that occurs when membrane potential remains depolarized for prolonged periods of time (68,69). Such automatic activity appears to be a cause of EAD-induced triggered activity.

The ionic mechanisms responsible for EADs and associated triggered activations are not completely clear and surely variable. Inward currents favor depolarization and movement to or maintenance of plateau membrane potential. Outward currents favor repolarization and movement back to resting membrane potential levels. Diminution of outward K^+ current or enhancement of inward window Na^+ currents, both of which overall favor inward depolarizing current, favor the phenomenon in general (as probably also does electrogenic Na-Ca exchange).

As for the ionic currents related to EAD-induced triggered activity, these depend on the take of potentials (Fig. 2.19). Activity occurring at more positive potentials probably result from slow inward Ca^+ current while that occurring at more negative potentials results from inward Na^+ current. Other mechanisms are also possible. It should also be noted that in some instances such as with aconitine (121), the inward current causing the triggered activation rather than the EAD appears to be the primary abnormality.

EADs can be caused by a wide variety of inciting agents,

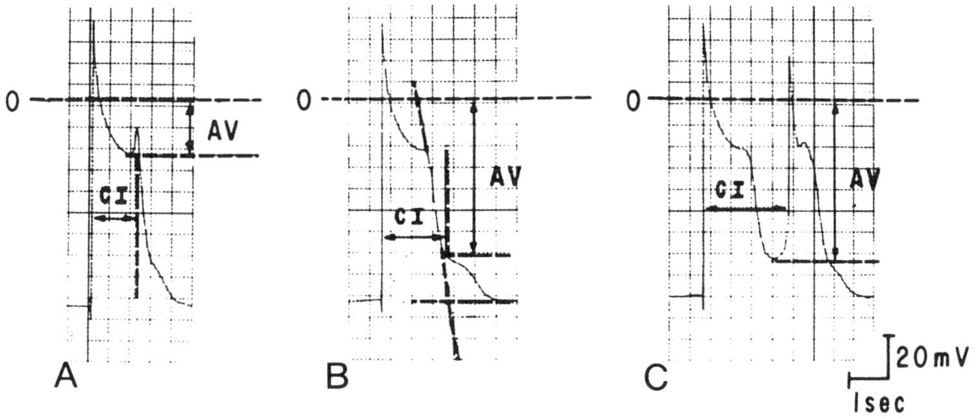

Figure 2.19. EADs and triggered activations at different levels of membrane potential. **A** shows a triggered activation arising from an EAD at "low membrane potential" level (i.e., more positive membrane potential). **B** shows a triggered activation arising from an EAD at a higher (more negative) membrane potential level. **C** shows an EAD occurring at a high membrane potential level. There is also a high membrane potential EAD in addition to the triggered activation in **A.** AV = activation voltage; CI = conduction interval from onset of action potential to onset of EAD or triggered activation. (From Damiano BP, Rosen M: Effects of pacing on triggered activity induced by early afterdepolarizations. Circulation 1984;69:1013–1025, by permission of the American Heart Association, Inc.)

many of them with clinical significance. These include aconitine (the active process in the poisonous plant hemlock; it inhibits deactivation of inward sodium current) (121–123), veratridine (124), hypoxia (113,114), hypercarbia (125), acidosis (114,125), catecholamines (113), hydrogen peroxide (126), cesium (which decreases potassium currents) (115,116), amiloride, injury (127) (possibly stretch) and toxicity with a number of antiarrhythmic drugs, i.e., Class IA and III drugs, including quinidine (128), *N*-acetylprocainamide (129), and sotalol (130,131). Amiodarone which prolongs action potential duration and can be associated with EADs, also suppresses Ca^+ current to inhibit the triggered activations arising from the EADs.

Characteristic Properties of EADs

The most characteristic property of EADs is exquisite rate sensitivity. Fast rates suppress them, and slow rates bring them on (in contrast to DADs which display the opposite characteristics). Thus, EADs display overdrive suppression. Even slight differences in cycle length and rate can have profound effects on action potential duration and the number of triggered activations (Fig. 2.20 and 2.21).

Clinical Criteria to Diagnose EAD-Induced Triggered Activity

With the above in mind, we can review the clinical criteria to diagnose arrhythmias due to EAD-induced triggered activity as follows.

1. EADs and associated increased triggered activations are enhanced at slow rates and suppressed at fast rates (unlike DADs) (113–116, 132). Longer pauses are followed by longer runs of triggered activity (Fig. 2.21). These responses are the most characteristic of EAD-induced triggered activity.
2. Overdrive pacing tends to suppress triggered activations for short periods of time, but then they reappear after cessation of pacing (as in Fig. 2.20).
3. Premature beats may (114,116) or may not (114) abolish tachycardias related to EAD-induced triggered activations. If it occurs, termination of the tachycardia is immediate, unlike in the case of DAD-induced triggered activity where "delayed termination" tends to occur. Premature beats may also reset the tachycardia (116).
4. At the same basic cycle length, triggered activations tend to have fixed coupling. The first beat of tachycardia also tends to (but not always) have a fixed coupling interval.
5. The first beat of the tachycardia tends to have a reasonably long coupling interval (more than in reentry). The next few coupling intervals should be somewhat shorter than the first (64).
6. There is a tendency for coupling interval of individual triggered activations to decrease with increasing bradycardia (116).
7. Tachycardias have a tendency to occur in bursts (which are prevented by rapid pacing) and to be self-limited. Triggered activity also tends to slow down prior to termination.
8. Use of special electrodes to record monophasic action potentials may elicit EADs and triggered activations (118,133,134). These have been recorded in patients with the long QT syndrome (135) (see Chapter 10). U-waves on the surface ECG have also been found to correlate with the phenomenon (118).

As can be seen, arrhythmias associated with the acquired long QT syndrome fit in very well with the above characteristics—emergence with bradycardia, suppression by overdrive, frequent nonsustained bursts of tachycardia, long QT interval reflecting the long action potentials, and frequent occurrence of

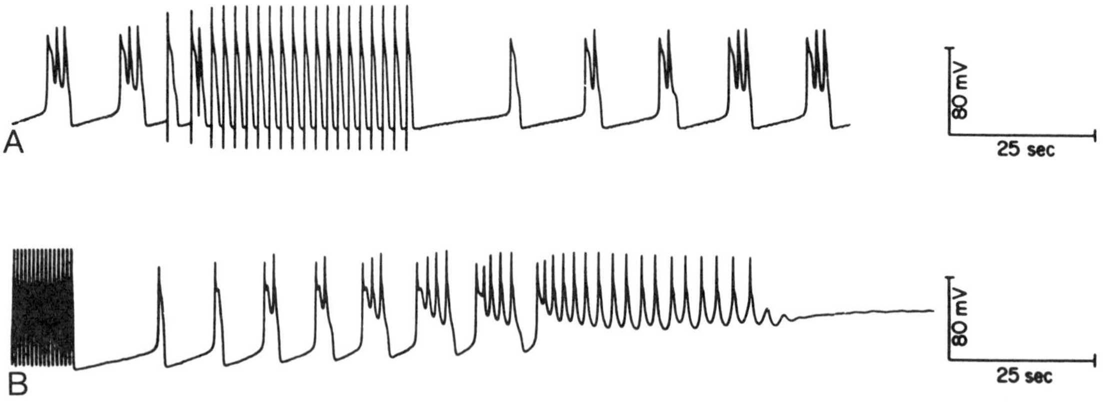

Figure 2.20. Effect of pacing on EADs and triggered activations. **A** shows first two action potentials with two triggered activations each, and then a train of rapid pacing, during which action potentials normalize. Following this, there is gradual return of EADs and triggered activations. **B** shows first a rapid train of pacing with normal action potentials. After termination of pacing action potentials gradually prolong and display triggered activations. Finally, there is an upstroke with a series of triggered activations followed by low-amplitude oscillations and then quiescence at a depolarized membrane potential. These recordings were made in hypoxic, acidic Tyrode's solution (pH 7.0) in sheep Purkinje fiber. (From Kupersmith J, Hoff P; Guo S: In vitro characteristics of repolarization abnormality—a possible cause of arrhythmias. J Electrocardiol 1986;19:361–370, with permission.)

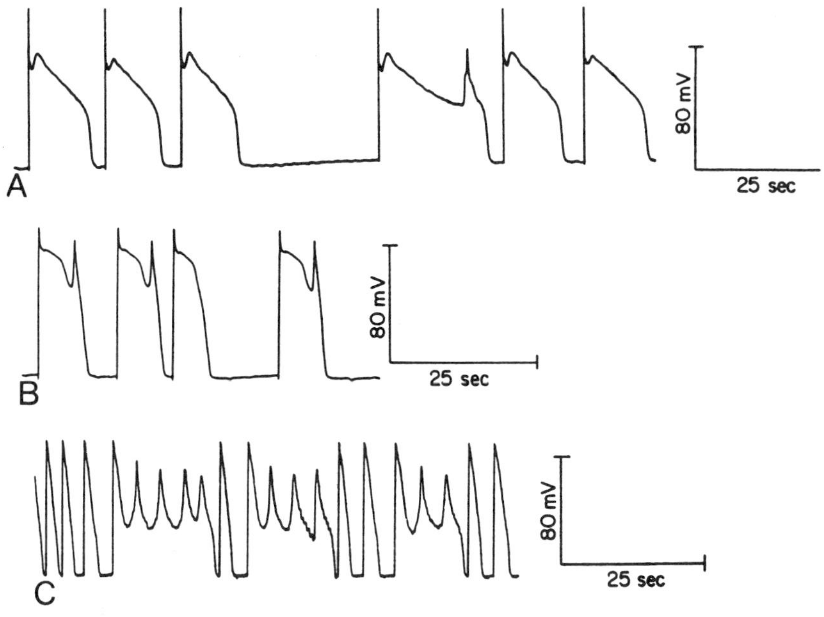

Figure 2.21. Effects of changes of diastolic interval on action potentials exhibiting EAD induced triggered activation. In **A,** there are three normally configured action potentials and then a pause following which there is an action potential with a triggered activation. In **B,** premature action potential uniquely does not display triggered activation, and in **C** slight changes in diastolic interval have a profound effect on action potential duration and the occurrence of triggered activations. (From Kupersmith J, Hoff P, Guo S: In vitro characteristics of repolarization abnormality—a possible cause of arrhythmias. J Electrocardiol. 1986; 19:361–370, with permission.)

ECG U waves which may represent EADs occurring in the His-Purkinje system (118). In addition, several of the previously noted causes of EADs (see above) are also known to cause long QT intervals and ventricular arrhythmias both in in situ experimental preparations (in the case of cesium and aconitine) (133) and in the clinic (118) (in the case of Class IA and III antiarrhythmic drugs). All of these observations make the case for EAD-induced triggered activity being the cause of arrhythmias associated with the acquired long QT syndrome (114,132,136). (See Chapter 10 for further discussion of the long QT syndrome.) It is also possible that some reperfusion arrhythmias are based on this mechanism. Torsade de pointe in which bursts of ventricular tachycardia display a twisting ECG pattern is an arrhythmia that accompanies the long QT syndrome. The twisting ECG pattern could represent triggered activations arising from two separate sites (137,138).

Effects of Drugs on EAD-induced Triggered Activity

To reverse EAD-induced triggered activity a drug might shorten action potential duration to completely reverse the EADs or might suppress the triggered activity directly leaving EADs intact. There are drugs that do either or both of these. Procainamide can suppress triggered activations directly, though EADs and action potential prolongation remain (127). Probably a number of other local anesthetic agents also act similarly (though some of them may induce EADs and EAD-induced triggered activity, the ever-present paradox with these types of drugs). Lidocaine, on the other hand, shortens action potential and thereby brings membrane potential to resting levels to reverse the phenomenon (113,127). Calcium channel blockers may either shorten action potential (130) or suppress the triggered activations directly (130).

Border Zone Automaticity Due to Injury Currents

As indicated above, border zone arrhythmias due to possible injury current have been a subject of speculation in various contexts over the years (50–52, 139). However, there is little experimental evidence for these postulates. We have elicited in a phenomenon which we call "border zone automaticity" (54). We have found that electrotonic transmission of injury current from the prolonged action potentials into the border zone causes membrane potential to be reduced and in this way enhances automatic activity (Fig. 2.22). (See Chapter 1 for discussion of

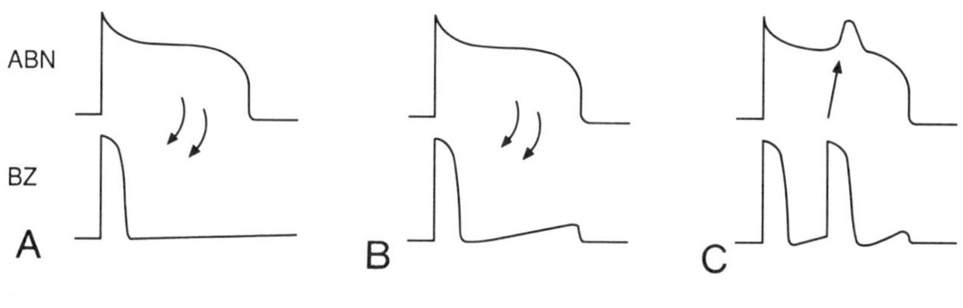

Figure 2.22. Schematic of border zone automaticity. In **A,** there is an abnormally prolonged (upper) and a normal (lower) action potential recorded at the border of a normal zone. Normal action potential is very slightly automatic. *Arrows* represent current flowing from the abnormally prolonged action potential into normal zone. In **B,** this current results in enhanced diastolic depolarization in the normal zone, and in **C** there is a resultant triggered activation arising at the border of the normal zone and conducting into the abnormal zone as indicated by the arrow. ABN = abnormal zone, BZ = normal zone border.

factors involved in automaticity.) The phenomenon is "triggered" in that it requires the initial upstroke of the long action potential to get it started (54). It is caused by "injury" current i.e., movement of current. As expected, selective addition of lidocaine to the border segment abolished the triggered activity as it would other automatic arrhythmias.

The border zone automaticity that we observed is a plausible clinical mechanism of arrhythmias in a number of situations including myocardial infarction and chronic fibrosis. One possible arrhythmia type is accelerated idioventricular rhythm. However the concept awaits further confirmation.

COMBINED AUTOMATICITY AND REENTRY

A number of situations could arise clinically in which there may be mixed or combined mechanisms of arrhythmias. For example, an automatic ventricular premature beat could trigger a run of reentrant ventricular tachycardia. Conversely, and perhaps less likely, a reentrant ventricular premature beat could induce triggered activity, secondary to DADs. Other combined mechanisms can be imagined.

References

1. McWilliam J: Fibrillar contraction of the heart. J. Physiol (Lond) 1887;8:296–310.
2. Mayer AG: Rhythmical pulsation in scyphomedusae. Publication 47 of the Carnegie Institution. Carnegie Institution of Washington, Washington, D.C., 1906:1–62.
3. Mines GR: On dynamic equilibrium in the heart. J Physiol (Lond) 1914;46:349–382.
4. Garrey WE: The nature of fibrillary contraction of the heart—its relation to tissue mass and form. Am J Physiol 1914;33:397–414.
5. Kent AFS: Observations on the auriculo-ventricular junction of the mammalian heart. Q J Exp Physiol 1913:7:193–197.
6. Mines GR: On circulating excitations in heart muscles and their possible relation to tachycardia and fibrillation. Trans R Soc Can 28 (Sect IV), 1914:43–52.
7. Lewis T: The mechanism and registration of the heart beat. ed. 3. Shaw & Sons, London, 1925.
8. Schmitt FO, Erlanger J: Directional differences in the conduction of the impulse through heart muscle and their possible relation to extrasystolic and fibrillary contractions. Am J Physiol 1928;87:326–347.
9. El-Sherif N, Mehra R, Gough WB, et al: Reentrant ventricular arrhythmias in the late myocardial infarction period. Interruption of reentrant circuits by cryothermal techniques. Circulation 1983;68:644–656.
10. Burchell HB, Fry RL, Anderson MW, et al.: Atrioventricular and ventriculo-atrial excitation in Wolff-Parkinson-White syndrome (type B). Temporary ablation at surgery. Circulation 1967;36:663–672.
11. Moe GK, Mendez C, Han J: Aberrant A-V impulse propagation in the dog heart: A study of functional bundle branch block. Circ Res 1965;16:261–286.
12. Moe GK, Preston JB, Burlington HJ: Physiologic evidence for a dual A-V transmission system. Circ Res 1956;4:357–375.
13. Wit AL, Hoffman BF, Cranefield PF: Slow conduction and reentry in the ventricular conducting system. I. Return extrasystole in canine Purkinje fibers. Circ Res 1972;30:1–10.
14. Sasyniuk BI, Mendez C: A mechanism for reentry in canine ventricular tissue. Circ Res 1971;28:3–15.
15. Frame, LH, Page RL, Boyden PA, *et al.*: Circus movement in the canine atrium around the tricuspid ring during experimental atrial flutter and during reentry in vitro. Circulation 1987;76:1155–1175.
16. Antzelevitch C, Jalife J, Moe GK: Characteristics of reflection as a mechanism of reentrant arrhythmias and its relationship to parasystole. Circulation 1980;61:182–191.
17. Waldo AL, Kaiser GA: A study of ventricular arrhythmias associated with acute myocardial infarction in the canine heart. Circulation 1973;47:1222–1228.
18. Josephson ME, Horowitz LN, Farshidi A, *et al.*: Sustained ventricular tachycardia: Evidence for protected localized reentry. Am J Cardiol 1978;42:416–426.
19. Simson MB: Use of signals in the terminal QRS complex to identify patients with ventricular tachycardia after myocardial infarction. Circulation 1981;64:235–242.
20. Kupersmith J Krongrad E, Waldo AL: Conduction intervals and conduction velocity in the human cardiac conduction system—studies during open heart surgery. Circulation 1973;47:776–787.
21. Janse MJ: Reentry rhythms. In Fozzard HA, Haber E, Jennings RB, *et al.* (eds): The Heart and Cardiovascular System. Raven Press, New York, 1986:1203–1238.
22. Han J, Moe GK: Nonuniform recovery of excitability of ventricular muscle. Circ Res 1964;14:44–60.
23. Kuo CS, Munakata K, Pratap Reddy C, *et al.* Characteristics and possible mechanisms of ventricular arrhythmias dependent on the dispersion of action potential durations. Circulation 1983;67:1356–1367.
24. Wellens HJJ: Value and limitations of programmed electrical stimulation of the heart in the study and treatment of tachycardias. Circulation 1978;57:845–853.
25. Freedman RA, Swerdlow CD, Echt DS, *et al.*: Facilitation of ventricular tachyrhythmia induction by isoproterenol. Am J Cardiol 1984;54:765–770.
26. MacLean WAH, Plumb VJ, Waldo AL: Transient entrainment and interruption of ventricular tachycardia. PACE 1981;4:358–365.
27. Waldo AL, MacLean WAH, Karp RB, *et al.*: Entrainment and interruption of atrial flutter with atrial pacing. Studies in man following open heart surgery. Circulation 1977;56:737–745.
28. Bigger JT, Goldreyer BN: The mechanism of supraventricular tachycardia. Circulation 1970;42:673–688.
29. Brugada P, Wellens HJJ: The role of triggered activity in clinical arrhythmias. In Rosenbaum MB, Elizari MV, (eds): Frontiers of Cardiac Electrophysiology. The Hague, Martinus Nijhoff, 1983:195.
30. Wellens HJJ, Lie KI, Durrer D: Further observation on ventricular tachycardia as studied by electrical stimulation of the heart. Circulation 1974; 49:647–653.
31. Wellens HJJ, Durer DR, Lie KI: Observation on mechanisms of ventricular tachycardia in man. Circulation 1976;43:237–244.
32. Disertori M, Inama G, Vergara G, *et al.*: Evidence of a reentry circuit in the common type of atrial flutter in man. Circulation 1983;67:435–440.
33. Janse MJ, van Capelle JL, Freud GE, *et al.*: Circus movement within the AV node as a basis for supraventricular tachycardia as shown by multiple microelectrode recordings in the isolated rabbit heart. Circ Res 1971;28:403–414.
34. Moak JP, Rosen MR: Induction and termination of triggered activity by pacing in isolated canine Purkinje fibers. Circulation 1984;69:149–162.
35. Kupersmith J, Antman EM, Hoffman BF: In vivo electrophysiologic effects of lidocaine in canine acute myocardial infarction. Circ Res 1975;36:84–91.
36. Allessie MA, Bonke FIM, Schopman FJG: Circus movement in rabbit atrial muscle as a mechanism of tachycardia. II. The role of non-uniform recovery of excitability in the occurrence of unidirectional block as studied with multiple microelectrodes. Circ Res 1976;39:168–177.
37. Allessie MA, Bonke FIM, Schopman FJG: Circus movement in rabbit atrial muscle as a mechanism of tachycardia. III. The "leading circle" concept: A new model of circus movement in cardiac tissue without the involvement of an anatomical obstacle. Circ Res 1977;41:9–18.
38. Allessie MA, Schalij MJ, Kirchhof CJHJ, *et al.*: Experimental electrophysiology and arrhythmogenicity. Anisotropy and ventricular tachycardia. Eur Heart J 1989;10:E2–E8.

39. Dillon S, Allessie MA, Ursell PC, *et al.*: Influences of anisotropic tissue structure on reentrant circuits in the epicardial border zone of subacute canine infarcts. Circ Res 1988;63:182–206.
40. Spach MS, Dolber PC, Heidlag JF: Interaction of inhomogeneities of repolarization with anisotropic propagation in dog atria: A mechanism for both preventing and initiating reentry. Circ Res 1989;65:1612–1631.
41. Kadish AH, Spear JF, Levine JH, *et al.*: The effects of procainimide on conduction in anisotropic canine ventricular myocardium. Circulation 1986;74:616–625.
42. Clerc L: Directional differences of impulse spread in trabecular muscle from mammalian Heart. J Physiol 1976;255:355–346.
43. Spach MS, Miller WT Jr, Geselowitz DB, *et al.*: The discontinuous nature of propagation in normal canine cardiac muscle. Evidence for recurrent discontinuities of intracellular resistance that affect the membrane currents. Circ Res 1981;48:39–54.
44. Hoffman BF, Rosen MR: Cellular mechanisms for cardiac arrhythmias. Circ Res 1981;49:1–15.
45. Malik M, Camm AJ: Termination of macro-reentrant tachycardia by single extrastimulus delivered during the effective refractory period. PACE 1990;13:103–109.
46. Akhtar M, Damato AN, Batsford WP, *et al.*: Demonstration of reentry within the His-Purkinje system in man. Circulation 1974;50:1150–1162.
47. Durrer D, Schoo L, Schuilenburg RM, *et al.*: The role of premature beats in the initiation and termination of supraventricular tachycardia in the Wolff-Parkinson-White syndrome. Circulation 1967;36:644–662.
48. Akhtar M, Gilbert C, Wolf FG, *et al.*: Reentry within the His-Purkinje system: elucidation of reentrant circuit using right bundle branch and His bundle recordings. Circulation 1978;58:295–304.
49. Josephson ME, Horowitz LN, Farshidi A: Continuous local electrical activity: A mechanism of recurrent ventricular tachycardia. Circulation 1978;57:659–665.
50. Hoffman BF: The genesis of cardiac arrhythmias. Prog Cardiovasc Dis 1966;8:319–329.
51. Singer D, Ten Eick RE: Pharmacology of cardiac arrhythmias. Prog Cardiov Dis 1969;11:488–514.
52. Trautwein W: Generation and conduction of impulses in the heart as affected by drugs. Pharmacol Rev 1963;15:277–332.
53. Duo GS, Hoff P, Kupersmith J: Repolarization interactions between cardiac segments of varying action potential duration. Am Heart J 1989;117:854–861.
54. Li Z, Noda T, Maldonado C, *et al.*: Junctional zone between segments of varying action potential duration appears to be a site of arrhythmogenesis (Abstr). J Am Coll Cardiol 1990;15:145A.
55. El-Sherif N, Mehra R, Gough WB, *et al.*: Ventricular activation pattern of spontaneous and induced rhythms in canine one-day-old myocardial infarction. Evidence for focal and reentrant mechanism. Circ Res 1982;51:152–166.
56. El-Sherif N, Gough WB, Zeiler RH, *et al.*: Reentrant ventricular arrhythmias in the late myocardial infarction period. 12. Spontaneous versus induced reentry and intramural versus epicardial circuits. J Am Coll Cardiol 1986;6:124–135.
57. Schuilenburg RM, Durrer D: Ventricular echo beats in the human heart elicited by induced ventricular premature beats. Circulation 1969;40:337–347.
58. Janse MJ, Van Capelle FJL, Morsink H, *et al.*: Flow of "injury" current and patterns of excitation during early ventricular arrhythmias in acute regional myocardial ischemia in isolated porcine and canine hearts. Evidence for 2 different arrhythmogenic mechanism. Circ Res 1980;47:151–165.
59. Moe GK: On the multiple wavelet hypothesis of atrial fibrillation. Arch Int Pharmacodyn Ther 1962;140:183–188.
60. Mendez C, Moe GK: Demonstration of a dual A-V nodal conduction system in the isolated rabbit heart. Circ Res 1966;19:378–393.
61. Denes P, Wu D, Dhingra RC, *et al.*: Demonstration of dual A-V nodal pathways in patients with paroxysmal supraventricular tachycardia. Circulation 1973;68:549–555.
62. Lewis T, Feil S, Stroud WD: Observations upon flutter and fibrillation. II. The nature of auricular flutter. Heart 1920;7:191–346.
63. Mahmud R, Denker S, Lehmann M, *et al.*: Functional characteristics of retrograde conduction in a pacing model of "Endless Loop Tachycardia." J Am Coll Cardiol 1984;3:1488–1499.
64. Cranefield PF, Aronson R: Cardiac Arrhythmias: The Role of Triggered Activity and Other Mechanisms. Futura, Mt. Kisco, NY, 1988.
65. Cranefield PF: The Conduction of the Cardiac Impulse. Futura, Mt. Kisco, NY, 1975.
66. Wit AL, Rosen MR, Hoffman BF: Electrophysiology and pharmacology of cardiac arrhythmias. I. Relationship of normal and abnormal electrical activity of cardiac fibers to the genesis of arrhythmia. B. Reentry. Am Heart J 1974;88:664–806.
67. Hauswirth O, Noble D, Tsien RW: Adrenaline: mechanism of action on the pacemaker potential in cardiac Purkinje fibers. Science 1968;162:916–917.
68. Katzung BG: Electrically induced automaticity in ventricular myocardium. Life Sci 1974;14:1133–1140.
69. Imanishi S, Surawicz B: Automatic activity in depolarized guinea pig ventricular myocardium. Characteristics and mechanisms. Circ Res 1976;39:751–759.
70. Hordof AJ, Edie R, Malm JR, *et al.*: Electrophysiologic properties and response to pharmacologic agents of fibers from diseased human atria. Circulation 1976;54:774–779.
71. Aronson RS, Cranefield PF: The effect of resting potential on the electrical activity of canine cardiac Purkinje fibers exposed to Na-free solution or to ouabain. Pflugers Arch 1974;347:101–116.
72. Lazzara R, El-Sherif N, Scherlag BJ: Electrophysiological properties of canine Purkinje cells in one-day-old myocardial infarction. Circ Res 1973;33:722–734.
73. Friedman PL, Stewart JR, Fenoglio JJ Jr, *et al.*: Survival of subendocardial Purkinje fibers after extensive myocardial infarction in dogs: In vitro and in vivo correlation. Circ Res 1973;33:597–611.
74. Dangman KH, Hoffman BG: Antiarrhythmic effects of ethmozine in cardiac Purkinje fibers: Suppression of automaticity and abolition of triggering. J Pharmacol Exp Ther 1983;227:578–586.
75. Imanishi S, McAllister RG Jr, Surawicz B: The effects of verapamil and lidocaine on the automatic depolarizations in guinea-pig ventricular myocardium. J Pharmacol Exp Ther 1978;207:294–303.
76. David LD: Effects of changes in cycle length on diastolic depolarization produced by ouabain in canine Purkinje fibers. Circ Res 1973;32:206–214.
77. Ferrier GR, Saunders JH, Mendez C: A cellular mechanism for the generation of ventricular arrhythmias by acetylstrophanthidin. Circ Res 1973;32:600–609.
78. Rosen MR, Gelband HB, Hoffman BF: Correlation between effects of ouabain on the canine electrocardiogram and transmembrane potentials of isolated Purkinje fibers. Circulation 1973;47:65–72.
79. Ferrier GR: Digitalis arrhythmias: role of oscillatory afterpotentials. Prog Cardiovas Dis 1977;19:459–474.
80. Mary-Rabine L, Hordof AJ, Danilo *et al.*: Mechanisms for impulse initiation in isolated human atrial fibers. Circ Res 1980;47:267–277.
81. Kano T, Nishi K: External Ph dependency of delayed afterdepolarization in rabbit myocardium. Am J Physiol 1986;251:H324–H330.
82. Levi R, Malm JR, Bowman FO, *et al.*: The arrhythmogenic actions of histamine on human atrial fibers. Circ Res 1981;49:545–550.
83. Pogwizd SM, Onufer JR, Kramer JB, *et al.*: Induction of delayed afterdepolarizations and triggered activity in canine Purkinje fibers by lysophosphoglycerides. Circ Res 1986;59:416–426.
84. Aronson RS: Afterpotentials and triggered activity in hypertrophied myocardium from rats with renal-hypertension. Circ Res 1981;48:720–727.
85. El-Sherif N, Gough WB, Zeiler RH, *et al.*: Triggered ventricular rhythms in one-day-old myocardial infarction in the dog. Circ Res 1983;52:566–579.
86. LeMarec H, Dangman KH, Danilo P, *et al.*: An evaluation of automaticity and triggered activity in the canine heart one to four days after myocardial infarction. Circulation 1985;71:1224–1236.

87. Eisner DA, Lederer WJ: Inotropic and arrhythmogenic effects of potassium depleted solutions on mammalian cardiac muscle. J Physiol (Lond) 1979;294:255–277.
88. Hiraoka M, Okamoto Y, Sano T: Effects of Ca^+ and K^+ on oscillatory afterpotentials in dog ventricular muscle-fibers. J Mol Cell Cardiol 1979;11:999–1015.
89. Cranefield RF, Aronson RS: Initiation of sustained rhythmic activity by single propagated action potentials in canine cardiac Purkinje fibers exposed to sodium free solution or to ouabain. Circ Res 1974;34:477–481.
90. Lederer WJ, Tsien RW: Transient inward current underlying arrhythmogenic effects of cardiotonic steroids in Purkinje fibers. J Physiol (Lond) 1976;263:73–100.
91. Mullins LJ: Ion Transport in Heart. Raven Press, New York, 1981.
92. Arlock P, Katzung BG: Effects of sodium substitutes on transient inward current and tension in guinea-pig and ferret papillary muscle. J Physiol (Lond) 1985;360:105–120.
93. Kass RS, Tsien RW, Weingart R: Ionic basis of transient inward current induced by strophanthidin in cardiac Purkinje fibers. J Physiol (Lond) 1978;281:209–226.
94. Hogan PM, Wittenberg SM, Klocke FJ: Relationship of stimulation frequency to automaticity in the canine Purkinje fiber during ouabain administration. Circ Res 1973;32:377–383.
95. Wit AL, Cranefield PF: Triggered activity in cardiac muscle fibers of the simian mitral valve. Circ Res 1976;38:85–98.
97. Wit AL, Rosen MR: Afterdepolarizations and triggered activity. In: Fozzard HA, Haber E, Jennings RB, *et al.*: (eds). The Heart and Cardiovascular System. Raven Press, New York, 1986:1449–1490.
98. Rosen MR, Fisch C, Hoffman BF *et al.*: Can accelerated AV junctional escape rhythms be explained by delayed afterdepolarization? Am J Cardiol 1980;45:1272–1282.
99. Brugada P, Wellens HJJ: The role of triggered activity in clinical ventricular arrhythmias. PACE 1984;7:260–271.
100. Wyndham CRC: Arnsdorf MF, Levitsky S, *et al.*: Successful surgical excision of focal paroxysmal atrial tachycardia: Observations in vivo and in vitro. Circulation 1980;62:1365–1372.
101. German LD, Packer DL, Bardy GH, *et al.*: Ventricular tachycardia induced by atrial stimulation in patents without symptomatic cardiac disease. Am J Cardiol 1983;52:1202–1207.
102. Rahily GT, Prystowsky EN, Zipes DP, *et al.*: Clinical and electrophysiologic findings in patients with repetitive monomorphic ventricular tachycardia and otherwise normal electrocardiogram. Am J Cardiol 1982;50:459–468.
103. Buxton AE, Waxman HL, Marchlinski FE, *et al.*: Right ventricular tachycardia: Clinical and electrophysiologic characteristics. Circulation 1967;36:663–672.
104. Mason JW, Swerdlow CD, Mitchell LB: Efficacy of verapamil in chronic recurrent ventricular tachycardia. Am J Cardiol 1983;51:1614–1617.
105. Wellens HJJ, Bar FW, Farre J, *et al.*: Initiation and termination of ventricular tachycardia by supraventricular stimuli: Incidence and electrophysiologic determinants as observed during programmed stimulation of the heart. Am J Cardiol 1980;46:576–580.
106. Palileo EV, Ashley WW, Swiryn S, *et al.*: Intrinsic deflections, local excitation, and transmembrane action potentials. Circ Res 1956;6:444–449.
107. Belhassen B, Shapria I, Pelleg A, *et al.*: Idiopathic recurrent sustained ventricular tachycardia responsive to verapamil: an ECG-electrophysiologic entity. Am Heart J 1984;108:1034–1037.
108. Lerman BB, Belardinelli L, West GA, *et al.*: Adenosine-sensitive ventricular tachycardia: Evidence suggesting cyclic AMP-mediated triggered activity. Circulation 1986;74:270–280.
109. Rosen MR, Danilo P: Effects of tetrodotoxin, lidocaine, verapamil and AHR-2666 on ouabain-induced delayed afterdepolarizations in canine Purkinje fibers. Circ Res 1980;46:117–124.
110. Ferrier GR, Moe GK: Effect of calcium on acetylstrophanthidin-induced transient depolarizations in canine Purkinje tissue. Circ Res 1973;33:508–515.
111. Rosen MR, Ilvento JP, Gelband H, *et al.*: Effect of verapamil on electrophysiologic properties of canine cardiac Purkinje fibers. J Pharmacol Exp Ther 1974;189:414–422.
112. Belardinelli L, Isenberg G: Actions of adenosine and isoproterenol on isolated mammalian ventricular myocytes. Circ Res 1983;287–297.
113. Kupersmith J, Hoff P: Occurrence and transmission of repolarization abnormalities in vitro. J Am Coll Cardiol 1985;6:152–160.
114. Kupersmith J, Hoff P, Guo S: In vitro characteristics of repolarization abnormality—a possible cause of arrhythmias. J Electrocardiol 1986; 19:361–370
115. Brachmann J, Scherlag BJ, Rosenshtraukh LV, *et al.*: Bradycardia-dependent triggered activity: Relevance to drug-induced multiform ventricular tachycardia. Circulation 1983;68:846–856.
116. Damiano BP, Rosen M: Effects of pacing on triggered activity induced by early afterdepolarizations. Circulation 1984;69:1013–1025.
117. Sleator W, Degubareff T: Transmembrane action potentials and contractions of human atrial muscle. Am J Physiol 1964;206:1000.
180. Habbab MA, El-Sharif N: Drug-induced Torsade de Pointes: role of early afterdepolarizations and dispersion of repolarization. Am J Med 1990; 69:241–247.
119. Li ZY, Zee-Cheng C, Maldonado C. *et al.*: Early afterdepolarizations in sheep Purkinje fiber–transmission and suppressive effects of magnesium (Abstr). Clin Res 1988;36:824A.
120. Li ZY, Zee-Cheng C, Maldonado C, *et al.*: Purkinje fiber papillary muscle interaction in the genesis of triggered activity (Abstr). Circulation 1988; (Suppl II):II–158.
121. Noda T, Maldonado C, Li ZY, *et al.*: The role of slow inward current in early afterdepolarization induced by aconitine (Abstr). Circulation 1989;80(Suppl):II–145.
122. Matsuda K, Hoshi T, Kameyama S: Effects of aconitine on the cardiac membrane potential of the dog. Jpn J Physiol 1959;9:419–429.
123. Schmidt RF: Versuche mit Aconitin zum Problem der spontanen Erregungsbildung im Herzen. Pflugers Arch 1960;526–536.
124. Matsuda K, Hoffman BF, Ellner CN, *et al.*: Veratridine-induced prolongation of repolarization in the mammalian heart. In Nineteenth International Physiological Congress. American Physiological Society, Bethesda, Maryland 1953;596–597.
125. Coraboeuf E, Deroubaix E, Coulombe A: Acidosis-induced abnormal repolarization and repetitive activity in isolated dog Purkinje fibers. J Physiol (Paris) 1980;76:97–106.
126. Li ZY, Wang YH, Maldonado C, *et al.*: Ionic mechanisms of reperfusion-induced triggered activity (Abstr). Clin Res 1991;39:713A.
127. Arnsdorf MF: The effect of antiarrhythmic drugs on triggered sustained rhythmic activity in cardiac Purkinje fibers. J Pharmacol Exp Ther 1977;201:689–700.
128. Roden DM, Hoffman BF: Action potential prolongation and induction of abnormal automaticity by low quinidine concentrations in canine Purkinje fibers. Relationship to potassium and cycle length. Circ Res 1985;56:857–867.
129. Dangman KH, Hoffman BF: In vivo and in vitro antiarrhythmic and arrhythmogenic effects of N-acetyl procainamide. J Pharmacol Exp Ter 1981;217:851–862.
130. Hiromasa S, Coto H, Li ZY, *et al.*: Dextrorotatory isomer of sotalol: Electrophysiologic effects and interaction with verapamil. Am Heart J 1988;116:1552–1557.
131. Carmeliet E: Electrophysiologic and voltage clamp analyses of the effects of sotalol on isolated cardiac muscle and Purkinje fibers. J Pharmacol Exp Ther 1985;232:817–825.
132. Brugada P, Wellens HJJ: Early afterdepolarizations: role in conduction/block, prolonged repolarization dependent resuscitation, and tachyarrhythmias. PACE 1984;7:260–271.
133. Levine JH, Spear JF, Guarnier T, *et al.*: Cesium chloride-induced long QT

syndrome: Demonstration of afterdepolarizations and triggered activity in vivo. Circulation 1985;72:1092–1104.

134. Priori SG, Mantica M, Napolitano C, *et al.*: Early afterdepolarizations induced in vivo by reperfusion of ischemic myocardium. A possible mechanism for reperfusion arrhythmias. Circulation 1990;81:1911–1920.

135. Bonatti V, Rolli A, Botti G: Recording of monophasic action potential of the right ventricle in the long QT syndrome complicated by severe ventricular arrhythmias. Eur Heart J:1983;4:168–172.

136. Schechter E, Freeman CC, Lazzara R: Afterdepolarizations as a mechanism for the long QT syndrome: electrophysiologic studies of a case. J Am Coll Cardiol 1984;3:1556–1567.

137. Leichter D, Danilo Jr P, Boyden P, *et al.*: A canine model of torsades de pointes. PACE 1988;11:2235–2245.

138. D'Aloncourt CN, Zierhut W, Luderitz B: "Torsades de pointes" tachycardia: re-entry or focal activity? Br Heart J 1982;48:213.

139. Sano T, Sawanobori T: Abnormal automaticity in canine Purkinje fibers focally subjected to low external concentrations of calcium. Circ Res 1972;16:423–430.

II

CLINICAL APPROACH TO ARRHYTHMIAS

3

CLINICAL APPROACH TO THE PATIENT WITH ARRHYTHMIA

Igor Singer, M.B.B.S., F.R.A.C.P., F.A.C.P., F.A.C.C., Marcus Stoddard, M.D.
and Joel Kupersmith, M.D., F.A.C.P., F.A.C.C.

PART I

CLINICAL EVALUATION

CLINICAL HISTORY

Proper elicitation of clinical history and physical examination, in a patient presenting with arrhythmias, subserves a dual purpose. It helps define the arrhythmia, and it identifies associated cardiac and noncardiac abnormalities. Arrhythmias can occur in isolation in patients with structurally normal hearts. More commonly, however, they may be a manifestation of an underlying structural heart disease. The need for a specific therapy hinges on the accurate assessment of the arrhythmia and identification of the associated cardiac problems.

Clinical history is always the fundamental starting point in establishing a correct diagnosis. Although it is never the only vehicle in a precise diagnosis of rhythm disturbance, symptom description provides valuable clues to the existence of such a disturbance. The most common symptoms caused by arrhythmias are listed in Table 3.1.

Clinical history is also important for examining underlying cardiac or other disease. Although arrhythmias may exist as primary condition, they are usually a feature of an underlying disease process. An arrhythmia may be a marker of an underlying structural cardiac problem or a manifestation of a pathophysiologic or metabolic disturbance.

Palpitation and syncope are two of the most prominent manifestations of arrhythmia. We will consider these first and then the symptoms of bradyarrhythmias and tachyarrhythmias.

Palpitations

Palpitations may be defined as an unpleasant awareness of the beating of the heart. Palpitations may be brought about by a variety of disorders involving changes in cardiac rhythm or rate, including all forms of tachycardias, ectopic beats, compensatory pauses, augmented stroke volume due to valvular regurgitation, or hyperkinetic states, e.g., anemia. However, they also normally occur with sinus tachycardia such as during exercise or emotional excitement. When palpitations begin and end abruptly, they are often due to a paroxysmal atrial or atrioventricular (AV) nodal tachycardia, atrial flutter or fibrillation, whereas a gradual onset suggests sinus tachycardia. A history of palpitations during or after strenuous physical effort may be normal, whereas palpitations (sinus tachycardia) during minimal activity suggests inadequate cardiac reserve, anemia, thyrotoxicosis, or poor exercise conditioning. When palpitations can be terminated by vagal maneuvers, e.g., gagging, or vomiting, AV nodal reentry tachycardia is suggested.

Palpitation, i.e., the subjective feeling of abnormal heart beats may occur with bradycardia as well as tachycardia. These conditions may be due to atrioventricular block or sinus node disease.

Patients should be asked to tap out the rhythm if possible, or the physician may be able to tap out typical rhythm cadences that the patient may recognize as being similar to his/her rhythm disturbance.

It should also be noted that ambulatory electrocardiogram (ECG) studies have shown that palpitation may occur in patients with established arrhythmia (e.g. in Wolff-Parkinson-White (WPW) syndrome) while the patient is in fact in sinus rhythm. This phenomenon may be due to anxiety or a sensitization to the subjective feeling of palpitation brought on by recurrent episodes of the arrhythmia.

Syncope

Syncope (see also Chapter 5) may be defined as a transient and sudden loss of consciousness. It is most commonly caused by reduced perfusion to the brain. A frequent cause of decreased cerebral perfusion is an arrhythmia, which may be due to either a bradyarrhythmia or a tachyarrhythmia. Other causes of syncope may be related to a reduction in systemic vascular resistance, hypovolemia, or other conditions that may result in sudden reduction of cardiac output. Loss of consciousness due to cardiac causes should be distinguished from primary seizure disorders by appropriate neurologic workup.

Table 3.1.
Presenting Symptoms

Tachyarrhythmias
- Palpitations
- Presyncope or syncope
- Dyspnea
- Fullness in the neck or a throbbing sensation
- Chest discomfort
- Angina
- Fatigue
- Seizures
- Post-tachycardia micturition

Bradyarrhythmias
- Syncope
- Presyncope
- Nausea with sudden urge to defecate
- TIAs
- Mental confusion
- Fatigue
- Dyspnea
- Seizures

Premature beats
- Palpitations
- "Flip-flops"
- Heart "stopping" for a second or two
- Pain in the chest or neck

Abbreviations: TIA, transient ischemic attack.

extremely slow ventricular rates (20–30 beats/min), or by rapid heart rates, e.g., ventricular tachycardia (VT), atrial fibrillation in a patient with WPW syndrome due to antegrade conduction through the accessory pathway. The occurrence of syncope depends on both the rate of bradycardia or tachycardia and on the patient's tolerance to alteration in heart rate. Such tolerance is in turn influenced by myocardial dysfunction, the status of the cerebral circulation, etc.

Syncope independent of body position suggests Stoke-Adams attacks or epilepsy, whereas vasodepressor syncope is often provoked by emotional or painful stimuli. Similarly, syncope that occurs during upright posture is usually associated with decreased peripheral vascular resistance, reduced circulatory volume or slow heart rates.

Syncope occurring during or immediately postexercise, suggests aortic stenosis, hypertrophic obstructive cardiomyopathy, or primary pulmonary hypertension.

A history of fainting during sudden movements of the head, wearing of a tight collar, or shaving suggests carotid sinus syncope.

Other diagnostic clues may be helpful. Consciousness is regained promptly in syncope of cardiovascular origin. When consciousness is regained in vasodepressor syncope, the patient is usually pale and diaphoretic with a slow heart rate. On the other hand, the patient with Stokes-Adams attacks is often flushed.

A history of syncope during childhood suggests the possibility of obstruction of the left or the right ventricular outflow, which may be valvular, subvalvular, or supravalvular. A family history of syncope or sudden cardiac death may suggest arrhythmias associated with long QT syndrome or hypertrophic cardiomyopathy.

A careful drug history should be sought, particularly with respect to antiarrhythmic drugs, digitalis, antihypertensives, and anxiolytic or sedative drugs.

Syncope as a symptom should never be dismissed. Careful evaluation is always indicated.

Tachyarrhythmias

Symptoms of tachyarrhythmias depend on the age of the patient, the duration of the rhythm disturbance, the ventricular rate during tachycardia, and presence of structural heart disease. For example, AV nodal reentry tachycardia may be tolerated for hours or days by a young athletic patient with only a subjective feeling of palpitations or fatigue. On the other hand, in an elderly patient with coronary artery disease, a similar arrhythmia may precipitate myocardial ischemia.

Ventricular tachycardia may present as loss of consciousness if the rate is rapid (>200 beats/min) or as dyspnea, palpitations, or fatigue, if the rate is less rapid (120–160 beats/min). The effective peripheral rate is important here. For example, a heart rate of 200 beats/min associated with marked alternans may be characterized by an effective peripheral rate of 100 beats/min.

The physician should encourage the patient to verbalize freely and avoid the temptation to dismiss symptoms even if they appear to be benign. Details of the time of onset of symptoms, association with activity, and precipitating and alleviating factors should be carefully sought. Relationship of symptoms to change in posture, emotional excitement, vagal maneuvers, meals, and sexual activity are frequently helpful clues. For example, AV nodal reentry tachycardia may be precipitated by a change in posture or an emotional upset. It may terminate with a vagal maneuver, e.g., straining.

Bradyarrhythmias

Maintenance of cardiac output is dependent on the stroke volume and heart rate. If heart rate decreases, a compensatory increase in the stroke volume can maintain an adequate cardiac output. However, with increased demand, an inadequate rate response may result in decreased cerebral perfusion. This in turn causes symptoms of fatigue, lightheadedness, or a transient loss of consciousness. If the interruption of cerebral perfusion is prolonged, i.e., in excess of several seconds, grand mal seizures may be the result (Stokes-Adams attacks). Elderly patients with coexistent cerebrovascular disease may also present with focal neurologic symptoms though this is not as common. In bedridden or sedentary patients, cerebral manifestations may either not be apparent or not occur, and signs and symptoms of congestive heart failure may predominate.

Vasovagal syncope should be suspected in patients in whom bradycardias are associated with intense pain, nausea, or vomiting. A witness or a clinical observer may be able to delineate a slow or absent pulse during an episode of decreased alertness or loss of consciousness.

Bradyarrhythmias may be subtle in their presentation. Thus, a careful inquiry is required to elicit the clinical history suggestive of bradyarrhythmias.

Premature Beats

Many patients consult their physicians because of a subjective feeling that the heart rhythm is not quite right. These patients often describe "skipped beats," "flip-flops," sudden "stopping" of heart beat, or chest "pounding" at night. Usually, but not always, these symptoms are benign. Premature atrial and ventricular beats may be a normal finding in the absence of structural heart disease. On the other hand, these symptoms may be associated with underlying disease processes, e.g., coronary artery disease or mitral valve prolapse.

Awareness of heart irregularities especially premature beats, is often heightened by anxiety. Such arrhythmias may also be more frequent in anxious patients due to heightened sympathetic tone (1–3).

PHYSICAL EXAMINATION

Clues to Underlying Cause of Arrhythmia

Since arrhythmias are frequently associated with underlying structural heart disease, search for associated cardiac abnormalities is pertinent to the diagnosis and important in formulating the treatment strategy.

Physical examination begins with the assessment of the general appearance. Skin color, presence of pallor or cyanosis, dyspnea at rest or orthopnea, marked weight loss, somnolence, and body habitus are helpful diagnostic clues.

Presence of exophthalmos may suggest thyrotoxicosis. Distinctive features of Marfan's syndrome, i.e., long extremities, arachnodactyly, and spinal and chest deformities may be noted. Other "spot" diagnoses may be made by the general observation, e.g., cushingoid appearance, pickwickian habitus, bobbing of the head (De Mussett's sign) associated with severe aortic regurgitation, are a few examples.

Other helpful diagnostic clues may be observed by the analysis of the pulse morphology. Examples include bisferiens pulse, characterized by two systolic peaks, which may be associated with aortic regurgitation or hypertrophic cardiomyopathy, pulsus parvus et tardus of aortic stenosis, pulsus alternans associated with severe myocardial depression, and pulsus paradoxus associated with pericardial tamponade.

Presence of left ventricular enlargement is suggested by the presence of a displaced apex beat. Sustained left ventricular lift is characteristic of pressure overload states as in hypertension, aortic stenosis and aortic coarctation. On the other hand, conditions associated with chronic volume overload result in hyperkinetic apex beat (e.g., aortic regurgitation). Dyskinetic anterior bulging may be detected with a left ventricular aneurysm.

Right ventricular enlargement may be detected by palpable anterior movement in the left parasternal area. Sustained lift in the parasternal area may be associated with conditions which cause right ventricular pressure overload, e.g., pulmonic stenosis. Pulmonary hypertension or increased pulmonary blood flow may result in prominent systolic pulsations of the pulmonary artery, in the second left intercostal space.

Auscultation of the heart also provides helpful bedside clues to the cause of the arrhythmia. Such clues include: (a) presence of systolic and diastolic murmurs, suggesting valvular dysfunction or congenital heart disease, (b) presence of a third heart sound, suggesting rapid ventricular diastolic inflow of blood, associated with a dilated, hyperdynamic, or failing ventricle, and (c) presence of a fourth heart sound, indicative of increased diastolic impedance to atrial systole in association with a noncompliant, hypertrophied ventricle.

Other auscultatory clues may be found, such as presence of a mid-systolic click in a patient with mitral valve prolapse or an ejection sound in a patient with mobile valvular obstruction, e.g., pulmonic stenosis. Fixed splitting of the second heart sound may be found in a patient with an atrial septal defect. Paradoxic splitting of S_2 may be found in patients with delayed left ventricular activation and contraction, e.g., left bundle branch block (LBBB), an artificial pacemaker in right ventricle, or a prolonged left ventricular mechanical systole in patients with left ventricular obstruction (e.g., aortic stenosis).

Signs of Arrhythmia

Examination of the pulse is, of course, an important part of arrhythmia assessment. In ventricular tachycardia, the pulse volume may be diminished and is sometimes barely detectable. However, variations in the amplitude of the pulse from beat to beat reflect a changing sequence of atrial and ventricular systole with augmentated beats designating well-timed AV sequence occurring due to the fusion beats (Dressler beats). In atrial fibrillation, on the other hand, a completely irregular rhythm is also noted with beat-to-beat change in the amplitude of the pulse.

Heart rate alone is inadequate to diagnose cardiac arrhythmias. However, some heart rates are more frequently associated with certain types of arrhythmias. For example, a heart rate of 150–160 beats/min is often associated with atrial flutter with 2:1 AV block, or with AV nodal reentry tachycardia. During AV nodal reentry tachycardia the rhythm is usually regular and has an abrupt onset. Similarly, heart rates in excess of 200 beats/min may be due to AV reciprocating tachycardias associated with WPW syndrome, atrial flutter with 1:1 conduction, or ventricular tachycardia.

Jugular venous pulsations may be helpful in elucidating the diagnosis. Atrial flutter is associated with rapid F waves of 280–320 beats/min. Ventricular tachycardia may be associated with intermittent cannon *a* waves as well as variable intensity of the first heart sound (with loud cannon sounds) (see below). Variation in intensity of the first heart sound may also occur in atrial fibrillation due to irregularity and variable diastolic filling (louder first sounds after shorter filling times), though this is less marked.

Causes of bradycardia (heart rates less than 60 beats/min) can sometimes be diagnosed on physical examination. In the presence of heart rates of 25–50 beats/min, cannon *a* waves along with cannon sounds are diagnostic of a complete heart block. Both cannon *a* waves and cannon sounds are due to contraction of the atrium against a closed AV valve in the presence of AV dissociation or block. Associated with cannon waves, cannon sounds may be heard during complete heart block. Second degree AV block can often be diagnosed by first observing "extra" *a* waves in the jugular venous pulse and then determining the *a* wave/*v* wave relationship. Cannon waves or sounds may also occur in second-degree block with close timing of ventricular and atrial waves.

PART II
EVALUATION OF VENTRICULAR FUNCTION

General evaluation of ventricular function is most important in the assessment of the arrhythmia patient. It provides (a) diagnostic information helpful in nonarrhythmia therapy (such as guiding the use of afterload reducing agents), (b) predictive information in assessing the likelihood of future arrhythmia or sudden death, (c) prognostic information, and (d) information of use in guiding specific antiarrhythmic therapy (e.g., regional contraction abnormalities may guide one to use surgical resection rather than another form of therapy). Thus, an accurate delineation of global and regional ventricular contraction has important impact in evaluating the arrhythmia patient in the clinic (4–9).

Of all the techniques discussed in this chapter, measures of ventricular function are probably the best predictor of future serious arrhythmia events. The left ventricular ejection fraction, or percentage of blood ejected by the left ventricle from end-diastole to end-systole, is the most commonly used but not the only index of global ventricular contraction. Measures of left ventricular ejection fraction as well as volumes can be made by several complementary techniques, such as contrast ventriculography, radionuclide ventriculography, and echocardiography. In addition to global systolic contraction, these modalities can be employed to assess segmental and regional wall motion abnormalities, although the various cardiac imaging techniques may give comparable information in many clinical situations. Each has specific advantages and disadvantages.

Diagnostic Utility of Cardiac Imaging Techniques

Impaired left ventricular contraction due to myocardial injury occurs from many types of cardiovascular diseases. Left ventricular injury may be regional or segmental. Assessment of ventricular size and wall thickness complements the analysis of ventricular contraction. Insight into the etiology of ventricular arrhythmia is often gained by the evaluation of ventricular contraction and size (e.g., coronary artery disease, dilated cardiomyopathy, aortic or mitral regurgitation, etc.) (10).

Therapeutic Utility of Cardiac Imaging Techniques

Treatment options for potential life-threatening ventricular tachyarrhythmias are often dictated by the specific anatomic and functional abnormalities of the left ventricle. For example, observation of a left ventricular apical aneurysm with otherwise preserved regional ventricular contraction, may make surgical resection a possible therapeutic option (11,12). On the other hand, diffuse impairment of ventricular contraction points to other treatment strategies.

Prognostic Utility of Cardiac Imaging Techniques

The prediction of arrhythmic events, sudden cardiac death and total cardiac mortality in subjects with coronary artery disease and cardiomyopathies is complicated by multiple independent and interacting dynamic determinants, such as myocardial ischemia, myocardial fibrosis, coronary anatomy, ventricular size and geometry, autonomic tone, intracardiac pressures, ventricular contraction, myocardial electrical stability, and conduction abnormalities (13–18). Thus, a multifaceted approach is necessary to assess arrhythmic risk and prognosis.

Left ventricular abnormalities are very important predictors of arrhythmic events (7,15,19–21). Both morphologic (variable size) and functional (regional vs. global) contraction abnormalities have been examined and found useful (22).

Ejection fraction is the most standard parameter (15,21). A left ventricular ejection fraction less than 40% in a subject with nonsustained VT and coronary artery disease or dilated cardiomyopathy is perhaps the most powerful predictor of risk for sudden cardiac death (7). Depressed left ventricular ejection fraction, when compared to segmental wall motion abnormality is a more important determinant of cardiac death in patients with nonischemic dilated cardiomyopathy (23). Cardiac imaging modalities are particularly useful when coupled with results of electrocardiographic (4–6) (see section on signal averaged ECG) or electrophysiologic studies.

METHODOLOGIES

Types of Imaging Modalities

CONTRAST VENTRICULOGRAPHY

Contrast vetriculography was one of the first cardiac imaging techniques employed to assess ventricular contraction. Although it has long been the "gold standard," newer and safer noninvasive imaging modalities have emerged and may, in some clinical situations, be preferable. Injection of iodinated contrast media opacifies the left ventricle. Ventricular contraction is recorded on x-ray cine film at rates of 30–60 frames/sec. End-systolic (ES) and end-diastolic (ED) ventricular volumes are calculated from tracings of the left ventricular silhouette in at least one or preferably two (i.e., biplane) views.

Ventricular volume calculations usually employ a geometric assumption about the shape of the left ventricle. An ellipsoid shape is assumed for biplane images and a prolated ellipsoid for single-plane views (24). Left ventricular ejection fraction is calculated as the difference between (ED) and (ES) volumes divided by ED volume, multiplied by 100% (([ED-ES]/ED) × 100). Regional wall motion abnormalities (i.e., hypokinesis, akinesis, dyskinesis, or aneurysm) are usually assessed by subjective visual inspection of cine film (Figure 3.1). However, quantitative analysis, such as the centerline method, is more reproducible when the influence of provocative maneuvers (e.g., postextrasystolic potentiation, catecholamine infusion, and pharmacologic alteration of loading conditions) on ventricular contraction are being determined (25).

The limitations of contrast ventriculography are well appreciated, but are often overlooked. These include alteration of contractility and loading conditions by contrast media, induction of extrasystolic beats which cannot be used to analyze ventricular contraction and inability to perform serial studies readily. Digital subtraction angiography, in lowering the amount of contrast media necessary, has minimized some of these problems (26).

RADIONUCLIDE VENTRICULOGRAPHY

Radionuclide ventriculography has become a primary procedure for evaluation of ventricular function. As it does not require geometric assumptions (inherent in contrast ventriculography), it is equally valuable for measurement of left ventricular ejection fraction in the presence of conditions that change ventricular shape. These include regional wall motion abnormalities and significant ventricular dilatation. Furthermore, its simplicity and noninvasive character permit serial studies to be performed easily.

Radionuclides which remain in the blood pool are used in this technique, e.g., technetium ^{99m}-labeled erythrocytes or albumin. The intracardiac radionuclide emits γ radiation which can be imaged during the initial transit from a peripheral intravenous injection (i.e., first-pass study) or after the radionuclide has reached an equilibrium blood pool concentration (i.e., equilibrium study). First-pass studies allow temporal separation of cardiac chambers in any projection.

The equilibrium technique is more widely used than the first-pass method. Imaging is performed in projections that attempt to minimize overlap of cardiac chambers. Background radioactivity is subtracted to calculate ejection fraction. Change in left ventricular activity is proportional to change in ventricular volume. Ejection fraction (EF) is calculated as follows: EF = EDC − ESC/EDC − BC, where EDC = end diastolic counts, ESC = end systolic counts, BC = background counts, and EF = ejection fraction. Ejection fraction may then be calculated without an assumption of ventricular shape. The background subtraction method may differ among laboratories and thus, the ejection fraction determinations may differ (27,28). Serial studies can be performed to assess the influence of provocative tests (e.g., exercise) (29).

Relative ventricular volume proportional to radioactive counts is easily measured using radionuclide ventriculography. Absolute volume can be determined but requires measurement of radioactivity in the blood and assumption of, or correction for, tissue attenuation (30,31). Regional ventricular contraction can also be assessed. Several hundred cardiac cycles of similar RR intervals are summed by a gating technique yielding an averaged

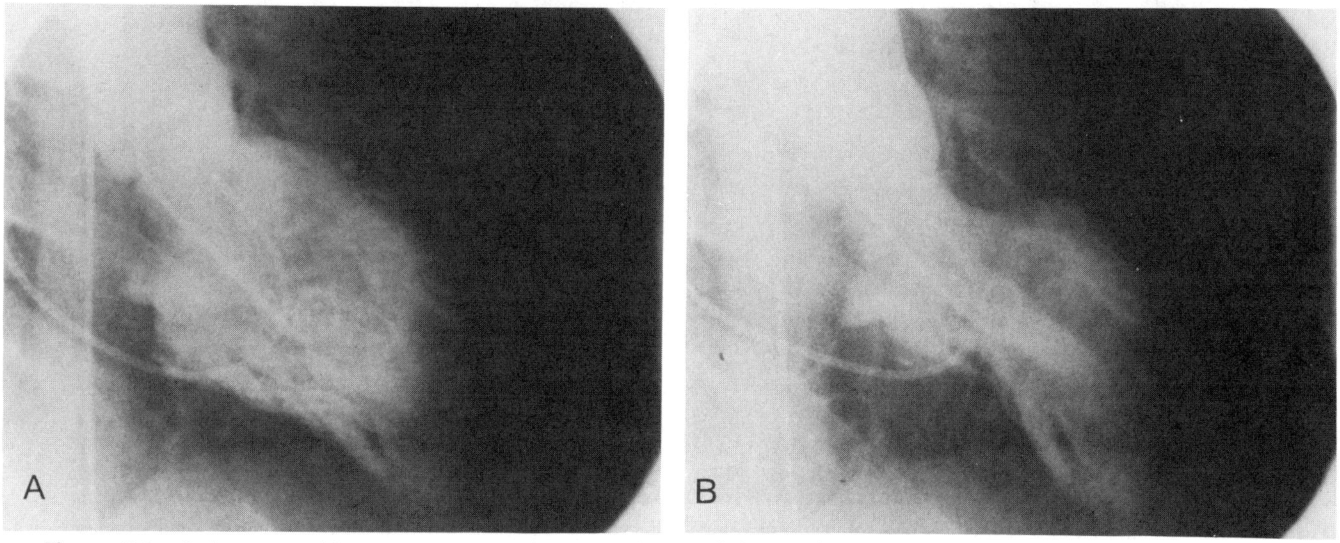

Figure 3.1. Right anterior oblique contrast ventriculograms in diastole (**left panel**) and systole (**right panel**) demonstrating an apical aneurysm.

cine cardiac cycle that is representative of ventricular contraction. Radionuclide ventriculography processed in this fashion is called a multiple-gated acquisition scan (MUGA). Because multiple regular beats for gating are required, chaotic rhythms such as atrial fibrillation may make MUGA impossible.

The technique tends to be precise though spatial resolution may diminish in several ways. Radioactive emissions from more superficial areas of the heart may obscure the overlying activity of deeper areas and thus contribute more to the final image (i.e., depth attenuation). For example, inferior wall motion abnormalities may be obscured in the left anterior oblique projection. The frame rate of radionuclide ventriculography is usually 16 frames/sec, typically slower than other imaging modalities. Frame rates of 30–60/sec can be achieved, but, at the cost of spatial resolution. Radionuclide techniques utilizing single-photon emission computed tomography (SPECT) allow for depth resolution in the determination of regional ventricular contraction and may eliminate the problems of depth attenuation and overlap seen with conventional radionuclide ventriculography. (32).

ECHOCARDIOGRAPHY

Transthoracic two-dimensional echocardiography, a completely noninvasive imaging technique which is devoid of risk, utilizes a mechanically or electronically steered ultrasound beam that transects the heart to construct potentially an infinite number of planar views. Standard orthogonal planar views of the heart have been devised by the American Society of Echocardiography (33). Two-dimensional echocardiography has emerged as an important cardiac imaging tool to assess regional wall motion abnormalities because multiple tomographic planes of the heart can be obtained and the degree of myocardial systolic thickening and inward excursion can be assessed (Fig. 3.2). Contrast and radionuclide studies assess the motion of the endocardial surface and not myocardial systolic thickening. Thus, they may be less well suited for assessing segmental wall motion abnormalities primarily due to abnormal conduction (e.g., LBBB) or thoracic surgery (e.g., postoperative paradoxic septal motion). On the contrary, optimal or complete imaging of the left ventricle by transthoracic two-dimensional echocardiography is not always possible, particularly in subjects with obesity or pulmonary disease. This remains the most significant limitation in the primary use of echocardiography to assess regional ventricular contraction.

Transesophageal two-dimensional echocardiography is a relatively new and promising semiinvasive technique which has practically eliminated suboptimal imaging of the left ventricle due to technical limitations which can be seen with transthoracic echocardiography (34).

Measures of left ventricular ejection fraction and volumes are

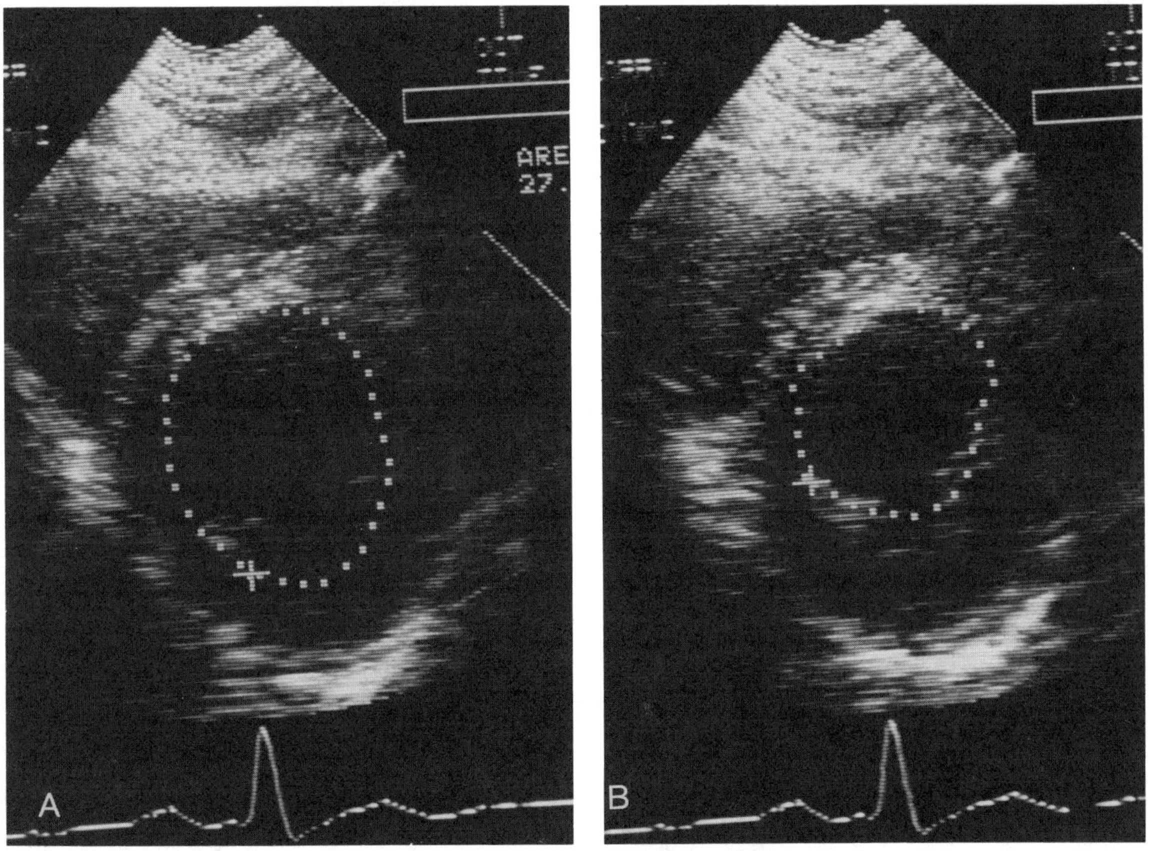

Figure 3.2. Two-dimensional short-axis view of left ventricle at papillary muscle (PM) level in diastole (**left panel**) and systole (**right panel**) demonstrating lack of systolic inward excursion and thickening of septum and anterior wall in subject with prior myocardial infarction.

usually deemed most reliable when derived from contrast or radionuclide ventriculography. However, the reliable calculation of left ventricular ejection fraction and volumes by transthoracic two-dimensional echocardiography has been demonstrated (32–39). Geometric assumptions of the shape of the left ventricle must be made to determine ventricular volume by conventional echocardiography.

Computed tomographic planes may eliminate the need for geometric assumptions (40). The widespread use of echocardiography to calculate ejection fraction and ventricular volumes has not occurred, primarily because of the inconvenience associated with the necessity for detailed analysis of multiple views in a videotape recording.

Overview

Each of the above-mentioned imaging techniques has some inherent advantages and disadvantages. Thus, the available techniques for assessment of left ventricular function may provide complementary information, though overall, costs are also important. The proper place of each imaging technique should be determined based on the clinical considerations and may in part be dictated by patient-related variables (e.g., body size, habitus).

PART III

ELECTROCARDIOGRAPHIC TECHNIQUES

ELECTROCARDIOGRAM

ECG is a cornerstone diagnostic tool for interpretation of arrhythmias, despite the availability of more sophisticated recording techniques. ECG is a simple technique. It is readily available and easily repeatable at the patient's bedside. Analysis of cardiac arrhythmias is directed at identifying the origin of the arrhythmia, the activation sequence and characterizing impulse conduction.

Fundamental to the interpretation of any rhythm disturbance is the identification of P waves and their relationship to the QRS complex. Every attempt to identify P waves should be made, including a careful examination of the rhythm strips, especially at the initiation and the termination of arrhythmias. Carotid sinus pressure may be helpful by slowing AV nodal conduction to expose P waves. An oesophageal recording may also be helpful to demonstrate the timing of atrial and ventricular activation (see below).

Whenever possible, a 12-lead ECG recording of the tachycardia should be obtained. This maximizes the chance that P waves will be accurately identified, as well as permitting the analysis of the activation sequence in the atrium (P wave axis) and the ventricle (QRS axis). Additionally, ST segments can be analyzed for repolarization changes and presence of concealed P waves. Additional Lewis leads such as in anteroposterior locations may be helpful.

Classification of arrhythmias into supraventricular or ventricular is useful. Both atria and ventricles may be components of the reentrant circuit. Atrioventricular reentrant tachycardias associated with WPW syndrome are such an example where both atria and ventricles are requisite components of the tachycardia circuit (41–48).

ECG is a useful tool for localizing the site of conduction disturbances. Both the type of block and the QRS morphology are used in assessing the site of AV block. First-degree AV block is usually due to prolonged AV nodal conduction, although it may be due to an isolated conduction delay in the atrium or infrequently, it may be due to an intra-His conduction delay (49). This is especially so, when QRS complex is normal. Type I second-degree AV block (Mobitz I) is also most likely located in the AV node when associated with a normal QRS complex, although less often it may be within the His bundle (49,50). The likelihood that the block is located in an infra-His location increases when the block is associated with a widened QRS complex, bundle branch block (BBB), although QRS complex duration > 0.12 sec, by itself, is an insufficient marker of the site of the block, since it may coexist in a given patient. When a wide QRS (BBB) is associated with Type II, second-degree AV block, a wide QRS complex favors the infra-Hisian site as the focus of the block (49,51). Alternating LBBB and right bundle branch block (RBBB) within the same recording or the presence of alternating fascicular block, left posterior fascicular block (LPFB) and left anterior fascicular block (LAFB), with RBBB similarly predicts the infra-Hisian site (52).

The ECG is also obviously of use in diagnosis and for determining prognosis of underlying cardiac disease in patients with arrhythmia. In addition, in some situations it is helpful in determining the future likelihood of arrhythmia.

Identification of Q waves on the 12-lead ECG and their distribution is helpful in establishing the diagnosis of a myocardial infarction (MI) and estimating the extent and the location of the infarct. For example, patients with a large anterior wall infarction, complicated by an infarct-related BBB are often at the highest risk of development of subsequent complications, including lethal ventricular arrhythmias (VT) and ventricular fibrillation (VF) or complete A-V block (53–55).

A well defined role of the ECG is identification of the long QT interval syndromes. ECG is also useful in localizing the site of an accessory pathway, in the presence of antegrade preexcitation (56–58).

ECG can also be helpful in monitoring the therapeutic and toxic effects of antiarrhythmic drugs by observing the serial changes in PR, QRS, and QT intervals.

Thus, a 12-lead ECG remains a fundamental and useful tool for the evaluation and interpretation of rhythm disturbances and is a useful adjunct in assessment of therapy and prognosis in patients with cardiac disorders.

SIGNAL-AVERAGED ELECTROCARDIOGRAPHY

Description of the Technique

Signal averaging is a recording technique which minimizes the extraneous random noise in order to detect signals of low (microvolt) amplitude in the ECG (59).

The purpose of signal averaging is to enhance the intrinsic cardiac electrical signals and reduce interference by noise such as muscle activity or outside AC current. In this way, one can noninvasively detect intrinsic cardiac electrical activity that is not apparent on routine ECGs.

There are a number of ways of achieving this goal. In *temporal* averaging, a number of beats are recorded, summed, and averaged. In *spatial averaging*, a number of leads in separate locations are recorded simultaneously and also averaged.

In *temporal averaging*, multiple samples of a repetitive waveform (e.g., multiple QRS complexes) are averaged. The complexes that are undergoing averaging are called "templated" beats. This process enhances those electrical signals that occur in every beat (i.e., cardiac electrical signals) and eliminate randomly occurring signals (i.e., random noise). By enhancing cardiac signals, the technique has the capacity to bring out electrical information that is not apparent in examining a simple ECG recording. Infrequently occurring beats (e.g., ectopic beats), are excluded, by comparing these to a templated beat (60,61).

The repetitive form that is being acquired has to have a reference time, so that the computer can average out appropriate points of the repetitive signal (61). The noise to be excluded from the signal must be nonrepetitive, i.e., random noise and must be independent in time from the signal of interest (59). Such noise would include muscle activity and AC current. Temporal averaging is the most frequently utilized clinical technique, because it achieves noise reduction, the easiest. However, one disadvantage is that in requiring averaging of many beats, it cannot evaluate beat-to-beat changes.

A second type of signal averaging is called *spatial averaging*. In this type of averaging, a number of independent electrode pairs are summed. The advantage of this technique is that beat-to-beat events can be analyzed, although the theoretical noise reduction is less (62).

After the ECG signal is averaged, it also usually undergoes high-pass filtering, to reduce large amplitude, low-frequency signals. Frequencies below 40 Hz are most frequently filtered, although some devices cut off at 25–100 Hz. However, muscle activity which is typically in the 5 to 20-μV range cannot be eliminated by filtering techniques since the frequency content is similar to the frequency content of the cardiac potentials (60).

Time domain analysis, i.e., analysis of electrical activity at a specific time window in the cardiac electrical cycles, is also used. For example, special digital filtering techniques have also been developed to detect and study ventricular late potentials (61).

Another technique to study the high-frequency domain is the fast Fourier transform (FFT) (63). This technique utilizes a mathematical transformation of the signal into fundamental and harmonic frequencies. This analysis displays amplitude against the frequency content. In this analysis, timing information is lost, however (64).

Signal-averaged ECG is easy to acquire at the patient's bedside. Orthogonal (XYZ) leads are generally employed. On the average, 300–400 beats are averaged. The leads are high-pass filtered and combined into a vector magnitude. The entire method is automated, with an analysis time of several minutes. Temporal averaged ECGs have been used in all clinical studies described here, though future technologic development may permit other techniques to be brought into this setting.

Detection of Ventricular Late Potentials

Several investigators have described small, high-frequency waveforms on temporal signal-averaged surface ECGs in patients with VT (65–68). Late potentials are related to the fragmented, delayed ventricular activation, which has also been detected on endocardial and epicardial electrograms recorded during invasive electrophysiologic studies or during intraoperative mapping in patient with VT (69–71). These potentials are thought to be associated with slowly conducing reentrant pathways. An example of an abnormal signal-averaged ECG is shown in Figure 3.3. For comparison, a normal signal averaged ECG is demonstrated in Figure 3.4.

Late potentials have the following characteristics: (a) Late potentials extend the duration of the filtered QRS complex (61), (b) they have low amplitude (61), and (c) they extend the terminal portion of the filtered QRS complex which remains below 40 μV (68).

The main use of the signal-averaging techniques to date has been the identification of patients at risk for subsequent VT or VF post-MI (65–68). There is no consensus about what constitutes the criteria for late potentials and the definitions are investigator specific. In general, however, for 40-Hz bidirectional filtering techniques, a late potential is said to exist if: (a) the filtered QRS complex is longer than 114 msec, (b) there is a less than 20-μV signal in the last 40 msec of filtered QRS complex, and (c) the terminal QRS complex remains below 40 μV for longer than 38 msec (4,68,72). In the presence of a bundle branch block and prolonged QRS duration, the terminal QRS cannot be subject to the same sort of analysis and Fourier transform analysis is preferred (73).

Clinical Utility of Signal-Averaged ECG

Signal averaging when combined with noninvasive or invasive assessment of left ventricular function can be a particularly powerful predictor of subsequent VT or VF events (75–79). For example, Breithardt *et al*. demonstrated late potentials in 46% of patients with left ventricular aneurysm or dyskinesis, patients more likely to have future arrhythmic event (VT/VF), but in only 9% of patients with normal LV function (74). Signal averaging has also been used as a screening tool prior to invasive electrophysiologic studies and has had other clinical purposes.

Several recent studies have evaluated the prognostic significance of late potentials after an acute MI. They have found that

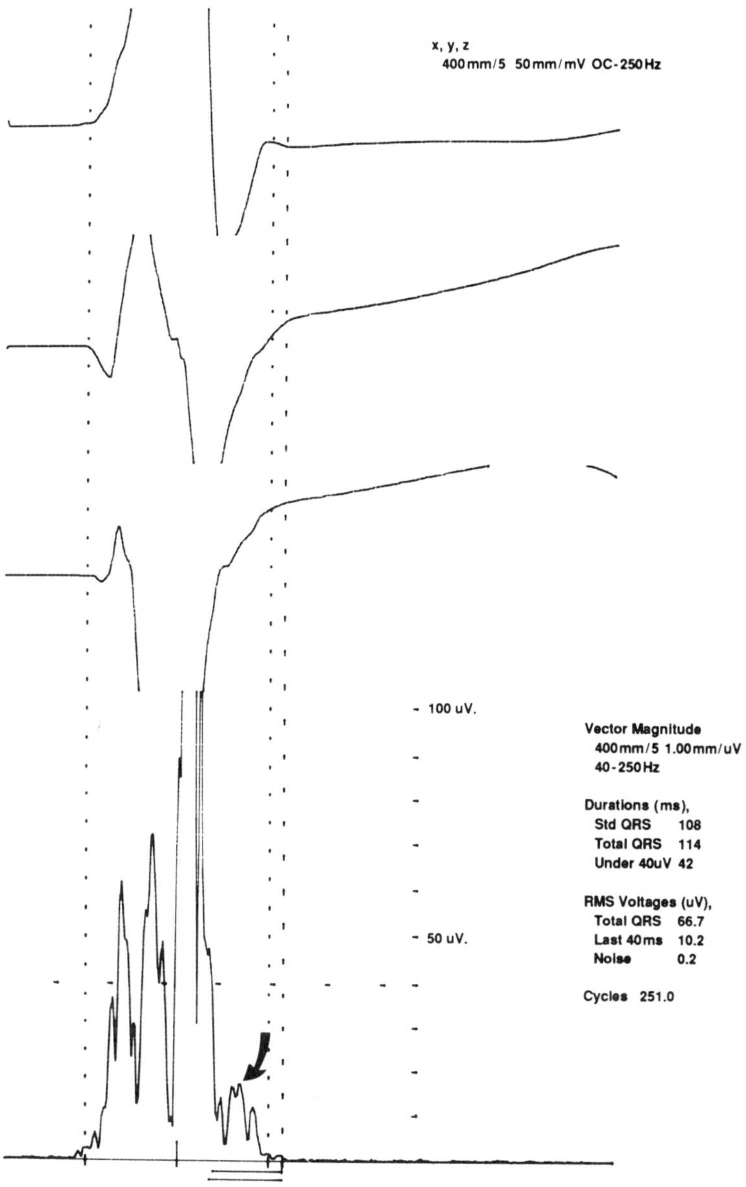

Figure 3.3. Abnormal signal-averaged ECG. Note the presence of late potentials (*arrow*).

the signal temporal averaged ECG has predictive value which is enhanced with the use of other diagnostic techniques. Prospective studies by Gomes, *et al.* and Kuchar, *et al.* evaluated the utility of the signal-averaged ECG, Holter monitoring, and radionuclide ventriculography in predicting subsequent VT or VF post-MI (4,5). Using multivariate analysis, both studies demonstrated that each of the three modalities had independent predictive value for identifying patients with subsequent events. Combining modalities enhanced predictive value.

The combination of a positive signal-averaged ECG and an ejection fraction of less than 40% had the highest predictive value for subsequent VT or VF (34–36%, over a mean follow-up period of 12–14 mo). In contrast, no patients with LV ejection fraction of >40% and a normal signal-averaged ECG had sustained VT or sudden death. A combination of an abnormal signal-averaged ECG and a low ejection fraction had a sensitivity of 80 and 100% and a specificity of 89 and 59% for subsequent VT or VF, respectively (4,5).

Borggrefe and Breithardt suggested that programmed electrical stimulation can also be used in conjunction with signal-averaged ECG to define high-risk patients (80).

Another role for signal-averaged ECG is to screen patients with syncope and nonsustained VT prior to undertaking invasive electrophysiologic studies. Several studies suggest that signal-averaged ECG is a sensitive and specific test for inducibility of VT by subsequent electrophysiologic study, and that it has an independent predictive value (81–84).

Abnormalities of signal-averaged ECG have been reported to

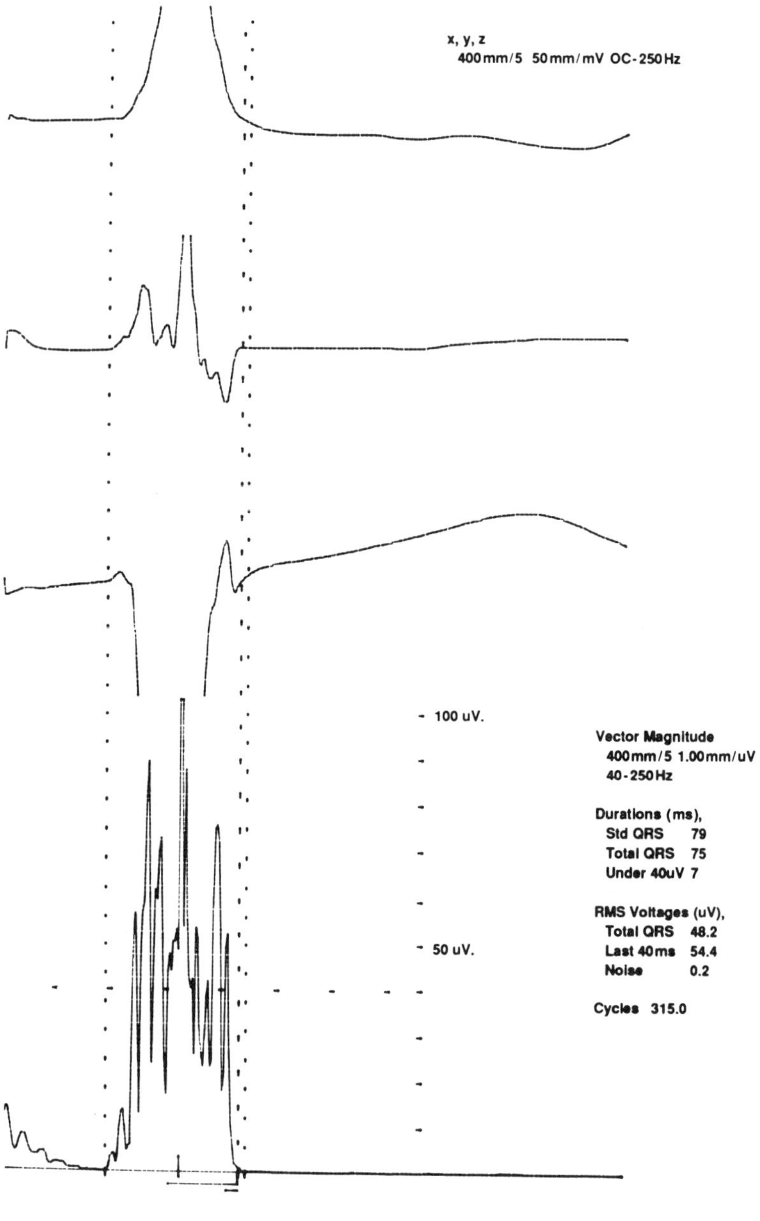

Figure 3.4. Normal signal-averaged ECG. Late potentials are absent.

disappear following a successful surgical ablation of VT (85,86). However, this is not a universal finding, suggesting that removal of all areas of abnormal myocardium where the late potentials originate is not a prerequisite for the abolition of VT.

Antiarrhythmic drugs do not abolish the late potentials. They prolong the filtered QRS duration and decrease the amplitude of the filtered QRS complex (87). At this time, it does not seem that signal-averaged ECG is a useful or a reliable way to assess either antiarrhythmic drug therapy or the results of surgery.

AMBULATORY ECG RECORDING

Continuous, ambulatory ECG recording provides the means to detect, record, and analyze spontaneous cardiac arrhythmias over an extended period of time.

Continuous ECG recording over a 24- or 48-hour period may be provided by tape recording (Holter). A small, battery-operated electromagnetic tape recorder stores the information from a bipolar lead system in either two or three channels of ECG data or reel to reel tape, tape cassette, or micro cassette. A patient-activated event marker is used to note specific clinical events or symptoms. The cassettes are analyzed using a playback instrument with a variable degree of operator interaction. ECG data may be displayed in tabular, trend, or real-time printouts.

Extended electrocardiographic monitoring (24 to 48-hr Holter recording) is particularly useful in examining the rhythm over a prolonged period and facilitating identification of relatively frequent events, e.g., ventricular ectopic beats (VEBs), nonsustained VT, or sinus pauses. Similarly, the effects of activity, or sleep on the clinical rhythm, or rate variability may be examined. Prolonged monitoring permits quantification of arrhythmia frequency and complexity, correlation with patient symptoms and evaluation of the effect of antiarrhythmic drugs on the arrhythmia (88–92).

In normal subjects and in patients with serious rhythm abnormalities, there is a considerable variability in arrhythmia frequency. To prove the efficacy of antiarrhythmic therapy, it is essential to demonstrate that the frequency of the abnormal rhythm disturbance is reduced by an antiarrhythmic drug in excess of that expected to occur by chance alone. Spontaneous reductions in frequency of VEBs of up to 90% have been demonstrated to occur between two 24-hr recording periods (90,93). Therefore, in order to demonstrate any efficacy, the frequency of VEBs must be reduced by greater than 85%, from the baseline to the 24-hr Holter recording while the patient is on an antiarrhythmic drug (94).

Holter directed antiarrhythmic therapy is therefore time consuming and requires prolonged clinical observation. On the other hand, Holter directed antiarrhythmic therapy may be reasonable if the patient is unwilling or unable to undergo electrophysiologic testing or when invasive electrophysiologic studies are not readily available to the clinician.

In certain circumstances, Holter technique may be preferable to invasive studies, e.g., in the assessment of patients with syncope of uncertain etiology prior to electrophysiologic study, identification of sinus nodal dysfunction, or in documenting suspected pacemaker or device (antitachycardia pacemaker or implantable cardioverter defibrillator) malfunction.

Ambulatory monitoring may be combined with electrophysiologic studies to assess antiarrhythmic drug efficacy. For example, complete suppression of sustained and nonsustained VT is required before reevaluating an antiarrhythmic drug by further electrophysiologic testing. Lack of suppression of sustained or nonsustained VT on a 24-hr Holter recording predicts drug failure.

Examination of heart rate variability and ST segment analysis, to document autonomic influence on heart rate and silent ischemia, is yet another potential application for continuous ECG recording and analysis. Heart rate variability is another powerful predictor of prognosis, independent of left ventricular function and ventricular arrhythmias in patients post-MI (95–97).

EVENT RECORDERS

Whereas the continuous recordings quantify and store the data for analysis over a 24- to 48-hr period, noncontinuous recorders take snapshots of arrhythmia events. In patients where the rhythm disturbances are transient and infrequent, the event recording devices may be particularly useful for arrhythmia documentation.

Transtelephonic transmission of an ECG signal permits an online identification and documentation of the arrhythmia. Event recorders are small, lightweight (cigarette package size) devices that are carried by the patients. The recording may be obtained by applying the device on to the precordial area, or with electrodes applied to the axilla or on the wrists (Fig. 3.5).

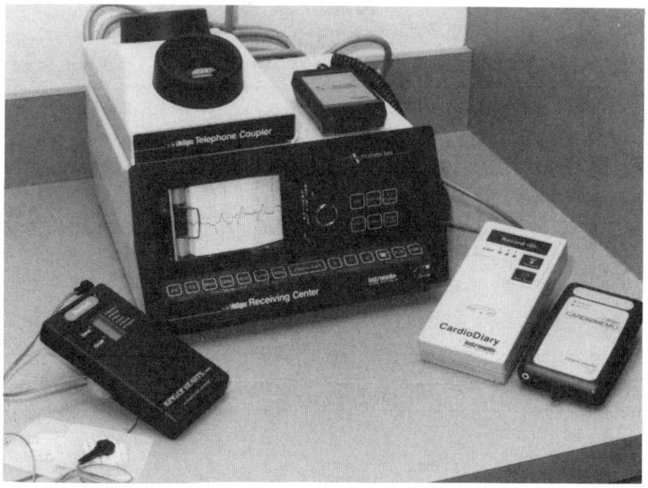

Figure 3.5. Event recorders and transtelephonic receiver.

Another type, the continuously applied event recorder, takes advantage of a memory loop circuitry by continuous monitoring of the applied bipolar electrodes (98). The advantage of a continuous recording is that it provides stored data before the event (60 secs) and following the event (approximately 60 secs). These data are subsequently available for analysis, transtelephonic transmission, or direct printout. The devices are particularly useful in infirm patients or in those patients in whom transient loss of consciousness may prevent the recording of an event.

Event recorders are particularly useful for follow up of patients with permanent pacemakers, antitachycardia devices and implantable cardioverter-defibrillators (ICDs) (Fig. 3.6). Special recording devices have become available for recording pacing artefacts in patients with permanent pacemakers (pacemaker Holter devices). These devices amplify and present the stimulus artefact in a separate channel to facilitate the analysis of paced rhythms (99,100). Such devices are reasonably reliable for the identification of the ventricular pacemaker artifact; however, they are less reliable for the atrial channel analysis (101).

TRANSESOPHAGEAL RECORDING AND PACING TECHNIQUES

Specialized esophageal recordings can be used to permit more accurate assessment of arrhythmias. They are used to record and distinguish atrial and ventricular depolarizations and to analyze the left atrial depolarization. This method is not only used to distinguish atrial from ventricular arrhythmia but also for more refined analysis such as distinguishing AV nodal reentry tachycardias from AV reciprocating tachycardias.

Successful esophageal recording requires optimal placement of the recording electrode in close proximity to the left atrium, which is located anterior to the esophagus. In general, either a

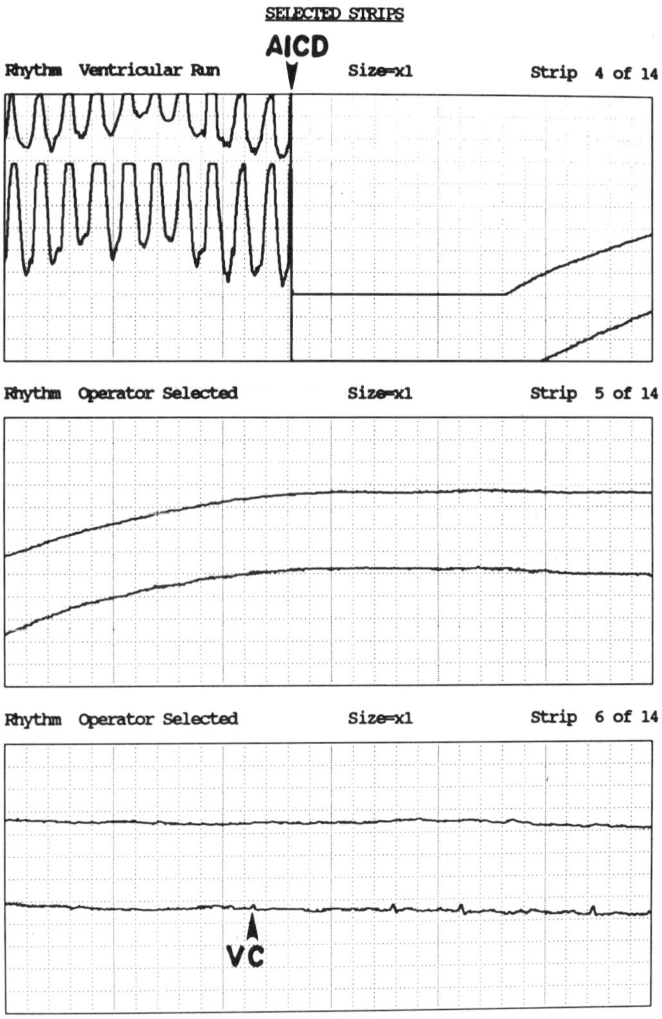

Figure 3.6. Recording of a termination of ventricular tachycardia by AICD shock (*arrow*), followed by a prolonged asystole. V.C. denotes ventricular capture.

bipolar (coronary sinus, nontined) lead (Fig. 3.7) or an esophageal "pill" electrode may be positioned transnasally (102). The "pill" electrode is a gelatin-coated capsule connected to a teflon-coated thin wire (103). The pill electrode is more suitable for prolonged (24-hr) Holter recordings. Bipolar signals are amplified and filtered (10–20 Hz) to exclude muscle artefact. An example of transesophageal recording is shown in Figure 3.8.

Stimulation of left atrium is also feasible using the transesophageal electrode though often pulse-widths of 5–15 msec are required to obtain successful capture (104,105). Transesophageal atrial pacing can be used to initiate and terminate AV nodal reentry tachycardias, and to study the antegrade refractory period of an accessory pathway in WPW syndrome patients (106). Similarly, transesophageal atrial pacing may be used to terminate atrial flutter (107).

The esosophageal technique is particularly useful in infants and children, where the advantages of avoiding invasive

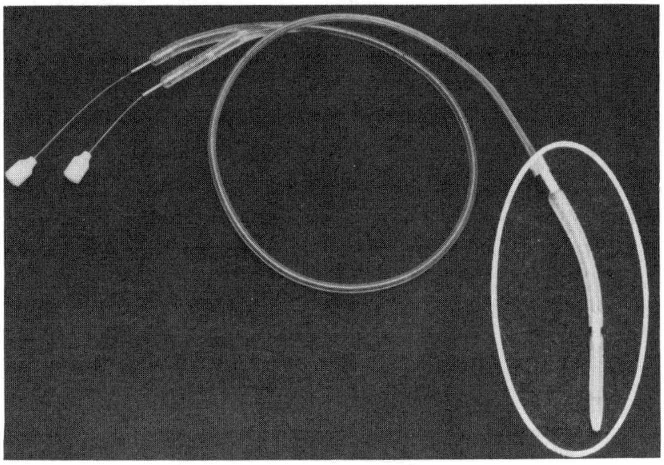

Figure 3.7. Esophageal lead (coronary nontined lead), courtesy of Medtronics, Minneapolis, MN.

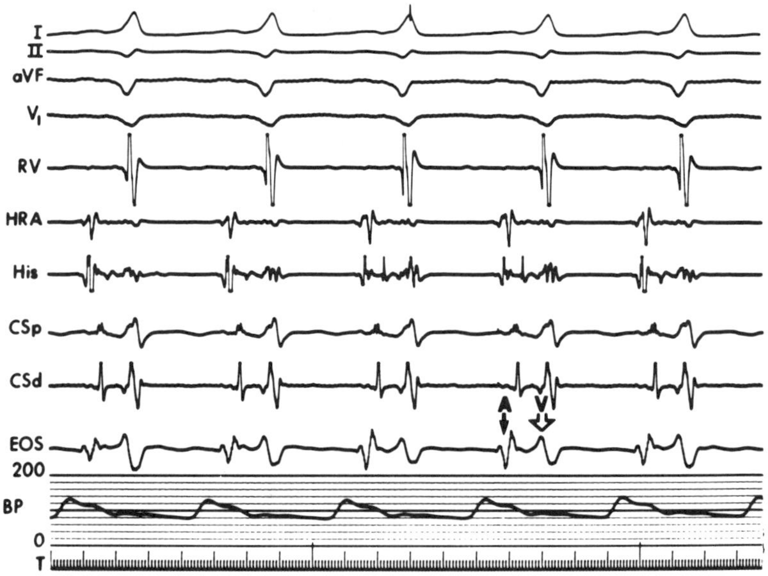

Figure 3.8. Example of a transesophageal recording in a patient with WPW syndrome during normal sinus rhythm. From **top** to **bottom:** leads I, II, aVF, and V_1, intracardiac leads: right ventricular (RV), right atrial (RA), His bundle (His), proximal coronary sinus (CSp), distal coronary sinus (CSd), esophageal (EOS), blood pressure (BP), and time lines (T). Note the high fidelity of esophageal recordings compared to coronary sinus recordings. Atrial depolarization (A) and ventricular depolarization (V) are noted on the esophageal recording.

catheterization for diagnostic or therapeutic reasons is obvious. Transesophageal recording and pacing is a simple and effective technique, with minimal risk, and one that can be accomplished without fluoroscopy.

CONCLUSION

Clinical history, physical examination, and the noninvasive techniques for evaluation of cardiac function and arrhythmias form the basis for therapeutic decisions, which is further enhanced by the invasive electrophysiologic techniques. Discussion of these techniques may be found elsewhere in the book (see Chapters 4–9).

References

1. Harvey WP, Levine SA: Paroxysmal ventricular tachycardia due to emotion. Possible mechanism of death due to fright. JAMA 1952;150:479–480.
2. Engle GL: Sudden and rapid death during psychologic stress. Folklore or folk wisdom? Ann Intern Med 1971;74:771–782.
3. Corbalan R, Vrerier R, Lown B: Psychologic stress and ventricular arrhythmias during myocardial infarction in the conscious dog. Am J Cardiol 1974;34(6):692–696.
4. Gomes JA, Winters SL, Stewart D, *et al*.: A new noninvasive index to predict sustained ventricular tachycardia and sudden death in the first year after myocardial infarction: based on signal-averaged electrocardiogram, radionuclide ejection fraction and Holter monitoring. J Am Coll Cardiol 1987; 10:349–357.
5. Kuchar DL, Thorburn DW, Sammel NL: Prediction of serious arrhythmic events after myocardial infarction: signal-averaged electrocardiogram. Holter monitoring and radionuclide ventriculography. J Am Coll Cardiol 1987;9:531–538.
6. Bigger TJ, Fleiss JL, Kleiger R, *et al*.: The relationships among ventricular arrhythmias, left ventricular dysfunction, and mortality in the 2 years after myocardial infarction. Circulation 1984;69:250–258.
7. Buxton AE, Marchlinski FE, Waxman HL, *et al*.: Prognostic factors in nonsustained ventricular tachycardia. Am J Cardiol 1984;53:1275–1279.
8. Hofmann T, Meinertz T, Kasper W, *et al*.: Mode of death in idiopathic dilated cardiomyopathy: a multivariate analysis of prognostic determinants. Am Heart J 1988;116:1455–1463.
9. Marcus FI, Cobb LA, Edwards JE, *et al*.: Mechanism of death and prevalence of myocardial ischemic symptoms in the terminal event after myocardial infarction. Am J Cardiol 1988;61:8–15.
10. Medina R, Panidis IPK, Morganroth J, *et al*.: The value of echocardiographic regional wall motion abnormalities in detecting coronary artery disease in patients with or without a dilated left ventricle. Am Heart J 1985;109:799–803.
11. Froehlich RT, Falsetti HL, Doty DB, *et al*.: Prospective study of surgery for left ventricular aneurysm. Am J Cardiol 1980;45:923–931.
12. Ryan T, Petrovic G, Anthony WF, *et al*.: Quantitative two-dimensional echocardiographic assessment of patients undergoing left ventricular aneurysmectomy. Am Heart J 1986;111:714–720.
13. Vlay SC, Reid PR, Griffith LS, *et al*.: Relationship of specific coronary lesions and regional left ventricular dysfunction to prognosis in survivors of sudden cardiac death. Am Heart J 1984;108:1212–1220.
14. Bonow RO, Kent KM, Rosing DR, *et al*.: Exercise-induced ischemia in mildly symptomatic patients with coronary artery disease and preserved left ventricular function. Identification of subgroups at risk of death during medical therapy. N Engl J Med 1984;311:1339–1345.
15. Fox RM, Nestico PF, Munley BJ, *et al*.: Coronary artery cardiomyopathy. Hemodynamic and prognostic implications. Chest 1986;89:352–356.
16. Unverferth DV, Magorien RD, Moeschberger ML, *et al*.: Factors influencing the one-year mortality of dilated cardiomyopathy. Am J Cardiol 1984; 54:147–1523.
17. Brandenburg RO: Cardiomyopathies and their role in sudden death. J Am Coll Cardiol 1985;5(Suppl 6):1858–1898.
18. Zimmermann M, Adamec R, Simonin P, *et al*.: Prognostic significance of ventricular late potentials in coronary artery disease. Am Heart J 1985;109:725–732.
19. von Olshausen K, Schafer A, Mehmel HC, *et al*.: Ventricular arrhythmias in idiopathic dilated cardiomyopathy. Br Heart J 1984;51:195–201.
20. Pryor DB, Harrell FE, Lee KL, *et al*.: Prognostic indicators from radionuclide angiography in medically treated patients with coronary artery disease. Am J Cardiol 1984;53:18–22.
21. Nestico PF, Hakki AH, Iskandrian AS: Left ventricular dilatation. Prognostic value in severe left ventricular dysfunction secondary to coronary artery disease. Chest 1985;88:215–220.
22. Shiina A, Tajik AJ, Smith HC, *et al*.: Prognostic significance of regional wall motion abnormality in patients with prior myocardial infarction: a prospective correlative study of two-dimensional echocardiography and angiography. Mayo Clin Proc 1986;61:254–262.
23. Schwartz F, Mall G, Munthey J, *et al*.: Determinants of survival in patients with congestive cardiomyopathy: quantitative morphologic findings and left ventricular hemodynamics. Circulation 1984;70:923–928.
24. Dogly MT, Sandler M, Ballew DW, *et al*.: The use of biplane angiocardiography for the measurement of left ventricular volume in man. Am Heart J 1960;60:762.
25. Sheehan FH, Bolson EL, Dodge HT, *et al*.: Advantages and applications of the centerline method for characterizing regional ventricular function. Circulation 1986;74(2):293–305.
26. Mancini GBJ, Higgins CB: Digital subtraction angiography: a review of cardiac applications. Prog Cardiovasc Dis 1985;28:111–141.
27. Pfisterer ME, Battler A, Zaret BL: Range of normal values of left and right ventricular ejection fraction at rest and during exercise assessed by radionuclide angiocardiography. Eur Heart J 1985;6:647–655.
28. Buda AJ, Dubbin JP, Meindok H: Radionuclide assessment of regional left ventricular function in acute myocardial infarction. Am Heart J 1986;111:36–41.
29. Iskandrian AS, Hatcki AH: Radionuclide evaluation of exercise left ventricular performance in patients with coronary artery disease. Am Heart J 1985;110:851–856.
30. Kronenberg MW, Parrish MD, Jenkins DW, *et al*.: Accuracy of radionuclide ventriculography for estimation of left ventricular volume changes and end-systolic pressure volume relations. J Am Coll Cardiol 1985;6:1064–1072.
31. Schiller NB, Acquatella J, Ports TA, *et al*.: Left ventricular volume from paired biplane two-dimensional echocardiography. Circulation 1979;60:547–555.
32. Caputo GR, Graham MM, Bruat KD, *et al*.: Measurement of left ventricular volume using single-photon emission computed tomography. Am J Cardiol 1985;56:781–786.
33. Sahn DJ, DeMaria A, Kisslo J, *et al*.: Recommendations regarding quantification in M-mode echocardiography: results of a survey of echocardiographic measurements. Circulation 1978;58:1072–1083.
34. Seward JB, Khandheria BK, Oh JK, *et al*.: Transesophageal echocardiography: Technique, anatomic correlations, implementation, and clinical applications. Mayo Clin Proc 1988;63:649–680.
35. Wyatt HL, Heng MK, Meerbaum S, *et al*.: Cross-sectional echocardiography: Analysis of mathematic models for quantifying volume of the formalin-fixed left ventricle. Circulation 1980;61:1119–1125.
36. Mercier JC, DiSessa TG, Jarmakani JM, *et al*.: Two-dimensional echocardiographic assessment of left ventricular volumes and ejection fraction in children. Circulation 1982;65:962–969.
37. Folland ED, Parisi AF, Moynihan PF, *et al*.: Assessment of left ventricular ejection fraction and volume by real-time, two-dimensional echocardiogra-

phy. A comparison of angiographic and radionuclide techniques. Circulation 1979;60:760–766.

38. Silverman NH, Ports TA, Snider AR, *et al.*: Echocardiographic and angiographic comparisons. Circulation 1980;60;548–557.
39. Stamm RB, Carabello BA, Mayers DL, *et al.*: Two-dimensional echocardiographic measurement of left ventricular ejection fraction: prospective analysis of what constitutes an adequate determination. Am Heart J 1982; 104:136–144.
40. Zoghbi WA, Buckley J, Massey MA, *et al.*: Determination of left ventricular volumes with use of a new nonconcentric echocardiographic method: Clinical validator and practical application. J Am Coll Cardiol 1990;15:610–617.
41. Bardy GH, Packer DL, Gernan LD, *et al.*: Preexcited reciprocating tachycardia in patients with Wolff-Parkinson-White syndrome: incidence and mechanisms. Circulation 1984;70:377–391.
42. Durrer D, Schuilenburg RM, Wellens HJ: Preexcitation revisited. Am J Cardiol 1970;25:690–697.
43. Gallagher JJ, Pritchett ELC, Sealy WC, *et al.*: The preexcitation syndromes. Progr Cardiovasc Dis 1978;20(4):285–327.
44. Bär FW, Brugada P, Dassen WRM, *et al.*: Differential diagnosis of tachycardia with narrow QRS complex (shorter than 0.12 seconds). Am J Cardiol 1984;54(6):555–560.
45. Coumel P, Attuel P, Mugica J: Junctional reciprocating tachycardia. The permanent form. In Kulbertus HE (ed): Reentrant Arrhythmias. Lancaster, MTP Press, 1977:170–183.
46. Wu D, Denes P, Amat-y-Leon F, *et al.*: An unusual variety of atrioventricular reentry due to retrograde dual atrioventricular nodal pathways. Circulation 1977;56(1):50–59.
47. Puech P, Grolleau R: L'onde P rétrograde négative en D1, signe de faisceau Kent postéro-latéral gauche. Arch Mal Coeur 1977;70(1):49–60.
48. Tchou P, Lehmann MH, Jazayeri M, *et al.*: Atriofascicular connection or a nodoventricular Mahaim fiber? Electrophysiologic elucidation of the pathway and associated reentrant circuit. Circulation 1988;77(4):837–848.
49. Narula OS, Scherlag BJ, Samet P, *et al.*: Atrioventricular block: localization and classification by His bundle recordings. Am J Med 1971;50:146–165.
50. Zipes DP: Second-degree atrioventricular block. Circulation 1979; 60(3):465–472.
51. Schuilenburg RM, Durrer D: Observations on atrioventricular conduction in patients with bilateral bundle branch block. Circulation 1970;41:967–979.
52. Rosenbaum MB, Elizari MV, Lazzari JO, *et al.*: Intraventricular trifascicular blocks. The syndrome of right bundle branch block wih intermittent left anterior and posterior hemiblock. Am Heart J 1969;78:306–317.
53. Lie KI, Liem KL, Schuilenburg RM, *et al.*: Early identification of patients developing late in-hospital ventricular fibrillation after discharge from the coronary care unit. A 5½ year retrospective and prospective study of 1897 patients. Am J Cardiol 1978;41(4):674–677.
54. Atkins JM, Leshin SJ, Blomquist G, *et al.*: Ventricular conduction blocks and sudden death in acute myocardial infarction. Potential indications for pacing. N Engl J Med 1973;288:281–284.
55. Dutch Ventricular Tachycardia Study Group: Determinants of mortality in 431 postinfarction patients with ventricular tachycardia or fibrillation: a multivariate analysis (Abstr). Circulation 1988;78:628.
56. Klein GJ, Gulamhusein SS: Intermittent preexcitation in the Wolff-Parkinson-White syndrome. Am J Cardiol 1983;52(3):292–296.
57. Wellens HJ, Bär FW, Gorgels AP, *et al.*: Use of ajmaline in patients with the Wolff-Parkinson-White syndrome to disclose short refractory period of the accessory pathway. Am J Cardiol 1980;45(5):130–133.
58. Wellens HJ, Braat S, Brugada P, *et al.*: Use of procainamide in patients with the Wolff-Parkinson-White syndrome to disclose a short refractory of the accessory pathway. Am J Cardiol 1982;50(5):1087–1089.
59. Hombach V, Hopp HW, Braun V, *et al.*: The applicability of the signal averaging technique in clinical cardiology. Clin Cardiol 1982;5(2):107–124.
60. Taylor TP, Macfarlane PW: Digital filtering of the e.c.g.—a comparison of low-pass digital filters on a small computer. Med Biol Eng 1974;12:493–502.
61. Simson MB: Use of signals in the terminal QRS complex to identify patients with ventricular tachycardia after myocardial infarction. Circulation 1981;64:235–242.
62. Flowers NC, Shvartsman V, Kennelly BM, *et al.*: Surface recording of His-Purkinje activity on an every-beat basis without digital averaging. Circulation 1981;63:948–952.
63. Cain ME, Ambos D, Witkowksi FX, *et al.*: Fast-Fourier transform analysis of signal-averaged electrocardiograms for the identification of patients prone to sustained ventricular tachycardia. Circulation 1984;69:711–720.
64. Haberl R, Jilge G, Pulter R, *et al.*: Comparison of frequency and time domain analysis of the signal-averaged electrocardiogram in patients with ventricular tachycardia and coronary artery disease: methodologic validation and clinical relevance. J Am Coll Cardiol 1988;2:150–158.
65. Uther JB, Dennett CJ, Tan A: The detection of delayed activation signals of low amplitude in the vectocardiogram of patients with recurrent ventricular tachycardia by signal averaging. In Sandor E, Julian DJ, Bell JW (eds): Management of Ventricular Tachycardia—Role of Mexiletine. Amsterdam-Oxford, Excerpta Medica, 1980;80.
66. Breithardt G, Becker R, Seipel L, *et al.*: Noninvasive detection of late potentials in man—a new marker for ventricular tachycardia. Eur Heart J 1981;2:1–11.
67. Rozanski JJ, Mortara D, Myerburg RJ, *et al.*: Body surface detection of delayed depolarization in patients with recurrent ventricular tachycardia and left ventricular aneurysm. Circulation 1981;63:1172–1178.
68. Denes P, Santarelli P, Hauser RG, *et al.*: Quantitative analysis of the high-frequency components of the terminal portion of the body surface QRS in normal subjects and in patients with ventricular tachycardia. Circulation 1983;67:1129–1138.
69. Josephson ME, Horowitz LN, Farshidi A: continuous local electrical activity. A mechanism of recurrent ventricular tachycardia. Circulation 1978;57:659–665.
70. Wiener I, Mindich B, Pitchon R: Determinants of ventricular tachycardia in patients with ventricular aneurysms: results of intraoperative epicardial and endocardial mapping. Circulation 1982;65:856–861.
71. Klein H, Karp RB, Kouchoukos NT, *et al.*: Intraoperative electrophysiologic substrate of ventricular arrhythmias. Circulation 1982;66:847–853.
72. Simson MB, Untereker WJ, Spielman SR, *et al.*: The relationship between late potentials on the body surface and directly recorded fragmented electrograms in patients with ventricular tachycardia. Am J Cardiol 1983;51:105–112.
73. Lindsay BD, Markham J, Schechtman KB, *et al.*: Identification of patients with sustained ventricular tachycardia by frequency analysis of signal-averaged electrocardiograms despite the presence of bundle branch block. Circulation 1988;77:122–130.
74. Breithardt G, Borggrefe M, Karbenn U, *et al.*: Prevalence of late potentials in patients with and without ventricular tachycardia: correlation and angiographic findings. Am J Cardiol 1982;49:1932–1937.
75. Denes P, Uretz E, Santarelli P: Determinants of arrhythmogenic ventricular activity detected on the body surface QRS in patients with coronary artery disease. Am J Cardiol 1984;523:1519–1523.
76. Freedman RA, Gillis AM, Keren A, *et al.*: Signal-averaged electrocardiographic late potentials in patients with ventricular fibrillation or ventricular tachycardia: correlation with clinical arrhythmia and electrophysiologic study. Am J Cardiol 1985;55:1350–1353.
77. Pollak SJ, Kertes PJ, Bredlau CE, *et al.*: Influence of left ventricular function on signal averaged late potentials in patients with coronary artery disease with and without ventricular tachycardia. Am Heart J 1985; 110:747–752.
78. Zimmerman M, Adamee R, Simonin P, *et al.*: Prognostic significance of ventricular late potentials in coronary artery disease. Am Heart J 1985; 109(4):725–732.
79. Gomes JA, Horowitz SF, Millner M, *et al.*: Relation of late potentials to ejection fraction and wall motion abnormalities in acute myocardial infarction. Am J Cardiol 1987;59:1071–1074.

80. Breithardt G, Borggrefe M: Pathophysiological mechanism and clinical significance of ventricular late potentials. Eur Heart J 1986;7:364–385.
81. Freedman RA, Gillis AM, Keren A, *et al.*: Signal-averaged electrocardiographic late potentials in patients with ventricular fibrillation or ventricular tachycardia: correlation with clinical arrhythmia and electrophysiologic study. Am J Cardiol 1985;55:1350–1353.
82. Denniss AR, Ross DL, Richards DA, *et al.*: Differences between patients with ventricular tachycardia and ventricular fibrillation as assessed by signal-averaged electrocardiogram, radionuclide ventriculography and cardiac mapping. J Am Coll Cardiol 1988;11:276–283.
83. Winters SL, Steward D, Gomes JA: Signal averaging of the surface QRS complex predicts inducibility of ventricular tachycardia in patients with syncope of unknown origin: a prospective study. J Am Coll Cardiol 1987;10:775–781.
84. Nalos PC, Gang EL, Mandel WJ, *et al.*: The signal-averaged electrocardiogram as a screening test for inducibility of sustained ventricular tachycardia in high risk patients: a prospective study. J Am Coll Cardiol 1987;9:539–548.
85. Breithardt G, Seipel L, Ostermeyer J, *et al.*: Effects of antiarrhythmic surgery on late ventricular potentials recorded by precordial signal averaging in patients with ventricular tachycardia. Am Heart J 1982;104:996–1003.
86. Marcus NH, Falcone RA, Harken AH, *et al.*: Body surface late potentials: effects of endocardial resection in patients with ventricular tachycardia. Circulation 1984;70:632–637.
87. Simson MB, Waxman HL, Falcone R, *et al.*: Effects of antiarrhythmic drugs on noninvasively recorded late potentials. In Breithardt G, Loogen F (eds): New Aspects in the Medical Treatment of Tachyarrhythmias. Munich, Urban & Schwarzenberg, 1983:80–86.
88. Kennedy HL: Comparison of ambulatory electrocardiography and exercise testing. Am J Cardiol 1981;47:1359–1365.
89. Holter NJ: New method for heart studies: Continuous electrocardiography of active subjects over long periods is now practical. Science 1961;134:1214–1220.
90. Harrison DC, Fitzgerald JW, Winkle RA: Ambulatory electrocardiography for diagnosis and treatment of cardiac arrhythmias. N Engl J Med 1976; 294:373–380.
91. Wenger NK, Mock MB, Ringquist I: Ambulatory Electrocardiographic Recording. Curr Probl Cardiol 1980;Part 1:5(6):1–42, Part II:5(7):1–46. Chicago, Year Book Medical Publishers, 1981.
92. Winkle RA: Recent status of ambulatory electrocardiography. Am Heart J 1981;102:757–770.
93. Winkle RA: Antiarrhythmic drug effect mimicked by spontaneous variability of ventricular ectopy. Circulation 1978;57:1116–1121.
94. Morganroth J, Michelson E, Horowitz LN, *et al.*: Limitations of routine long-term ambulatory electrocardiographic monitoring to assess ventricular ectopy frequency. Circulation 1978;58:408–414.
95. Kleiger RE, Miller JP, Bigger JT, *et al.*: Heart rate variability: a variable predicting mortality following acute myocardial infarction (Abstr). J Am Coll Cardiol 1984;3(2):547.
96. Kleiger RE, Miller JP, Bigger JT Jr, *et al.*: Decreased heart rate variability and its association with increased mortality after acute myocardial infarction. Am J Cardiol 1987;59:256–262.
97. Bigger JT, Kleiger RE, Fleiss JL, *et al.*: Components of heart rate variability measured during healing of acute myocardial infarction. Am J Cardiol 1988;61:208–215.
98. Brown AP, Dawkins KD, Davies JG: Detection of arrhythmias: use of a patient-activated ambulatory electrocardiogram device with a solid-state memory loop. Br Heart J 1987;58(3):251–253.
99. Famularo MA, Kennedy HL: Ambulatory electrocardiography in the assessment of pacemaker function. Am Heart J 1982;104(5 Pt 1):1086–1094.
100. Kelen GJ, Bloomfield DA, Hardage M, *et al.*: A Clinical evaluation of an improved Holter monitoring technique for artificial pacemaker function. PACE 1980;3(2):192–197.
101. Ludmer PL, Goldschlager N: Cardiac pacing in the 1980s. N Engl J Med 1984;311:1671–1680.
102. Schnittger I, Rodrigues IM, Winkle RA: Esophageal electrocardiography: a new technology revives an old technique. Am J Cardiol 1986;57(8):604–607.
103. Harte MT, Teo KK, Horgan JH: The diagnosis and management of supraventricular tachycardia by transesophageal cardiac stimulation and recording. Chest 1988;93(2):339–344.
104. Gallagher JJ, Smith WM, Kerr CR, *et al.*: Esophageal pacing: a diagnostic and therapeutic tool. Circulation 1982;65:336–341.
105. Benson DW, Sanford M, Dunnigan A, *et al.*: Transesophageal atrial pacing threshold: role of interelectrode spacing, pulse width, and catheter insertion depth. Am J Cardiol 1984;53(1):63–67.
106. Critelli G, Grassi G, Perticone F, *et al.*: Transesophageal pacing for prognostic evaluation of preexcitation syndrome and assessment of protective therapy. Am J Cardiol 1983;51:513–518.
107. Montoyo JV, Angel J, Valle V, *et al.*: Cardioversion of tachycardias by transesophageal atrial pacing. Am J Cardiol 1973;32:85–90.

4

ELECTROPHYSIOLOGIC STUDY

Igor Singer, M.B.B.S., F.R.A.C.P., F.A.C.P., F.A.C.C.

INTRODUCTION

Invasive techniques to study normal intracardiac activation and abnormalities occurring during spontaneous and provoked arrhythmias are a reasonably recent development. The era of clinical electrophysiology was opened by the successful recording of human His bundle activation via catheter in 1969 by Scherlag *et al.* (1) Since that time, the technique of recording the intracardiac electrical signals has been enhanced by the technique of the programmed electrical stimulation. In the last two decades invasive electrophysiologic (EP) study has evolved from a purely diagnostic study to include interventional techniques for therapy of specific arrhythmias as well.

Electrophysiologic studies permit a detailed analysis of normal and abnormal cardiac activation and arrhythmia mechanisms in a controlled clinical environment. The techniques involved permit a careful and methodical study of the disorders of the cardiac rhythm. More recently, insights into the mechanisms of arrhythmias has stimulated the development of interventional techniques such as transcatheter ablation, antitachycardia pacing and the development of automatic cardioversion/defibrillation devices.

INDICATIONS

Electrophysiologic studies are performed to evaluate electrophysiologic properties such as automaticity, conduction, and refractoriness. During EP studies, tachycardias are initiated and terminated and may be mapped to determine the sequence of activation. Perhaps the most important indication for EP studies is to evaluate patients' response to various forms of therapy. Evaluation of drug therapy was one of the earliest uses of the technique. Subsequently, EP studies were used in preparation for interventional therapies such as antitachycardia pacemakers, implantable cardioverter defibrillators, and catheter ablation. Studies are modified in accordance with the problem investigated, to provide the information to a specific diagnostic or therapeutic problem.

Recently, a task force was set up to review the guidelines for performance of clinical electrophysiologic studies (2). The task force has identified three separate subclasses for consideration: (a) Class 1—conditions for which there is a general agreement among experts that the information provided by the EP study is useful and important in patient management, (b) Class 2—conditions for which EP studies are frequently performed, but where there is less certainty regarding the usefulness of information obtained, and (c) Class 3—conditions where there is a general agreement that EP studies provide no useful information.

Currently accepted indications for electrophysiologic study are listed in Table 4.1. Therapeutic applications will be discussed in subsequent chapters (20–24) of this book.

Aborted Sudden Cardiac Death

All patients who are resuscitated from an aborted sudden cardiac arrest without a new Q wave myocardial infarction or a reversible acute ischemia or another clearly identifiable cause (e.g. aortic stenosis), should undergo EP studies unless the clinical circumstances dictate otherwise. It is generally recognized that patients who are resuscitated successfully, have a significant risk of a recurrent cardiac arrest if left untreated (3). Most commonly, the initiating rhythm at the time of the cardiac arrest is ventricular tachycardia (VT), which may degenerate into ventricular fibrillation (VF) (4). Less frequently, VF is the initiating rhythm. In the minority (10–20%) of patients, the initial documented rhythm is a bradyarrhythmia (5). The purpose of the EP study in these patients is to: (a) establish the mechanism of the cardiac arrest, and (b) to initiate therapy to prevent a recurrence of cardiac arrest.

Approximately 80% of patients with aborted sudden cardiac death have inducible ventricular tachyarrhythmia on programmed electrical stimulation (PES). Polymorphic VT or VF are more readily inducible than is monomorphic VT (6). The induction protocols in most centers include the use of up to three ventricular extrastimuli and left ventricular programmed stimulation (7). Independent predictive value of EP testing for subse-

Table 4.1.
Indications for Electrophysiologic Study

Diagnosis
• Aborted sudden cardiac death
• Syncope of undetermined cause
• Recurrent wide complex tachycardias
• Ventricular tachycardia
• Recurrent tachycardias or syncope associated with Wolff-Parkinson-White syndrome
• Symptomatic narrow QRS tachycardia refractory to therapy
• Bundle branch block, bifascicular block, or second-degree A-V block with syncope
• Preoperative evaluation prior to surgical ablation e.g., VT, WPW
Therapy
• To guide antiarrhythmic drug therapy for tachycardias: e.g., VT
• Catheter ablation: for AV nodal reentry tachycardia, WPW, VT
• Prior to device implant and for device testing (antitachycardia pacemakers, ICDs)
• Acute termination of a hemodynamically destabilizing tachycardia

Abbreviations: ICD, implantable cardioverter-defibrillator.

quent events in these patients has been established (8–13). In those patients in whom a monomorphic VT is induced, and in whom an antiarrhythmic drug prevents VT reinduction, prognosis is more favorable (13). When polymorphic VT or VF are induced, the endpoint is less clear cut. Certain studies suggest that polymorphic VT or VF may have similar prognostic implications to inducible monomorphic VT (14).

Controversy exists about patients who are noninducible. Some studies suggest low risk in noninducible patients (9,14,15), but others suggest risk similar to the inducible patients (12,16). In summary, electrophysiologic studies are recommended in patients surviving an episode of cardiac arrest without an evidence of an acute Q wave myocardial infarction or in patients surviving an episode of cardiac arrest occurring ≥ 48 hrs after acute myocardial infarction.

Syncope of Undetermined Cause

In patients who present with syncope of undetermined origin, where the noninvasive studies, e.g., 24-hr Holter, event recorders, tilt table studies or exercise testing are nondiagnostic, EP studies may be helpful in establishing the cause. The yield is higher in patients with structural heart disease or a prior myocardial infarction, and relatively low in patients with a normal resting electrocardiogram (ECG) and no evidence of structural heart disease (17).

Sinus node, atrioventricular (AV) node or infranodal disease, or tachycardia (ventricular or supraventricular), can be identified when noninvasive testing is unhelpful. In patients with bifascicular block or bundle branch block, measurement of HV interval and its response to atrial pacing are helpful to guide further therapy (18).

Electrophysiologic studies, in patients with unexplained syncope, are therefore recommended when noninvasive studies are unhelpful and known or suspected structural heart disease exists. Patients with no abnormalities noted during electrophysiologic studies have a low incidence of sudden death during follow-up, suggesting a possible prognostic value of a negative test.

Recurrent Wide QRS Complex Tachycardias (QRS Complex > 0.12 sec)

In patients with recurrent wide QRS tachycardias, EP study may be used to determine the origin and the presumptive mechanism of the tachycardia and to differentiate ventricular from AV reciprocating tachycardias and supraventricular tachycardias with aberrant conduction. Using PES, reentrant arrhythmias are readily initiated and terminated. Arrhythmias in which reentry is not the underlying mechanism are not readily inducible by PES. For example, a sustained VT is generally not inducible in patients with long QT syndrome (19).

Electrophysiologic study is mandatory for evaluation of patients prior to the implantation of an antitachycardia device or an implantable cardioverter-defibrillator (20–22). Information regarding tachycardia morphology, cycle length, modes of induction and termination, and the hemodynamic consequences of the tachycardia are critical to program the devices appropriately.

If surgical or catheter ablation is contemplated, endocardial EP mapping is used to identify the zone of slow onduction in the reentrant circuit and to guide the ablative therapy (23).

Electrophysiologic study is useful in distinguishing VT from AV reciprocating tachycardias where antegrade conduction occurs via the accessory tract (24). Supraventricular tachycardias with pre-existing bundle branch block or those utilizing the Mahaim fiber (left bundle branch (LBBB) morphology) can also be distinguished from VT (24,25).

In patients with frequent, symptomatic and recurrent wide complex tachycardias, EP studies can be helpful to establish the mechanism and suggest possible avenues for therapy. PES may also be used to guide antiarrhythmic therapy (26,27).

To distinguish wide QRS complex tachycardias, one needs to record a His deflection during the tachycardia or during the sinus rhythm either before the onset or after the tachycardia conversion, to insure that His deflection is being recorded. Analysis of the timing and sequence of atrial activation during the tachycardia and the response of the His deflection to ventricular stimulation (during tachycardia) is essential to distinguish the nature of the tachycardia. Advancement of the atrial activation by a premature ventricular extrastimulus during the His refractoriness indicates a presence of an accessory pathway, for example.

Electrophysiologic studies are recommended in patients with wide QRS complex tachycardias that are sustained or symptomatic, or both, and where the correct diagnosis cannot be established by less invasive means.

Ventricular Tachycardia

The use of electrophysiologic studies to diagnose and treat patients with known sustained VT is well established. Further discussion of this important subject may be found in subsequent chapters (6, 8, 10, 20, 21, 23).

However, controlled prospective studies utilizing EP studies for risk stratification in patients with nonsustained VT are lacking. Two retrospective studies suggest that patients with high-grade ventricular ectopy and inducible VT have worse prognosis, with increased incidence of sudden cardiac death (28,29). It is likely that the presence of left ventricular dysfunction enhances the predictive value of EP studies as well as the presence of a positive signal-averaged ECG (30).

In patients with a dilated, nonischemic cardiomyopathy, who have nonsustained VT, the incidence of inducible VT on programmed electrical stimulation is relatively low (<30%) (31–34). Thus, at the present time, EP study cannot be recommended in this patient population, unless the patient presents with sustained VT or sudden cardiac death. The yield is higher in patients with hypertrophic cardiomyopathy (35–37).

Prospective studies are required in order to improve the understanding of the role of PES in these subsets of patients.

Preexcitation Syndromes

Wolff-Parkinson-White (WPW) and other preexcitation syndromes (see also Chapter 9) may be associated with troubling and recurrent tachycardias. These tachycardias may be difficult and potentially hazardous to treat by empiric antiarrhythmic therapy. Often these patients are referred for EP studies to evaluate recurrent symptomatic tachycardias or for evaluation of syncope.

The purpose of the EP studies in patients with WPW syndrome is to: (a) confirm the diagnosis, (b) establish the location of the accessory pathways, (c) prove their participation in the tachycardia, (d) estimate the risk of sudden cardiac death from VF, and (d) assess the utility of various treatment strategies, e.g., ablation (surgical and nonsurgical).

Localization of the atrial and the ventricular sites of insertion of the accessory pathways is determined by retrograde mapping of orthodromic tachycardia or during ventricular pacing, (atrial insertion) and antegrade mapping during differential atrial pacing (ventricular insertion) (38). Direct recordings of accessory pathway potentials are also sometimes possible (39). Precise localization is particularly important if surgical or catheter ablation is contemplated (40).

Atrial fibrillation in patients with WPW syndrome may be life-threatening in the setting of an accessory pathway with a short antegrade refractory period. In these patients, VF may occur during atrial fibrillation. The EP properties of the accessory pathways are an important determinant of the incidence and rate of AV reciprocating tachycardia and the ventricular rate during atrial fibrillation.

The risk for sudden cardiac death may be estimated by observing the shortest interval between successive ventricular depolarizations (RR interval) during spontaneous or induced atrial fibrillation. Retrospective analyses have suggested that RR intervals of less than 250 msec during atrial fibrillation, are associated with an increased risk of sudden cardiac death (41). Unfortunately, measurements obtained at rest, in the supine position do not necessarily reflect the conduction rates occurring during exercise. The sensitivity may be enhanced by the administration of isoproterenol during an EP study (42).

Electrophysiologic studies are indicated in patients with WPW syndrome who are considered for non-pharmacologic therapy (surgical or nonsurgical accessory pathway ablation) because of life-threatening or incapacitating arrhythmias or drug intolerance (Class 1 indication) (2).

Electrophysiologic studies may be useful in patients in whom information about the type of arrhythmia, localization, and the number of accessory pathways and the information regarding the effect of antiarrhythmic therapy on accessory pathways, may influence the selection of the most optimal therapy (Class 2 indication) (2).

Other patients in whom an EP study may be useful are asymptomatic patients who present with ECG evidence of preexcitation during sinus rhythm, who have an occupation where the risk of sudden cardiac death is important to determine (e.g., in athletes or pilots). Similarly, EP study may be useful establishing the risk in patients with WPW syndrome and a family history of premature sudden cardiac death (Class 2 indication) (2).

In asymptomatic patients with WPW syndrome who do not fall into the previously discussed categories, EP studies are generally not recommended.

Narrow Complex Tachycardia (QRS complex <0.12 sec)

A narrow QRS tachycardia (see also Chapter 7) may be caused by sinus tachycardia, atrial tachycardia, atrial flutter or fibrillation, AV junctional tachycardia, AV node reentrant tachycardia, or AV reciprocating tachycardia. Rarely, VT originating high in the interventricular conduction system may manifest as narrow QRS tachycardia.

Twelve-lead ECG is often sufficient to establish the correct diagnosis. Rate and relation of atrial activity to the ventricular activity is essential to establish the correct diagnosis.

PR and RP interval relationships on 12-lead ECG may be helpful in establishing a correct diagnosis. Atrial tachycardias are usually characterized by a PR interval that is shorter than the RP interval. During a typical AV node reentrant tachycardia, the atrium and the ventricle are activated simultaneously, so that the P wave is hidden in the QRS complex. In atypical AV reentrant tachycardia, RP interval may be longer than the PR interval, due to retrograde conduction over an accessory pathway during the tachycardia.

Rarely, AV disassociation may be present during a narrow QRS tachycardia. Such tachycardias may originate in the AV node, His bundle, or fascicle or utilize a fasciculoventricular fiber retrograde and AV node-His bundle antegrade.

Atrioventricular nodal reentrant tachycardia is a regular "narrow complex" tachycardia frequently seen in the general population. The EP substrate is the presence of functionally dissociated AV nodal pathways. This type of tachycardia is inducible by either atrial or ventricular programmed stimulation (43). The common type of reentrant AV nodal tachycardia is characterized by antegrade conduction utilizing the "slow" pathway, and retrograde conduction via the "fast" pathway. Occasionally, the conduction is reversed, so that the "fast" pathway forms the antegrade limb of the circuit and the "slow" pathway, the retrograde limb (44). This type of tachycardia must be distinguished from an orthodromic tachycardia utilizing the accessory pathway for retrograde conduction.

Current understanding of the mechanisms of the AV nodal reentrant tachycardia suggests that perinodal tissue is involved in the reentrant circuit. Cryoablation or surgical resection has resulted in the surgical cure of this arrhythmia, presumably by interrupting the perionodal connections (45,46).

Atrial tachycardias with reentrant mechanism may be induced by programmed electrical stimulation. These arrhythmias are characterized by abnormal P wave axis and morphology. Surgical and catheter ablation approaches are available for this type of arrhythmia. Therefore, atrial mapping may be indicated in refractory cases (47).

The availability of atrial ablation techniques as well as techniques for modification of AV nodal conduction extend the usefulness of EP study techniques to patients who present with atrial flutter and fibrillation with rapid AV conduction and who are refractory to pharmacologic therapy.

Electrophysiologic studies are indicated for patients who present with frequent episodes of narrow complex tachycardia and are refractory to drug therapy. In these patients, information regarding the origin, mechanism, and electrophysiologic properties of the pathways involved in the tachycardia is essential for guiding therapy (pharmacologic, ablative, or antitachycardia pacing). In those patients who may prefer ablative to pharmacologic therapy, EP studies are essential (Class 1 indication) (2).

Assessment of antiarrhythmic drug effects on the sinus node or on AV conduction in symptomatic patients with frequent episodes of narrow complex tachycardia requiring pharmacologic therapy, constitutes a less well-defined indication (Class 2 indication) (2).

Electrophysiologic studies are not indicated for patients with infrequent episodes of tachycardia or where less invasive techniques (e.g., a 12-lead ECG) provides a sufficient information to establish the diagnosis or guide the therapy (Class 3 indication).

Patients with Bundle Branch Block or Bifascicular Block and Syncope

Progression to complete heart block in patients with bifascicular block or bundle branch block is infrequent (48). In symptomatic patients (syncope or presyncope), EP study may be helpful if a markedly prolonged HV interval (>100 msec) is demonstrated or an infra-His block is present during atrial pacing. These patients have a higher propensity to develop complete heart block and should have permanent pacemakers implanted (48,49). Exclusion of other inducible tachyarrhythmias as a cause of syncope is also warranted in this group of patients, e.g., VT. Sinus node disease should also be excluded in these patients.

His bundle recordings allow differentiation of the anatomic site of block to above the bundle of His (proximal), intra-Hisian (within the His bundle), and infra-Hisian (distal), which may be located either within the distal His bundle or within the bundle branches.

Prognosis of patients with AV block depends on the site of the block. Patients with chronic first-degree AV block usually have a good prognosis. Prognosis in patients who have a second-degree AV node block depends on the presence and the severity of the associated heart disease. Untreated second-degree block below the His bundle and acquired complete AV block require pacing (48,49).

Electrophysiologic studies are recommended in symptomatic patients (syncope or near syncope), and in patients in whom distal (His-Purkinje) block is suspected but unproven with continuous ECG recordings (Class 1 indication) (2).

Those patients who remain symptomatic with second- or third-degree A-V block, despite a pacemaker therapy, require exclusion of VT as a cause of syncope.

In patients with concealed junctional extrasystoles in whom pseudo AV block is suspected, EP study may also be helpful to clarify the diagnosis. Similarly, if the site of block is unclear, EP study may be of benefit to establish its precise site (Class 2 indication) (2).

Sinus Node Function

Sinus node dysfunction may be manifested by extreme sinus bradycardia, sinus arrest, or sinoatrial exit block. Sinus node dysfunction may be related to intrinsic sinus node disease or may be brought about by extrinsic influences (e.g., drugs that depress sinus node function).

Evaluation of sinus node function (see Chapter 5) is facilitated by continuous ECG monitoring, exercise testing, and the effects of carotid sinus massage. The use of pharmacologic perturbations, e.g., atropine, isoproterenol and propranolol, may also be helpful.

When the diagnosis of sinus node dysfunction is unclear from the noninvasive testing, EP study may be of further help in evaluating the sinus node function (see Chapter 5). Sinoatrial conduction time (50), sinus node recovery time (51) or direct measurement of sinoatrial conduction time may be helpful (52).

The sensitivity and the specificity of the corrected sinus node recovery time for detecting sinus node dysfunction is 54% and of the sinoatrial conduction time 51% approximately, with a combined sensitivity of 64% (53,54). The sensitivity of the combined tests is 88% (54,54).

Electrophysiologic studies are recommended in symptomatic patients (with syncope or presyncope) in whom sinus node dysfunction is suspected, but in whom the diagnosis cannot be established by noninvasive techniques (Class 1 indication) (2).

Exclusion of other arrhythmias as a cause of syncope, evaluation for the most appropriate form of pacing therapy and exclusion of extrinsic from intrinsic causes of sinus nodal dysfunction, constitute other recognized indications for EP studies (Class 2 indication) (2). However, it should be noted that in most patients with sinus node dysfunction, therapeutic decisions are made mainly on clinical grounds.

ELECTROPHYSIOLOGIC STUDY

Technical Aspects

Electrophysiologic studies should be performed in clinical centers where a trained electrophysiologist, nursing personnel, and technical support staff are readily available. Since electrophysiologic study involves induction and termination of potentially lethal arrhythmias, often in patients with impaired cardiac function, appropriate resuscitative equipment and trained staff must be available.

Laboratory Organization

The general organization of a clinical EP laboratory is shown in Figure 4.1. The components of the EP laboratory are the following: (a) Imaging equipment (multiple-plane cine fluoroscopy); (b) EP station which consists of a stimulator, tape recorder, storage oscilloscope, junction box (Fig. 4.2), (c) recording apparatus (12–16 channels), including three to five surface ECG leads (standard and augmented leads for the determination of frontal plane axis and P wave polarity and frontal leads V_1 and V_5, for timing simultaneously with multiple intracardiac signals) (Fig. 4.3), (d) 12-lead ECG machine for on-line recording of tachycardias during the course of an EP study, (e) standby defibrillator, connected to the patient by means of R_2 pads or similar, and a backup defibrillator.

Staff should include, at a minimum, an EP-trained physician, a nurse trained in resuscitation, and a recording technician.

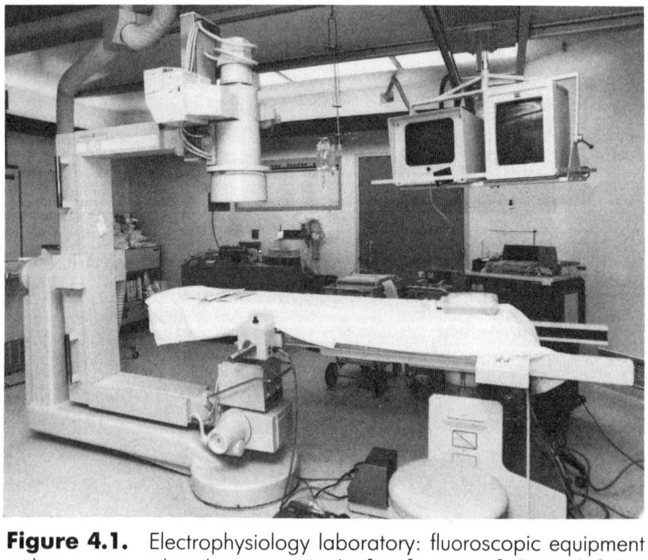

Figure 4.1. Electrophysiology laboratory: fluoroscopic equipment with remote overhead monitors. In the **background:** from **right** to **left:** defibrillators (2), 12-lead ECG, resuscitative equipment.

EQUIPMENT

Junction box

The junction box consists of a number of multiple-pole switches matched to each recording and stimulation channel. A ready selection of any pair of electrodes is available for stimulation or recording (Fig. 4.2 and 4.3). The junction box is connected to

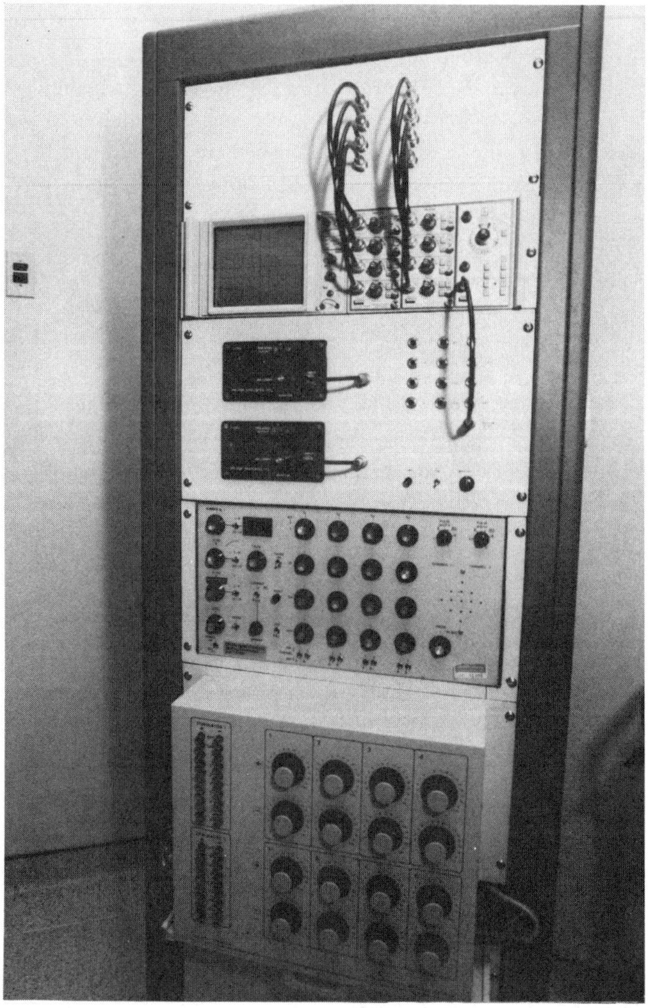

Figure 4.2. EP station: mobile electrophysiology console used for intraoperative mapping procedures. **Top** to **bottom:** storage oscilloscope, isolation boxes for stimulation and synchronization to external input, stimulator, and junction box.

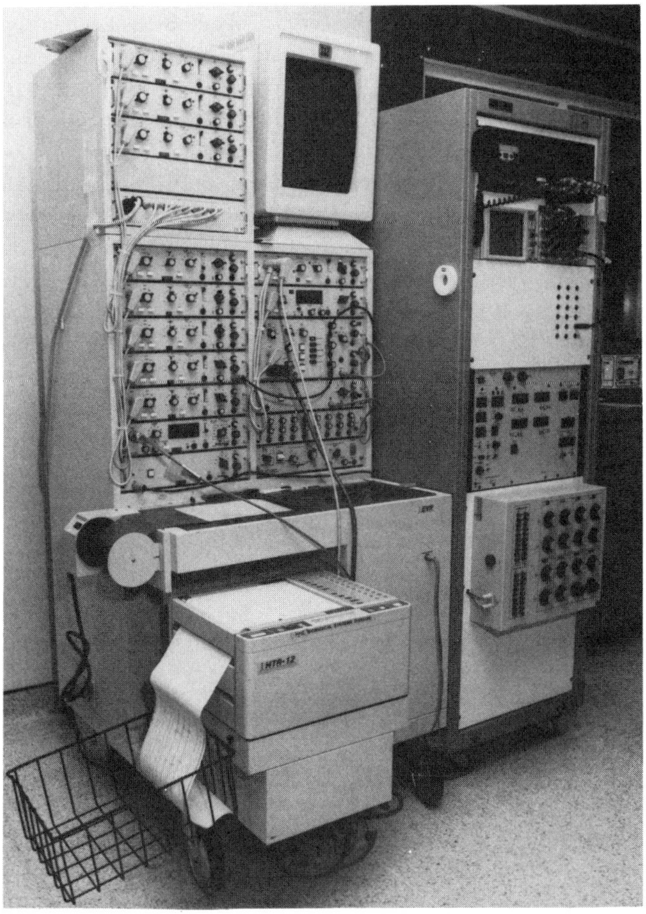

Figure 4.3. Recording apparatus (**left**), next to the EP station (**right**).

the intracardiac catheters by means of a cable, permitting simultaneous display of several intracardiac channels and pacing from any selected pair of electrodes.

Recording Apparatus

The signal processor (filters and amplifiers), switch beam oscilloscope, and recorder are incorporated into a single unit (Fig. 4.3).

Signals are filtered using low-band and high-band filters. The bipolar signal is usually conditioned at 30-Hz (low-band) and 500-Hz (high-band) filtering, amplified, and displayed. Unipolar filtering is accomplished by using a low-pass filtering (less than 10 Hz). The recorder must be capable of providing a hard copy with a frequency response of greater than 500 Hz and a paper speed of at least up to 150 mm/sec.

Stimulator

Stimulator is essentially a complex pacemaker capable of external programming and able to deliver multiple, timed extrastimuli into a spontaneous rhythm or after a paced sequence of stimuli. It

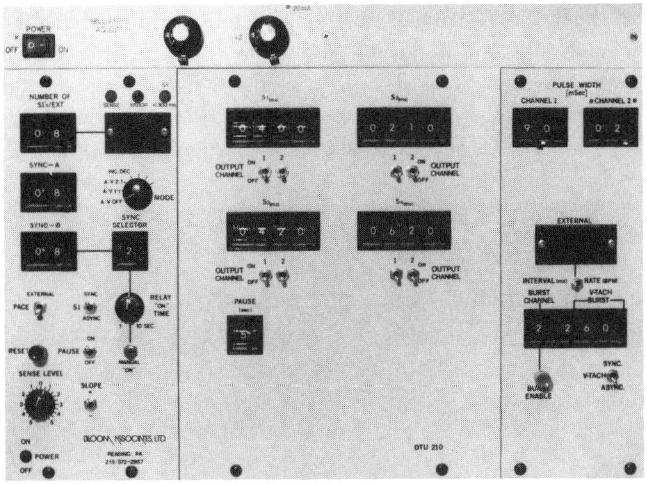

Figure 4.4. Stimulator (Bloom Associates, Reading, PA)—a closeup. **Left panel:** synchronization selectors; **middle panel:** switches for timing of extrastimuli; **right panel:** pulse width selectors for pacing channels and overdrive burst module.

provides a constant current source with a variable pulse width, with minimal current leakage. It should have an ability to accurately pace at a wide range of cycle lengths, from at least two sites, simultaneously. The stimulator must be capable of introducing multiple extrastimuli (at least three), with a programming accuracy of 1 msec. The stimulator should have an ability to be synchronized to an external signal (intrinsic or paced rhythm) and be able to deliver a calibrated burst of extrastimuli (Fig. 4.4).

CATHETERIZATION TECHNIQUES

Performance of invasive electrophysiologic studies requires placement of intracardiac electrode catheters to record intracardiac electrical activity and deliver electrical stimulation to the cardiac cells. The most common catheterization approach utilizes the femoral vein access. Alternative approaches are available, including the internal jugular, subclavian, or antecubital veins.

Femoral Approach

The approach to the femoral vein is guided by the femoral artery pulsation. Ipsilateral femoral artery is palpated at midpoint between an imaginary line connecting the superior iliac spine and the symphysis pubis and 1–2 cm inferior to the femoral crease. The femoral vein lies parallel to and medial to the femoral artery (1–2 cm). A small amount of anesthetic (1% nesacaine or equivalent) is infiltrated first superficially, then deeply and syringe slowly withdrawn until dark venous blood is aspirated. When the vein has been located, a dermotomy is made utilizing a no. 11 blade. A small curved hemostat is used to spread the superficial tissues. An 18-gauge single-pass needle is advanced with a saline-filled, 10-cc syringe, at the end of the aspirating needle while advancing the aspirating needle or during withdrawal of the needle (Fig. 4.5).

Entry into the femoral vein is signaled by easy and abundant, nonpulsatile flow of dark blood into the syringe. The syringe is then carefully removed, with care taken not to displace the needle position, and a short J-tipped guidewire is advanced (Fig. 4.6). The guidewire should encounter no resistance. If resistance is encountered, the syringe should be reattached and the vein again identified by aspirating blood. Assuring that the angle between the skin and the needle is less acute (approximately 30°), facilitates the entry and passage of the guidewire. Once the guidewire is advanced, the needle is removed and pressure is applied using the third and the fourth finger of the left hand, while the thumb and the forefinger steady and support the guidewire (Fig. 4.6). The wire is cleaned with a wet sponge and a 6 or a 7F sheath is advanced over the guidewire (Fig. 4.7). The guidewire and the dilator are then removed, leaving the sheath in the vein. The side-arm is then aspirated for a free flow of blood and flushed with heparinized saline. The side-arm of the sheath can be connected to fluids and for the administration of medications.

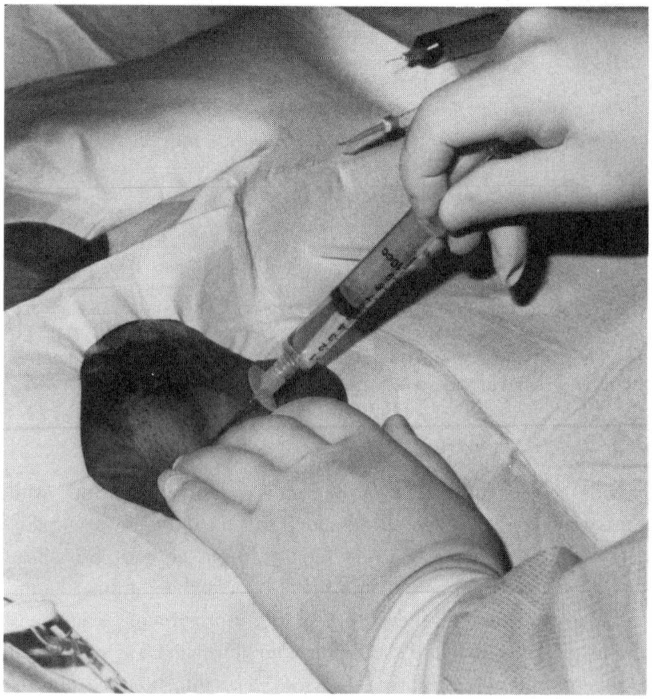

Figure 4.5. Localization of the femoral vein. Fingers of the left hand are palpating the right femoral artery. The needle is introduced parallel and medial to the femoral artery, below the inguinal ligament (see text).

Up to three separate sheaths may be placed in a single femoral vein for a routine EP study. Each sheath is positioned approximately 1 cm caudal to the initial site (Fig. 4.8).

Femoral Artery Puncture

Continuous blood pressure monitoring is routine in our laboratory. Monitoring of arterial pressure provides a number of advantages: (a) better patient monitoring during EP study, (b) correlation of patient's arrhythmia with blood pressure, and (c) a ready access for retrograde left heart catheterization, if required. Disadvantages include the recognized complications of arterial catheterization (see below). With careful technique, however, complications resulting from arterial puncture may be minimized and are infrequent.

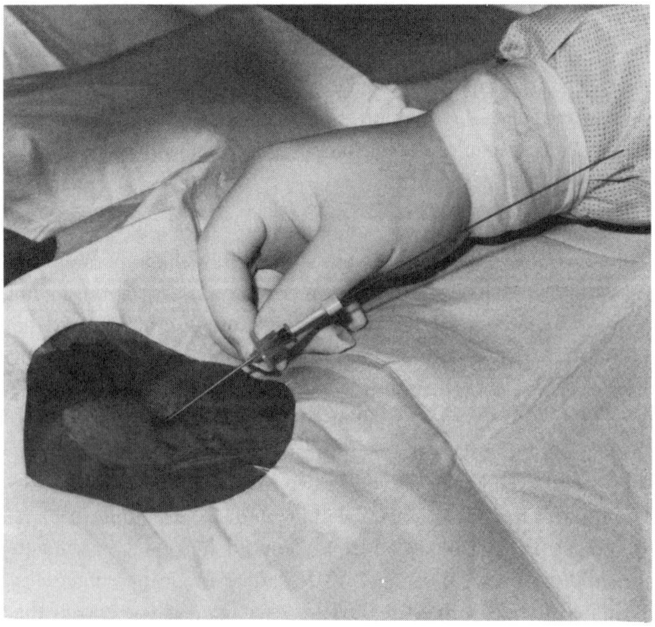

Figure 4.6. J-tipped, short guidewire is advanced through the lumen of the introducer needle (see text).

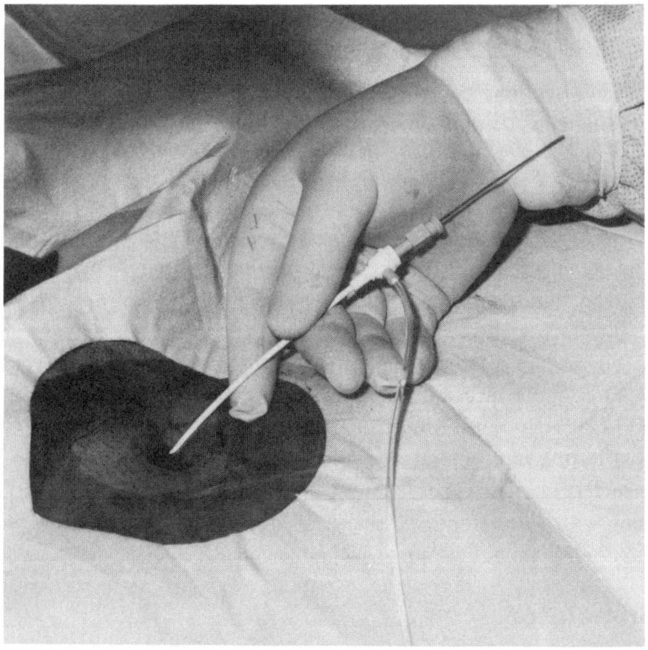

Figure 4.7. A 6F sheath is advanced over the guidewire. The introducer and the guidewire are then removed and the side arm flushed with heparinized saline.

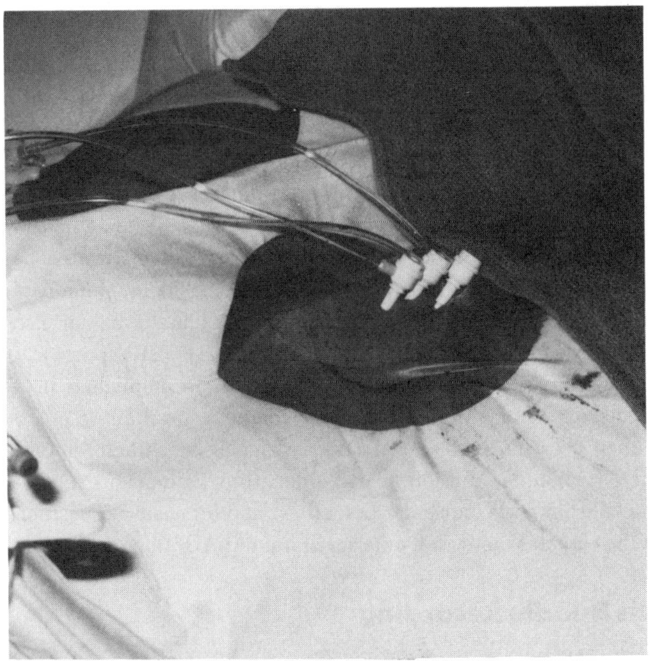

Figure 4.8. Three venous sheaths positioned in the right femoral vein.

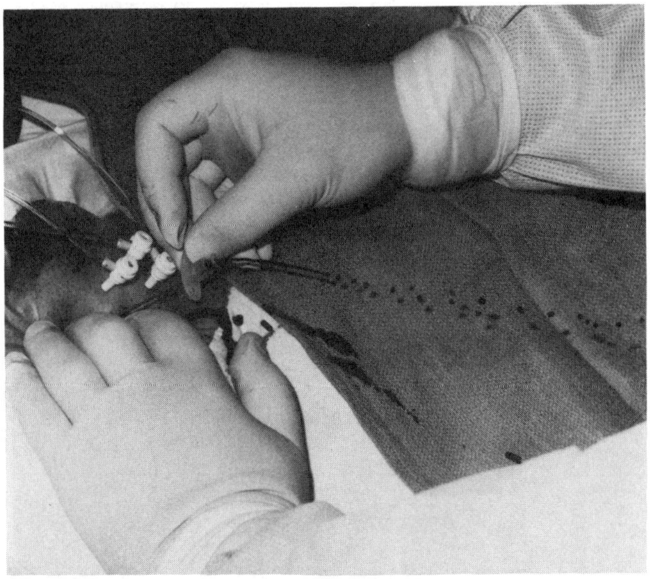

Figure 4.9. Femoral artery puncture with a pulsatile flow of blood.

We generally utilize a small-gauge cannula (no. 19 gauge longdwell) which is continuously flushed with heparinized saline. Throughout the study, blood pressure waveform should be carefully monitored and damping of the pulse waveform promptly investigated and corrected. Usually, kinking of the line is the most common cause of damping of the pressure pulse waveform. Catheter repositioning or slight withdrawal of the catheter is all that is usually required. Patients should be encouraged to report any discomfort in the ipsilateral leg. If this occurs, distal pulses should be palpated and auscultated using a Doppler probe. If signs of distal ischemia develop, cannula should be removed.

The catheterization technique is similar to the venous puncture technique. When femoral artery is entered, pulsatile flow of blood indicates that the needle lumen is intravascular (Fig. 4.9).

A no. 36 J-guidewire should be advanced using fluoroscopy, with **no** resistance. The needle is removed and a longdwell cannula advanced over the guidewire. The guidewire is then removed and the longdwell cannula attached to the pressure tubing with heparinized saline. Continuous flushing with heparinized saline is recommended throughout the procedure (Fig. 4.10).

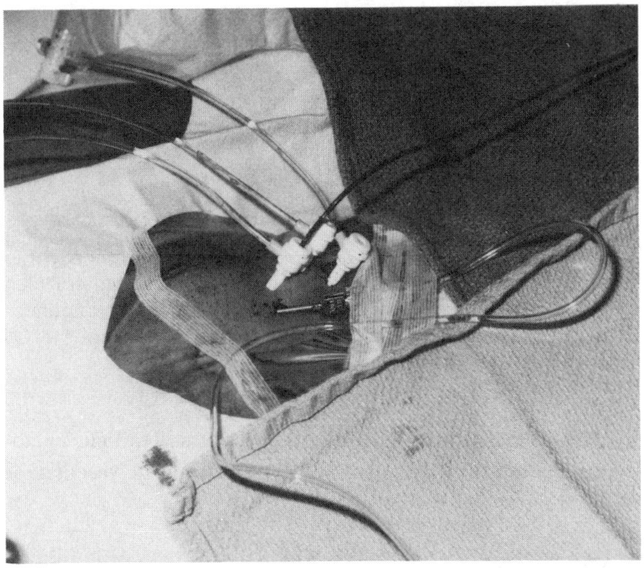

Figure 4.10. The arterial longdwell cannula is continuously flushed with heparinized saline. The tubing is secured using Steristrips or similar adhesive. An electrode catheter within the sketch is shown.

Jugular or Subclavian Approaches

The principles of venipuncture are similar as with the femoral approach, although the anatomic landmarks are clearly different. We do not recommend these approaches for routine EP studies unless coronary sinus catheter placement is required, or if bilateral femoral vein disease precludes their use, since the potential for complications is greater. These include the following: (a) pneumothorax; (b) brachial plexus injury (with subclavian approach), or carotid artery injury (with jugular approach); (c) superficial hematoma or hemothorax; (d) periosteal pain (subclavian puncture); and (e) air embolus. When these approaches are contemplated, the potential benefits should outweigh the risks.

POSITIONING OF CATHETERS

Fluoroscopic guidance is used to position the electrode catheters (Fig. 4.11). Advancing of the catheters should be painless.

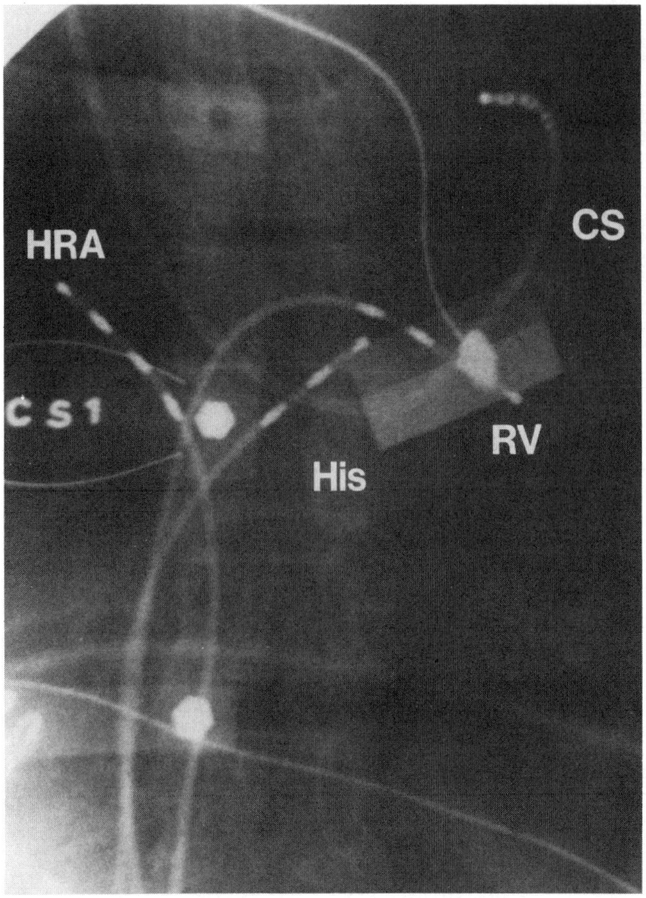

Figure 4.11. Positioning of the electrode catheters: From **right** to **left:** right atrial (quadripolar) catheter (HRA), His (tripolar) catheter, right ventricular (quadripolar) catheter, and coronary sinus (quadripolar) catheter. CS_1 designates the first mapping position of the CS catheter. The R_2 pad is overlying the CS catheter.

Since the electrode catheters are generally stiffer than angiographic catheters, care must be taken to prevent vascular or cardiac injury.

Right Atrium

Catheters are usually positioned at the junction of the superior vena cava and the right atrium close to the site of the sinoatrial node. Other stable sites for stimulation are atrial appendage and atrial septum, at the fossa ovalis. Positioning of the catheters in the right atrium requires special care, since the atrial wall is thin and more readily perforated. Undue catheter tip pressure and manipulation must be avoided.

Right Ventricle

The most common sites for the electrode positioning in the right ventricle are the apex and the outflow tract, but other accessible sites include the intramuscular septum and the anterior right ventricular wall.

Left Atrium

Left atrial recording is usually accomplished from the coronary sinus. The catheterization of the coronary sinus is most easily accomplished from the left subclavian or jugular veins. Alternatively, left atrial electrograms may, on occasion, be recorded by passing an electrode catheter from the right atrium into the left atrium via a patent foramen ovale or by a trans-septal catheterization technique (55). Left atrial electrograms may also be recorded by advancing the catheter into the main pulmonary artery (56). The potentials from the posterior left atrium may also be recorded by transesophageal electrode (57) (see Chapter 3).

Coronary sinus (CS) recording may be accomplished in a bipolar or in an unipolar fashion. Adequate positioning of CS catheter is confirmed by: (a) easy passage of the catheter toward the left shoulder and left heart border, (b) simultaneous recording of atrial and ventricular potentials, and (c) posterior position of the catheter on the left anterior oblique (LAO) fluoroscopy.

His Bundle Recording

His bundle recording is most easily accomplished from the right femoral vein. The catheter is advanced to the right ventricle and then withdrawn until it assumes a curved profile. On the anteroposterior (AP) fluoroscopy (Fig. 4.11), the tip should point to the left side of the heart. Clockwise torque is generally helpful in snuggling the catheter close to the septum. His bundle recording may be accomplished using a low-pass filter at 30 Hz and high-pass filter at 500 Hz settings. A large atrial potential should be recorded, as well as a large right ventricular potential, together with the His-bundle electrogram (58). If the atrial potential is small, and HV interval is less than 30 msec, it is likely that the distal His or the right bundle branch potential are being recorded. As a rule, the most proximal pair of electrodes that clearly identify the His potential and a large atrial potential simultaneously, should be monitored (58).

Left ventricle

Left ventricular recording and stimulation may be required in selected patients. This is especially true in patients who are being considered for VT ablation or in patients who are considered for left freewall or left posteroseptal accessory pathway transcatheter ablation.

Retrograde passage of the left ventricular catheter is most easily accomplished by using a steerable electrode catheter where the curvature of the catheter tip may be altered (Polaris, Bard Corporation, Tewksbury, MA or similar). Patients should be fully heparinized (100 units/kg body weight), prior to the retrograde left heart catheterization. Passage of the catheter is best accomplished by using biplane fluoroscopy or a single plane right anterior oblique (RAO) or left anterior oblique (LAO) fluoroscopy. Various sites in the left ventricle may be defined on fluoroscopy.

ELECTROPHYSIOLOGIC STUDY

Recording

Electrophysiologic study is a technique for systematic evaluation of electrical activation of the cardiac tissues and of the specialized cardiac cells (e.g., sinoatrial, AV nodal, and His-Purkinje cells). The technique provides a method for evaluation and therapy of selected rhythm disorders. The approach to the patient should be individualized based on the presenting problem. A general discussion of a typical sequence of an EP study will be discussed here. However, specific approaches to supraventricular tachycardia, VT evaluation, antiarrhythmic drug selection, device evaluation, and interventional aspects may be found elsewhere in this book (Chapters 7–9, 11, 12, and 20–24).

Basic Intervals

Elecrophysiologic study begins with the measurement of the basic intervals (Fig. 4.12). The accuracy of measurements depends on the paper speed at which the recordings are made. For routine recordings, paper speed of 100 mm/sec is generally adequate. However, for detailed endocardial mapping, paper speeds of >200 mm/sec are preferable.

His Bundle Recording

His deflection is a triphasic or a biphasic deflection of 15 to 25-msec duration which is recorded at least 35 msec or more proximal to the ventricular depolarization signal and after the right atrial depolarization (Fig. 4.12). The most proximal signal recorded which is associated with a large atrial depolarization represents the proximal His recording. His bundle pacing is sometimes possible to validate the His bundle. However, His bundle capture may be difficult to achieve. During pacing of the His bundle, QRS and T waves on the surface ECG should be identical to those observed during the normal sinus rhythm (58). Furthermore, stimulus-to-V interval should be identical to the HV interval measured during the sinus rhythm (59–62).

AH Interval

AH interval is measured from the earliest rapid deflection of the atrial electrogram to the onset of the His bundle deflection in the His bundle electrogram (Fig. 4.12). The AH interval represents conduction time from the lower right atrium through the AV node to the His bundle. AH interval is affected by the autonomic nervous system (enhanced sympathetic tone results in AH shortening, and increased vagal tone in AH interval prolongation). The response of AH interval to pacing and vagolytic or sympathomimetic drugs may be helpful in assessment of the AV nodal conduction. In our laboratory, the normal range of values for the AH interval is 60–120 msec.

HV Interval

The HV interval is measured from the earliest deflection of the His potential to the earliest onset of ventricular depolarization (beginning of the QRS complex in any surface lead) (Fig. 4.12). The HV interval represents the conduction time from the His bundle to the ventricular myocardium (63). The normal value in our laboratory is 35–55 msec.

PA Interval

PA interval measures the time interval from the onset of P wave to the onset of the atrial activation in the His bundle electrogram.

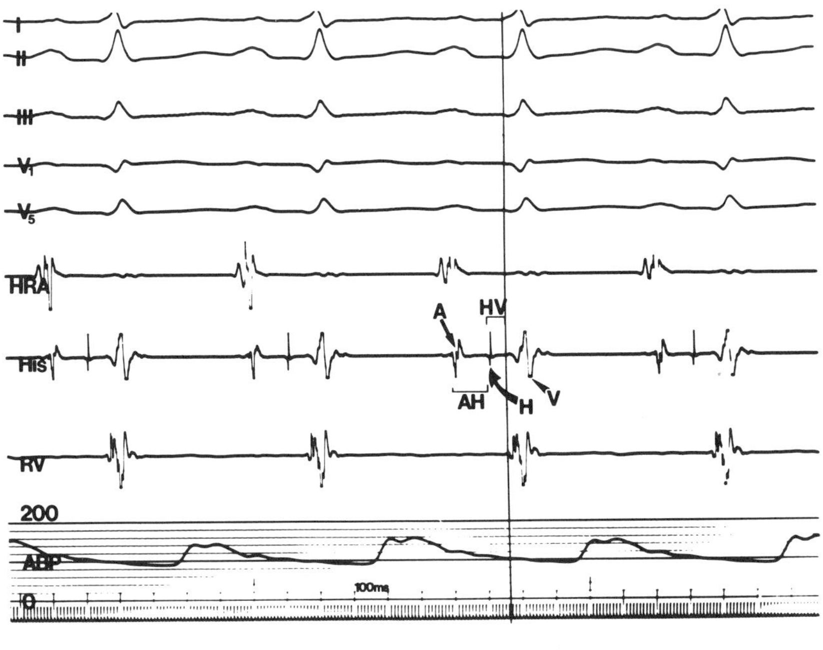

Figure 4.12. Recording from **top** to **bottom:** surface leads I, II, AVF, V_1, and V_5, intracardiac leads high right atrium (HRA), proximal His bundle (His), right ventricular apex (RV), intra-arterial blood pressure (ABP), and time lines (T). *Arrows* point to the atrial depolarization (A), His bundle depolarization (H), and ventricular depolarization (V). Note AH and HV intervals.

Most investigators have used this measurement as an indicator of intraatrial conduction (64–69).

A number of considerations, however, make the measurement of PA interval of questionable utility in measuring the intra-atrial conduction. These include the following: (a) the endocardial activation may precede P wave (70), (b) PA interval correlates poorly with P wave duration in patients with left atrial enlargement (69–72), (c) distal positioning of the His bundle catheter can result in a prolonged PA interval (71). Thus, PA interval may be used only as an indirect measure of right atrial conduction.

Other Useful Measurements

PR, QRS, QT_c, and RR intervals may be measured using the 12-lead ECG. However, they are more accurately measured during an EP study, due to the higher speed of recording (100–150 mm/sec).

PR interval is the time from the earliest atrial depolarization determined by the surface recording to the onset of the ventricular depolarization. Thus, PR measurement incorporates intra-atrial, AV nodal, and His bundle-ventricular conduction times.

QRS interval measures the total time required for the ventricles to depolarize. QRS prolongation may be due to delay in the ventricular depolarization (intraventricular conduction delay), or may be due to the effect of the antiarrhythmic drugs on depolarization, e.g., Type IA drugs.

QT_c interval measures the time from the onset of the ventricular depolarization to the end of the ventricular repolarization. Long QT_c may be congenital as well as acquired, usually due to drug-induced prolongation of the QT_c interval. Long QT_c interval may be associated with "torsade de pointes." QT_c interval is calculated as follows: $QT_c = QT/\sqrt{RR}$ (Bazett's formula).

Programmed Electrical Stimulation

Programmed electrical stimulation PES is a technique that utilizes constant or intermittent cardiac pacing. Critically timed premature extrastimuli may be introduced into the spontaneous rhythm, or after a paced train of stimuli. Critically timed extrastimuli may be used to test the properties of the specialized cardiac cells, e.g., sinus node, AV node, His bundle, and ventricle, or used to elicit and reproduce arrthymias in which reentry or triggered activity are the underlying mechanisms.

Atrial Pacing

Atrial pacing provides a method of analyzing the antegrade functional properties of the AV conduction system.

Atrial pacing is accomplished typically from the high right atrial position, but may also be performed from the other sites in certain circumstances, e.g., coronary sinus. Atrial pacing begins at the cycle lengths of 50–100 msec shorter than the spontaneous rhythm. Each paced cycle length is maintained for 30–60 sec to ensure stability. The paced cycle length is then progressively decreased in 20 to 50-msec steps until the cycle length of 400 msec is reached, and then smaller increments (10–20 msec each). The normal response to incremental atrial pacing is the prolongation of the AH interval until AV nodal (Wenckebach) block is reached. The HV interval is usually unaffected. Because of the autonomic influences on the AV node, there is a wide range of normal responses. In the absence of enhanced AV nodal conduction, or pre-excitation, AV nodal block is usually seen at paced cycle lengths of 350–500 msec (Fig. 4.13). Prolongation of the HV interval or infra-His block at paced cycle lengths of greater than 400 msec is abnormal. It signifies impaired or abnormal infranodal conduction.

Ventricular Pacing

Ventricular pacing provides information about retrograde ventriculoatrial (VA) conduction. Ventricular pacing is usually performed from the right ventricular apex and begun at a cycle lengths 50–100 msec shorter than the intrinsic rhythm and

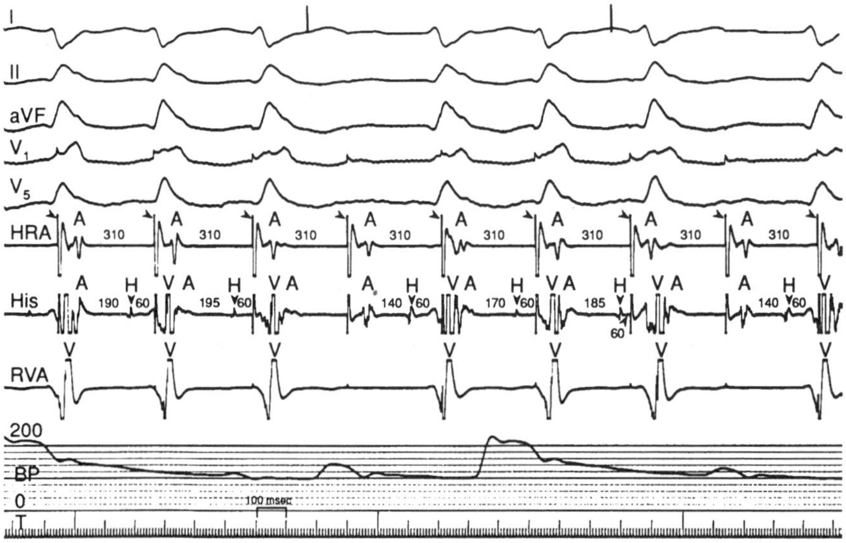

Figure 4.13. Lead arrangement is as for Figure 4.12. "Typical" Type I second-degree block in the AV node induced by atrial pacing. The paced cycle length is 310 msec. Note that each atrial depolarization (A) is followed by progressive lengthening of AH interval, until third and seventh A are not followed by His bundle (H) deflection. Note that an intraventricular conduction delay is also present (left posterior hemiblock (LPHB) and right bundle branch block (RBBB) and that HV interval is slightly prolonged (60 msec).

progressively decremented, as during the atrial pacing. The normal response is a gradual VA prolongation as the paced cycle length is decreased. Retrograde Wenckebach block is observed in 40–80% of those patients in whom retrograde conduction is present. In only 10% of patients, retrograde His deflection can be identified (73,74). In patients in whom His deflection cannot be readily identified, the site of block may be inferred by pharmacologic interventions (e.g., atropine administration) which only affect the AV node conduction.

Refractory Periods

Temporary refractoriness of cardiac cells to depolorization is the fundamental property common to all excitable cells. Three types of refractoriness are recognized in clinical studies: (a) *relative refractory period* (RRP), which may be defined as the longest coupling interval of a premature impulse that results in prolonged conduction of that impulse; (b) *effective refractory period* (ERP), the longest coupling interval that fails to propagate; and (c) *functional refractory period* (FRP), the minimum interval between the two consecutively conducted impulses (e.g., FRP of the AV node is the shortest H_1–H_2 interval in response to any A_1–A_2 interval).

Refractory periods are determined by utilizing the extrastimulus techniques, whereby a single atrial or a ventricular extrastimulus is introduced at progressively shorter coupling intervals (75). Extrastimuli are delivered following a fixed train of 8–10 beats (e.g., at 600 or 450 msec). Extrastimuli may also be introduced into a spontaneous sinus rhythm (e.g., to determine sinoatrial conduction times).

Refractory periods of the atrium, ventricle, and His bundle are cycle length dependent, i.e., they tend to decrease with decreasing drive cycle lengths (76). The opposite is true of the AV nodal tissue, i.e., the effective refractory period is inversely related to the cycle drive. Atrioventricular node refractory periods are also dependent on the autonomic tone (77).

Since the ERP of the atrial or the ventricular muscle is inversely related to the current used, PES is standardized with the current applied at twice the diastolic threshold.

Programmed Atrial Stimulation

Programmed atrial stimulation is usually performed at two or more cycle drives (e.g., 600 and 450 msec). An 8- to 10-beat drive is utilized with coupling intervals decremented initially by 20 msec, until A_2–H_2 interval begins to prolong, then at 10-msec intervals. Sustained tachycardia (AV nodal reentry tachycardia or reciprocating A-V tachycardia) may be induced during programmed atrial stimulation in patients with functionally dissociated AV nodal pathways or with an accessory tract. Induction of AV nodal reentrant tachycardia or reciprocating AV tachycardias may be facilitated by the administration of atropine or isoproterenol. Refractoriness of the AV node, His bundle, and atrial tissues and antegrade refractory properties of accessory pathways may be determined using this technique.

Several different types of responses to programmed atrial extrastimuli have been described (78). Type I response is characterized by progressive delay in the AV node without a change in infranodal conduction (Fig. 4.14). Type II response is characterized by an initial delay in the AV node with subsequent delay in conduction in the His-Purkinje system. Block may occur first in the AV node or in the atrium, or on occasion in the His-Purkinje system. With Type III response, the initial slowing occurs in the AV node, but at the critical coupling interval,

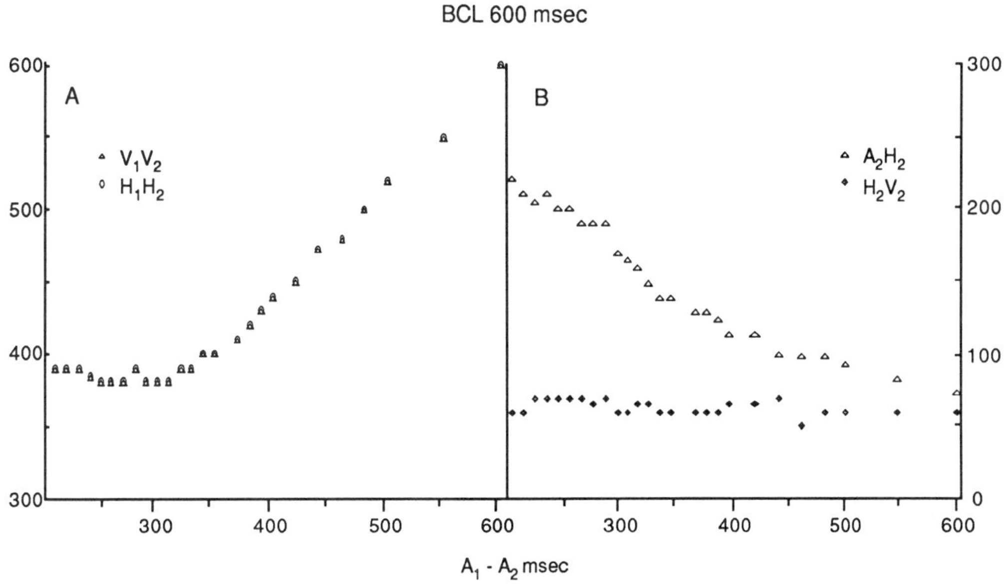

Figure 4.14. Panel A: A_1–A_2 relationship to V_1–V_2 and H_1–H_2. **Panel B:** A_1–A_2 versus A_2–H_2 and H_2–V_2. Type I pattern of response to atrial extrastimuli is demonstrated (see text).

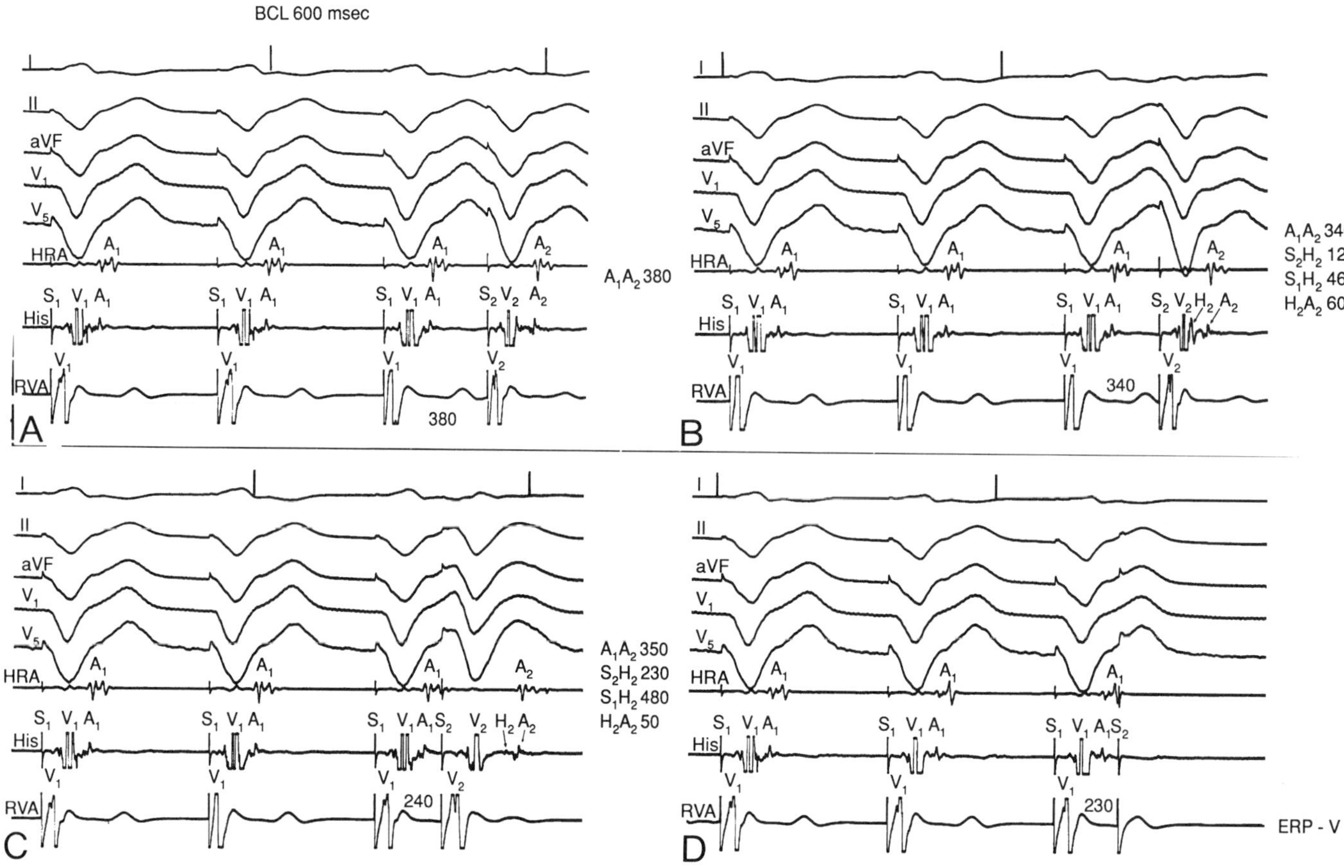

Figure 4.15. Ventricular extrastimulus technique: **Panels A–D** show the effects of shortening of premature right ventricular extrastimulus (S_2). Basic drive (S_1–S_1) is 600 msec. At long coupling intervals **(panel A),** there is no retrograde delay. **Panels B** and **C** demonstrate delay in the His-Purkinje system (S_2–H_2 prolongation). At the coupling interval (S_1–S_2 = 230 msec), the effective refractory period of the ventricle is reached (ERP-V).

sudden prolongation occurs in the His-Purkinje system. Eventual block typically appears in the His-Purkinje system in Type III block. The pattern of conduction may be modified by pharmacologic perturbations, altering the pattern of responses in the same patient (78).

The pattern of A-V conduction may be expressed by plotting refractory curves in one of two ways: (a) by plotting functional input-output relationship, e.g., A_1–A_2 versus H_1–H_2 and V_1–V_2, or (b) by plotting the actual conduction times, e.g., A_1–A_2 versus A_2–H_2 and H_2–V_2 (Fig. 4.14).

The ERP of the atrium is not infrequently encountered earlier than that of the AV node, particularly when the basic drive is slow (by lengthening the atrial refractoriness) and/or when the sympathetic tone is enhanced (by shortening the AV node refractoriness).

Assessment of Retrograde Conduction

The use of ventricular extrastimulus technique provides a method for systematic evaluation of retrograde V-A conduction (78). The technique is similar to the techniques used to study antegrade conduction and utilizes introduction of progressively more premature ventricular extrastimuli after an 8- to 10-beat drive, until ventricular refractoriness is reached. Detailed assessment of retrograde conduction is limited by the fact that His deflection is often not visualized during a wide range of ventricular coupling intervals. Therefore, the evaluation of the His-Purkinje and AV nodal conduction is often incomplete.

In the absence of a recorded His bundle deflection during ventricular drive (H_1), the functional refractory period of the His-Purkinje system may be approximated by using S_1–H_2 interval (S_1 is stimulus artifact of the basic drive). The rationale underlying this approach relies on the observation that over a wide range of ventricular paced rates, S_1–H_1 interval remains constant, so that S_1–H_2 approximates H_1–H_2, minus a fixed (S_1–H_1) interval (79,80). The typical response may be schematically expressed by plotting S_1–S_2 versus S_2–H_2, S_2–A_2 and H_2–A_2 or by plotting S_1–H_2 versus A_1–A_2.

His-Purkinje refractoriness is cycle length dependent. Consistent shortening of S_2–H_2 at any given S_1–S_2 is noted at decreasing cycle lengths (79). The V-A conduction time (S_2–A_2) is determined by the His-Purkinje conduction delay (S_2–H_2). As

S_1–S_2 interval is decreased, either block within the His-Purkinje system appears or ventricular refractoriness is reached. Thus, in most patients, the major site of delay during retrograde conduction is in the His-Purkinje system (Fig. 4.15).

During programmed ventricular stimulation, ventricular echo beats may be seen due to reentry within the AV node when a critical degree of retrograde AV nodal conduction delay is reached. Atrial activity always precedes the His bundle deflection before the QRS complex (80). A second type of reentry may occur within the bundle branch, resulting in a reentry beat of similar morphology to the stimulated complex. Finally, reentry may occur within the ventricular myocardium (81,82).

Programmed Ventricular Stimulation

The purpose of the programmed ventricular stimulation is to: (a) examine the retrograde properties of the conduction system and (b) to elicit ventricular tachycardia. Other reentrant tachycardias, e.g., AV nodal reentry or A-V reciprocating tachycardias may be initiated during programmed ventricular stimulation.

PES is performed typically at at least two cycle lengths (e.g., 600 and 400 msec) using single, then double and triple extrastimuli. Some EP laboratories also utilize a technique of programmed ventricular stimulation during the spontaneous rhythm. This technique has a somewhat lower yield for induction of VT and is not routinely utilized in our laboratory.

At least two ventricular sites are stimulated, typically the right ventricular apex and the right ventricular outflow tract. In selected patients, left ventricular programmed stimulation is also utilized.

Premature impulse (S_2) is used to scan the diastole. S_2 is introduced in late diastole and the extrastimulus scanned from late diastole to ventricular refractoriness. If a single extrastimulus (S_1, S_2) is ineffective, a second extrastimulus is introduced (S_2, S_3) and subsequently, the third (S_3, S_4).

Double extrastimuli (S_2, S_3) are introduced with S_1–S_2 initially positioned 50–100 msec beyond the point of refractoriness and S_2–S_3 equal to the S_1–S_2 interval. The S_2–S_3 interval is shortened until S_3 no longer evokes a ventricular response. At that point, the S_1–S_2 interval is decreased by 10-msec steps until S_3 is able to elicit a ventricular response. This method is used until both S_2 and S_3 are refractory. Similar sequence is followed with triple extrastimuli (S_1, S_2, S_3, S_4).

Care should be exercised that the coupling interval between the extrastimuli is not shorter than the ventricular refractory period. The ease of induction of nonspecific polymorphic VT is enhanced by using close coupling intervals. Whenever PES is performed, resuscitation equipment must be available and a standby defibrillator attached to the patient, to enable prompt defibrillation.

Administration of isoprenaline (1–4 μg/min) facilitates the induction of ventricular tachycardia. In patients with long QT syndrome, isoprenaline may provoke "torsade de pointes."

Once VT is induced, it may be terminated, in most cases by using timed single, double, and triple extrastimuli or more efficiently, by bursts of synchronized ventricular pacing. Ability to initiate and to terminate VT by PES suggests reentry or triggered arrhythmia as the mechanism of the VT.

Sinus Nodal Function

Evaluation of sinus nodal function will be discussed separately in Chapter 5.

COMPLICATIONS

Electrophysiologic study is a safe technique and in experienced hands the complications are infrequent. In a recent review of the subject, the most frequently reported complications are related to the catheterization technique per se and not the induced arrhythmias (83). The most common complications were: (a) hypotension due to drug infusion or vagal reaction (1%); (b) vascular complications (hemorrhage, arterial injury, thrombophlebitis) (0.7%); (c) emboli (0.2%); (d) cardiac perforation (0.15%); and (e) proarrhythmia due to antiarrthythmic drugs. The mortality is reported to be 0–0.6%, which is comparable or lower than the mortality associated with coronary angiography (83).

CONCLUSION

Electrophysiologic study is an invasive technique used to study clinical arrhythmias in a controlled clinical environment. The information provided by the EP study enables the physician to formulate the treatment strategy. Specialized applications of electrophysiologic studies for therapy will be discussed in subsequent chapters of the book (see Chapters 20–24).

References

1. Scherlag BJ, Lau SH, Helfant RA, *et al.*: Catheter technique for recording His bundle activity in man. Circulation 1969;39:13–18.
2. Zipes DP, Akhtar M, Denes P, *et al.*: ACC/AHA Task Force Report—Guidelines for clinical intracardiac electrophysiologic studies. A report of the American College of Cardiology/American Heart Association Task Force on assessment of diagnostic and therapeutic cardiovascular procedures (Subcommittee to assess clinical intracardiac electrophysiologic studies). J Am Coll Cardiol 1989;14:1827–1842.
3. Baum RS, Alvarez H, Cobb LA: Survival after resuscitation from out-of-hospital ventricular fibrillation. Circulation 1974;50:1231–1235.
4. Liberthson RR, Nagel EL, Hirschman JC, *et al.*: Prehospital ventricular fibrillation. Prognosis and follow-up course. N Engl J Med 1974;291:317–321.
5. Myerburg RJ, Kessler KM, Zaman L, *et al.*: Survivors of prehospital cardiac arrest. JAMA 1982;247:1485–1490.
6. Buxton AE, Waxman HL, Marchlinski FE, *et al.*: Role of triple extrastimuli during electrophysiologic study of patients with documented sustained ventricular tachyarrhythmias. Circulation 1984;69:532–540.
7. Morady F, DiCarlo L, Winston S, *et al.*: A prospective comparison of triple extrastimuli and left ventricular stimulation in studies of ventricular tachycardia induction. Circulation 1984;70:52–57.
8. Ruskin JM, DiMarco JP, Garan H: Out-of-hospital cardiac arrest: electrophysiologic observations and selection of long-term antiarrhythmic therapy. N Engl J Med 1980;303:607–613.
9. Morady F, Scheinman MM, Hess DS, *et al.*: Electrophysiologic testing: the

management of survivors of out-of-hospital cardiac arrest. Am J Cardiol 1983;51:85–89.

10. Benditt DG, Benson DW Jr, Klein GJ, *et al.*: Prevention of recurrent sudden cardiac arrest: role of provocative electropharmacologic testing. J Am Coll Cardiol 1983;2:418–425.
11. Skale BT, Miles WM, Heger JJ, *et al.*: Survivors of cardiac arrest: prevention of recurrence by drug therapy as predicted by electrophysiologic testing on electrocardiographic monitoring. Am J Cardiol 1986;57:113–119.
12. Eldar M, Suave JJ, Scheinman MM: Electrophysiologic testng and follow up of patients with aborted sudden death. J Am Coll Cardiol 1987;10:291–298.
13. Wilber DJ, Garan H, Finkelstein D, *et al.*: Out of-hospital cardiac arrest use of electrophysiologic testing in the prediction of long-term outcome. N Engl J Med 1988;318:19–24.
14. Freedman RA, Swerdlow CD, Soderholm-Difatte V, *et al.*: Prognostic significance of arrhythmia inducibility or non-inducibility at initial electrophysiologic study in survivors of cardiac arrest. Am J Cardiol 1988;61:578–582.
15. Zheutlin TA, Steinman RT, Mattioni TA, *et al.*: Long-term arrhythmic outcome in survivors of ventricular fibrillation with absence of inducible ventricular tachycardia. Am J Cardiol 1988;62:1213–1217.
16. Roy D, Waxman HL, Kienzle MG, *et al.*: Clinical characteristics and long-term follow up in 119 survivors of cardiac arrest: relation to inducibility on electrophysiologic testing. Am J Cardiol 1983;52:969–974.
17. Krol RB, Morady F, Flaker GC, *et al.*: Electrophysiologic testing in patients with unexplained syncope: clinical and noninvasive predictors of outcome. J Am Coll Cardiol 1987;10:358–363.
18. McAnulty J, Rahimtoola SH, Murphy E, *et al.*: Natural history of "high risk" bundle branch block. Final report of a prospective study. N Engl J Med 1982;307:137–143.
19. Bhandari AK, Shapiro WA, Morady F, *et al.*: Electrophysiologic testing in patients with the long QT syndrome. Circulation 1985;71:63–71.
20. Klein GJ, Guiraudon GM, Sharma AJ, *et al.*: Surgery for tachycardia: indications and electrophysiologic assessment. Circulation (Suppl) 1987; 75:186–189.
21. Kelly PA, Cannom DS, Garan H, *et al.*: The automatic implantable cardioverter-defibrillator: efficacy, complications and survival in patients with malignant ventricular arrhythmias. J Am Coll Cardiol 1988;11:1278–1286.
22. Parsonnet V, Bernstein AD: Techniques for implanation of antitachyarrhythmia devices. Circulation (Suppl) 1987;75:169–177.
23. Morady F, Frank R, Kou WH, *et al*: Identification of a zone of slow conduction in the reentrant circuit in humans. J Am Coll Cardiol 1988;11:775–782.
24. Bardy GH, Packer DL, German LD, *et al.*: Preexcited reciprocating tachycardia in patients with Wolff-Parkinson-White: incidence and mechanisms. Circulation 1981;70:377–391.
25. Smith WM, Broughton A, Reiter MJ, *et al.*: Bystander accessory pathway participation during AV node reentrant tachycardias. PACE 1983;6:537–547.
26. Wu D, Amat-y-Leon F, Simpson RJ, *et al.*: Electrophysiological studies with multiple drugs in patients with atrioventricular reentrant tachycardias utilizing an extranodal pathway. Circulation 1977;56:727–736.
27. Bauernfeind RA, Wyndham CR, Dhingra RC, *et al.*: Serial electrophysiological testing of multiple drugs in patients with atrioventricular nodal reentrant paroxysmal tachycardia. Circulation 1980;62:1341–1349.
28. Gomes JA, Hariman RI, Kang PS, *et al.*: Programmed electrical stimulation in patients with high-grade ventricular ectopy: electrophysiologic findings and prognosis for suvival. Circulation 1987;75:1178–1185.
29. Buxton AE, Marchlinski FE, Flores BT, *et al.*: Nonsustained ventricular tachycardia in patients with coronary artery disease: role of electrophysiologic study. Circulation 1987;75:1178–1185.
30. Winters SL, Stewart D, Targonski A, *et al.*: Role of signal averaging of the surface QRS complex in selecting patients with nonsustained ventricular tachycardia and high grade ventricular arrhythmias for programmed ventricular stimulation. J Am Coll Cardiol 1988;12:1481–1487.
31. Meinertz T, Treese N, Kasper W, *et al.*: Determinants of prognosis in idiopathic dilated cardiomyopathy as determined by programmed electrical stimulation. Am J Cardiol 1985;56:337–341.
32. Poll DS, Marchlinski FE, Buxton AE, *et al.*: Usefulness of programmed stimulation in idiopathic dilated cardiomyopathy. Am J Cardiol 1986;58: 992–997.
33. Das SK, Morady F, DiCarlo L Jr, *et al.*: Prognostic usefulness of programmed ventricuclar stimulation in idiopathic dilated cardiomyopathy without symptomatic ventricular arrhythmias. Am J Cardiol 1986;58:998–1000.
34. Stamato NJ, O'Connell JB, Murdock DK, *et al.*: The response of patients with complex ventricular arrhythmias secondary to dilated cardiomyopathy to programmed electrical stimulation. Am Heart J 1986;112:505–508.
35. Anderson KP, Stinson EB, Derby N, *et al.*: Vulnerability of patients with obstructive hypertrophic cardiomyopathy to ventricular arrhythmias induction on the operating room. Am J Cardiol 1983;9:476–481.
36. Schiavone WA, Maloney JD, Lever HM, *et al.*: Electrophysiologic studies in patients with hypertrophic cardiomyopathy presenting with syncope of undetermined etiology. PACE 1986;9:476–481.
37. Watson RM, Schwartz JL, Maron BJ, *et al.*: Inducible polymorphic ventricular tachycardia and ventricular fibrillation: a subgroup of patients with hypertrophic cardiomyopathy at high risk for sudden death. J Am Cardiol 1987;10:761–774.
38. Gallagher JJ, Pritchett ELC, Benditt DG, *et al.*: New catheter techniques for analysis of the sequence of retrograde atrial activation in man. Eur J Cardiol 1977;6:1–14.
39. Jackman WM, Friday KJ, Yeung-Lai-Wah JA, *et al.*: New catheter technique for recording left free-wall accessory atrioventricular pathway activation. Identification of pathway fiber orientation. Circulation 1988;78:598–611.
40. Warin JF, Haissaguerre M, Lemetayer P, *et al.*: Catheter ablation of accessory pathways with a direct approach. Circulation 1988;78:800–815.
41. Klein GJ, Bashore TM, Sellers TD, *et al.*: Ventricular fibrillation in the Wolff-Parkinson-White syndrome. N Engl J Med 1979;301:1080–1085.
42. German LD, Gallagher JJ, Broughton A, *et al.*: Effects of exercise and isoproterenol during atrial fibrillation in patients with Wolff-Parkinson-White syndrome. Am J Cardiol 51:1983;1203–1206.
43. Wu D, Denes P, Dhingra R, *et al.*: Determinants of fast-and-slow-pathway conduction in patients with dual atrioventricular nodal pathways. Circ Res 1975;36:782–790.
44. Wu D, Denes P, Amat-y Leon F, *et al.*: An unusual variety of atrioventricular nodal reentry due to retrograde dual atrioventricular nodal pathways. Circulation 1977;56:50–59.
45. Ross DL, Johnson DC, Denniss AR, *et al.*: Curative surgery for atrioventricular junctional ("AV nodal") reentrant tachycardia. J Am Coll Cardiol 1985;6:1383–1392.
46. Cox JL, Holman WL, Casin ME: Cryosurgical treatment of atrioventricular node reentrant tachycardia. Circulation 1987;76:1329–1336.
47. Anderson KP, Stinson EB, Mason JW: Surgical excision of focal paroxysmal atrial tachycardia. Am J Cardiol 1982;49:869–874.
48. Dhingra RC, Amat-y-Leon F, Pouget JM, *et al.*: Infranodal block: diagnosis, clinical significance and management. Med Clin North Am 1976;60:175–192.
49. Scheinman MM, Peters RW, Suave MJ, *et al.*: Value of the H-Q interval in patients with bundle branch block and the role of prophylactic permanent pacing. Am J Cardiol 1982;50:1316–1322.
50. Yee R, Strauss HC: Electrophysiologic mechanisms: sinus node dysfunction. Circulation 1987;75 (Suppl III):III-12-8.
51. Mandel WH, Hayakawa H, Danzig R, *et al.*: Evaluation of sino-atrial node function in man by overdrive suppression. Circulation 1971;44:59–66.
52. Hariman RJ, Krongrad E, Boxer RA, *et al.*: Method of recording electrical activity of the sinoatrial node and automatic atrial foci during cardiac catheterization in human subjects. Am J Cardiol 1980;45:775–81.
53. Breidthardt G, Speipel L, Loogen F: Sinus node recovery time and calculated sinoatrial conduction time in normal subjects and patients with sinus node dysfunction. Circulation 1977;56:43–50.

54. Gann D, Tolentino A, Samet P: Electrophysiologic evaluation of elderly patients with sinus bradycardia. A long-term follow-up study. Ann Intern Med 1979;90:24–9.
55. Ross J: Considerations regarding the technique for transseptal left heart catheterization. Circulation 1966;34:391–399.
56. Amat-y-Leon F, Deedwaric P, Miller RM, *et al.*: A new approach for indirect recording of anterior left atrial activation in man. Am Heart J 1977;93:408–410.
57. Puech, P: The P wave: correlation of surface and intraatrial electrograms. Cardiol Clin 1974;6:43–68.
58. Kupersmith J, Krongrad E, Waldo AL: Conduction intervals and conduction velocity in the human cardiac conduction system—studies during open heart surgery. Circulation 1973;47:776–787.
59. Kupersmith J, Krongrad E, Gowman FO Jr, *et al.*: Pacing the human specialized conduction system during open heart surgery. Circulation 1974;50:449–506.
60. Narula OS, Scherlag BJ, Samet P: Pervenous pacing of the specialized conduction system in man: His bundle and AV nodal stimulation. Circulation 1970;41:77–87.
61. Narula OS, Samet P: Pervenous pacing of the A-V juncton in man. Fed Proc 1969;28:269, AB#58.
62. Scherlag BJ, Samet P, Helfant RH: His bundle electrogram—a critical appraisal of its uses and limitations. Circulation 1972;46:601–613.
63. Damato AN, Lau SH, Helfant R, *et al.*: Study of heart block in man using His bundle recordings. Circulation 1969;39:297–305.
64. Narula OS, Cohen LS, Samet P, *et al.*: Localization of A-V conduction defects in man by recording of the His bundle electrogram. Am J Cardiol 1970;25:228–237.
65. Damato AN, Lau SH: Clinical value of the electrogram of the conduction system. Prog Cardiovasc Dis 1970;13:119–140.
66. Narula OS, Scherlag BJ, Samet P, *et al.*: Atrioventricular block: localization and classification by His bundle recordings. Am J Med 1971;50:146–165.
67. Castellanos A Jr, Castillo C, Agha A: Contribution of His Bundle recording to the understanding of clinical arrhythmias. Am J Cardiol 1971;28:499–508.
68. Schuilenburg RM, Durrer D: Conduction disturbances located within the His bundle. Circulation 1972;45:612–628.
69. Rosen KM: Evaluation of cardiac conduction in the cardiac catheterization laboratory. Am J Cardiol 1972;30:701–703.
70. Josephson ME, Scharf DL, Kastor JA, *et al.*: Atrial endocardial activation in man. Electrode catheter technique for endocardial mapping. Am J Cardiol 1977;39:972–981.
71. Wyndham CRC, Shantha N, Dhingra RC, *et al.*: PA interval: lack of clinical electrocardiographic and electrophysiologic correlations. Chest 1975; 68:533–537.
72. Bekheit S, Murtagh G, Morton P, Fletcher E: His bundle electrogram in P mitrale. Br Heart J 1972;34:1057–1061.
73. Akhtar M, Damato AN, Batsford WP, *et al.*: A comparative analysis of antegrade and retrograde conduction patterns in man. Circulation 1975;52:766–778.
74. Josephson ME, Kastor JA: His-Purkinje conduction during retrograde stress. J Clin Invest 1978;61:171–177.
75. Damato AN, Lau SH, Patten RD, *et al.*: A study of atrioventricular conduction in man using premature atrial stimulation and His bundle recordings. Circulation 1969;40:61–69.
76. Denes P, Wu D, Dhingra R, *et al.*: The effects of cycle length on cardiac refractory periods in man. Circulation 1974;49:32–41.
77. Reddy, CP, Damato AN, Akhtar M, *et al.*: Time dependent changes in the functional properties of the atrioventricular conduction system in man. Circulation 1975;52:1012–1022.
78. Wit AL, Weiss MB, Berkowitz WD, *et al.*: Patterns of atrioventricular conduction in the human heart. Circ Res 1970;27:345–359.
79. Akhtar M, Damato AN, Caracta AR, *et al.*: Unmasking and conversion of gap phenomenon in the human heart. Circulation 1974;49:624–630.
80. Schuilenburg RM, Durrer D: Ventricular echo beats in the human heart elicited by induced ventricular premature beats. Circulation 1969;40:337–347.
81. Akhtar M, Damato AN, Ruskin JN, *et al.*: Characteristics and coexistence of two forms of ventricular echo phenomenon. Am Heart J 1976;92:174–182.
82. Castillo C, Castellanos A Jr: Retrograde activation of the His bundle in the human heart. Am J Cardiol 1971;27:264–271.
83. Horowitz LN, Kay HR, Kutalek SP, *et al.*: Risks and complications of clinical cardiac electrophysiologic studies: a prospective analysis of 1,000 consecutive patients. J Am Coll Cardiol 1987;9:1261–1268.

5

EVALUATION OF SYNCOPE

Antonio Asso, M.D., Stephen Remole, M.D., and David G. Benditt, M.D.

INTRODUCTION

Syncope, broadly defined as sudden transient loss of both consciousness and postural tone with prompt spontaneous recovery, is a common medical problem, accounting for about 3% of emergency room visits and 1–6% of general hospital admissions in the United States (1,2). According to the Framingham Study (3) at least one syncopal spell can be anticipated in 3% of men and in 3.5% of women during their lifetime, with recurrences occurring in roughly one third of cases.

Following a complete history and physical examination it is often said that a correct etiologic basis for syncopal spells can be ascertained in approximately one-half of patients. However, the medical history may be misleading (4,5), and the presence of certain common findings such as atrial or ventricular ectopy, sinus bradycardia, or bundle branch block may predispose the attending physician toward certain diagnoses, despite failure to confirm the precise origin of the symptoms. A careful diagnostic evaluation although often difficult and occasionally unrewarding, is mandatory in all cases. In particular, assessment of the presence of structural cardiac and vascular causes of syncope should receive highest priority due to the increased mortality associated with syncope occurring in this setting (6–9).

ETIOLOGY

Many conditions can cause syncope or closely "mimic" a syncopal spell. From the perspective of planning diagnostic studies and assessing prognosis, it is useful to classify causes of syncope as being of either cardiovascular—including neurally mediated (vasovagal) reflex syncope, or noncardiovascular origin (Table 5.1).

Cardiovascular Disorders

CARDIAC/PULMONARY DISEASE

Both left ventricular outflow and inflow obstruction may cause syncope, and in general carry a grave prognosis unless recognized and treated promptly. In the case of left ventricular outflow obstruction (e.g., aortic stenosis, hypertrophic obstructive cardiomyopathy), the mechanism of syncope is believed to be in part the result of inadequate blood flow secondary to mechanical obstruction and partly the result of reflex bradycardia and vasodilation. The latter is considered a manifestation of the Bezold-Jarish reflex (10). Other conditions commonly associated with acute alterations of flow, possibly aggravated by neural effects as well, include atrial myxoma, pulmonary embolus, pericardial effusion, and acute myocardial infarction. In regard to the latter, syncope occurs frequently, being a presenting symptom in 7% of patients with acute myocardial infarction over 65 yr of age in one series (11). In this setting syncope is probably multifactorial in origin, including transient reductions of cardiac output, neural reflex mechanisms, and cardiac arrhythmias.

Rhythm Disturbances

Arrhythmias associated with structural heart disease are among the most common causes of syncope, and invasive electrophysiologic studies can be highly effective in defining the etiology and directing appropriate therapy (12,13). In these studies, electrode catheters are placed at specific sites within the heart to assess both cardiac conduction measurements, and evaluate susceptibility to arrhythmias—either being potential causes of syncope.

Sinus node dysfunction

Sinus node dysfunction (SND) is another frequent cause of dizziness and syncope, especially in the elderly. Patients may manifest both periods of bradyarrhythmia and bouts of tachycardia (particularly atrial fibrillation/flutter) either of which can produce transient cerebral hypoperfusion (Fig. 5.2). Chronotropic incompetence is another manifestation of SND which can lead to exertional syncope/dizziness.

Bradycardias

Bradyarrhythmias are among the most common arrhythmic causes of syncope. These may occur as a result of cardiac conduction system disease, sinus node disease (see below), or in conjunction with neurally mediated hypotension/bradycardia episodes. With

Table 5.1.
Major Clinical Conditions Associated with Syncope

I Cardiovascular disorders
- Cardiac/pulmonary disease
  - Mechanical disturbances (obstruction/inadequate flow)
    - Cardiac valvular disease (aortic stenosis, mitral stenosis, prosthetic valve malfunction)
    - Acute myocardial infarction/ischemia (possibly "neurally mediated"/arrhythmogenic mechanisms)
    - Hypertrophic cardiomyopathy with obstruction
    - Pericardial disease/tamponade
    - Pulmonary embolus
    - Primary pulmonary hypertension
  - Rhythm disturbances
    - Sinus node dysfunction (brady- and tachycardia)
    - AV conduction system disease
    - Supraventricular tachycardias
    - Ventricular tachycardia (including torsade de pointes)
    - Pacemaker malfunction/pacemaker-mediated tachycardia
  - Vascular disturbances
    - Cerebrovascular disorders (spinal cord/vertebrobasilar ischemia)
    - Noncerebral vessels (subclavian steal, aortic dissection)
    - Autonomic neuropathies
  - Neurally mediated reflex syncope
    - Vasovagal syncope (emotional, situational)
    - Carotid sinus syncope
    - Syncope related to increased intrathoracic pressure (e.g., cough)
    - Syncope of gastrointestinal, pelvic, or urologic origin (swallowing, postmicturition, defecation, etc.)
    - Drug-induced (e.g., vasodilators)

II Noncardiovascular disorders
- Central nervous system substrates (syncope and "syncope mimics")
  - Epilepsy (with or without seizure-like activity)
  - Hydrocephalus
  - Third ventricular colloid cyst
  - Atlantoaxial spine instability
  - Foramen magnum tumors
  - Narcolepsy
- Metabolic/endocrine disturbances
  - Hypoglycemia
  - Hyperventilation (hypocapnia)
- Psychiatric disorders
  - Panic attacks
  - Hysteria/conversion reaction
  - Cataplexy

respect to the first of these, the causes are most commonly underlying ischemic heart disease, cardiomyopathy, or age-related degenerative disease. The most serious manifestations are Mobitz II atrioventricular (AV) block, high-grade AV block, or complete heart block. Sinus node dysfunction and neurally mediated causes of bradycardia are discussed more fully below.

Tachycardias

Syncope is not a prominent clinical feature in patients with supraventricular tachycardia. However, several factors need to be considered: the rate and mechanism of the tachycardia, the posture at the onset of the episode, the presence of structural heart disease, and the role of compensatory autonomic reflexes (Fig. 5.1). Not unexpectedly ventricular tachycardias are frequent causes of syncope in patients with heart disease, and on average (depending on the nature of the referral population) account for about 20% of diagnoses among syncope patients referred for electrophysiologic study (14). Presumably, the frequent occurrence of structural heart disease in these patients plays a role in both the cause and the hemodynamic consequence of the tachycardia. Furthermore, susceptibility to ventricular tachycardia often coexists with evident abnormalities of cardiac conduction, due to common underlying disease processes. Thus, in many syncope patients with electrocardiographic evidence of AV conduction system disease, ventricular tachycardia may in fact be responsible for symptoms. For example, in patients with chronic bifascicular block, Dhingra, *et al.* showed (15) that a conduction disorder accounted for syncope in 17% of cases while ventricular tachycardia was identified as the likely cause in 30% of patients.

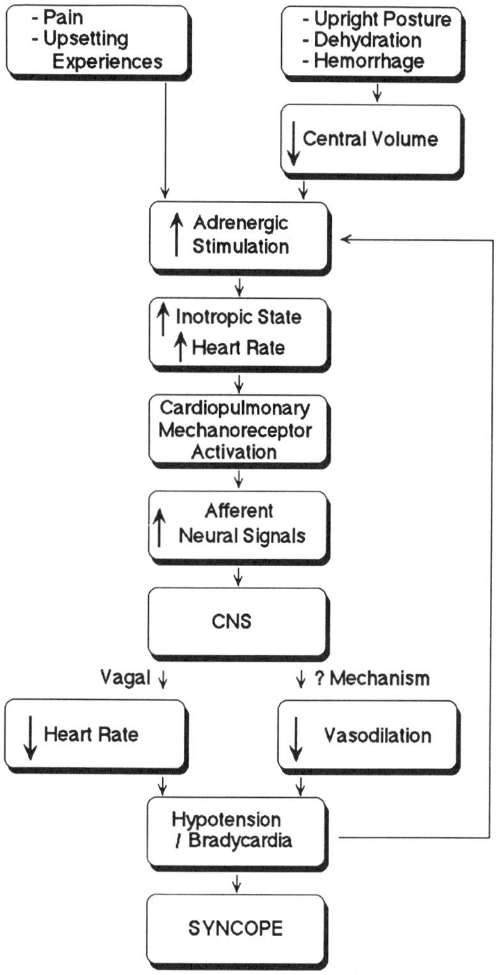

Figure 5.1. Proposed pathophysiology of neurally mediated syncope (see text for discussion).

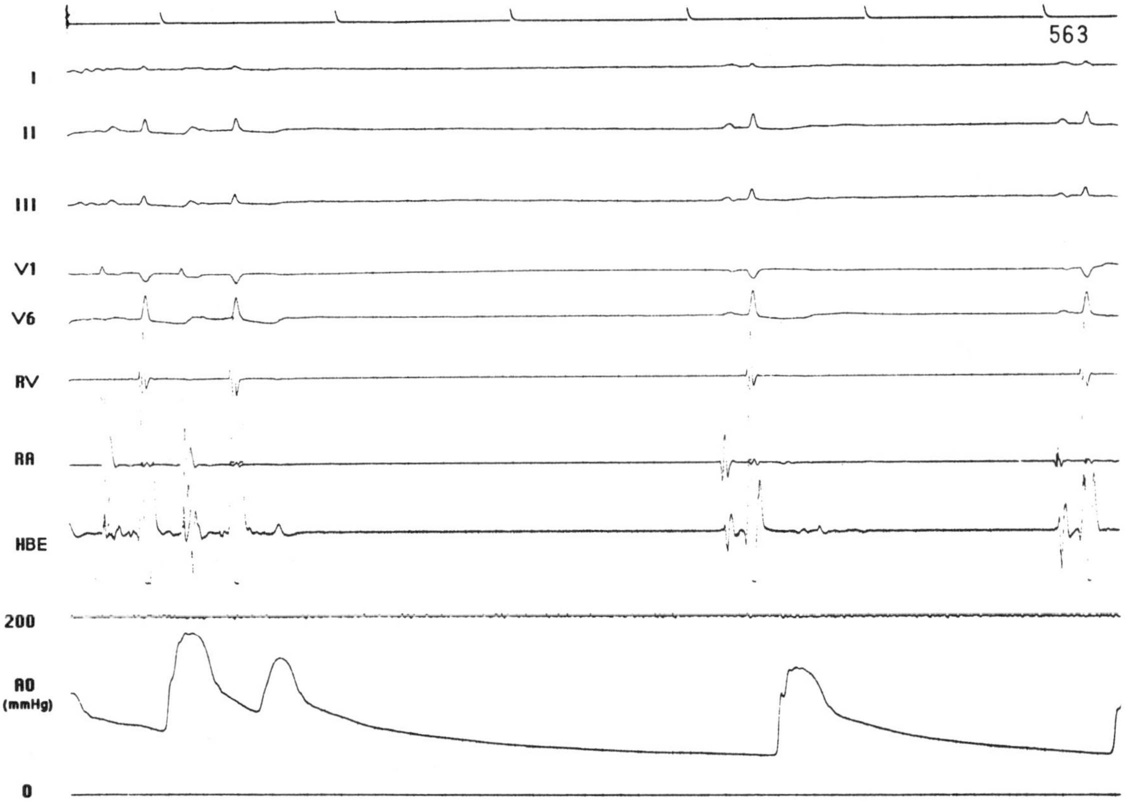

Figure 5.2. Recordings illustrating a prolonged sinus node recovery time in a patient with sick sinus syndrome and syncope. From **top** to **bottom** the traces are ECG leads I, II, III, V1, and V_6, intracardiac electrograms from the right ventricle (RV), right atrium (RA), His bundle region (HBE), and arterial pressure (AO mm Hg). The postpacing recovery time (SNRT) is 3060 msec, followed by a secondary pause in the rhythm. These findings are abnormal.

VASCULAR DISTURBANCES

Several vascular disorders should be considered in the differential diagnosis of syncope. Cerebrovascular disease (e.g., vertebral-basilar insufficiency) is of particular concern, and may necessitate invasive studies in selected patients. However, such studies should be undertaken only if clinical circumstances are highly suggestive of the diagnosis.

NEURALLY MEDIATED REFLEX SYNCOPE

Neurally mediated reflex syncope may be considered as a group of apparently related conditions or syndromes (Table 5.1). These syndromes are believed to be the most common source of spontaneous syncope in all age groups. However, only a few of these syndromes occur frequently (e.g., the vasovagal faint/syncope) 16–19), while most (e.g., carotid sinus syndrome (20,21), postmicturition syndrome (22), cough syncope (23)) are relatively rare.

Several factors may contribute to the development of neurally-mediated syncope, in susceptible patients (e.g., drug therapy, hypovolemia, venous insufficiency), with the elderly patient being particularly at risk since they are often treated with multiple drugs and are more likely to exhibit structural heart disease and neurologic disorders (24). Of importance, while the presence of concomitant conditions may increase susceptibility to syncope, they may also complicate recognition of the actual etiologic diagnosis and thereby lead to selection of inappropriate therapies.

In susceptible individuals, the so-called vasovagal form of neurally mediated syncope can be initiated by a wide variety of factors (25,26): emotional upset, anxiety, pain, heat, dehydration, unpleasant sights. Usually, the episode is marked by a premonitory period of symptomatic hypotension, diaphoresis, and nausea, followed by progressive and often severe bradycardia (19). Clearly, "vasovagal" syncope is by far the most common mechanism of syncope in humans. On the other hand, although carotid sinus hypersensitivity is relatively common, especially in older individuals, carotid sinus syndrome is only infrequently the cause of syncope. Estimates suggest that only 5–10% of patients exhibiting carotid hypersensitivity actually have syncope of carotid sinus origin (20,27,28). Clinically, the diagnosis is suspected if the attack is triggered by or associated with (21,29) turning or extending the neck, tight collars, and previous neck surgery/irradiation. Additionally, although even less common than carotid sinus syndrome, syncope may be the result of neurally mediated mechanisms, in several other situations: increased intrathoracic pressure (cough syncope) (23,30,31); postmicturition (22); defecation and other forms of pelvic stimulation (32); and swallowing (33–36) (Table 5.1).

Noncardiovascular Causes of Syncope

As a rule, noncardiovascular causes of transient loss of consciousness, such as hypoglycemia, seizure disorder, or hemorrhage are suggested by the medical history, physical examination, and/or biochemistry profile. In such cases selected additional diagnostic studies may confirm the diagnosis. However routine use of an array of hematologic, biochemical, imaging, and neurologic test are rarely productive. In particular, it should be kept in mind that generalized tonic/clonic movements can be the result of syncope (cerebral hypoperfusion), rather than the cause (epilepsy) of it.

Psychiatric conditions causing situations that mimic syncope can cause particular diagnostic difficulties. In such cases, establishing the correct diagnosis may be extremely frustrating, although witnessing a spontaneous episode may prove helpful.

PATHOPHYSIOLOGY

In the healthy individual cerebral blood flow is maintained over a wide range of perfusion pressures by the autoregulatory features of the cerebral vascular bed. Diminution of oxygen delivery to the brain below minimum requirements—3.5 ml O_2/100 g tissue min—for 10 sec or longer may be accompanied by loss of both consciousness and postural tone. Any condition causing a derangement in oxygen delivery can lead to syncope. Additionally, in elderly and/or hypertensive patients, the range over which autoregulation occurs may be altered, thereby further increasing susceptibility to transient cerebral hypoperfusion.

The mechanisms by which diminished cerebral blood flow occurs as a consequence of underlying cardiac or vascular disease are often multifactorial. Thus patients with aortic valvular stenosis or hypertrophic subaortic stenosis may become syncopal as a result of both diminished forward flow, as well as a consequence of neurally mediated vasodilatation. A similar complex of events may be associated with acute myocardial infarction. On the other hand, syncope occurring as a result of left atrial myxoma may be attributed primarily to intermittent inflow obstruction, while subclavian steal syndrome is thought to be exclusively the consequence of diversion of cerebral blood flow to the exercising arm in the setting of a proximal subclavian artery stenosis. Finally, recent evidence suggests that in certain forms of neurally-mediated syncope, cerebral vasospasm of vasoconstriction may contribute to reduced cerebral blood flow (37).

The mechanisms responsible for neurally mediated syncope are only incompletely understood (Fig. 5.1). Currently, excessive or inappropriate stimulation of certain receptors (particularly mechanoreceptors) located in various organ systems is believed to account for many of these syndromes. Carotid sinus syncope can be considered a prototype of the neurally mediated syncopal syndromes in that the origin of the hypotension and bradycardia is either excessive stimulation of presumably abnormally sensitive carotid sinus baroreceptors, or an inordinate response to stimulation of otherwise normal receptor sites (27,28). In a similar way, hypersensitivity of cardiac and cardiopulmonary mechanoreceptors might be implicated as trigger sites in other neurally mediated syndromes (10,38). Furthermore, in susceptible individuals a reduction of central circulatory volume (39–44) (e.g., due to upright posture, dehydration) in conjunction with marked elevation of circulatory catecholamines, perhaps secondary to volume depletion, anxiety, or an idiosyncratic reaction may play a key role in sensitizing receptors and enhancing afferent neural traffic from ventricular mechanoreceptors. Alternatively, since these receptors respond to mechanical force and thereby to inotropic state, enhancement of the force applied to these mechanoreceptors may result in greater afferent neural traffic in parasympathetic nerves to the medulla (so-called C-fibers) (45). In general, abundant afferent neural traffic from these receptors promotes efferent neural signals which elicit reflex bradycardia and peripheral vascular dilatation.

The frequent observation of relative tachycardia preceding hypotension and bradycardia, as well as measured increases of circulating catecholamine levels, and the favorable results of β-adrenergic blockade therapy in some patients, support the view that sympathetic enhancement of receptor sites with a consequent greater than normal parasympathetic afferent neural traffic from central vascular receptor sites is key to the initiation of many forms of neurally mediated syncope. Similar receptors in other organ systems (e.g., bladder, bowel) may also participate in initiation of other forms of syncope (e.g., postmicturition, defecation-induced). Additionally, according to several recently published studies, these same pathophysiologic mechanisms may also be responsible for some cases of asystolic cardiac arrest leading to sudden death or near-sudden death in otherwise healthy individuals (46,47).

EVALUATION

Initial Assessment

HISTORY AND PHYSICAL EXAMINATION

A detailed medical history and thorough physical examination are crucial first steps in the initial evaluation of syncope. The information obtained provides the groundwork for establishing an effective strategy for subsequent laboratory studies (48). In all cases of syncope it should be kept in mind that on average 30% of untreated patients manifest recurrence of syncope within 2–3 yr, and that syncope patients with structural cardiovascular disease are at a higher mortality risk then control subjects or syncope patients without cardiovascular disease (8). Thus, thorough evaluation of each case is prudent. A patient presenting with syncope without exhibiting other apparent illness may be an optimal candidate for tilt-table testing as an initial procedure, while an individual with findings suggestive of structural heart disease may best be evaluated with invasive electrophysiologic studies in conjunction with necessary anatomic and functional cardiac studies.

Assessment of a syncopal event requires information from both the patient and witnesses. The circumstances surrounding the episode, prodromal symptoms, the rapidity with which the loss of consciousness occurred, its duration, and the speed of recovery are all important information. For example, neurally mediated syncopal syndromes (e.g., the vasovagal faint) are often associated with certain specific situations or emotionally upsetting experiences, and preceded by prodromal symptoms such as nausea, diaphoresis, and a general sense of impending collapse. Alternatively, since tachycardias are a common cause of syncope, a history of palpitations should be sought, although absence of such a history should not exclude the search for symptomatic tachyarrhythmias. In one study this symptom was reported to be absent in 43% of patients with ventricular tachycardia, many of whom (30%) had lightheadedness, and reported syncope (15%) (49). Presumably many patients are unaware of rapid heart beating due to relatively ineffective cardiac mechanical activity (in those circumstances).

Routine batteries of hematologic and biochemical studies, rarely pay dividends in syncope patients (50). Selective testing based on history and physical examination is more cost effective. In such cases testing will confirm a diagnosis already suspected on clinical grounds (anemia in a peptic ulcer patient, hypoglycemia in a diabetic, etc.). Similarly, routine neurologic studies—electroencephalogram (EEG), computed tomography (CT), and magnetic resonance imaging (MRI)—are not warranted as an initial step when the history or physical findings are not clearly suggestive of a neurologic condition as cause of syncope. On the other hand, a suspicion of vertebrobasilar or carotid vessel disease may warrant proceeding with noninvasive and invasive vascular studies.

Noninvasive Cardiovascular Studies

Ultrasonic studies are among the most useful noninvasive tools for assessment of the presence and severity of underlying cardiac and vascular disease. An echocardiogram should be obtained in all syncope patients, since it is a far more reliable means of identifying and quantifying structural heart disease than is either the history or physical examination. Ultrasonic studies of the carotids and other vascular beds (including transcranial Doppler studies) may also play a role in selected cases.

A baseline 12-lead ECG rarely provides a specific diagnosis for syncope. However, certain findings may suggest possible causes and thereby warrant proceeding with additional testing. For instance, the presence of Q waves, a prolonged QT interval, or ventricular preexcitation suggest susceptibility to tachyarrhythmias. An inappropriate bradycardia and/or evidence of sinus arrest or sinoatrial exit block are presumptive of SND. On the other hand, a normal baseline electrocardiogram (ECG) may suggest that conventional electrophysiologic testing will be of relatively low yield compared to, for example tilt-table testing. In one study of 104 patients with syncope, only 6% of those with a normal baseline ECG had diagnostic findings during conventional electrophysiologic study (6).

Obtaining ECG documentation of symptomatic arrhythmia may be achieved by "long-term" ECG recording techniques (51,52) in the outpatient setting. The diagnostic yield of the monitoring techniques is highest in suspected sinus node dysfunction and in conduction disturbances. In any case, a clear relation between symptoms and findings must be established, since minor nonspecific abnormalities occur commonly, particularly in the elderly (53). When syncopal symptoms are infrequent, conventional magnetic-tape electrocardiographic monitoring techniques (e.g., Holter monitoring) are rarely cost-effective. In these instances, event recorder monitoring may prove more useful (54). These systems can be employed in a continuous loop mode for patients whose symptoms are brief. However event recorders do require patients to be able to respond appropriately when the episode begins. Exercise testing is not routinely helpful in the evaluation of syncope, but may be a useful diagnostic procedure (55,56) in selected circumstances (Table 5.2).

The role of the signal-averaged ECG (SAECG) in assessment of syncope is incompletely defined (57,58). A positive SAECG in a patient with structural heart disease raises suspicion of the substrate for ventricular tachyarrhythmias and suggests the need for electrophysiologic study. For example, Winters, *et al.* (59) noted an abnormal SAECG in 92% of patients with syncope who had ventricular tachycardia induced at electrophysiologic study. However, the sensitivity and specificity of SAECG in a broader range of syncope patients is unclear, and its overall utility is likely to be limited to those cases in which it may be helpful to stratify patients with respect to ventricular tachycardia risk (i.e., patients with structural heart disease).

Invasive Cardiac Studies

Depending on the clinical circumstances, the evaluation of syncope may necessitate coronary angiography, left ventriculo-

Table 5.2.
Circumstances in which Exercise Testing May Contribute to Establishing a Basis for Syncope

Myocardial ischemia (substrate for ventricular tachycardia, exacerbation of LV dysfunction)
Catecholamine-sensitive (exercise-induced) tachycardias
Supraventricular (particularly certain fastidious reentrant SVT)
Ventricular (particularly the syndrome of VT with a LBBB + inferior axis morphology in the setting of a "normal" heart)
Exercise-induced AV block (rate-dependent block, distal to His)
Chronotropic incompetence (in sinus node dysfunction)

Abbreviations: LBBB, left bundle branch block; LV, left ventricular; SVT, supraventricular tachycardia; VT, ventricular tachycardia.

graphy, cerebrovascular angiography, and radiographic assessment of other vascular beds. However, among all invasive studies, conventional cardiac electrophysiologic testing is the most frequently employed and the most productive, especially in the setting of structural heart disease. In general, these studies utilize cardiac recording and stimulation techniques (by means of predominantly transvenous, but occasionally intra-arterial electrode catheters) to assess both intracardiac conduction intervals and susceptibility to inducible tachy- and bradyarrhythmias. Table 5.3 summarizes findings from a number of published reports examining the efficacy of electrophysiologic studies in referred patients with recurrent syncope. As noted above, it is clear that the utility of electrophysiologic testing is greatest when underlying structural heart disease is present (Table 5.3). In the absence of cardiac abnormalities, head-up tilt testing (HUT) is more useful (see below), and should probably be undertaken prior to considering invasive electrophysiologic study. Overall, based on our own experience (60) and the recent report by Sra, *et al.* (61) the combination of electrophysiologic studies and upright tilt test can be expected to identify the cause of symptoms in approximately 75% of patients evaluated for unexplained syncope.

Invasive electrophysiologic testing is indicated in the setting of structural heart disease whenever an arrhythmia is considered a probable cause of syncope (12,62–66). When positive, such testing will prove helpful not only for establishing a diagnosis but also for guiding therapy and in assessing prognosis. The diagnostic yield of this technique in the evaluation of syncope has been reported to be widely variable 18–96% (65,67–69). The wide range is primarily due to differences in patient groups (particularly the presence of structural heart disease) and in endpoints among these studies. Additionally, technical considerations may be a factor. In particular, placement of an arterial line may be essential in order to assess the hemodynamic consequences of an observed arrhythmia adequately. Noninvasive blood pressure monitoring may not be sufficient in some cases, given the transient nature of many arrhythmias. Furthermore, a tachyarrhythmia tolerated in the supine position (in the laboratory) may cause profound hypotension with syncope if the patient were in the upright posture. On the other hand, the induction of a well-tolerated arrhythmia requires that the evaluation be pursued in an attempt to uncover other mechanisms of tachycardia and/or other causes of syncope (5).

ELECTROPHYSIOLOGIC LABORATORY TECHNIQUES

The following discussion deals briefly with various electrophysiologic testing approaches in patients with syncope of various suspected underlying causes. The reader is referred to the references provided for more detailed treatments of the techniques. See also Chapters 4; 7–9.

Sinus Node Dysfunction (Sick Sinus Syndrome)

The diagnosis of SND (70) is rarely based on electrophysiologic findings alone. In most cases the correlation of symptoms with ECG monitoring results provides the diagnosis. The importance of such correlation (although often difficult to obtain) cannot be over emphasized. For example, SND patients may exhibit marked bradyarrhythmias, intermittent tachyarrhythmias, or both. Syncope in patients with the bradycardia-tachycardia variant of SND (bradycardia-tachycardia syndrome) may occur as a result of bradycardia (e.g., sinus bradycardia, sinus pausses, or sinoatrial exit block), intermittent tachyarrhythmia (usually atrial flutter or fibrillation), or asystolic periods occurring after cessation of a tachycardia episode. Clearly the appropriate treatment depends on establishing an accurate diagnosis.

Measurement of sinus node recovery times (SNRT) (Fig. 5.2) and sinoatrial conduction times (SACT) are the principal electrophysiologic techniques available to assist in establishing the diagnosis of SND. SNRT is primarily thought to assess the recovery of automaticity in the sinus node after brief periods (usually 1 min) of rapid atrial pacing at different cycle lengths (71). After subtracting the basic sinus cycle length, the corrected SNRT usually has a value of <525 msec. SACT is primarily an indirect estimation of the time required for a sinus impulse to exit the node and access atrial myocardium. The latter is mainly a function of conduction properties of the node/perinodal tissues. Two principal methods have been developed to estimate SACT (atrial extrastimulus technique (72) and constant pacing method (73)). Normal values for SACT are typically <206 msec. Taken together, SNRT, corrected SNRT, and SACT are fairly specific (about 90%) for SND, but lack sensitivity (about 70%). Additionally, for a proper interpretation of these findings the assessment of autonomic influences on sinus node function must be undertaken. To this end, atropine 0.04 mg/kg IV is administered and normally the heart rate increases to more than 90 beats/min while corrected SNRT and SACT shorten.

Table 5.3.
Electrophysiologic Testing in Syncope of Unknown Origin

Reference	No. Patients	No. Patients With Heart Disease	Overall EP-Positive	EP-Positive With Structural HD	EP-Positive Without Structural HD
Akhtar, *et al.* (1983) (65)	30	18	16 (53%)	15 (83%)	1 (8%)
Morady, *et al.* (1983) (67)	53	38	30 (57%)	27 (71%)	3 (20%)
Teichman, *et al.* (1985) (68)	150	75	112 (75%)	64 (85%)	48 (64%)
Crozier, *et al.* (1986) (69)	94	42	26 (28%)	16 (38%)	10 (20%)
Total	327	173	184 (56%)	122 (71%)	62 (36%)

Abbreviations: HD, heart disease.

Failure of atropine to produce such an effect suggests intrinsic sinus node disease. Normalization of SNRT and SACT after atropine suggests that observed initial abnormalities were related to hypervagotonia. The evaluation of the observed intrinsic heart rate (IHR) after total autonomic blockade has similar implications. In addition to atropine, estimation of IHR requires concomitant administration of propranolol 0.2 mg/kg IV (74). Normal values are approximately 118 − (0.57 × age).

Conduction System Disease

Transient high-grade AV block is an important cause of syncope. In many instances the diagnosis is established during ECG monitoring, and consequently electrophysiologic testing is not required. In other instances, however, establishing intermittent AV block as a cause of syncope may prove elusive, even in the presence of ECG evidence of conduction system disease (e.g., bifascisular block). In such cases a complete electrophysiologic study of AV conduction may permit establishing the diagnosis. In particular, evaluation of the distal conduction system (HV interval, normal <55 msec) may require maneuvers to uncover "latent" disease such as the use of incremental atrial pacing (75) (with atropine if AV nodal block (Wenckebach) occurs <120 beats/min), and pharmacologic stress with Class IA antiarrhythmics (e.g., procainamide (76), usual dosage 15–20 mg/kg at 50 mg/min). Additionally, since patients with intraventricular conduction abnormalities typically also have underlying heart disease, a complete protocol of programmed ventricular stimulation should also be performed. In many cases a ventricular tachyarrhythmia may be proven to be the true cause of syncope, with the conduction disorder being an epiphenomenon (77).

Supraventricular and Ventricular Tachyarrhythmias

During electrophysiologic study, multiple attempts should be made to induce a tachycardia with associated hypotension severe enough to account for the clinical symptoms (78). Again, the factors of posture (79), and underlying heart disease should be noted. The induction protocol minimally includes (80) programmed atrial and ventricular stimulation with up to two extrastimuli in both chambers, incremental pacing, and specific protocols to exclude or characterize the existence of accessory AV pathway(s), nodoventricular connections, enhanced AV nodal conduction, and dual AV node physiology. When negative, the protocol should be repeated following initiation of isoproterenol infusion. The latter drug is usually used in doses of 1–5 μg/min depending on patient tolerance (81). In specific instances, other pharmacologic interventions (e.g., atropine, antiarrhythmic drugs) may be appropriate. Sustained ventricular tachycardia, or reciprocating tachycardias incorporating an accessory pathway or due to AV node reentry in this setting may be diagnostic. On occasion, more than one tachycardia, each with different hemodynamic repercussions will be noted (Fig. 5.3) (4).

Ventricular tachycardia is the most frequently induced arrhythmia in patients with organic heart disease undergoing electrophysiologic study for evaluation of unexplained syncope (82,83). Although the optimal protocol for ventricular programmed stimulation has not been defined (84), the introduction of up to three extrastimuli at two ventricular sites is warranted when suspicion is high, such as in the setting of a prior myocardial infarction or if the SAECG shows late potentials. Induction of polymorphic ventricular tachycardia generally represents a nonspecific response (85). However in selected cases polymorphic ventricular tachycardia may represent a clinically signifi-

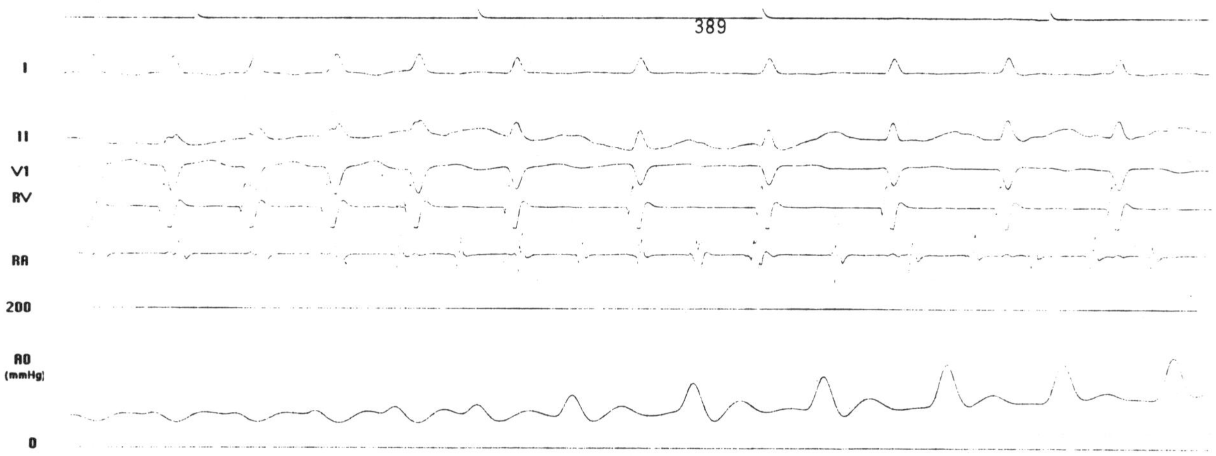

Figure 5.3. Electrocardiograms and intracardiac recordings during two forms of tachycardia in one patient evaluated for syncope. Traces are arranged in the same format as in Figure 5.2. The first four beats show a short ventriculo atrial (VA) interval, and proved to be atrioventricular (AV) node reentrant tachycardia. Subsequently, atrial flutter spontaneously develops as evidenced by the increased atrial rate. Nevertheless, since there is 2:1 AV block during atrial flutter, the ventricular rate decreases compared to AV node reentry, accounting for better tolerance of this tachycardia (note the improved blood pressure). The first tachycardia—due to AV node reentry—was the real cause of syncope.

cant response, especially when the result of a "nonaggressive" protocol (one to two extrastimuli), or if obtained during "pause-dependent" (long-short) stimulation protocols.

TESTING AUTONOMIC NERVOUS SYSTEM RESPONSES

Head-up Tilt Test

Evaluation of the relationship between the autonomic nervous system and cardiovascular function is particularly important in those syncope patients who do not have evidence of underlying cardiac disease. In recent years, the response to upright posture during head-up tilt table testing (HUT) has been the subject of particular interest for assessing susceptibility to spontaneous neurally mediated reflex syncopal syndromes (86–88). Several reports confirm the reproducibility of HUT (89–91). Since it is believed that the reflexes responsible for neurally-mediated syncope are universally present in humans (10,38–46) (Pathophysiology, above), false-positive responses to HUT may occur, especially the longer the duration and the greater angle of tilt used. Currently we utilize a protocol comprising 80° tilt for 25 min; if neither syncope nor presyncope is reproduced, an infusion of isoproterenol is started at 1 μg/minute. The procedure is repeated at successive stages of 3 and 5 μg/min as needed.

Using a protocol similar to our current one (10 min duration) we reported HUT to exhibit a sensitivity of 82% and a specificity of 88% in reproducing symptoms in patients with suspected neurally mediated syncope (45). Furthermore, HUT alone yielded no false-positive results in 18 control subjects, and HUT plus isoproterenol resulted in only 2 false positive tests. When necessary, HUT can be undertaken after completion of the electrophysiologic study (EPS) although a reasonable period of time (e.g., 45–60 min) should be permitted between procedures, and fluid replacement is essential if the patient has been fasted. In either case, an arterial line to monitor blood pressure is advantageous, as is a quiet atmosphere while the test is in progress. In susceptible individuals, a slight but characteristic variability in heart rate and blood pressure is usually detected prior to symptom development. Typically, in the HUT-positive patient, blood pressure falls first, following which bradycardia ensues and accentuates the hemodynamic derangement (Fig. 5.4). In some cases the abnormal response in rate predominates over pressure, but the pathophysiology is the same. Whenever symptoms are reproduced, both heart rate

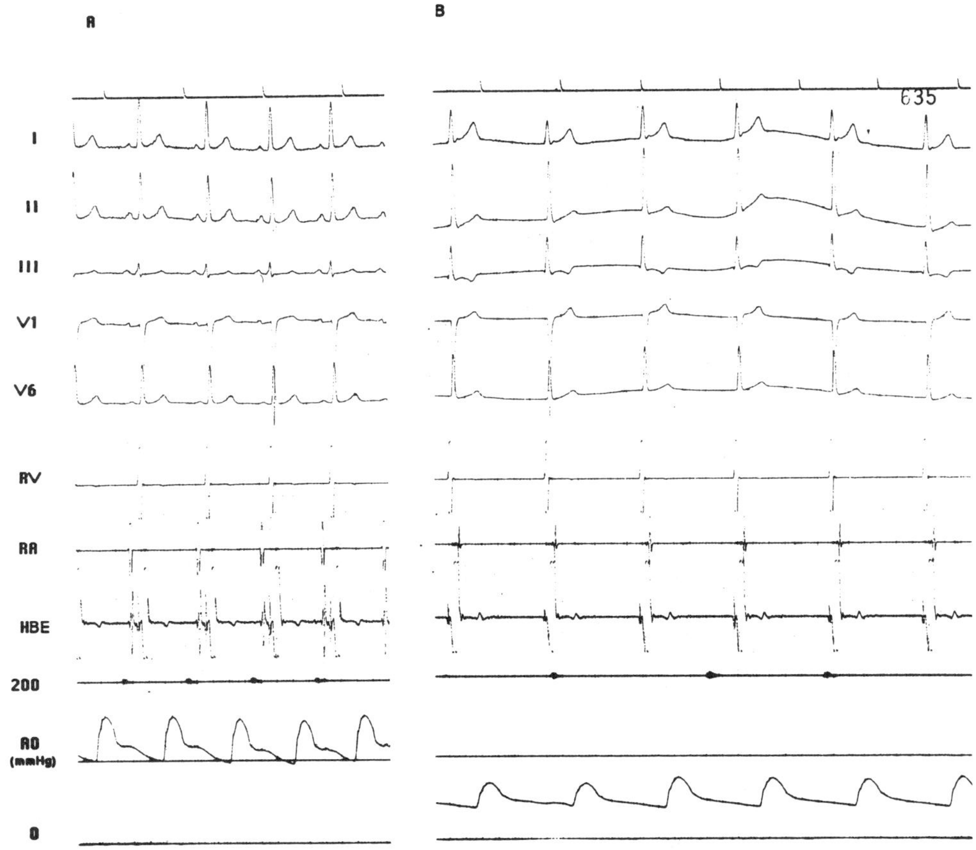

Figure 5.4. A positive response to upright tilt table testing. Traces are similar to those used in Figure 5.2. **Panel A:** Baseline conditions showing normal heart rate and blood pressure (150/95 mm Hg). **Panel B:** After several minutes in the upright tilt posture there was evident heart rate slowing accompanied by relatively severe hypotension (70/40 mm Hg). Note that during bradycardia the cardiac rhythm is no longer of sinus origin but comes from the AV junction with retrograde atrial activation.

and blood pressure promptly return to normal upon resumption of supine position.

Other Autonomic Testing Maneuvers

Carotid sinus stimulation and the Valsalva maneuver provide additional means for assessing cardiac autonomic neural control. The role of the latter is as yet uncertain. Carotid sinus massage, on the other hand, provides a direct means of initiating afferent neural activity from one set of mechanoreceptors known to be capable of inducing neurally mediated hypotension and bradycardia (27,92). After carotid artery obstruction is ruled out, the left and right carotid sinuses should be individually massaged for 5–10 sec. Although controversial, an abnormal response (carotid sinus hypersensitivity) is said to be present when asystole for more than 3 sec and/or a fall in systolic blood pressure greater than 40–50 mm Hg are obtained. In any event, interpretation of the significance of the findings must be done with caution. In most cases evident carotid sinus hypersensitivity is unrelated to the symptoms. True carotid sinus syncope is much less frequent and its diagnosis depends on both demonstrating the presence of carotid sinus hypersensitivity and obtaining a compatible medical history (93,94). The latter might be, for instance, syncope in association with head movements, or in association with tight collars, previous neck surgery, or neck irradiation.

TREATMENT

Overview

The appropriate treatment for prevention of recurrent syncope is entirely dependent on establishing the underlying cause (95,96). Thus, syncope of cardiovascular origin may necessitate addressing a structural abnormality, e.g., valvular stenosis, or the prevention of arrhythmia recurrences through use of drugs, ablation, or implanted devices (particularly pacemakers). In certain instances an implanted cardioverter/defibrillator will be required.

The treatment value of cardiac pacemakers is well established when a symptomatic bradycardia, whose origin is related to structural conduction system disease or intrinsic SND, is the cause of symptoms. On the other hand, when the slow heart rate is associated with a neurally mediated syndrome, the prevention of bradycardia alone may not be completely effective. In these syndromes peripheral vasodilation is an almost universal feature and this "vasodepressor component" (92) may be the principal cause of the syncopal spell. Typically, it is unusual for a pacemaker to be curative in this setting, but on occasion pacing may be necessary as adjunctive therapy.

NEURALLY MEDIATED SYNDROMES

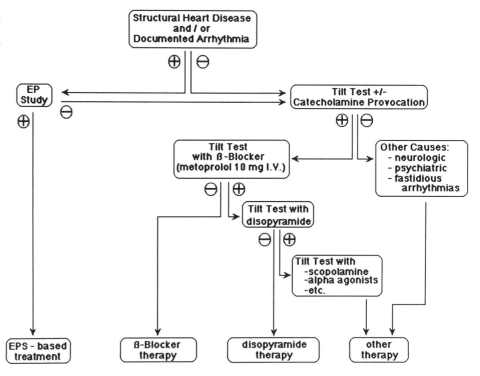

Recent insights into the pathophysiology of these syndromes (38–46,97,98) have opened new perspectives for pharmacologic treatment (99). The β-adrenergic blockers have been used in preventing hypotension-bradycardia of reflex origin, presumably based in part on their negative inotropic action (100). We prefer a cardioselective agent (e.g., metoprolol 50–200 mg/day), although nonselective agents and beta blockers with intrinsic sympathomimetic action have been similarly effective. Similar good results are accumulating with disopyramide (101), an antiarrhythmic drug with prominent anticholinergic and negative

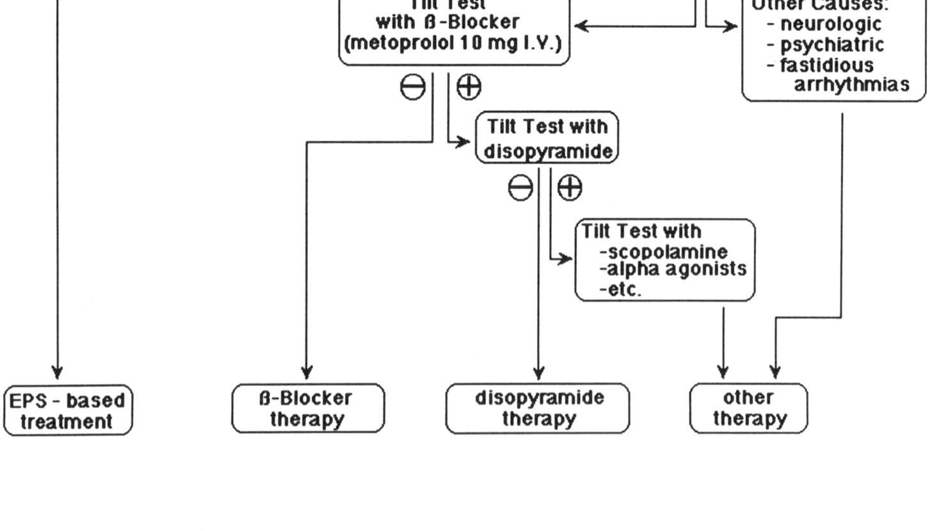

Figure 5.5. Block diagrams depicting one practical approach to the management of patients in whom syncope remains of unknown origin despite preceding noninvasive evaluation. EP = electrophysiologic.

inotropic actions. By virtue of these effects, disopyramide presumably reduces parasympathetic outflow and decreases stretch on central mechanoreceptors. The usual dose of disopyramide for this purpose is 150 mg t.i.d. Only rarely are side effects a limitation in therapy at that dosage (102). Other drugs, including theophilline, ephedrine, and scopolamine have also been used in selected cases (103). In all cases, the most appropriate management has to be individualized (8,9,104). Our current general approach is depicted in Figure 5.5 as a guideline. It should be emphasized, however, that the need for treatment must take into consideration: the number of recurrences, severity of episodes, situations related to symptom onset, associated medical conditions, and secondary effects of medication (105).

CONCLUSION

Syncope is a common medical problem with multiple causes. Although single syncopal events may not elicit alarm in young individuals without underlying cardiovascular disease, such episodes should be considered as a potentially serious matter in older patients and in individuals with structural cardiovascular disorders. In particular, in the latter group, syncope is known to be associated with higher mortality rates. In the elderly, syncope can result in substantial physical injury.

Attention to the history, to events surrounding the syncopal episode, and to the physical examination may often lead to a presumptive basis for syncopal symptoms. However, noninvasive and invasive testing is usually needed in order to substantiate the diagnosis with sufficient confidence to permit initiation of a course of therapy. Given the broad array of tests available, the most effective strategy is one of careful selection based on the medical history and physical examination. Currently, judicious use of diagnostic procedures permits substantiation of the cause of syncope in more than three quarters of patients with syncope of unknown origin, with highly effective therapies being readily available for most of these patients.

Acknowledgment

The authors would like to thank Barry L.S. Detloff and Renee Haugh for valuable technical assistance, and Wendy Markuson and Stephanie Wiebke for preparing the manuscript.

References

1. Kapoor WN, Hammill SC, Gersh BJ: Diagnosis and natural history of syncope and the role of invasive electrophysiologic testing. Am J Cardiol 1989;63:730–734.
2. Doherty JU, Pembrook-Rogers D, Grogan E, *et al.*: Electrophysiologic evaluation and follow-up characteristics of patients with recurrent unexplained syncope and presyncope. Am J Cardiol 1985;55:703–708.
3. Savage DD, Corwin L, McGee DL, *et al.*: Epidemiologic features of isolated syncope: The Framingham Study. Stroke 1985;16:626–629.
4. Ezri MD, Jacobs LG, Denes P: Unexpected coexistence of supraventricular and ventricular tachycardia in patients with syncope. PACE 1985;8:329–340.
5. Leitch J, Klein G, Tee R, *et al.*: Neurally mediated syncope and atrial fibrillation. N Engl J Med 1991;324:495–496.
6. Krol RB, Morady F, Flaker CG, *et al.*: Electrophysiologic testing in patients with unexplained syncope, clinical and noninvasive predictors of outcome. J Am Coll Cardiol 1987;10:358–363.
7. Kapoor WN, Hammill SC, Gersh BJ: Diagnosis and natural history of syncope and the role of invasive electrophysiologic testing. Am J Cardiol 1989;62:730–734.
8. Kapoor WN, Karpf M, Wieand S, *et al.*: A prospective evaluation and follow-up of patients with syncope. New Engl J Med 1983;309:197–204.
9. Kapoor WN, Peterson J, Wieand HS, *et al.*: Diagnostic and prognostic implications of recurrences in patients with syncope. Am J Med 1987; 83:700–708.
10. Mark AL: The Bezold-Jarish reflex revisited: Clinical implications of inhibitory reflexes originating in the heart. J Am Coll Cardiol 1983;1:90–102.
11. Pathy MS: Clinical presentation of myocardial infarction in the elderly. Br Heart J 1967;29:190–199.
12. Borbola J, Denes P: Electrophysiologic evaluation of syncope of unexplained origin. In El-Sherif N, Samet PH (eds): Cardiac Pacing and Electrophysiology,3rd ed. WB Saunders, Philadelphia, 1991:293–302.
13. Di Marco JP: Electrophysiologic studies in patients with unexplained syncope. Circulation (Suppl III) 1987;75:140–143.
14. Camm AJ, Lau CP: Syncope of undetermined origin: diagnosis and management. Prog Cardiol 1988;1:139–156.
15. Dhingra RC, Denes P, Wu D, *et al.*: Syncope in patients with chronic bifascicular block. Significance, positive mechanisms and clinical implications. Ann Intern Med 1974;81:302–306.
16. Weissler AM, Warren JV, Estes EH Jr, *et al.*: Vasodepressor syncope. Factors influencing cardiac output. Circulation 1957;15:875–882.
17. Hickler RB: Orthostatic hypotension and syncope. N Engl J Med 1977; 296:336–337.
18. Johnson RH, Lambie DG, Spalding JMK: Neurocardiology. The Interrelationships Between Dysfunction in the Nervous and Cardiovascular Systems. WB Saunders, London, 1984.
19. Ross RT: Syncope, WB Saunders, London, 1988.
20. Weiss S, Baker JP: The carotid sinus reflex in health and disease. Its role in the causation of fainting and convulsions. Medicine 1933;12:297–354.
21. Thomas JE: Hyperactive carotid sinus reflex and carotid sinus syncope. Mayo Clin Proc 1969;44:127–139.
22. Kapoor WN, Peterson JR, Karpf M: Micturition syncope: a reappraisal. JAMA 1985;253:796–798.
23. Sharpey-Schafer EP: The mechanism of syncope after coughing. Br Med J 1953;2:860–863.
24. Lipsitz LA, Wei JY, Rowe JW: Syncope in an elderly, institutionalized population: prevalence, incidence, and associated risk. QJ Med 1985; 55:45–55.
25. Sharpey-Schafer EP, Hayter CJ, *et al.*: Mechanism of acute hypotension from fear and nausea. Br Med J 1958;2:878–880.
26. Engel GL: Psychologic stress, vasodepressor (vasovagal) syncope and sudden death. Ann Intern Med 1978;89:403–412.
27. Sugrue DD, Wood DL, McGoon MD: Carotid sinus hypersensitivity and syncope. Mayo Clin Proc 1984;59:637–640.
28. Strasberg B, Sagie A, Erdman S, *et al.*: Carotid sinus hypersensitivity and the carotid sinus syndrome. Prog Cardiovasc Dis 1989;31:379–391.
29. Leatham A: Carotid sinus syncope. Br Heart J 1982;47:409–410.
30. Faulkner M, Sharpey-Schafer EP: Circulatory effects of trumpet playing. Br Med J 1959;1:685–686.
31. Klein LJ, Saltzman AJ, Heyman A, *et al.*: Syncope induced by the valsalva maneuver. Am J Med 1964;37:263–268.
32. Menzies DN: Syncope on pelvic examination (letter). Br Med J 1970; 716:221.
33. Levin B, Posner JB: Swallow syncope-report of a case and review of the literature. Neurology (Minneap) 1972;22:1086–1093.
34. Palmer ED: The abnormal upper gastrointestinal vasovagal reflexes that affect the heart. Am J Gastroenterology 1976;66:513–522.

35. Garretson HD, Elvidge AR: Glossopharyngeal neuralgia with asystole and seizures. Arch Neurol 1963;8:26–31.
36. Armstrong PW, McMillan DG, Simon JB: Swallow syncope. Can Med Assoc J 1985;132:1281–1284.
37. Grubb BP, Gerard G, Temesy-Armos P, *et al.*: Cerebral vasoconstriction during upright tilt induced syncope (Abstr). PACE 1991;14:662.
38. Abboud FM: Ventricular syncope. is the heart a sensory organ? (editorial). N Engl J Med 1989;320:390–392.
39. Come PC, Pitt B: Nitroglycerin-induced severe hypotension and bradycardia in patients with acute myocardial infarction. Circulation 1976;54:624–628.
40. Scherrer U, Vissing S, Morgan BJ, *et al.*: Vasovagal syncope after infusion of a vasodilator in a heart-transplant recipient. N Engl J Med 1990;322:602–604.
41. Waxman MB, Yao L, Cameron DA, *et al.*: Isoproterenol induction of vasodepressor-type reaction in vasodepressor-prone persons. Am J Cardiol 1989;63:58–65.
42. Barcroft H, Edholm OG, McMichael J, *et al.*: Posthaemorrhagic fainting. Lancet 1944;i:489–491.
43. Barcroft H, Edholm OG: On the vasodilatation in human skeletal muscle during posthemorrhagic fainting. J Physiol (Lond) 1945;104:161–175.
44. Oberg B, Thoren P: Increased activity in left ventricular receptors during hemorrhage or occlusion of caval veins in the cat. A possible cause of the vaso-vagal reaction. Acta Physiol Scand 1972;85:164–173.
45. Almquist A, Goldenberg IF, Milstein S, *et al.*: Provocation of bradycardia and hypotension by isoproterenol and upright posture in patients with unexplained syncope. N Engl J Med 1989;320:346–351.
46. Milstein S, Buetikofer J, Lesser J, *et al.*: Cardiac asystole: a manifestation of neurally mediated hypotension-bradycardia. J Am Coll Cardiol 1989;14: 1626–1632.
47. Maloney JD, Jaeger FJ, Fouad-Tarazi FM, *et al.*: Malignant vasovagal syncope: prolonged asystole provoked by head-up tilt. Cleve Clin J Med 1988;55:542–548.
48. Blanc JJ, Genet L, Forneiro I, *et al.*: Perte de connaissance breve: etiologie et demarche. Resultats d'une etude prospective. Presse Med 1989;18:923–926.
49. Morady F, Shen EN, Bhandari A, *et al.*: Clinical symptoms in patients with sustained ventricular tachycardia. West J Med 1985;142:341–344.
50. Radack KL: Syncope. Cost-effective patient workup. Postgrad Med 1986;80:169–178.
51. Gibson JC, Heitzman MR: Diagnostic efficacy of 24-hour electrocardiographic monitoring for syncope. Am J Cardiol 1984;53:1013–1017.
52. Winkle RA: Ambulatory electrocardiography. Mod Concepts Cardiovasc Dis 1980;49:7–12.
53. Camm AJ, Evans KE, Ward DE, *et al.*: The rhythm of the heart in active elderly subjects. Am Heart J 1981;99:598–603.
54. Linzer M, Pritchett ELC, Pontinen M, *et al.*: Incremental diagnostic yield of loop electrocardiographic recorders in unexplained syncope. Am J Cardiol 1990;66:214–219.
55. Palileo EV, Ashley WW, Swiryin S, *et al.*: Exercise provocable right ventricular outflow tract tachycardia. Am Heart J 1982;104:185–193.
56. Woelfel AK, Simpson RJ, Gettes LS, *et al.*: Exercise-induced distal atrioventricular block. J Am Coll Cardiol 1983;2:578–581.
57. Kuchar DL, Thorburn CW, *et al.*: Signal-averaged electrocardiogram for evaluation of recurrent syncope. Am J Cardiol 1986;58:949–953.
58. Gang ES, Peter T, Rosenthal ME, *et al.*: Detection of late potentials on the surface electrocardiogram in unexplained syncope. Am J Cardiol 1986;58:1014–1020.
59. Winters SL, Steward D, Gomes JA: Signal averaging of the surface QRS complex predicts inducibility of ventricular tachycardia in patients with syncope of unknown origin: a prospective study. J Am Coll Cardiol 1987;10:775–781.
60. Johnson WB, Milstein S, Reyes WJ, *et al.*: Head-up tilt testing for diagnostic evaluation of syncope of unknown origin. (Abstr). Circulation 1989(Pt II) 80:656.
61. Sra JS, Anderson AJ, Shabbir HS, *et al.*: Unexplained syncope evaluated by electrophysiologic studies and head-up tilt testing. Ann Intern Med 1991; 114:1013–1019.
62. Brooks R, Garan H, Ruskin JN: Evaluation of the patient with unexplained syncope. In Zipes DP, Jalife J (eds): Cardiac Electrophysiology: From Cell to Bedside. WB Saunders, Philadelphia, 1990:646–666.
63. Gulamhusein S, Naccarelli GV, Ko PT, *et al.*: Value and limitations of clinical electrophysiologic study in assessment of patients with unexplained syncope. Am J Med 1983;73:700–705.
64. Bass EB, Elson JJ, Fogoros RN, *et al.*: Long-term prognosis of patients undergoing electrophysiologic studies for syncope of unknown origin. Am J Cardiol 1988;62:1186–1191.
65. Akhtar M, Shenasa M, Denker S, *et al.*: Role of cardiac electrophysiologic studies in patients with unexplained recurrent syncope. PACE 1983;6:192–201.
66. Sharma AD, Klein GJ, Milstein S: Diagnostic assessment of recurrent syncope. PACE 1984;7:749–759.
67. Morady F, Shen E, Schwartz A, *et al.*: Long term follow-up of patients with recurrent unexplained syncope evaluated by electrophysiologic testing. J Am Coll Cardiol 1983;2:1053–1059.
68. Teichman SL, Felder SD, Matos JA: The value of electrophysiologic studies in syncope of undetermined origin: report of 150 cases. Am Heart J 1985;110:469–479.
69. Crozier IG, Ikram H: Electrophysiological evaluation and natural history of unexplained syncope (Abstr). Aust N Z J Med 1986;16:587.
70. Benditt DG, Milstein S, Goldstein MA, *et al.*: Sinus node dysfunction: pathophysiology, Clinical features, evaluation and treatment. In Zipes DP, Jalife J (eds): Cardiac Electrophysiology: From Cell to Bedside. WB Saunders, Philadelphia, 1990:708–734.
71. Mandel WJ, Hayakawa H, Allen HN, *et al.*: Assessment of sinus node function in patients with sick sinus syndrome. Circulation 1972;46:761–769.
72. Strauss HC, Saroff AL, Bigger JT Jr, *et al.*: Premature atrial stimulation as a key to the understanding of sinoatrial conduction in man. Circulation 1973;47:86–93.
73. Narula OS, Shanttha N, Vasquez M, *et al.*: A new method for measurement of sinoatrial conduction time. Circulation 1978;58:706–714.
74. Jose AD, Collison D: The normal range and the determinants of the intrinsic heart rate in man. Cardiovasc Res 1970;4:160–167.
75. Dhingra RC, Wyngham C, Bauernfeind R, *et al.*: Significance of block distal to the His bundle induced by atrial pacing in patients with chronic bifascicular block. Circulation 1979;7:1455–1464.
76. Twidale N, Heddle WF, Tonkin A: Procainamide administration during electrophysiologic study; utility as a provocative test for intermittent atrioventricular block. PACE 1988;11:1388–1397.
77. McAnulty JH, Rahimtoola SH, Murphy E, *et al.*: Natural history of "high risk" bundle branch block. Final report of a prospective study. N Engl J Med 1982;307:137–143.
78. Goldreyer BN, Kastor JA, Kershbaum KL: The hemodynamic effects of induced supraventricular tachycardia in man. Circulation 1976;54:783–789.
79. Curry PVL, Rowland F, Fox KM, *et al.*: The relationship between posture, blood pressure, and electrophysiologic properties in patients with supraventricular tachycardia. Arch Mal Coeur 1978;71:293–299.
80. Morady F: The spectrum of tachyarrhythmias in preexcitation syndromes. In Benditt DG, Benson DW (eds): Cardiac Preexciation Syndromes. Martinus Nijhoff, Boston, 1986:119–139.
81. Brownstein SL, Hopson RC, Martins JB, *et al.*: Usefulness of Isoproterenol in facilitating atrioventricular nodal reentry tachycardia during electrophysiologic testing. Am J Cardiol 1988;61:1037–1041.
82. Denes P, Ezri MD: The role of electrophysiologic studies in the management of patients with unexplained syncope. PACE 1985;8:424–435.
83. Olshansky B, Meir M, Martins JB: Significance of inducible tachycardia in patients with syncope of unknown origin: a long term follow-up. J Am Coll Cardiol 1985;5:216–223.

84. Wellens HJJ, Brugada P, Stevenson WG: Programmed electrical stimulation of the heart in patients with life-threatening ventricular arrhythmias: what is the significance of induced arrhythmias, and what is the correct stimulation protocol? Circulation 1985;72:1–7.
85. Brugada P, Green M, Abdollah H, *et al.*: Significance of ventricular arrhythmias initiated by programmed ventricular stimulation: the importance of the type of ventricular arrhythmia induced and the number of premature stimuli required. Circulation 1984;69:87–92.
86. Kenny RA, Bayliss J, Ingram A, *et al.*: Head-up tilt: a useful test for investigating unexplained syncope. Lancet 1986;1:1352–1355.
87. Milstein S, Reyes WJ, Benditt DG: Upright body tilt for evaluation of patients with recurrent, unexplained syncope. PACE 1989;12:117–123.
88. Abi-Samra F, Maloney JD, Fouad-Tarazi M, *et al.*: The usefulness of head-up tilt testing and hemodynamic investigations in the workup of syncope of unknown origin. PACE 1988;11:1202–1214.
89. Chen XC, Milstein S, Dunnigan A, *et al.*: Reproducibility of upright tilt testing for eliciting neurally-mediated syncope (Abstr). Circulation 1988 (Pt II):78:951.
90. Blanc JJ, Genet L, Mansourati J, *et al.*: Interet du test d'inclination dans le diagnostic etiologique des pertes de connaissance. Presse Medi 1990; 19:857–859.
91. Raviele A, Gasparini G, Di Pede F, *et al.*: Sincopi di natura indeterminata dopo studio elettrofisiologico. Utilita dell'head-up tillt test nella diagnosi di origine vaso-vagale e nella scelta della terapia. G Ital Cardiol 1990;20:185–194.
92. Almquist A, Gornick CC, Benson DW Jr, *et al.*: Carotid sinus hypersensitivity: evaluation of the vasodepressor component. Circulation 1985;67:927–936.
93. Huang SKS, Ezri MD, Hauser DR, *et al.*: Carotid sinus hypersensitivity in patients with unexplained syncope: clinical, electrophysiologic, and long term follow-up observations. Am Heart J 1988;116:989–996.
94. Lown B, Levine JA. The carotid sinus. Clinical value of its stimulation. Circulation 1961;23:766–789.
95. Moazez F, Peter T, Simonson J, *et al.*: Syncope of unknown origin: clinical, noninvasive, and electrophysiologic determinants of arrhythmia induction and symptom recurrence during long term follow-up. Am Heart J 1991;121:81–88.
96. Kapoor WN: Evaluation and outcome of patients with syncope. Medicine 1990;69:160–175.
97. Chen MY, Goldenberg I, Milstein S, *et al.*: Cardiac electrophysiologic and hemodynamic correlates of neurally mediated syncope. Am J Cardiol 1989;63:66–72.
98. Perry JC, Garson A: The child with recurrent syncope: autonomic function testing and beta-adrenergic hypersensitivity. J Am Coll Cardiol 1991; 17:1168–1171.
99. Ferguson DW, Thames MD, Mark AL: Effects of propranolol on reflex vascular responses to orthostatic stress in humans; Role of ventricular baroreceptors. Circulation 1983;67:802–807.
100. Goldenberg IF, Almquist A, Dunbar D, *et al.*: Prevention of neurally-mediated syncope by selective beta-1 adrenoreceptor blockade (Abstr). Circulation 1987;76(Suppl IV): 133.
101. Milstein S, Buetikofer J, Lesser J, *et al.*: Usefulness of Disopyramide for prevention of upright tilt induced hypotension-bradycardia. Am J Cardiol 1990;65:1339–1344.
102. Brogden LM, Tod PA: Focus on disopyramide. Drugs 1987;34:151–187.
103. Benditt DG, Benson DW, Kreitt J, *et al.*: Electrophysiologic effects of theophyline in young patients with recurrent symptomatic bradyarrhythmias. Am J Cardiol 1983;52:1223–1229.
104. Raviele A, Proclemer A, Gasparini G, *et al.*: Long-term follow-up of patients with unexplained syncope and negative electrophysiologic study. Eur Heart J 1989;10:127–132.
105. McAnulty JH: Syncope. In Nacarelli GV (ed): Cardiac Arrhythmias: A Practical Approach. Futura Publishing Co. Mt. Kisco, NY, 1991.

6

EVALUATION OF A RESUSCITATED PATIENT WITH ABORTED SUDDEN CARDIAC DEATH

Igor Singer, M.B.B.S., F.R.A.C.P., F.A.C.P., F.A.C.C.

INTRODUCTION

Although the overall mortality from cardiovascular disease has been decreasing steadily, sudden cardiac death remains a major epidemiologic problem (1). It is estimated that over 400,000 persons die annually in the United States from sudden cardiac death each year (2,3). A major cause of sudden cardiac deaths in the Western Hemisphere is coronary artery disease (80%), with a smaller proportion of cases accounted for by cardiomyopathies (10–15%), valvular heart disease (5%), and infrequently, other cardiac diseases (4).

Most patients who die suddenly have significant coronary artery disease, often a previous history of myocardial infarction, angina pectoris or hypertension, and evidence of impaired left ventricular function (3). Rarely, sudden death is the first manifestation of coronary heart disease. In the coronary artery population group, certain patients are at a higher risk of sudden cardiac death: survivors of recent myocardial infarction (5–8), patients who have been resuscitated from aborted sudden cardiac death due to ventricular fibrillation (VF) unassociated with acute myocardial infarction (9–11) and patients with recurrent sustained ventricular tachycardia (VT) (12–13). Prior healed myocardial infarction has been observed in up to 75% of patients presenting with sudden cardiac death (14–16). Left ventricular and occasionally right ventricular hypertrophy have also been identified as independent risk factors of fatal ventricular arrhythmias (17).

Incidence of malignant ventricular arrhythmias is high also in patients with dilated cardiomyopathy (18,19). Approximately 50% of deaths in this patient population are due to sudden and unexpected cardiac death, resulting from VT or VF (20).

Another group includes patients without structural heart disease in whom electrical instability occurs as a result of congenital abnormalities, e.g., Wolff-Parkinson-White syndrome (21), or some acquired abnormality, e.g., conduction system disease (4).

PATHOPHYSIOLOGY

Ventricular fibrillation is the most common mechanism of sudden unexpected cardiac death in persons with asymptomatic or symptomatic coronary artery disease. No single mechanism or factor can explain all types of spontaneous or experimentally produced fibrillation. Ventricular fibrillation requires presence of: (a) a critical mass of myocardium to sustain fibrillation, (b) some excitable stimulus to initiate the arrhythmia and (c) a critical relationship between conduction velocity and refractory period duration in the entire myocardium, or parts of myocardium, to produce and maintain disorganized electrical activity. Factors that increase vulnerability to fibrillation include increased automaticity, electrical currents resulting from differences in the membrane potential during activity or at rest, and dispersion of refractoriness. Extensive discussion of VF is beyond the scope of this chapter. It is further discussed in Chapter 19.

It is now well recognized that the initiating mechanism of out-of-hospital VF is usually sustained VT, which subsequently degenerates into VF. The underlying mechanism of VT and VF is currently believed to be reentry (see Chapter 2). Reentry can occur only in a nonhomogeneous tissue in which conduction velocity and dispersion of refractoriness differ in various areas of myocardium. Slow conduction and depolarized myocardium may result from either activation of inward current flowing through the "slow channel," or depression of the Na^+ current flowing through the "rapid channel."

Various conditions may facilitate spontaneous VF. These include: (a) slow heart rate, (b) long QT syndrome (22), (c) hypokalemia (23), (d) acidosis (24), (e) proarrhythmia due to antiarrhythmic drugs (25,26), (f) digitalis intoxication (27), (g) sympathetic stimulation (28,29), (h) myocardial ischemia (30–32), and (i) reperfusion arrhythmias post–myocardial infarction (33–35).

In patients with coronary artery disease, fixed or variable obstruction resulting from coronary artery spasm leads to increased myocardial oxygen demand in the region of myocardium subserved

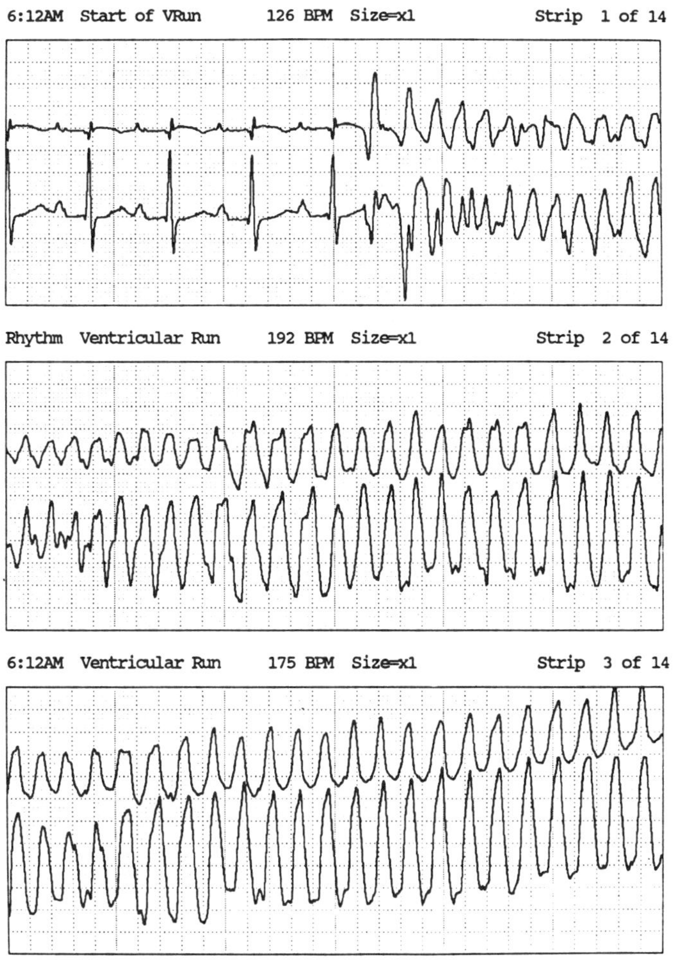

Figure 6.1. Holter recording in a patient with aborted sudden death documenting onset of a fast ventricular tachycardia resulting in syncope and ultimately in cardiac arrest.

by the affected vessel. Spasm of coronary arteries may lead to transient ischemia with subsequent reperfusion (36). Platelet aggregation and thrombosis may both be important in the initiation of the lethal arrhythmias (37–39). Endothelial damage leads to plaque fissuring and platelet activation and aggregation, followed by thrombosis. In addition, platelet activation produces a series of biochemical events that may enhance susceptibility to VF (40).

Transient ischemia may alter vulnerability to the initiation of fatal arrhythmias by generation of substances injurious to the cell membranes and lead to disturbances in ionic homeostasis. Reperfusion of ischemic myocardium may be important in altering the ionic fluxes subsequent to ischemic membrane damage. Metabolic changes include increases in interstitial potassium levels during ischemia, regional decreases in potassium levels in border cells of healed infarctions (41), changes in autonomic tone (42), elevation of myocardial cyclic adenosine monophosphate (cyclic-AMP), accumulation of free fatty acids and their metabolites, and impaired myocardial lypolisis (43).

Autonomic responses during acute myocardial ischemia may influence outcome, i.e., occurrence of VF (42). Experimental evidence suggests antifibrillatory effect of vagal activation and the reverse effects of sympathetic stimulation.

The pathophysiologic mechanisms in nonischemic cardiomyopathy are less well studied. Reentry, triggered activity and other mechanisms have been proposed as possible mechanisms of VF and ventricular tachycardia.

CLINICAL PRESENTATION

Sudden cardiac death has been defined as "natural death from cardiac causes, heralded by an abrupt loss of consciousness within one hour of the onset of acute symptoms in an individual with no known pre-existing heart disease, but in whom the time and the mode of death are unexpected" (4). Another commonly used definition of sudden death is death occurring within an hour of onset of symptoms. Rarely, a clinical prodrome consisting of nonspecific cardiovascular symptoms is seen prior to the sudden cardiac death. Usually, however, the onset of symptoms is abrupt with lightheadedness, dyspnea, and loss of consciousness. Cardiac arrest ensues, with abrupt loss of systemic perfusion and cerebral blood flow. In the majority of patients, ventricular fibrillation is preceded by ventricular tachycardia (Fig. 6.1), but occasionally ventricular fibrillation may be the initial dysrhythmia. In a minority of cases, bradyarrhythmias are the cause of the cardiac arrest (44).

Successful resuscitation depends on the setting in which the arrest occurs, the mechanism of the arrest and the underlying clinical status of the patient (45). The eventual outcome depends on the speed and the effectiveness of cardiac resuscitation (46). If VF is allowed to persist without intervention beyond 3–4 min, irreversible brain damage and death ensues.

Prognosis is dismal even in the individuals who are successfully resuscitated, if appropriate therapy designed to prevent further recurrence is not implemented. Of those patients who are successfully resuscitated, 40–60% die during initial hospitalization (46).

EVALUATION OF PATIENTS PRESENTING WITH ABORTED SUDDEN CARDIAC DEATH

The purpose of the clinical evaluation is to identify the cause, the precipitating and contributing factors, and to correct the underlying condition (when possible), and to protect the patient from a subsequent cardiac arrest. In general, both noninvasive and invasive studies may be helpful in the clinical evaluation (Table 6.1).

NON-INVASIVE STUDIES

Serum Electrolytes and Cardiac Enzymes

Exclusion of acute myocardial infarction is important. This may be accomplished by serial measurements of serum cardiac isoenzymes (creatine kinase (CK)-MB fractions and lactic dehydrogenase (LDH) isoenzymes) and serial 12-lead electrocardiogram

Table 6.1.
Tests Useful in Evaluating Patients Who Present with Aborted Sudden Cardiac Death

Noninvasive tests
Serum electrolytes: Na^+, Ca^{2+}, Mg^{2+}, arterial blood gas (pH)
Serial cardiac isoenzymes (CK-MB, LDH isoenzymes)
12-lead ECG
Holter monitoring, ambulatory ECG, telemetry
Signal-averaged ECG
Noninvasive tests of LV and RV function: 2D echo, radionuclide angiography, nuclear resonance imaging, fast CT scanning
Invasive tests
Coronary arteriography, left ventriculography
Right ventriculography (selected cases)
Right ventricular biopsy (selected cases)
Electrophysiologic studies
Initial diagnostic study
To guide antiarrhythmic drug therapy
To localize VT focus (preoperative and intraoperative mapping)
To test suitability for ICD therapy
To test ICD function (intraoperative and postoperative)

Abbreviations: CK-MB = creatine kinase-myocardial band; CT = computed tomography; ECG = electrocardiogram; ICD = implantable cardioverter-defibrillator; LDH = lactic dehydrogenase; LV = left ventricular; RV = right ventricular; 2D echo = two-dimensional echocardiography; VT = ventricular tachycardia.

(ECG) analysis. If the diagnosis is still in doubt, scintigraphic imaging with technetium-99m (Tc^{99m}) pyrophosphate or a combined (computed enhanced) technetium-99m (Tc^{99m}) pyrophosphate and thallium-201 ($thallium^{201}$) subtraction imaging, may be helpful.

Serum electrolyte disturbances may precipitate or cause cardiac arrest and therefore, should be sought and excluded. Disturbances in potassium, magnesium, calcium, and acid-base balance are of particular clinical importance. Digitalis toxicity and proarrhythmia due to antiarrhythmic drugs should also be excluded. Appropriate serum assays may be helpful in this regard.

12-Lead ECG

An abnormal ECG in an adult is most often associated with an acquired abnormality indicative of clinically evident or silent myocardial disease. The electrocardiographic abnormalities may include evidence of acute myocardial infarction or ischemia, intraventricular conduction defects, especially left bundle branch block, ST segment, and T wave changes associated with left ventricular hypertrophy or a prolonged QT interval.

The importance of a 12-lead ECG as a marker of risk has been emphasized by the Framingham study (46). Of the 234 deaths attributed to coronary heart disease in the Framingham study, 109 were sudden. Of these, 60% of patients had prior incidence of coronary heart disease. It was suggested that electrocardiographic pattern of left ventricular hypertrophy with both voltage and ST-T segment changes with presence of one or more conventional risk factors of coronary artery disease, suggests presence of ischemic heart disease. Such patients have a fivefold greater risk of sudden death than do those without such an electrocardiographic pattern (46).

The significance of bundle branch block as an independent marker for sudden death is controversial. Presence of bundle branch block, with or without an accompanying fascicular block is associated with higher mortality rate and incidence of sudden death (47). Prognostic value of bundle branch block in survivors of acute myocardial infarction differs from that of patients with other forms of heart disease. There is considerable evidence that bundle branch block appearing during acute myocardial ischemia, either transient or persistent, is accompanied by a significantly increased incidence of sudden cardiac deaths (47).

Role of Exercise Testing in Prediction of Sudden Death

Exercise testing has been utilized extensively to identify patients with coronary heart disease who are at increased risk of subsequent cardiac mortality, primarily due to coronary ischemia. The sensitivity of the exercise test may be enhanced by using scintigraphic imaging with thallium-201 ($thallium^{201}$) or newer imaging agents. In this clinical setting, exercise testing is of limited utility. However, exercise testing may provide prognostic information that is independent of other clinical variables and may have clinical utility for assessment of functional significance of coronary disease, particularly when combined with $thallium^{201}$ scintigraphy.

For patients unable to exercise, persantine or adenosine may be administered intravenously or orally with $thallium^{201}$ to assess functional significance of coronary disease.

24-Hr Holter Monitoring and Ambulatory Monitoring

Cardiac arrhythmias may be detected and quantified using ambulatory electrocardiographic monitoring. The technique has the advantage of being noninvasive and relatively inexpensive. It may be utilized to document the mechanism of sudden cardiac death (Fig. 6.1). Presence of advanced ventricular arrhythmias identifies patients with coronary heart disease who are at a relatively higher risk for sudden death in contrast to those without such arrhythmias. Presence of high-grade ventricular arrhythmias appears also to increase the risk of sudden death in patients with hypertrophic and dilated cardiomyopathy.

Left ventricular dysfunction is an independent and additive risk factor for subsequent development of sudden cardiac death. In all studies in which left ventricular function was assessed, either clinically or with noninvasive testing, ventricular arrhythmias were strongly associated with the presence of ventricular dysfunction. This has led some investigators to conclude that, although associated with increased risk of sudden death, ventricular ectopy is more a marker of left ventricular dysfunction than an independent prognostic indicator. However, more recent studies have suggested that arrhythmias and left ventricular dysfunction may be independent variables in conferring an increased risk for sudden death (48–54).

Twenty-four-hour Holter monitoring may also be helpful in identifying bradyarrhythmias, as a cause of cardiac arrest in patients with sinus node dysfunction or intermittent conduction abnormalities. Ambulatory monitoring has been used by some investigators for monitoring efficacy of antiarrhythmic therapy. However, the usefulness of this technique to monitor antiarrhythmic drug therapy in patients who present with aborted sudden cardiac death, is limited (see below).

Signal-Averaged ECG

Signal-averaged ECG has emerged as an important noninvasive test for assessment of risk for development of VT or VF. Detailed discussion of this diagnostic technique may be found in chapter 3.

The prognostic significance of late potentials, post–acute myocardial infarction, has been evaluated in several studies. Prospective studies by Gomes (55) *et al.* and Kuchar (56) *et al.* have examined the usefulness of signal-averaged ECG, Holter monitoring, and radionuclide ventriculography to predict VT and sudden cardiac death post–myocardial infarction. Multivariate analysis demonstrated that signal-averaged ECG, ejection fraction (EF) of <40%, or complex ventricular ectopic activity had independent predictive value for serous arrhythmic events after acute myocardial infarction.

These tests could be combined to more accurately identify the high-risk patients. Combination of signal-averaged ECG and low EF, for example, had the highest sensitivity and specificity in these studies. No patients with a normal signal-averaged ECG and an EF >40% had sustained VT or sudden cardiac death on follow-up, which ranged from 12 ± 6 mo (55) to 6–24 mo (56). In contrast, 34–36% of patients with an abnormal signal-averaged ECG and EF <40% had a life-threatening arrhythmic events during follow-up. A combination of an abnormal signal-averaged ECG and low EF had sensitivity of 80–100% and a specificity of up to 89% for predicting sudden death or sustained VT (55,56).

A more recent prospective study by Breithardt and Borgreffe (57) suggested that programmed electrical stimulation combined with signal-averaged ECG may be used to define the highest risk of development of sustained VT after an acute myocardial infarction. Patients at the highest risk were characterized by the presence of ventricular late potentials and an inducible sustained VT at a rate <270 beats/min.

Signal-averaged ECG may also prove useful in selecting patients who could benefit from more intense, prolonged monitoring after an acute myocardial infarction. The natural history of late potentials after myocardial infarction has been reported in several studies (58). Late potentials can be detected as early as 3 hr after the onset of chest pain. Prevalence of late potentials increases in the first week following acute myocardial infarction. In patients without late potentials, soon after myocardial infarction, the late potentials rarely develop after 12 months in the absence of reinfarction (59).

Many studies support the notion that signal-averaged ECG is a sensitive and a specific test for predicting inducibility of sustained VT during electrophysiologic study and has an independent predictive value (60–65). Signal-averaged ECG appears to be a useful screening test prior to electrophysiologic study to detect patients in whom sustained VT is likely to be inducible.

The role of signal-averaged ECG in predicting sudden cardiac death in patients with nonischemic cardiomyopathies, is less well defined. Late potentials have been detected in patients with arrhythmogenic right ventricular dysplasia (66). Relatively little information is available, however, on signal-averaged ECG in hypertrophic cardiomyopathy (67), and no prospective data are available on the value of signal-averaged ECG as a predictor of sudden cardiac death in patients with dilated cardiomyopathies.

Noninvasive Studies of Left Ventricular Function

Noninvasive studies of left ventricular infarction include two-dimensional (2D) echocardiography, transesophageal echocardiography, radionuclide angiography, and magnetic resonance imaging. These modalities are discussed in Chapter 3. The purpose of the noninvasive studies is to examine the cardiac structures, evaluate global ventricular function, and quantify the extent and the distribution of regional myocardial dysfunction.

Appropriate Selection of Noninvasive Studies

Selection of noninvasive tests to evaluate a specific patient or clinical problem should be based on clinical considerations and cost-effectiveness of individual studies. For example, gated blood pool scan provides a better estimate of global left ventricular systolic function, the echocardiogram may be better suited for diagnosis of valvular heart disease, hypertrophic cardiomyopathy, or right ventricular dysplasia. Therefore, when evaluation of valvular function is critical, 2D echocardiographic and Doppler techniques are preferred.

Similarly, if a patient has critical coronary artery disease by coronary arteriography necessitating coronary bypass surgery, scintigraphic thallium^{201} imaging may be superfluous. On the other hand, if the coronary artery lesions are of intermediate severity (50–70% stenoses) thallium^{201} exercise imaging or adenosine thallium^{201} imaging may be helpful to evaluate specific coronary artery lesions.

Sequencing and the choice of noninvasive testing is based on the clinical considerations.

Coronary Arteriography and Left Ventriculography

The majority of patients presenting with aborted sudden cardiac death have underlying coronary disease. Coronary arteriography is therefore, mandatory for evaluation of such patients. Presence of multivessel or segmental coronary artery disease identifies ischemia as a possible cause or the contributing factor in cardiac arrest. In such patients, reversal of ischemia, by percutaneous angioplasty or surgical revascularization, should be considered in the overall treatment strategy.

Contrast left ventriculography helps identify segmental wall motion abnormalities associated with coronary disease, presence of focal left ventricular infarct or aneurysm, regional akinesis or hypokinesis, and global hypokinesis associated with diffuse cardiomyopathies. In selected individuals, in whom right ventricular dysplasia is suspected, right ventriculography may also be useful.

Cardiac catheterization may also provide valuable information and hemodynamic data for assessment of severity of valvular stenosis and regurgitation, and may be helpful in evaluation of congenital heart disease.

Role of Electrophysiologic Studies

Patients who are resuscitated from cardiac arrest without a new Q-wave myocardial infarction are at a high risk for recurrent cardiac arrest and sudden death after discharge (67–72). In this subgroup of patients, recurrence is frequent. One- and 2-yr recurrence rates of cardiac arrest have been estimated to be 30 and 45%, respectively (68,72).

In the absence of antiarrhythmic drug therapy, ventricular arrhythmias can be initiated during electrophysiologic (EP) studies in 70–80% of patients resuscitated from cardiac arrest (73–78). In most instances, sustained monomorphic ventricular tachycardia may be initiated. In the remaining patients, polymorphic VT degenerating to VF or nonsustained VT may be initiated. Sustained monomorphic VT or polymorphic VT degenerating into VF are accepted therapeutic endpoints, whereas nonsustained VT as a guide to therapy is a more controversial endpoint.

Aggressive stimulation protocols, using up to three extrastimuli increase the likelihood of inducing sustained VT or VF. The reproducibility of inducing sustained VT in patients with coronary disease is high (up to 95%) (79–81). Furthermore, induction of sustained VT provides an objective endpoint by which to evaluate prospective therapeutic modalities including antiarrhythmic drugs. Induction of VF at EP study in this setting is an acceptable endpoint. Inducible VF may be related to ischemia or reentry or a combination of both mechanisms.

Identification of an effective drug regimen, which suppressed induced VT or VF, has been reported in 26–80% of survivors of cardiac arrest (73–78). Those patients whose arrhythmias remain inducible at the time of hospital discharge are at a substantially higher risk for recurrent cardiac arrest and sudden death. Those patients in whom arrhythmias have been suppressed, have an estimated risk of recurrence of sudden cardiac death of 6% at 1 yr and 15% at 3 yr (73–78). Cardiac arrest survivors whose arrhythmias remain electrically inducible despite drug therapy should be considered for nonpharmacologic therapy, including arrhythmia surgery and automatic implantable defibrillators (see Chapters 20 and 23). Inducible VF may be supressed by coronary artery revascularization and VT by endocardial map-directed surgery in approximately 20% of patients (73–77).

Occasionally, ventricular arrhythmias may not be induced during baseline electrophysiologic studies. Noninducibility is observed in 20–30% of survivors of cardiac arrest and is associated with variable prognosis. Patients with depressed left ventricular function, in whom reversible cause of arrhythmia cannot be identified (e.g., ischemia), remain at a significant risk for recurrent cardiac arrest despite noninducibility (73–78). Those patients should also be considered for implantation of an automatic defibrillator. On the other hand, patients with reversible ischemia and preserved left ventricular function have a favorable prognosis when treated by revascularization (78).

Patients with nonischemic heart disease who have survived cardiac arrest have less favorable prognosis even when left ventricular function is well preserved (73–77). Patients without structural heart disease and those with the long QT interval syndrome are rarely inducible by programmed cardiac stimulation (73–77), but their prognosis is nevertheless not benign.

The American College of Cardiology/American Heart Association (ACC/AHA) task force (82) recommends that EP studies be performed in all patients surviving an episode of cardiac arrest without evidence of an acute Q-wave myocardial infarction and in patients surviving an episode of cardiac arrest occurring more than 48 hr after acute myocardial infarction (Class I indications).

Class II indication for EP study (conditions for which EP studies are frequently performed but where there is less certainty regarding the usefulness of the information that is obtained) includes patients surviving cardiac arrest due to bradyarrhythmias.

Electrophysiologic studies are not recommended in patients with cardiac arrest occurring within the first 48 hr of acute myocardial infarction, or in patients with cardiac arrest resulting from acute reversible ischemia or another clearly identifiable cause.

Details of electrophysiologic study techniques are discussed further in Chapter 4 with specific emphasis on assessment of VT in Chapter 8. Briefly, the purpose of the EP study is: (a) to identify the underlying EP mechanism underlying cardiac arrest, (b) to document associated EP abnormalities (e.g., presence of supraventricular arrhythmias, conduction abnormalities, or sinus node disease), and (c) to characterize the nature of the underlying arrhythmia. Electrophysiologic studies may be used to guide antiarrhythmic drug therapy, or to select patients who are likely to benefit from automatic implantable defibrillator therapy and may be used to guide surgical interventions, including subendocardial resection, with or without aneurysectomy. In rare instances, mechanism of sudden death may be identified as long QT syndrome or atrial fibrillation associated with Wolff-Parkinson-White syndrome with rapid antegrade conduction through an accessory tract.

For patients with suspected but undocumented atrioventricular (AV) conduction abnormality as the cause of sudden cardiac death invasive electrophysiologic studies are helpful for assessment of sinus node, AV node function, and infranodal conduction. His bundle recording may be helpful. An HV interval ≥ 100 msec (83) or intermittent AV block distal to the His during atrial pacing, is associated with a strong propensity for development of complete heart block. Presence of complete heart block, without an effective escape rhythm, may result in sudden death.

In patients in whom sinus node dysfunction is suspected, sinus node testing may provide evidence of mechanism of bradyarrhythmic cardiac arrest. For example, sinus node recovery testing (see Chapter 5) may unmask prolonged asystolic pauses following overdrive suppression of sinus node by rapid atrial pacing. The sensitivity of sinus node testing however, is relatively low and normal results do not exclude sinus node dysfunction.

TREATMENT OF ABORTED SUDDEN CARDIAC DEATH

Treatment of aborted sudden cardiac death depends on the EP mechanism and associated cardiac disease. If the underlying mechanism of cardiac arrest is ischemia, therapy should be directed toward reversal of ischemia, which may be achieved by catheter directed methods, e.g., percutaneous angioplasty, atherectomy, or combined procedures, or by surgical revascularization techniques. However, long-term results with revascularization alone, in patients with left ventricular dysfunction and ventricular dysrhythmias, is disappointing (85–87). Recurrence of VT or occurrence of sudden cardiac death is more likely in patients with depressed left ventricular function and documented VT, particularly when VT presents with hemodynamic collapse (88–92).

Antiarrhythmic drug therapy has been the cornerstone of therapy for patients presenting with malignant VT or VF. Both Holter guided therapy and EP testing have been used to monitor and assess appropriate antiarrhythmic drug therapy.

Holter guided antiarrhythmic drug therapy in this subset of patients has a number of possible disadvantages: (a) control of ventricular ectopy in patients with significant left ventricular dysfunction (left ventricular ejection fraction (LVEF) < 30%) does not significantly improve outcome with respect to risk of sudden cardiac death (88), (b) approximately one half of patients with VF do not have significant baseline ectopy to use as a guide for antiarrhythmic therapy (93) (c) hemodynamic consequences of arrhythmias cannot be assessed by this method, even though hemodynamic collapse during VT has been identified as a significant predictor of worse outcome (91), and (d) no information regarding the location of the tachycardia focus or the usefulness of pacing and defibrillation therapy can be assessed by this technique.

Selection of antiarrhythmic drugs for therapy of VT is based on serial drug testing (see Chapters 4 and 11). Type IA antiarrhythmic drugs are usually tested initially. Inability to induce VT after intravenous procainamide appears to be predictive of subsequent drug efficacy during serial drug testing (93).

Type IA drugs are often combined with Type IB drugs when ventricular tachycardia remains inducible on a single drug (94). Type IC drugs are generally tested next, but must be used with caution in patients with left ventricular dysfunction, since they significantly depress left ventricular function and have somewhat greater propensity to be proarrhythmic (95–97).

Amiodarone has the greatest efficacy of all antiarrhythmic drugs, but unfortunately it also has long-term side effects which may be serious (98). Noninducibility on amiodarone is associated with better prognosis than continued VT inducibility (99–101). Easier inducibility during therapy, compared to baseline EP study or induction of hemodynamically unstable VT on amiodarone, predicts drug failure (102). The effectiveness of long-term therapy with amiodarone has not been compared directly with efficacy of automatic implantable defibrillators in prospective randomized trials, though such trials are currently being contemplated or are underway. Combination of amiodarone with other antiarrhythmic drugs (Type IA or Type IB) has also been employed with encouraging results (103–105).

It is important to note that antiarrhythmic drugs can be given as primary therapy to prevent recurrences of VT or VF or as a secondary therapy to prevent arrhythmias, e.g., non-sustained VT or atrial fibrillation in patients with implanted implantable cardiac defibrillators (ICDs). Primary antiarrhythmic drug therapy should be reserved for patients with inducible hemodynamically stable VT and an ejection fraction (EF) of > 30%, or patients who refuse ICD or are not candidates for surgical therapy. Coronary revascularization should be performed in all patients with significant ischemia even when drug therapy is employed primarily.

A successful drug regimen may be found in about 20–30% of patients using EP testing, with worse outcome in patients with pronounced left ventricular dysfunction (106).

The role of EP studies in predicting long-term outcome of out-of-hospital cardiac arrest survivors, not associated with myocardial infarction, was examined by Wilber *et al.* (78) Ventricular arrhythmias were inducible in 79% of baseline studies and were suppressed by antiarrhythmic drugs or surgery (or both) in 72% of patients. During a median follow-up period of 21 months, recurrent cardiac arrest occurred in 12% of patients in whom the arrhythmias were suppressed, 33% of patients in whom arrhythmias remained inducible, and 17% of patients in whom arrhythmias could not be induced at the baseline EP study. Independent predictors of recurrent cardiac arrest were persistence of ventricular arrhythmias, left ventricular dysfunction (LVEF < 30%) and absence of cardiac surgery. Thus, although noninducibility on EP study confers better prognosis, the noninducible patients still remain at significant risk of sudden cardiac death. This consideration has led some investigators to argue that antiarrhythmic therapy alone is insufficient to guarantee freedom from subsequent cardiac arrhythmic death and to conclude that ICD therapy alone, or in combination with antiarrhythmic drugs or surgery, should be considered in this patient population (107).

The enthusiasm for ICD therapy is based on over a decade of clinical experience demonstrating ICD efficacy in preventing sudden deaths due to VT/VF. The reported sudden death mortality in ICD-treated patients reported in one of the largest clinical

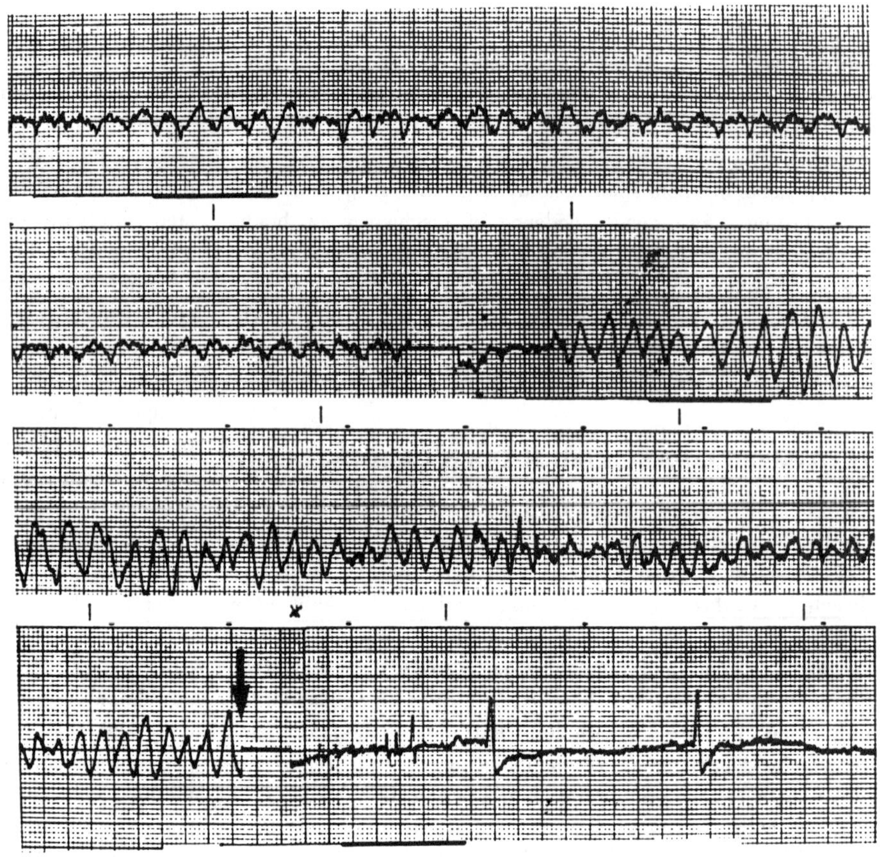

Figure 6.2. Patient with implanted ICD. Ventricular fibrillation is noted on telemetry. The arrhythmia is appropriately recognized by the ICD and treated (*arrow* denotes the ICD discharge) with resumption of sinus rhythm.

series by Winkle *et al.*, is 1% at 1 yr and 4% at 5 yr, with a total mortality of 7% at 1 yr and 26% at 5 yr, despite significant LV dysfunction (108). Similarly, favorable results have been reported by other independent investigators (109–112). These data are further corroborated in the Cardiac Pacemakers, Inc. (CPI) (St. Paul, MN) registry (the largest worldwide registry of patients with implanted ICDs (see Chapter 20)).

The critical factor influencing survival and subsequent recovery in patients who present with aborted sudden cardiac death episode, is the rapidity with which they are resuscitated. Since ICDs can deliver the defibrillation shock within 10–20 sec of the onset of VT or VF, cerebral damage and indeed even syncope due to hypoperfusion may be prevented effectively. Irrespective of how efficient the resuscitation effort might be, even within an intensive care setting with immediate availability of experienced trained personnel, this goal cannot be rivaled (Fig. 6.2).

Only a fraction of patients who present with aborted sudden cardiac death are successfully resuscitated and transported to clinical centers where further intervention is available to treat and prevent subsequent recurrences (1,2,4). These discouraging statistics have inspired a search for ways of identifying the high-risk patient before sudden cardiac death occurs so that effective therapy is instituted prior to the event (48–56).

Cardiac Arrhythmia Suppression Trial (CAST) demonstrated that despite considerable suppression of spontaneous ventricular arrhythmias in a high-risk postinfarction group (patients with low EF and ventricular arrhythmias) mortality was increased substantially during treatment with encainide or flecainide compared to the placebo-treated group, with no benefit in the moricizine-treated group (13,114). This was the first large-scale controlled clinical trial to attempt to evaluate whether suppression of ventricular arrhythmias post–myocardial infarction would improve survival. The increased mortality with antiarrhythmic drugs with Class I action prompted a review of smaller trials with analysis further supporting the findings of the CAST trial (115,116).

The evidence of lack of efficacy of antiarrhythmic drugs in "completely" preventing arrhythmia events and sudden cardiac death has stimulated interest in ICD therapy. Some of the extensions of ICD therapy, which have been proposed for patients with established ventricular arrhythmias have included the following: (a) earlier use of ICD in treatment sequence (107), (b) ICD treatment for patients with malignant VT and who have LVEF <0.40 and whose inducible sustained VT is unresponsive to intravenous procainamide (78), and (c) proposals to evaluate ICD therapy in several high-risk groups of patients (117,118). Since ICD therapy has been demonstrated to be very effective for therapy of recurrent VT and VF (107–113), the idea that arrhythmic cardiac death may be prevented by implantation of an ICD prior to such an event, so-called prophylactic ICD implantation, was conceived. A number of large-scale, multicenter, prospective studies of prophylactic use of ICDs in high-risk patient populations are underway to establish the role of this preventive treatment strategy. These include "CABG Patch" (coronary artery disease patients with positive late potentials and left ventricular EF below 0.36 who are already scheduled for bypass surgery) (119,120), "MUSTT" (asymptomatic nonsustained ventricular tachycardia, late potentials, and LVEF below 0.40), and "MADIT" (coronary artery disease patients with nonsustained VT, inducible and not suppressed by procainamide, and LVEF below 0.36, who are not suitable for bypass) (121).

Another potential area for prophylactic ICDs has been suggested for patients with congestive heart failure, who are known to have malignant ventricular dysrrhythmias, and who will ultimately undergo heart transplantation, as a bridge, to prevent sudden arrhythmic death prior to the transplantation. Scientific studies are now being developed and are expected to get underway in the near future (122).

It is anticipated that the results of these and possibly other prospective randomized studies will become available in the next 3–5 yr. If clear advantage of prophylactic ICD therapy is demonstrated in these high-risk patients, it is possible that prophylactic ICD implantation will become the therapy of choice for prevention of sudden cardiac death due to VT and VF. As technology advances, and smaller devices (<120 g) become available, coupled with the development of the endocardial defibrillation electrodes (some are already in the clinical trials), it is conceivable that implantation of the future devices will be simplified, so that the endocardial leads and the ICD generator may be implanted in the electrophysiology laboratory without a need for thoracotomy (see Chapter 20).

The role of ablative surgery for therapy of ventricular tachycardia is discussed in detail in Chapter 23. In general, patients most suitable for surgical ablation (endocardial resection, aneurysmectomy, cryoablation, or laser assisted surgical ablation) are patients with a single morphology, monomorphic ventricular tachycardia refractory to pharmacologic therapy, associated with a focal scar or ventricular aneurysm, with moderately well-preserved left ventricular function. Most postoperative deaths are due to heart failure. The highest risk for postoperative mortality is associated with left ventricular dysfunction (EF <20%) patients with both previous anterior and inferior myocardial infarctions and with prior heart surgery (123). Localized resection of sites of VT guided by endocardial mapping in selected patients, in experienced clinical centers, have resulted in 90% cure rate and operative mortality of 5–15% (124,125). Patients who remain inducible postoperatively should be considered for implantation of an implantable defibrillator. The role of arrhythmia surgery alone, or in combination with ICD therapy, versus ICD therapy, for patients with malignant ventricular dysrhythmias, has not been studied in a prospective randomized fashion. Since arrhythmic surgery is most beneficial for a specific subgroup of patients (especially those with a localized scar or aneurysm), it is less likely that arrhythmia surgery would be found to be more beneficial than ICD therapy.

Therapy for documented bradyarrhythmias due to sinus node dysfunction or conduction disease resulting in complete heart block or Mobitz 2 AV block is treated by pacemaker implantation. This subject is discussed at length in Chapters 14–18.

CONCLUSION

Sudden cardiac death is an important clinical problem. Electrophysiologic techniques and evolution of antiarrhythmic drug therapy, implantable defibrillators, and effective surgical therapies for ventricular dysrhythmias have improved the overall survival of patients presenting with aborted sudden cardiac death. Further improvements in survival may be anticipated if prophylactic ICD implantation for high-risk patients proves to be beneficial in the ongoing clinical trials (118–122). Studies to identify and treat high-risk patients with implantation of an automatic defibrillator prior to the occurrence of cardiac arrest are currently in progress. In the next 3–5 yr, the results of these randomized prospective trials will become available, establishing the role of prophylactic ICD implantation for prevention of sudden cardiac death.

References

1. Lown B: Sudden cardiac death: the major challenge confronting contemporary cardiology. Am J Cardiol 1979;43:313–328.
2. National Center for Health Statistics: Advance Report, Final Mortality Statistics, 1981. Monthly Vital Statistics, Vol. 33 (Suppl 3): DHHS Pub. No. (PHS) 84-1120:4–5.
3. Gordon T, Kannel WB: Premature mortality from coronary heart disease. The Framingham Study. JAMA 1971:215:1617–1625.
4. Myerburg RJ, Castellanos A: Cardiac arrest and sudden cardiac death. In Braunwald E (ed): Heart Disease: A Textbook of Cardiovascular Medicine, 3rd ed. Philadelphia, WB Saunders, 1987:742–777.
5. Cobb LA, Werner JA: Predictors and prevention of sudden cardiac death. In: The Heart, 5th ed. Hurst JW (ed): McGraw-Hill, New York, 1982;32:599–610.
6. Bigger JT Jr, Fleiss JL, Kleiger RE, *et al.*: The Multicenter Post-Infarction Research Group. The relationships among ventricular arrhythmias, left ventricular dysfunction and mortality in the 2 years after myocardial infarction. Circulation 1984;69:250–258.
7. Moss AJ, Davis HT, DeCamilla J, *et al.*: Ventricular ectopic beats and their relation to sudden and nonsudden cardiac death after myocardial infarction. Circulation 1978;60:998–1003.
8. Maisel AS, Scott N, Gilpin E, *et al.*: Complex ventricular arrhythmias in patients with Q wave versus non-Q wave myocardial infarction. Circulation 1985;72:963–970.
9. Cobb LA, Baum RS, Alvarez H III, *et al.*: Resuscitation from out-of-hospital ventricular fibrillation: 4 year follow-up. Circulation 1975;52(Suppl III):III-223–8.
10. Schaffer WA, Cobb LA: Recurrent ventricular fibrillation and modes of death in survivors or aborted sudden cardiac death.
11. Baum RS, Alvarez H, Cobb LA: Survival after resuscitation from out-of-hospital ventricular fibrillation. Circulation 1974;50:1231–1235.
12. Mason JW, Winkle RA. Accuracy of ventricular tachycardia-induction study for predicting long-term efficacy and inefficacy of antiarrhythmic drugs. N Engl J Med 1980;303:1073–1077.
13. The Cardiac Arrhythmia Suppression Trial (CAST) Investigators: Preliminary report: effect on encainide and flecainide on mortality in a randomized trial of arrhythmia suppression after myocardial infarction. N Engl J Med 1989;321:406–412.

14. Friedman M, Manwaring JH, Rosenman RH, *et al.*: Instantaneous and sudden deaths: Clinical and pathological differentiation in coronary artery disease. JAMA 1973;225:1319–1328.
15. Reichenbach DD, Moss NS, Meyer E: Pathology of the heart in sudden cardiac death. Am J Cardiol 1977;39:865–872.
16. Newman WP, Strong JP, Johnson WD, *et al.*: Community pathology of atherosclerosis and coronary heart disease in New Orleans: Morphologic findings in young black and white men. Lab Invest 1981;44:496–501.
17. Gordon T, Kannel WB: Premature mortality from coronary heart disease. The Framingham Study. JAMA 1971;215:1617–1625.
18. Meinertz T, Hoffmann T, Kasper W, *et al.*: Significance of ventricular arrhythmias in idiopathic dilated cardiomyopathy. Am J Cardiol 1984; 53:902–907.
19. Chakko CS, Gheorghiade M: Ventricular arrhythmias in severe heart failure: Incidence, significance, and effectiveness of antiarrhythmic therapy. Am Heart J 1985;109:497–504.
20. Packer M: Sudden unexpected death in patients with congestive heart failure: A second frontier. Circulation 1985;72:681–685.
21. Kline GJ, Bashore TM, Sellers TD, *et al.*: Ventricular fibrillation in the Wolff-Parkinson-White syndrome. N Engl J Med 1979;301:1080–1085.
22. James TN: Congenital deafness and cardiac arrhythmias. Am J Cardiol 1967;19:627–643.
23. Surawicz B: Arrhythmias and electrolyte disturbances. Bull NY Acad Med 1967;43:1160–1180.
24. Gerst PH, Fleming WH, Malm JR: Increased susceptibility of the heart to ventricular fibrillation during metabolic acidosis. Circ Res 1966;19:63–70.
25. Koster RW, Wellens HJJ: Quinidine-induced ventricular flutter and fibrillation. Am J Cardiol 1976;38:519–523.
26. Ruskin JM, McGovern B, Garan H, *et al.*: Antiarrhythmic drugs: a possible cause of out-of-hospital cardiac arrest. N Engl J Med 1983;309:1302–1306.
27. Vassalle M, Karis J, Hoffman BF: Toxic effects of ouabain on Purkinje fibers and ventricular muscle fibers. Am J Physiol 1962;203:433–439.
28. Verrier RL, Thompson PL, Lown B: Ventricular vulnerability during sympathetic stimulation: role of heart rate and blood pressure. Cardiovasc Res 1974;8:602–610.
29. Verrier RL, Calvert A, Lown B: Effect of posterior hypothalamic stimulation on ventricular fibrillation threshold. Am J Physiol 1975;228:923–927.
30. Russell DC, Oliver MF. Ventricular refractoriness during acute myocardial ischemia and its relationship to ventricular fibrillation. Cardiovasc Res 1978;12:221–227.
31. Naimi S, Avitall B, Mieszala J, *et al.*: Dispersion of effective refractory period during abrupt reperfusion of ischemic myocardium in dogs. Am J Cardiol 1977;39:407–412.
32. Battle WE, Naimi S, Avittal B, *et al.*: Distinctive time course of ventricular vulnerability to fibrillation during and after release of coronary ligation. Am J Cardiol 1974;34:42–47.
33. Murdock DK, Loeb JM, Euler DE, *et al.*: Electrophysiology of coronary reperfusion a mechanism for reperfusion arrhythmias. Circulation 1980;61:175–182.
34. Levine HJ, Avitall B, Pauker SG, *et al.*: Sequential unipolar strength-interval curves and conduction times during myocardial ischemia and reperfusion in the dog. Circ Res 1978;43:63–72.
35. Corbalan R, Verrier RL, Lown B: Differing mechanisms for ventricular vulnerability during coronary artery occlusion and release. Am Heart J 1976;92:223–230.
36. Schamroth L: Mechanism of lethal arrhythmias in sudden death. Possible role of vasospasm and release. Pract Cardiol 1981;7:105–115.
37. Haerem JW: Mural platelet microthombi and major acute lesions of main epicardial arteries in sudden coronary death. Atherosclerosis 1974;19:529–541.
38. Baroldi G, Faizi G, Mariana F: Sudden coronary death: A post-mortem study in 208 selected cases compared to 97 "control" subjects. Am Heart J 1979;98:20–31.
39. Mehta J, Mehta P: Role of platelets and prostaglandins in coronary artery disease. Am J Cardiol 1981;48:366–373.
40. Hammon JW, Oates JA: Interaction of platelets with the vessel wall in the pathophysiology of sudden cardiac death. Circulation 1986;73:224–226.
41. Kimura S, Bassett AL, Gaide MS, *et al.*: Regional changes in intracellular potassium and sodium activity after healing of experimental myocardial infarction in cats. Circ Res 1986;58:202–208.
42. Surawicz B: Ventricular fibrillation. J Am Coll Cardiol (Suppl B) 1985; 51:43–54.
43. Opie LH: Products of myocardial ischemia and electrical instability of the heart. J Am Coll Cardiol (Suppl B) 1985;5:161–165.
44. Myerburg RJ, Conde CA, Sung RJ, *et al.*: Clinical, electrophysiologic, and hemodynamic profile of patients resuscitated from prehospital cardiac arrest. Am J Med 1980;68:568–576.
45. Standard and guidelines for cardiopulmonary resuscitation (CPR) and emergency cardiac care (ECC). Part II Adult Basic Life Support Product of National Conference Cardiopulmonary Resuscitation (CPR) and Emergency Cardiac Care. JAMA 1986;255:2915–2954.
46. Myerburg KJ, Kessler KM, Zaman, *et al.*: Factors leading to decreasing mortality among patients resuscitated from out-of-hospital cardiac arrest. In Bruguda P, Weller MJJ (eds): Cardiac Arrhythmias: Where Do We Go from Here? Mt. Kisco, NY, Futura Publishing Co., 1987:505–552.
47. Fisch GR, Zipes DP, Fisch C: Bundle branch block and sudden death. Prog Cardiovasc Dis 1980;23:187–224.
48. Moss AJ, Davis HT, DeCamilla J, *et al.*: Ventricular ectopic beats and their relation to sudden and nonsudden cardiac death after myocardial infarction. Circulation 1979;60:998–1003.
49. Ruberman W, Weinblatt E, Goldberg JD, *et al.*: Ventricular premature complexes and sudden death after myocardial infarction. Circulation 1981;64:297–305.
50. Bigger JT, Weld FM, Rolnitzky LM: Prevalence, characteristics and significance of ventricular tachycardia (three or more complexes) detected with ambulatory electrocardiographic recording in the late hospital phase of acute myocardial infarction. Am J Cardiol 1981;48:815–823.
51. Bigger JT, Weld FM, Rolnitzky LM: Which postinfarction ventricular arrhythmias should be treated? Am Heart J 1982;103:660–665.
52. Multicenter Postinfarction Research Group: Risk stratification and survival after myocardial infarction. N Engl J 1983;309:331–336.
53. Bigger JT, Fleiss JL, Kleiger R, *et al.*: Multicenter postinfarction research group. The relationships among ventricular arrhythmias, left ventricular dysfunction, and mortality in the 2 years after myocardial infarction. Circulation 1984;69:250–258.
54. Bigger JT: Patients with malignant or potentially malignant ventricular arrhythmias: opportunities and limitations of drug therapy in prevention of sudden death. J Am Coll Cardiol 1985;5:23B–26B.
55. Gomes JA, Winters SL, Stewart D, *et al.*: A new noninvasive index to predict sustained ventricular tachycardia and sudden death in patients in the first year after myocardial infarction: based on signal averaged electrocardiogram, radionuclide ejection fraction and Holter monitoring. J Am Coll Cardiol 1987;10:349–357.
56. Kuchar DL, Thorburn CW, Sammel NL: Predictor of serious arrhythmic events after myocardial infarction: signal-averaged electrocardiogram, Holter monitoring and radionuclide ventriculography. J Am Coll Cardiol 1987; 9:531–538.
57. Breithardt G, Borgreffe M: Pathophysiological mechanisms and clinical significance of ventricular late potentials. Eur Heart J 1986;7:364–385.
58. McGuire M, Kuchar D, Gamis J, *et al.*: Natural history of late potentials in the first ten days after acute myocardial infarction and relation to ventricular arrhythmias. Am J Cardiol 1988;61:1187–1190.
59. Kuchar DL, Thorburn CW, Sammel NL: Late potentials detected after myocardial infarction: natural history and prognostic significance. Circulation 1986;74:1280–1289.
60. Buckingham TA, Thessen CC, Stevens RM, *et al.*: Effects of conduction defects on the signal-averaged electrocardiographic determination of late potentials. Am J Cardiol 1988;61:1265–1271.
61. Freedman RA, Gillis AM, Karen A, *et al.*: Signal-averaged electrocardiogra-

phic late potentials in patients with ventricular fibrillation or ventricular tachycardia: correlation with clinical arrhythmia and electrophysiologic study. Am J Cardiol 1985;55:1350–1353.
62. Denniss AR, Ross DL, Richards DA, *et al.*: Differences between patients with ventricular tachycardia and ventricular fibrillation as assessed by signal-averaged electrocardiogram, radionuclide ventriculography and cardiac mapping. J Am Coll Cardiol 1988;11:276–283.
63. Denniss AR, Richards DA, Cody DV, *et al.*: Prognostic significance of ventricular tachycardia and ventricular fibrillation induced by programmed stimulation and delayed potentials detected on the signal-averaged electrocardiogram of survivors of acute myocardial infarction. Circulation 1986;74:731–745.
64. Lindsay BD, Ambos HD, Schechtner KB, *et al.*: Improved selection of patients for programmed ventricular stimulation by frequency analysis of signal-averaged electrocardiograms. Circulation 1986;73:675–683.
65. Kapoor WN, Karpf M, Wieard S, *et al.*: A prospective evaluation and follow up of patients with syncope. N Engl J Med 1983;309:197–204.
66. Abboud S, Belhasser B, Laniado S, *et al.*: Non-invasive recording of late ventricular activity using an advanced method in patients with damaged mass of ventricular tissue. Electrocardiology 1983;16:245–252.
67. Garaghan TP, Kelly RP, Kuchar DL, *et al.*: The prevalance of arrhythmias in hypertrophic cardiomyopathy: role of ambulatory monitoring and signal-averaged electrocardiography. Aust NZ J Med 1986;16:666–670.
68. Liberthson RR, Nagel EL, Hirschman JC, *et al.*: Prehospital ventricular defibrillation: prognosis and follow-up course. N Engl J Med 1974;291:317–321.
69. Baum RS, Alvarez H III, Cobb LA: Survival after resuscitation and out-of-hospital ventricular fibrillation. Circulation 1974;50:1231–1235.
70. Schaffer WA, Cobb LA: Recurrent ventricular fibrillation and modes of death in survivors of out-of-hospital ventricular fibrillation. N Engl J Med 1975;293;259–262.
71. Weaver WD, Lorch GS, Alvarez HA, *et al.*: Angiographic findings and prognostic indicators in patients resuscitated from sudden cardiac death. Circulation 1976;54:895–900.
72. Josephson ME, Horowitz LN, Spielman SR, *et al.*: Electrophysiologic and hemodynamic studies in patients resuscitated from cardiac arrest. Am J Cardiol 1980;46:948–955.
73. Ruskin JN, DiMarco JP, Garan H: Out-of-hospital cardiac arrest. Electrophysiologic observations and selection of long-term antiarrhythmic therapy. N Engl J Med 1980;303:607–612.
74. Morady F, Scheinman MM, Hess DS, *et al.*: Electrophysiologic testing in the management of survivors of out-of-hospital cardiac arrest. Am J Cardiol 1983;51:85–89.
75. Roy D, Waxman HL, Kienzle MG, *et al.*: Clinical characteristics and long-term follow-up in 119 survivors of cardiac arrest: relation to inducibility at electrophysiologic testing. Am J Cardiol 1983;52:969–974.
76. Benditt DG, Benson DW Jr, Klein GJ, *et al.*: Prevention of recurrent sudden cardiac arrest: role of provocative electropharmacologic testing. J Am Coll Cardiol 1983;2:418–425.
77. Skale BT, Miles WM, Heger JJ, *et al.*: Survivors of cardiac arrest: prevention of recurrence by drug therapy as predicted by electrophysiologic testing or ECG monitoring. Am J Cardiol 1986;57:113–119.
78. Wilber DJ, Garan H, Finklestein D, *et al.*: Out-of-hospital cardiac arrest: role of electrophysiologic testing in prediction of long term oucome. N Engl J Med 1988;318:19–24.
79. Schoenfield MH, McGovern B, Garan H, *et al.*: Long-term reproducibility of responses to programmed cardiac stimulation in spontaneous ventricular tachyarrhythmias. Am J Cardiol 1984;54:564–568.
80. Cooper MJ, Koo CC, Skinner MP, *et al.*: Comparison of immediate versus day to day variability of ventricular tachycardia induction of programmed stimulation. J Am Coll Cardiol 1989;13:1599–1607.
81. Kudenchuk PJ, Kron J, Walance CG, *et al.*: Reproducibility of arrhythmia induction with intracardiac testing: Patients with clinical sustained ventricular tachyarrhythmias. J Am Coll Cardiol 1986;7:819–828.
82. ACC/AHA Task Force Report: Guidelines for clinical intracardiac electrophysiologic studies. J Am Coll Cardiol 1989;14:1827–1842.
83. Scheinman MM, Peters RW, Suave MJ, *et al.*: The value of the H-Q interval in patients with bundle branch block and the role of prophylactic permanent pacing. Am J Cardiol 1982;50:1316–1322.
84. Dhingra RC, Wyndham C, Bauernfeind R, *et al.*: Significance of block distal to the His bundle induced by atrial pacing in patients with chronic bifascicular block. Circulation 1979;60:1455–1464.
85. Shearn DL, Brent BB: Coronary artery bypass surgery in patients with left ventricular dysfunction. Am J Med 1986;80:405–411.
86. Kron IL, Lerman BB, Haines DE, *et al.*: Coronary artery bypass grafting in patients with ventricular fibrillation. Ann Thorac Surg 1989;48:85–89.
87. Kron IL, Flanagan TL, Blackbourne LH, *et al.*: Coronary revascularization rather than cardiac transplantation for chronic ischemic cardiomyopathy. Ann Surg 1989;210:348–354.
88. Lampert S, Lown B, Graboys TB, *et al.*: Determinants of survival in patients with malignant ventricular arrhythmia associated with coronary artery disease. Am J Cardiol 1988;61:791–797.
89. Swerdlow CD, Winkle RA, Mason JW: Determinants of survival in patients with ventricular tachyarrhythmias. N Engl J Med 1983;308:1436–1442.
90. Gottlieb CD, Berger MD, Miller JM, *et al.*: What is an acceptable risk for cardiac arrest patients treated with amiodarone? (Abstr) Circulation 1988; 78(11):500.
91. DiCarlo LA, Morady F, Sauve MJ, *et al.*: Cardiac arrest and sudden death in patients treated with amiodarone for sustained ventricular tachycardia or ventricular fibrillation: risk stratification based on clinical variables. Am J Cardiol 1985;55:372–374.
92. Graboys T: Long-term survival of patients with malignant ventricular arrhythmia treated with antiarrhythmic drugs. Am J Cardiol 1982;50:437–443.
93. Swerdlow CD, Peterson J: Prospective comparison of Holter monitoring and electrophysiologic study in patients with coronary artery disease and sustained ventricular tachyarrhythmias. Am J Cardiol 1985;56:577–585.
94. Greenspan AM, Spielman SR, Webb CR, *et al.*: Efficacy of combination therapy with mexiletine and a type IA agent for inducible ventricular tachyarrhythmias secondary to coronary artery disease. Am J Cardiol 1985;56:277–284.
95. Podrid PJ, Lown B: Propafenone: new therapy for a tough, old arrhythmia. J Am Coll Cardiol 1988;12:1012–1014.
96. Josephson MA, Ikeda N, Singh BN: Effects of flecainide on ventricular function: Clinical and experimental correlations. Am J Cardiol 1984; 53:95B–100B.
97. Mason JW, Peters FA: Antiarrhythmic efficacy of encainide in patients with refractory recurrent ventricular tachycardia. Circulation 1981;63:670–675.
98. Greene HL: The efficacy of amiodarone in the treatment of ventricular tachycardia or ventricular fibrillation. Prog Cardiovasc Dis 1989;31:319–354.
99. Horowitz LN, Greenspan AM, Spielman SR, *et al.*: Usefulness of electrophysiologic testing in evaluation of amiodarone therapy for sustained ventricular tachyarrhythmias associated with coronary heart disease. Am J Cardiol 1985;55:367–371.
100. Fisher JD, Kim SG, Waspe LE, *et al.*: Amiodarone: value of programmed electrical stimulation and Holter monitoring. PACE 1986;9:422–435.
101. Borggrefe M, Breithardt G: Predictive value of electrophysiologic testing in the treatment of drug-refractory ventricular arrhythmias with amiodarone. Eur Heart J 1986;7:735–742.
102. Klein LW, Fineberg N, Heger JJ, *et al.*: Prospective evaluation of a discriminant function for prediction of recurrent symptomatic ventricular tachycardia or ventricular fibrillation in coronary artery disease patients receiving amiodarone and having inducible ventricular tachycardia at electrophysiologic study. Am J Cardiol 1988;61:1024–1030.
103. Marchlinski FE, Buxton AE, Miller JM, *et al.*: Amiodarone versus amiodarone and a type IA agent for treatment of patients with rapid ventricular tachycardia. Circulation 1986;74:1037–1043.

104. Waleffe A, Mary-Rabine L, Legrand V, *et al.*: Combined mexiletine and amiodarone treatment of refractory recurrent ventricular tachycardia. Am Heart J 1980;100:788–793.
105. Marchlinski FE, Buxton AE, Kindwall KE, *et al.*: Comparison of individual and combined effect of procainamide and amiodarone in patients with sustained ventricular tachyarrhythmia. Circulation 1988;78:583–591.
106. Meissner MD, Kay HR, Horowitz LN, *et al.*: Relation of acute antiarrhythmic drug efficacy to left ventricular function in coronary artery disease. Am J Cardiol 1988;61:1050–1055.
107. Lehmann MH, Steinman RT, Schuger CD, *et al.*: The automatic implantable cardioverter defibrillator as antiarrhythmic treatment of choice for survivors of cardiac arrest unrelated to acute myocardial infarction. Am J Cardiol 1988;62:803–805.
108. Winkle RA, Mead RH, Guadiani VA, *et al.*: Long-term outcome with the automatic implantable cardioverter-defibrillator. J Am Coll Cardiol 1989; 13:1353–1361.
109. Mirowski M, Reid PR, Winkle RA, *et al.*: Mortality in patients with implanted automatic defibrillators. Ann Intern Med 1983;98:585–588.
110. Echt DS, Armstrong K, Schmidt P, *et al.*: Clinical experience, complications and survival in 70 patients with the automatic implantable cardioverter-defibrillator. Circulation 1985;104;481–488.
111. Thomas AC, Moser SA, Smutka ML, *et al.*: Implantable defibrillation: eight years of clinical experience. PACE 1988;11:2035–2058.
112. Tchou PJ, Kadri N, Anderson J, *et al.*: Automatic implantable cardioverter defibrillators and survival of patients with left ventricular dysfunction and malignant ventricular arrhythmias. Ann Intern Med 1988;109:529–534.
113. Fogoros RN, Elson JJ, Bonnet CA, *et al.*: Efficacy of the automatic implantable cardioverter-defibrillator in prolonging survival in patients with severe underlying cardiac disease. J Am Coll Cardiol 1990;16:381–386.
114. Echt DS, Liebson PR, Mitchell LB, *et al.*: Mortality and morbidity in patients receiving encainide, flecainide, or placebo. N Engl J Med 1991;324:781–788.
115. May GS, Eberlein KA, Furberg CD, *et al.*: Secondary prevention after myocardial infarction: a review of long-term trials. Prog Cardiovasc Dis 1982;24;331–352.
116. Furberg CD: Effect of antiarrhythmic drugs on mortality after myocardial infarction. Am J Cardiol 1983;52:32C–36C.
117. Bigger JT Jr: Prophylactic use of implantable cardioverter defibrillators: Medical, technical, and economic considerations. PACE 1991;14:376–380.
118. Bigger JT Jr, Morganroth J: Treatment algorithms, including the role of implantable cardioverter defibrillators, for management of ventricular arrhythmias after the Cardiac Arrhythmia Suppression Trial. Am J Cardiol 1991;67:332–333.
119. Proceedings of the prospective randomized studies program. Ninth Annual AICD Clinical Symposium, CPI, May 28, 1991, Washington, DC.
120. Bigger JT: A discussion of CABG patch trial. CPI AICD Advances, First Quarter, 1991:6–7.
121. Moss AJ: MUSTT and MADIT trials examine role of antiarrhythmic therapy in nonsustained VT patients. CPI AICD Advances, Fourth Quarter, 1991.
122. Lehmann M, for Defibrillator Study Group: A critical risk of sudden death while awaiting cardiac transplantation in patients with atherosclerotic heart disease. Am J Cardiol 1991;68:545–546.
123. Miller JM, Gottfred CD, Hargrove WC, *et al.*: Factors influencing operative mortality in surgery for ventricular tachycardia. Circulation 1988;78:II–44.
124. Josephson ME, Harken AM, Horowitz LM: Endocardial excision: a new surgical technique for the treatment of recurrent ventricular tachycardia. Circulation 1987;76:332–342.
125. Hanes DE, Lerman BB, Kron IL, *et al.*: Surgical ablation of ventricular tachycardia with sequential map guided subendocardial resection: electrophysiologic assessment and long term follow up. Circulation 1988;7:131–141.

7

NARROW QRS COMPLEX TACHYCARDIA

Tibor S. Szabo, M.D., and Igor Singer, M.B.B.S., F.R.A.C.P., F.A.C.P., F.A.C.C.

NARROW QRS TACHYCARDIAS

Several features of tachyarrhythmias may be useful for classification. One common approach is to use the anatomic site of origin. Tachycardias are considered supraventricular when the site of impulse formation is within the atrium or within the normal conduction system, but above the bifurcation of the His bundle. This definition was extended later to include tachycardias in which the "atrium or atrioventricular junction above the bifurcation of the His bundle is the origin or a critical link in the perpetuation of tachycardia" (1). The mechanism of a given rhythm may not be readily appreciated from the clinical presentation or electrocardiographic (ECG) appearance. Some arrhythmias are difficult to classify on anatomic basis, since both atrial and ventricular myocardium is involved in their mechanism. A classification based on ECG morphology, i.e., narrow QRS morphology versus wide QRS morphology may be more practical. Classification of arrhythmias on a purely descriptive basis does not involve any presumption regarding the underlying mechanism. The ECG presentation, along with the clinical picture, indicates what diagnostic and therapeutic steps may have to be taken. The clinical approach to diagnose and treat tachycardias, that present with a narrow QRS complex morphology, is presented in this chapter.

By definition, a wide QRS complex is one that lasts 0.12 sec or longer (2,3). Any QRS complex shorter than that (i.e., $\leq$ 0.11 sec) is considered narrow (4). This classification is descriptive and the spectrum of arrhythmias (Table 7.1) represents a variety of underlying mechanisms that may develop in normal or diseased hearts. It is therefore important to remember that several different underlying mechanisms may result in an identical ECG presentation. The terminology of these arrhythmias is evolving. Terms like supraventricular tachycardia or paroxysmal atrial tachycardia are gradually replaced by more specific terms that imply the underlying mechanism, e.g., orthodromic atrioventricular (AV) reciprocating tachycardia. The term "narrow QRS tachycardia" includes arrhythmias that are usually classified as supraventricular or a narrow QRS ventricular tachycardia. Accordingly, the underlying electrophysiologic (EP) mechanism varies greatly.

The predominant underlying mechanism of these rhythms is reentry. The best studied model of reentrant arrhythmias is AV reentry utilizing an accessory AV pathway. The nature of AV nodal reciprocating tachycardias is also well studied, but the anatomical location of the circuit is not known. The mechanism of several tachycardias (e.g., multifocal atrial tachycardia) is not known. In the presence of aberrant AV nodal conduction all of the supraventricular narrow QRS tachycardias can present with wide QRS complexes, entering the differential diagnosis of wide QRS rhythms, which are discussed elsewhere in this book (see Chapters 3, 4, 8, 9).

The clinical presentation varies considerably. Symptoms depend on the underlying mechanism and the rate of the tachycardia, associated heart disease, patient's age, general health and fitness, and presence of noncardiac disease. Some patients may be unaware of having tachyarrhythmias, while others complain only about occasional palpitations. Chest pain, shortness of breath, dizziness, lightheadedness, congestive heart failure, weakness with diaphoresis may interfere with the patient's daily activities. Systemic embolization may accompany atrial fibrillation (AF). Near-syncope and syncope may occur, as well as sudden cardiac death.

DIAGNOSTIC TECHNIQUES

History and Physical Examination

Asymptomatic arrhythmias may be discovered fortuitously during a routine physical examination. When the patient is symptomatic, the history reveals important clues about the frequency and length of the arrhythmia episodes, the mode of spontaneous onset and termination, the regularity of the rhythm, possible triggering factors, and type and severity of symptoms. Sudden onset and termination suggest reentry mechanism. Gross irregularity of the rhythm is characteristic of atrial fibrillation.

Infrequent, mildly symptomatic tachycardias may not require aggressive treatment. Treatment of arrhythmias occurring predictably on a daily basis may be guided by symptomatic relief or noninvasive tests, e.g., Holter monitoring. Frequent or severely symptomatic tachycardias require treatment guided by either noninvasive tests (e.g., Holter monitoring) or by EP studies.

Table 7.1.
Narrow QRS Tachyarrhythmias

Tachycardias originating in the atrial myocardium (the AV node is an "innocent bystander")
Sinus tachycardia
Sinoatrial reentry
Atrial tachycardia
Atrial flutter
Atrial fibrillation
Multifocal atrial tachycardia
Tachycardias incorporating the AV junction
AV nodal reciprocating tachycardia
Nonparoxysmal junctional tachycardia
Orthodromic AV reciprocating tachycardia
Permanent form of junctional reciprocating tachycardia (PJRT)
Narrow QRS ventricular tachycardia

Physical examination during arrhythmia may provide important clues. Diagnostic features such as the regularity of the rhythm, presence of pulse deficit, and signs of AV dissociation are easy to appreciate and are helpful in differentiating the rhythm disturbance (see Chapter 3). Physical signs may also reveal underlying cardiac or systemic disorders.

Chest Radiograph, Echocardiogram, Cardiac Catheterization, Radionuclide Angiogram, and Myocardial Perfusion Scan

The results of these tests can support the diagnosis and quantitate the physiologic impairment resulting from underlying cardiac disorders. They also provide information about anatomic, physiologic, and angiographic characteristics of associated cardiac conditions which may either be the cause of, or may be associated with the arrhythmias. This information may be crucial regarding the prognosis and treatment of arrhythmias (e.g., atrial dimension, presence of an atrial septal defect or an atrial thrombus in patients with AF).

Twelve-Lead Electrocardiogram

Surface electrocardiogram is the most important clinical diagnostic technique that is readily available. Tracings taken during normal sinus rhythm may identify underlying organic or physiologic abnormalities. The electrocardiogram during the arrhythmias may establish, or at least suggest one or more likely diagnoses. The following features of the narrow QRS rhythms are analyzed: (a) regularity or irregularity of the rhythm, (b) presence or absence of signs of organized atrial activity (P or F waves), (c) P wave (F wave) morphology (when present) and its relationship to ventricular activity, and (d) rate. All of these features must be interpreted in the light of the clinical setting. Electrocardiographic recordings of the onset and termination of an arrhythmia are especially informative.

Esophageal Recordings

Electrode catheters can readily be passed down the esophagus to record left atrial electrical activity. This technique may identify atrial electrical activity and its relationship to the QRS complexes, when this activity is not readily apparent on the surface electrocardiogram. The technique of recording esophageal electrograms is described in detail elsewhere in this book (see Chapter 3).

Physiologic and Pharmacologic Maneuvers

Vagal maneuvers may terminate some reentrant supraventricular tachycardias (e.g., AV nodal reentry). In case of atrial tachycardias development of transient AV nodal block may reveal atrial activity not apparent on a rhythm strip (e.g., in the case of atrial flutter with 2:1 AV conduction). For this purpose carotid sinus massage is used most commonly, in patients in the absence of significant carotid artery disease. Among available pharmacologic agents, the recently released drug adenosine is particularly useful as a diagnostic agent. A rapid intravenous bolus of adenosine induces transient AV nodal block, interrupting a reentrant circuit that includes the AV node, or revealing previously hidden P or F waves in the case of atrial tachycardias. A major advantage of adenosine is its short half-life, limiting potential side effects to less than 30 sec.

Long-Term Electrocardiographic Monitoring Techniques

Assessment of the relationship between symptoms and clinical arrhythmias is crucial in the diagnostic process, as clinical manifestations are not specific for the underlying rhythm. Frequently occurring arrhythmias can readily be recorded by 24-hr Holter monitoring. However, most of these tachycardias occur infrequently, without a predictable pattern. When Holter monitor or telemetry recordings do not record arrhythmias over a 24- to 48-hr period, further continuous monitoring may be impractical. In this case a patient-activated event recorder, that can be carried by the patient for an extended period, may be more successful in documenting the heart rhythm and coinciding with the symptoms (5). Apart from being dependent on the unpredictable occurrence of arrhythmias, Holter monitoring has other limitations, e.g., only two leads are usually recorded which may not show discernible P waves, making the differential diagnosis more difficult.

Exercise Test

Supraventricular tachycardias are infrequently induced by exercise. However, stress tests are routinely performed to assess cardiopulmonary status and to exclude underlying heart disease. Although various arrhythmias can be induced by exercise, the reproducibility of this technique as a means of guiding therapy has not been established (6).

Invasive Electrophysiologic Testing

Severely symptomatic, frequently recurring or incessant life-threatening narrow QRS tachycardias, require EP testing to determine the arrhythmia mechanism and to guide medical, surgical, or catheter ablation therapy. The technique of the EP study is described in detail in Chapter 4. Briefly, three multipolar electrode catheters are introduced percutaneously into the femoral vein (usually on the right side) and positioned in the high right atrium (close to the sinus node), in the right ventricular apex, and across the tricuspid valve to record His bundle electrogram. A fourth multipolar catheter is introduced in the subclavian or internal jugular vein and positioned in the coronary sinus to facilitate atrial activation mapping. Three to five leads of the surface electrocardiogram (usually a combination of leads I, II, III, V_1, and V_6) are also displayed. The distal electrode pair of the multipolar catheters is used for pacing and the proximal electrode pair for recording. Bipolar electrograms from the right ventricular apex, high right atrium, and His bundle region are recorded, as well as multiple unipolar or bipolar electrograms from the coronary sinus. Special catheters may be used to facilitate certain maneuvers, e.g., Gallagher catheter for right atrial mapping, Jackman catheter for recording of accessory pathway AP potentials.

The stimulation protocol depends on the presumptive diagnosis. In arrhythmias that are likely to be of supraventricular origin, ventricular stimulation is performed first in an attempt to avoid premature induction of AF. Incremental pacing and extrastimulus testing at multiple cycle lengths are performed from both the right ventricle and the right atrium to determine ventricular, AV nodal, and atrial refractory periods and to induce arrhythmias. Sinus node function is tested including sinus node recovery times and sino-atrial conduction times (7). Specific details of the EP study are discussed under the sections describing the individual arrhythmias.

CHARACTERISTIC FEATURES OF NARROW QRS TACHYCARDIAS

Sinus Tachycardia

A rhythm that originates in the sinus node with rates exceeding 100 beats/min is sinus tachycardia. The rate is usually below 160 beats/min, but occasionally, especially in younger individuals during peak exercise, reaches 180–200 beats/min or even higher. The rhythm is regular, with slight irregularities only. It accelerates and slows down gradually. The QRS complexes are preceded by P waves of normal morphology, duration, and axis. The P waves are identical with those observed during "normal sinus rhythm" at rest, among baseline conditions. Atrial activation mapping during EP studies shows an activation from the high lateral right atrium toward the low septum and to the left, i.e., the normal atrial activation pattern originating in the sinus node. Sinus tachycardia can exist in the presence of AV block. Most commonly, however, the PR interval is normal or shorter than, but definitely not longer than the one recorded during normal sinus rhythm. Vagal maneuvers may slow the tachycardia transiently, but a faster rate gradually resumes as soon as the maneuver is terminated. A more rapid pacemaker, e.g., junctional rhythm or an artificial pacemaker can suppress the sinus tachycardia temporarily (overdrive suppression), but does not terminate it. As soon as the more rapid rhythm slows down or terminates, the sinus tachycardia resumes.

Sinus tachycardia is due to an increased rate of phase 4 spontaneous diastolic depolarization in the normal pacemaker cells. Accordingly, an increase in the rate of spontaneous depolarization or a decrease in the threshold will result in sinus tachycardia. Changes in the autonomic nervous system, namely, sympathetic activation and parasympathetic withdrawal and increase in circulating catecholamines result in sinus tachycardia.

Sinus tachycardia can occur under physiologic conditions (Table 7.2). The normal, resting heart rate in infants and young children is higher than in older children and in adults. Both emotional and physical stress normally results in sinus tachycardia. The peak heart rate in response to exercise and circulating catecholamines declines with age. Sinus tachycardia developing among pathologic conditions is almost always a secondary arrhythmia, i.e., a nonspecific manifestation of various disease processes. Therefore, the presence of sinus tachycardia warrants a thorough search for the underlying disorder. Fever and pain of any origin, cardiac causes including acute myocardial infarction, congestive heart failure, tamponade, pulmonary embolism, and various systemic illnesses all can result in sinus tachycardia. Nicotine, caffeine, and alcohol, as well as sympathomimetic and vagolytic medications are frequently the underlying cause of sinus tachycardia.

The symptoms caused by sinus tachycardia are variable. Young and healthy individuals usually tolerate this rhythm well.

Table 7.2.
Causes of Sinus Tachycardia

Physiologic
Infants, young children
Emotional stress, anxiety
Exercise
Pathologic
Hypermetabolic states (fever, thyrotoxicosis, etc.)
Pain
Cardiac causes: congestive heart failure, acute myocardial infarction, bacterial endocarditis, cardiac tamponade, aortic dissection
Infections
Anemia
Pulmonary embolism
Hypovolemia, shock
Postoperative states
Pheochromocytoma
Drugs
Catecholamines, sympathetic agonists
Parasympatholytic agents
Alcohol, caffeine, nicotine

Older individuals, or those with severe coronary artery disease or diastolic dysfunction of the left ventricle may develop symptoms of myocardial ischemia or left ventricular failure. Sinus tachycardia in the setting of acute myocardial infarction is particularly ominous, indicating severe ventricular dysfunction.

Sinus tachycardia by itself, does not require treatment. When the underlying disorder is recognized and treated, the sinus rate will slow. Occasionally, when myocardial ischemia is induced by the rapid rhythm, and when no apparent underlying cause is recognized in the setting of myocardial infarction, patient may benefit from slowing the heart rate with β-adrenergic blocking agents.

Sinoatrial Reentrant Tachycardia

A paroxysmal tachycardia that has an ECG appearance indistinguishable from sinus tachycardia is thought to be the result of a reentry circuit localized in the high lateral right atrium, i.e., the region that includes the sinus node. The tachycardia is regular, with relatively slow rates between 100 and 160 beats/min. When the rate is below 100 beats/min, it usually represents a relative tachycardia in patients with a baseline bradycardia. The P wave morphology is identical with, or similar to that recorded during normal sinus rhythm.

Several features distinguish sinoatrial reentry from sinus tachycardia. The PR interval is prolonged, as the inappropriately high rate induces AV nodal conduction delay. In sinus tachycardia the PR interval is equal to or shorter than the PR interval during baseline sinus rhythm. Usually the RP/PR ratio is higher than 1. In contrast to the gradual initiation and termination of sinus tachycardia, the onset and termination of sinoatrial reentry is sudden. Spontaneous initiation of the tachycardia does not usually require premature beats. The tachycardia cycle length usually prolongs before sudden termination. Carotid sinus massage and verapamil may terminate the tachycardia. The mechanism of the arrhythmia is thought to be reentry of the leading circle type (8).

The localization of the reentrant circuit is uncertain. It may be within the sinus node or may involve the surrounding myocardium, as well. Alternative arrhythmia mechanism, namely triggered activity, has also been proposed.

Sinoatrial reentry can exist in the presence of AV block. During EP investigations sinoatrial reentry tachycardias are usually reproducibly induced and terminated by critically timed atrial extrastimuli or rapid atrial pacing. Stimulation is most effectively performed in the high lateral right atrium. The induction of the tachycardia does not require development of a critical AV or intra-atrial conduction delay. The sequence of anterograde atrial activation is identical with that recorded during sinus rhythm (8–12). Single sinoatrial echo beats are frequently induced, but the induction of sustained episodes is uncommon.

The incidence of sinoatrial reentry is not known. Reports indicate that this is a relatively rare tachycardia occurring in about 1.8–3.0% of patients referred for assessment of tachyarrhythmias (9–13). Patients with this arrhythmia often have organic heart disease, mainly coronary artery disease. Sinoatrial tachycardia is frequently symptomatic, with palpitations, lightheadedness, near-syncope, or frank syncope.

When the onset or termination of the arrhythmia is not recorded, electrocardiographic differentiation of sinoatrial reentry from sinus tachycardia may be impossible. A prolonged PR interval may indicate that the rhythm is not sinus. The characteristic paroxysmal presentation, the effects of vagal and pharmacologic maneuvers may support the diagnosis. Invasive EP studies may occasionally be needed to establish the diagnosis.

Reassurance is the only treatment necessary in most cases. When sinoatrial reentry is sustained, recurrent, or symptomatic, it may require treatment. Carotid sinus massage may terminate the arrhythmia. Intravenous administration of verapamil or adenosine (14) was also reported to be successful. Chronic administration of digitalis or verapamil may prevent further episodes (13). The effect of β-adrenergic blocking agents is not uniform (10–13). Other agents, e.g., amiodarone can be effective, but may not be justified when antiarrhythmic agents with less potential for adverse effects are available. In a few select cases, other treatment modalities, e.g., antitachycardia pacing, cryosurgical ablation, were used successfully (15,16).

Atrial Tachycardia

Atrial tachycardias originate in the atrial myocardium excluding the area of the sinoatrial node and the AV junction. Traditionally, arrhythmias with cycle lengths between 600 and 250 msec (most commonly between 400 and 300 msec) belong to this category. Atrial flutter and fibrillation, which are also atrial tachyarrhythmias, have shorter atrial cycle lengths and are discussed later. According to the underlying EP mechanism, atrial tachycardias can be automatic or reentrant. In some cases triggered activity appears to be the most likely mechanism. An uncommon tachycardia, which has been called paroxysmal atrial tachycardia (PAT) with block, is characteristic of digitalis intoxication.

Atrial tachycardias share some common electrocardiographic features and it may be impossible to identify the underlying mechanism based on the surface electrocardiogram. Neither the rate nor the P wave morphology is specific for the arrhythmia mechanism. The P wave axis and the PR interval are variable, according to the location of the arrhythmia focus within the atria. Atrial activation sequence differs from the sequence recorded during normal sinus rhythm. The rate is usually regular, and there is one-to-one AV conduction. The PR interval may exceed the PR interval recorded during sinus rhythm and it is usually rate dependent. Variability of the PR interval when the P-P intervals are regular strongly suggests an atrial tachycardia. The presence of AV block does not affect the tachycardia. Vagal maneuvers may slow the ventricular rate but usually do not terminate the tachycardia.

Spontaneous onset and termination of intraatrial reentry

tachycardias is sudden. The morphology of the first P wave is different from the morphology of the previous P waves. The tachycardia can be initiated by programmed atrial stimulation and is dependent on a critical intra-atrial conduction delay. Critically timed atrial extrastimuli and rapid atrial pacing can terminate the tachycardia. Single premature stimuli may also reset or accelerate the reentry tachycardia (17,18).

Automatic atrial tachycardias can neither be initiated nor terminated by programmed stimulation. After onset, they usually show the "warm-up" phenomenon, i.e., the cycle length gradually shortens for several cycles, before the stable tachycardia rate is reached (Fig 7.1). The onset is not preceded by a critical intraatrial conduction delay. Initiation does not require premature beats. If the arrhythmia starts with a premature beat, it occurs usually late in the diastole. The morphology of the first and subsequent tachycardia P waves is identical. Single premature complexes reset the automatic rhythm. Overdrive pacing at fast cycle lengths suppresses the automatic focus temporarily, which is indicated by the pause observed after cessation of rapid pacing (overdrive suppression) (17,19).

Intraatrial reentry is the underlying mechanism in about 5–7% of patients studied for supraventricular tachycardias. The majority of these patients have organic heart disease. In children it is frequently associated with corrected congenital malformations (e.g., atrial septal defect and transposition of the great arteries). Surgery may set up the necessary requirements for the atrial conduction delay needed for the development of these rhythms.

Automatic atrial tachycardia is the least frequent form of atrial tachycardias. Repetitive automatic tachycardia develops in normal hearts and it is usually asymptomatic. Incessant automatic atrial tachycardia occurs in children. When the tachycardia persists for a long time, it leads to impairment of the left ventricular function, i.e., tachycardia-induced cardiomyopathy. Atrial tachycardias that develop in the setting of digitalis intoxication are presumed to be the result of triggered activity. A rare form of atrial tachycardia, i.e,. PAT with AV block, may be associated with digitalis intoxication. Atrial tachycardias presenting in short episodes or developing in normal hearts are frequently asymptomatic. In more symptomatic cases the severity of symptoms depends on the tachycardia rate and the underlying cardiac or noncardiac diseases.

Atrial tachycardias are frequently resistant to medical treatment. Digitalis, calcium channel blocking, and β-adrenergic blocking agents may control the ventricular rate, but usually do not terminate the tachycardia. Class IA and IC agents may suppress intraatrial reentry. Class IA antiarrhythmic medications do not have a consistent effect on automatic atrial rhythms. Flecainide, encainide, propafenone, and moricizine were reported to be effective in some cases. Amiodarone can be effective, but its long-term use, especially in younger patients, is limited by its side effects.

Nonpharmacologic therapeutic modalities were successfully used in selected cases. Surgical or cryosurgical ablation of an arrhythmia focus is feasible in the atrium (20). As scar tissue created by surgical or cryosurgical interventions behaves as an electrical insulator, parts of the atria can be isolated electrically from the rest of the heart with these methods. Isolation of an automatic focus in the left atrium allows normal sinus rhythm to emerge.

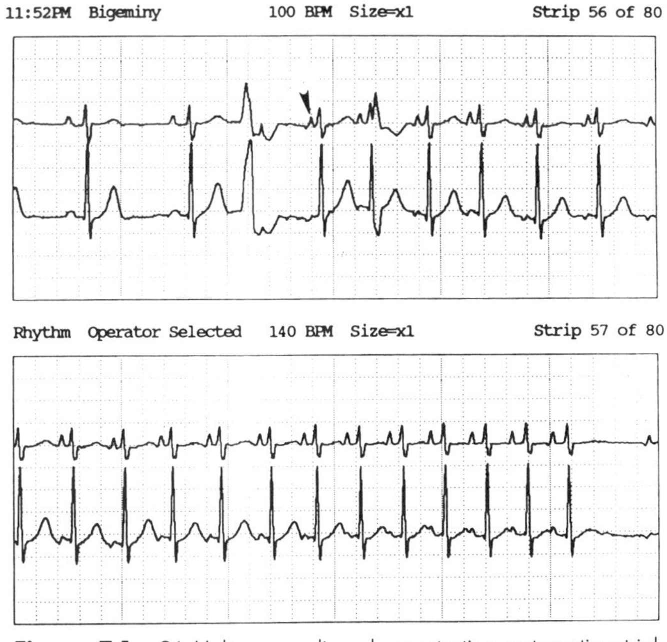

Figure 7.1. 24 Holter recording demonstrating automatic atrial tachycardia. Note the sudden onset (*arrow*) and acceleration, with a distinct P wave morphology (different from the sinus rhythm).

Atrial Flutter

Atrial flutter is a rapid, regular atrial rhythm with atrial cycle lengths usually between 240 and 170 msec (250–350 beats/min). This atrial rhythm is conducted to the ventricles with a variable AV block. Usually, in untreated flutter, the conduction ratio is 2:1, with a resultant ventricular cycle length of around 400 msec (150 beats/min) (Fig. 7.2). The conduction ratio may be changing from 2:1 to 4:1, or higher multiples. Higher conduction ratios can occur (e.g., 6:2, 8:3, etc.) especially in patients treated with antiarrhythmic drugs that slow AV nodal conduction or prolong AV nodal refractoriness. Odd number ratios (3:1, 5:1) are unusual. Atrial flutter with 1:1 conduction is a poorly tolerated arrhythmia. One-to-one AV conduction can occur in children, in individuals with enhanced AV nodal conduction, thyrotoxicosis, and in the presence of AV accessory pathways.

Regular, distinct electrocardiographic deflections, called F waves, with a characteristic "sawtooth" morphology in the inferior leads represent atrial activity during flutter. Usually, there is no isoelectric line separating individual F waves, but there are exceptions. In the "common" type of atrial flutter the axis of the F waves is directed leftward, resulting in dominant negative

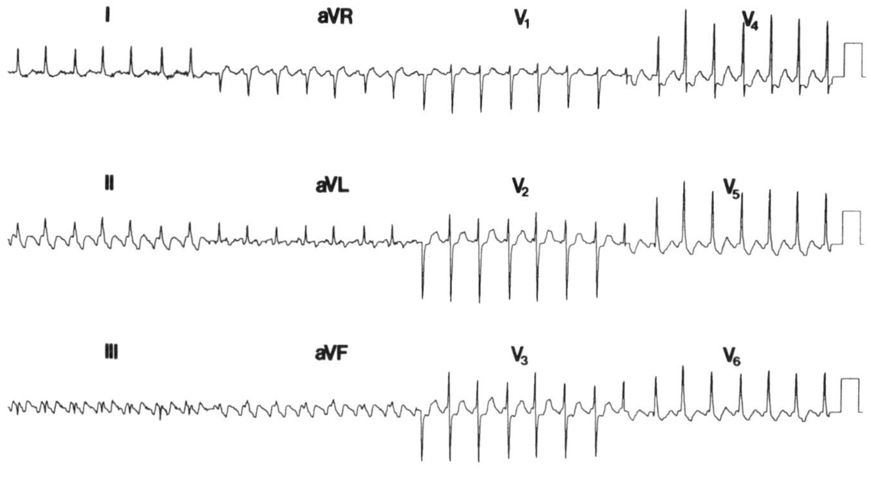

Figure 7.2. Twelve-lead electrocardiogram demonstrates atrial flutter, with flutter waves particularly prominent in II, III, and aVF.

deflections in the inferior leads. The F waves are best discernible in leads II and V_1. The "uncommon" type of flutter includes all other possible F wave morphologies. These differences in F wave morphology were thought to be the result of differences in right atrial activation pattern. The common type was thought to be the result of a counterclockwise activation from the distal low septal area toward the left atrium and the high right atrium (21). A more recent classification of the subtypes of atrial flutter is based on the rate and the response to rapid stimulation in the high right atrium (22). Type I or "classic" atrial flutter has an atrial cycle length of 240–180 msec (250–340 beats/min) and it can be converted to sinus rhythm, AF, or Type II flutter by rapid pacing from the high right atrium. Type II atrial flutter has faster atrial cycle lengths of 180–140 msec (340–430 beats/min), and is not affected by rapid pacing from the high right atrium. This latter classification is independent of F wave morphology and axis.

All types of atrial flutter have remarkably constant atrial cycle lengths, morphology, polarity and axis of the local atrial electrograms when recorded by intracardiac electrodes (22). These features help distinguish atrial flutter from fibrillation. More than one mechanism may be responsible for different types of atrial flutter. Most experimental and clinical observations support a reentrant mechanism. It has been suggested, that Type I, or classic atrial flutter, is due to a macroreentrant circuit localized in the right atrium (23–25). The critical area of slow conduction appears to be in the posteroseptal area, in the vicinity of the coronary sinus. Surgical or catheter ablation of this area resulted in the abolition of atrial flutter (25,26). Transient entrainment and interruption of Type I flutter by rapid atrial pacing supports the presence of a reentrant circuit with an excitable gap (27,28) (Table 7.3).

The mechanism of Type II atrial flutter is speculative. A microreentrant circuit of the leading circle type, i.e., without an anatomic obstacle, is thought to be the most likely mechanism resulting in a reentry circuit lacking an excitable gap.

In the electrophysiology laboratory atrial flutter can be initiated by rapid atrial pacing or closely coupled atrial extrastimuli

Table 7.3.
Criteria of Transient Entrainment of a Reentry Tachycardia

1. Constant fusion beats on the electrocardiogram with rapid pacing with a constant rate during the spontaneous tachycardia, with the exception of the last captured beat (the last entrained beat has the morphology of the spontaneous tachycardia)
2. Progressive fusion, i.e., rapid pacing with different constant rates during the tachycardia results in different degrees of constant fusion at any given pacing rate
3. Localized conduction block to one or more sites for one beat when the tachycardia is interrupted, followed by subsequent activation of those sites from a different direction, manifested by a change of morphology of the electrogram and a shorter conduction time
4. A change in electrogram morphology and conduction time at a given recording site, when pacing from another site at two different constant pacing rates, which are faster than the spontaneous tachycardia rate but fail to interrupt the tachycardia (the electrogram equivalent of progressive fusion)

Demonstration of any of these four criteria establishes the presence of transient entrainment.

with short basic drive cycle lengths. An intra-atrial conduction delay is frequently demonstrated and appears to be a necessary precondition in patients with spontaneously occurring or induced atrial flutter. Induction of atrial flutter is uncommon in patients who do not have this arrhythmia occurring spontaneously. The recording of low-amplitude, prolonged, and fractionated local electrograms is thought to identify the zone of slow conduction. Pacing capture of the reentry circuit of type I atrial flutter, i.e., transient entrainment of the flutter circuit supports the theory of reentry with an excitable gap.

Atrial flutter is a common arrhythmia occurring usually in the setting of cardiac disease. The underlying medical conditions are generally the same as those which result in AF (Table 7.4). Usually acute conditions responsible for the initiation of atrial flutter can be identified. These conditions may include atrial distention of any cause, infection, ischemia, pulmonary embolism, pericarditis, blood gas, and acid-base disturbances, postoperative states, exacerbation of cor pulmonale due to worsening chronic obstructive pulmonary disease, or other lung disease

Table 7.4.
Common Causes of Atrial Fibrillation and Flutter

Cardiovascular
Hypertensive heart disease
Congestive heart failure
Rheumatic heart disease
Coronary artery disease
Sinus node dysfunction (tachycardia-bradycardia syndrome)
Pericarditis
Cardiac surgery
Wolff-Parkinson-White syndrome
Other heart diseases (atrial septal defect, mitral valve prolapse, cardiomyopathies)
Systemic diseases
Thyrotoxicosis
Lung diseases (chronic obstructive lung diseases, pulmonary embolism, pneumonia, etc.)
Metabolic or drug related (alcohol, electrolyte abnormalities)
Cardioversion-defibrillation
Miscellaneous (hypovolemia, atrial pacing, electrical injury, trauma)

processes. Most often, atrial flutter is a transient arrhythmia, but it can be recurrent, paroxysmal, or chronic. It causes a variety of symptoms, ranging from symptomatic palpitations to acute left ventricular failure, and sudden cardiovascular collapse.

The diagnosis of atrial flutter may be evident from the surface ECG. A narrow QRS rhythm with a cycle length around 400 msec (150 beats/min), especially when "P waves" (F waves) are located in the middle portion of the RR intervals, should always suggest the possibility of atrial flutter. The identification of the characteristic F waves is crucial. At times maneuvers causing AV nodal block (vagal maneuvers, adenosine, verapamil, etc.) help identify F waves. Special electrocardiographic leads may be needed (e.g., right-sided precordial leads), or recording of the left atrial electrogram with an esophageal electrode. Placement of an esophageal lead also allows bipolar pacing to terminate atrial flutter. Invasive EP studies are seldom needed for diagnosis. If surgical or catheter ablation procedures are contemplated, an EP study with detailed atrial mapping is necessary.

Atrial flutter which results in a hemodynamic compromise may be best treated with direct current cardioversion. One may start at 5–50 J, while 100 J is almost uniformly successful. When the patient is hemodynamically stable, administration of antiarrhythmic medications, or preferably rapid atrial pacing may be tried. When appropriate techniques are used, type I atrial flutter can always be terminated by pacing.

Currently a ramp atrial pacing technique is recommended in the high right atrium. The starting pacing rate is about 10 beats/min faster than the flutter's atrial rate (29). Esophageal pacing may also be successful. Transformation of flutter to AF is another possible outcome of pacing. Atrial fibrillation is easier to control medically.

Digitalis, verapamil, β-adrenergic blocking agents may all slow the ventricular rate, but do not terminate flutter. Quinidine, a Type IA antiarrhythmic, may also slow AV conduction, usually without terminating the flutter. As this effect may be accompanied by enhancement of AV nodal conduction due to parasympatholytic effects, drugs slowing AV nodal conduction should be administered concomitantly. More recently intravenous type IC antiarrhythmic agents (flecainide or propafenone) were reported to successfully terminate atrial flutter. For chronic prevention of recurrence of atrial flutter Type IA, IC, and Type III antiarrhythmic agents can be used.

Catheter ablation of the AV node-His bundle system with the implantation of a permanent pacemaker is an effective method to control severely symptomatic atrial flutter refractory to medical therapy. Catheter ablation of the reentry circuit itself is possible, but it remains an investigational technique (25). The same is true for surgical ablation of the reentrant circuit. Surgical or catheter ablation of an accessory AV pathway eliminates AF and flutter in patients with Wolff-Parkinson-White syndrome.

Atrial Fibrillation

Atrial fibrillation is disorganized electrical, and consequently mechanical, activity of the atria. Irregular, disordered, and unsynchronized electrical activity has very rapid cycle lengths of 170–100 msec (350–600 cycles/min). This chaotic atrial activity is manifested by an undulating baseline on the surface electrocardiogram, without discernible P waves, (Fig. 7.3). Low-amplitude irregular f waves are frequently seen, but in many cases the baseline may be entirely flat. The morphology, amplitude, presence, or absence of fibrillatory waves correlates neither with the type of the underlying heart disease nor with the atrial size. Local endocardial electrograms vary in amplitude, width, polarity and shape, in addition to constantly changing cycle lengths. The fast, irregular atrial rate is conducted to the ventricles through the AV node. The physiologic conduction delay of the AV node does not allow 1:1 conduction. Normally, in an untreated person, recent-onset AF has an average ventricular cycle length between 600 and 370 msec (100–160 beats/min). The ventricular rhythm in AF is irregularly irregular. In fact, this irregularity is so characteristic, that AF can be diagnosed based on the degree of irregularity of the rhythm. With faster ventricular rates the rhythm may appear more regular. Regular, slow ventricular rates may occur if AF coexists with high-degree or complete AV block, in the presence of a junctional or ventricular escape rhythm.

The ventricular response during AF is determined by the conduction characteristics of the AV node, the presence or absence of an accessory AV pathway, the status of the autonomic nervous system, presence of concealed conduction into the AV node, and possibly other, as yet unknown factors. The ventricular rate is slower in individuals with diseases of the conduction system, in the elderly, and in those who take medications that impair AV nodal conduction. Younger patients may have enhanced AV nodal conduction or take sympathomimetic medications which enhance AV nodal conduction, resulting in faster

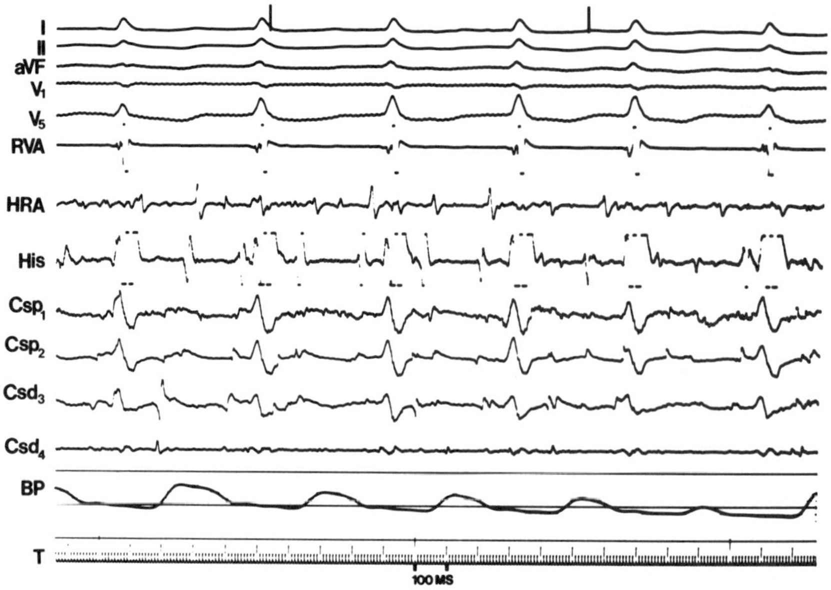

Figure 7.3. Atrial fibrillation. From **top** to **bottom:** surface leads I, II, aVF, V_1, and V_5, intracardiac electrocardiograms from right ventricular apex (RV_A), high right atrium (HRA), His bundle electrocardiogram (HIS), coronary sinus proximal to distal (1–4), blood pressure (BP), and time scale (T).

ventricular rates. Ventricular response during AF can be characterized by measuring the average and the shortest RR intervals. Accurate assessment of the average and shortest RR intervals during AF requires ECG samples of at least 30 sec and 2 min long, respectively (30).

The mechanism of AF is unknown. The presence of multiple reentrant circuits of the leading circle type is the most likely explanation (31,32). Conditions that facilitate AF include high vagal tone, rapid atrial pacing, dilatation of the atria, and the presence of intra-atrial conduction disturbances. A relatively short atrial refractory period, heterogeneity of atrial refractory periods, and a critical mass of atrial myocardium were found to be necessary conditions in the animal models (33). Spontaneous AF can be initiated by very early premature atrial beats. The phenomenon of premature atrial stimuli, falling in the relative refractory period of the atria, producing repetitive responses, nonsustained or sustained atrial tachyarrhythmias, is called atrial vulnerability (21). In normal hearts sustained AF (i.e. an episode lasting longer than 5 minutes) is usually not induced by single premature stimuli. Rapid atrial pacing with cycle lengths below 200 msec can induce and maintain AF. However, sinus rhythm almost always returns immediately or shortly after the stimulation is stopped. Atrial vulnerability is more common in patients with a history of AF-flutter (21).

Atrial fibrillation may be chronic and established or paroxysmal and recurrent. Physiologically, it results in a loss of normal chronotropic competence provided by the sinus node, AV synchrony, and the "booster pump" function of atrial systole. This function may be crucial in patients with organic heart disease. It is not unusual for acute left ventricular failure to develop shortly after the onset of new AF. While an enlarged left atrium itself may be a major contributor to AF, chronic AF itself produces progressive atrial enlargement (34).

The prevalence of AF and flutter in healthy individuals is very low. In an unselected population of adults less than 60 yr old the prevalence was found to be 0.28–0.40%. The prevalence in people older than 60 yr was found to be higher, between 1.7 and 5.0%, and among those older than 75 yr it was 11.6 % (35). Atrial fibrillation is much more common in the presence of coexistent heart disease. The most common conditions resulting in AF are hypertensive heart disease, congestive heart failure, and rheumatic heart disease. The association with coronary artery disease is not as strong as with the above conditions. Among the noncardiac diseases the association is strongest with hyperthyroidism (Table 7.4). In the absence of an apparent underlying heart or systemic disease the arrhythmia is called "lone atrial fibrillation". The reported occurrence of lone fibrillation widely varies between 2.7 and 32% of chronic AF cases (35). At least some of these cases may represent early, subclinical cardiovascular diseases. Some patients remain asymptomatic after the onset of AF. This may be more common in lone fibrillators. Others have palpitations, fatigue, dyspnea, or any other symptom of tachycardias. A common scenario is when acute left ventricular failure develops soon after the onset of AF, due to rapid ventricular rates and the loss of the atrial booster pump function. With rapid ventricular rates, e.g., in the presence of Wolff-Parkinson-White syndrome, ventricular fibrillation and cardiac arrest may develop.

A significant consequence of AF is peripheral arterial embolization, resulting most often in a stroke. The Framingham study suggests that the risk of stroke in patients with chronic AF is markedly increased compared to the population with sinus rhythm (36). The increased risk of stroke is present in patients with chronic AF due to valvular and nonvalvular heart disease, and to a lesser degree in those with paroxysmal AF or lone fibrillator syndrome (35).

History, physical examination, and a search for symptoms and signs of possible underlying heart disease are important.

Thyroid function tests should always be performed, as otherwise asymptomatic thyrotoxicosis may be the underlying cause. The echocardiogram is particularly useful in the assessment of AF. An enlarged left atrium is usually associated with AF. Findings associated with an increased risk of embolization in a recent study included an echocardiographic left atrial size in excess of 4 cm, female sex, and the presence of organic heart disease (36). Anticoagulation is recommended in any patient who presents with at least two of the three features (37). Long-term ECG recordings or patient activated event recording may be necessary to document paroxysmal AF as the cause of a patient's symptoms. Chronic AF is associated with an increased mortality in patients with hypertensive, mitral valve, and coronary artery disease.

Depending on the mode of presentation and hemodynamic consequences of AF the therapeutic approach varies. In recent-onset AF, restoration of sinus rhythm and prevention of further paroxysms of AF is desirable. When the ventricular rate is rapid and hemodynamic deterioration is expected or already present, prompt treatment is necessary. Slowing the ventricular rate can be achieved by one or more antiarrhythmic drugs that act on the AV node, i.e., digitalis, beta blockers, and verapamil. Intravenous digitalization is the time-honored treatment in this situation, but it may take several hours to take effect. Intravenous verapamil or beta blockers, when tolerated, will provide prompt effect. These medications cannot be expected to restore the sinus rhythm. They are also ineffective in Wolff-Parkinson-White syndrome, since they do not affect accessory pathway (AP) conduction. Frequently, paroxysmal AF terminates spontaneously, without further intervention. When pharmacologic conversion of AF is needed, type IA antiarrhythmic medications (quinidine, procainamide, disopyramide) are used traditionally. Reported conversion to sinus rhythm varies widely between 43 and 88% (38). Type IC medications (flecainide, propafenone) were also reported to be effective. When antiarrhythmic agents fail to restore sinus rhythm, elective direct current cardioversion can be attempted under sedation or short term intravenous anesthesia. The recommended starting energy is 100 J.

When AF has been present for less than about a week, the risk of peripheral embolization is minimal and anticoagulation is not necessary before cardioversion. Exceptions are patients with mitral valve disease, prosthetic valves, and those with a history of peripheral embolization. Unstable situations, e.g., very rapid rates during AF in the Wolff-Parkinson-White syndrome, may require prompt cardioversion. Once sinus rhythm is restored, prevention of recurrence is the main concern. If AF was caused by a transient underlying disorder, prophylactic antiarrhythmic treatment for 1–3 mo may be satisfactory. With an established underlying disorder long-term prophylaxis is necessary. Type IA, IC, and III drugs (amiodarone, sotalol) are used for this purpose (39–41).

Patients presenting with chronic AF may be candidates for elective pharmacologic or electrical cardioversion. The underlying, predisposing, or initiating disorders have to be treated (e.g., congestive heart failure, thyrotoxicosis) and the patient may have to be anticoagulated. The likelihood of restoration and preservation of sinus rhythm decreases markedly when AF has been present for more than 3–6 mo, and when left atrial dimensions are significantly enlarged. If AF persists despite efforts to restore sinus rhythm, antiarrhythmic medications can be discontinued and the purpose of further treatment is to control the ventricular rate. Digitalis, verapamil, diltiazem, or beta blockers alone or in combination are used to slow the ventricular response. Low-dose amiodarone can also slow the ventricular rate, with relatively infrequent adverse effects. Atrioventricular block may also be produced by surgical or catheter ablation, with subsequent implantation of a rate-responsive ventricular pacemaker. It is an effective nonpharmacologic treatment in patients who do not tolerate or respond to drugs.

Experimental surgical methods have been devised and used in a few selected patients with AF refractory to drug therapy to restore the sinus rhythm (42,43). Atrial "corridor" operation has been described by Guiradon (42) and more recently, the "maze" procedure was developed by Cox *et al* (43). Early results with these surgical techniques appear promising.

Patients with chronic AF, especially with associated left atrial enlargement, have to be anticoagulated to prevent peripheral embolization, if specific contraindication does not exist. Low-dose warfarin (prothrombin time ratio 1.2–1.5) has been advised for nonrheumatic disease (44). Aspirin prophylaxis also appears to be beneficial (45). The use of anticoagulants should be weighed against the potential risk of bleeding.

Multifocal Atrial Tachycardia

An atrial tachycardia with distinct P waves of at least three different, nonsinus morphologies recorded on the same ECG lead is called multifocal atrial tachycardia (MAT). The PP, PR and RR intervals are all variable, the PP cycle lengths shorter than 600 msec on the average (a rate exceeding 100 beats/min). Isoelectric baseline separates the P waves. The P-QRS relationship is usually 1:1, but the tachycardia is not interrupted by AV block. The electrophysiologic mechanism of MAT is unknown, although triggered activity has been proposed.

MAT is an infrequent arrhythmia appearing in about 0.32–0.36% of electrocardiograms of a general hospital population (46–48). Most commonly it occurs in elderly, critically ill patients. About 60% of patients have pulmonary disorders, most frequently chronic obstructive lung disease. Pulmonary infections or infrequently, pulmonary embolism may be the underlying cause. Factors that contribute to the genesis of MAT in these patients include blood gas, acid-base, and electrolyte abnormalities related to severe respiratory disease, right atrial enlargement, and medications used to treat pulmonary conditions, e.g., β-agonists and aminophylline. When heart disease is the cause, coronary artery disease is the most common etiology, followed by congestive heart failure and valvular heart disease. In the presence of severe lung disease, the assessment of cardiac function may be very difficult. Metabolic disorders in diabetes and chronic renal insufficiency and diuretic induced hypokalemia have also been associated with MAT. A combination of the above causes can contribute to MAT developing in the postoperative period. The prognosis of these critically ill elderly patients is often poor, with mortality rates as high as 29–55% (46). The prognosis of MAT occurring in infants, children, and young adults is less serious.

MAT is generally secondary to an underlying critical illness, improving, or worsening with the course of the underlying disorder. When rapid ventricular rates result in myocardial ischemia, congestive heart failure, or ventricular arrhythmias, verapamil or beta blockers (when lung disease is not present) may be used to slow the tachycardia. Magnesium and potassium replacement may also be helpful. Type I antiarrhythmic agents and digitalis are generally not effective. Cardioversion is not recommended, as it usually does not terminate the tachycardia.

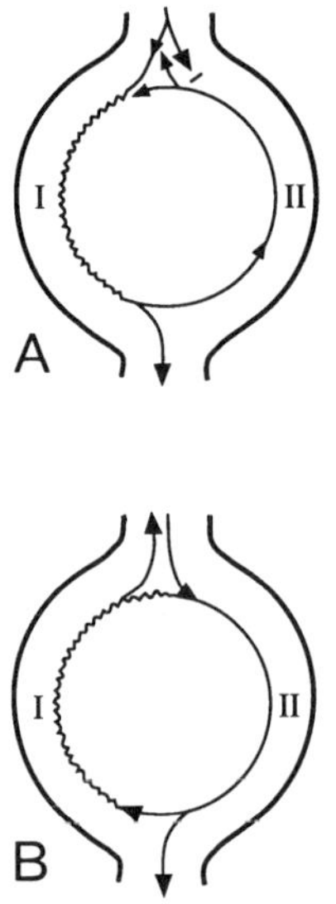

Figure 7.4. Diagrammatic representation of AV node reentry tachycardia demonstrating "slow-fast" reentry (**A**) and "fast-slow" reentry (**B**). For discussion see text.

Atrioventricular Nodal Reentry Tachycardia

Reentry within the AV node is a common mechanism of paroxysmal supraventricular tachycardias. Two (or more) functionally distinct pathways with different refractoriness, called slow and fast pathways according to their respective conduction characteristics, serve as the anterograde and the retrograde limbs of the circuit (49). When unidirectional block develops in one of the pathways, accompanied by a critical conduction delay in the other pathway, reentry becomes possible (Fig. 7.4). In the common type of AV nodal reentry the slow pathway conducts in the anterograde direction and the fast pathway conducts retrogradely, resulting in a "slow-fast" tachycardia (Fig. 7.5). Arrhythmias due to a reentry circuit with the opposite direction of activation, i.e., a "fast-slow" circuit, are much less common. Atrioventricular nodal reentry of the common or slow-fast type is a regular narrow QRS tachycardia with cycle lengths of 550–240 msec (110–250 beats/min). There is usually a 1:1 relationship between atrial and ventricular activity. The atria are activated in the retrograde direction, from the AV nodal area, resulting in negative P waves in leads II, III, and aVF. The P waves are usually in the proximity of the QRS complexes closely preceding or following them. Frequently, the atrial and ventricular activities are simultaneous and the P wave is "buried" within the QRS complex, resulting in the apparent absence of P waves on the surface electrocardiogram (Fig. 7.6). In the case of the uncommon or fast-slow type of AV nodal reentry the retrograde P wave presents with a PR interval that is shorter than the RP interval. This latter arrhythmia has to be differentiated from ectopic atrial tachycardias and AV reentry using a concealed posteroseptal AP as the retrograde limb. Sustained fast-slow tachycardia is rare. When it develops, it can be incessant. Echo beats due to fast-slow reentry are not uncommon.

Diagnosis of AV nodal reentrant tachycardias may be difficult even with invasive EP techniques. Evidence that suggests the diagnosis includes demonstration of dual AV nodal physiology by programmed stimulation or incremental pacing, in either anterograde or retrograde directions (Fig. 7.7). Dual AV nodal pathways appear on anterograde AV nodal conduction curves relating H_1–H_2 or A_2–H_2 intervals to A_1–A_2 intervals as discontinuities or "jumps." A "jump" is considered to be diagnostic when a sudden prolongation of the H_1–H_2 or A_2–H_2 interval of at least 50 msec accompanies a 10-msec shortening of the A_1–A_2 coupling interval. The sudden prolongation of H_1–H_2 or A_2–H_2 interval represents a shift of conduction from the fast to the slow pathway following the development of block in the former (50). Both the fast and the slow pathways exhibit conduction delay characteristic of AV nodal conduction. Vagal maneuvers and drugs usually affecting AV nodal conduction (beta blockers, calcium channel blockers, adenosine) also affect both pathways and may terminate the arrhythmia. Local anesthetic agents also frequently affect the fast pathway. Dual-pathway physiology may be present in the absence of arrhythmias. In approximately 30% of patients with AV nodal reentry, dual pathways cannot be demonstrated.

Atrioventricular node reentry tachycardia can be initiated and terminated by critically timed premature stimuli, indicating the reentrant nature of the rhythm. The slow-fast rhythm is easier to induce from the atrium, while the fast-slow tachycardia is easier to induce from the ventricle. Tachycardias can only be induced after one of the pathways is blocked and a critical AV nodal conduction delay (AH or HA delay), i.e., conduction delay in the other pathway, has been attained. The conduction delay on the surface ECG appears as a prolonged PR interval, following a premature atrial complex. The first P wave and PR interval differ from the subsequent ones during the tachycardia.

Atrial and/or ventricular activity may be transiently dissociated from the tachycardia, without affecting the tachycardia cycle length. Premature stimuli that capture either the atrium or

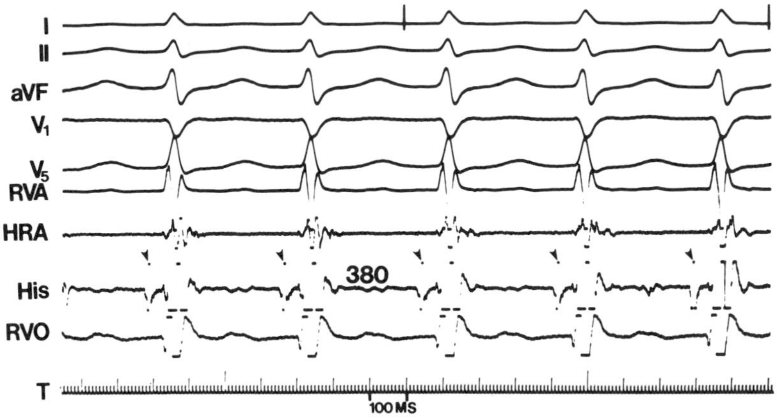

Figure 7.5. Atrioventricular node reentry tachycardia of "slow-fast" type. Displayed from **top** to **bottom** are surface leads I, II, aVF, V_1 and V_5, intracardiac electrograms right ventricular apex (RVA), high right atrium (HRA), His bundle (His), and time scale (T). Note that His deflection precedes the ventricular activation. His is labeled with an *arrowhead,* with short V-A time, so that the P waves are "buried" in the QRS complex (surface leads).

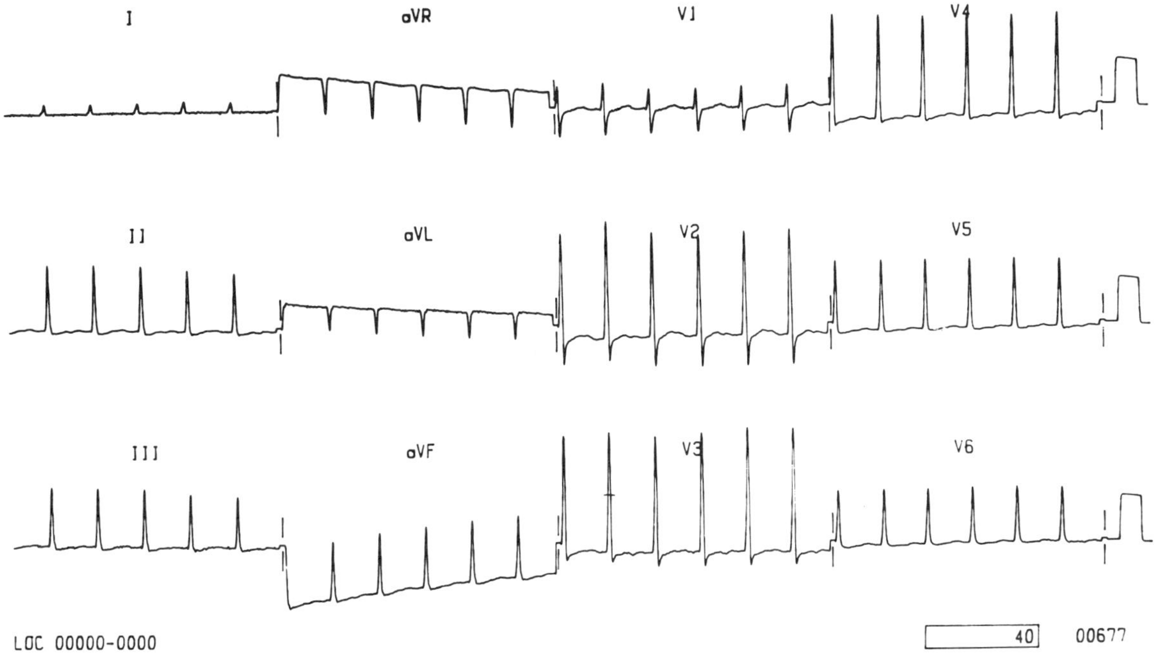

Figure 7.6. Twelve-lead electrocardiogram displaying a typical AV node tachycardia of the "slow-fast" type. Note "absence" of P waves, which are buried in the QRS complexes.

the ventricle and advance the respective electrical activity without affecting the tachycardia, suggest that the captured chamber is not a part of the arrhythmia circuit and localizes the reentry to the AV junction. Atrioventricular nodal reentry may continue in the presence of either anterograde or retrograde conduction block. Premature ventricular stimuli delivered at a time when the His bundle is refractory do not advance atrial activity (Fig. 7.8). This finding rules out the participation of a concealed accessory AV pathway as a retrograde limb of the circuit. Atrial activation is only rarely advanced by ventricular premature stimulation during the tachycardia.

Retrograde atrial activation during the tachycardia is usually concentric, i.e., the earliest site of activation is found in the low septum (the His bundle electrogram) (17). However, the proximal coronary sinus may also be the first site of retrograde atrial activation when conduction is over the AV node (Fig. 7.9).

Ventriculoatrial (VA) conduction times are short, ruling out the participation of an accessory AV pathway as the retrograde limb of the reentrant circuit. The VA conduction time does not exceed 60 to 90 msec as measured on the His bundle and high right atrial electrograms, respectively. Development of functional bundle branch block affects neither the VA conduction time nor the tachycardia cycle length. The temporal relationship between atrial and ventricular activity is dependent on the relative conduction times in the anterograde and retrograde directions. At times, it may be impossible to distinguish between AV nodal reentry and orthodromic AV reentry incorporating a posteroseptal accessory AV pathway as a retrograde limb.

Atrioventricular nodal reentry has been reported to be present in approximately 38% of patients referred for EP studies for symptomatic supraventricular tachycardias (51). The arrhythmia can be present both with and without organic heart disease. It

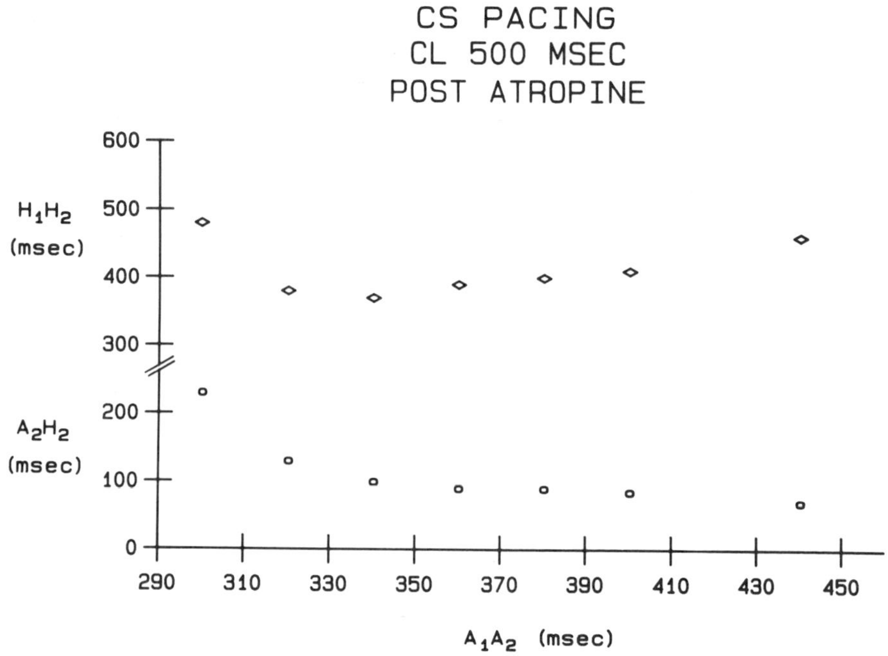

Figure 7.7. Patient with dual AV node pathways. After atropine administration, programmed atrial stimulation is performed from the proximal coronary sinus at the basic cycle drive of 500 msec, with progressive shortening of A_1A_2 coupling intervals (*abscissa*). A_2H_2 (open circles) and H_1H_2 (*diamonds*) are plotted, in response to A_1A_2, (*ordinate*). Discontinuous curves are demonstrated typical of dual AV node pathways. "Jumps" in A_2H_2 and H_1H_2, in response to shortening A_1A_2 interval from 320 to 300 msec, are noted (100-msec increment).

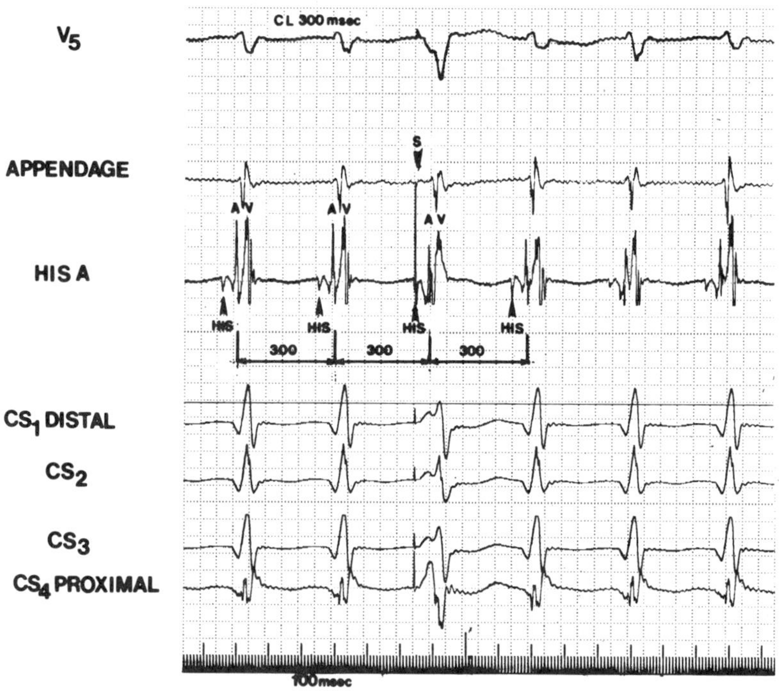

Figure 7.8. Premature ventricular stimulus delivered at the time when the His is refractory fails to advance the atrial activity, thus ruling out the participation of a concealed accessory AV pathway as the retrograde limb of the circuit. From top to bottom: surface lead V_5, intracardiac recordings from right atrial appendage, His (His A), distal coronary sinus (CS_1 distal), CS_2, CS_3, and proximal coronary sinus (CS_4 proximal).

may coexist with an accessory AV pathway. In this case the diagnosis may be impossible until after the ablation of the AP.

A typical patient with AV nodal reentry is a young, otherwise healthy person with a history of recurrent palpitations. The episodes usually start and terminate abruptly. Young and healthy individuals tolerate even prolonged episodes of tachycardia well, but with time, symptoms of weakness, lightheadedness, shortness of breath, chest discomfort, presyncope, or syncope may develop. Frequent, symptomatic episodes may interfere with the patient's usual activities, but the arrhythmia is usually not life-threatening. The surface electrocardiogram may show significant ST depression, which usually does not indicate underlying ischemia in association with coronary disease, when it develops during narrow QRS tachycardia (52).

Atrioventricular reentrant tachycardia may be diagnosed from the surface electrocardiogram. Causal relationship between the

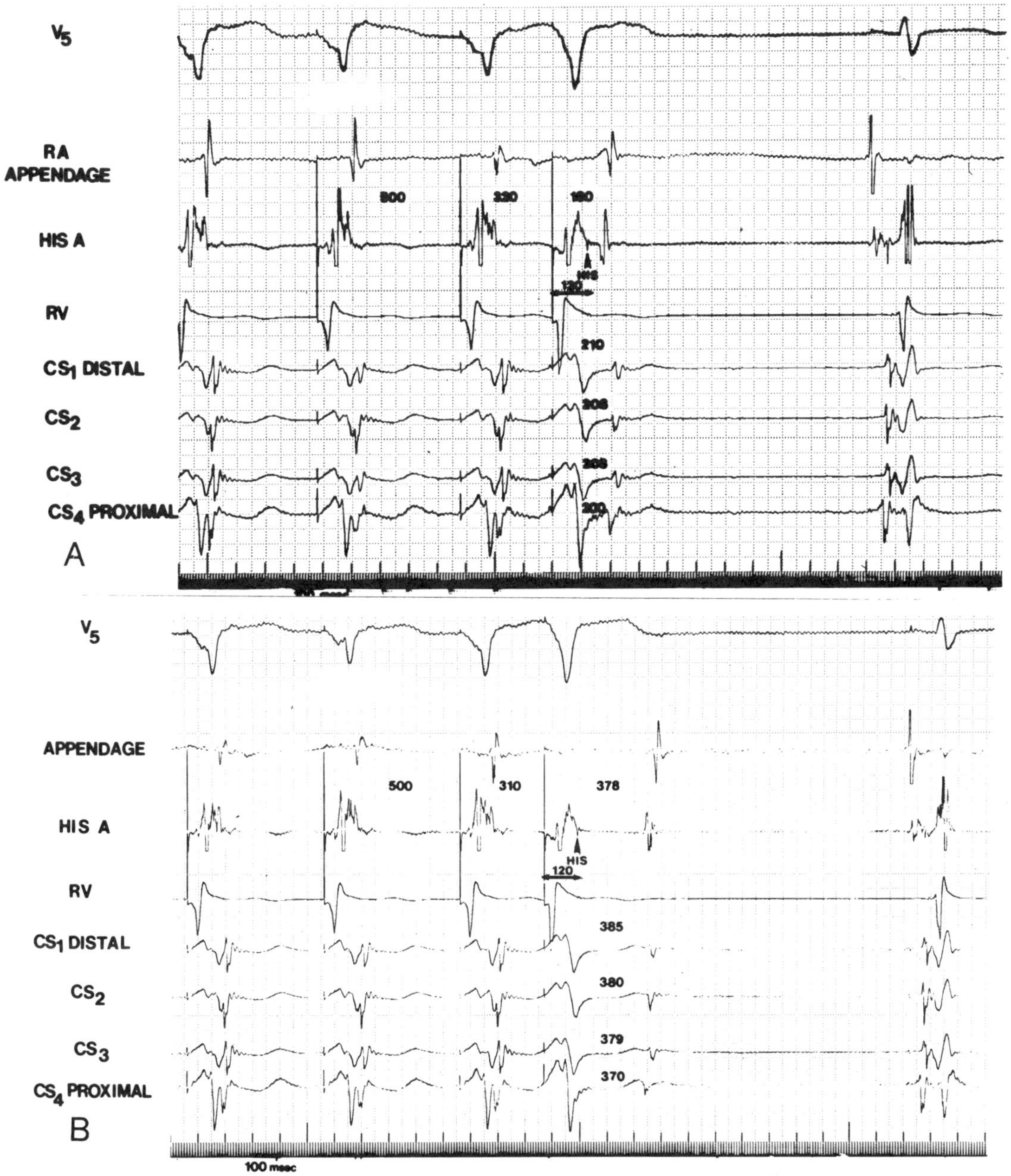

Figure 7.9. Alternating sequence of retrograde activation in a patient with dual AV node pathways. Note the shift from the earliest (His A) activation to proximal coronary sinus (CS_4 proximal) with decrementing of V_1V_2 intervals. Electrograms are arranged as in Fig. 7.8. (Reproduced from Singer I, *et al.* PACE 1989;12:80–85, with publisher's permission.)

tachycardia and symptoms can be documented by long-term ECG monitoring. Invasive EP studies are indicated when the arrhythmia mechanism needs to be elucidated, in case of frequently recurring, symptomatic tachycardias to guide antiarrhythmic therapy, and when antitachycardia pacing, surgical, or catheter ablation of the tachycardia circuit are contemplated.

Patients may be able to terminate AV nodal reentrant tachycardia episodes by using vagal maneuvers. Valsalva maneuver, assumption of supine position, carotid sinus massage or immersion of the face in cold water may terminate the tachycardia, especially immediately after the onset.

Pharmacologic agents acting on the AV node can be administered intravenously if vagal maneuvers fail. Verapamil, beta blockers, adenosine, and adenosine triphosphate may be used. If these drugs fail, intravenous administration of Type IA or IC drugs may be tried. In the case of infrequent, mildly symptomatic episodes, an oral dose of an appropriate antiarrhythmic agent may hasten conversion to sinus rhythm.

Antitachycardia pacing using a transvenous or an esophageal electrode may effectively terminate the arrhythmia. Occasional older patients with organic heart disease may not tolerate the tachycardia hemodynamically and may require prompt cardioversion.

A variety of antiarrhythmic drugs can be used for long term prophylaxis of tachycardia recurrence, including Type IA and IC drugs, β-adrenergic blocking agents, calcium channel blockers, and amiodarone. Drug treatment guided by repeated electrophysiologic studies is helpful in identifying an effective treatment regimen.

Antitachycardia pacing is another option available for long term management. This modality does not prevent arrhythmia recurrences, but terminates the tachycardia effectively and quickly in selected patients. Atrial antitachycardia pacing carries the risk of induction of AF.

Surgical, cryosurgical, and catheter ablation of the AV node with the implantation of a permanent ventricular pacemaker was an option in the past to treat severely symptomatic, therapy-resistant arrhythmias. More recently, modification of AV nodal conduction, i.e., selective ablation of one or the other of the dual pathways with preservation of normal AV conduction is used to eliminate AV nodal reentry. This can be achieved with surgical, cryosurgical, and more recently catheter techniques using radiofrequency energy delivery (see Chapters 22 and 24).

Nonparoxysmal Junctional Tachycardia

Junctional tachycardias with a mechanism other than reentry are much less common than AV nodal reentrant rhythms. A rapid automatic junctional tachycardia (cycle length 450–240 msec, rate 110–250 beats/min) occurs in infants and as a perioperative tachycardia in infants or children. This rhythm is usually irregular and is accompanied by AV dissociation (53,54).

Automatic junctional tachycardia is very unusual in adults. It is thought to be caused by catecholamine-sensitive or catecholamine-dependent abnormal automaticity and responds to treatment with beta adrenergic blockers (55). Another form of nonreentrant junctional tachycardia, called nonparoxysmal junctional tachycardia, is more common in adults. It is characterized by regular narrow QRS tachycardia with cycle lengths of 860–460 msec (70–130 beats/min). When the cycle length is between 860 and 600 msec (70–100 beats/min) the arrhythmia is called an accelerated junctional rhythm. When a retrograde P wave is visible, it can occur as early as 100 msec prior to the QRS complex or it can follow the QRS complex by up to 200 msec. After initial acceleration ("warm-up") the RR interval is usually stable. The underlying mechanism is thought to be either enhanced automaticity or triggered activity.

Atrioventricular dissociation occurs more commonly than in AV nodal reentry. When AV dissociation is present, the atria may be driven by the sinus node or by another atrial pacemaker. Nonparoxysmal junctional tachycardia is usually a transient arrhythmia that develops in the setting of digitalis intoxication, acute inferior or posterior myocardial infarction, viral or rheumatic carditis, hypokalemia, or in the postoperative period following open heart surgery.

Electrophysiologic investigations are seldom performed in patients with this tachycardia. Intracardiac recordings are indistinguishable from those recorded during AV nodal reentry, i.e., ventricular electrograms are preceded by His electrograms with a normal HV interval. The first site of retrograde atrial activation is either the low septum or the orifice of the coronary sinus. Atrial overdrive pacing may suppress the tachycardia and result in 1:1 AV conduction.

The diagnosis is suggested by the electrocardiogram and by the clinical presentation. In the absence of digitalis intoxication the arrhythmia is usually self-limiting and does not need antiarrhythmic treatment. When the hemodynamic status is compromised, temporary atrial or AV sequential pacing may improve the cardiac output. Beta blockers may slow the tachycardia rate making overdrive pacing more feasible. Digitalis intoxication is treated in the usual manner.

Orthodromic Atrioventricular Reciprocating Tachycardia

The regular narrow QRS tachycardia resulting from a macroreentrant circuit, that incorporates the normal conduction system as anterograde and an accessory AV pathway as retrograde limb, is called orthodromic AV reciprocating tachycardia. This arrhythmia can develop in the setting of Wolff-Parkinson-White syndrome or in the presence of a concealed AP. It is discussed in more detail in Chapter 9. This arrhythmia and AV node reentry tachycardia are the most common causes of regular narrow QRS tachycardia.

Orthodromic AV reentry can be initiated and terminated with critically timed extrastimuli. Stimulation from both the atrium and the ventricle can start or terminate the tachycardia, demonstrating the participation of atrial and ventricular myocardium in the macroreentrant circuit. Arrhythmia initiation is related to a critical AV delay, not necessarily confined to the AH interval. Retrograde conduction time is longer than the one observed with AV nodal reentry, manifesting in a retrograde P wave located close to the mid-point of the RR interval, with an RP interval shorter than the PR interval. Retrograde atrial activation is eccentric, the earliest activation site being other than the low septum (His bundle electrogram), dependent on the AP location. Premature ventricular extrastimuli delivered during the tachycardia, at a time when the His bundle is refractory, may advance the atrial activation, demonstrating the participation of an AP as the retrograde limb of the tachycardia circuit. Acutely or chronically, the tachycardia may be treated with Type IA, IC, and III antiarrhythmic medication, acutely with verapamil and adenosine and chronically by surgical or catheter ablation of the macroreentrant circuit.

The Permanent Form of Junctional Reciprocating Tachycardia

The differential diagnosis of a regular narrow QRS complex tachycardia with discernible "retrograde" P waves (i.e., negative P waves in leads II, III and aVF) and an RP interval longer than the PR interval includes ectopic atrial tachycardias, the uncommon (fast-slow) form of AV nodal reentry and PJRT (56). The latter two arrhythmias may present as incessant tachycardias and may be unresponsive to medical treatment. The permanent form of junctional reciprocating tachycardia (PJRT) is caused by a macroreentrant circuit analogous with that described in orthodromic AV reciprocating tachycardia (57,58). The concealed accessory pathway involved in this circuit, however, is atypical. It has AV node–like conduction properties with a long retrograde conduction time. It is responsive to autonomic tone, catecholamines, beta blockers, and digoxin. The AP is usually located in the posteroseptal area and its unique EP properties are thought to be the result of a long and tortuous course (59). Initiation of PJRT is usually related to a critical shortening of the sinus cycle length without AV conduction delay. The P to QRS relationship is always 1:1. Therefore, AV block terminates the tachycardia.

PJRT is more common in infants and children than in adults. When the rapid rhythm is present for a sufficiently long time, left ventricular dilatation and tachycardia-induced cardiomyopathy may develop (60). Treatment of the tachycardia before the development of irreversible damage is important. In adults, PJRT may be asymptomatic or may present with congestive heart failure (60). As PJRT is frequently unresponsive to antiarrhythmic drug treatment, surgical and more recently catheter ablation is the treatment (61,62).

Narrow QRS Ventricular Tachycardia

A narrow QRS complex (<120 ms) does not exclude the diagnosis of ventricular tachycardia. A recent study of 106 patients who had inducible ventricular tachycardia on EP study identified 5 patients (4.7%) whose QRS duration in any ECG lead did not exceed 110 ms (63). These arrhythmias are presumed to originate in the vicinity of the bundle branches (64,65). The features that helped diagnose ventricular tachycardia included documentation of AV dissociation, an HV interval shorter than the one recorded during normal sinus rhythm, and morphologic clues (precordial concordance of QRS polarity, etc.) It is important to include narrow QRS ventricular tachycardia in the differential diagnosis, especially when the clinical picture is suggestive of the presence of ventricular arrhythmias.

Conclusion

Narrow QRS tachycardias encompass a spectrum of different arrhythmias. Management of these arrhythmias depends on the understanding of the underlying mechanisms. Electrophysiologic techniques are helpful in providing physiologic and anatomic information to guide pharmacologic, AV ablative therapy, or the use of antitachycardia pacing modalities in selected patients.

References

1. Klein GJ, Sharma AD, Yee R, *et al.*: Classification of supraventricular tachycardias. Am J Cardiol 1987;60:27D–31D.
2. Wellens HJJ, Bar FWHM, Lie KI: The value of the electrocardiogram in the differential diagnosis of a tachycardia with a widened QRS complex. Am J Med 1978;64:27–33
3. Brugada P, Brugada J, Mont L, *et al.*: A new approach to the differential diagnosis of a regular tachycardia with a wide QRS complex. Circulation 1991;83:1649–1659.
4. Bar FW, Brugada P, Dassen WRM, *et al.*: Differential diagnosis of tachycardia with narrow QRS complex (Shorter than 0.12 second). Am J Cardiol 1984;54;555–560.
5. Pratt CM, Eaton T, Francis M, *et al.*: Ambulatory electrocardiographic recordings: The Holter monitor. Curr Prob Cardiol 1988;13:549–552.
6. Shenasa M, Nadeau R, Savard P, *et al.*: Noninvasive evaluation of supraventricular tachycardias. Cardiol Clin 1990;8:443–464.
7. Leitch J, Klein GJ, Yee R, *et al.*: Invasive electrophysiologic evaluation of patients with supraventricular tachycardia. Cardiol Clin 1990;8:465–477.
8. Kirchhoff CJHJ, Bonke FIM, Allessie MA.; Sinus node reentry: fact or fiction? In Brugada P, Wellens HJJ (eds): Cardiac arrhythmias: Where to Go from Here? Futura Publishers, Mt. Kisco, NY, 1987:53–65.
9. Huycke EC, Sung RJ: Atrial tachycardias. In Zipes DP, Rowland DJ (eds): Progress in Cardiology. Lea & Febiger, Philadelphia, 1988:313–325.
10. Curry PVL, Shenasa M: Atrial arrhythmias: clinical concepts. In Mandel WJ (ed): Cardiac Arrhythmias: Their Mechanism, Diagnosis and Management. J.B. Lippincott, Philadelphia, 1987:208–234.
11. Wu D, Amat-y-Leon F, Denes P, *et al.*: Demonstration of sustained sinus and atrial re-entry as a mechanism of paroxysmal supraventricular tachycardia. Circulation 1975;51:234–243.
12. Gomes JA, Hariman RJ, Kang PS, *et al.*: Sustained symptomatic sinus node reentrant tachycardia: incidence, clinical significance, electrophysiologic observations and the effects of antiarrhythmic agents. J Am Coll Cardiol 1985;5:45–57.
13. Gomes JA, Hariman RJ, Kang PS, *et al.*: Sustained symptomatic sinus node reentrant tachycardia: incidence, clinical significance, electrophysiologic observations and the effects of antiarrhythmic agents. J Am Coll Cardiol 1985;5:45–57.
14. Griffith MJ, Garratt CJ, Ward DE, *et al.*: The effects of adenosine on sinus node reentrant tachycardia. Clin Cardiol 1989;17:409–411.
15. Kerr CR, Klein GJ, Guiraudon GM, *et al.*: Surgical therapy for sinoatrial reentrant tachycardia. PACE 1986;11:776–783.
16. Friehling TD, Marinchak RA, Kowey PR: Role of permanent pacemakers in the pharmacologic therapy of patients with reentrant tachycardias. PACE 1988;11:83–92.
17. Josephson, ME, Seides SF: Supraventricular tachycardias. Clinical Cardiac Electrophysiology. Techniques and Interpretations. Lea & Febiger Philadelphia, 1979:147–190.
18. Swerdlow CD, Liem LB. Atrial and junctional tachycardias: clinical presentation, course and therapy. In Zipes DP, Jalife J (eds); Cardiac Electrophysiology. From Cell to Bedside. W.B. Saunders, Philadelphia, 1990:742–755.
19. Goldreyer BN, Gallagher JJ, Damato AN: The electrophysiologic demonstration of atrial ectopic tachycardia in man. Am Heart J 1973;85:205–215.
20. Josephson ME, Spear JF, Harken AH, *et al.*: Surgical excision of automatic atrial tachycardia: anatomic and electrophysiologic correlates. Am Heart J 1982;104:1076–1085.
21. Josephson ME, Sedies SF: Atrial flutter and fibrillation. Clinical Cardiac Electrophysiology. Techniques and Interpretations. Lea & Febiger, Philadelphia, 1979:194–206.

22. Wells JL, MacLean WAH, James TN, *et al.*: Characterization of atrial flutter. Studies in man after open heart surgery using fixed atrial electrodes. Circulation 1979;60:665–673.
23. Olshansky B, Okumura K, Henthorn RW, *et al.*: Atrial mapping of human atrial flutter demonstrates reentry in the right atrium. J Am Coll Cardiol 1986;7:194A.
24. Cosio FG, Arribas F, Barbero JM, *et al.*: Validation of double spike electrograms as markers of conduction delay in block in atrial flutter. Am J Cardiol 1988;61:775–780.
25. Klein GJ, Guiraudon GM, Sharma AD, *et al.*: Demonstration of macroreentry and feasibility of operative therapy in the common type of atrial flutter. Am J Cardiol 1986;57:587–591.
26. Saoudi N, Atallah G, Kirkorian G, *et al.*: Catheter ablation of the atrial myocardium in human type I atrial flutter. Circulation 1990;81:762–771.
27. Henthorn RW, Okumura K, Olshansky B, *et al.*: A fourth criterion for transient entrainment: the electrogram equivalent of progressive fusion. Circulation 1988;77:1003–1012.
28. Waldo AL, Carlson MD, Henthorn RW: Atrial flutter: transient entrainment and related phenomena. In Zipes DP, Jalife J (eds): Cardiac Electrophysiology. From Cell to Bedside. W.B. Saunders, Philadelphia, 1990:530–537.
29. Waldo AL: Clinical evaluation in therapy of patients with atrial fibrillation or flutter. Cardiol Clin 1990;8:479–490.
30. Watt JHM, Donner AP, McKinney CM, *et al.*: Atrial fibrillation: minimal sampling interval to estimate average rate. J Electrocardiol 1984;17:153–156.
31. Moe GK: On the multiple wavelet hypothesis of atrial fibrillation. Arch Int Pharmacodyn Ther 1962;140:183–188.
32. Allessie MA, Lammers WJEP, Bonke FIM, *et al.*: Experimental evaluation of Moe's multiple wavelet hypothesis of atrial fibrillation. In Zipes DP, Jalife J (eds): Cardiac Arrhythmias. Grune & Stratton, Philadelphia, 1985:265–276.
33. Allessie MA, Bonke FIM, Kirchhof CJHJ: Atrial reentry. In Rosen MR, Janse MJ, Wit AL (eds): Cardiac Electrophysiology: A Textbook. Futura Publishing Co., Mt. Kisco, NY, 1990:555–571.
34. Sanfilippo AJ, Abascal VM, Sheehan M, *et al.*: Atrial enlargement as a consequence of atrial fibrillation. A prospective echocardiographic study. Circulation 1990;82:792–797.
35. Cairns JA, Connolly SJ. Nonrheumatic atrial fibrillation. Risk of stroke and role of antithrombotic therapy. Circulation 1991;84:469–481.
36. Wolf PA, Dawber TR, Thomas E Jr, *et al.*: Epidemiologic assessment of chronic atrial fibrillation and risk of stroke: The Framingham Study. Neurology 1978;28:973–977.
37. Cabin HS, Clubb KS, Hall C, *et al.*: Risk for systemic embolization of atrial fibrillation without mitral stenosis. AM J Cardiol 1990;65:1112–1116.
38. Lewis RV: Atrial fibrillation. The therapeutic options. Drugs 1990;40:841–853.
39. Coplen SE, Antman EM, Berlin JA, *et al.*: Efficacy and safety of quinidine therapy for maintenance of sinus rhythm after cardioversion. A meta-analysis of randomized control trials. Circulation 1990;82:1106–1116.
40. Petersen P: Thromboembolic complications of atrial fibrillation and their prevention: a review. Am J Cardiol 1990;65:24C–28C.
41. Karlson BW, Herlitz J, Edvardsson N, *et al.*: Prophylactic treatment after electroconversion of atrial fibrillation. Clin Cardiol 1990;13:279–286.
42. Leitch JW, Klein GJ, Yee R, *et al.*: Sinus node-Atrioventricular node isolation: long-term results with the "corridor" operation for atrial fibrillation. J Am Coll Cardiol 1991;17:970–975.
43. Cox JL, Schuessler RB, D'Agostino HJ, *et al.*: The surgical treatment of atrial fibrillation. III. Development of a definitive surgical procedure. J Thorac Cardiovasc Surg 1991;101:569–583.
44. The Boston Area Anticoagulation Trial for Atrial Fibrillation Investigators: The effect of low-dose warfarin on the risk of stroke in patients with nonrheumatic atrial fibillation. N Engl J Med 1990;323:1505–1511.
45. Preliminary report of the stroke prevention in atrial fibrillation study. N Engl J Med 1990;322:863–868.
46. Habibzadeh MA: Multifocal atrial tachycardia:a 66 month follow-up of 50 patients. Heart Lung 1980;9:328–335.
47. Scher DL, Arsura EL: Multifocal atrial tachycardia: mechanisms, clinical correlates, and treatment. Am Heart J 1989;118:574–580.
48. Kastor JA: Multifocal atrial tachycardia. N Engl J Med 1990;322:1713–1717.
49. Wu D: Dual atrioventricular nodal pathways: a reappraisal. PACE 1982;5:72–88.
50. Sung RJ, Huycke EC, Keung EC, *et al.*: Atrioventricular node reentry: evidence of reentry and functional properties of fast and slow pathways. In Zipes DP, Jalife J (eds): Cardiac Electrophysiology. From Cell to Bedside. W.B. Saunders, Philadelphia, 1990:513–525.
51. Sharma AD, Yee R, Guiraudon GM, *et al.*: AV nodal reentry—current concepts and surgical treatment. Prog Cardiol 1988;1:129–145.
52. Imrie JR, Yee R, Klein GJ, *et al.*: Incidence and clinical significance of ST segment depression in supraventricular tachycardia. Can J Cardiol 1990;6:323–326.
53. Brechenmacher C, Coumel P, James TN: Intractable tachycardia in infancy. Circulation 1976;53:377–381.
54. Garson A, Gillette PC: Junctional ectopic tachycardia in children: electrocardiography, electrophysiology and pharmacologic response. Am J Cardiol 1979;44:298–302.
55. Ruder MA, Davis JC, Eldar M, *et al.*: Clinical and electrophysiologic characterization of automatic junctional tachycardia in adults. Circulation 1986;73:930–937.
56. Castellanos A, Myerburg RJ: The wide electrophysiologic spectrum of tachycardias having R-P intervals longer than the P-R intervals. PACE 1987;10:1382–1384.
57. Gallagher JJ, Sealy WC: The permanent form of junctional reciprocating tachycardia: further elucidation of the underlying mechanism. Eur J Cardiol 1978;8:413–430.
58. Coumel P: Junctional reciprocating tachycardias. The permanent and paroxysmal forms of A-V nodal reciprocating tachycardias. J Electrocardiol 1975;8:79–90.
59. Critelli G, Gallagher JJ, Monda V, *et al.*: Anatomic and electrophysiologic substrate of the permanent form of junctional reciprocating tachycardia. J Am Coll Cardiol 1984;4:601–610.
60. McLaran CJ, Gersh BJ, Sugrue DD, *et al.*: Tachycardia-induced myocardial dysfunction: a reversible phenomenon. Br Heart J 1985;53:323–327.
61. O'Neill BJ, Klein GJ, Guiraudon GM, *et al.*: Results of operative therapy in the permanent form of junctional reciprocating tachycardia. Am J Cardiol 1989;63:1074–1079.
62. Smith RT, Gillette PC, Massumi A, *et al.*: Transcatheter ablative techniques for treatment of the permanent form of junctional reciprocating tachycardia in young patients. J Am Coll Cardiol 1986;8:385–390.
63. Hayes JJ, Stewart RB, Greene HL, *et al.*: Narrow QRS ventricular tachycardia. Ann Intern Med 1991;114:460–463.
64. Cohen HC, Gozo EG, Pick A: Ventricular tachycardia with narrow QRS complexes (left posterior fascicular tachycardia). Circulation 1972;45:1035–1043.
65. Weiss J, Stevenson WG: Narrow QRS ventricular tachycardia. Am Heart J 1986;112:843–847.

8

VENTRICULAR TACHYCARDIA

Igor Singer, M.B.B.S., F.R.A.C.P., F.A.C.P., F.A.C.C.

INTRODUCTION

Sustained ventricular tachycardia is an unstable rhythm associated with significant morbidity and mortality. It is most commonly associated with coronary artery disease in the setting of a prior myocardial infarction. However, other pathologic entities may on occasion cause ventricular tachycardia. These entities include dilated and hypertrophic cardiomyopathies, mitral valve prolapse, congenital heart disease, myocarditis, and right ventricular dysplasia. Rarely, ventricular tachycardia may occur in a patient with a structurally normal heart.

VENTRICULAR TACHYCARDIA ASSOCIATED WITH CORONARY ARTERY DISEASE

MECHANISMS OF VENTRICULAR TACHYCARDIA[a]

Reentry

Reentry is the most common mechanism of clinically recognized ventricular tachycardia (1,2). Evidence for reentry comes from electrophysiologic (EP) catheter mapping and intraoperative mapping studies. These have suggested that the reentrant circuit of ventricular tachycardia originates in the subendocardial layer and is associated with previous myocardial infarction (2–5). Catheter and endocardial mapping studies during surgery have utilized the earliest site of continuous diastolic activity to identify the site of origin of ventricular tachycardia. Support for this approach is derived from cryoablation studies. When a cryolesion or cooling is applied to the site of the earliest activation, ventricular tachycardia is promptly terminated (5).

Initiation of reentrant ventricular tachycardia requires that a circuit exists that is capable of sustaining the tachycardia. The prerequisites are the presence of an unidirectional block and slow conduction in another part of the circuit permitting recovery of excitability within the circuit. Indirect clinical evidence for slow conduction is derived from the observation of low-amplitude, fractionated potentials during sinus mapping (6) and pace mapping (7). Anisotropic conduction and dispersion of refractoriness are necessary requirements for certain types of reentry (8).

Results of programmed ventricular stimulation provides further support for reentry as the underlying mechanism of most ventricular tachycardias associated with coronary artery disease. The ability of extrastimuli to start, stop, and reset ventricular tachycardia suggests reentry.

Automatic rhythms cannot be reliably initiated or terminated by programmed electrical stimulation. Presence of these features, however, does not always mean that the mechanisms of the tachycardia is reentry. Automatic foci and triggered arrhythmias may on occasion also be started, stopped, and reset by extrastimuli (9–11).

Automaticity

The role of automatic rhythms in ventricular tachycardia is less well defined. Automatic rhythms occur spontaneously as the result of phase 4 depolarization (12). Normal automaticity may be defined as spontaneous depolarizations occurring within cells with relatively high diastolic membrane potentials. Abnormal automaticity, on the other hand, results from spontaneous depolarizations in tissues with more positive resting membrane potentials. These potentials are calcium dependent and are less amenable to overdrive pacing suppression. The onset of abnormal automatic rhythms is usually associated with a gradual increase in rate—a "warm-up" phenomenon (12). It is characteristic of automatic rhythms that although they may be reset transiently or abolished, they cannot be reliably initiated or terminated by programmed electrical stimulation (13).

Triggered Activity

Triggered activity is caused by transient oscillations in membrane potentials called afterdepolarizations. When these small-amplitude potentials reach a threshold, an action potential may be generated. If sustained and repetitive action potentials result, sustained rhythmic or triggered activity may follow.

Early afterdepolarizations occur before a complete repolariza-

[a]See also Chapter 2 for more complete discussion of mechanisms.

tion has taken place. This can occur under a variety of circumstances, including acidosis, hypoxia, hypokalemia, or antiarrhythmic drug toxicity (14). Initiation of triggered activity is bradycardia dependent. (15). It has been suggested that early afterdepolarizations may be the underlying mechanism of polymorphic ventricular tachycardia associated with acquired and congenital QT prolongation (16).

Delayed afterdepolarizations are oscillations that occur after the repolarization of the action potential has occurred. The mechanism of delayed afterdepolarizations is thought to be calcium loading within the cell leading to electrogenic Na-Ca exchange or possibly a secondary increase in the sodium conductance (17). Triggered rhythms secondary to delayed afterdepolarizations may be initiated and terminated by programmed electrical stimulation. Rapid pacing is the most efficacious method for initiation of triggered rhythms. Triggered rhythms frequently exhibit gradual acceleration or a "warm-up" phenomenon and a gradual deceleration before termination (17).

Differing responses to programmed electrical stimulation may provide clues as to the mechanism of underlying ventricular tachycardia, although a conclusive proof is often difficult and incomplete.

INCIDENCE OF VENTRICULAR TACHYCARDIA

Most commonly, ventricular tachycardia is associated with prior myocardial infarction in a patient with coronary artery disease. Significant numbers of patients are asymptomatic post–myocardial infarction even in the presence of moderately severe ventricular dysfunction. Sometimes the first presentation of a malignant ventricular tachycardia is sudden cardiac death. Unfortunately, only a minority of patients presenting in this manner are successfully resuscitated. On the other hand, patients presenting with sustained ventricular tachycardia post–myocardial infarction, are more easily identified and are therefore more likely to be referred for further EP evaluation (18).

High-risk subgroups of patients can be identified by noninvasive studies (19–21). The markers of increased risk of development of ventricular tachycardia are significant left ventricular dysfunction (ejection fraction < 40%) (22) and presence of late potentials on a signal-averaged electrocardiogram (ECG) (22–25). Other recognized risk factors associated with higher risk of ventricular tachycardia development are a new bundle branch block (with anterior infarction), congestive heart failure, primary ventricular fibrillation, and hypotension during myocardial infarction requiring pressor support (26,27).

Although coronary artery disease is by far the most important cause of sustained ventricular tachycardia, other conditions are less frequently associated with ventricular tachycardia. These include dilated cardiomyopathies (28–30), arrhythmogenic right ventricular dysplasia (31), and congenital heart disease with sequelae or corrective surgical therapy (e.g., ventricular scar following repair of tetralogy of Fallot) (32–34). Occasionally, ventricular tachycardia may arise in an apparently structurally normal heart (35–40). Rarely, ventricular tachycardia may be associated with systemic disease processes that cause focal muscle infiltration, e. g., sarcoidosis or cardiac tumors.

DIAGNOSIS

Ventricular tachycardia is most often identified by continuous electrocardiographic recordings (Fig. 8.1). Electrocardiographic

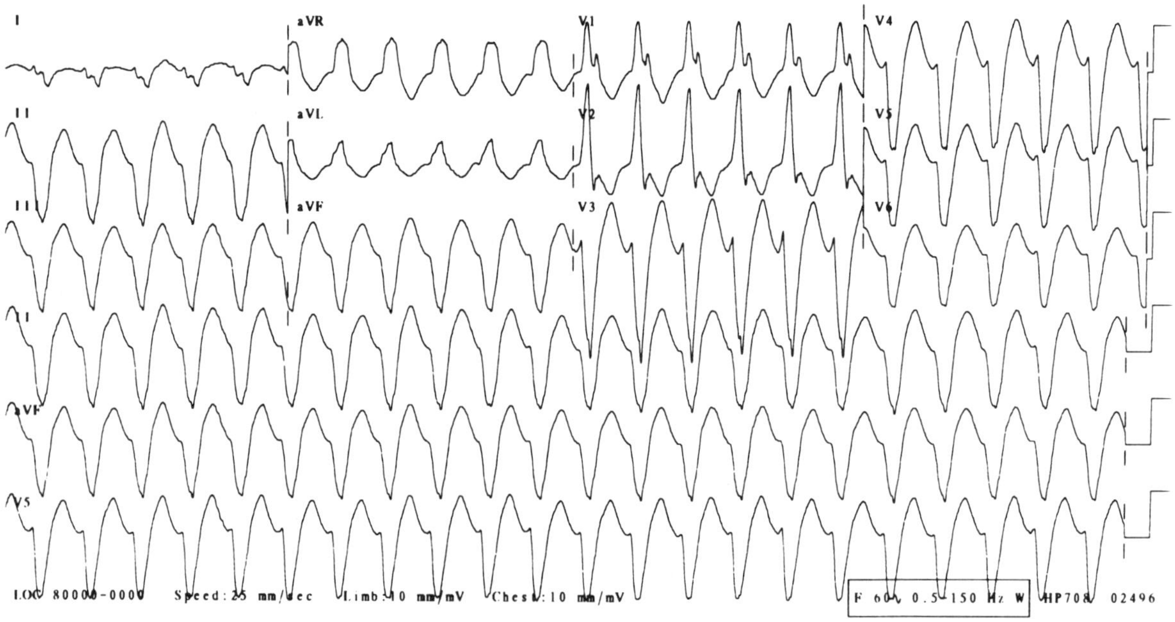

Figure 8.1. Twelve-lead ECG of ventricular tachycardia. Note: Indeterminate frontal axis, right bundle branch block morphology, and a markedly prolonged QRS duration. QRS prolongation is secondary to amiodarone effect.

features that suggest ventricular tachycardia are: (a) wide QRS tachycardia, (b) QRS duration > 0.14 sec, (c) monophasic or biphasic QRS complex in V_1, (d) left bundle branch block pattern, (e) superior and rightward frontal axis, (f) atrioventricular (AV) dissociation, (g) precordial concordance, and (h) presence of fusion complexes (41). Although these electrocardiographic clues are helpful, the diagnosis can often be established with certainty only by intracardiac recording techniques.

Frequent episodes of nonsustained or sustained ventricular tachycardia are best diagnosed by continuous 24-hr Holter monitoring, but relatively infrequent episodes of tachycardia may be documented by the use of event recorders.

Ventricular tachycardia may be asymptomatic or may cause sudden loss of consciousness and death. A spectrum of possible symptomatology between these two extremes exists, including frequent episodes of "palpitations," "skipped" beats, momentary "light-headedness," and potentially more serious symptoms, such as near-syncope or syncope (Chapter 3).

Physical findings associated with ventricular tachycardia have already been described elsewhere (Chapter 3). Physical examination should focus on the identification of the underlying cardiac pathology, e.g., valvular or congenital heart disease, presence of left ventricular aneurysm, and exclusion of other disease processes that may affect the management of the patient.

ELECTROPHYSIOLOGIC STUDY

Indications

The value of EP study to diagnose and treat patients with malignant ventricular tachycardia is well established. Patients with ventricular tachycardia may present in one of several ways: (a) frequent premature beats, (b) wide QRS tachycardia, (c) aborted sudden cardiac death, and (d) established diagnosis of ventricular tachycardia.

FREQUENT PREMATURE COMPLEXES

Presence of high-grade ventricular ectopy in patients with coronary artery disease and left ventricular dysfunction is associated with an increased risk of sudden cardiac death (42–45). However, to date no studies have demonstrated that suppression of ventricular premature complexes with antiarrhythmic agents reduces the incidence of sudden cardiac death. To the contrary, data from the Cardiac Arrhythmia Suppression Trial (CAST) indicate that treatment designed to suppress ventricular ectopy with some antiarrhythmic drugs (Type IC agents) after myocardial infarction was harmful (46). At present, no prospective randomized trials exist to corroborate the usefulness of EP studies to detect inducible ventricular tachycardia or guide therapy in patients with frequent ventricular ectopy. Electrophysiologic testing in this subgroup of patients is thus not recommended.

WIDE QRS TACHYCARDIA

The indications for EP testing in patients presenting with wide QRS tachycardia have already been discussed (Chapter 4).

ABORTED SUDDEN CARDIAC DEATH

Patients resuscitated from cardiac arrest, without evidence of a new myocardial infarction, are at a significant risk for recurrent sudden death postdischarge (46–50). In this high-risk group, the 1- and 2-yr recurrence rate of cardiac arrest is reported to be 30 and 45%, respectively (46,48).

Ventricular tachycardia or ventricular fibrillation may be initiated during EP studies in 70–80% of patients resuscitated from cardiac arrest. In the majority, monomorphic ventricular tachycardia is inducible. In others, polymorphic ventricular tachycardia, nonsustained ventricular tachycardia, or ventricular fibrillation are inducible (51–56).

Effective drug therapy may be identified in up to 80% of survivors (51–56). Patients who remain inducible are at a significantly higher risk for recurrent cardiac arrest (estimated risk of 23% at 1 yr and 30% at 3 yr) (42, 56). Patients whose arrhythmias have been successfully suppressed by antiarrhythmic drugs or surgery or a combination of therapies have a reduced risk (6% at 1 yr and 15% at 3 yr) (56). Cardiac arrest survivors who remain inducible should be considered for nonpharmacologic therapies, including surgery and implantable cardioverters-defibrillators (ICDs).

Failure to induce ventricular tachycardia or ventricular fibrillation at the baseline study does not necessarily signify a good prognosis in patients with depressed left ventricular function. These patients remain at a substantial risk for subsequent arrhythmic events or recurrent cardiac arrest (56,57).

Since the risk of subsequent cardiac arrest is high in patients presenting with an aborted sudden cardiac death who do not have evidence of an acute myocardial infarction (< 48 hr) and who have no identifiable reversible factors (e.g., ischemia, aortic stenosis), these patients should undergo further EP evaluation. Presence of advanced multisystem or terminal disease or inability of patients to cooperate may preclude EP testing in some patients.

Established Diagnosis of Ventricular Tachycardia Where Electrophysiologic Studies Are Used for Management

The available data suggest that EP studies are the method of choice to assess drug efficacy in patients with inducible ventricular tachycardia but insufficient spontaneous ventricular arrhythmias to allow assessment by serial long-term ECG recordings (58,59).

All patients who are considered candidates for device therapy (cardioverter/defibrillator) or an antitachycardia pacemaker/defibrillator must undergo EP studies prior to the device implantation. The goals of EP studies in these patients are to: (a) define the rate of tachycardia, (b) to identify the most appropriate site for stimulation to terminate ventricular tachycardia, (c) to demonstrate the most effective stimulation sequence(s) to terminate ventricular tachycardia, (d) to document the safety and reproducibility of cardiac pacing and defibrillation therapy, and (e) to ascertain the appropriateness of automatic arrhythmia detection by the device.

All patients undergoing surgery for recurrent ventricular tachycardia require preoperative EP studies. Localization of the tachycardia circuit should take place both prior to (preoperative) and during the surgical intervention (intraoperative electrophysiologic study) (60–62). Localization by catheter techniques in the EP laboratory is necessary since the arrhythmia may not be inducible in the operating room or because surgical complications may preclude operative mapping.

Mapping of the site of origin of the ventricular tachycardia may be difficult in some patients. Therefore, alternative surgical techniques that do not rely on mapping have been proposed. Encircling endocardial ventriculotomy or cryoablation and total subendocardial resection have been developed as alternative approaches (63–65). However, mapping and localization of ventricular tachycardia focus is preferred, because resection of unnecessary tissue (e.g., papillary muscles) may thereby be avoided. Furthermore, lack of anatomic landmarks (e.g., identifiable scar or aneurysm) may render such surgery impossible.

Patients who undergo surgical therapy should also undergo postoperative EP studies to evaluate the surgical results.

ELECTROPHYSIOLOGIC STUDY

The general principles of EP study are discussed in Chapter 4. The discussion here will focus on the evaluation of ventricular tachycardia.

A minimum of three to four catheters are used to record and to stimulate for a typical ventricular tachycardia study. These catheters are positioned in the high right atrium (HRA), the right ventricular apex (RVA), His-bundle region (His), and the left ventricle (LV). The techniques for catheter positioning are discussed in Chapter 4.

The left ventricular catheter is utilized for left ventricular mapping (see below) or occasionally for programmed electrical stimulation in selected patients. Simultaneous recordings of intracardiac and surface ECG are obtained.

The following represents the minimal protocol for a ventricular tachycardia study: (a) incremental atrial pacing, (b) programmed atrial stimulation, (c) incremental ventricular pacing, and (d) programmed ventricular stimulation before and after pharmacologic intervention.

Programmed ventricular stimulation may be performed during sinus rhythm and/or following a ventricular pace drive (S_1–S_1). Programmed stimulation is initiated with a single extrastimulus (S_2), which is scanned from late diastole to ventricular refractoriness (Fig. 8.2). If S_2 does not initiate ventricular tachycardia, a second extrastimulus is introduced (S_3). Double premature extrastimuli (S_2–S_3) are introduced with S_1–S_2 coupling interval 50–100 msec longer than ventricular effective refractory period (ERP), with S_2–S_3 equal to the S_1–S_2 interval. The S_2–S_3 interval is shortened in 10-msec steps until S_3 is no longer able to evoke a ventricular response. At that point, the S_1–S_2 interval is shortened until S_3 is once again able to elicit a ventricular response. S_2 and S_3 are sequentially decremented until S_2 stimulus becomes refractory.

If S_2–S_3 is unable to initiate ventricular tachycardia, a third extrastimulus is introduced (S_4). Sequence of stimulation is analogous to that previously described, again starting with S_2 at 50–100 msec beyond ventricular refractoriness and S_2–S_3 and S_3–S_4 intervals equal to S_1–S_2 interval. Sequential shortening of coupling intervals is performed similar to the previously described sequence.

Programmed electrical stimulation is typically performed from two right ventricular sites: right ventricular apex and right ventricular outflow, and in selected cases left ventricle (patients with documented aborted sudden cardiac death, who are not inducible from the right ventricular sites, or patients in whom left ventricular mapping is required to guide ablative therapy). Programmed electrical stimulation is usually performed using 2- to 3-cycle drives (e.g., 600, 500, and 400 msec).

If programmed stimulation does not induce ventricular tachycardia, infusion of isoproterenol may be used to facilitate induction. Isoproterenol infusion is usually begun at 1 μg/min and increased every 3 min to a maximum rate of 4–5 μg/min or until sinus rate increases to 125–150 beats/min. Programmed electrical stimulation is then repeated during isoproterenol infusion.

Once ventricular tachycardia is induced, it may be terminated by single, double or triple ventricular extrastimuli or by bursts of rapid ventricular pacing. Infrequently, when ventricular tachycardia rates are rapid (cycle length < 250 msec), synchronized cardioversion may be required to terminate the tachycardia.

In patients with coronary artery disease with prior myocardial infarctions or in patients with a ventricular aneurysm, greater than 90% of ventricular tachycardias are inducible (66). In approximately 10% of patients with ventricular tachycardia originating in the left ventricle, programmed electrical stimulation of the left ventricle is required to initiate the tachycardia.

Occasionally, infusion of isoproterenol is required to facilitate the induction of ventricular tachycardia. Possible mechanisms involved in facilitation of induction by isoproterenol include localized ischemia, shortening of ventricular refractoriness, facilitation of conduction, or increased abnormal automaticity (Chapter 4).

Termination of Ventricular Tachycardia

Once the ventricular tachycardia is initiated, ability to terminate the tachycardia using premature stimuli should be tested, provided that the tachycardia is hemodynamically stable and well

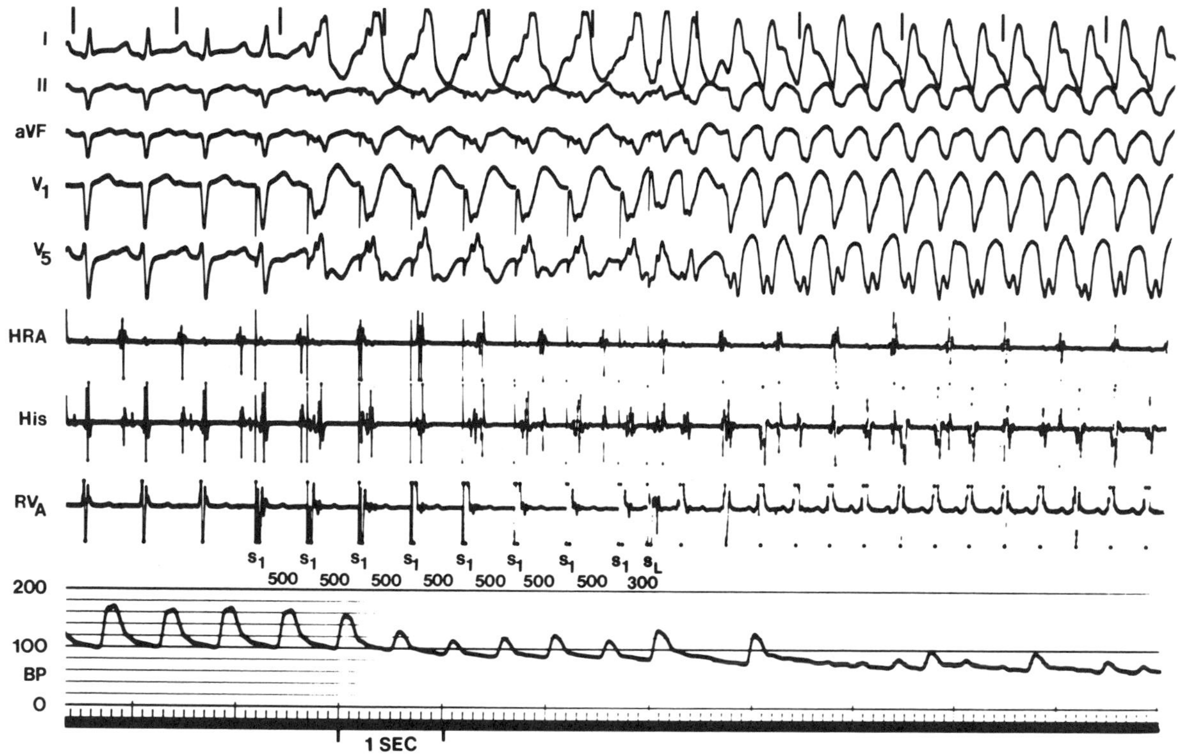

Figure 8.2. Induction of ventricular tachycardia using a single ventricular extrastimulus (S_2) at the coupling interval S_1–S_2 of 300 msec, following an eight-beat S_1–S_1 drive at S_1–S_1 interval of 500 msec. From top to bottom: surface leads I, II, aVF, V_1, and V_5 and intracardiac electrograms HRA, His, RV_A, blood pressure (BP), and time scale.

tolerated. Using a right or left ventricular electrogram as reference to trigger the stimulator, premature ventricular extrastimuli are introduced at progressively more premature intervals, until the tachycardia is terminated or ventricular refractoriness is encountered. If single extrastimuli are ineffective, second and third extrastimuli may be added (Fig. 8.3). If ventricular tachycardia is rapid ($\geq$ 175 beat/min), overdrive pacing may be required to terminate the tachycardia. Overdrive pacing is attempted at 30- to 50-msec intervals shorter than the tachycardia cycle length and maintained for 5–20 beats. Burst cycle length is progressively decremented (in 10- to 20-msec steps) until the tachycardia is entrained and terminated. In approximately 10–15% of patients, overdrive pacing results in ventricular tachycardia acceleration or degeneration to ventricular fibrillation, requiring external cardioversion.

Use of Programmed Ventricular Stimulation to Evaluate Therapy

In patients in whom ventricular tachycardia can be reproducibly initiated and terminated in the baseline drug-free state, the effect of antiarrhythmic drugs can be assessed by comparing the ability to initiate the tachycardia before and after drug administration.

The most frequently chosen drug for testing is procainamide (Type IA drug). The rationale for testing procainamide first is ready availability of intravenous preparation, permitting a repeat programmed stimulation at the initial electrophysiologic study. Comparable electrophysiologic effects are seen with intravenous and oral procainamide (67,68). Patients who do not respond to procainamide are generally also unresponsive to other Type IA drugs (69). If a patient is inducible on procainamide, the efficacy of Type IB drug (mexiletene) or Type IC drugs (flecainide, encainide, or propoferone) may be tested next. Type IC drugs should be avoided in patients with severe left ventricular dysfunction (left ventricular ejection fraction $<$ 30%) (70–72).

A combination of Type IA drug (quinidine or procainamide) with a IB agent (mexiletene) may be tried next, since the combination of these agents is usually more effective than either class of drugs used separately (73). If this combination is unsuccessful, amiodarone or an experimental antiarrhythmic drug may be tried next.

Amiodarone loading for at least 2 wks should precede any repeat testing. Slowing of ventricular tachycardia or noninducibility may be used as indices of positive therapeutic outcome. Since chronic administration of amiodarone results in further slowing of ventricular tachycardia, repeat programmed electrical stimulation at 6 wks post–amiodarone administration may be helpful (74–76).

Addition of Type IB drug (mexiletene) and Type IA drug

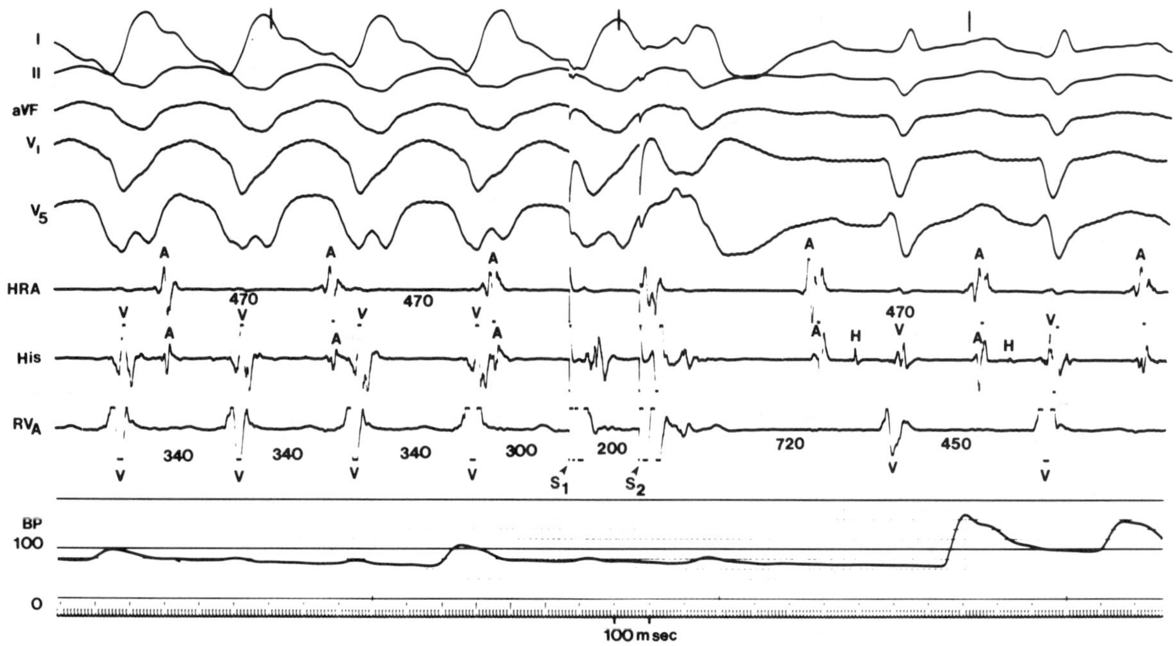

Figure 8.3. Termination of ventricular tachycardia by timed extrastimuli. From **top** to **bottom:** surface leads I, II, aVF, V_1, and V_5 intracardiac electrograms HRA, His, RV_A, blood pressure (BP), and time scale. Ventricular tachycardia (cycle length 340 msec) is terminated by two extrastimuli at the coupling intervals of 300 and 200 msec (QRS-S_1-S_2).

(e.g., quinidine) may further enhance the amiodarone effect by slowing ventricular tachycardia or preventing ventricular tachycardia reinduction (77,78).

A successful drug regimen to prevent ventricular tachycardia reoccurrence may be found in 20–30% of patients with chronic ventricular tachycardia (79). If ventricular tachycardia reinduction is prevented during programmed electrical stimulation using a selected antiarrhythmic drug regimen, suppression of ventricular tachycardia may be anticipated in greater than 90% of patients over a 2-yr follow-up (80).

Inducibility of ventricular tachycardia by programmed electrical stimulation following antiarrhythmic drug administration tends to overpredict drug failure. Therefore, additional criteria, other than noninducibility of ventricular tachycardia at EP study, have been proposed. These include: (a) increased difficulty of induction of ventricular tachycardia, (b) marked slowing of ventricular tachycardia (>100 msec), and (c) improved hemodynamic tolerance (81,82). However, these criteria do not have as complete justification as noninducibility.

Therapeutic response to pharmacologic therapy, as assessed by programmed electrical stimulation, does not assure freedom from subsequent arrhythmic events or sudden cardiac death. The context within which ventricular tachycardia presents is also important and should be considered carefully before choosing pharmacologic therapy exclusively. Patients who present with aborted sudden cardiac death or patients who present with hemodynamically unstable ventricular tachycardia should be considered for ablative therapy or ICD implantation (83). In contrast, patients who have relatively slow ventricular tachycardia that is well tolerated hemodynamically are less likely to present with sudden cardiac death. These patients may be considered for pharmacologic therapy initially.

Alternative Methods to Assess Pharmacologic Therapy for Ventricular Tachycardia

Holter recordings may also be used to assess therapy for ventricular tachycardia. Success of antiarrhythmic therapy is judged by abolition of nonsustained and sustained ventricular tachycardia and >85% suppression of spontaneous frequent ventricular ectopy on 24-hr Holter monitoring during drug therapy compared to the baseline Holter recording. Holter guided therapy has a number of potential limitations: (a) frequency of spontaneously occurring ventricular ectopy may be low, precluding the use of Holter criteria as therapeutic endpoints, (b) hemodynamic tolerance of ventricular tachycardia cannot be assessed during Holter monitoring, (c) serial Holter monitoring is time consuming, and (d) suppression of ventricular ectopy in patients with impaired left ventricular function (left ventricular ejection fraction <30%) may not predict improved outcome or freedom from sudden cardiac death (84–86). If EP studies are not readily available, or the patient is reluctant or unable to undergo EP studies, Holter guided therapy provides an alternative method of monitoring drug therapy. Holter guided therapy may also be used as an adjunct to invasive EP testing (68). For example, the presence of nonsustained ventricular tachycardia on Holter monitoring with adequate serum levels of an antiarrhythmic drug would predict drug failure, thus obviating the need for a repeat EP study.

Localization of Site of Origin of Ventricular Tachycardia

If surgical or catheter ablation of ventricular tachycardia is contemplated, localization of the presumed site of origin of the tachycardia is mandatory. Surgical or catheter ablation should be considered in patients with frequent recurrences of ventricular tachycardia despite pharmacologic therapy, or incessant ventricular tachycardia, or in patients with discreet left ventricular aneurysm. Localization of ventricular tachycardia is established by the combination of the following techniques: (a) analysis of the 12-lead ECG, (b) endocardial mapping during ventricular tachycardia, and (c) endocardial pace mapping.

12-LEAD ECG

Scalar 12-lead ECG is helpful for localizing the site of origin of ventricular tachycardia (87). For example, left bundle branch block (LBBB) pattern suggests the origin of ventricular tachycardia to the left of the intraventricular septum in the setting of coronary artery disease. Presence of persistent R waves in the precordial leads suggests the basal origin. Q waves in leads I, V_1, V_2, and V_6 suggest an apical site (88).

ENDOCARDIAL MAPPING

The "gold standard" for localization of ventricular tachycardia is endocardial mapping during ventricular tachycardia. Standard sites for mapping have been suggested by Josephson, et al. and are listed in Table 8.1 (89,90).

Mapping is used to systematically record multiple endocardial sites within the right and the left ventricles during ventricular tachycardia and establish the site of the earliest ventricular activation (Fig. 8.4). His-bundle and right ventricle apical

Table 8.1.
Mapping Sites for Ventricular Tachycardia

Left Ventricle	Right Ventricle
Apex	His (A-V junction)
Septum	Apex
High	Outflow tract
Middle	Inflow tract
Low	Anterior
Anterior	
Lateral	
Low	
High	
Posterobasal	

Abbreviations: A-V = atrioventricular.

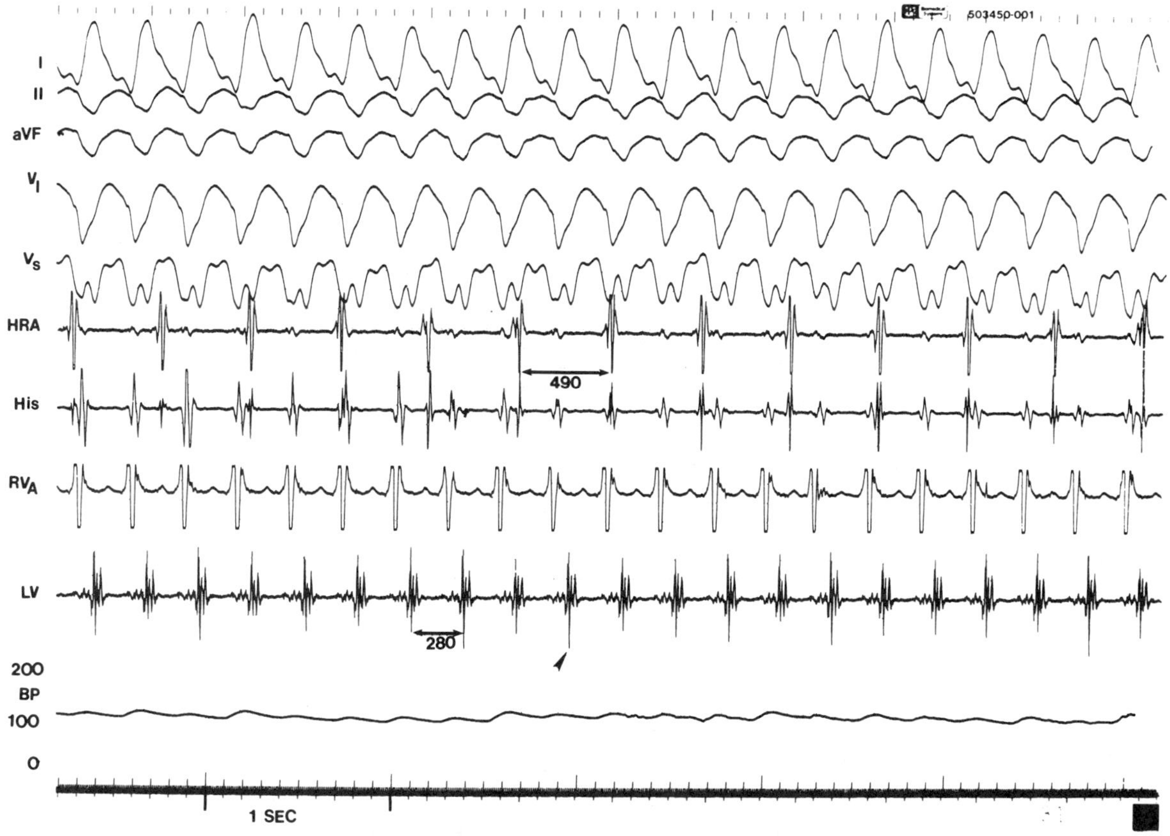

Figure 8.4. Left ventricular mapping. Surface leads I, II, aVF, V_1, and V_5 are displayed simultaneously with intracardiac electrograms in the high right atrium (HRA), His bundle (His), right ventricular apex (RV_A), and left ventricle (LV). Blood pressure (BP) and time scale are also displayed. Note fragmented systolic activity of the LV electrogram (marked with arrowhead).

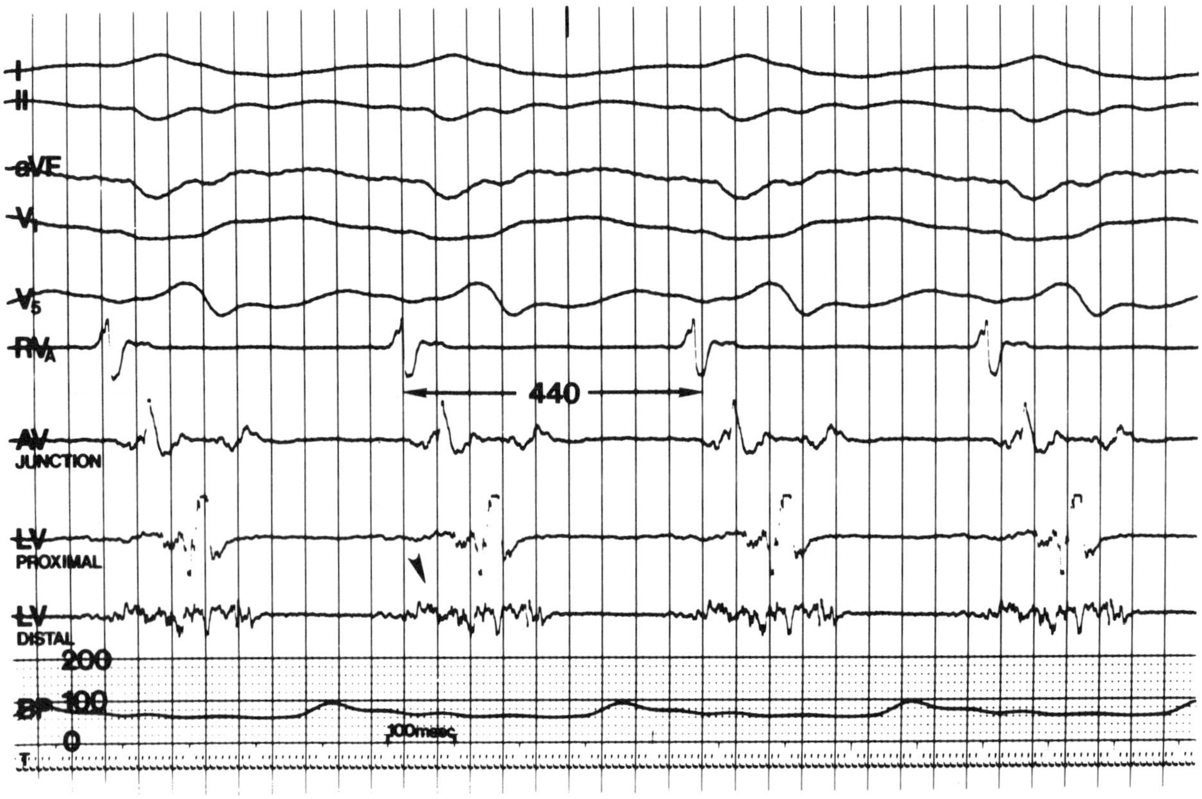

Figure 8.5. Ventricular tachycardia. From **top** to **bottom:** Surface leads I, II, aVF, V_1, and V_5 and intracardiac electrograms right ventricle (RV) apex, RV (AV junction), left ventricle (LV) proximal and LV distal (quadripolar catheter), blood pressure (BP), and time lines (T). Note: fractionated electrical activity during systole. The electrogram precedes the QRS (*arrow*) and extends beyond its terminal inscription.

catheters are held in fixed positions and used as the reference points to compare the activation timing of the sampled sites. Sites that are recorded are listed in Table 8.1. In addition, left ventricular aneurysm sites are carefully mapped. Fluoroscopy in multiple views is used to assess and to record the position of the catheters during mapping. Left ventricular mapping should be performed with full systematic heparinization.

In many patients, fragmented diastolic and systolic activity can also be recorded and may persist throughout the diastole (Fig. 8.5). Such activity is considered to represent continuous localized reentry. An example of earliest site of endocardial activation during mapping of a ventricular tachycardia is shown in Figure 8.6.

ENDOCARDIAL PACE MAPPING

Endocardial pace mapping may be used to confirm the results of endocardial mapping during ventricular tachycardia, or in patients in whom ventricular tachycardia is not readily inducible or sustainable. The goal of pace mapping is to find the site that corresponds to the site of reentry, by comparing the 12-lead ECG during ventricular pacing to the clinically recorded or induced ventricular tachycardia (91). Pacing close to the site of origin of ventricular tachycardia should theoretically yield a morphology similar to the clinically observed tachycardia. However, small changes in catheter positioning may result in dramatic changes in QRS morphology. Another disadvantage of this technique is that it is time consuming. Thus, pace mapping is most useful as a confirmatory technique, once an endocardial site has been localized by endocardial mapping techniques.

OPERATIVE TECHNIQUES FOR TREATMENT OF VENTRICULAR TACHYCARDIA[b]

Direct cardiac mapping during cardiac surgery has been shown to increase the effectiveness of surgery for recurrent ventricular tachycardias (92). Preoperative and intraoperative mapping may be performed with a hand-held probe to guide the surgical ablation (92–97). Because it is often difficult to sustain ventricular tachycardia in the operating room, multichannel data acquisition systems have been developed for experimental and clinical use (98–100). Many types of sensing electrodes have been designed and developed for experimental and clinical mapping including plunge electrodes (101), electrodes embedded in socks or plaques (102), intracavitary probes, and balloons (103).

Multiple signal acquisition and display of isopotential maps enables the electrophysiologist and surgeon to construct an instantaneous activation map which can be used to locate and guide surgical therapy. Epicardial mapping is generally performed first and provides some useful information. However, the site of the arrhythmia epicardial breakthrough may be removed from the endocardial site. Therefore, this technique is generally

[b]See also Chapter 23.

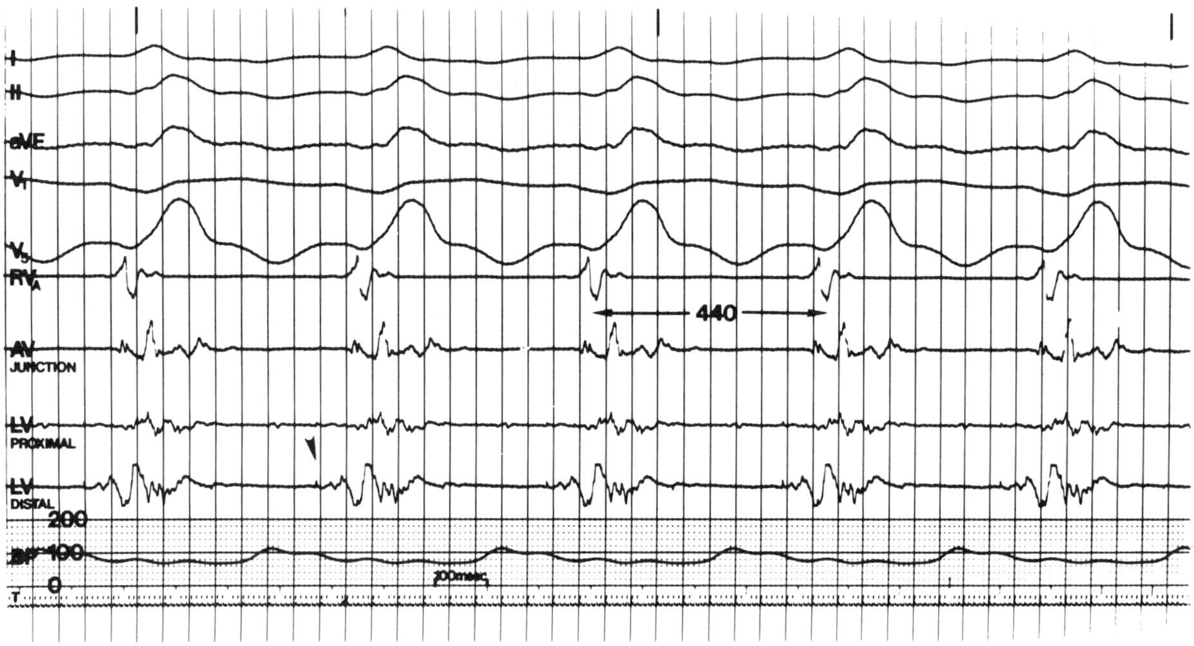

Figure 8.6. The earliest site of ventricular activation (arrow) was localized to the basal septum. Note that left ventricle (LV) distal electrogram precedes the surface QRS activation. Leads are arranged as in Figure 8.5.

complemented by endocardial mapping using either an endocardial balloon with multiple electrodes with a computerized acquisition system, or by using a single roving probe mapping after a ventriculotomy is made. Detailed discussion of the surgical techniques for ventricular tachycardia ablation is beyond the scope of this chapter and is discussed elsewhere in this book (see Chapter 23).

TREATMENT OF VENTRICULAR TACHYCARDIA

Therapy of ventricular tachycardia may be pharmacologic, ablative (surgical and nonsurgical), or electrical (ICDs and antitachycardia pacemakers). It should be emphasized, however, that these therapeutic approaches are not mutually exclusive and may be combined to enhance the therapeutic efficacy.

The most important decision of all is to decide which patients to treat. Several clinical features may be helpful in this regard. It has been established that patients with depressed left ventricular function (left ventricular ejection fraction <40%), multiple documented ventricular tachycardia episodes, or patients who present with aborted sudden cardiac death should be vigorously treated, since their prognosis is generally poor without therapy (83,104–107). On the other hand, patients with normal left ventricular function and nonsustained ventricular tachycardia generally have good prognosis and may not require therapy.

Antiarrhythmic Drug Therapy

Antiarrhythmic drug therapy remains the initial therapeutic modality of choice for most patients with sustained ventricular tachycardia. Drug therapy guided by programmed electrical stimulation is currently preferred by most electrophysiologists. This is especially true for patients who present with life-threatening symptoms, since recurrences of arrhythmia may be fatal in these patients (80,84,86,107). The likelihood that these patients will require ablative or device therapy is relatively high. The use of noninvasive testing to guide drug therapy should be reserved for patients who have sustained ventricular tachycardia without life-threatening symptoms, or as an adjunct to the electrophysiologic assessment of drug therapy (87,108).

The use of EP testing for drug selection is based on two assumptions: (a) that ventricular tachycardia initiated in the electrophysiologic laboratory is the same as the clinically observed tachycardia, and (b) that the response to antiarrhythmic drugs in the electrophysiology laboratory predicts the clinical outcome. In our laboratory, an *effective drug* is defined as one that is capable of suppressing the induction of sustained ventricular tachycardia (>30 sec or requiring intervention, e.g., antitachycardia pacing or cardioversion to terminate the tachycardia) or nonsustained ventricular tachycardia (>10 beats). Slowing of ventricular tachycardia, improved hemodynamic tolerance, or increased difficulty of induction are considered favorable prognostic signs.

Baseline EP study is performed following discontinuation of all antiarrhythmic drugs for a period of ≥5½ half-lives. Antiarrhythmic agent is then administered intravenously or orally and patient restudied when steady-state levels of the antiarrhythmic drug are achieved. Since procainamide and quinidine are available in both the intravenous and oral form, these drugs are commonly tested first. The list of commonly used antiarrhythmic drugs and their usual dosages in EP studies are listed in Table

Table 8.2.
Commonly Utilized Antiarrhythmic Drugs in the Electrophysiology Laboratory for Treatment of Ventricular Tachycardia

Drugs (Class)	Intravenous	Oral Loading
Type IA Drugs		
Quinidine	6–10 mg/kg	300–600 mg q6–8hr
Procainamide	10–20 mg/kg	1.0–1.5 g q6hr
Disopyramide	2 mg/kg	150–300 mg q6–8hr
Moricizine (Ethmozine)		75–200 mg q8hr
Type IB Drugs		
Lidocaine	1–2 mg/kg bolus followed by 20–40 μg/kg/min infusion	—
Mexiletene		150–300 mg q6–8hr
Type IC drugs		
Flecainide		100–200 mg q12hr
Encainide		25–75 mg q6–8hr
Propafenone (also has beta blocking effects)		100–300 mg q8hr
Type III drugs		
Amiodarone	5–10 mg/kg bolus over 5–15 min, then 800–1600 mg/24 hr infusion	1200–1600 mg qd × 2 wk, then 200–600 mg qd
Bretylium	5–10 mg/kg bolus over 10–30 min, then 1–4 mg/min	—

8.2 (see also Chapters 11 and 12 for more complete discussion of drugs).

Antiarrhythmic drug serum levels must be correlated with drug efficacy. A serum level should always be obtained prior to the EP study to confirm therapeutic serum levels of the drug and during, or following the induction protocol. Patients who do not respond to antiarrhythmic drug(s) (i.e., in whom induction of ventricular tachycardia cannot be suppressed) should be considered for ablative or device therapy. Factors which predict poor outcome to antiarrhythmic drug therapy include: (a) lack of significant slowing of ventricular tachycardia following drug administration, (b) hemodynamic collapse requiring cardioversion, and (c) repeated inductions of ventricular fibrillation or rapid polymorphic ventricular tachycardia on drug therapy.

Induction of a well-tolerated ventricular tachycardia during treatment is associated with low risk (4–6% at 1–2 yr) of sudden cardiac death, but not of arrhythmia recurrence (109–111). However, in patients who present with poorly tolerated ventricular tachycardias, slowing of the tachycardia during EP study does not necessarily predict good outcome (83). Therefore, in the author's opinion, in these patients ICDs should be considered in addition to, or instead of antiarrhythmic drug therapy.

Ablative Therapy

SURGICAL

Many patients have ventricular tachycardias refractory to antiarrhythmic drug therapy. Ablative therapy is considered the preferred therapeutic alternative in patients with frequent episodes of ventricular tachycardia despite drug therapy, particularly in patients who present with a single morphology tachycardia and a discreet resectable left ventricular aneurysm. Ablative therapy is aimed at destroying the critical part of the reentrant circuit that participates in the ventricular tachycardia.

Successful ablation is critically dependent on the ability to localize the involved myocardium which is necessary to initiate and perpetuate the ventricular tachycardia (112). Diagnostic techniques used to localize the reentry circuit include an analysis of the 12-lead ECG, catheter mapping during ventricular tachycardia, and pace mapping (see above).

Once the site of origin of ventricular tachycardia is localized, ablative procedures (surgical or catheter directed) can be performed. The techniques used for surgical and for catheter ablation are discussed elsewhere (see Chapters 23 and 24).

The largest surgical experience to date has been with localized subendocardial resection guided by preoperative and intraoperative endocardial mapping (113,114). Cryoablation or laser ablation may be combined with subendocardial resection or used instead of subendocardial resection to destroy the reentrant tissues. These techniques are particularly useful in the area of the mitral valve apparatus and papillary muscles (115).

The operative mortality of electrophysiologically guided subendocardial resection has been reported to be between 5 and 15% in experienced clinical centers (114). Because of significant immediate operative risk, subendocardial resection should be considered only in drug refractory ventricular tachycardia or in patients with a discreet resectable LV aneurysm. Predictors of poor outcome (perioperative heart failure or death) are left ventricular ejection fraction of <20%, history of prior cardiac surgery, and evidence of prior anterior and inferior myocardial infarctions (116). In experienced centers, cure rates have been reported to be as high as 90% (115,116).

NONSURGICAL (CATHETER ABLATION)

Catheter ablation theoretically offers an attractive alternative for ventricular tachycardia ablation. However, a number of technical problems limit the usefulness of this technique at the present time. These include the following: (a) limited ability to localize the arrhythmia site origin by the single catheter technique, (b) inability to fixate the catheter to the ablation site, and (c) limited size of the lesions generated by direct current (DC) shock and radiofrequency energy, in particular. In addition, significant morbidity and mortality may be associated with the procedure (particularly by DC ablation) which limits the usefulness of this technique at present.

Results of catheter ablation are difficult to evaluate and to

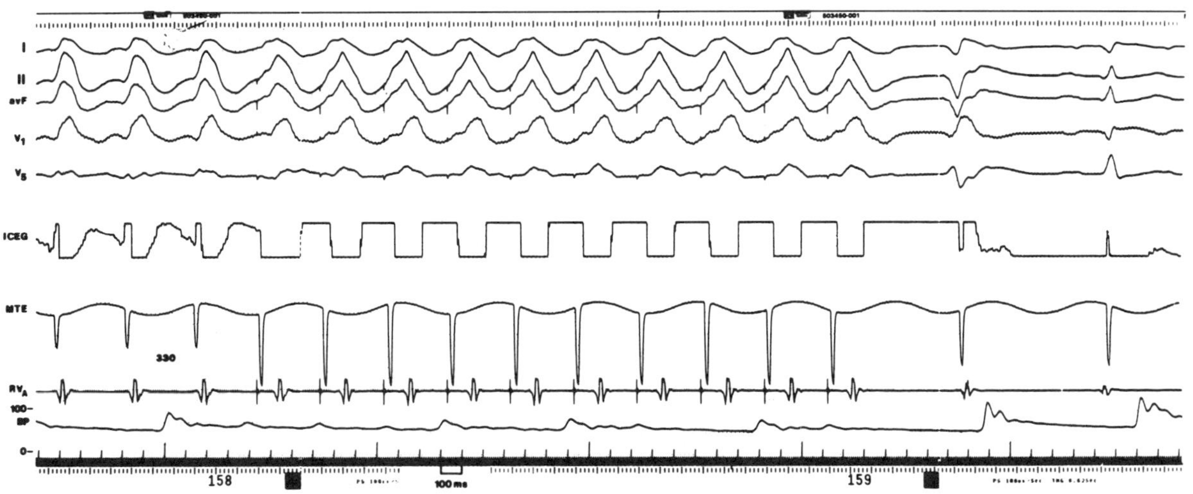

Figure 8.7. Antitachycardia pacing with successful ventricular tachycardia termination (Guardian ATP 4210). From **top** to **bottom:** surface leads I, II, AVF, V_1, and V_5, intracardiac electrogram (ICEG), monitored telemetry event marker (MTE), and right apical ventricular electrogram (RVA). (Reproduced from Singer I, *et al.*, PACE 1991; 14:1119–1128, with publisher's permission.)

compare among different investigators and clinical investigative sites since the technique is not standardized. Therefore, it is not possible to provide precise data on the success of this procedure. Response rates have been variously reported to be 25–50% (defined as noninducibility of ventricular tachycardia postablation) (117,118). Unfortunately, long-term results are difficult to evaluate since no true control group exists, and many patients remain on antiarrhythmic drugs following catheter ablation.

We have found this technique particularly useful in patients with incessant ventricular tachycardia who are not surgical candidates and who are unresponsive to vigorous antiarrhythmic therapy. In such patients, termination of ventricular tachycardia can be regarded as clear therapeutic success, since all other attempts at ventricular tachycardia termination have already failed. The associated morbidity and mortality risks in such patients are therefore justified. It is likely that further improvements in catheter mapping techniques and radiofrequency ablation will improve the outlook for catheter directed ablative therapy. A detailed discussion of catheter ablation techniques can be found elsewhere (see Chapter 24).

Device Therapy[c]

Electrical therapy is designed to terminate ventricular tachycardia by creating a block in the reentrant circuit (antitachycardia pacing) or by uniformly depolarizing the tissue involved in the tachycardia circuit (cardioversion/defibrillation). ICDs have revolutionized the approach to patients who present with an aborted sudden cardiac death or with hemodynamically unstable ventricular tachycardias. ICD therapy is the treatment of choice for patients who have poorly tolerated ventricular tachycardia, who are unresponsive to antiarrhythmic drug therapy and are not candidates for ablative therapy.

Antitachycardia pacing as well as cardioversion and defibrillation is available in the newest (third-generation) devices (Fig. 8.7). Further advancements in this technology, particularly development of transvenous endocardial electrodes for defibrillation, will simplify the implantation techniques and lead to even wider applications of this therapeutic approach.

VENTRICULAR TACHYCARDIA UNASSOCIATED WITH CORONARY ARTERY DISEASE

Ventricular Tachycardia in a Structurally Normal Heart

Some patients have ventricular tachycardia without identifiable structural heart abnormalities. Sudden cardiac death has been reported rarely in association with ventricular tachycardia in these patients (119). The hallmark of this type of ventricular tachycardia is the absence of slow conduction with a generally normal signal-averaged ECG (35), noninducibility by programmed electrical stimulation (119), and inducibility by atrial or ventricular pacing, exercise testing, or beta stimulation (36).

These arrhythmias are frequently responsive to beta blockade or verapamil administration, suggesting a mechanism other than reentry (120). Response to a calcium channel blocking drug (verapamil) suggests triggered activity as the underlying mechanism (35).

Tachycardias originating in the left ventricle have a right bundle branch block QRS morphology, and superior frontal plane axis (38,39). These tachycardias are usually responsive to verapamil and occasionally, to beta-blockade (120).

Another type of tachycardia can be localized to the right ventricular outflow tract (36). This tachycardia typically has a left bundle branch block QRS morphology and an inferior frontal plane axis. Repetitive salvos of a monomorphic ventricular tachycardia are usually noted. This ventricular tachycardia is

[c]See also Chapters 20 and 21.

critically dependent on the heart rate and is often initiated by exercise or exertion (121). It usually cannot be initiated by programmed electrical stimulation (36) though it can be initiated by atrial or ventricular pacing or with isoproterenol infusion (119). The arrhythmia is usually responsive to beta-blocking drugs and occasionally verapamil (119). If it can be terminated with adenosine, a cylic adenosine monophosphate (cyclic AMP)–mediated triggered activity is suggested as the underlying mechanism (121). Localization of the arrhythmia to right ventricular outflow makes this arrhythmia particularly amenable to catheter ablation techniques or surgical cryoablation (see Chapters 23 and 24).

Arrhythmogenic Right Ventricular Dysplasia

Arrhythmogenic right ventricular dysplasia is a rare disorder caused by infiltration of the right ventricle with fatty tissue and fibrosis (31,122). This abnormality tends to occur in young adults, but can be found at any age and is more common in males. The disorder is characterized by right ventricular dilatation and diffuse or localized disease. Histopathologic data demonstrate fatty tissue with strands of surviving or partially degenerating myofibrillar fascicles. Pseudodiverticular or aneurysmal appearance may be observed grossly in the right ventricle with focal ventricular thinning. Signal-averaged ECG is usually positive and the patients are frequently inducible by programmed ventricular stimulation, suggesting reentry as the underlying mechanism (123). Ventricular tachycardia usually has a left bundle branch block QRS morphology. This particular ventricular tachycardia is amenable to antiarrhythmic drug therapy. Alternatively, ablative approaches are available, including surgical resection or isolation procedures (124) or catheter directed ablation (125).

Dilated Cardiomyopathy

Sustained ventricular tachycardia is uncommon in dilated cardiomyopathies. However, nonsustained ventricular tachycardias, frequent ventricular ectopic beats, and sudden cardiac death are relatively frequent occurrences in patients with dilated cardiomyopathies (28). Signal-averaged ECG is usually positive and most patients are inducible with programmed electrical stimulation (28). Frequently, multiple ventricular tachycardia morphologies are elicited during programmed electrical stimulation. Because antiarrhythmic drugs are frequently ineffective in suppressing inducibility of ventricular tachycardia, ICD therapy should be considered early. Most patients have severe left ventricular dysfunction. When left ventricular dysfunction is marked and heart failure symptoms predominate, cardiac transplantation should be considered as a therapeutic alternative.

Mitral Valve Prolapse (MVP)

Mitral valve prolapse (MVP) is generally a benign disease of young adults, predominantly females. Palpitations and frequent premature beats are common occurrence, although syncope and cardiac arrest have been reported rarely (126–129). The mechanism of ventricular tachycardia in these patients is not established, but triggered activity (130) and adrenergic hyperresponsiveness have been suggested as the possible mechanisms (131). Reentry has also been suggested as a mechanism. The use of beta-blockers and electrophysiologically guided antiarrhythmic therapy has been suggested in the inducible patients. In patients who present with aborted sudden cardiac death, ICD implantation should be considered.

Hypertrophic Cardiomyopathy

Hypertrophic cardiomyopathy is a relatively infrequent disorder which usually presents in young adults and may cause sudden death (132). The mechanism of sudden death in this disorder is complex and may be related to a number of factors, including myocardial ischemia due to impaired coronary reserve, conduction abnormalities, or ventricular tachycardia related to reentry. Although beta-blocker and calcium channel blocker therapy usually relieves the hemodynamic symptoms, they do not prevent ventricular tachycardia or ventricular fibrillation (133, 134).

Electrophysiologic studies are useful in guiding antiarrhythmic drug therapy. Polymorphic ventricular tachycardia is usually induced during the EP study (135–138).

In patients at risk for sudden cardiac death (patients who present with near-syncope or syncope), ICD therapy should be considered.

CONCLUSION

Although most ventricular tachycardias occur within the setting of coronary artery disease in the adult population, ventricular tachycardia may also occur in a variety of other cardiac disorders. Evaluation is indicated in patients who present with recurrent sustained or nonsustained ventricular tachycardia. Particular attention should be paid to hemodynamic tolerance of ventricular tachycardia, the mode of presentation, the status of LV function and presence of reversible factors, e.g., ischemia or drug toxicity.

Advances in therapy have altered significantly the natural history of disease in patients with ventricular tachycardia, resulting in improved survival and quality of life in these patients.

References

1. Josephson ME, Almendral JM, Buxton AE, *et al.*: Mechanisms of ventricular tachycardia. Circulation 1987;75:41–47.
2. Josephson ME, Horowitz LN, Farshidi A, *et al.*: Recurrent sustained ventricular tachycardia, 2. Endocardial mapping. Circulation 1978;57: 440–470.
3. Horowitz LN, Josephson ME, Harken AH: Epicardial and endocardial activation during sustained ventricular tachycardia in man. Circulation 1980;61:1227–1238.
4. deBakke JMT, Janse MJ, van Capelle, *et al.*: Endocardial mapping by simultaneous recording of endocardial electrograms during cardiac surgery for ventricular tachycardia. J Am Coll Cardiol 1983;2:947–953.

5. Miller JM, Harken AH, Hargrove WC, *et al.*: Patterns of activation during sustained ventricular tachycardia. J Am Coll Cardiol 1985;5:1280–1287.
6. Cassidy DM, Vasallo JA, Buxton AE, *et al.*: The value of sinus rhythm catheter mapping to localize ventricular tachycardia site of origin. Circulation 1984;69:1103–1110.
7. Morady F, Frank R, Kou WH, *et al.*: Identification and catheter albation of a zone of slow conduction in the reentrant circuit of ventricular tachycardia in humans. J Am Coll Cardiol 1988; II:755–782.
8. Gough WB, Mehra R, Restivo M, *et al.*: Reentrant ventricular arrhythmias in the late MI period in the dog: correlation of activation and refractory maps. Circ Res 1985;57:422–432.
9. Damiano BP, Rosen MR: Effects of pacing on triggered activity induced by early afterdepolarizations. Circulation 1984;69:1013–1025.
10. Wellens HJJ, Durrer DR, Lie KJ: Observations on mechanisms of ventricular tachycardia in man. Circulation 1984;69:149.
11. Waldo AL, Olshansky B, Okumura K, *et al.*: Current perspective on entrainment of tachyarrhythmias. In Brugada P, Wellens HJJ (eds): Cardiac Arrhythmias: Where to Go from Here? Futura Publishing Co., New York, 1987:171–189.
12. Cranefield PF: The Conduction of the Cardiac Impulse. Futura Publishing Co., New York, 1975.
13. Jalife J, Antzelevitch C: Pacemaker annihilation: diagnostic and therapeutic implications. Am Heart J 1980;100:128–130.
14. Cranefield PF: Action potentials, after potentials, and arrhythmias. Circ Res 1977;41:415–423.
15. Brachman J, Scherlag BJ, Rosenshtraukh LV, et al.: Bradycardia-dependent triggered activity: relevance to drug induced multiform ventricular tachycardia. Circulation 1983;68:846–856.
16. Jackman WM, Friday KL, Anderson JL, *et al.*: The long QT syndromes: a critical review, new clinical observations and a unifying hypothesis. Prog Cardiovasc Dis 1988;31:115–172.
17. Moak JP, Rosen MR: Induction and termination of triggered activity by pacing in isolated canine Purkinje fibers. Circulation 1984;69:149–162.
18. Richards DA, Cody DV, Denniss AR, *et al.*: Ventricular electrical instability: A predictor of death after myocardial infarction. Am J Cardiol 1983; 51:75–80.
19. Kuchar DL, Thorburn CW, Sammel WL: Prediction of serious arrhythmic events after myocardial infarction: signal averaged electrogram, Holter monitoring, and radionuclide ventriculography. J Am Coll Cardiol 1987;9:531–538.
20. Gomes JA, Winters JL, Stewart D, *et al.*: A new noninvasive index to predict sustained ventricular tachycardia and sudden death in the first year after myocardial infarction: based on signal-averaged electrocardiogram, radionuclide ejection fraction and Holter monitoring. J Am Coll Cardiol 1987;10:349–357.
21. Breithardt G, Borggrefe M, Haerten K: Role of programmed ventricular stimulation and noninvasive recording of ventricular late potentials for the identification of patients at risk of ventricular tachyarrhythmias after acute myocardial infarction. In Zipes DP, Jalife J (eds): Cardiac Electrophysiology and Arrhythmias. Grune & Stratton, Orlando, FL, 1985, pp. 553–561.
22. Denniss AR, Ross DL, Richards DA, *et al.*: Differences between patients with ventricular tachycardia and ventricular fibrillation as assessed by signal-averaged electrocardiogram, radionuclide ventriculography and cardiac mapping. J Am Coll Cardiol 1988;11:276–283.
23. Stevenson WG, Brugada P, Waldecker B, *et al.*: Clinical, angiographic and electrophysiologic findings in patients with aborted sudden death as compared with patients with sustained ventricular tachycardia after myocardial infarction. Circulation 1985;71:1146–1152.
24. Freedman RA, Gillis A, Keren A, *et al.*: Signal-averaged electrocardiographic late potentials in patients with ventricular fibrillation or ventricular tachycardia: correlation with clinical arrhythmia and electrophysiologic study. Am J Cardiol 1985;55:1350–1353.
25. Simson MB: Use of signals in the terminal QRS complex to identify patients with ventricular tachycardia after myocardial infarction. Circulation 1981; 64:235–242.
26. Denniss AR, Richards DA, Cody DV, *et al.*: Prognostic significance of ventricular tachycardia and fibrillation induced at programmed stimulation and delayed potentials detected on the signal-averaged electrocardiograms of survivors of acute myocardial infarction. Circulation 1986;74:731–745.
27. Marchlinski FE, Waxman HL, Buxton AE, *et al.*: Sustained ventricular arrhythmias during the early postinfarction period: electrophysiologic findings and prognosis for survival. J Am Coll Cardiol 1983;2:240–250.
28. Poll DS, Marchlinski FE, Buxton AE, *et al.*: Sustained ventricular tachycardia in patients with idopathic dilated cardiomyopathy: electrophysiologic testing and lack of response to antiarrhythmic drug therapy. Circulation 1984;70:451–456.
29. Poll DS, Marchlinski FE, Falcone RA, *et al.*: Abnormal signal-averaged electrocardiogram in nonischemic congestive cardiomyopathy: relationship to sustained ventricular arrhythmias. Circulation 1985;72:1308–1313.
30. Poll DS, Marchlinski FE, Buxton AE, *et al.*: Usefulness of programmed stimulation in idiopathic dilated cardiomyopathy. Am J Cardiol 1986; 58:992–997.
31. Marcus FI, Fontaine GH, Guiraudon G, *et al.*: Right ventricular dysplasia: a report of 24 adult cases. Circulation 1982;65:384–398.
32. Horowitz LN, Vetter VL, Harken AH, *et al.*: Electrophysiologic characteristics of sustianed ventricular tachycardia occurring after repair of tetralogy of Fallot. Am J Cardiol 1980;46:446–452.
33. Kugler JD, Pinsky WW, Cheatham JP, *et al.*: Sustained ventricular tachycardia after repair of tetralogy of Fallot: new electrophysiologic findings. Am J Cardiol 1983;51:1137–1143.
34. Garson A Jr, Porter CJ, Gillette PC, *et al.*: Induction of ventricular tachycardia during electrophysiologic study after repair of tetralogy of Fallot. J Am Coll Cardiol 1983;1:1494–1502.
35. Ohe T, Shimomura K, Aihara N, *et al.*: Idiopathic sustained left ventricular tachycardia: clinical and electrophysiologic characteristics. Circulation 1988;77:560–568.
36. Palileo EV, Ashley WW, Swiryn S, *et al.*: Exercise provocable right ventricular outflow tract tachycardia. Am Heart J 1982;104:185–193.
37. Belhassen B, Shapira I, Pelleg A, *et al.*: Idiopathic recurrent sustained ventricular tachycardia responsive to verapamil: an ECG-electrophysiologic entity. Am Heart J 1983;106:1034–1037.
38. German LD, Packer DL, Bardy GH, *et al.*: Ventricular tachycardia induced by atrial stimulation in patients without symptomatic cardiac disease. Am J Cardiol 1983;52:1202–1207.
39. Lin F-C, Finley CD, Rahimtoola SH, *et al.*: Idiopathic paroxysmal ventricular tachycardia with a QRS pattern of right bundle branch block and left axis deviation: a unique clinical entity with specific properties. Am J Cardiol 1983;52:95–100.
40. Buxton AE, Marchlinski FE, Doherty JU, *et al.*: Repetitive, monomorphic ventricular tachycardia clinical and electrophysiologic characteristics in patients with and patients without organic heart disease. Am J Cardiol 1984;54:997–1002.
41. Wellens HJJ, Bär FWHM, Lie KI: The value of the electrocardiogram in the differential diagnosis of tachycardia with a widened QRS complex. Am J Med 1978;64:27–33.
42. ACC/AHA Task Force Report: Guidelines for Clinical Intracardiac Electrophysiologic Studies. J Am Coll Cardiol 1989;14:7:1827–1842.
43. Moss AJ, Davis HT, DeCamilla J, *et al.*: Ventricular ectopic beats and their relation to sudden and nonsudden cardiac death after myocardial infarction. Circulation 1979;60:998–1003.
44. Ruberman W, Weinblatt E, Goldberg JD, *et al.*: Ventricular premature complexes and sudden death after MI. Circulation 1981;64:297–305.
45. Bigger JT Jr, Webb FM, Rolnitzky LM: Prevalence, characteristics and significance of ventricular tachycardia (three or more complexes) detected with ambulatory ECG recording in the late hospital phase of acute MI. Am J Cardiol 1981;48:815–823.
46. Cardiac Arrhythmia Suppression Trial Investigators: Preliminary report: effect of encainide and flecainide on mortality in a randomized trial of

arrhythmia suppression after myocardial infarction. N Engl J Med 1989; 321:406–412.
47. Bigger JT Jr, Webb FM, Rolnitzky LM: Prevalence, characteristics and significance of ventricular tachycardia (three or more complexes) detected with ambulatory ECG recording in the late hospital phase of acute MI. Am J Cardiol 1981;48:815–823.
48. Baum RS, Alvarez H III, Cobb LA: Survival after resuscitation from out-of-hospital ventricular fibrillation. Circulation 1974;50:1231–1235.
49. Schaffer WA, Cobb LA: Recurrent ventricular fibrillation and modes of death in survivors of out-of-hospital ventricular fibrillation. N Engl J Med 1975;293:259–262.
50. Weaver WD, Lorch GS, Alvarez HA, *et al.*: Angiographic findings and prognostic indicators in patients resuscitated from sudden cardiac death. Circulation 1976;54:895–900.
51. Ruskin JN, DiMarco JP, Garan H: Out-of-hospital cardiac arrest. Electrophysiologic observations and selection of long-term antiarrhythmic therapy. N Engl J Med 1980;303:607–612.
52. Morady F, Scheinman MM, Hess DS, *et al.*: Electrophysiologic testing in the management of survivors of out-of-hospital cardiac arrest. Am J Cardiol 1983;51:85–89.
53. Roy D, Waxman HL, Kienzle MG, *et al.*: Clinical characteristics and long-term follow up in 119 survivors of cardiac arrest: relation to inducibility at electrophysiologic testing. Am J Cardiol 1983;52:969–974.
54. Benditt DG, Benson DW Jr, Klein GJ, *et al.*: Prevention of recurrent sudden cardiac arrest: role of provocative electropharmacologic testing. J Am Coll Cardiol 1983;2:418–425.
55. Skale BT, Miles WM, Heger JJ, *et al.*: Survivors of cardiac arrest: prevention of recurrence by drug therapy as predicted by electrophysiologic testing or ECG monitoring. Am J Cardiol 1986;57:113–119.
56. Wilber DJ, Garan H, Kelly E, *et al.*: Out-of-hospital cardiac arrest: role of electrophysiologic testing in prediction of long term outcome. N Engl J Med 1988;318:19–24.
57. Wilber DJ, Kelly E, Garan H, *et al.*: Determinants of inducible ventricular arrhythmias in survivors of out-of-hospital cardiac arrest (Abstr). Circulation 1985;72(Suppl III):III–45.
58. Ruskin JN, DiMarco JP, Garan H: Out-of-hospital cardiac arrest. Electrophysiologic observations and selection of long term antiarrhythmic therapy. N Engl J Med 1980;303:607–613.
59. Buxton AE, Marchlinski FE, Flores BT, *et al.*: Nonsustained ventricular tachycardia in patients with coronary artery disease: role of electrophysiologic study. Circulation 1987;75:1178–1185.
60. Gallagher JJ, Kassell JH, Cox JL, *et al.*: Techniques of intraoperative mapping. Am J Cardiol 1982;49:221–240.
61. Miller JM, Marchlinski FE, Harken AH, *et al.*: Subendocardial resection for sustained ventricular tachycardia in the early period after acute MI. Am J Cardiol 1985;55:980–984.
62. Gallagher JJ, Pritchett ELC, Sealy WC, *et al.*: The preexcitation syndromes. Prog Cardiovasc Dis 1978;20:285–327.
63. Josephson ME, Harken AH: Surgical therapy of arrhythmias. In Rosen MR, Hoffman BF (eds): Cardiac Therapy. Martinus Nijhoff, Boston; 1983:337–385.
64. Cox JL: The status of surgery for cardiac arrhythmias. Circulation 1985;71:413–417.
65. Moran JM, Kehoe RF, Loeb JM, *et al.*: Extended endocardial resection for the treatment of ventricular tachycardia and ventricular fibrillation. An Thorac Surg 1982;34:538–552.
66. Cooper MJ, Hust LJ, Richards DA, *et al.*: Effect of repetition of extrastimuli on sensitivity and reproducibility of mode of induction of ventricular tachycardia by programmed ventricular stimulation. J Am Coll Cardiol 1986;11:1260–1267.
67. Marchlinski FE, Buxton AE, Vassallo JA, *et al.*: Comparative electrophysiological effects of intravenous and oral procainamide in patients with sustained ventricular arrhythmias. J Am Coll Cardiol 1984;4:1247–1254.
68. Kim AG: The management of patients with life-threatening tachyarrhythmias: programmed stimulation or Holter monitoring (either or both). Circulation 1987;76:1–5.
69. Waxman HL, Buxton AE, Sadowski LM, *et al.*: The response to procainamide during electrophysiologic study for sustained ventricular tachyarrhythmias predicts the response to other medication. Circulation 1982;67:30–37.
70. Mason JW, Peters FA: Antiarrhythmic efficacy of encainide in patients with refractory recurrent ventricular tachycardia. Circulation 1981;63:670–675.
71. Josephson MA, Ikeda N, Singh BN: Effects of flecainide on ventricular function: Clinical and experimental correlations. Am J Cardiol 1984; 53:95B–100B.
72. Podrid PJ, Lown B: Propafenone: a new agent for ventricular arrhythmia. J Am Coll Cardiol 1984;4:117–125.
73. Greenspan AM, Spielman SR, Webb CR, *et al.*: Efficacy of combination therapy with mexiletene and a Type IA agent for inducible ventricular tachyarrhythmias secondary to coronary artery disease. Am J Cardiol 1985; 56:277–284.
74. Kadish AH, Marchlinski FE, Josephson ME, *et al.*: Amiodarone: correlation of early and late electrophysiologic studies with outcome. Am Heart J 1986;112:1134–1140.
75. Greenspan AJ, Volosin KJ, Greenberg RM, *et al.*: Amiodarone therapy: role of early and late electrophysiologic studies. J Am Coll Cardiol 1988;11:117–123.
76. Waleffe A, Mary-Rabine L, Legrand V, *et al.*: Combined mexiletine and amiodarone treatment of refractory recurrent ventricular tachycardia. Am Heart J 1980;100:788–793.
77. Marchlinski FE, Buxton AE, Miller JM, *et al.*: Amiodarone versus amiodarone and a type IA agent for treatment of patients wish rapid ventricular tachycardia. Circulation 1986;74:1037–1043.
78. Marchlinski FE, Buxton AE, Kindwall KE, *et al.*: Comparison of individual and combined effect of procainamide and amiodarone in patients with sustained ventricular tachyarrhythmia. Circulation 1988;76:583–591.
79. Kuchar DL, Rottman J, Berger E, *et al.*: Prediction of successful suppression of sustained ventricular tachyarrhythmias by serial drug testing from data derived at the initial electrophysiologic study. J Am Coll Cardiol 1988; 12:982–988.
80. Horowitz LN, Borggrefe M: Many things are not found in books or journals . . . but some things are! Value of electrophysiologic testing in patients with malignant ventricular arrhythmias. Am J Cardiol 1988;62:1292–1294.
81. Borggrefe M, Hans-Joachim T, Gunter B: Reappraisal of criteria for assessing drug efficacy in patients with ventricular tachyarrhythmias: complete versus partial suppression of inducible arrhythmias. J Am Coll Cardiol 1988;12:140–149.
82. Klein LS, Fineberg N, Heger JJ, *et al.*: Prospective evaluation of a discriminant function for prediction of recurrent symptomatic ventricular tachycardia or ventricular fibrillation in coronary artery disease patients receiving amiodarone and having inducible ventricular tachycardia at electrophysiologic study. Am J Cardiol 1988;61:1024–1030.
83. Gottlieb CD, Berger MD, Miller JM, *et al.*: What is an acceptable risk for cardiac arrest patients treated with amiodarone? Circulation 1988; 78(II):500.
84. Swerdlow CD, Peterson J: Prospective comparison of Holter monitoring and electrophysiologic study in patients with coronary artery disease and sustained ventricular tachyarrhythmias. Am J Cardiol 1985;56:577–585.
85. Marchlinski FE: Value of Holter monitoring in identifying risk for sustained ventricular arrhythmia recurrence on amiodarone. Am J Cardiol 1985; 55:709–712.
86. Mitchell LB, Duff HJ, Manyari DE, *et al.*: A randomized clinical trial of the noninvasive and invasive approaches to drug therapy of ventricular tachycardia. N Engl J Med 1987;317:1681–1687.
87. Miller JM, Marchlinski FE, Buxton AE, *et al.*: Relationship between 12

lead electrocardiogram during ventricular tachycardia and endocardial site of origin in patients with coronary artery disease. Circulation 1986; 77(41):759–766.

88. Berger MD, Waxman HL, Buxton AE, *et al.*: Spontaneous compared with induced onset of sustained ventricular tachycardia. Circulation 1988; 78:885–892.
89. Josephson ME, Horowitz LN, Spielman SR, *et al.*: Comparison of endocardial catheter mapping with intraoperative mapping of ventricular tachycardia. Circulation 1980;61:395–404.
90. Josephson ME, Horowitz LN, Spielman SR, *et al.*: The role of catheter mapping in the preoperative evaluation of ventricular tachycardia. Am J Cardiol 1982;49:207–220.
91. Waxman HL, Josephson ME: Ventricular activation during ventricular endocardial pacing: I. Electrocardiographic patterns to the site of pacing. Am J Cardiol 1982;50:1–10.
92. Mason JW, Stinson EB, Winkle RA, *et al.*: Surgery for ventricular tachycardia: efficacy of left ventricular aneurysm resection compared with operation guided by electrical activation mapping. Circulation 1982;65:1148–1155.
93. Josephson ME, Horowitz LN, Spielman SR, *et al.*: Role of catheter mapping in the preoperative evaluation of ventricular tachycardia. Am J Cardiol 1982;49:207–220.
94. Hauer RNW, deZwart MT, deBakker JMT, *et al.*: Endocardial catheter mapping: wire skeleton technique for representation of computed arrhythmogenic sites compared to intraoperative mapping. Circulation 1986;74:1346–1356.
95. Waspe LE, Brodman R, Kim SG, *et al.*: Activation mapping in patients with coronary artery disease with multiple ventricular tachycardia configurations: occurrence and therapeutic implications of widely separate apparent sites of origin. J Am Coll Cardiol 1985;5:1075–1086.
96. Saksena S, Hussain SM, Gieldinsky I, *et al.*: Intraoperative mapping—guided Argon laser ablation of malignant ventricular tachycardia. Am J Cardiol 1987;59:78–83.
97. Caceres J, Werner P, Jazayeri M, *et al.*: Efficacy of cryosurgery alone for refractory monomorphic sustained ventricular tachycardia due to inferior wall infarction. J Am Coll Cardiol 1988;11:1254–1259.
98. deBakker JMT, Janse MJ, van Capelle FJL, *et al.*: Endocardial mapping by simultaneous recording of endocardial electrograms during cardiac surgery for ventricular aneurysm. J Am Coll Cardiol 1983;2:947–953.
99. Downar E, Harris L, Mickleborough LL, *et al.*: Endocardial mapping of ventricular tachycardia in the intact human ventricle: evidence for reentrant mechanisms. J Am Coll Cardiol 1988;11:783–791.
100. Harris L, Downar E, Mickleborough LL, *et al.*: Activation sequence of ventricular tachycardia: endocardial and epicardial mapping studies in the human ventricle. J Am Coll Cardiol 1987;10:1040–1047.
101. Kassell J, Gallagher JJ: Construction of multipolar needle electrode for activation study of the heart. Am J Physiol 1977;233:H312–H317.
102. Wit AL, Allessie MA, Bonke FIM, *et al.*: Electrophysiologic mapping to determine the mechanisms of experimental ventricular tachycardia initiated by premature impulses: Experimental approach and initial results demonstrating reentrant excitation. Am J Cardiol 1982;49:166–185.
103. Taccardi B, Arisi G, Macchi E, *et al.*: A new intracavitory probe for detecting the site of origin of ventricular ectopic beats during one cardiac cycle. Circulation 1987;75:272–281.
104. Lampert S, Lown B, Graboys TB, *et al.*: Determinants of survival in patients with malignant ventricular arrhythmia associated with coronary artery disease. Am J Cardiol 1988;61:791–797.
105. Swerdlow CD, Winkle RA, Mason JW: Determinants of survival in patients with ventricular arrhythmias. N Engl J Med 1983;308:1436–1442.
106. DiCarlo LA, Morady F, Sauve MJ, *et al.*: Cardiac arrest and sudden death in patients treated with amiodarone for sustained ventricular tachycardia or ventricular fibrillation: risk stratification based on clinical variables. Am J Cardiol 1985;55:372–374.
107. Wilber DJ, Garan H, Finkelstein D, *et al.*: Out-of-hospital cardiac arrest. Use of electrophysiologic testing in the prediction of long term outcome. N Engl J Med 1986;318:19–24.
108. Graboys T: Long-term survival of patients with malignant ventricular arrhythmia treated with antiarrhythmic drugs. Am J Cardiol 1982;50:437–443.
109. Waller TJ, Kay HR, Spielman SR, *et al.*: Reduction in sudden death and total mortality by antiarrhythmic therapy evaluated by electrophysiologic drug testing: criteria of efficacy in patients with sustained ventricular tachyarrhythmia. J Am Coll Cardiol 1987;10:1083–1089.
110. Horowitz LN, Greenspan AM, Spielman SR, *et al.*: Usefulness of electrophysiologic testing in evaluation of amiodarone therapy for sustained ventricular tachyarrhythmias associated with coronary heart disease. Am J Cardiol 1985;35:367–371.
111. Kadish AH, Buxton AE, Waxman HL, *et al.*: Usefulness of electrophysiologic study to determine the clinical tolerance of arrhythmia recurrences during amiodarone therapy. J Am Coll Cardiol 1987;10:90–96.
112. Marchlinski FE, Josephson ME: Appropriate diagnostic studies for arrhythmia surgery. PACE 1984;7:902–916.
113. Josephson ME, Harken AH, Horowitz LN: Endocardial excision: a new surgical technique for the treatment of recurrent ventricular tachycardia. Circulation 1987;76:332–342.
114. Haines DE, Lerman BB, Kron IL, *et al.*: Surgical ablation of ventricular tachycardia with sequential map-guided subendocardial resection: electrophysiologic, assessment and long term follow up. Circulation 1988;7:131–141.
115. Caceres J, Werner P, Jazayeri M, *et al.*: Efficacy of cryosurgery alone for refractory monomorphic sustained ventricular tachycardia due to inferior wall infarction. J Am Coll Cardiol 1988;11:1254–1259.
116. Miller JM, Gottlieb CD, Hargrove WC, *et al.*: Factors influencing operative mortality in surgery for ventricular tachycardia. Circulation 1988;78:II–44.
117. Morady F, Scheinman MM, DiCarlo LA, *et al.*: Catheter ablation of ventricular tachycardia with intracardiac shocks: results in 33 patients. Circulation 1987;75:1037–1049.
118. Fontaine G, Frank R, Tonet J, *et al.*: Fulguration of chronic ventricular tachycardia: Results of forty-seven consecutive cases with follow-up ranging from 11 to 65 months. In Zipes DF, Jalife J (eds): Cardiac Electrophysiology (from Cell to Bedside). W.B. Saunders, Philadelphia, 1990:978–985.
119. Buxton AE, Waxman HL, Marchlinski FE, *et al.*: Right ventricular tachycardia: clinical and electrophysiologic characteristics. Circulation 1983;68:917–927.
120. Sung RJ, Keung EC, Nguyen NX, *et al.*: Effects of beta-adrenergic blockade on verapamil-responsive and verapamil-irresponsive sustained ventricular tachycardias. J Clin Invest 1988;81:688–699.
121. Zimmerman M, Masonblanche P, Cauchemez B, *et al.*: Determinants of the spontaneous ectopic activity in repetitive monomorphic idiopathic ventricular tachycardia. J Am Coll Cardiol 1986;7:1219–1227.
122. Blomstrom LC, Sabel KG, Olsson SB: A long term follow up of 15 patients with arrhythmogenic right ventricular dysplasia. Br Heart J 1987;58:477–488.
123. Belhassen B, Caspi A, Miller H, *et al.*: Extensive endocardial mapping during sinus rhythm and ventricular tachycardia in a patient with arrhythmogenic right ventricular dysplasia. J Am Coll Cardiol 1984;4:1302–1306.
124. Giuraudon GM, Klein GJ, Gulamhusein SS, *et al.*: Total disconnection of the right ventricular free wall: surgical treatment of right ventricular tachycardia associated with right ventricular dysplasia. Circulation 1983;67:463–470.
125. Leclercq JF, Chouty F, Cauchemez B, *et al.*: Results of electrical fulguration in arrhythmogenic right ventricular disease. Am J Cardiol 1988;62:220–224.
126. Roy D, Waxman HL, Kienzle MG, *et al.*: Clinical characteristics and long term follow up in 119 survivors of cardiac arrest: relation to inducibility in electrophysiologic testing. Am J Cardiol 1983;52:969–974.

127. Morady F, Shen E, Bhandari A, *et al.*: Programmed ventricular stimulation in mitral valve prolapse: analysis of 36 patients. Am J Cardiol 1984;53:135–137.
128. Rosenthal ME, Hamer A, Gang ES, *et al.*: The yield of programmed ventricular stimulation in mitral valve prolapse patients with ventricular arrhythmias. Am Heart J 1985;110:970–976.
129. Duren DR, Becker AE, Dunning AJ: Long term follow up of identifying mitral valve prolapse in 300 patients: a prospective study. J Am Coll Cardiol 1988;11:42–47.
130. Wit AL, Fenoglio JJ, Hordof AJ, *et al.*: Ultrastructure and transmembrane potentials of cardiac muscle in the human anterior mitral valve leaflet. Circulation 1979;59:1284–1292.
131. Boudoulas H, Wooley CF: Mitral valve prolapse syndrome. Evidence of hyperadrenergic state. Postgrad Med 1988;152–162.
132. Maron BJ, Savage DD, Wolfson JK, *et al.*: Prognostic significance of 24 hour ambulatory electrocardiographic monitoring in patients with hypertrophic cardiomyopathy: a prospective study. Am J Cardiol 1987;48:252–257.
133. McKenna WJ, Harris L, Percy G, *et al.*: Arrhythmia in hypertrophic cardiomyopathy. II. Comparison of amiodarone and verapamil in treatment. Am Heart J 1981;46:173–178.
134. McKenna WJ, Chetty S, Oakley CM, *et al.*: Arrhythmia in hypertrophic cardiomyopathy: exercise and 48 hour ambulatory electrocardiographic treatment with and without beta adrenergic blocking therapy. Am J Cardiol 1980;45:1–5.
135. Nicod P, Polikar R, Peterson KL: Hypertrophic cardiomyopathy and death. N Engl J Med 1988;318:1255–1256.
136. Anderson KP, Stinson EB, Derby G, *et al.*: Vulnerability of patients with obstructive hypertrophic cardiomyopathy to ventricular arrhythmia induction in the operating room. Am J Cardiol 1983;51:811–816.
137. Schiavone WA, Maloney JD, Lever HM, *et al.*: Electrophysiologic studies of patients with hypertrophic cardiomyopathy presenting with syncope of undetermined etiology. PACE 1986;476–481.
138. Watson RM, Schwartz JL, Maron BJ, *et al.*: Inducible polymorphic ventricular tachycardia and ventricular fibrillation in a subgroup of patients with hypertrophic cardiomyopathy at high risk for sudden death. J Am Coll Cardiol 1987;10:761–774.

9

WOLFF-PARKINSON-WHITE AND OTHER PREEXCITATION SYNDROMES

Tibor S. Szabo, M.D., and Igor Singer, M.B.B.S., F.R.A.C.P., F.A.C.P., F.A.C.C.

DEFINITION OF THE PREEXCITATION SYNDROMES

Preexcitation was defined by Ohnell in 1944 as anomalous ventricular excitation, whereby a portion of the ventricle was depolarized prior to any conduction through the atrioventricular (AV) node-His bundle system (1). According to Durrer's modified definition in 1970, preexcitation is present "if in the relation to atrial events, the whole or some part of the ventricular muscle is activated earlier by the impulse originating from the atrium than would be expected if the impulse reached the ventricles by way of the normal specialized conduction system only" (2). Later, to accommodate the variants of preexcitation, this definition was extended by Gallagher to include any case in which activation, either anterograde or retrograde, arrived at an area distal to the site of impulse formation earlier than could be explained by conduction over the normal conduction system (3).

By far the most common of the clinical preexcitation syndromes, of which there are several, is the Wolff-Parkinson-White (WPW) syndrome. This review will focus on the pathophysiology, clinical features, diagnosis, and treatment of the WPW syndrome, with reference to the less common variants of preexcitation syndromes.

DEFINITION OF THE WOLFF-PARKINSON-WHITE SYNDROME

In 1930, Wolff, Parkinson, and White described the syndrome that was named after them, as a functional bundle branch block and a short PR interval occurring in healthy young people who also had paroxysms of tachycardia (4). The two elements of the definition, the characteristic electrocardiographic pattern and the history of symptomatic tachyarrhythmias, were the essential diagnostic criteria. The electrocardiogram (ECG) demonstrates typical features: short PR intervals and prolonged QRS complex duration (Fig. 9.1). The initial portion of the QRS has a characteristic slurring, which is called the delta wave. The extent of the delta wave and consequently the width of the QRS complex, is variable due to differing levels of preexcitation and AV node conduction at any one time. The QRS complex is followed by ST segment and T wave changes.

Most patients with WPW syndrome have recurrent episodes of tachyarrhythmias, though many are asymptomatic. Some patients have infrequent, mildly symptomatic arrhythmia episodes, whereas others have almost incessant tachycardia causing serious symptoms.

MECHANISM OF VENTRICULAR PREEXCITATION AND THE ACCOMPANYING ARRHYTHMIAS

The anatomic basis of ventricular preexcitation in the WPW syndrome is an accessory atrioventricular (A-V) connection. This consists of a band of myocardium connecting the atria and the ventricles at a site where normally there is no muscular continuity. The anomalous conduction system can be located anywhere around the mitral or tricuspid rings. In the majority of cases, there is only a single accessory connection, but in approximately 5–15% of WPW patients, two or more accessory connections may be present (5–7). The accessory connections are most commonly located close to the epicardial surface, or in the fat pad in the AV groove. Some connections, however, are intramural or subendocardial. The accessory AV connections represent alternative pathways of impulse conduction, in addition to the AV node-His bundle system.

Several different anatomic types of accessory pathways are now recognized. A classification of these pathways was suggested by the European Study Group for Preexcitation (8). According to this classification, a "tract" is an accessory pathway (AP) that inserts into specialized conduction tissue. A "connection" is a pathway that terminates in the working myocardium, e.g., nodoventricular or fasciculoventricular (Mahaim) fibers. Accessory AV connections, which are the substrate of the WPW syndrome, are by far the most common APs, however.

The electrophysiologic (EP) properties of an accessory connection differ markedly from those of the AV node. Atrioventric-

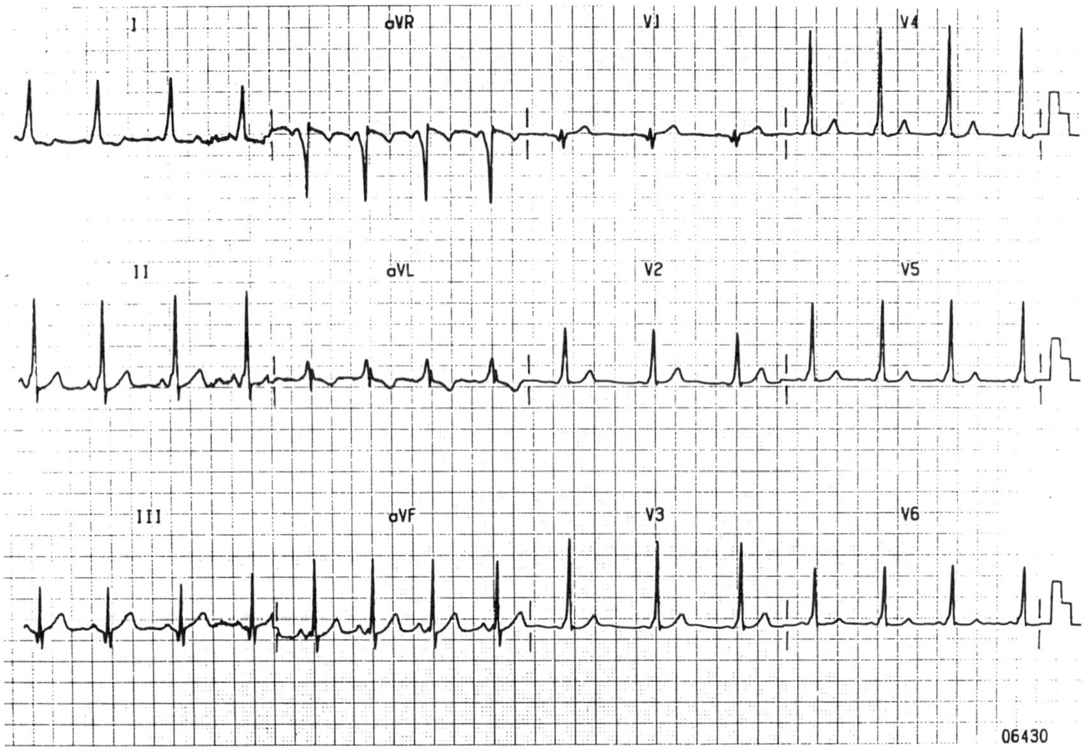

Figure 9.1. Twelve-lead electrocardiogram of a patient with Wolff-Parkinson-White syndrome. The electrocardiographic features of ventricular preexcitation are short PR interval, wide QRS complex, and the characteristic delta wave.

ular node conduction is rate-dependent, i.e., with faster atrial pacing rates or shorter atrial coupling intervals during atrial extrastimulus testing, a delay of electrical conduction develops in the AV node. This delay is manifested by gradual prolongation of the AV node conduction time (first-degree AV block), followed by the development of second-degree AV block at critical atrial rates (9). In the AV node, Type I second-degree block is usually noted at atrial pacing cycle lengths of 500–300 msec, following a gradual prolongation of AV node conduction times (AH interval prolongation) (9–10).

In contrast to the AV node, conduction over the accessory AV connection is faster and is independent of the rate. This is manifested by shorter conduction times over the accessory connections, which do not lengthen as a function of increasing atrial rates. One to one impulse conduction may be maintained to cycle lengths up to 200 msec (300 beats/min). Characteristically, Type II second-degree AV block (Mobitz II) develops suddenly and is not preceded by the prolongation of AP conduction times (9). This distinction between AV node and AP conduction patterns is valid in both anterograde and retrograde directions.

The AV node-His bundle system and the accessory AV connections conduct the impulse originating in the sinus node in a parallel fashion. Consequently, the ventricular myocardium is activated from two directions. One is the normal conduction system, which would result in a normal, narrow QRS complex. The other is the activation through the AP. Since the accessory pathways insert in the ventricular myocardium far from the normal specialized conduction tissue, conduction is in part, via the working ventricular myocardium. The result is a slower spread of electrical activation which is manifested as a wide QRS complex. This is analogous to the ventricular activation from an ectopic ventricular focus. The resulting QRS complex is a product of fusion of the two distinct activation wavefronts. Since the conduction over the AP is faster than that which occurs over the normal conduction system, the initial part of the QRS complex represents ventricular activation over the AP (delta wave). The terminal part of the QRS represents the late ventricular activation via the normal conduction system (Fig. 9.2). Secondary repolarization changes, i.e., the abnormal ST segments and T waves, are a result of the abnormal ventricular activation sequence.

The relative contribution of the separate activation wavefronts determines the width of the QRS complex. Factors that determine the degree of this contribution include: (a) conduction velocity via the AV node relative to that via the AP, (b) site of the AP in relation to the mitral or the tricuspid ring, (c) site of the atrial pacemaker and the size of the atria, and (d) conduction velocity via the atrial and the ventricular myocardium.

Based on the above considerations, it is possible that an AP is present even in the absence of the classic ECG criteria of the WPW syndrome (9). When the AP is close to the site of impulse formation, the pathway is reached by the impulse earlier than the AV node. The proximity of the AP and faster conduction in

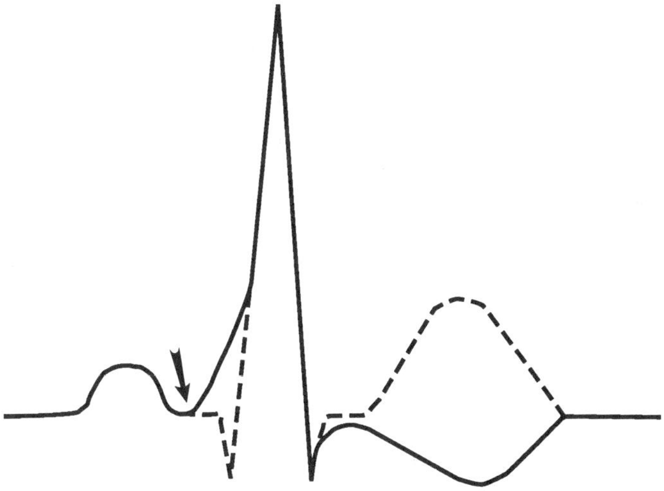

Figure 9.2. A preexcited QRS complex is superimposed on the normal QRS complex. The *arrow* points to the onset of the delta wave. This point represent the earliest ventricular activation via the accessory pathway.

relation to the AV nodal conduction, result in predominant ventricular activation over the AP. The resultant wide QRS complex is therefore, maximally preexcited. On the other hand, an AP located in left lateral free wall, may be reached by the sinus impulse much later than the AV node. This may result in ventricular activation predominantly over the normal conduction system, resulting in a narrow QRS complex with an inconspicuous delta wave. In this case, minimal ventricular preexcitation is present. When the QRS complex is normal, in the presence of an accessory connection that is capable of anterograde conduction, ventricular preexcitation is said to be latent. Thus, minimal preexcitation is a useful clue suggesting presence of left-sided accessory pathways (11).

Table 9.1.
Characteristic Features of Atrioventricular Reciprocating Tachycardias

- Initiation and termination with critically timed extrastimuli
- Initiation and termination by pacing from the atrium and/or ventricle (both the atrium and the ventricle participate in the reentry circuit)
- Arrhythmia initiation requires a critical AV/VA conduction delay
- AV/VA block always terminates the tachycardia
- Premature ventricular stimuli delivered during the tachycardia at a time when the His bundle is refractory advance the atrial activation (preexcite the atrium)
- Retrograde atrial activation is eccentric during the tachycardia (atrial activation in the His bundle electrogram is late)

A "concealed" accessory AV connection is one that conducts only in the retrograde (VA) direction. In this case, the QRS complex is normal, as anterograde ventricular activation occurs exclusively over the normal conduction system. However, the patient may suffer from paroxysmal supraventricular tachycardia due to reentry involving the retrogradely conducting AP.

Tachyarrhythmias in Wolff-Parkinson-White Syndrome

A variety of tachyarrhythmias have been described in patients with WPW syndrome. Reentry tachycardias and atrial fibrillation (AF) are the most common and the most important of these tachycardias. The presence of an alternative conduction pathway together with the AV node, provides the anatomic and physiologic substrate for development of reentry. The following structures participate in the reentry circuit: (a) the normal AV con-

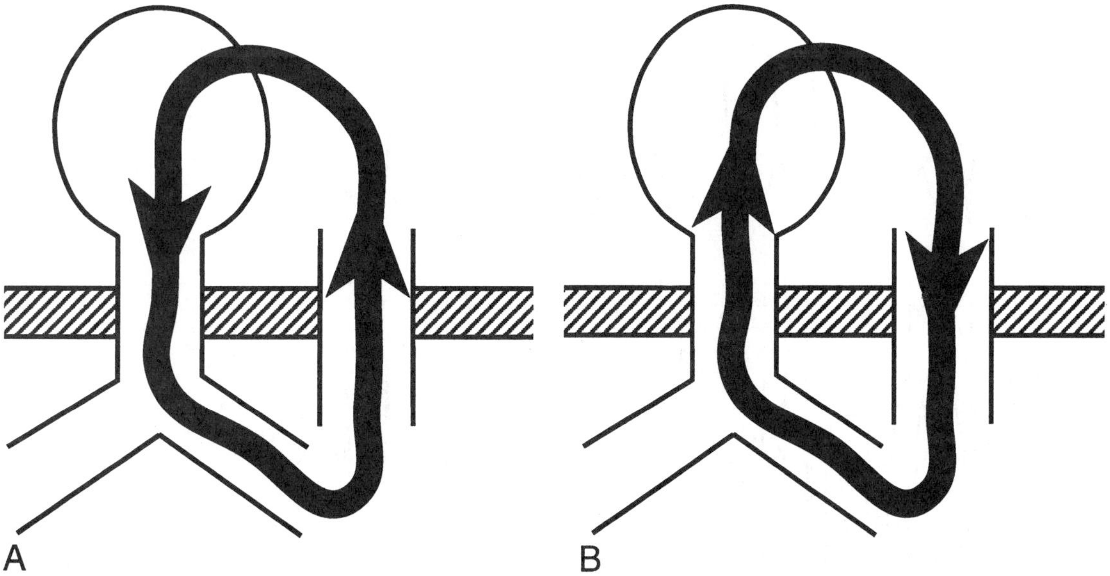

Figure 9.3. Mechanism of atrioventricular (AV) reentry. **A.** The diagram of orthodromic AV reciprocating tachycardia. Anterograde conduction is over the AV node - His bundle, resulting in a narrow QRS morphology. **B.** The diagram of antidromic AV reciprocating tachycardia. The wide QRS complex is the result of ventricular activation exclusively via the accessory pathway.

duction system (AV node-His bundle), (b) the accessory AV connection, (c) atrial myocardium, and (d) ventricular myocardium. Reentry circuits utilizing multiple APs have also been reported. During AF and flutter the accessory pathway is not part of the arrhythmia mechanism, but acts as a passive bystander and may become a conduit for rapid conduction to the ventricle.

The reentry tachycardia involving all of the above structures is called AV reciprocating (reentrant) tachycardia, (Table 9.1). Activation can spread in two directions around this circuit. Distinction is made according to the direction of conduction through the normal conduction system. When the impulse spreads from the atrium to the ventricle anterogradely over the AV node-His bundle system, the resulting tachycardia is called orthodromic AV reciprocating tachycardia (RT) (Fig. 9.3). The AP participates as the retrograde limb of the reentry circuit. In the absence of preexistent or functional bundle branch block, the QRS complex in orthodromic reentry is narrow, since the ventricular activation occurs exclusively through the normal conduction system. The ability to sustain orthodromic AVRT is independent of the anterograde AP properties. When the normal conduction system participates as the retrogradely conducting limb of the reentry circuit, anterograde ventricular activation occurs exclusively over the accessory connection. The resulting QRS morphology is maximally preexcited, and the tachycardia is called antidromic AVRT (Fig. 9.3). Antidromic AVRT is much less frequent than the orthodromic type. In one study, it was induced only in 6% of 374 patients with a single accessory AV pathway. However, it was induced in 32% of 60 patients with multiple APs (12). These RT's are generally regular and have a cycle length between 420 and 220 msec (13).

The cycle length of the AV reciprocating tachycardia depends on the conduction time over each component of the circuit. Variability of the cycle length of tachycardia is mainly due to alterations in the AV node-His bundle conduction. This is the segment of the reentry circuit that is most sensitive to autonomic changes. With faster tachycardia rates, electrical alternans may be present. Repolarization changes are observed frequently during normal QRS tachycardia. A "retrograde" P′ wave is usually discernible on the surface ECG, with a P′R interval longer than the RP′ interval.

During atrial flutter or AF the normal conduction system with its characteristic AV nodal conduction delay and the resulting physiologic AV block protects the ventricles from rapid rates. Accessory AV connections do not exhibit conduction delay and usually develop second-degree block at rapid atrial rates. Consequently, dangerously rapid ventricular rates may occur during AF-flutter, (Fig. 9.4). Atrial flutter may be conducted with a one to one ratio to the ventricles over an AP. The resulting ventricular rates can be as rapid as 250–350 beats/min. Exceedingly rapid ventricular rates occurring during atrial fibrillation-flutter

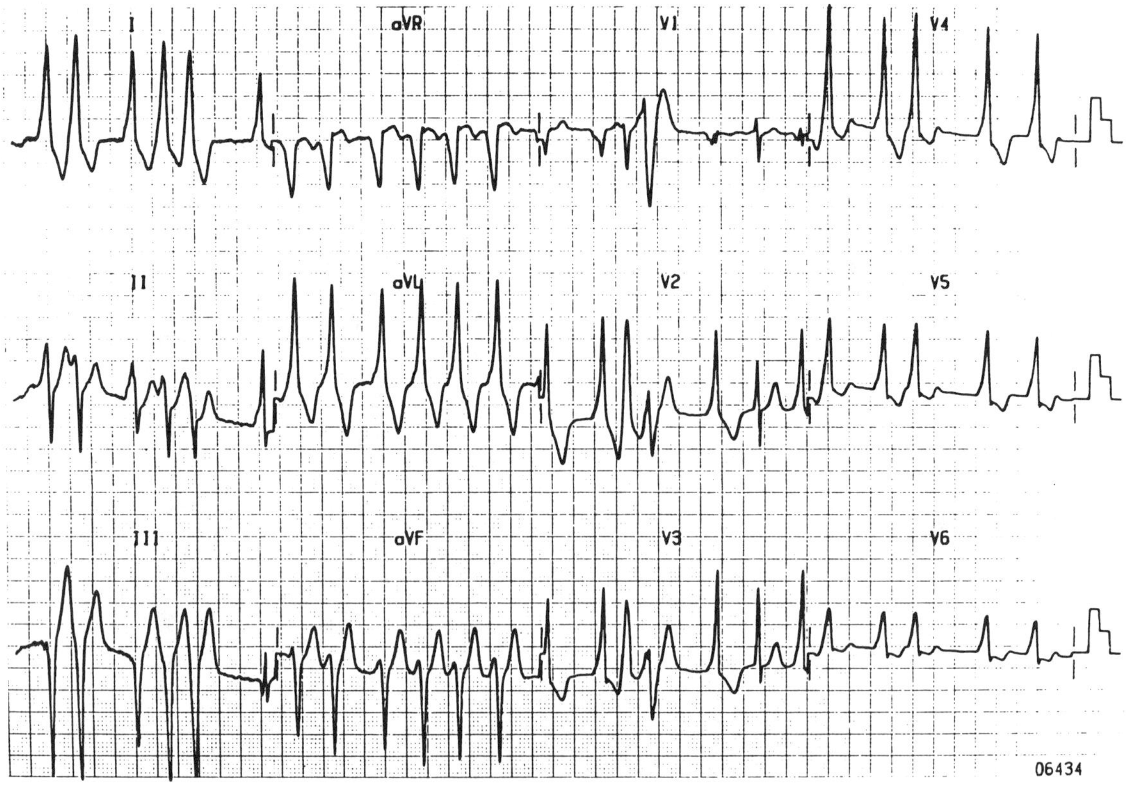

Figure 9.4. Twelve-lead electrocardiogram of a patient with an accessory AV pathway and atrial fibrillation (same patient as in Fig. 9.1). QRS morphologies range from completely normal, narrow QRS morphology, to maximal preexcitation. The shortest RR interval between two consecutively, preexcited QRS complexes is 200 msec.

in the setting of the WPW syndrome may induce ventricular fibrillation (VF). This is the presumed mechanism of sudden cardiac death occurring in this setting.

Ventricular fibrillation develops in patients who are able to sustain AF and have accessory pathways capable of rapid conduction (14). In one study, only 1 of 19 patients with WPW syndrome and documented AF had recurrent AF during a 1.9-yr follow-up period following a successful surgical AP ablation (15). Patients with WPW syndrome and inducible AF were found to have significantly longer PA intervals, shorter atrial functional refractory periods, and shorter AP refractoriness than patients in the control group (16). The reported incidence of AF in WPW syndrome is between 11.5 and 39% (17,18).

The reason why AF occurs more frequently in patients with accessory pathways than in individuals with normal hearts, is unknown. Presence of both a functioning AP and certain EP features of the atrial myocardium appear to be necessary prerequisites for the development of AF in the WPW syndrome (15–20). Atrial vulnerability, i.e., repetitive atrial responses or paroxysms of AF or atrial flutter in response to a single closely coupled trial extrastimulus, is observed frequently in WPW patients with AF (21). Klein, *et al.* found that patients with a history of documented VF had a significantly higher incidence of multiple accessory pathways than those without such a history. The shortest RR interval between two consecutive, preexcited QRS complexes (SRR-PX) during AF was significantly shorter in patients with VF as well (14). The SRR-PX during AF did not exceed 250 msec in any of the patients in the VF group. An SRR-PX of 250 msec or less has traditionally been used as an indicator of high risk for sudden death.

The determinants of the ventricular rate during AF in the presence of ventricular preexcitation include the anterograde refractory period of the AP and the AV node-His bundle system, ventricular refractoriness, degree of concealed retrograde conduction in the accessory pathway and the AV node, adrenergic tone, and possibly other, as yet unknown factors (22–25). Some patients exhibit only preexcited QRS complexes during AF, while others may have a mixture of preexcited and normal QRS complexes, or exclusively "normal" QRS complexes, despite having a characteristic WPW pattern when they are in sinus rhythm.

One possible explanation for exclusive ventricular activation via the normal conduction system during AF is thought to be retrograde concealed conduction in the AP. Electrical impulses conducted anterogradely via the normal conduction system would activate the ventricle and the ventricular insertion of the AP, rendering it refractory. Variable degrees of ventricular preexcitation are usually present during AF, reflecting varying degrees of fusion. If more than one AP is present, the appearance of preexcited QRS complexes of different morphologies during AF may be the only clue indicating the presence of multiple accessory pathways (Fig. 9.5) (26).

Atrial fibrillation in the WPW syndrome can be appropriately characterized using the following parameters: (a) average ventricular cycle length (ARR), (b) average RR interval between consecutive preexcited QRS complexes (ARR-PX), (c) shortest RR interval between two consecutive preexcited QRS complexes (SRR-PX), and (d) the percentage of preexcited QRS complexes (PX%).

The shortest RR interval between consecutive, preexcited QRS complexes indicates the fastest possible rate that can be conducted anterogradely to the ventricle. This parameter correlates well with the anterograde effective refractory period (ERP) of the AP, and should always be determined in a symptomatic WPW patient (27). It was demonstrated, that analyzing a 2-min-long sample is sufficient to obtain data that accurately represents a particular episode of AF (28).

The Incidence of Preexcitation

The true incidence of WPW syndrome is unknown. Reported figures in the literature estimate that approximately 1–3/1000 ECGs show ventricular preexcitation (29,30). The incidence of concealed accessory connections and that of inconspicuous delta waves or latent preexcitation is not known. The incidence of tachyarrhythmias in patients who exhibit preexcited QRS complexes during sinus rhythm on their ECG is also unknown. Reported incidence of symptoms varies widely, between 4.3% and 90% depending on patient population studied (18). In one study of 514 patients with WPW syndrome 337 had documented AVRT, 101 patients had AF, and 86 patients had experienced both of these arrhythmias (31).

Syncope occurs relatively frequently in patients with the WPW syndrome. The reported incidence in referred patients is 19–22%, but it may be as high as 36% according to a more recent report (32,33). No distinct clinical features or a more malignant EP profile could be identified in WPW patients who had at least one syncopal episode, compared to those who had no such episodes (32). It was suggested that other, perhaps extracardiac factors, may play a role in the genesis of syncope. Considering the sporadic incidence of sudden death in this population, a relatively frequent event like syncope cannot be used as a specific marker to identify patients at risk.

APPROACH TO PATIENTS WITH WOLFF-PARKINSON-WHITE SYNDROME

Clinical investigations of WPW patients have several important objectives: (a) demonstration of the presence of ventricular preexcitation, (b) determination of the mechanism of the patient's tachyarrhythmias and proof of the participation of the AP in the tachycardia circuit, (c) diagnosis of multiple accessory pathways and other possible coexistent arrhythmia mechanisms, (d) assessment of the risk for sudden cardiac death and the change in risk due to therapy, (e) testing of the efficacy of antiarrhythmic medications and other therapeutic modalities (e.g., antitachycardia pacing) and (f) anatomic localization of the APs when surgical or other ablative procedures are contemplated.

The complete diagnostic evaluation includes noninvasive clinical tests and in a selected group of patients, invasive EP studies. The strategy for the investigation is determined by the clinical presentation. Some patients have an asymptomatic WPW pattern on the ECG, while others may have infrequent, mildly symptomatic tachycardias, and still others may have frequent episodes of life-threatening, severely symptomatic arrhythmias and even sudden death. Noninvasive tests are therefore crucial in the selection of those patients, who may require further electrophysiologic studies or ablative therapy.

At present, aggressive investigation of asymptomatic patients with WPW pattern is not indicated. If EP testing is contemplated, risk stratification based on induced AF is suggested (34). The extent of diagnostic studies and treatment of symptomatic patients is generally dictated by the severity of symptoms.

History and Physical Examination

Based on the history, WPW patients may be classified as asymptomatic or symptomatic. Individuals with persistent ventricular preexcitation on their surface ECG, who had neither documented arrhythmias nor sustained symptomatic palpitations requiring medical attention are considered asymptomatic (35). They are thought to have a deficient reentrant circuit that cannot sustain AVRT and to lack atrial vulnerability. In these patients, it is difficult to induce AF. When induced, by rapid atrial pacing, AF is always self-terminating. Apart from the above features, no other EP differences were detected between asymptomatic and symptomatic patients.

One potential problem is that a relatively high incidence (17%) of rapidly conducting accessory pathways was reported in asymptomatic WPW pattern (SRR-PX $\leq$ 250 msec) (36). If these patients develop AF as a result of some concomitant medical problem, (e.g. thyrotoxicosis, congenital or ischemic heart disease, etc.) they may be at risk for developing VF and sudden death. The short-term prognosis of asymptomatic WPW is excellent, despite the presence of short SRR-PX in 17–23% of these patients. However, long-term prognosis is not known at present. In one natural history study of asymptomatic ventricular preexcitation, 9 of 29 patients followed for a mean of 54 months lost the delta wave, possibly due to fibrosis of the AP (36).

The indications for further diagnostic workup and invasive EP studies in asymptomatic patients are not clearly defined due to lack of long-term follow-up data. Since VF and sudden death may be the initial clinical manifestation of the WPW syndrome even in these individuals, assessment of the anterograde refractory period of the AP may be advisable in certain situations. Even so, the overall incidence of sudden death in WPW patients is low (approximately 1 in 1000 patient-yr of follow-up). In adults, an anterograde ERP of the AP $<$270 msec indicates that the AP is capable of conducting rapidly during AF (27). Noninvasive testing (see below) is capable of identifying the patients with short AP refractoriness (37). In symptomatic patients, further investigation is indicated. Patients in the high-risk category should have invasive EP assessment.

Physical examination is primarily useful to assess and to exclude accompanying cardiac or medical abnormalities. Certain congenital malformations are more common in patients with accessory AV connections. For example, an accessory pathway is present in approximately 10% of patients with Ebstein's anomaly. Mitral valve prolapse (MVP) is also a commonly associated abnormality with left-sided pathways (18). Particular attention should be paid to any disorder that may result in the development of AF, with a mechanism independent from ventricular preexcitation.

Electrocardiogram

A 12-lead surface ECG is an important diagnostic tool for the assessment of ventricular preexcitation. Characteristic delta wave is evidence of the presence of an AP conducting in the anterograde direction. The ECG also provides valuable information for localization of the AP.

Rosenbaum (38) introduced a descriptive classification of the WPW electrocardiographic pattern according to the QRS morphology in leads V_1 and V_2. Those with a predominantly positive QRS deflection in leads V_1 and V_2 were classified as type A WPW pattern, while those with a predominantly negative deflection in these leads were classified as type B pattern. This classification was developed before the present techniques of AP localization were introduced. It has subsequently been demonstrated that type A pattern is almost invariably found with left free-wall or posteroseptal accessory pathways. On the other hand, type B pattern is less specific, but it is most commonly associated with right-sided pathways (39).

Subsequently, it was recognized that the initial QRS vector, i.e., the vector of the delta wave, may be used to characterize the location of the APs. Delta waves may be positive, isoelectric, or negative in individual leads, depending on the main vector of ventricular activation via the AP. Negative delta waves may mimic pathologic Q waves associated with transmural myocardial infarction.

Gallagher, *et al*. proposed surface electrocardiographic delta wave vector analysis to help localize accessory pathways (18). Ten separate AP locations were distinguished, but there was considerable overlap between electrocardiographic features of adjacent locations. Sealy, *et al*. (39) proposed a simplified classification distinguishing four major locations which are important for planning ablative surgery: left and right ventricular free wall, and anterior or posterior septal regions. Based on this surgical classification and previously tabulated electrocardiographic criteria, Milstein, *et al*. (40) developed a simple algorithm to approximate the location of APs (Fig. 9.6). The AP can be localized to one of the four surgical locations with the help of four simple decisions based on surface electrocardiographic features. Using this method, APs were correctly localized in 90% of 141 WPW patients (40). However, there are some limitations that apply to all AP localization techniques based on the surface ECG. To be accurate, prominent preexcitation must be present. Body habitus, concomitant cardiac pathology, conduction disturbances, and the presence of multiple APs may produce overlapping electrocardiographic patterns.

The site of the AP does not predict its EP properties. However, particular locations may suggest the presence of multiple APs or associated cardiac pathology. It has been described, for example, that posteroseptal pathways may be associated with multiple APs, which are usually located in the right free wall (6,41). The association of right-sided accessory pathways with Ebstein's anomaly is also well recognized (6).

Ambulatory Electrocardiography

Ambulatory electrocardiographic recordings are useful in documenting recurrent arrhythmia episodes, and correlating these events with symptoms. Serial ECGs or continuous ambulatory electrocardiographic recordings may also be helpful in detecting sudden or unexpected loss of preexcitation.

Patients with intermittent ventricular preexcitation are thought to have "precarious" conduction over the AP and are considered to be at low risk for sudden death (42). The prevalence of intermittent preexcitation in the WPW population has been reported to occur in 25–76% of patients. Klein, *et al.* demonstrated intermittent preexcitation in 50% of 52 WPW patients by using ECG, 24-hr ambulatory ECG recordings, and exercise tolerance tests (42). The ECG alone diagnosed 27% of the patients. ECG and exercise tolerance test provided the diagnosis in 46% of the patients (42). These patients usually do not require further invasive investigations.

Acceleration of conduction in the normal conduction system may result in more subtle preexcitation and narrow QRS complexes. This "pseudonormalization" usually develops gradually, and is not accompanied by a prolongation of the PR (P-delta) interval. This may occur as a result of junctional or His bundle extrasystoles. Beats that originate in the sinus node may not manifest preexcitation if they are preceded by a ventricular extrasystole. This may not represent a true normalization of the QRS complex (i.e., anterograde block in the AP), but is rather a consequence of concealed retrograde conduction in the AP.

Exercise Testing

Acceleration of the heart rate during exercise may expose intermittent preexcitation. Again, disappearance of the delta wave is usually abrupt and accompanied by a PR prolongation to indicate a long anterograde ERP of the AP. Paroxysmal tachyarrhythmias are infrequently provoked by exercise. During exercise it is common to develop more subtle preexcitation, as conduction over the AV node-His bundle system accelerates more markedly than that over the AP. Recording of multiple

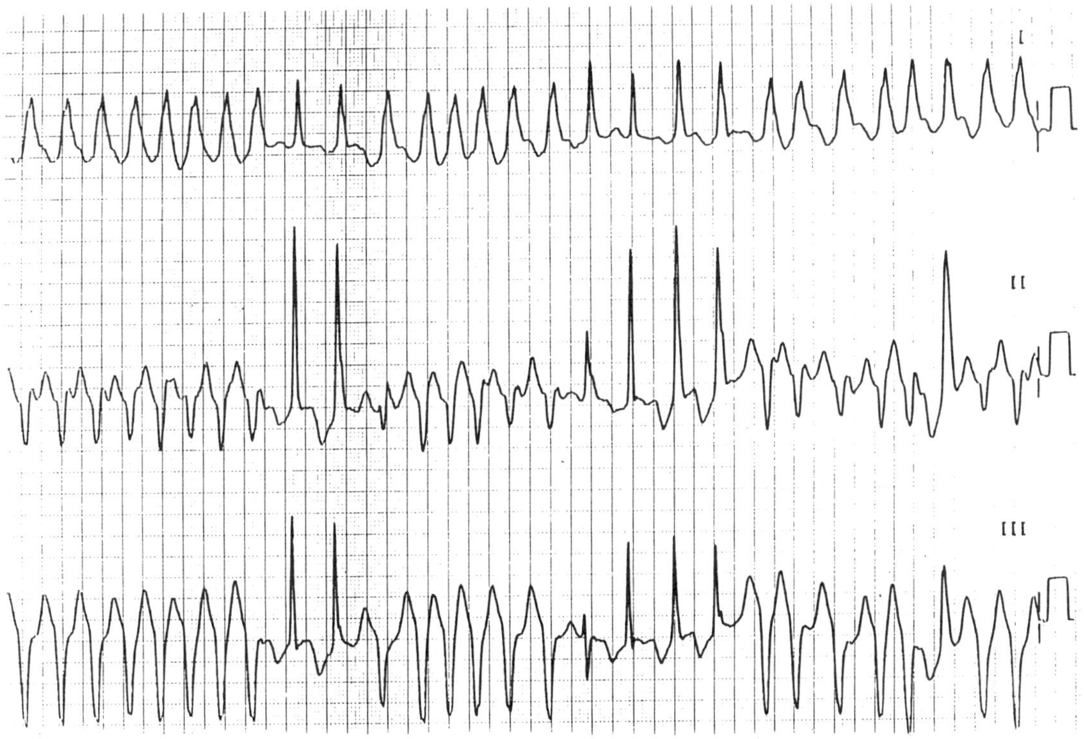

Figure 9.5. Rhythm strip (limb leads I, II, and III) of a patient with Wolff-Parkinson-White syndrome and atrial fibrillation. This patient has two accessory pathways. The striking difference in the frontal axis of the wide QRS complexes represents anterograde conduction over separate accessory pathways.

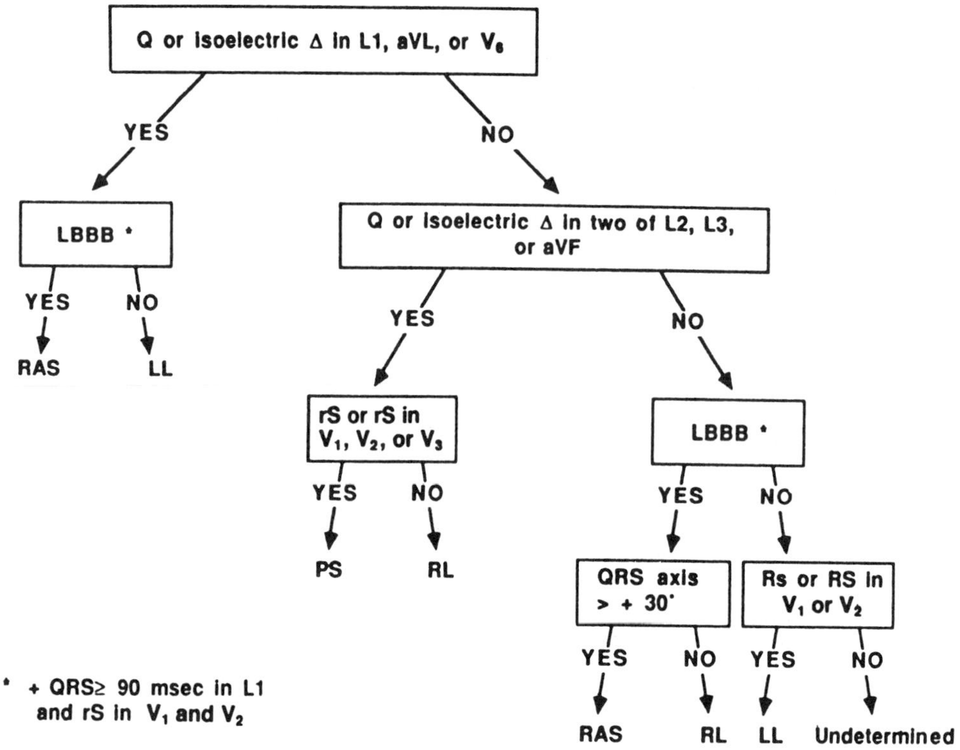

Figure 9.6. An algorithm designed by Milstein, *et al.* to help determine accessory pathway location based on the surface electrocardiogram. (Reproduced from Milstein S, Sharma AD, Guiraudon GM, Klein GJ: An algorithm for the electrocardiographic localization of accessory pathways in the Wolff-Parkinson-White syndrome. PACE 1987;10:555–563 with permission.)

surface leads facilitates the recognition of ventricular preexcitation.

Pharmacological Tests Used in the Noninvasive Diagnosis of the WPW Syndrome

Latent or subtle ventricular preexcitation may require additional techniques to demonstrate the presence and anterograde conduction of an AP. Vagal maneuvers or medications that slow impulse propagation in the normal conduction system, while leaving the AP conduction unaffected may unmask preexcitation (43). Verapamil and β-adrenergic blockers slow AV nodal conduction selectively when administered intravenously, separately or in combination. These medications are also useful for postoperative assessment following AP ablation (44). More recently, adenosine has been used for this purpose, administered as a rapid intravenous bolus (45). The advantage of adenosine is its very short half-life, limiting the occurrence of potential side effects to a period of less than 30–60 sec. The appearance of marked or maximal ventricular preexcitation with these agents is an evidence of the presence of an AP.

Other pharmacologic tests have been used in an attempt to estimate the anterograde effective refractory period of accessory pathways. Wellens, *et al.* demonstrated, that intravenous injection of class I antiarrhythmic agents, ajmaline or procainamide, produced complete anterograde block in APs with a long anterograde ERP (ERP > 270 ms) (46,47). Failure to lose preexcitation following these pharmacologic interventions classifies patients to a high-risk group for development of rapid ventricular rates during AF. Boahene, *et al.* (48) administered intravenous procainamide in incremental boluses. They found, that a relatively low dose of 550 mg procainamide provided the best sensitivity (60%) and specificity (89%) in identifying patients with an SRR-PX longer than 250 msec during AF (low-risk group). Specificity decreased with higher doses of the drug.

Esophageal Pacing

Esophageal pacing provides a convenient noninvasive technique for recording epicardial electrograms and for pacing (49). With rapid atrial pacing using esophageal techniques, latent or subtle ventricular preexcitation can be exposed. Rapid atrial pacing from the esophagus at cycle lengths between 100 and 200 msec can be used to induce and maintain AF. The average ventricular cycle length during AF and the shortest RR interval between two consecutive, preexcited QRS complexes should be recorded. As mentioned above, an SRR-PX 250 msec or shorter classifies a patient in the high-risk category for sudden death and warrants further, invasive testing. The sustained or nonsustained nature of the induced AF should also be noted. Atrial fibrillation is considered to be sustained if it lasts longer than 5 min.

Other Noninvasive Tests

Other tests may be useful in the assessment of patients with ventricular preexcitation. A two-dimensional echocardiogram or transesophageal echocardiogram may reveal concomitant structural heart disease, e.g., Ebstein's anomaly, MVP, etc. Wall motion abnormalities caused by the anomalous ventricular activation may also be noted. Vectorcardiogram, body surface map, and radionuclide ventriculography may all be useful for localization of APs, although the resolution of these techniques is insufficient at present to guide surgical ablation.

Conclusion

Based on the information provided by noninvasive methods, further decision to proceed to invasive EP studies may be made. Asymptomatic patients with a WPW electrocardiographic pattern, patients with intermittent ventricular preexcitation on serial ECGs, Holter monitor recordings of sudden normalization of a previously preexcited QRS pattern during an exercise tolerance test, or patients who have an AP with a long anterograde ERP demonstrated by loss of the delta wave after intravenous administration of Class I antiarrhythmic agents, do not require invasive EP studies.

All symptomatic patients should, at the minimum, have AF induced to measure the shortest RR interval between consecutive, preexcited beats for risk stratification. Those, who are markedly symptomatic with frequent or prolonged arrhythmia episodes, or who are capable of conducting at rapid rates during AF, need further EP testing.

Based on the American College of Cardiology/American Heart Association (ACC/AHA) Task Force Report guidelines (see Chapter 4 for further discussion) patients considered for non-pharmacologic treatment (e.g., AP interruption) because of incapacitating arrhythmias should undergo EP testing prior to the ablation procedure (Class 1 indication).

In patients with arrhythmias requiring treatment, in whom information about the type of arrhythmia, localization, number, and EP properties of one or more accessory AV pathways and the effect of antiarrhythmic drugs may influence the selection of the most appropriate treatment, EP study is indicated. Asymptomatic patients with electrocardiographic evidence of WPW syndrome in high-risk occupations (e.g., pilots, athletes) or patients with family history of premature sudden cardiac death may also benefit from an EP study to determine the risk of sudden death (see below). In patients who are undergoing other cardiac surgery and may benefit from a concurrent AP surgical ablation (preoperative EP study is also indicated) (Class 2).

Asymptomatic patients without arrhythmias who are determined to have low risk by noninvasive studies should not be subjected to an EP study.

ELECTROPHYSIOLOGIC STUDY

Since the development of catheter EP techniques, ventricular preexcitation has been one of the best-studied arrhythmic phenomena. Atrioventricular reciprocating tachycardias serve as a prototype of the reentry phenomenon. A general description of the EP study protocol for WPW syndrome is presented below (Table 9.2) (18,50–51).

Placement of at least four multipolar electrode catheters is required to study arrhythmias associated with ventricular preexcitation and to map APs. The techniques of catheterization and positioning of intracardiac electrode catheters are described in Chapter 4.

The catheters are positioned as follows: (a) lateral high right atrial wall, (b) right ventricular apex, (c) His bundle region, and (d) coronary sinus. The coronary sinus catheter is usually quadripolar, with 10 mm separation between the electrodes. It is introduced through the left subclavian, brachial, or internal jugular veins, to facilitate its positioning within the coronary sinus. The position of the coronary sinus catheter should be noted carefully, since the distance of each recording site from the orifice is important for accurate mapping. Other catheters are usually introduced through the right femoral vein. Quadropolar catheters are generally used, with the distal pair of electrodes used for pacing and the proximal pair for recording. Both unipolar and bipolar electrograms are recorded from the coronary sinus. Bipolar electrograms recorded from the right ventricle, right atrium, and His bundle region are filtered at 30–500 Hz. The unipolar electrograms obtained from each electrode of the quadripolar coronary sinus catheter are filtered at 0.05–40 Hz. Multiple surface electrocardiographic leads are also recorded along with the intracardiac electrograms. A typical recording setup would display the surface ECG leads 1, 2, 3, V_1 and V_5, and electrograms from the right ventricular apex, high right atrium, His bundle region, and multiple sites from the coronary sinus.

New catheters have been introduced to facilitate catheter placement in the coronary sinus (22). Jackman developed an orthogonal electrode system that facilitates mapping by direct recording of AP potentials (53). The Jackman orthogonal catheter has three sets of four electrodes arranged at 90° around the perimeter of the catheter. Low-gain bipolar recording between adjacent electrodes of the same set enhances the recording of an AP potential (54,55).

Minimal study protocol includes incremental atrial and ven-

Table 9.2.
Information That Can Be Obtained by Invasive Electrophysiologic Testing

- Evidence of the presence of an accessory atrioventricular connection
- Electrophysiologic properties of normal and accessory conduction pathways
- Identification of the mechanism of the clinical tachycardias, demonstration of accessory pathway participation in the arrhythmias
- Induction of atrial fibrillation, assessment of atrial vulnerability
- Diagnosis of multiple accessory pathways
- Detection of any other coexistent arrhythmia mechanism (e.g., AV nodal reentry)
- Anatomic localization of the accessory pathway(s)
- Effects of pharmacologic agents

tricular pacing and extrastimulus testing from the high right atrium and right ventricle at multiple drive cycle lengths (usually 600, 500, and 400 msec). Stimulation is usually performed from the ventricle first, to avoid inadvertent induction of AF early in the study. Pacing and extrastimulus testing from the coronary sinus may also be helpful. Other stimulation techniques (e.g., multiple premature stimuli, etc.) and autonomic maneuvers (administration of atropine or isoporterenol) may be needed for the induction of the clinical arrhythmias.

Atrial fibrillation should electively be induced by rapid atrial pacing at the end of the study, if AF was not observed during the study. Careful analysis of the cycle lengths during AF is crucial for the assessment of the conduction characteristics of the AP (see above). Recording previously undetected preexcited QRS morphologies during AF may be the only clue to indicate the presence of multiple APs (Fig. 9.5). A typical diagnostic EP study is described below in further detail.

Evidence for the Presence of an Accessory Atrioventricular Pathway

The following findings provide evidence for the presence of an accessory AV pathway conduction in the anterograde direction: (a) presence of delta waves on the surface ECG; (b) short HV interval, which becomes progressively shorter as the AV interval prolongs during increasingly rapid atrial stimulation or with increasing prematurity of atrial extrastimuli. With the prolongation of the AH interval the H deflection moves into the QRS complex, and the QRS becomes wider (more preexcited), while the interval from the stimulus to the delta wave remains unchanged; (c) normalization of the QRS complex with His bundle extrasystoles and during orthodromic AV RT.

Differential Atrial Pacing

During atrial pacing the stimulus to delta wave interval and the degree of ventricular preexcitation is dependent on the location of the AP relative to the site of impulse generation (56). The time from the stimulus to the onset of the delta wave represents the sum of the intra-atrial conduction time from the site of the pacemaker to the atrial insertion of the AP and the conduction time over the AP. This latter interval is usually stable and rate-independent. Accordingly, the closer the pacing site is to the atrial insertion of the AP, the shorter the stimulus to delta wave interval. This phenomenon can be used to localize accessory pathways and may also be used to expose latent or minimal preexcitation with left free-wall APs, or in the presence of multiple APs (Fig. 9.7). Pacing is usually performed at multiple cycle lengths and at multiple sites in the atria. The most useful positions for this purpose in the atria are the lateral right atrial wall, the proximal and distal coronary sinus (representing posteroseptal and left atrial sites, respectively). The 12-lead surface ECG is usually recorded during pacing, in addition to the intracardiac recordings.

Incremental Atrial and Ventricular Pacing

This particular pacing technique utilizes continuous pacing with gradually decreasing cycle lengths (increasing rates). During pacing, each cycle length is maintained for about 8–10 beats or longer, to allow time for the conduction system to adapt. Usually, pacing in the ventricle is terminated at 250 msec cycle length, to avoid the induction of ventricular tachycardia or VF. This pacing modality tests the EP properties of the AV conduction system. Anterograde conduction is tested with atrial pacing and retrograde conduction is tested with ventricular pacing. Both the normal conduction system and the accessory connections have characteristic conduction properties. Conduction over the AV node-His bundle system is rate-dependent. With increasing pacing rates progressive conduction delay develops in the AV node, manifested as a gradual and smooth prolongation of the AH interval in the His bundle electrogram. This conduction delay develops to a point where one-to-one conduction cannot be maintained any further and a physiologic second-degree AV block of the Wenckebach type develops. The shortest pacing cycle length still maintaining one-to-one conduction is a characteristic feature of any conduction system. In contrast, the AP conducts in a rate-independent manner. This is manifested as a constant AV interval relative to pacing with decreasing pacing cycle lengths. The anterograde and retrograde conduction properties may differ, even in the case of the same conduction pathway.

Infrequently, conduction over an AP may be rate-dependent, resembling AV nodal conduction (57,58). In this case, the only clue indicating that conduction is over an anomalous pathway may be the retrograde activation sequence.

Murdock, *et al.* reported that about 7.6% of accessory pathways will conduct in a rate-dependent manner (59). An AP has "decremental" conduction when there is rate-dependent conduction, i.e., prolongation of VA or atrial to delta wave intervals by more than 30 msec as measured in the electrograms nearest to the AP, or when type I second-degree AV block (Wenckebach block) can be demonstrated over the AP in the anterograde or retrograde direction (59).

Some AV nodes exhibit "enhanced conduction," that should be differentiated from rate-independent conduction over an AP. Enhanced AV nodal conduction is said to be present when: (a) AH interval in sinus rhythm is less then or equal to 60 msec, (b) one-to-one conduction between the atrium and His bundle is maintained during right atrial pacing at cycle lengths less than 300 msec, and (c) an interval prolongation is less than or equal to 100 msec at the shortest cycle length associated with one-to-one conduction compared to the value measured during sinus rhythm. When there is uncertainty about the substrate of conduction, e.g., following ablation of an AP, incremental pacing may have to be complemented with pharmacologic testing (verapamil, propranolol, adenosine). Enhanced AV nodal conduction is slowed by these medications, while AP conduction is not.

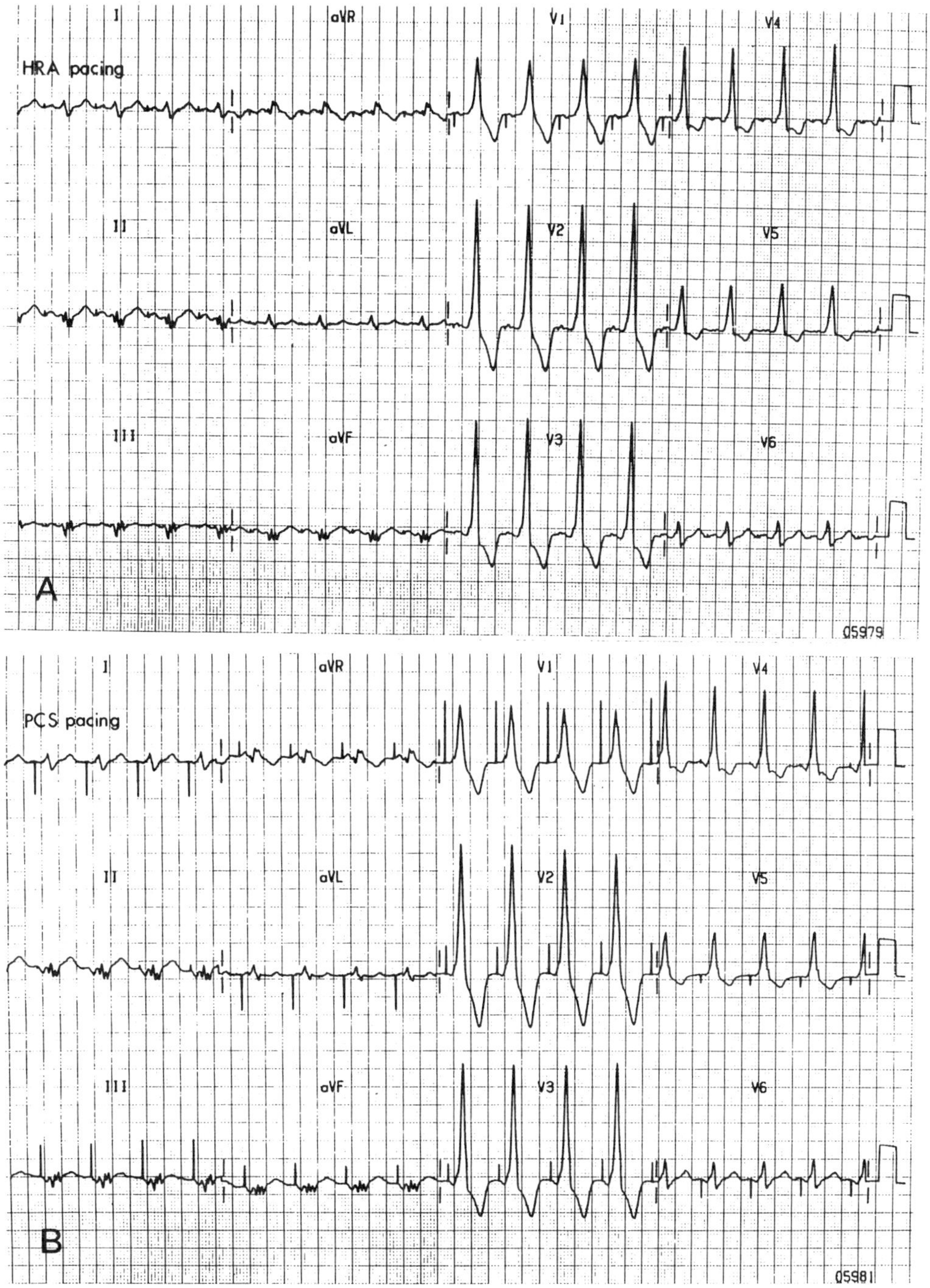

Figure 9.7. Differential atrial pacing in the presence of a left posteroateral accessory atrioventricular pathway. The stimulus to delta wave interval is 160 msec with high right atrial pacing (HRA) pacing **(A)**, while it is only 80 msec with proximal coronary sinus pacing (PCS) **(B)**. This indicates that the accessory pathway is close to the coronary sinus pacing site.

During EP studies the retrograde atrial activation pattern also helps identify the conducting pathway.

Atrioventricular reciprocating tachycardias or AF may also be induced by rapid atrial pacing. Atrial fibrillation may be induced inadvertently at relatively long pacing cycle lengths, or else it has to be induced purposefully. Short atrial pacing cycle lengths between 100 and 200 msec are used to induce and maintain AF. Rapid pacing can be maintained for about 1 min. Should AF not be sustained after discontinuation of pacing, ventricular rates can still be measured during AF maintained by rapid atrial pacing. Atrial capture has to be constantly monitored during incremental atrial pacing.

Atrial and Ventricular Extrastimulus Testing

Extrastimulus testing is performed during pacing and during sinus rhythm. Usually, a short train of paced beats is delivered at a constant pacing cycle length (S_1–S_1), followed by a single premature stimulus with a gradually decreasing coupling interval (S_1–S_2) scanning the electrical diastole up to the point of refractoriness. The refractoriness of the conduction tissue is dependent on the length of the preceding cycles. The short train of paced beats (generally eight beats) is used to avoid possible variation in these parameters and to facilitate the reproducibility of measurements. Extrastimulus testing is usually performed at multiple drive cycle lengths (usually 600, 500, and 400 msec).

Extrastimulus testing is performed: (a) to determine the electrical refractoriness of various segments of the conduction system and working myocardium, (b) to describe the EP properties of the conduction system(s), and (c) to reproduce the patient's clinical arrhythmias. Electrophysiologic properties of the conduction system can be visualized by plotting the intervals measured distal to a segment of the conduction system ("output"), as a function of the intervals measured proximal to the same conduction system segment ("input") (Fig. 9.8). The intervals should be measured at the closest possible sites to the studied segment of the conduction system. For example, if the AV node is to be studied, the H_1–H_2 intervals ("output" of the AV node) are plotted against the A_1–A_2 coupling intervals measured on the His bundle electrogram that represents low right atrial-septal recording ("input" of the AV node). The resulting AV nodal functional curve, relating H_1–H_2 to A_1–A_2, is characteristic of the AV node, displaying conduction delay in the AV node. In the case of APs the use of different recording sites is logical. The resultant functional curve will be different (Fig. 9A and B), as the AP does not usually exhibit conduction delay. Similar measurements can be obtained during retrograde conduction over the conduction systems.

Since the normal and accessory conduction systems differ with respect to their EP properties, their conduction features can be manipulated independently with pacing. When block is achieved with a critically timed extrastimulus (ERP) in one conduction system, while the other is still conducting with some conduction delay, the basic requirements for a reentry circuit are fulfilled. During atrial stimulation, if block in the AP is reached earlier than block in the AV node-His bundle system, the QRS complex "normalizes" when anterograde block develops in the AP. At that point significant conduction delay is usually present in the AV node, allowing the AP to recover and be available for retrograde conduction. This is the manner in which orthodromic AVRT is initiated from the atrium. More commonly, however, AV nodal refractoriness is reached earlier. This event is not visible, as QRS complexes remain maximally preexcited, masking any conduction or block in the AV node. The stimulus conducted anterogradely through the AP may return to the atrium over the His bundle-AV node giving a rise to an antidromic reentrant circuit. Antidromic tachycardias rarely sustain. Usually only a few echo beats are seen. The way induced or spontaneous reentrant arrhythmias terminate provides important information about the "weak link" in the tachycardia circuit.

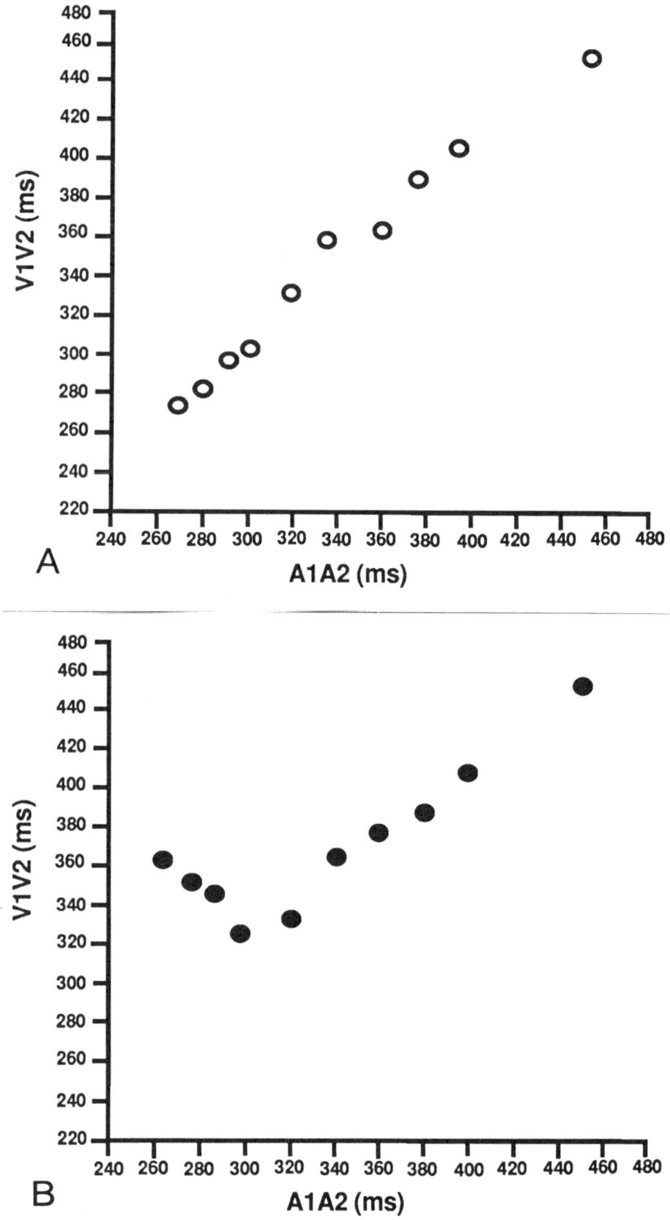

Figure 9.8. Conduction curves of an accessory AV pathway **(A)**, and the AV node **(B)** as determined by atrial extrastimulus testing. The AV node shows conduction delay with shorter coupling intervals, while conduction over the accessory pathway is rate-independent, and ventricular intervals vary directly with atrial intervals (see text). A_1A_2 = paced intraatrial interval; V_1V_2 = recorded intraventricular intervals.

Pacing from the ventricle results in appearance of AV block, usually in the AV node. Retrograde conduction then takes place exclusively over the AP followed by anterograde conduction over the normal conduction system resulting in an orthodromic AVRT. This is the most common way of initiating an orthodromic AVRT. Antidromic AV reentry can also be induced from the ventricle. Block in the AP, which is generally the conduction system that conducts more rapidly, is seen in the functional curves as an abrupt prolongation of the measured intervals coinciding with the induction of tachycardia. If reentry tachycardias cannot be induced with single premature stimuli, different techniques using multiple extrastimuli or autonomic drugs (atropine, isoproterenol) may still be successful.

Techniques Used for Localization of Accessory Pathways

Electrophysiologic investigations provide information regarding the location of accessory AV connections. The procedure used to obtain this information is called "mapping." During catheter mapping in the WPW syndrome, local myocardial activation times are measured at multiple endocardial sites, close to the AV groove. Mapping is done on the ventricular side during sinus rhythm, atrial pacing, or antidromic RT, to locate the ventricular insertion site of the AP. Atrial activation is mapped during ventricular pacing, but preferably, during orthodromic AVRT. Mapping should be performed, when conduction is over a known single pathway. This condition is met during orthodromic AVRT, when retrograde conduction, and consequently retrograde atrial activation occurs exclusively through the AP. The same is true during antidromic AVRT, when ventricular activation is exclusively the result of anterograde conduction over the AP. In these situations the site of the earliest atrial or ventricular activation (representing the shortest local VA or AV conduction interval) is closest to the atrial or ventricular insertion of the AP. During sinus rhythm, atrial pacing, and ventricular pacing, the impulse spreads through both the normal and the accessory conduction systems. The resulting activation therefore represents fusion between different activation fronts, making it more difficult to localize the AP. Rapid pacing and drugs that only affect the AV node (verapamil, propranolol, adenosine) may promote conduction over the AP, thus improving the accuracy of mapping.

Ventricular activation mapping during sinus rhythm may be particularly useful when the AP conducts only in the anterograde direction. Ventricular activation mapping should be done during maximal preexcitation. A steerable catheter design facilitates coronary sinus mapping. Mapping from the ventricular side of the tricuspid valve is more complicated, as not all sites are readily accessible for the presently available mapping catheters. Standard catheter positions reproducibly attainable in the right ventricle are the right ventricular apex and the outflow tract. The ventricular deflection of the His bundle electrogram also originates in the right ventricle.

Mapping of retrograde atrial activation, during ventricular pacing, has similar limitations to ventricular mapping during normal sinus rhythm. Pacing in the vicinity of the ventricular insertion of the AP, pacing at a cycle length favoring AP conduction (rapid pacing), and pharmacologic procedures affecting the AV node selectively may all facilitate mapping in this situation.

Atrial mapping during orthodromic AVRT still remains one of the most important techniques of AP localization (Fig. 9.9). The atrial endocardium close to the AV groove is readily accessible to transvenous electrode catheters to determine the site of the atrial insertion of accessory AV pathways. Mapping around the mitral annulus is possible with a catheter positioned in the coronary sinus. This represents locations in the left ventricular free wall and in the posteroseptal region. The coronary sinus is located in the epicardial fat pad filling the AV groove around the posterior and left lateral aspect of the mitral annulus. Close to the AV ring both atrial and ventricular electrograms are easily discernible. Electrode catheters, usually quadripolar or multipolar, with 1 cm interelectrode spacing are used for coronary sinus mapping. The orifice of the coronary sinus is relatively easy to negotiate with a catheter inserted from the left subclavian or brachial vein. An appropriate curve of the catheter tip or a deflectable catheter tip greatly facilitates catheter placement. On the AP fluoroscopic projection the orifice is located approximately in the middle of the spine (Fig. 9.10). The catheter is first positioned in the most distal position and is later sequentially

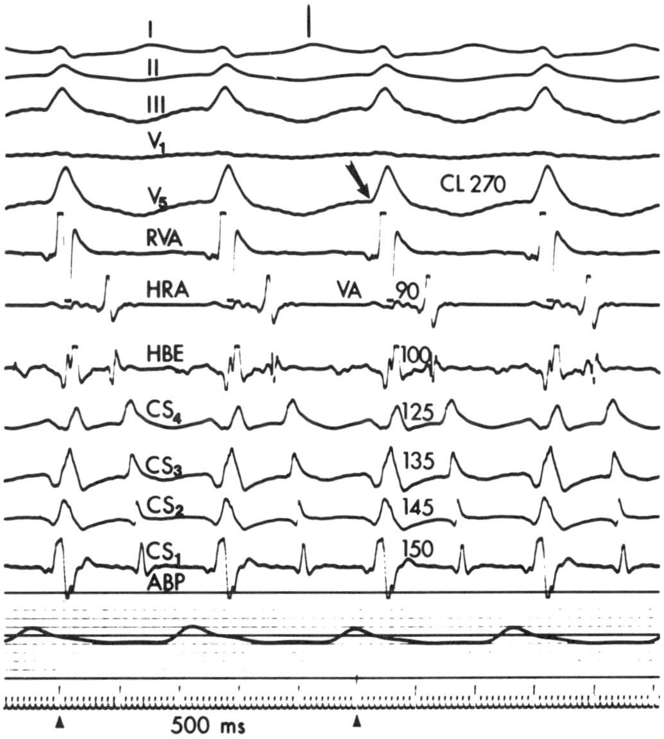

Figure 9.9. "Eccentric" retrograde atrial activation pattern during orthodromic AV reciprocating tachycardia which utilizes the right-sided accessory pathway as the retrograde limb of the reentry circuit. The earliest activation was recorded on the right atrial electrogram. I, II, III, V1, V5 -surface ECG leads; intracardial electrograms: ABP = systemic arterial blood pressure; CS = coronary sinus, #4: most proximal, #1 = most distal; HBE = His bundle electrogram; HRA = high lateral right atrium; RVA = right ventricular apex; VA = local ventriculoatrial activation time; arrow = earliest ventricular activation time on the surface ECG (point of reference for VA measurement).

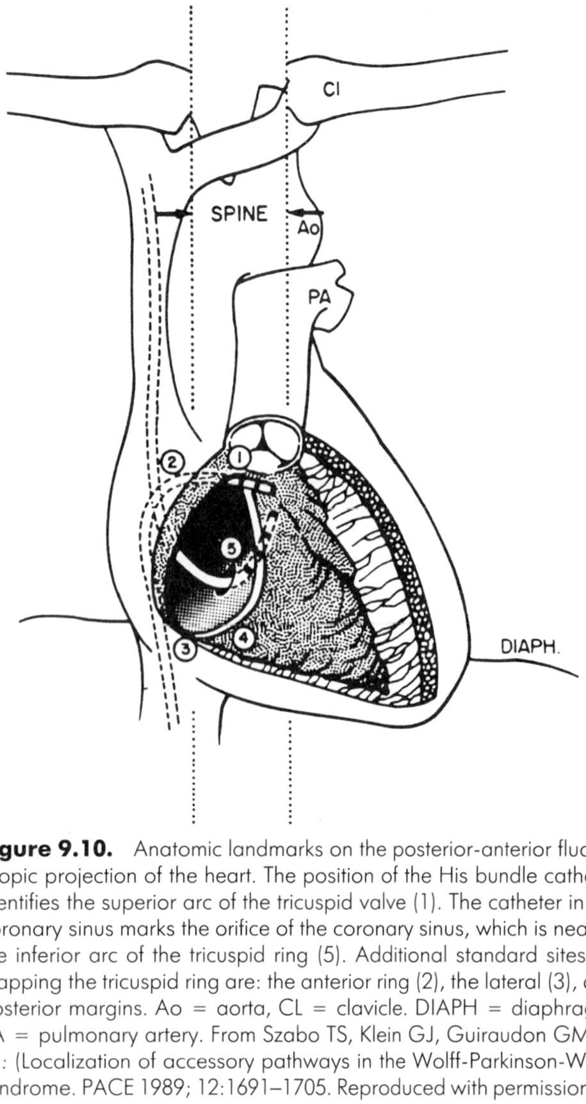

Figure 9.10. Anatomic landmarks on the posterior-anterior fluoroscopic projection of the heart. The position of the His bundle catheter identifies the superior arc of the tricuspid valve (1). The catheter in the coronary sinus marks the orifice of the coronary sinus, which is near to the inferior arc of the tricuspid ring (5). Additional standard sites for mapping the tricuspid ring are: the anterior ring (2), the lateral (3), and posterior margins. Ao = aorta, CL = clavicle. DIAPH = diaphragm. PA = pulmonary artery. From Szabo TS, Klein GJ, Guiraudon GM, *et al.*: (Localization of accessory pathways in the Wolff-Parkinson-White syndrome. PACE 1989; 12:1691–1705. Reproduced with permission).

withdrawn to the orifice. Recordings at each position are taken at high recording speed (250 mm/sec). To provide accurate anatomic information during catheter "pullback" the position of the catheter has to be adequately recorded. Usually the distal electrode is moved to the previous position of a proximal electrode, resulting in some overlap of electrode positions. It may be difficult to maneuver a standard electrode catheter around the lateral margin of the heart, in the great cardiac vein. This is greatly facilitated by a steerable catheter with a deflectable tip, designed by Gallagher for this purpose (52). The point of reference for the measurement of the VA conduction time is the earliest ventricular activation on the surface ECG (Fig. 9.9).

The use of the Jackman orthogonal catheter provided new insight in the conduction characteristics of the accessory pathways (53,54). Conventional catheters with narrow interelectrode spacing (1.5–2.0 mm) may also facilitate the recording of AP potentials. Direct catheter recording of AP potentials may improve the resolution of mapping. This is particularly important if radiofrequency ablation of the AP is contemplated. For routine preoperative mapping, determination of the earliest site of retrograde atrial activation with "conventional" techniques provides adequate localization.

Mapping of the right side of the heart, around the tricuspid ring, is technically more difficult. The right-sided mapping technique was described by Gallagher, *et al.* (60). Mapping is performed using an electrode catheter that has a central lumen. A semirigid preformed stylet can be introduced in the catheter lumen to facilitate catheter positioning. The shape of the stylet is similar to that of the Brockenbrough transseptal catheter. This stylet provides the necessary torque control. The direction of the catheter tip can be monitored by the help of an arrow-shaped directional indicator located at the proximal end of the stylet. Precise localization of the mapping electrode pair at the tip of the catheter is possible with the help of fluoroscopy and the directional indicator.

Right-sided mapping requires an understanding of the localization of the tricuspid valve and its fluoroscopic projection. The tricuspid ring is a circular structure fitting a plane that is oriented anteriorly and medially. This circle is projected in the anteriopposterior fluoroscopic view as an ellipsoid, with a long axis oriented vertically (Fig. 9.10). The projection of the tricuspid valve is superimposed on the right side of the spine. Key landmarks identify certain aspects of the tricuspid ring. The tip of the catheter recording the His bundle electrogram is at the superior-medial margin of the tricuspid annulus ("1 o'clock"). The other landmark is the coronary sinus catheter, the position of which identifies the site of the coronary sinus orifice. The orifice is located in the middle region of the spine, and indicates the inferomedial aspect of the tricuspid ring ("5 o'clock"). Using these landmarks, the mapping catheter can be moved around the rim of the tricuspid annulus. The left anterior oblique projection may further facilitate catheter positioning, as the tricuspid valve projects en face in this plane (Fig. 9.11). The appearance of the electrogram also helps catheter positioning. In the vicinity of the AV ring, both atrial and ventricular deflections should be recorded. If only atrial deflections are recorded, the electrode is most likely further away from the AV ring. The main directions used for recording are anterior, anteromedial, and anterolateral. Posterior and lateral electrode orientation represent mapping sites located away from the AV ring (61,62).

Other Findings that Help Accessory Pathway Localization

The development of a functional bundle branch block during orthodromic AVRT, usually at the onset of the tachycardia, is not uncommon. This finding has a localizing value when the AP is localized to the left or the right ventricular free wall. With the development of block in the bundle branch ipsilateral with a free-wall AP, the reentry circuit is lengthened and the tachycardia cycle length is prolonged (Fig. 9.12). In the case of free-wall

APs, this VA interval prolongation was found to be 25 msec or more, while in the case of septal or contralateral accessory pathways it never exceeded 20 msec (63–65). It is important to measure the AH and HV intervals, as well. Although AV conduction time does not change usually, changes in the AH and HV intervals may lead to cycle length prolongation. This phenomenon can also be observed in the presence of concealed APs.

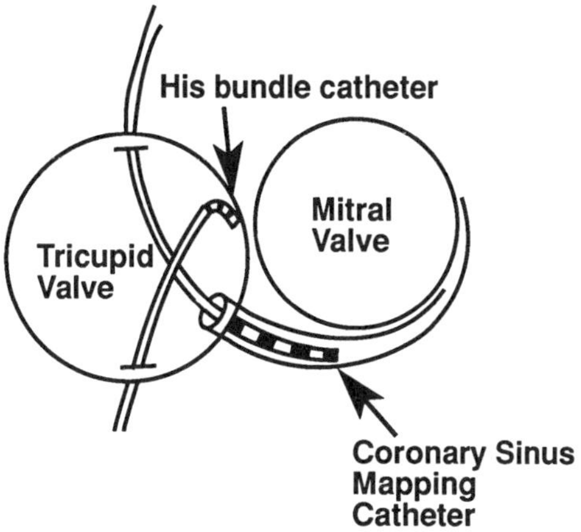

Figure 9.11. Diagram of the mitral and tricuspid valve regions as shown in the left anterior oblique projection on fluoroscopy. The coronary sinus-great cardiac vein, which are major mapping landmarks, are shown around the posterior and lateral aspect of the mitral valve. Mitral = mitral annulus. Tricuspid = tricuspid annulus. (After Jackman *et al.*, PACE, 1989;12:204–214, with permission from the author and the publisher.)

Preexcitation of the atrium by ventricular extrastimuli delivered during RT at a time when the His bundle is refractory indicates that the AP participates in the reentrant circuit as a retrograde limb (Fig. 9.13) (66). A "preexcitation index" can be calculated by subtracting the longest ventricular coupling interval that results in atrial preexcitation from the baseline tachycardia cycle length ($PI = [V_1–V_1] - [V_1–V_2]$). It was found that atrial preexcitation was achieved at longer coupling intervals (relatively late extrastimuli) when the pacing site was located closer to the reentrant circuit. This is indeed the case when right ventricular extrastimulation results in atrial preexcitation at significantly longer coupling intervals in case of reentrant circuits utilizing a right free-wall AP, as compared to circuits utilizing a left ventricular free-wall AP. The preexcitation index was found to be useful in distinguishing left free-wall accessory pathways that were always associated with a preexcitation index > 50 msec, from septal and right-sided accessory pathways which were associated with an index < 45 msec. Tachycardias due to AV nodal reentry could either not be preexcited at all or when atrial preexcitation was achieved, the preexcitation index was long, indicating that a short ventricular coupling interval was required for atrial preexcitation. This finding can be helpful in distinguishing between AV nodal reentry and a posteroseptal AP (67).

VARIANTS OF THE PREEXCITATION SYNDROMES

A variety of anatomic structures have been described and theoretically related to various types of preexcitation. In the majority

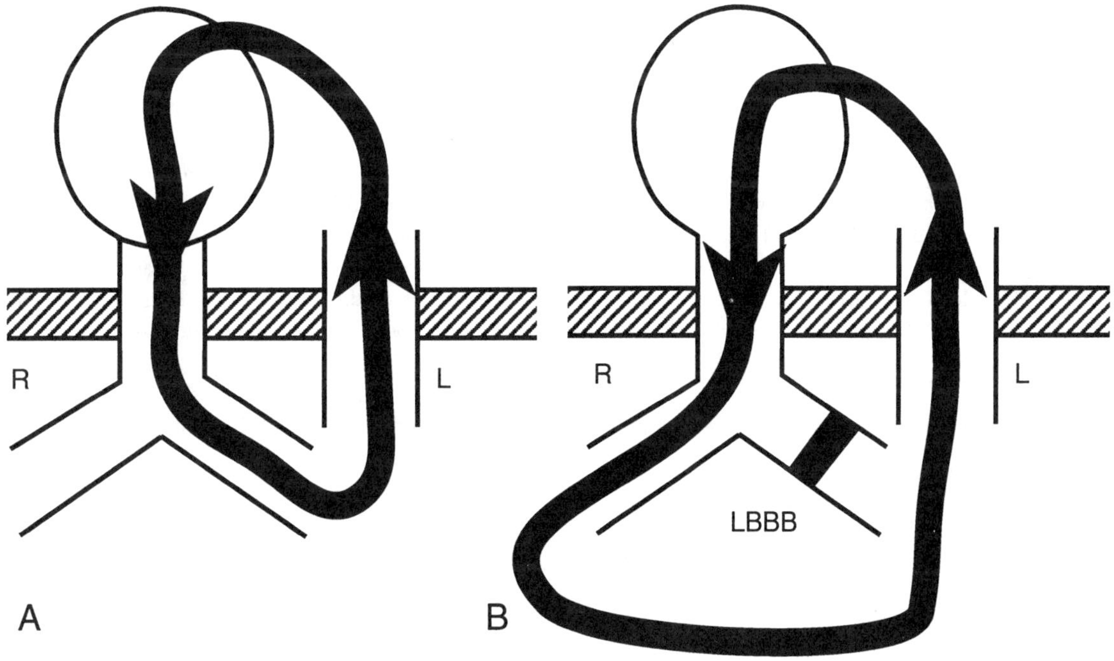

Figure 9.12. Functional bundle branch block in the ipsilateral bundle branch during orthodromic AV reciprocating tachycardia will result in prolongation of the tachycardia cycle length due to a longer ventriculo-atrial conduction time in the presence of a free-wall accessory pathway. **A,** Diagram of the tachycardia circuit with orthodromic AV reentry. **B,** Diagram of the lengthened tachycardia circuit, due to left bundle branch block, in the presence of a left free-wall accessory pathway. L = left, LBBB = left bundle branch block; R = right.

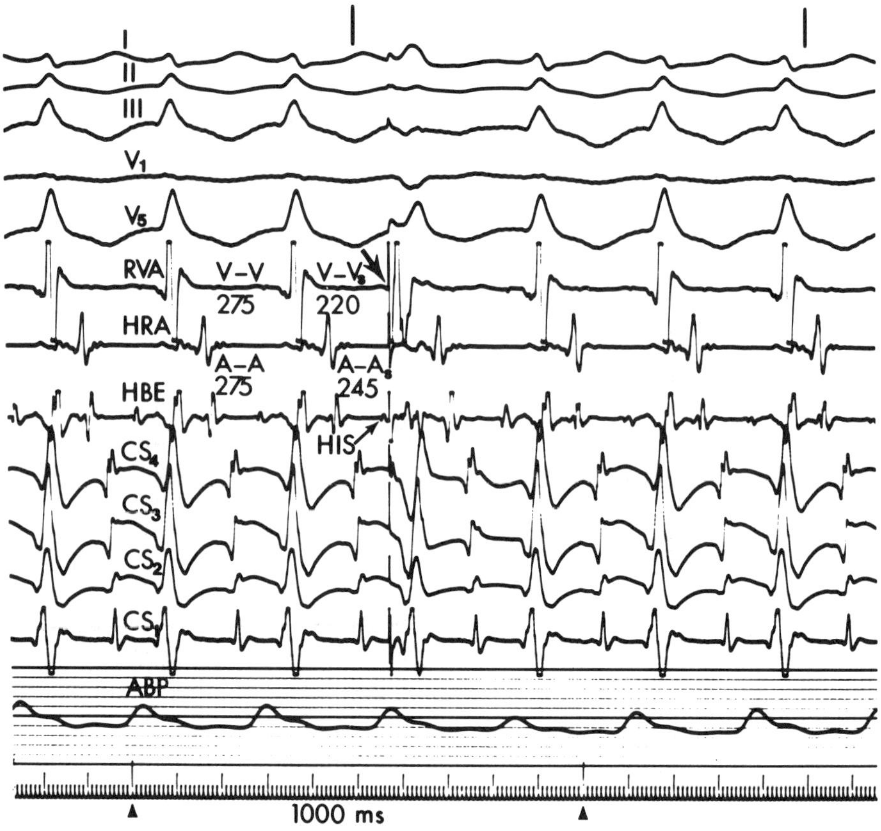

Figure 9.13. Preexcitation of the atrium by a ventricular extrastimulus delivered during orthodromic AV reciprocating tachycardia, at a time when the His bundle was refractory. This finding indicates that an accessory pathway participates as the retrograde limb of the tachycardia circuit. Lead arrangement is identical to Figure 9.9. A-A = atrial cycle length during the tachycardia; A-As = coupling interval of the atrial activation conducted from the premature ventricular stimulus; His = H deflection on the His bundle electrogram; V-V = ventricular cycle length during the tachycardia; V-Vs = coupling interval of the premature ventricular stimulus.

of these structures the functional role of the anatomic substrate has never been proven.

Preexcitation based on the so-called Mahaim tracts is a fascinating variant of the preexcitation syndromes. The tract, as it was described, was proposed to connect the specialized conduction system, either the AV node (nodoventricular fibers) or the His bundle (fasciculoventricular fibers) with the ventricular myocardium (18,68,69). The resultant electrocardiographic picture is characteristic (70). The RP interval and the QRS morphology can be normal during sinus rhythm but when AV nodal conduction delay develops, the QRS complexes will gradually show increasing preexcitation with a characteristic left bundle branch block–like QRS morphology. Wide QRS tachycardias can develop as part of this syndrome (68). Occasionally, AV dissociation is observed during these tachycardias. The underlying abnormality of this syndrome may not be uniform. Few cases of proven Mahaim pathways have been reported. In many cases, a right-sided AP with AV node–like properties was identified as the underlying disorder. This latter mechanism was confirmed by several successful surgical ablations (71).

Another relatively common variant of the preexcitation syndromes has the somewhat confusing name of the permanent form of junctional reciprocating tachycardia (PJRT). This arrhythmia was described by Coumel, and its mechanism was only elucidated later (72). The arrhythmia usually affects children, is usually incessant, i.e., present most of the time (69). If present for a sufficiently long time, it may result in the impairment of myocardial function and eventually may lead to a dilated cardiomyopathy.

The ECG in this syndrome shows a narrow QRS tachycardia with an abnormal "retrograde" P wave, with a PR interval shorter than the RP interval. The initiation of tachycardia does not require premature beats. At times it starts at a critical sinus rate. The mechanism of this tachycardia is similar to that of an orthodromic AVRT. During PJRT an AP with AV node–like properties is utilized as the retrograde limb of the reentry circuit (73,74). The pathway is located to the posteroseptal area. The conduction delay characteristic of this pathway is thought to be the result of a peculiar anatomy: some of these pathways were described as long and tortuous fibers of anomalous conduction tissue (74).

PJRT is usually resistant to medical treatment. Surgical or catheter ablation may result in permanent cure, thus preventing myocardial impairment.

The syndrome of a short PR interval with a normal QRS morphology was described by Lown, Ganong, and Levine (75, 76). This syndrome appears to be the results of several different underlying mechanisms, including enhanced AV nodal conduction, and possibly partial AV nodal bypass tracts (75,76).

TREATMENT OF PATIENTS WITH PREEXCITATION SYNDROMES

The goal of treatment of patients with preexcitation syndromes is to terminate tachycardia episodes, and prevent the development

Table 9.3.
Schematic Approach to the Investigation and Treatment of Patients with the Wolff-Parkinson-White Syndrome

1. Asymptomatic patients
   a. No investigations/treatment
   b. Risk assessment (at patient's request)
      (1) Low risk: no treatment
      (2) High risk: prophylactic medications, ablation (?)

2. Symptomatic patients: risk assessment by noninvasive methods and induction of atrial fibrillation
   a. Infrequent, mild symptoms and low risk
      (1) No treatment
      (2) Vagal maneuvers/drugs only with arrhythmias
   b. Frequent, more severe symptoms and low risk
      (1) Invasive EPS
         (a) EPS-guided medical therapy
         (b) Ablation

3. High-risk patients
   a. EPS-guided medical therapy
   b. Ablation

Low risk = SRR-PX > 250 ms during AF; high risk = SRR-PX ≤ 250 ms during AF.
Abbreviations: EPS = Electrophysiologic study.

of arrhythmias. Successful arrhythmia prevention is also expected to eliminate the risk of sudden death in those who are considered to be at risk.

The first question regarding therapy is whether to treat at all (Table 9.3). At present, asymptomatic patients are generally neither investigated nor treated. However, these individuals should be informed about the nature of their condition and the possible outcome. Investigations may be performed at the patient's request. Medical prophylaxis with antiarrhythmic agents may be offered to those at the highest risk (SRR-PX < 250 msec). In special situations ablation of the AP may be considered (competitive athletes, airplane pilots, etc.) (34).

The need for therapy in symptomatic patients is determined by consideration of multiple factors: (a) type of tachycardia, (b) frequency of the episodes, (c) severity of the accompanying symptoms, and (d) age and myocardial function of the patients. A low-risk patient with infrequent, hemodynamically stable arrhythmias may not need any treatment. Some patients can be taught to use vagal maneuvers (Valsalva maneuver, carotid sinus massage, dive reflex) to terminate their tachycardias, others may benefit from taking oral medications intermittently, only when they have a tachycardia episode (e.g., verapamil 120 mg).

Patients with frequent, symptomatic tachycardias may be treated with antiarrhythmic medications. High-risk symptomatic patients or patients with hemodynamically unstable arrhythmias may be referred for surgical or catheter ablation. For arrhythmia termination and prevention, several treatment modalities are available. If a hemodynamically stable AVRT is present, vagal maneuvers may first be tried. If the arrhythmia is hemodynamically unstable, direct current (DC) cardioversion/defibrillation is the treatment of choice.

Medical Treatment

Antiarrhythmic medications are used both to terminate and prevent AVRT and AF. Medications that prolong refractoriness and slow the conduction of the AP (Class IA, IC, and III) are used in patients who have rapid ventricular rates (SRR-PX < 250 msec) and predominantly preexcited QRS complexes during AF (51, 77–79).

The most commonly used medications are class IA agents, e.g., procainamide, quinidine, and disopyramide. Class IC and III drugs affect both the AP and the AV node-His bundle system. Flecainide and encainide, although effective, should be used with caution because of the results of the Cardiac Arrhythmia Suppression Trial (CAST). They are mainly used if other medications have failed, and in absence of coronary artery disease.

Amiodarone is an effective drug for therapy of both AF and AVRT. However, its frequent and potentially serious side effects limit its use in this patient population.

Atrioventricular RT may be treated with the medications listed above or with drugs acting on the AV node-His bundle system only (verapamil, digoxin, adenosine). Medications slowing the AV node-His bundle conduction may result in predominant conduction over the AP if AF develops (an increase in the proportion of preexcited complexes). Thus, the risk of developing VF may increase. Verapamil should not be given to WPW patients with AF and predominantly preexcited QRS complexes (80). Digoxin can only be used in patients with a known and relatively long anterograde AP refractoriness (e.g., > 300 msec). Adenosine may become the drug of choice in termination of AVRT because of its short lasting effect (81). Beta blockers may be useful if enhanced sympathetic tone contributes to the development of the arrhythmias.

The effect of lidocaine on AP conduction is unpredictable, and its use is not recommended in ventricular preexcitation. All antiarrhythmic medications may cause serious side effects, including a proarrhythmic effect. Since the majority of patients with WPW syndrome are young, lifelong antiarrhythmic therapy may increase the risk of possible side effects (Table 9.4).

Table 9.4.
Medications Commonly Used in the Treatment of Wolff-Parkinson-White Syndrome

Hemodynamically stable atrial fibrillation
   Procainamide: IV: 10 mg/kg body weight, 50 mg/min

Hemodynamically stable reciprocating tachycardia
   Verapamil: IV: 5–10 mg, with ECG and blood pressure monitoring the same dose can be repeated once
   Adenosine: IV: 5 mg as a rapid bolus; if ineffective, 10 mg can be given
   Procainamide: IV: 10 mg/kg body weight, 50 mg/min

Prevention of arrhythmias
   Type IA: procainamide, quinidine, disopyramide
   Type IC: propafenone, flecainide, encainide
   Type III: amiodarone

In patients who present with sustained, hemodynamically stable AVRT vagal maneuvers should be tried first. The next step is the use of intravenous verapamil or adenosine. Adenosine may be safer in patients who have a potential to develop AF. Intravenous procainamide may also be used. In hemodynamically stable AF, intravenous procainamide or other Class IA medications might be tried first. The effectiveness of chronic drug treatment should be demonstrated with follow-up EP studies. Suppression of tachycardia induction and prolongation of SRR-PX beyond the high-risk range during AF should be documented. If these endpoints cannot be achieved with medications, alternative treatments should be considered.

Ablation of the Accessory Atrioventricular Pathways

Ventricular preexcitation is permanently cured by successful surgical or catheter ablation of accessory AV connections. These techniques eliminate the anatomic substrate of the tachyarrhythmias. Surgical and catheter procedures used for ablation of APs are discussed in detail in Chapters 22 and 24, respectively. These more invasive treatment modalities are considered for patients at high risk for sudden death and for patients who have frequent, symptomatic arrhythmias that do not respond to medical treatment. The indications used at different institutions vary considerably depending on the local experience with the available techniques. Surgical ablation was first performed in 1968 by Sealy (82). During the last decade, reported success rates were higher than 90%, with very low mortality and morbidity. However, surgical ablation requires open heart or open chest surgery. More recently, catheter ablation techniques have been developed. Direct current shocks were first used for AP ablation. A distinct potential for serious side effects limited the usefulness of this technique.

Intracardiac use of radiofrequency energy is currently thought to be a safe alternative. Success rates of over 90% have recently been reported from major U.S. and European centers. Complications are infrequent and usually minor. Radiofrequency catheter ablation may become the treatment of choice of ventricular preexcitation in the future.

Antitachycardia Pacing

Reentrant tachycardias can be terminated reliably with antitachycardia pacing (see Chapter 21). A major concern in WPW patients, however, is the inadvertent induction of AF during atrial antitachycardia pacing. Therefore, this modality may be used in only a few selected patients with concealed APs. Generally, antitachycardia pacing is not used as the first line therapy of ventricular preexcitation syndromes.

CONCLUSIONS

WPW syndrome presents a fascinating model of macro reentry in humans. Much has been learned in the past decade about this syndrome and a variety of therapeutic modalities have evolved. It is likely that further diagnostic and therapeutic advancements will evolve in the future.

References

1. Ohnell RF: Preexcitation, a cardiac abnormality. Acta Med Scand (Suppl) 1944;152:1–167.
2. Durrer D, Schuilenberg RM, Wellens HJJ: Preexciation revisited. Am J Cardiol 1970;25:690–697.
3. Gallagher JJ: Variants of preexciation: Update 1984, In Zipes DP, Jalife J (eds): Cardiac Electrophysiology and Arrhythmias. Grune and Stratton, Orlando, FL 1984:419–433.
4. Wolff L, Parkinson J, White PD: Bundle-branch block with short P-R interval in healthy young people prone to paroxysmal tachycardia. Am Heart J 1930;5:685–704.
5. Wellens HJJ, Atie J, Smeets JLRM, *et al.*: The electrocardiogram in patients with multiple accessory atrioventricular pathways. J Am Coll Cardiol 1990;16:745–751.
6. Colavita PG, Packer DL, Pressley JC, *et al.*: Frequency, diagnosis and clinical characteristics of patients with multiple accessory atrioventricular pathways. Am J Cardiol 1987;59:601–606.
7. Gallagher JJ, Sealy WC, Kasell J, *et al.*: Multiple accessory pathways in patients with the pre-excitation syndrome. Circulation 1976;54:571–591.
8. Anderson RH, Becker AE, Brechenmacher C, *et al.*: Ventricular preexcitation: a proposed nomenclature for its substrates. Eur J Cardiol 1975;3:27–36.
9. Wellens HJJ: Contribution of cardiac pacing to our understanding of the Wolff-Parkinson-White syndrome. Br Heart J 1975;37:231–241.
10. Ross TF, Mandel WJ: Invasive cardiac electrophysiologic testing, In Mandel WJ (ed): Cardiac Arrhythmias. Their Mechanism, Diagnosis and Management, 2nd ed. JB Lippincott, Philadelphia, 1987;101–142.
11. Teo WS, Klein GJ, Yee R, *et al.*: Significance of minimal preexcitation in Wolff-Parkinson-White syndrome. Am J Cardiol 1991;67:205–207.
12. Bardy GH, Packer DL, German LD, *et al.*: Preexcited reciprocating tachycardia in patients with Wolff-Parkinson-White syndrome: incidence and mechanisms. Circulation 1984;70:377–391.
13. Akhtar M, Shenasa M, Tchou PJ, *et al.*: Role of electrophysiologic studies in supraventricular tachycardia, In Brugada P, Wellens HJJ (ed): Cardiac Arrhythmias: Where to Go from Here? Futura Publishing Co., Mt. Kisco, NY, 1987:233–242.
14. Klein GJ, Bashore TM, Sellers TD, *et al.*: Ventricular fibrillation in the Wolff-Parkinson-White syndrome. N Engl J Med 1979;301:1080–1085.
15. Sharma AD, Klein GJ, Guiraudon GM, *et al.*: Atrial fibrillation in patients with Wolff-Parkinson-White syndrome: incidence after surgical ablation of the accessory pathway. Circulation 1985;72:161–169.
16. Fujimura O, Klein GJ, Sharma AD, *et al.*: The mode of onset of atrial fibrillation in the Wolff-Parkinson-White syndrome: how important is the accessory pathway? J Am Coll Cardiol 1990;15:1082–1086.
17. Campbell RWF, Smith RA, Gallagher JJ, *et al.*: Atrial fibrillation in the preexcitation syndrome. Am J Cardiol 1977;40:514–520.
18. Gallagher JJ, Pritchett ELC, Sealy WC, *et al.*: The preexcitation syndrome. Prog Cardiovasc Dis 1978;20:285–327.
19. Waspe LE, Brodman R, Kim SG, *et al.*: Susceptibility to atrial fibrillation and ventricular tachyarrhythmia in the Wolff-Parkinson-White syndrome: role of the accessory pathway. Am Heart J 1986;112:1141–1152.
20. Bauernfeind RA, Wyndham CR, Swiryn SP, *et al.*: Paroxysmal atrial fibrillation in the Wolff-Parkinson-White syndrome. Am J Cardiol 1981;47:562–568.
21. Sung RJ, Tai DY: Electrophysiologic characteristics of accessory connections: an overview. In Benditt DG, Benson DW (ed): Cardiac Preexcitation Syndromes. Martinus Nijhoff, The Hague, 1986:165–199.
22. Wellens HJJ, Durrer D: Wolff-Parkinson-White syndrome and atrial fibrillation. Relation between refractory period of accessory pathway and ventricular rate during atrial fibrillation. Am J Cardiol 1974;34:777–784.

23. Castellanos A, Myerburg RJ, Craparo K, *et al.*: Factors regulating ventricular rates during the atrial flutter and fibrillation in pre-excitation. (Wolff-Parkinson-White) syndrome. Br Heart J 1973;35:811–816.
24. Klein GJ, Yee R, Sharma AD: Concealed conduction in accessory atrioventricular pathways: an important determinant of the expression of arrhythmias in patients with Wolff-Parkinson-White syndrome. Circulation 1984;70:402–411.
25. Milstein S, Klein GJ, Rattes MF, *et al.*: Comparison of the ventricular response during atrial fibrillation in patients with enhanced atrioventricular node conduction and Wolff-Parkinson-White syndrome J Am Coll Cardiol 1987;10:1244–1248.
26. Fananapazir L, German LD, Gallagher JJ, *et al.*: Importance of preexcited QRS morphology during induced atrial fibrillation to the diagnosis and localization of multiple accessory pathways. Circulation 1990;81:578–585.
27. Wellens HJJ, Durrer D: Wolff-Parkinson-White syndrome and atrial fibrillation. Relation between refractory period of the accessory pathway and ventricular rate during atrial fibrillation. Am J Cardiol 1974;34:777–782.
28. Watt JH, Donner AP, McKinney CM, *et al.*: Atrial fibrillation: minimal sampling interval to estimate average rate. J Electrocardiol 1984;17:153–156.
29. Chung KY. Walsh TJ, Massie E: Wolff-Parkinson-White syndrome. Am Heart J 1965;69:1–8.
30. Bellet S: Clinical Disorders of the Heart Beat, 3rd ed., Lea & Febiger, Philadelphia, 1971.
31. Wellens HJJ, Penn OC, Gorgels APM, *et al.*: Diagnosis and treatment of patients with accessory pathways. Cardiol Clin 1990;8:503–521.
32. Yee R, Klein GJ: Syncope in the Wolff-Parkinson-White syndrome: incidence and electrophysiologic correlates. PACE 1984;7:381–388.
33. Auricchio A, Klein H, Trappe HJ, *et al.*: Lack of prognostic value of syncope in patients with Wolff-Parkinson-White syndrome. J Am Coll Cardiol 1991;17:152–158.
34. Klein GJ, Prystowsky EN, Yee R, *et al.*: Asymptomatic Wolff-Parkinson-White syndrome: should we intervene? Circulation 1989;80:1902–1905.
35. Milstein S, Sharma AD, Klein GJ: Electrophysiologic profile of asymptomatic Wolff-Parkinson-White pattern. Am J Cardiol 1986;57:1097–1100.
36. Klein GJ, Yee R, Sharma AD: Longitudinal electrophysiologic assessment of asymptomatic patients with the Wolff-Parkinson-White electrocardiographic pattern. N Engl J Med 1989;320:1229–1233.
37. Klein GJ, Sharma AD, Milstein S: Initial evaluation of patients with the Wolff-Parkinson-White syndrome. In Benditt DG, Benson DW (eds): Cardiac Preexcitation Syndromes. Martinus Nijhoff, Boston, 1986:305–319.
38. Rosenbaum FF, Hecht HH, Wilson FN, *et al.*: The potential variations of the thorax and esophagus in anomalous atrioventricular excitation (Wolff-Parkinson-White Syndrome). Am Heart J 1945;29:281.
39. Sealy WC, Hattler BG Jr, Blumenshein SD, *et al.*: Surgical treatment of Wolff-Parkinson-White syndrome. Ann Thorac Surg 1969;8:1–11.
40. Milstein S, Sharma AD, Guiraudon GM, *et al.*: An algorithm for the electrocardiographic localization of accessory pathways in the Wolff-Parkinson-White syndrome. PACE 1987;10:555–563.
41. Morady F, Scheinman MM, DiCarlo LA, *et al.*: Coexistent posteroseptal and right sided atrioventricular bypass tracts. J Am Coll Cardiol 1985;5:640–646.
42. Klein GJ, Gulamhusein SS: Intermittent preexcitation in the Wolff-Parkinson-White syndrome, Am J Cardiol 1983;52:292–296.
43. Przybylski J, Chiale P, Halper S, *et al.*: Unmasking of ventricular preexcitation by vagal stimulation or isoproterenol administration. Circulation 1980;61:1030–1037.
44. Milstein S, Dunnigan A, Beutikofer J, *et al.*: Usefulness of combined propranolol and verapamil for evaluation of surgical ablation of accessory atrioventricular connections in patients without structural heart disease. Am J Cardiol 1990;66:1216–1221.
45. Garratt CJ, Antoniu A, Griffith MJ, *et al.*: Use of intravenous adenosine in sinus rhythm as diagnostic test for latent preexcitation. Am J Cardiol 1990;65:868–873.
46. Wellens HJJ, Bar FW, Gorgels APM, *et al.*: Use of ajmaline in identifying patients with the Wolff-Parkinson-White syndrome and a short refractory period of their accessory pathway. Am J Cardiol 1980;45:130–133.
47. Wellens HJJ, Braat S, Brugada P, *et al.*: Use of procainamide in patients with the Wolff-Parkinson-White syndrome to disclose a short refractory period of the accessory pathway. Am J Cardiol 1982;50:1087–1089.
48. Boahene KA, Klein GJ, Sharma AD, *et al.*: Value of a revised procainamide test in the Wolff-Parkinson-White syndrome. Am J Cardiol 1990;65:195–200.
49. Critelli G, Grassi G, Perticone F, *et al.*: Transesophageal pacing for prognostic evaluation of preexcitation syndrome and assessment of protective therapy. Am J Cardiol 1983;51:513–518.
50. Waldo AL, Akhtar M, Benditt DG, *et al.*: Appropriate electrophysiologic study and treatment of patients with the Wolff-Parkinson-White syndrome. J Am Coll Cardiol 1988;11:1124–1129.
51. Prystowsky EN: Diagnosis and management of the preexcitation syndromes. Curr Prob Cardiol 1988;13:227–310.
52. Gallagher JJ: Facilitation of atrial mapping by a new "steerable" catheter electrode (Abstr). Circulation 1988;78:II-154.
53. Jackman W, Friday K, Bizouati G, *et al.*: New catheter system for recording accessory AV pathway potentials from the coronary sinus. J Am Coll Cardiol 1984;3:512.
54. Jackman W, Friday KJ, Yeung-Lai-Wah JA, *et al.*: New catheter technique for recording left free-wall accessory atrioventricular pathway activation. Identification of pathway fiber orientation. Circulation 1988;78:598–610.
55. Jackman WM, Kuck KH, Friday KJ, *et al.*: Catheter recordings of accessory atrioventricular pathway activation. In Zipes DP, Jalife J (eds): Cardiac electrophysiology. From Cell to Bedside. WB Saunders, Philadelphia, 1990:491–502.
56. Denes P, Wyndham CR, Amat-y-Leon F, *et al.*: Atrial pacing at multiple sites in the Wolff-Parkinson-White syndrome. Br Heart J 1977;39:506–514.
57. Klein GJ, Prystowsky EN, Pritchett ELC, *et al.*: Atypical patterns of retrograde conduction over accessory atrioventricular pathways in the Wolff-Parkinson-White syndrome. Circulation 1979;60:1477–1486.
58. Klein GJ, Hackel DB, Gallagher JJ: Anatomic substrate of impaired antegrade conduction over an accessory atrioventricular pathway in the Wolff-Parkinson-White syndrome. Circulation 1980;61:1249–1256.
59. Murdock CJ, Leitch JW, Teo WS, *et al.*: Characteristics of accessory pathways exhibiting decremental conduction. Am J Cardiol 1991;67:506–510.
60. Gallagher JJ, Pritchett ELC, Benditt DG, *et al.*: New catheter techniques for analysis of the sequence of retrograde atrial activation in man. Eur J Cardiol 1977;6(1):1–14.
61. Szabo TS, Klein GJ, Guiraudon GM, *et al.*: Localization of accessory pathways in the Wolff-Parkinson-White syndrome. PACE 1989;12:1691–1705.
62. Packer DL, Stanton MS, Hammill SC, *et al.*: Improved accuracy of right freewall accessory pathway localization using a modified catheter mapping technique (Abstr). Circulation 1990;82:III-318.
63. Pritchett ELC, Tonkin AM, Dugan FA, *et al.*: Ventriculo-atrial conduction time during reciprocating tachycardia with intermittent bundle-branch block in Wolff-Parkinson-White syndrome. Br Heart J 1976;38:1058–1064.
64. Broughton A, Gallagher JJ, German LD, *et al.*: Differentiation of septal from free wall accessory pathway location: observations during bundle branch block in reciprocating tachycardia in the presence of type I antiarrhythmic drugs. Am J Cardiol 1983;52:751–754.
65. Kerr CR, Gallagher JJ, German LD: Changes in ventriculoatrial intervals with bundle branch block aberration during reciprocating tachycardia in patients with accessory atrioventricular pathways. Circulation 1982;66:196–201.
66. Sellers TD, Gallagher JJ, Cope GD, *et al.*: Retrograde atrial preexcitation

following premature ventricular beats during retrograde reciprocating tachycardia in the Wolff-Parkinson-White syndrome. Eur J Cardiol 1976;4(3):283–294.
67. Miles WM, Yee R, Klein GJ, *et al.*: The preexcitation index: An aid in determining the mechanism of suprventracular tachycardia and localizing accessory pathways. Circulation 1986;74:493–500.
68. Gallagher JJ: Role of nodoventricular and fasciculoventricular connections in tachyarrhythmias. In Benditt DG, Benson DW (eds): Cardiac Preexcitation Syndromes. Martinus Nijhoff, Boston, 1986;201–213.
69. Gallagher JJ, Selle JG, *et al.*: Variants of pre-excitation: Update 1989. In Zipes DP, Jalife J (eds): Cardiac Electrophysiology: From Cell to Bedside. WB Saunders, Philadelphia, 1990;480–490.
70. Bardy GH, Fedor JM, German LD, *et al.*: Surface electrocardiographic clues suggesting presence of a nodofascicular Mahaim fiber. J Am Coll Cardiol 1984;3:1161–1168.
71. Klein GJ, Guiraudon GM, Kerr CR, *et al.*: "Nodoventricular" accessory pathway: evidence for a distinct accessory pathway with atrioventricular node-like properties. J Am Coll Cardiol 1988;11:1035–1040.
72. Coumel P, Cabrol C, Fabiato A, *et al.*: Tachycardie permanente par rhythm reciproque. Arch Mal Coeur 1967;60:1830–1840.
73. Gallagher JJ, Sealy WC: The permanent form of junctional reciprocating tachycardia: further elucidation of the underlying mechanism. Eur J Cardiol 1978;8:413–430.
74. Critelli G, Gallagher JJ, Monda V, *et al.*: Anatomic and electrophysiologic substrate of the permanent form of junctional reciprocating tachycardia. J Am Coll Cardiol 1984;4:601–610.
75. Gornick CC, Benson DW: Electrocardiographic aspects of the preexcitation syndromes. In Benditt DG, Benson DW (eds): Cardiac Preexcitation Syndromes. Martinus Nijhoff, Boston, 1986;43–73.
76. Castellanos A, Zaman L, Luceri RM, *et al.*: The wide spectrum of tachyarrhythmias occurring in patients with short PR intervals and narrow QRS complexes. In Levy S (ed): Cardiac Arrhythmias: From Diagnosis to Therapy. Futura Publishing, Mt. Kisco, NY, 1984:255–278.
77. Boahene KA, Klein GJ, Yee R, *et al.*: Termination of acute atrial fibrillation in the Wolff-Parkinson-White syndrome by procainamide and propafenone: importance of atrial fibrillatory cycle length. J Am Coll Cardiol 1990;16:1408–1414.
78. Kunze KP, Schluter M, Kuck KH: Sotalol in patients with Wolff-Parkinson-White syndrome. Circulation 1987;75:1050–1057.
79. Prystowsky EN: Antiarrhythmic drug therapy in patients with preexcitation syndromes. In: Benditt DG, Benson DW (eds): Cardiac Preexcitation Syndromes. Martinus Nijhoff, Boston, 1986:447–463.
80. Gulamhusein S, Ko P, Carruthers G, *et al.*: Acceleration of the ventricular response during atrial fibrillation in the Wolff-Parkinson-White syndrome after verapamil. Circulation 1982;65:348–354.
81. DiMarco JP, Sellers TD, Berne RM, *et al.*: Adenosine: electrophysiological effects and therapeutic use for terminating supraventricular tachycardia. Circulation 1983;68:1254–1263.
82. Cobb FR, Blumenschein SD, Sealy WC, *et al.*: Successful surgical interruption of the bundle of Kent in a patient with Wolff-Parkinson-White syndrome. Circulation 1968;38:1018–1029.

10

LONG QT SYNDROME

Joel Kupersmith, M.D., F.A.C.P., F.A.C.C.

BACKGROUND

The long QT syndrome (LQTS) has intrigued cardiologists for many years. It is a clinically interesting and dangerous syndrome that may in addition be a revealing natural experiment about fundamental electrophysiologic process.

In 1957, Jervell and Lange-Nielsen (1) described a family with a long QT interval, nerve deafness, and a high incidence of sudden death which they attributed to asystole. In the early 1960s Ward (2) and Romano (3,4) independently described a similar syndrome of familial prolonged QT intervals and sudden death without nerve deafness. Sudden death was now correctly attributed to ventricular arrhythmias.

Shortly thereafter Dessertenne (5) reported a case of an 80-yr-old female with complete heart block, a long QT interval, and a strange form of ventricular arrhythmia which he labeled torsade de pointes (TdP). In this arrhythmia, QRS complexes seemed to twist around a point, as if, he thought, there were two sites of origin of the ventricular pacemaker. It soon became apparent that this sort of arrhythmia was characteristic of LQTS.

In the 1960s and 1970s there was considerable interest in the relationship between QT interval and the autonomic nervous system and the thought arose that familial or congenital LQTS was in fact due to autonomic imbalance (6,11).

Also beginning in the 1970s, a toxic syndrome was described with many of the same electrocardiographic and other features as congenital LQTS. Causes included antiarrhythmic and other drugs, electrolyte imbalance, and starvation diets (12–18). While this syndrome had many similarities to congenital LQTS there were also important differences and the fit between two syndromes has not as yet been completely resolved.

QT INTERVAL

The QT interval reflects both ventricular depolarization and repolarization. All cardiac cells have action potentials with phases of depolarization and repolarization (Chapter 1). The QRS complex of the ECG represents depolarization. Specifically, it represents membrane potential differences between cells across the heart as the wave of ventricular depolarization spreads in a subendocardial (where the His-Purkinje system inserts) to epicardial direction.

The T wave of the electrocardiogram (ECG) reflects potential differences across the heart during ventricular repolarization. If all ventricular cells repolarized at the same time there would be no T wave. However, the cells repolarize at different times and do so in an apparent epicardial to endocardial direction (opposite to that of depolarization). This normally leads to generation of a positive T wave in virtually all surface ECG leads (Fig. 10.1A).

Conditions that prolong ventricular action potential duration (APD) prolong QT interval (Fig. 10.1B). Conditions that cause greater dispersion of repolarization also influence the size, polarity, and duration of the T wave and QT interval. (Longest QT intervals recorded are in elephants who presumably have the most dispersion (19).)

However, one more point concerning the T wave is somewhat confusing. Some ventricular repolarization seems to occur after the T wave has terminated. It is usually silent due to cancellation of repolarization forces. That is ventricular repolarization is still proceeding in some parts of the heart but potential differences are not great enough to generate surface ECG waves (20). The significance of this phenomenon will be further discussed below.

The T wave may be followed by another deflection, the U wave (Fig. 10.1C). This wave may occur normally, especially in precordial leads, but it is especially prominent in LQTS. There is some evidence that the normal U wave (21,22) represents repolarization of Purkinje fibers which have longer APDs than ventricular muscle. In abnormal states such as LQTS, U waves may represent afterdepolarizations or possibly localized increases in APD (23) (Chapter 2).

The QT interval measurement is generally thought of as a measure of ventricular repolarization but in fact includes both depolarization (QRS) and repolarization (ST segment and T wave). The JT interval (the "J" point is the junction of the QRS and ST segment) (Fig. 10.1B) is a more precise measure of repolarization, but it is not routinely used.

The problem of rate correction of QT is much discussed

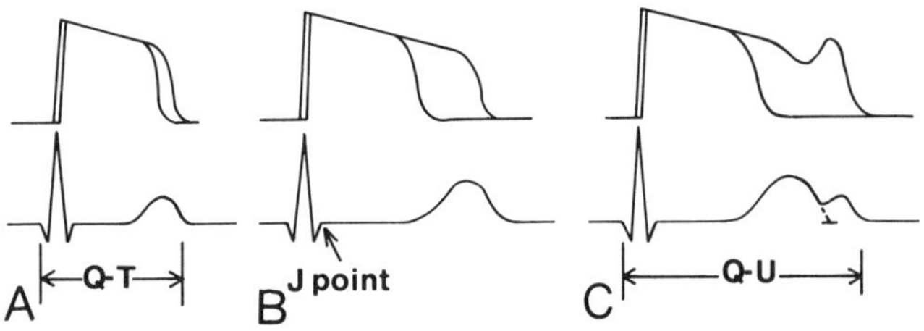

Figure 10.1. Relationship of ventricular action potentials (**upper**) to QT and QU intervals in the ECG (**lower**). **A** shows normal action potentials and ECG, **B** shows prolongation of APD, and **C** shows EAD and triggered activation. In **A**, QRS occurs due to potential differences across the heart during depolarization and T wave occurs due to potential differences during repolarization. In **B** there is prolongation and increased disparity of APD. This causes T wave to become larger and Q-T interval to prolong. **C** shows the development of a U wave when an EAD and triggered activation occur. Measurement of QT interval and QU interval are shown in **A** and **C** in location of J point in **B**. Note also in **C** that, because of the U wave it is difficult to measure a QT interval. One method is to draw a line continuous with the downslope of the T wave, as shown, to facilitate measurement of QT rather than QU.

(24–30). Normally, APD and QT interval shorten as the heart rate increases. A number of formulas were devised for determination of a rate-corrected QT interval (QT_c) (24-30) but the oldest, Bazett's 1920 formula (25), is the one that remains in use:

$$QT_c = \frac{QT}{\sqrt{RR}}$$

Studies on the accuracy of this formula have yielded variable results (31). Its error is probably to undercorrect (i.e., overestimate) QT at fast rates and overcorrect (underestimate) it at slow heart rates.

QT_c intervals prolong with interventions that prolong ventricular APD as expected. QT_c is also under autonomic control and responds to beta blockade (prolongation), cognitive effort, sleep (prolongation), biofeedback, and other autonomic interventions (32–35), but variably to strictly parasympathetic interventions (31,36,37).

Other issues regarding QT_c that are pertinent to its proper evaluation are (30,38,39).

1. The normal QT_c range of 0.35–0.44 sec is frequently used in published series but it has little experimental justification (30). Table 10.1 shows recently derived upper limits of QT_c corrected for age and gender and based on 578 healthy subjects (40,41).

2. Downslope of the T wave is gradual and therefore its termination is hard to define (Fig. 10.1C) particularly when QT is prolonged and at faster rates. Some electrocardiographers in fact measure a "QU" interval while others make an attempt to measure QT. One suggestion is that a line be drawn on the downslope of the T wave to estimate its time of termination (39,42) (Fig. 10.1C).

3. Some reports use uncorrected QT while others use QT_c, creating confusion in interpretation.

Table 10.1.
Upper Limits of QT_c Intervals

	QT_c Intervals—Upper Limits[a]		
Status	1–15 yr	Men[b]	Women[b]
Normal	<0.44	<0.43	<0.45
Borderline	0.44–0.46	0.43–0.45	0.45–0.46
Prolonged	>0.46	>0.45	>0.46

From Moss AJ, Robinson J: Identification of high-risk population: clinical features of the idiopathic long QT syndrome. Circulation 1992;85:140–144.
[a]Based on 578 healthy subjects.
[b]Above age 15 yr.

4. An ECG machine that meets American Heart Association standards should be used (40,43).

CLASSIFICATION OF LQTS

There are two distinct varieties of LQTS that converge in a very similar appearance of baseline ECGs and polymorphic VT. These distinct syndromes have been classified as "idiopathic" and "acquired" LQTS. Idiopathic LQTS includes familial LQTS as well as nonfamilial, sporadic cases with the same features (except nerve deafness).

The most characteristic feature of congenital LQTS is that VTs distinctively emerge with heightened adrenergic tone such as during exercise or intense emotion. Acquired LQTS does not display adrenergic responsiveness. Here ventricular tachycardias (VTs) emerge with bradycardia and pauses.

This classification is not perfect and there are borderline and mixed forms. Acquired LQTS with autonomic features may, for example, occur due to central nervous system diseases (typically subarachnoid hemorrhage) (44) and following surgery involving the autonomic nervous system (45). Conversely, however, a congenital nonadrenergic form of LQTS has not been described.

Jackman, *et al.* (39), suggested classifying LQTS as either "adrenergic-dependent" or "pause-dependent." In this chapter, however, LQTS will be classified "idiopathic" or "acquired" though the Jackman classification is attractive.

IDIOPATHIC LONG QT SYNDROME

In 1857, Meisner (46) described the following patient in his textbook on deaf mutism. A young girl had stolen a trifle from another child and was called before the director of her school in the presence of the other pupils. She was so struck by repentance and grief that she fell dead to the floor. The other children apparently interpreted this as an act of God punishing her for her transgression and reminding them never to stray. Her parents, however, were not surprised as two other deaf mute children in their family had died, one from fright and the other after a fit of rage.

The Jervell-Lange-Nielsen syndrome (1) of congenital LQTS includes nerve deafness and has autosomal recessive inheritance (47). The Romano-Ward syndrome (2,4) has normal hearing and autosomal dominant inheritance (48,49). Recently a deoxyribonucleic acid (DNA) marker in a family with Romano-Ward Syndrome has been placed at the Harvey-ras-1 locus, chromosome 11 (11 p 15.5) (49) that may be involved with K^+ rectifier current (40). Sporadic forms (about 10% of cases) (40) are not associated with nerve deafness and may at times be transient. All of these are rare syndromes.

Electrocardiographic Features

Besides prolongation of QT_c or QU intervals, patients with congenital LQTS have striking T wave aberrations including large, wide-based biphasic, inverted, peaked, or otherwise atypical T waves; long ST segments with normal T waves; large or inverted U waves (sometimes called "slow" or "late" waves to distinguish them from normal U waves) that may merge with the T waves; and T or U wave alternans (10,39,40,50,51). Examples are shown in Figs. 10.2 and 10.3 (40). A specific family may display a specific ST-T-U configuration (suggesting genetic heterogeneity of this syndrome) (40). These repolarization abnormalities may vary over minutes, hours, or even from beat to beat (Fig. 10.4) and can be elicited by adrenergic provocative testing.

Using computer analysis, Benhorin, *et al.* (52) described a number of more refined electrocardiographic features that occur in idiopathic LQTS. There was greater beat-to-beat variation in T wave and more symmetric T waves (52,53) in LQTS patients as well as other characteristics. Signal-averaged ECG has been reported as normal (54).

The QT and/or TU wave changes tend to display a delayed, diminished or absent response to heart rate very different to what occurs in the acquired syndrome (55,56). However, this response is not consistent and TU changes may be bradycardia and pause-dependent as in acquired LQTS.

Abrupt occurrence of many of the more striking TU changes may indicate impending ventricular arrhythmias. These prodromes include large and unusual-appearing or inverted T or U waves and especially T wave alternans (Fig. 10.3) which may result from abrupt sympathetic discharge (7). When observed on ambulatory ECG, T wave alternans indicates a poorer prognosis.

QT_c prolongation in congenital LQTS can be blunted by beta blockers (36,57–59) (which have no effect on or lengthen QT_c in normals (5,8,60) and lengthen APD in normal tissue in situ (61)), atropine (62), intravenous KCl, and digitalis (which does not alter the exercise response (62)).

ECGs in idiopathic LQTS also commonly display bradycardia and sinus pauses and atrioventricular (AV) dissociation.

Arrhythmias

Both idiopathic and acquired LQTS have similar characteristic patterns of VTs. The difference is in the critical trigger, i.e., sympathetic stimulation (idiopathic) versus bradycardia (acquired).

Some of the confusion regarding characteristic arrhythmias of

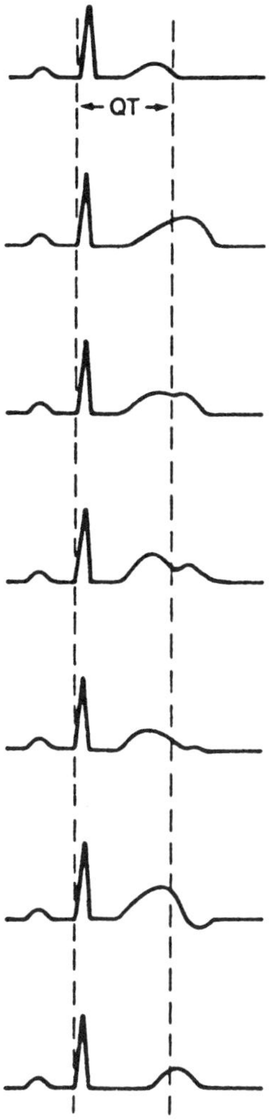

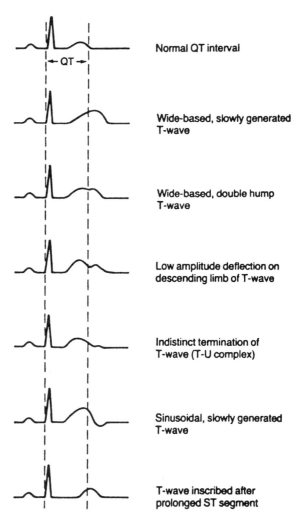

Figure 10.2. Examples of ST-U wave changes that are observed in patients with congenital LQTS. A given family may have one specific pattern (From Moss AJ, Robinson J: Identification of high-risk population: clinical features of the idiopathic long QT syndrome. Circulation 1992;85:140–144, by permission of the American Heart Association, Inc.)

LQTS is reflected in many other names that have been applied: cardiac ballet (63), atypical VT (64), multiform VT (65), ventricular fibrillo-flutter (66), pseudo fibrillation (67), paroxysmal ventricular fibrillation VF (68), and transient (recurrent) VF (69). In presently used terminology the characteristic arrhythmias of LQTS are called torsade de pointe (TdP) (5,17,70) and/or polymorphous VT (poly VT) (71).

TdP or poly VT (Figs. 10.5 and 10.6) is a nonsustained wide complex (usually greater than 0.16 sec) tachycardia which tends to occur in repetitive bursts of 4–20 complexes at fast rates, generally 200–250 beats/min (39,71,72). Typically there are clusters of activity, sometimes occurring in crescendo fashion and then often subsiding. The first beat of the tachycardia is usually late in the cycle, after the T wave (Figs. 10.6 and Fig. 10.7B). In idiopathic LQTS, VT generally but not always occurs

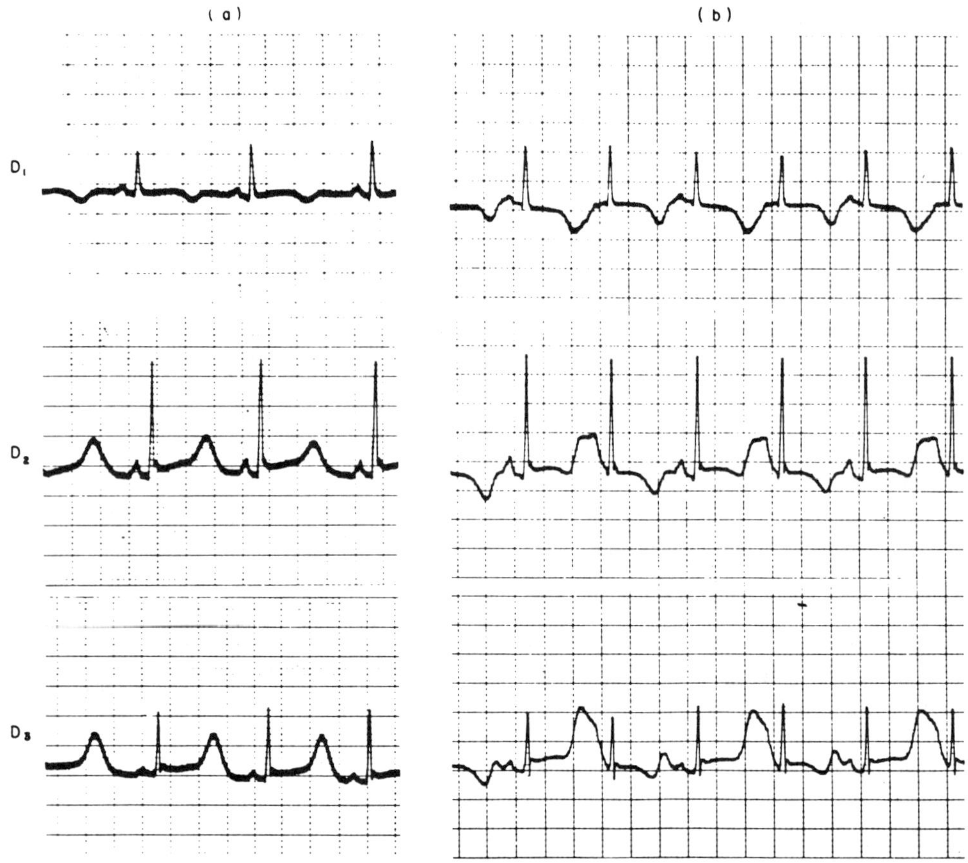

Figure 10.3. Example of T wave alternans in a 9-yr-old female. ECGs are at rest (**A**) and during unintentionally induced fear (**B**). QT_C is prolonged at rest but is even more prolonged and TU alternans occurs during fear. TU alternans is considered a sign of impending arrhythmia and may as in this example be elicited with provocative maneuvers such as exercise or fright. (From Schwartz PJ, Locati E: The idiopathic long QT syndrome: pathogenetic mechanisms and therapy. Eur Heart J 1985;6:103–114, with permission.)

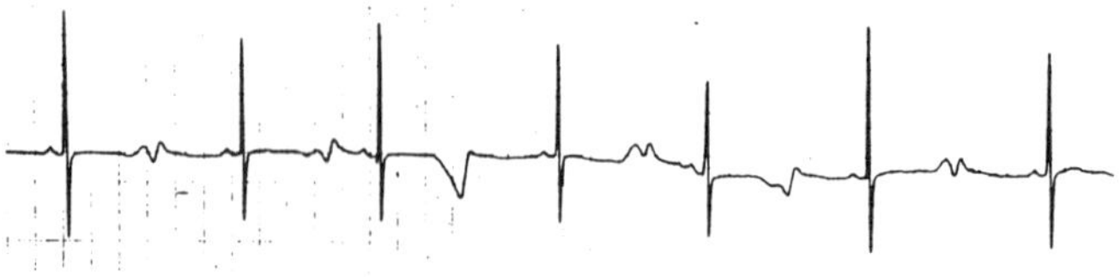

Figure 10.4. Marked beat-to-beat variation in TU wave and QT interval in a 6-year-old female and with congenital LQTS. (From Schwartz PJ: Autonomic modulation of arrhythmias in patients, in Rosen MR, Janse MJ, Wit AL. (eds): Cardiac Electrophysiology. Futura Publishing Co., Mt. Kisco, NY, 1990:951–966, with permission.)

when there are relatively rapid underlying sinus rates (Fig. 10.6).

During the characteristic tachycardia QRS complexes in LQTS display progressive changes in amplitude and axis. Torsade de pointe (translated this means "twist of the point") refers to complexes that are least in one lead appear to be twisting around an isoelectric baseline (17,73) (Figs. 10.5 and 10.6). To observe this pattern one generally needs multiple-lead recordings.

More generally, tachycardias in LQTS display multiple and highly variable wave forms, may not or only transiently have the twisting appearance, or may be so bizarre as to resemble VF (69).

Poly VT may also progress to true VF or conversely, change to sustained monomorphic VT (examples of these in acquired LQTS are discussed below). Monomorphic VT may occur for one of several reasons—it may be the primary rhythm of patients with LQTS, it may be triggered by the poly VT or it may appear monomorphic when only one or two ECG leads are recorded (74). Thus, in LQTS there can be monomorphic or polymorphic VT and also VF.

As can be seen, criteria for TdP and poly VT are somewhat imprecise depending on wave forms more than precise numeric indices. This can create uncertainty in individual cases as well as in evaluating published series of LQTS. Presently used criteria for VT in LQTS are in Table 10.2.

Clinical Features

Symptoms of idiopathic LQTS begin early in life with mean age of onset of 21–24 yr (75,76) (first months to the 30s). Primary clinical manifestations are palpitation, syncope, seizures, or

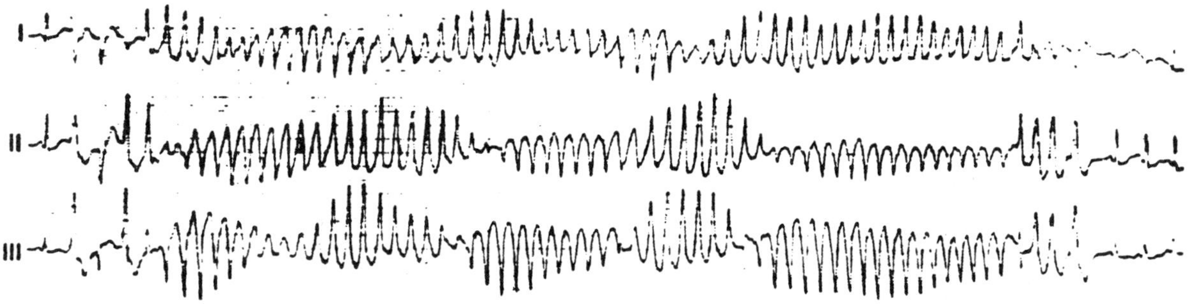

Figure 10.5. Typical torsades de pointe (TdP) showing "twisting of the point." Note that QRS complexes during the ventricular tachycardia gradually change in size and then reverse their polarity and axis. This creates a concertina-like effect. (From Krikler DM, Curry PVL: Torsade de pointes, an atypical ventricular tachycardia. Br Heart J 1976;38:117–120, with permission.)

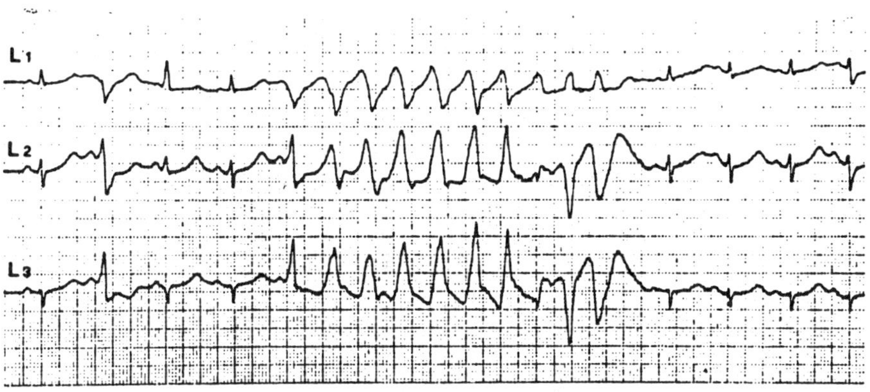

Figure 10.6. Ventricular tachycardia in idiopathic LQTS. Note that there is a "twisting" TdP-like pattern. Note also that pauses do not precede the onset of ventricular arrhythmia in this patient and that first beat of tachycardia occurs late in the cycle. Recording is from a 36-year-old female with idiopathic LQTS. (From Schwartz PJ: Autonomic modulation of arrhythmias in patients. In Rosen MR, Janse MJ, Wit AL (eds): Cardiac Electrophysiology. Futura Publishing Co., Mt. Kisco, NY, 1990:951–966, with permission.)

sudden death, all due to poly VT. Typically, episodes begin and end abruptly as in other arrhythmia situations (7,47,58,75–79). Cases may be dangerously misdiagnosed as primary epilepsy for many years, sometimes with tragic consequences, underscoring the need for careful analysis of ECGs in epileptics (76,80,81). In infancy and early childhood attacks can be difficult to diagnose. The child may stop moving, grab the breast or stomach, moan and cry, or have chest pain (78).

Symptoms occur in clusters with intervals of months or years. They are typically triggered by states of sympathetic arousal such as extreme emotional upset, e.g., fright, grief, pain, exertion (especially sudden exertion), loud noises, delirium tremors, and menses (2,10,47,58,75,76,78,82–86). There are vivid descriptions of patients with tachycardia or sudden death after being awakened by thunder, telephone, or the alarm clock (86) (Figs. 10.8 and 10.9) or with extreme upset such as learning of the death of a relative (sometimes the sudden death of a relative who also has LQTS) or other adverse news. These are often specific in a given individual. Cocaine has also been a trigger (87).

In the International Registry of familial LQTS, a worldwide prospective follow-up study and the most comprehensive data available, triggers for syncopal episodes sorted out as follows (75): acute emotion (anger, fright)—58%, vigorous physical activities (exclusive of swimming)—45%, swimming—16%, awakening—15%, mild noises—9%, menses—9%.

Nerve deafness does not occur commonly in congenital LQTS. In the International Registry of familial LQTS, it occurred in 7% of probands, 1% of affected, and less than 1% of nonaffected family members (75,76). Conversely, in 6557 births with congenital nerve deafness from ten reports, incidence of LQTS was 0.25% (82).

Sinus bradycardia is common in idiopathic LQTS (31%) and sinus pauses of greater than 1.2 secs occur in about 2% (76). Mean heart rates are slower than normal, especially below age 3 (88) and there is a blunted heart rate response to exercise and atropine (1,78,82,89). These findings lend credence to the hypothesis that there is autonomic dysfunction in the syndrome.

A-V dissociation has also been reported in idiopathic LQTS (90). It may be related to adrenergic dysfunction or, an interesting possibility for which there is some evidence, prolonged APD in the His-Purkinje system. Consistent with this notion, LQTS patients may have an abnormal infra-Hisian response to pacing (91,92).

Provocative Testing

Arrhythmias in idiopathic LQTS are not inducible by programmed premature stimulation and the standard electrophysiologic test is not useful. However, a number of adrenergic provocative maneuvers elicit or worsen the typical findings of LQTS and are used as provocative tests to diagnose or confirm the syndrome (39,85,93). These include treadmill exercise (58,82,85), infusion of catecholamine, epinephrine (58,94), isoproterenol (58,77,83), or phenylephrine (58,77,94), cold

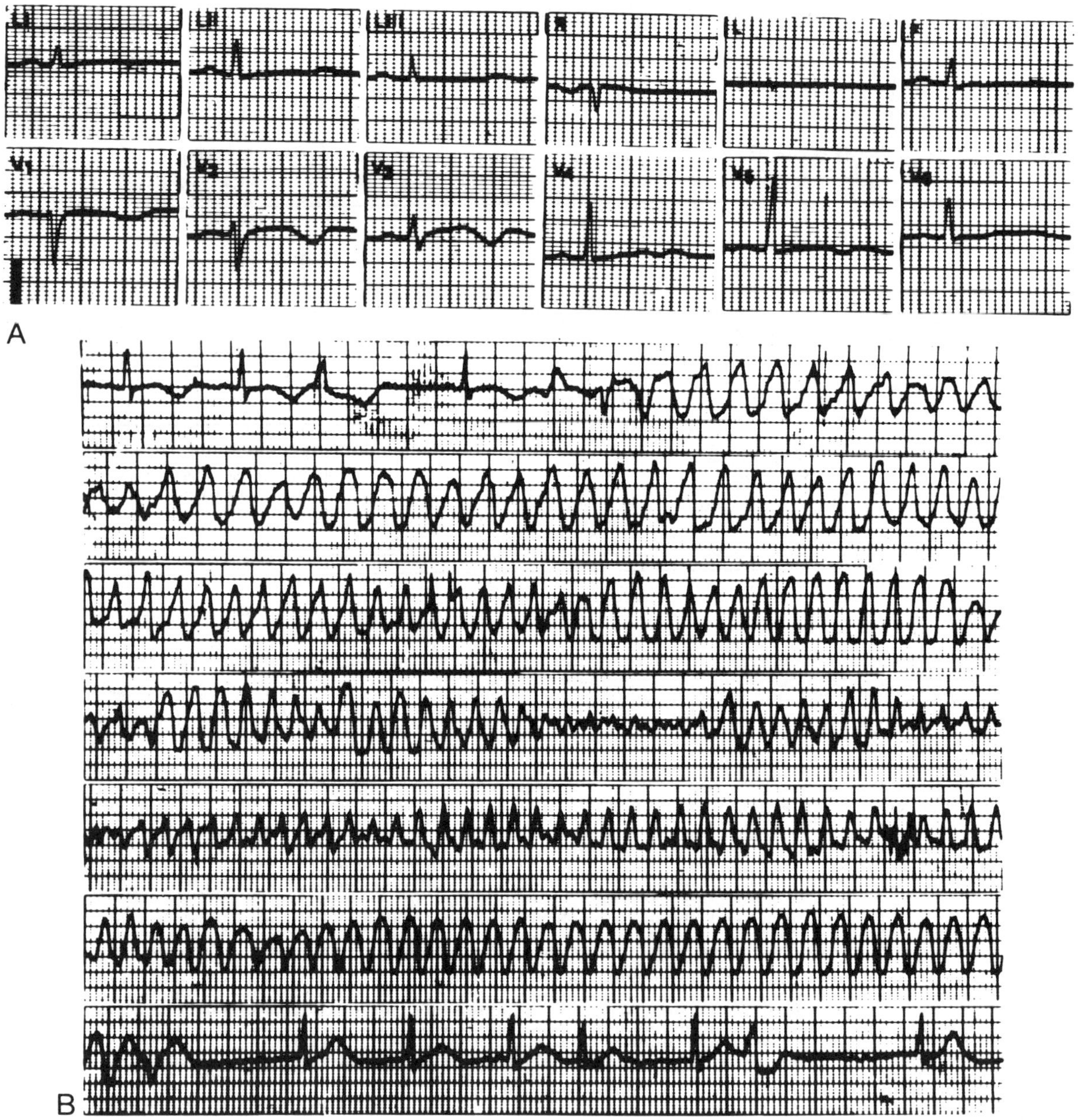

Figure 10.7. Twelve-lead ECG (**A**) and poly VT in lead V_1 (**B**) in a 19-year-old female with congenital LQTS. **B** is a continuous recording. ECG shows markedly prolonged QT interval with T wave and U wave aberration. Ventricular tachycardia starts with a late ventricular beat; note that VT rate is very rapid (sixth trace) and ventricular flutter-like but still terminates spontaneously. ECGs are kindly supplied by Dr. Park Willis III.

Table 10.2.
Ventricular Tachycardia in Long QT Syndrome

Wide complex,
often >0.16 sec
Nonsustained,
usually 4–20 complexes
Fast Rates
generally >200/min
Repetitive bursts,
often in clusters
Late T_1,[a]
typically TQ > 600 msec[b]
Varying waveform,
twisting pattern frequent but not universal

[a]T_1 = first beat of tachycardia.
[b]See ref. 55.

pressor (95), Valsalva maneuver (95,96), and auditory stimulation (86) (Figs. 10.10 and 10.11). Cognitive effort can change QT interval (32) but it has not yet been organized into a test.

Observation of typical QT or TU wave changes, failure of QT to shorten, or exaggerated QT prolongation in the recovery phase (40,79,97) constitute positive responses. Propranolol blunts or blocks these responses (39,86,96).

It is important to note that these tests do not have a rigorously standardized protocols, endpoints or, because of the rarity of LQTS, any precise information on sensitivity or specificity as, for example, does treadmill exercise testing in the diagnosis of ischemic heart disease. Another limitation is the imperfect QT rate correction formula though an absent QT response to increased rate leaves no doubt as to the diagnosis.

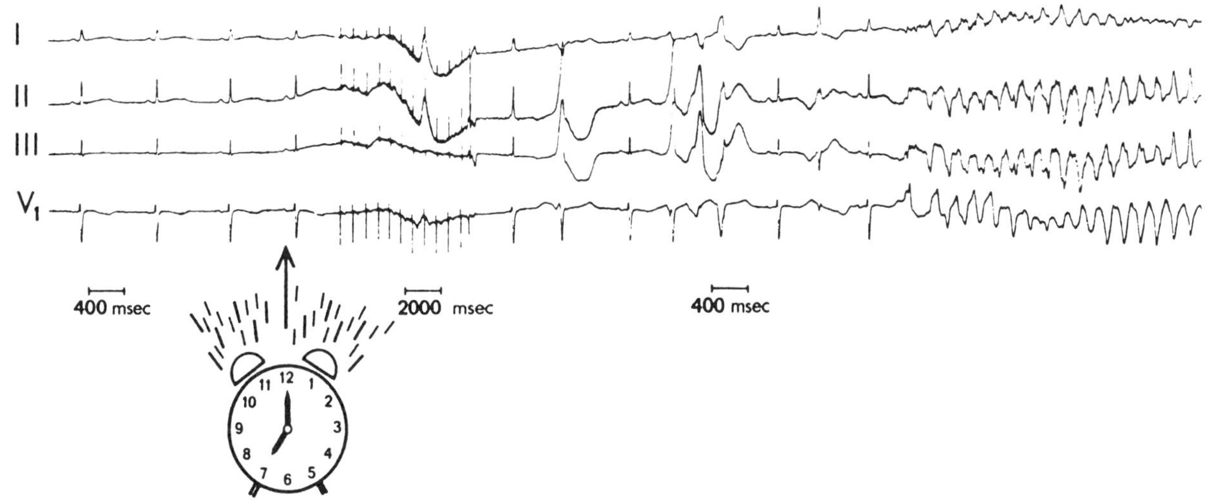

Figure 10.8. Auditory stimulus from an alarm clock initiating ventricular fibrillation in a 14-yr-old girl with idiopathic LQTS. The patient had carried the diagnosis of epilepsy for 4 yr. (From Wellens HJJ, Vermuelen A, Durrer D: Ventricvular fibrillation occurring on arousal from sleep by auditory stimuli. Circulation 1972;46:661–665, by permission of the American Heart Association, Inc.)

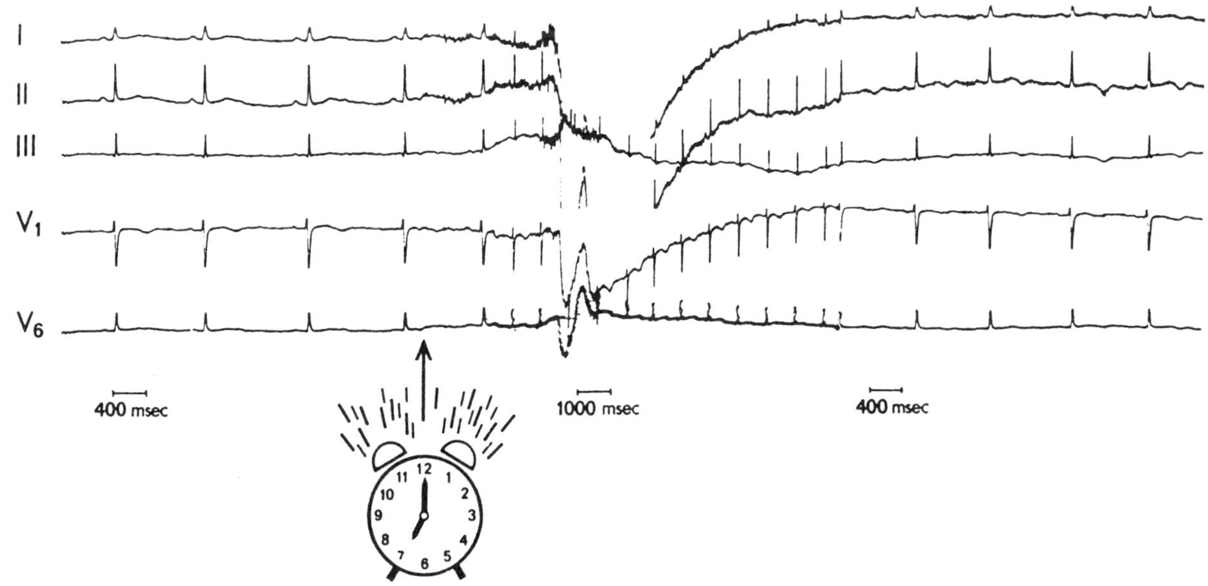

Figure 10.9. Same patient as in Figure 10.8. After propranolol treatment, the alarm clock no longer provokes ventricular arrhythmia. (From Wellens HJJ, Vermuelen A, Durrer D: Ventricular fibrillation occurring on arousal from sleep by auditory stimuli. Circulation 1972;46:661–665, by permission of the American Heart Association, Inc.)

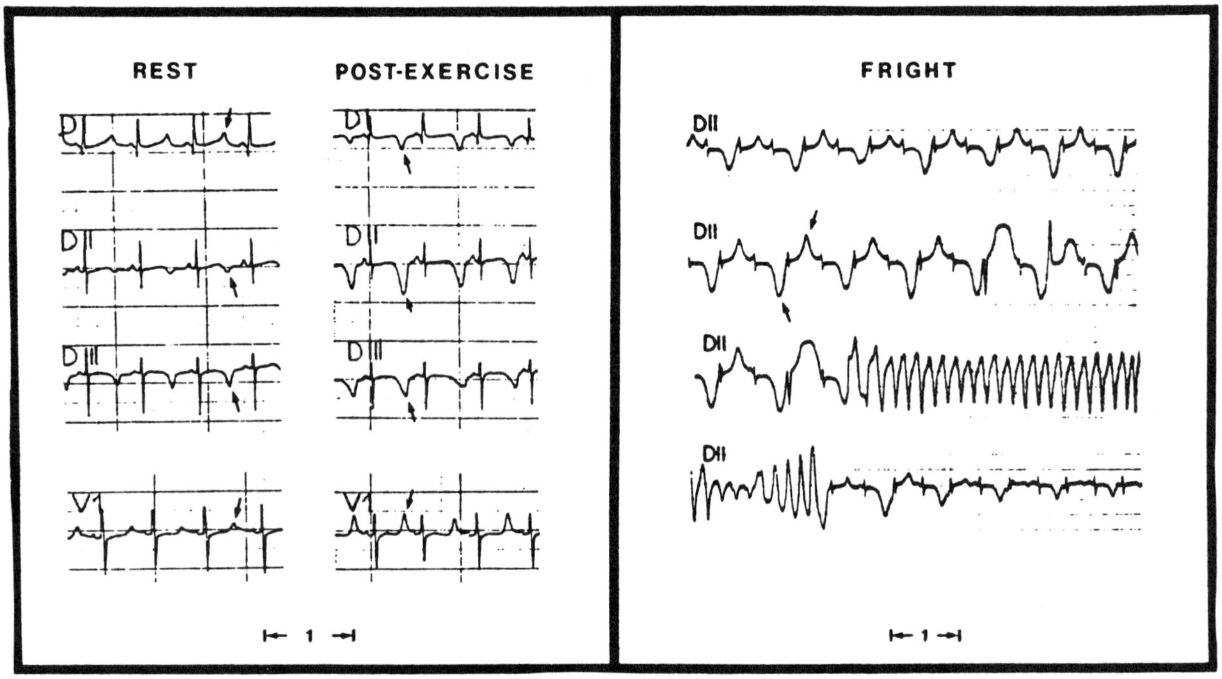

Figure 10.10. Provocative test in a patient with Jervell Lange-Nielsen syndrome. ECG at rest displayed QT_C prolongation and T wave inversion. Following exercise, QT_C becomes greatly prolonged with TU wave inversion. Fright elicits a stronger response with TU alternans (*arrows*) and VT. (From Jackman WM, Friday KJ, Anderson JL, *et al.*: Long QT syndromes: a critical review, new clinical observations and unified hypothesis. Prog Cardiovasc Dis 1988;31:115–172, with permission.)

Patients may be stimulus-specific in their responses to provocation. For example, the patient shown in Figs. 10.9 and 10.10 had ventricular fibrillation after ringing of the alarm clock but no response to other stimuli such as fright, exercise, or Valsalva maneuver while awake (86). For this reason careful history as to possible trigger is important.

Provocative testing for LQTS must only be done with resuscitation equipment ready and defibrillator patches in place as recalcitrant VT or VF may occur (85). Of all tests, the exercise stress test for LQTS has the most use and infusion of catecholamine is probably the most sensitive. Recording of adrenergic-enhanced early afterdepolarizations (EADs) in monophasic action potentials directly from the heart (see below) is a promising test for the future when more data becomes available. EADs have been observed via this technique in both congenital and acquired LQTS (98,99).

Diagnosis

The diagnosis of idiopathic LQTS is based on the findings listed in Table 10.3. Fig. 10.12 is a suggested algorithm (40) for sorting and managing these patients.

Prognosis

Prognosis in untreated idiopathic LQTS varies from asymptomatic patients with QT_c prolongation and rare event rates to highly virulent forms, especially in certain families. The International Registry report of 1991 (76) gives data on familial LQTS probands ($N = 328$) and what they termed affected ($QT_c > 0.44$ sec) ($N = 688$—note high number) and unaffected ($QT_c \leq 0.44$ sec) ($N = 1004$) family members. Fig. 10.13 shows cumulative probability of experiencing a cardiac event (76) (syncope or sudden death). After 10 yr of follow-up, 37% of probands, 5% of affected but notably rare if any (<1%) unaffected family members had experienced a cardiac event (76).

For probands annual incidence of syncope was 5% and sudden death 0.9%. This was a better prognosis than in the previous Registry report of 1985 (8.6%/yr syncope, 1.34%/yr sudden death) (75) and other data (82,100), attributed to treatment of milder forms with beta blockers (76). Of patients with history of syncope marked increase in QT and no antiadrenergic therapy, 57% were dead by age 20 yr (76).

Tables 10.4 and 10.5 show the particular features of congenital LQTS that are associated with a poor prognosis and are based on International Registry and other reports (39,75,76,79). Faster heart rate is a newly reported risk but may in part be due to a relative increase in heart rate when compared to beta blocker therapy, which both slows heart rate and improves prognosis. However, patients tend to have symptoms at fast rates. Certain risk factors in Table 10.4 are for probands and family members combined and these are distinguished in Table 10.5. Note also that children have a more virulent form of the disease (79).

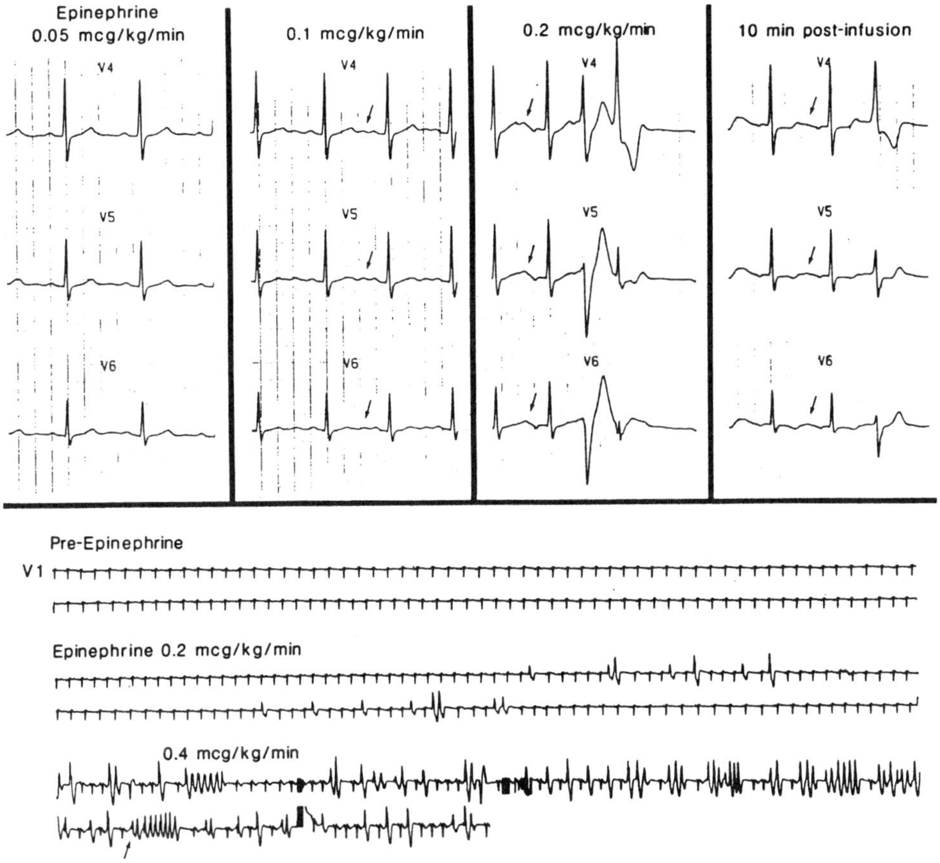

Figure 10.11. Example of provocative testing with epinephrine in gradually increasing concentrations in a 40-yr-old asymptomatic male with idiopathic LQTS. Note that as the epinephrine doses increased, TU wave abnormalities become more prominent and ventricular arrhythmia appears. This is particularly apparent in a lower portion of the trace where 0.2 μg/kg/min of epinephrine induced VPCs and couplets while 0.4 μg/kg/min induced runs of VT. (From Jackman WM, Friday KJ, Anderson JL, *et al.*: Long QT Syndromes: a critical review, new clinical observations, and unified hypothesis. Prog Cardiovasc Dis 1988;31: 115–172, with permission.)

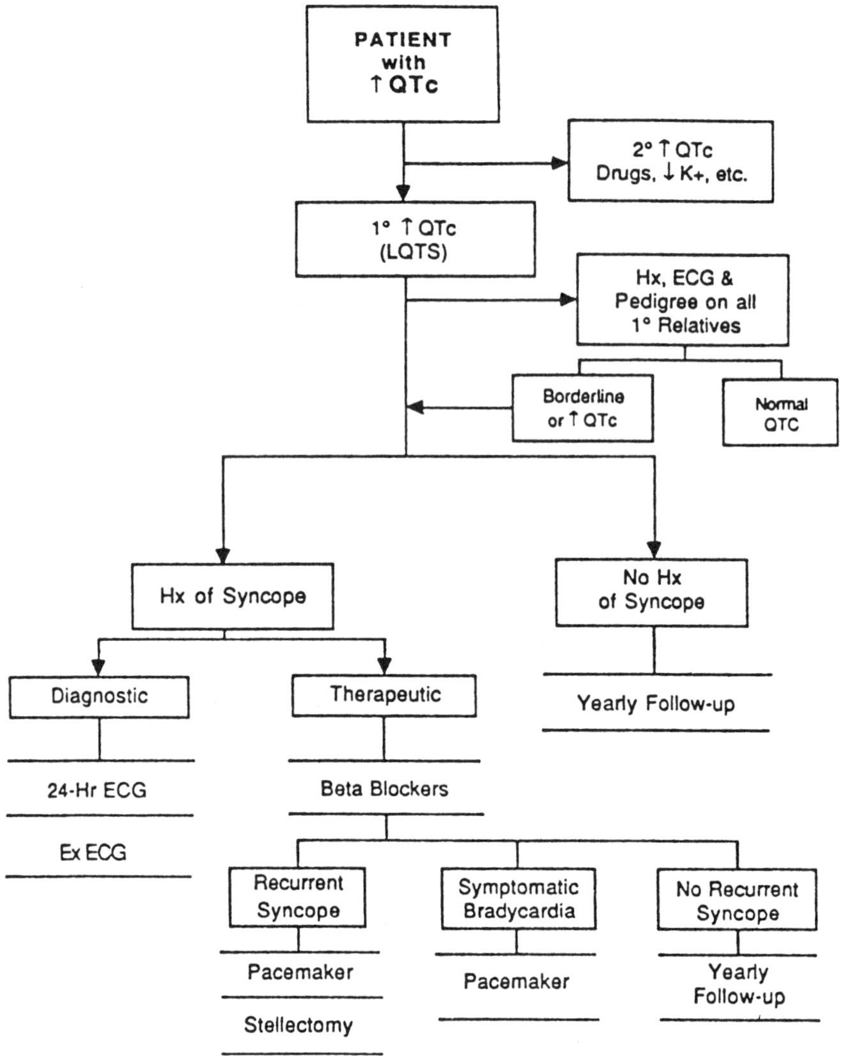

Figure 10.12. Algorithm for sorting and managing patients with familial LQTS. Hx = history. (From Moss AJ, Robinson J: Identification of high-risk population: Clinical features of the idiopathic long QT syndrome. Circulation 1992;85:140–144, by permission of the American Heart Association, Inc.)

Table 10.3.
Clinical Diagnosis of Idiopathic Long QT Syndrome

12-lead and ambulatory[a] ECGs
↑ QT_c, TU abnormalities, poly VT, bradycardia
History of cardiac events consistent with LQTS
Syncope, cardiac arrest, palpitations
Autonomic trigger and abrupt onset and offset are typical
Family history
Exclusion of acquired causes of LQTS
Adrenergic provocative testing
Genetic marker (future)

[a]12-lead ECG is important for accurate measure of QT_c and also helps in establishing TU abnormalities (especially alternans), poly VT, or TdP.

Atypical and Borderline Cases of Idiopathic LQTS

While there is little doubt about the diagnosis, when LQTS appears in the classic form, problems arise in patients with mixed, atypical and borderline features. These include the following:

1. Familial or sporadic cases with normal QT_c and poly VT (101). These are very rare. In fact in the International Registry, a normal QT_c interval in a family member of a proband with LQTS virtually assured the absence of a cardiac event (76).
2. Patients with adrenergic responsive monomorphic VT and prolonged QT_c. As monomorphic VT may occur in LQTS for various reasons (74) these cases should be classified along with LQTS.
3. Patients with prolonged QT interval, poly VT, no adrenergic responsiveness but inducibility via programmed premature stimulation. This is a well-described group of patients with arrhythmias that respond to Class IA and similar antiarrhythmic agents (102) (considered particularly harmful and contraindicated in idiopathic LQTS), rather than beta blockers. These patients should not be classified as LQTS.
4. Patients with borderline QT_c prolongation and a questionable history of cardiac event (39). Approach to and classification of these patients would depend on other diagnostic features (Tables 10.3 and 10.4). Asymptomatic patients with intermittent QT_c prolongation should be approached similarly (39).

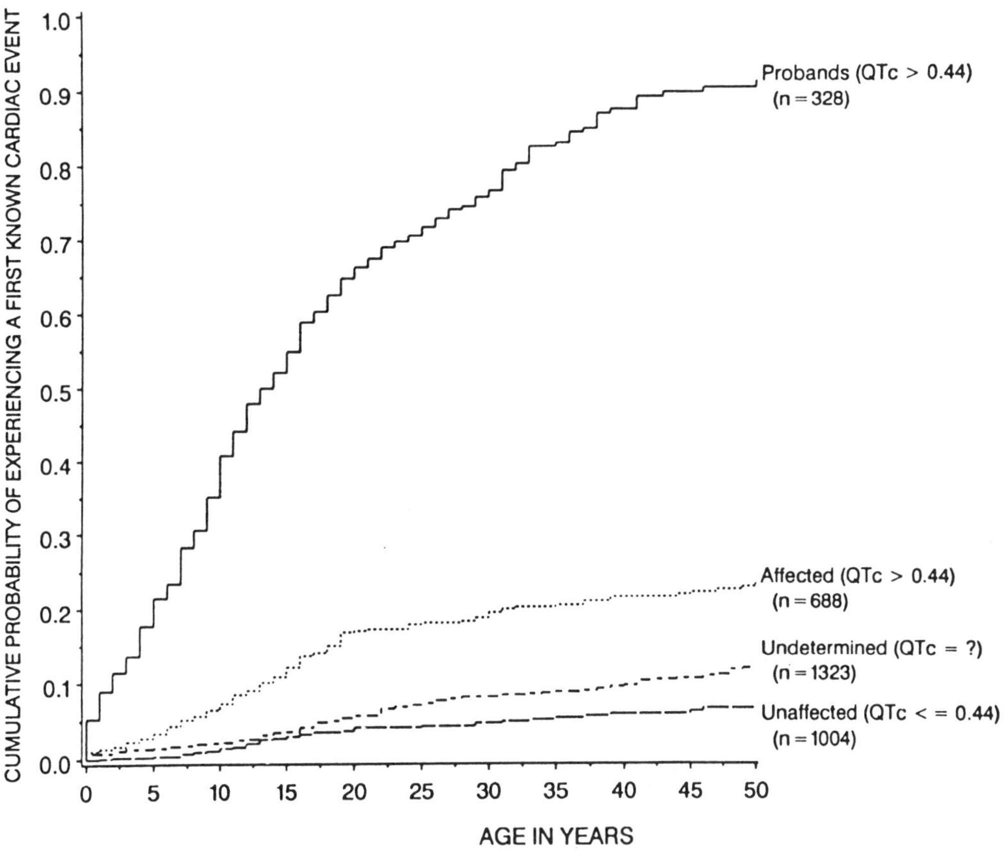

Figure 10.13. Cumulative probability of experiencing a first known cardiac event (syncope or probable LQTS-related death) from time of birth in probands ($QT_C > 0.44$ sec), affected (QT_C) > 0.44 sec), unaffected ($QT_C \leq 0.44$ sec), and undetermined (unknown QT_C) family members enrolled in the International Registry of idiopathic LQTS. (From Moss AJ, Schwartz PJ, Crampton RS, *et al.*: The long QT syndrome: prospective longitudinal study of 328 families. Circulation 1991;84:1136–1144, by permission of the American Heart Association, Inc.)

Table 10.4.
Risk Factors for Cardiac Events in Idiopathic Long QT Syndrome

Female sex
History of cardiac event[a,b]
$QT_c > 0.54$ sec[a,b]
Faster heart rate[a,b]
Virulent family history
Onset in childhood (especially at younger age)
Congenital deafness[c]
History of repetitive ventricular arrhythmia
Neonatal A-V block
T wave alternans
No antiadrenergic therapy

Adapted from Moss AJ, Robinson J: Identification of high-risk population: clinical features of the idiopathic long QT syndrome. Circulation 1992;85:140–144; Moss AJ, Schwartz PJ, Crampton RS, *et al.*: The long QT syndrome: a prospective international study. Circulation 1985;71:17–21; Moss AJ, Schwartz PJ, Crampton RS, *et al.*: The long QT syndrome: prospective longitudinal study of 328 families. Circulation 1991;84:1136–1144; Weintraub RG, Gow RM, Wilkinson J: The congenital long QT syndromes in childhood. J Am Coll Cardiol 1990;16:674–680.

[a]In probands and family members combined. See Table 10.3 for risk in probands, probands vs. family member.

[b]Hazard rates (risk per unit time vs. not having factor) is 1.052/0.01 units for QT_c, 1.017/beat for heart rates, and 3.1 for history of cardiac event (76).

[c]Risk ratio (risk vs. not having factor) 9.9 (75).

ACQUIRED LONG QT SYNDROME

Electrocardiographic Features and Arrhythmias

ECGs in acquired LQTS have the same striking TU wave abnormalities and arrhythmias as the congenital form. The fundamental difference is that abnormalities (15,34,64,72,103,105) emerge or are associated with bradycardia or even one pause (Figs. 10.14 and 10.15). Adrenergic excess and specifically emotion have not been observed as triggers for arrhythmias in acquired LQTS.

ECG findings include lability, prominence, broadness, and inversion of TU waves as well as QT and TU wave alternans. QT_c prolongation not present at baseline may be apparent only after a pause (15,39,64,72,103,104) (Fig. 10.14) and QT_c shortens substantially with tachycardia (15,103). QRS prolongation is not an integral part of the syndrome but may result as an independent feature with certain inciting agents such as Class IA antiarrhythmic drugs.

Ventricular tachycardia also has the same morphology as in congenital LQTS. It may be monomorphic as well as polymorphic

Table 10.5.
Individual Risk Factors in Probands and Family Members

Subjects	Hazard ratio
Probands	
Heart rate (per beat)	1.055
QT_c (per 0.01 units)	1.018
Family members	
History of cardiac event	6.2
Female sex	3.9

From Moss AJ, Schwartz PJ, Crampton RS, *et al.*: The long QT syndrome: prospective longitudinal study of 328 families. Circulation 1991;84:1136–1144.

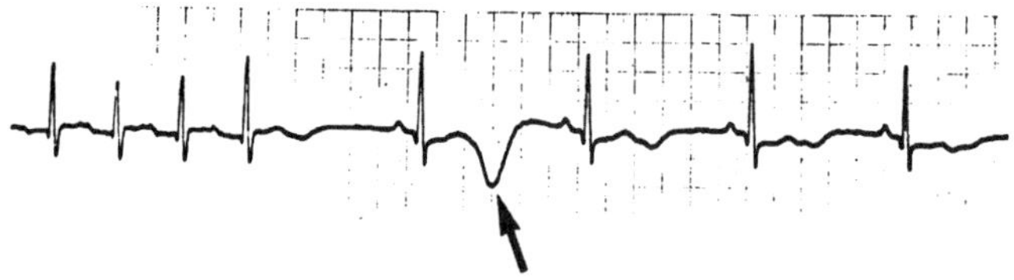

Figure 10.14. Marked postpause increase in QT interval and inversion of TU wave in a patient taking quinidine (*arrows*). Note that QT and T waves appear relatively normal in beats without pauses. (From Jackman WM, Clark M, Friday KJ, *et al.*: Ventricular tachyarrhythmias in the long QT syndromes. Med Clin North Am 1984;65:1079–1109, with permission.)

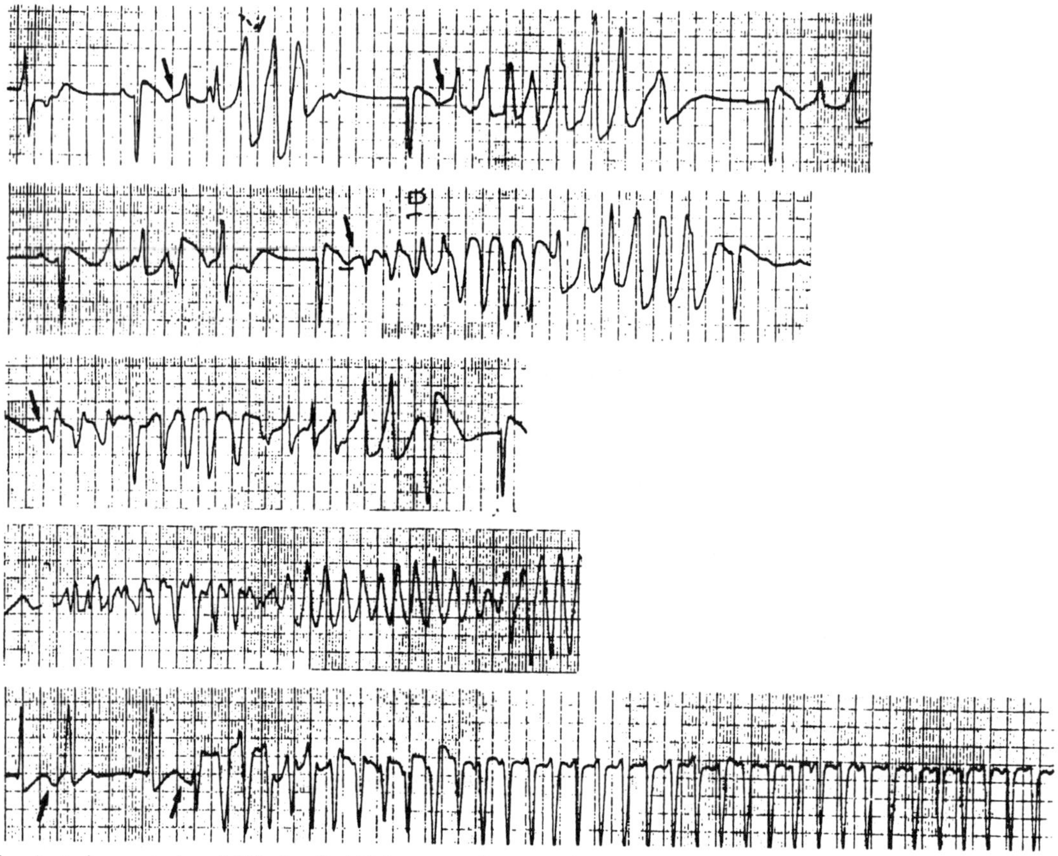

Figure 10.15. Amiodarone-induced VT. An **A**, VT begins with "long-short" sequences. In **B-D** tachycardia has the "twisting" TdP pattern though in parts of **D** it resembles VF. *Arrows* indicate large U waves in the supraventricular beat preceding the tachycardia. In **E** tachycardia is monomorphic. Note varying pattern of tachycardia in this sequence of tracings—twisting TdP type (**A-C**), VF-like—**D**; monomorphic—**E**. Note also that first beat of tachycardias are late in the cycle and rates of tachycardia vary. (From Jackman WM, Friday KJ, Anderson JL, *et al.*: Long QT syndromes: a critical review, new clinical observations, and unified hypothesis. Prog Cardiovasc Dis 1988;31:115–172, with permission.)

(Fig. 10.15) and may progress to VF (Fig. 10.16) (74,105). Typically it begins with a long coupling interval after the T wave (0.27–0.88 sec, mean 0.497 sec in one study (103)) and often in association with the U wave (15,39,64,72,103–105). Ventricular tachycardia rates are fast (170–300 beats/min, mean 227 beats/min in one study (103)).

Ventricular tachycardias tend to occur in bursts which are clustered. They tend to have fixed coupling to the preceding sinus beat and to slow down prior to termination (Fig. 10.15). These features plus the bradycardia dependence are reminiscent of EAD-induced triggered activity (see especially Fig. 2.21, Chapter 2 for marked pause-dependent changes that occur with EADs (106,107)).

In an individual patient the more prolonged the pause or bradycardia, the more striking subsequent TU change (including U wave amplitude) and the more prolonged the VT tends to be (Fig.

10.18). A typical (perhaps predominant) way for poly VT to begin is after long-short pauses with VPCs (39,103) (Fig. 10.17). Ventricular tachycardias then occur in crescendo clusters in a self-perpetuating fashion with a pause, short-long cycle lengths, then VT followed by another pause, and then further and longer runs of tachycardia (15,39,64,72,103–105) (Fig. 10.18). Ventricular tachycardias may also occur in association with T wave alternans.

While the above premonitory signs are helpful, they are not sensitive or specific enough or necessarily associated with sufficient lead time to predict arrhythmias in a given patient on an inciting agent. For example, bradycardia does not always precede VT which in one series initiated at mean sinus rates of 72 beats/min (39). QT intervals ≥ 0.60 sec (uncorrected) have been alleged to indicate impending arrhythmia (15) but there is in fact considerable overlap of QT in patients who do and do not have arrhythmias (108,109).

Programmed premature stimulation does not induce arrhythmias in acquired LQTS and is not useful. Monophasic action potential recordings may detect EADs in acquired as in congenital LQTS (98) but are probably not diagnostically helpful. Diag-

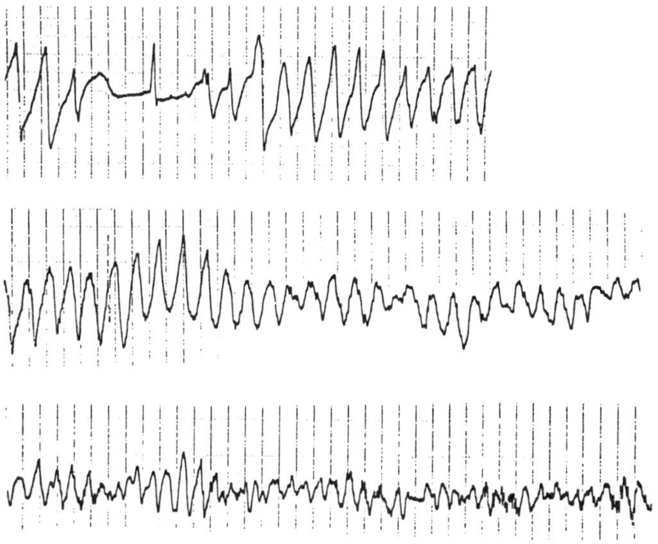

Figure 10.16. Quinidine-induced polymorphic VT progressing to VF. Although poly-VT may mimic VF it may also degenerate into VF. (From Roden DM: The long QT syndrome and torsades de pointes: basic and clinical aspects. In El-Sherif N, Samet P (eds); Cardiac Pacing and Electrophysiology, WB Saunders, Philadelphia, 1991:265–284, with permission.)

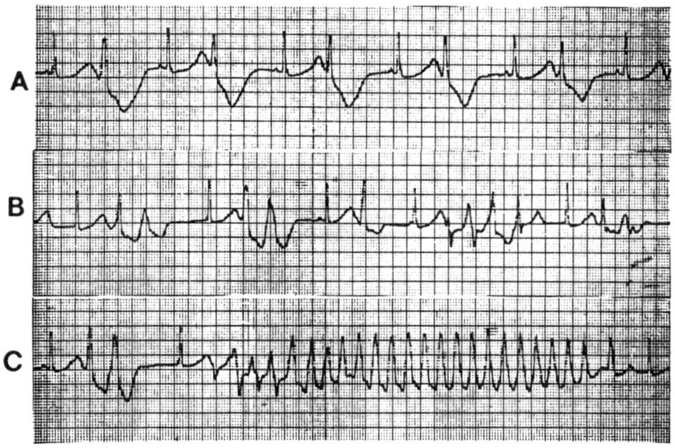

Figure 10.17. Recordings from a patient with acquired LQTS due to prenylamine. **A** shows ventricular bigeminy. **B** and **C** show onsets of VT which occur with typical long-short sequences. (From Kahn MM, Logan KR, McComb JM, *et al.*: Management of recurrent ventricular tachyarrhythmias associated with QT prolongation. Am J Cardiol 1981;45:1301–1308, with permission.)

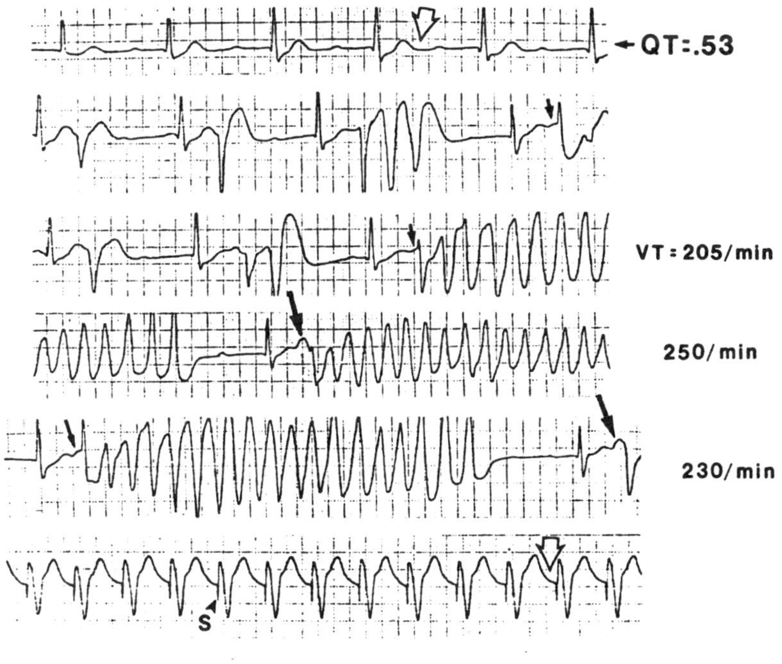

Figure 10.18. Imipramine-induced poly VT after 3 mo of drug administration in a patient with "therapeutic" serum drug levels. Tracings display several features: (a) There is AV dissociation with junctional escape rhythm, rate 46 beats/min. QT interval during this rhythm is 0.53 sec. (b) There is initiation of long-short cycle lengths due to, at first, VPCs (in second trace) and then progression to and longer runs of poly VT. (c) Postpause U waves (*arrows*) are prominent and vary with the length of the preceding pause rate. Duration of VT also increases with both the length of preceding pause and the amplitude of the U waves. (d) Pacing (lower trace) completely suppresses the tachycardia. (From Jackman WM, Clark M, Friday KJ, *et al.*: Ventricular tachyarrhythmias in the long Q-T syndromes. Med Clin North Am 1984;65: 1079–1109, with permission.)

nosis is generally clear-cut with typical ECG, typical arrhythmias and a known or suspected inciting agent.

Clinical Features

Table 10.6 lists causes of acquired LQTS (12,13,15–17,39,68, 72,73,84,93,103,104,109–139). They are rather numerous but have a common thread: most are associated with known prolongation of APD, including psychotropic drugs that apparently do not cause LQTS via central nervous system (CNS) effects.

Among electrolyte deficiencies, hypokalemia, and hypomagnesemia (or both) (15,39,84,103,105) appear frequently in series of acquired LQTS while hypocalcemia is a rare cause though it often induces ST segment prolongation without arrhythmias (140). Nutritional deficiencies cause LQTS in the absence of electrolyte imbalance for unknown reasons. They are also associated with myocardiopathies (12).

Sinus bradycardia and complete heart block, including the congenital form, may be associated with LQTS in the absence of the other known factors, even after many years.

Often multiple factors are associated with acquired LQTS, in particular hypokalemia and/or one or more inciting antiarrhythmic drugs (15,103).

Antiarrhythmic Drug-Induced Long QT Syndrome

Antiarrhythmic drugs associated with APD prolongation are the most widely reported causes of acquired LQTS. These include, Class IA and III agents (104,111,123,126–128,136) (see Chapter 12 for drug classification). Quinidine was first reported to cause ventricular arrhythmias in the 1920s (141) and then in a widely read report in 1964 (142), and is the most analyzed cause of poly VT (104,123,124,128,143).

Beta and calcium channel blockers do not cause LQTS except for sotalol (126,127) which also has Class III effects and bepridil which also has Class IA effects (139). Drugs in Class IB are probably not causes of LQTS even though there have been unsubstantiated claims (e.g., for lidocaine). These agents shorten APD and have, in fact, been used to treat TdP (73,103).

Class IC drugs are associated with a dangerous form of incessant VT due to profound suppression of I_{Na} (inward sodium current) rather than poly VT due to APD prolongation. The VT is not bradycardia pause-dependent or responsive to interventions that ordinarily suppress poly VT. Occasionally, however, Class IC agents may cause LQTS and poly VT (39), e.g., encainide via its metabolite, 3 methoxy-*o*-desmethyl encainide, which prolongs APD (129).

Patients with LQTS due to antiarrhythmic drugs have a wide variety of underlying diseases and arrhythmias to prompt the initial therapy. Many have poor ventricular function and/or structural heart disease (especially children) (124) but this may merely reflect the most likely patients to require such therapy.

Frank or near-hypokalemia (39,104,124) hypomagnesemia, bradycardia, and possibly hypothyroidism contribute to drug-induced LQTS while digitalis preparations, contrary to long-held beliefs, do not seem to play an important role (39,74,104,124). Patients under treatment for atrial fibrillation appear to develop poly VT after conversion to normal sinus rhythm (39,74,104) (Fig. 10.19) and not as previously thought in relation to long pauses during the atrial fibrillation.

For quinidine, the incidence of poly VT and sudden death was 8–9% in two prospective (109,144) and 1.5%/yr in one retrospective study (104). Time of onset of poly VT is within 4 days in about half the cases (39,73), the rest dividing between about a week and months or years later. Reasons for late onset are often not clear. Serum levels of drug (and metabolites) are predominantly in or below the therapeutic range (39,103,104,145) (Fig. 10.20). The lack of correlation of poly VT with "toxic" drug levels combined with the almost universal absence of other signs of drug toxicity has led observers to consider acquired LQTS as an idiosyncratic reaction.

Unfortunately, there is no reliable way to predict which patients on antiarrhythmic drug therapy will develop poly VT. Patients may develop the arrhythmia with previous uncomplicated administration of the drug; normal or prolonged QT_c prior to therapy (104); variable degree of QT_c prolongation with drug (sometimes normal, at time of arrhythmia or only abnormal after a pause (39,108) (Fig. 10.14); presence or absence of prodromal ECG signs described above, e.g., long-short sequences (these are not entirely specific or may precede arrhythmias by seconds or minutes so as to render them useless for prediction); therapeutic or even low drug levels (Fig. 10.20); previous uncomplicated treatment with the same or similar drug.

One reason why predictions are so difficult are the many contributing factors to acquired LQTS. For example, slight changes in heart rate or ionic milieu may bring on the syndrome when it would not have occurred otherwise. Thus, close observation of patients is necessary when starting agents with a potential for LQTS even if the same agent had been administered uneventfully in the past. The fact that half of the cases of poly VT occur within 4 days of drug initiation (39) makes for a useful, though imperfect window for in-hospital observation.

If a patient previously had LQTS due to an antiarrhythmic drug, it is not wise to use another possibly inciting agent, even if there had been a clear contributing factor such as hypokalemia. However, Class IB agents can be used in such patients (73,103,146).

The prognosis of drug-induced LQTS is variable. Removal of inciting agent will uniformly cause the arrhythmias to subside. However, early recognition of the syndrome is most important to prevent its lethal consequences.

OTHER CLINICAL STATES ASSOCIATED WITH A PROLONGED QT INTERVAL

Acquired Central Nervous System Disease

Certain central nervous system (CNS) diseases can cause acquired adrenergic syndromes similar to idiopathic LQTS. These

Table 10.6.
Causes of Pause-Dependent Long QT Syndrome

Antiarrhythmic drugs	Toxins
Class IA: quinidine, procainamide, disopyramide, bepridil[a]	Organophosphate insecticides
Class III: amiodarone, sotalol,[b] NAPA, bretylium	Heavy metals (Arsenic)
Other — encainide	Radiographic contrast media
Psychotropic drugs	Hypothyroidism
Phenothiazides (thioridazine most commonly reported)	Severe bradycardia
Tricyclic antidepressants	Nutritional deficiencies
Antibiotics	Anorexia nervosa
Ampicillin anaphylaxis	Liquid protein diets
Erythromycin	Electrolyte abnormalities
Trimethoprim sulfa	Hypokalemia
Pentamidine	Hypomagnesemia
Anthracyclines	Hypocalcemia (rarely)
Other drugs	Other
Doxorubicin	Coxsackie B3 myocarditis
Papaverine (intracoronary)	Idiopathic
Ketanserin (a selective S_2 serotonin antagonist)	
Lidoflazine	
Probucol	
Prenylamine	
Terfenadine (Seldane)	
Indoramin (an alpha blocker)	
Chloral hydrate	
Chui-feng-su-ho-wan (a Chinese herbal remedy)	

From Isner JM, Sours HE, Paris AL, *et al.*: Sudden, unexpected death in avid dieters using the liquid-protein-modified-fast diet: observations in 17 patients and the role of the prolonged QT interval. Circulation 1979;60:1401–1412; Fowler NO, McCall D, Chou T, *et al.*: Electrocardiographic changes and cardia arrhythmias in patients receiving psychotropic drugs. Am J Cardiol 1976;37:223–230; Karen A, Tzioni D, Davish A, *et al.*: Etiology of warning signs and therapy of torsades de pointes: a study of 10 patients. Circulation 1981;64:1167–1174; Koster RW, Wellens HJJ: Quinidine-induced ventricular flutter and fibrillation without digitalis therapy. Am J Cardiol 1976;38:519–523; Krikler DM, Curry PVL: Torsade de pointes, an atypical ventricular tachycardia. Br Heart J 1976;38:117–120; Jackman WM, Friday KJ, Anderson JL, *et al.*: Long QT syndromes: a critical review, new clinical observations and unified hypothesis. Prog Cardiovasc Dis 1988;31:115–172; Loeb HS, Pietras RJ, Gunnar RM, *et al.*: Paroxysmal ventricular fibrillation in two patients with hypomagnesemia: treatment by transvenous pacing. Circulation 1968;37:210– 215; Soffer J, Dreifus LS, Michelson EL: Polymorphous ventricular tachycardia: associated with normal and long Q-T intervals. Am J Cardiol 1982;49:2021–2029; Nguyen PT, Scheinman MM, Seger J: Polymorphous ventricular tachycardia: clinical characterization, therapy, and the QT interval. Circulation 1986;74:340–349; Bhandari AK, Scheinman M: The long QT syndrome. Mod Concepts Cardiovascular Dis 1985;54:45–50; Jackman WM, Clark M, Friday KJ, *et al.*: Ventricular tachyarrhythmias in the long Q-T syndromes. Med Clin North Am 1984;65:1079–1109; Kay GN, Plumb VJ, Archiniegas JG, *et al.*: Torsades de pointes: the long-short initiating sequence and other clinical features: observations in 32 patients. J Am Coll Cardiol 1983;2:806–817; Roden DM, Woosley RL, Primm RK: Incidence and clinical features of the quinidine-associated long QT syndrome: implications for patient care. Am Heart J 1986;111:1088–1093; Ejvinsson G, Prinius E: Prodromal ventricular premature beats preceded by a diastolic wave. Acta Med Scand 1980;208:445–450; Steinbrecher UP, Fitchett DH: Torsade de pointes: a cause of syncope with atrioventricular block. Arch Intern Med 1980;140:1223–1226; Chow MJ, Piergies AA, Bowsher DJ, *et al.*: Torsade de pointes induced by n-acetylprocainamide. J Am Coll Cardiol 1984;4:621–624; Bender KS, Shematek JP, Leventhal BG, *et al.*: QT interval prolongation associated with anthracycline cardiotoxicity. J Pediatr 1984;105:442; Abinader EG, Shahar J: Possible female preponderance in prenylamine-induced 'torsade de pointes' tachycardia. Cardiol 1983;70:37–40; Mehta D, Warwick GL, Goldberg MJ: QT prolongation after ampicillin anaphylaxis. Br Heart J, 1986;55:308–310; VanderMotten M, Verhaeghe R, DeGeest H: Ventricular arrhythmias and QT-prolongation during therapy with ketanserin: report of a case. Acta Cardiol 1989;44:431–437; Kern MJ, Deligonul U, Serota H, *et al.*: Ventricular arrhythmia due to intracoronary papaverine: analysis of QT intervals and coronary vasodilatory reserve. Cath Cardiovasc Diag 1990;19:229–236; Matsuhashi H, Onodera S, Kawamura Y, *et al.*: Probucol-induced QT prolongation and torsades de pointes. Jpn J Med 1989;28:612–615; Freedman RA, Anderson KP, Green LS, *et al.*: Effect of erythromycin on ventricular arrhythmias and ventricular repolarization in idiopathic long QT syndrome. Am J Cardiol 1987;59:168–169; Aunsholt NA: Prolonged Q-T interval and hypokalemia caused by haloperidol. Acta Psychiatr Scand 1989;79:411–412; Little RE, Kay GN, Cavender JB, *et al.*: Torsade de pointes and T-U wave alternans associated with arsenic poisoning. PACE 1990;13:164–170; Eiferman C, Chanson P, Cohen A, *et al.*: Torsades de pointes and Q-T prolongation in secondary hypothyroidism. Lancet 1988;1:170–171; Bryer-Ash M, Zehnder J, Angelchik P, *et al.*: Torsades de pointes precipitated by a Chinese herbal remedy. Am J Cardiol 1987;60:1186–1187; Nattel S, Ranger S, Talajic M, *et al.*: Erythromycin-induced long QT syndrome: concordance with quinidine and underlying cellular electrophysiologic mechanism. Am J Med 1990;89:235–238; Webb CL, Dick II M, Rocchini AP, *et al.*: Quinidine syncope in children. J Am Coll Cardiol 1987;9:1031–1037; James MA, Culling W, Jones JV: Polymorphous ventricular tachycardia due to alpha-blockade. Int J Cardiol 1987;14:225; McKibbin JK, Pocock WA, Barlow JB, *et al.*: Sotalol hypokalemia, syncope, and torsade de pointes. Br Heart J 1984;51:157; Neuvonen PJ, Elonen E, Vuorenmaa T, *et al.*: Prolonged Q-T interval and severe tachyarrhythmias, common features of sotalol intoxication. Eur J Clin Pharmacol 1981;20:85; Kennelly BM: Comparison of lidoflazine and quinidine in prophylactic treatment of arrhythmias. Br Heart J 1977;39:540; Barbey JT, Thompson KA, Echt DS, *et al.*: Antiarrhythmic activity, electrocardiographic effects and pharmacokinetics of the encainide metabolites O-desmethyl encainide and 3-meth-oxy-O-desmethyl encainide in man. Circulation 1988;77:380–388; Curry P, Fitchett D, Stubbs W, *et al.*: Ventricular arrhythmia and hypokalemia. Lancet 1976;2:231–233; Ludomirsky A, Klein HO, Sarelli P, *et al.*: Q-T prolongation and polymorphous ("torsade de pointes") ventricular arrhythmias associated with organophosphorus insecticide poisoning. Am J Cardiol 1982;49:1654–1658; Herrmann HC, Kaplan LM, Bierer BE: Q-T prolongation and torsades de pointes ventricular tachycardia produced by the tetracyclic antidepressant agent maprotiline. Am J Cardiol 1983;51:904–906; Luomanmaki K, Heikkila J, Hartikainen M: T-wave alternans associated with failure and hypomagnesemia in alcoholic cardiomyopathy. Eur J Cardiol 1975;3:167–170; Strasbuerg B, Sclarvsky S, Erdberg A, *et al.*: Procainamide-induced polymorphous ventricular tachycardia. Am J Cardiol 1981;47:1309–1314; Wald RW, Waxman MB, Coman JM; Torsade de pointes ventricular tachycardia: A complication of disopyramide shared with quinidine. J Electrocardiol 1981;14:301–308; Olshansky B, Martins J, Hunt S: N-acetylprocainamide causing torsades de pointes. Am J Cardiol 1982;50:1439–1441; Rothman MT: Prolonged QT interval, atrioventricular block, and torsade de pointes after antiarrhythmic therapy. Br Med J 1980;280:922–923; Tzivoni D, Keren A, Stern S, *et al.*: disopyramide-induced torsade de pointes. Arch Intern 1981;141:946–947; Leclercq JF, Kural S, Valere PE: Bepridil et torsades de point. Arch Mal Coeur 1983;76:341–348.

[a]Bepridil has both calcium channel blocking and Class IA antiarrhythmic properties.

[b]Sotalol has both beta blocking and Class III antiarrhythmic properties.

Abbreviations: NAPA = N-acetyl procainamide.

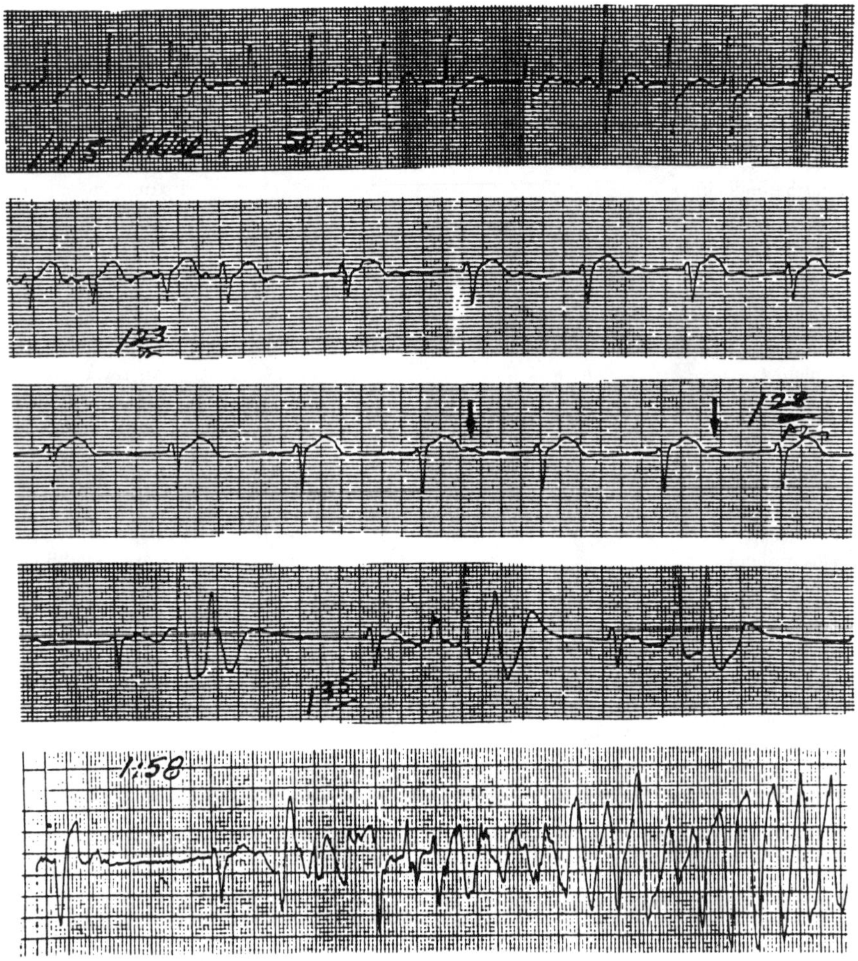

Figure 10.19. Poly VT developing in a 77-year-old female treated with quinidine and digitalis for atrial fibrillation. The *upper trace* shows atrial fibrillation. The *second* and *third traces* show sinus rhythm and junctional bradycardia following electroconversion. Note that in the *third trace* there is development of U wave (*arrows*), in the *fourth* and *fifth traces* there is development of poly VT preceded by short-long-short cycles. Note that poly VT has begun following and not before conversion of atrial fibrillation. (From Roden DM: The long QT syndrome and torsades de pointes: basic and clinical aspects. In El-Sherif N, Samet P (eds): Cardiac Pacing and Electrophysiology, WB Saunders, Philadelphia, 1991:265–284, with permission.)

include head injury (147,148), subarachnoid hemorrhage (44,149,150), cerebrovascular accident (151,152), surgical injuries to the autonomic nervous system (including those from radical neck dissection (45), carotid endarterectomy, and transabdominal truncal vagotomy (153)) and diabetic neuropathy (154). These conditions display many typical ECG features of LQTS except that severe arrhythmias are not common (usually just ventricular premature contractions (VPCs) but occur.

Mitral Valve Prolapse

Patients with mitral valve prolapse (MVP) may display typical LQTS with poly VT (155) and a therapeutic response to beta blockers or may have ventricular arrhythmias that are provocable by programmed stimulation and respond to the usual antiarrhythmic agents. Since MVP is so common, its association with LQTS may be coincidental (156). However, there is some evidence of autonomic dysfunction in MVP and beta blockers have been anecdotally advocated for ventricular arrhythmias in general in this condition (157).

Reported incidence of QT_c prolongation in mitral valve prolapse has been variable, i.e., has not been increased (158) or has been about 10–15% (159,160) with few patients displaying significant arrhythmia. Also, QT_c prolongation has been reported as either not associated with arrhythmia at all (156) or with a higher incidence when $QT_c \geq 0.51$ sec (161).

Diagnostic factors in Tables 10.3 and 10.5 plus electrophysiologic testing to distinguish more usual types of VT should be of help in properly assessing the MVP patient with significant ventricular arrhythmia.

Acute Myocardial Infarction

Some studies have shown that a prolonged QT interval following myocardial infarction predicts the occurrence of arrhythmias (162) and/or indicates a poor prognosis for total or sudden death (19,30) while others have not (163). The positive observations have fueled speculation that LQTS has wide implications for the problem of sudden death.

Interestingly patients with ischemic heart disease may have a blunted QT response to increased rate along with exercise induced arrhythmias (42). Also, QT_c prolongation may correlate with the number of vessels involved and poor ventricular function (164).

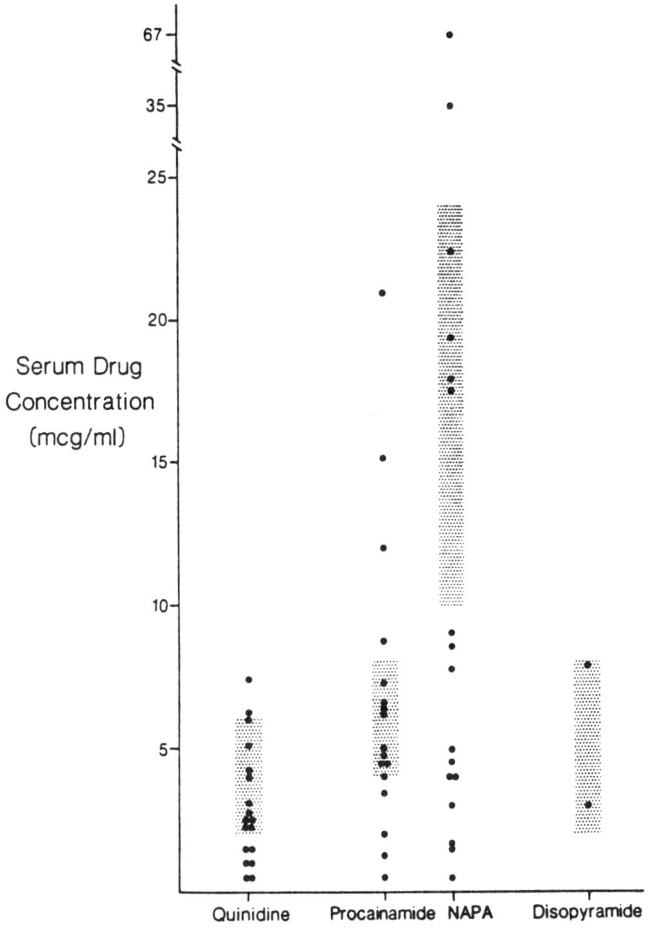

Figure 10.20. Drug levels of inciting "antirhythmic" drugs at time of TdP. *Stippled bars* represent the usually accepted therapeutic range. *Filled circles* represent 37 drug regimens in 30 patients. Note that in most patients with poly VT, drug levels were within or below the usually accepted therapeutic range. (From Jackman WM, Friday KJ, Anderson JL, *et al.*: Long QT syndromes: a critical review, new clinical observations, and unified hypothesis. Prog Cardiovasc Dis 1988;31:115–172, with permission.)

Sudden Infant Death Syndrome

An intriguing theory of the origin of sudden infant death syndrome (but with little evidence) is that it is due to (probably transient) LQTS (165). A long QT interval has been recorded in some (165) surviving patients and family members but not in others (166). LQTS probably does not account for most sudden infant deaths but may account for a few.

MECHANISMS OF LQTS

Although their ECG and arrhythmia appearances are rather similar, acquired and idiopathic LQTS seem to have different mechanisms. The adrenergic nervous system appears to be the key factor in idiopathic LQTS while certain cellular mechanisms related to afterdepolarizations appear the key to understanding acquired LQTS.

Acquired LQTS

There is considerable circumstantial evidence that arrhythmias in acquired LQTS are due to EAD-induced triggered activity. This phenomenon is described in Chapter 2, including clinical criteria that enable one to diagnose the abnormality. Briefly, EADs are afterdepolarizations that interrupt or prolong repolarization and triggered activations are new "activations" i.e., action potentials that arise in association with them (Fig. 2.13, Chapter 2). EADs and triggered activations may account for surface ECG changes such as prolonged QT intervals, T wave abnormalities, and the presence of U waves as well as poly VT (Fig. 10.1).

Circumstantial evidence in favor of EAD-induced triggered activity causing poly VT includes:

1. Poly VT displays the characteristics considered typical of early EAD-induced triggered activity including exquisite cycle length sensitivity, tendency for VT to occur in nonsustained bursts with a long first cycle length, some shortening of cycle lengths of subsequent ventricular beats and a later slowing down just prior to termination (Figs. 10.15–10.18; also see Chapter 2).
2. Long-short sequences described earlier as a prodrome for poly VT are also very typical of EAD-induced triggered activity.
3. Many of the same agents that prolong APD and cause typical EADs in vitro have also been found to cause poly VT in situ in both clinical and experimental studies, e.g., quinidine in the presence of low K^+, *N*-acetyl procainamide, aconitine, and cesium (23,57,106,107,167–170).
4. The same agents that suppress EADs and triggered activity in vitro, also suppress poly VT, e.g., magnesium and lidocaine.
5. Monophasic action potential recordings in both acquired and idiopathic LQTS (98,99,171) have displayed EADs.
6. EADs have been correlated with ECG U waves (23). In addition, postpause U wave changes and TU alternans that are highly typical of acquired LQTS are also consistent with the behavior of EADs.
7. Poly VT in acquired LQTS does not display features suggestive of reentry such as inducibility with programmed premature stimulation.

The "twisting" polymorphic pattern of TdP may be due to foci of triggered activation arising at two separate sites with "accrochage" (synchronization and fusion beats) (6,172). More complex patterns may be due to three or more foci. With monomorphic VT there is only one focus of origin of the arrhythmia. However, varying exit conduction patterns from one site could also explain TdP pattern (173). Studies of possible factors that influence the likelihood of a triggered activation conducting out from its site of origin, e.g., its amplitude, may add to our understanding of the origin of the poly VT pattern (174,176).

Antiarrhythmic drugs may impact on EADs and triggered activations in various ways either in a pro- or antiarrhythmic direction (Chapter 2). Drugs that prolong APD such as Class IA and III agents induce or favor the phenomenon. Drugs that suppress inward Ca^{2+} (Class IV agents) or Na^{+} current (Class IA, B, and C agents) tend to suppress triggered activations which are based on these currents. This may explain why a Class IA drug like disopyramide can either cause or suppress the phenomenon. It could, for example, induce EADs and consequent QT_c prolongation but suppress any triggered activations that might result from the EADs (Chapter 2). This concept may explain why poly VT occurs at only modest drug levels of the Class IA agents. These levels may be high enough to prolong repolarization and induce EADs but not high enough to suppress the triggered activations.

Drugs that shorten APD, such as the Class IB agents, suppress or reverse LQTS. Ca^{2+} channel blockers should also suppress the phenomenon by suppressing triggered activations and sometimes by shortening APD (177).

Amiodarone is interesting. It should favor the phenomenon by prolonging APD. On the other hand, it suppresses inward Na^{2+} and Ca^{2+} currents and thus suppresses triggered activations. This may explain why LQTS has been unusual (but possible) (18,103,178) with amiodarone and why the drug has, at times, been successfully used to treat this arrhythmia.

Idiopathic LQTS

Idiopathic LQTS is harder to explain than is the acquired syndrome. In particular, it is not clear just how the autonomic nerve system plays its crucial role (39).

The two general lines of thinking have been: (a) There is an imbalance of sympathetic input to the heart causing a disparity in refractoriness which in turn leads to reentrant arrhythmias (100,179,180) (see also Chapter 2); (b) Patients with congenital LQTS have a cellular defect in repolarization that is intensified or unmasked by sympathetic stimulations.

The sympathetic imbalance hypothesis (100) was originally based on the observation by Yanowitz, *et al.* (20) that right stellate ganglion interruption or left stellate stimulation in dogs caused QT_c prolongation. How an intervention that shortens APD (left stellate sympathetic stimulation) also prolongs QT_c was explained as follows. As indicated earlier, repolarization in some parts of the heart continues after the end of the T wave and is ECG silent because of cancellation of electrical forces to the body surface. Left stellate stimulation by shortening APD in one zone of the heart would unmask the previously canceled forces, extend the T wave, and thereby prolong QT_c (9,20).

It should be noted that in this study only one ECG lead was recorded; the converse sympathetic maneuvers, i.e., right stimulation and left interruption, did not prolong QT_c; there were no arrhythmias (20); and QT_c prolongation was transient and was in fact followed by QT_c shortening (181).

Other evidence for the sympathetic balance hypothesis have been uncertain. Later results with sympathetic stimulation in animals have been inconsistent with variable ECGs and induction of arrhythmias which were usually mild in any case (8,182–185). Evidence in humans for sympathetic imbalance can otherwise be explained. Favorable results of left-sided sympathetic denervation (equivalent to stellectomy in animals) in patients with idiopathic LQTS usually do not result in QT_c normalization (186). Locally varying monophasic APD, refractory periods, or repolarization on body surface maps in patients with LQTS are consistent with but do not prove the sympathetic imbalance (55,99,180,198), and one case of congenital LQTS did not benefit from complete sympathetic denervation by auto transplantation (188). In addition, as indicated earlier, evidence in LQTS arrhythmias does not favor a reentrant mechanism which is the postulated result of sympathetic imbalance.

Most observers are now moving to explain idiopathic LQTS as a defect in cellular repolarization, perhaps via a K^{+} channel, leading to EADs and triggered activations that are enhanced or elicited by adrenergic stimulation. This would explain the inconsistent findings on ECGs and arrhythmias of adrenergic interventions in humans and animals noted above as well as a number of other observations including:

1. ECGs and arrhythmias are similar in congenital and acquired LQTS.
2. Pacing has been effective in suppressing some arrhythmias in idiopathic (79,189) as it is in acquired LQTS suggesting an EAD mechanism.
3. Magnesium (190) and lidocaine (73) which shorten APD and suppress EADs also suppress arrhythmias in both idiopathic and acquired LQTS.
4. EADs have been recorded in both congenital and acquired LQTS (98,171).
5. Catecholamines can enhance EADs in vitro (106,176).
6. Intravenous catecholamines which cause generalized and not localized adrenergic stimulation, induce typical abnormalities in congenital LQTS (58,99).

Two recent studies are helpful here. Shimuzu, *et al.* (99) found that the β-agonist isoproterenol prolonged monophasic APD and QT_c interval and induced EADs not present at baseline in patients with congenital LQTS (Fig. 10.21). These EADs appeared in both right and left ventricles, i.e., in the distribution of both right and left sympathetic ganglia, and they occurred in fast rates. In normal controls, isoproterenol shortened APD and QT_c and did not induce EADs. This study provides substantial evidence for the adrenergic enhanced EAD hypothesis (for which there had been some direct experimental evidence earlier (57)).

Ben David and Zipes (191) found in dogs that cesium-induced EADs were enlarged and arrhythmias were induced more by bilateral or left than right ansa subclavia stimulation and were also enlarged by intravenous catecholamines. Enlargement of EAD amplitude would favor transmission of triggered activations

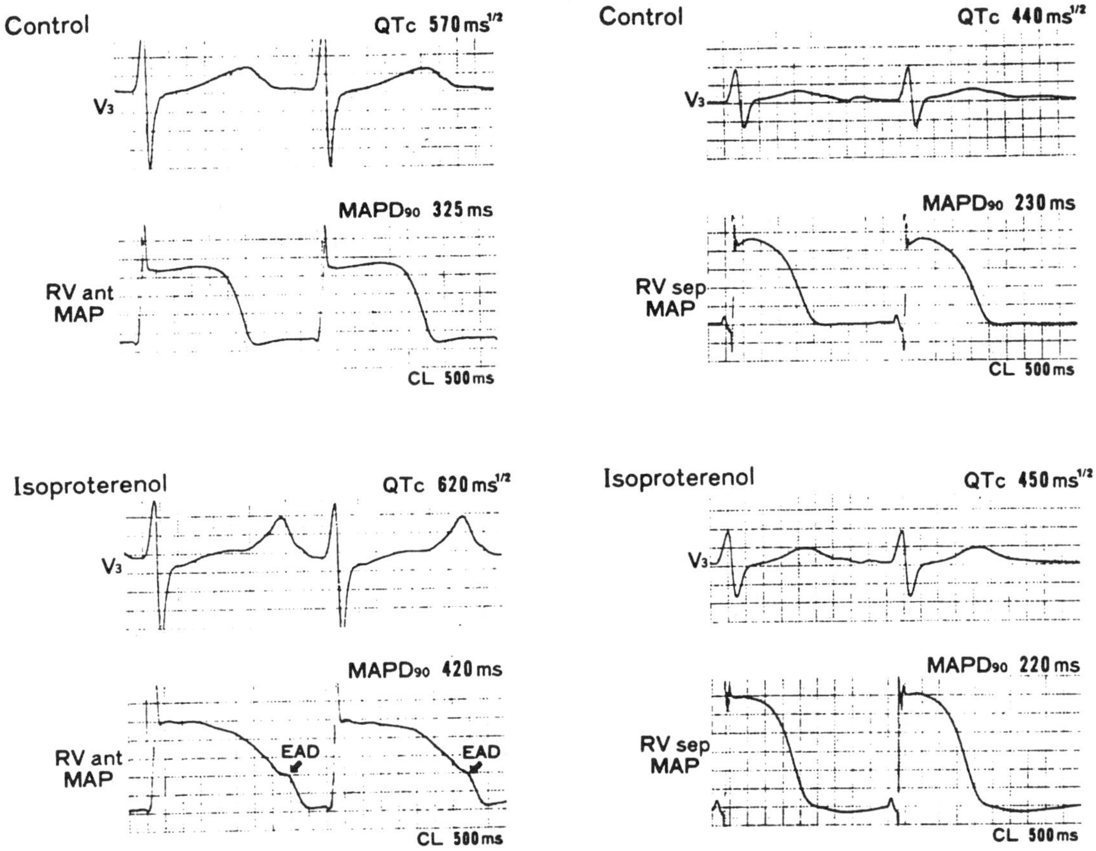

Figure 10.21. Effect of isoproterenol on QT_C interval and monophasic APD in patients with (**left**) and without (**right**) idiopathic LQTS. In the patient with LQTS (**left**), isoproterenol infusion increases both QT_C and monophasic APD and induces an EAD. In the normal patient (**right**), QT_C and monophasic APD did not change significantly after isoproterenol and EAD does not develop. $MAPD_{90}$ = monophasic action potential duration at 90% of repolarization; RV ant MAP = right ventricular anterior monophasic action potential; RV sep MAP = RV septal MAP; V_3 = ECG. (From Shimizu W, Ohe T, Kurita T, *et al.*: Early afterdepolarizations induced by isoproterenol in patients with congenital long QT syndrome. Circulation 1991;84:1915–1923, by permission of the American Heart Association, Inc.)

from localized abnormal zones and thus favor arrhythmias (174). Greater effect of left-sided sympathetic stimulation was attributed to innervation of a greater mass of the heart (191) rather than sympathetic imbalance.

Thus findings in LQTS appear to be explicable by EADs that are enhanced by or may have a particular sensitivity to adrenergic stimulation and that are perhaps caused by a genetic defect in the cellular membrane K^+ channel (49). Left-sided sympathetic interruption is thus especially effective because the left ganglia innervate a substantial part of the heart.

This explanation leaves some interesting unanswered questions.

1. Why is sympathetic denervation more effective than beta blockade (see below)? This suggests a role for α-adrenergic stimulation which has been shown to prolong APD and enhance EADs and ventricular arrhythmias while alpha blockade (specifically alpha-2 blockade) suppresses them (193). In addition, difficulty in long-term compliance, less than complete beta blockade, and varying serum levels which at times may fall below minimum effective concentration with oral agents may be other factors in the better results of surgery.

2. Why is there a tendency for arrhythmias to be initiated at fast basic rates in idiopathic but not acquired LQTS? One possibility is that heightened sympathetic stimulation serves to both induce EADs and speed the heart rate, especially if for some reason EADs in congenital LQTS are especially sensitive to catecholamine. However, it is also true that slow rates and pauses not uncommonly precede arrhythmias in idiopathic LQTS and pacemaker therapy may be beneficial (see below). Another possibility is that delayed afterdepolarizations (DADs), which are induced or enhanced at fast rates and by catecholamines (194) are also involved in LQTS but there is thus far no evidence for this.

3. Why do sinus bradycardia, pauses, and a blunted heart rate response to exercise and atropine occur in idiopathic LQTS suggesting sympathetic dysfunction? This question is difficult to answer via the EAD hypothesis. One possibility is that prolongation of APD in the sinus node (180) or transitional atrial cells adjacent to the sinus node rather than autonomic dysfunction creates the bradycardia or pauses. A similar abnormality in the AV conduction system could explain AV blocks and condition delays that occur in congenital LQTS (91,195).

4. Why does heightened adrenergic activity not appear to play a role in acquired LQTS? Perhaps it has not been tested adequately since administration of adrenergic agents would be most dangerous and patients are probably at any rate in a heightened sympathetic state at times of poly VT. Interestingly, the postelectroconversion state is one of heightened sympathetic stimulation and TdP seems prone to occur at this time (39,74) (Fig. 10.19).

TREATMENT OF LONG QT SYNDROME

Idiopathic Long QT Syndrome

MEASURES

Antiadrenergic measures are the logical therapy for congenital LQTS. The primary antiadrenergic therapy is beta blockade, usually propranolol (75,76,100). Beta blockade should be as complete as possible; reduction of maximum heart rate to 130 beats/min on excise testing has been suggested as an endpoint (40). In patients who develop excessive bradycardia or in whom ventricular arrhythmias emerge at slow rates, pacemakers are advised (40).

Beta blockers are usually taken alone. However, Class IB drugs (lidocaine acutely and mexiletine, tocainide, and phenytoin chronically) may be adjunctively used (10,86,146, 196) as may magnesium sulfate (197,198) (acutely) and primidone (chronically) (199). In one report, propranolol along with phenytoin was successfully administered via a drug reservoir infusion pump system in a patient refractory to oral therapy (196). The pump overcame the problem of missed doses and varying serum levels.

Left sympathectomy was first reported for LQTS by Moss and McDonald (11) and has been used in patients who are refractory to beta blockers, especially those at high risk patients.

There are three types of procedures used to achieve cardiac sympathetic denervation (186). Left stellectomy refers to ablation of the left stellate ganglion which is a fusion of the eighth cervical and first thoracic ganglia. Since ocular nerve fibers cross the upper part of the stellate ganglia, this procedure causes an obligatory Horner's syndrome and leads to only limited cardiac sympathetic denervation.

The other two procedures are called left cervical thoracic sympathectomy and high thoracic left sympathectomy (186). Both of these involve removal of the first four to five thoracic ganglia providing adequate cardiac sympathetic denervation (these are equivalent to stellectomy in animals). However, in the former there is an addition complete left stellectomy and an obligatory Horner's syndrome while in high thoracic left sympathectomy there is an ablation of lower part of the stellate and no or a minimal Horner's syndrome. Thus, though Horner's syndrome is common, it is neither obligatory nor an index of successful denervation.

In the above procedures the surgeon generally utilizes the supraclavicular extrapleural approach. Prior testing with local pharmacologic blockade is no longer used. Operative mortality has been virtually zero (186).

Beta blockers are maintained after sympathetic denervation for several months since surgical success is not assured, circulating catecholamines are still present, and arrhythmias may recur for many months. In some patients, refractoriness of arrhythmias to beta blockade prior to surgery changes to responsiveness afterwards (75,82).

Permanent pacemakers of various types appear to be effective in suppressing ventricular arrhythmias (with and without adrenergic provocation) (79,189,200,201) and in preventing syncopal episodes in idiopathic LQTS. They are generally used adjunctively when beta blockers and/or cardiac sympathetic denervation are not sufficiently effective alone or when there is spontaneous or drug induced bradycardia or A-V block. Pacemakers have been set in the 70–90 beats/min range (189). Use of a QT-sensitive cybernetic pacemaker is an interesting suggestion but remains untested (202).

Implantable cardioverter defibrillator therapy is now reserved for "last resort" therapy (203). However, one can expect more widespread use in idiopathic LQTS especially as more sophisticated devices become available. Coexisting pharmacologic therapy and/or sympathetic denervation to reduce episodes and avoid frequent shocks must accompany this form of therapy as well.

In addition to the above measures, conditions and agents that exacerbate the abnormalities should be curtailed. Avoidance of stimuli that cause adrenergic arousal such as loud noises (e.g., phone ringing, rock concerts, and firearm shooting) is recommended in high-risk groups (39). Also to be avoided are alcohol, which can cause adrenergic stimulation, tobacco, adrenergic decongestants, etc. as well as Class I and Class III antiarrhythmic agents (amiodarone has been used as treatment but is not generally recommended) and agents which lower serum K^+ or Mg^{2+} such as diuretics.

The question of recreational exercise or professional sports can in this, as in other situations be a difficult one (39). It should generally be avoided, especially competitive sports, but this, of course, depends on the risk level of the patient and the results of exercise tests. These and other adrenergic provocative tests have also been suggested as an evaluation for sensitive occupations, such as commercial airline pilot (30). Pregnancy does not exacerbate LQTS but beta blockers should be continued (40).

Regarding anesthesia for surgery performed in idiopathic LQTS, thiopental, vecuronium, fentanyl, isoflurane (204), and spinal (205) and epidural (206) anesthesia have been used safely.

Immediate endpoints for evaluating treatment are somewhat of a problem. Shortening of QT_c may not occur even when treatment is successful especially with beta blockade; after surgical sympathectomy QT_c returns to normal in only 11% of patients (186,207). Adrenergic provocative measures, especially exercise stress tests or, when appropriate, patient-specific stimuli are helpful. Intravenous catecholamines induce an adrenergic state of an intensity that will never occur naturally (39) and thus may not be of practical use as an endpoint for therapy.

It is also difficult to assess the long-term results of therapy. While there is no doubt of the efficacy of antiadrenergic therapy, the small numbers of patients with LQTS, lack of randomized studies (which would be most difficult to do), and reliance on observational data hamper precise evaluation. Also data on children, who may have a more virulent pathologic process (79), is especially scanty.

In 1985, Moss, *et al.* reported that risk ratio (i.e., relative risk with vs without therapy) of syncope/mortality was lowered to 0.41 by propranolol and to 0.25 by left cardiac sympathectomy (75).

Recently, in a data base of 85 high-risk congenital LQTS patients treated from 1969 to 1985, left sympathectomy markedly reduced cardiac events (syncope and sudden death). The number of patients without symptoms increased from 1 to 55% and mean number of cardiac events decreased from 22 to 1 (186). These encouraging, though nonrandomized results may place sympathectomy at a higher notch in the treatment hierarchy.

Overall, it has been said that aggressive triple therapy (beta blockers, surgical sympathectomy, and pacemakers) suppress malignant arrhythmias in 95% of patients (39).

SELECTION OF PATIENTS FOR THERAPY

Because of the variable nature of idiopathic LQTS, selection of patients for and hierarchy of therapy presents a problem. It is clear that patients in higher-risk categories (see Tables 10.4 and 10.5) should be treated maximally (including implantable defibrillators if triple therapy is not successful). For family members and borderline cases, careful history, ECGs, and exercise tests with attention to factors that convey risk is a practical approach. One should note that family members with normal QT_c are at extremely low risk. Fig. 10.12 is an algorithm for patient evaluation and care suggested by Moss and Robinson (39).

Acquired LQTS

Early recognition and observation on monitoring units is crucial to the management of acquired LQTS. Arrhythmias are dangerous, tend to be repetitive and progressive, and may continue on to VF (or sustained VT). However, about half of the patients never have hemodynamic compromise or symptoms (105).

Removal of the offending cause will cause arrhythmias to subside in acquired LQTS but there is a time lag as the agent or condition (e.g., electrolyte imbalance) and its effects are cleared from the body.

Acceleration of heart rate suppresses the arrhythmias and ECG abnormalities. This is accomplished most rapidly by an infusion of isoproterenol, 1–4 μg/min (15,84) to maintain rate at about 90 beats/min. (Note isoproterenol is therapeutic in acquired while provocative in idiopathic LQTS.) Adverse affects of isoproterenol include increased myocardial oxygen demand, a problem in patients in ischemic heart disease, possible undue acceleration of heart rate, and hypotension. Isoproterenol is generally but not uniformally effective.

If arrhythmias persist for any length of time temporary pacing is the next step (15,72,84) (Fig. 10.18). Generally, ventricular rather than atrial pacing is performed because of the stability of the electrode placement, the ability to control heart rate at the precise level to suppress the arrhythmia and the occasional occurrence of blocks with atrial pacing. However, an atrial contribution to cardiac output is not provided and placement of the ventricular electrode may cause ventricular irritability.

Patients generally do well with these measures. Other therapies include magnesium (190,208) and Class IB antiarrhythmic agents (73).

Magnesium sulfate which has been previously used for digitalis-toxic, alcoholic, and other ventricular arrhythmias (209) suppresses EADs, triggered activations, and TdP, and shortens QT_c in animal models (174,210). The mechanism may be enhancement of NaK adenosinetriphosphatase (ATPase) (Na-K pump) or inward calcium current (I_{Ca}) blockade (210).

Dose of magnesium sulfate in TdP is 1–2 g intravenously followed in some cases by another infusion of 2–4 g or continuous infusion of 3–20 mg/min (190). Effectiveness of magnesium has been variable (190) but does not depend on an initially low serum magnesium level. The drug dissipates quickly and adverse effects are minimal (flushing) (190,208).

Intravenous lidocaine, which is administered in the usual clinical doses (see Chapter 12), is occasionally effective (73,211) in acquired LQTS. Bretylium tosylate has been reported to be both anti (16,212) and proarrhythmic (73).

It should be noted that it is always difficult to distinguish drug effectiveness against arrhythmia versus spontaneous regression in acute arrhythmia situations, especially when concurrent measures have been taken.

Beta blockers are generally considered deleterious in acquired LQTS because of bradycardia although there are occasional reports of effectiveness (16). Ca^{2+} channel blockers may be deleterious if they slow heart rate, but they have been reported to be effective (213) and have some theoretical (diminished slow inward current) and experimental (177) justification.

References

1. Jervell A, Lange-Nielsen F: Congenital deaf-mutism functional heart disease with prolongation of the QT interval and sudden death. Am Heart J 1957;54:59–68.
2. Ward OC: A new familial cardiac syndrome in children. J Irish Med Assoc 1964;54:103–106.
3. Romano C, Gemme G, Pongiglione R: Aritmie cardiache rare dell'eta pediatrica. Clin Pediatr 1963;45:656–661.
4. Romano C: Congenital cardiac arrhythmias. Lancet 1965;1:658–659.
5. Dessertenne F: La tachycardia ventricular à deux foyers opposés variables. Arch Mal Coeur 1966;59:263–272.
6. Schwartz PJ, Stone HL, Brown AM: Effects of unilateral stellate ganglion blockade on the arrhythmias associated with coronary occlusion. Am Heart J 1976;92:589–599.

7. Schwartz PJ, Malliani A: Electrical alternation of the T wave: clinical and experimental evidence of its relationship with the sympathetic nervous system and with the long QT syndrome. Am Heart J 1975;89:45–50.
8. Schwartz PJ, Verrier RL, Lown B: Effect of stellectomy and vagotomy on ventricular refractoriness in dogs. Circ Res 1977;40:536–546.
9. Burgess MJ, Millar K, Abildskov JA: Cancellation of electrocardiographic effects during ventricular recovery. J Electrocardiol 1969;2:101–108.
10. Crampton R: Preeminence of the left stellate ganglion in the long Q-T syndrome. Circulation 1979;59:769–778.
11. Moss AJ, McDonald J: Unilateral cervicothoracic sympathetic ganglionectomy for the treatment of long QT interval syndrome. N Engl J Med 1971;285:903–904.
12. Isner JM, Sours HE, Paris AL, *et al.*: Sudden, unexpected death in avid dieters using the liquid-protein-modified-fast diet: observations in 17 patients and the role of the prolonged QT interval. Circulation 1979;60:1401–1412.
13. Fowler NO, McCall D, Chou T, *et al.*: Electrocardiographic changes and cardiac arrhythmias in patients receiving psychotropic drugs. Am J Cardiol 1976;37:223–230.
14. Kember AJ, Dunlap R, Pietro DA: Thioridazine-induced torsade de pointes. JAMA 1983;249:2931–2934.
15. Keren A, Tzioni D, Davish A, *et al.*: Etiology, warning signs and therapy of torsades de pointes: a study of 10 patients. Circulation 1981;64:1167–1174.
16. Koster RW, Wellens HJJ: Quinidine-induced ventricular flutter and fibrillation without digitalis therapy. Am J Cardiol 1976;38:519–523.
17. Krikler DM, Curry PVL: Torsade de pointes, an atypical ventricular tachycardia. Br Heart J 1976;38:117–120.
18. Nicholson WJ, Martin LE, Gracey JG, *et al.*: Disopyramide-induced ventricular fibrillation. Am J Cardiol 1979;43:1053–1055.
19. Puddu PE, Bourassa MG: Prediction of sudden death from QT_c interval prolongation in patients with chronic ischemic heart disease. J Electrocardiol 1986;19:203–212.
20. Yanowitz R, Preston JB, Abildskov JA: Functional distribution of right and left stellate innervation to the ventricles: Production of neurogenic electrocardiographic changes by unilateral alteration of sympathetic tone. Circ Res 1966;18:416–428.
21. Wantanabe Y, Toda H: The U wave and aberrant intraventricular conduction: Further evidence for the Purkinje repolarization theory on the genesis of the U wave. Am J Cardiol 1978;41:23–31.
22. Hoffman BF, Cranefield P: Electrophysiology of the Heart. McGraw-Hill, New York, 1960.
23. Habbab MA, El-Sherif N: Drug-induced torsades de pointes: role of early afterdepolarizations and dispersion of repolarization. Am J Med 1990;89: 241–246.
24. Ahnve S: Correction of the QT interval for heart rate: Review of different formulas and the use of Bazett's formula in myocardial infarction. Am Heart J 1985;109:568–574.
25. Bazett HC: An analysis of the time-relations of electrocardiograms. Heart 1920;7:353–370.
26. Hodges M, Salerno D, Erlien D: Bazett's QT correction reviewed: Evidence that a linear QT correction for heart rate is better. (Abstract) J Am Coll Cardiol 1983;1:694.
27. Manion CV, Whitsett TL, Wilson MF: Applicability of correcting the QT interval for heart rate. Am Heart J 1980;99:678.
28. Ashman R: The normal duration of the QT interval. Am Heart J 1942; 23:522–534.
29. Kovacs SJ: The duration of the QT interval as a function of heart rate: a derivation based on physical principles and a comparison to measured values. Am Heart J 1985;110:872–878.
30. Ward DE: Prolongation of the QT interval as an indicator of risk of cardiac event. Eur Heart J 1988;9:139–144.
31. Browne KF, Zipes DP, Heger JJ, *et al.*: Influence of the autonomic nervous system on the Q-T interval in man. Am J Cardiol 1982;50:1099–1103.
32. Huang MH, Ebey J, Wolf S: Manipulating the QT interval of the ECG by cognitive effort. Pav J Biol Sci 1989;24:102–108.
33. Bexton RS, Fallin HO, Camm AJ: Diurnal variation of the QT interval—influence of the autonomic nervous system. Br Heart J 1986;55:253–258.
34. Browne KF, Prystowksy E, Heger JJ, *et al.*: Prolongation of the QT interval in man during sleep. Am J Cardiol 1983;3:55–59.
35. Gillis AM, MacLean KE, Guilleminault C: The QT interval during wake and sleep in patients with ventricular arrhythmias. Sleep 1988;11:333–339.
36. Solti F, Szatmary L, Vecsey T, *et al.*: The effect of sympathetic and parasympathetic activation on QT duration: clinical study in patients with normal and prolonged QT time. Cor Vasa 1989;31:9–15.
37. Ahnve S, Vallin H: Influence of the heart rate and inhibition of autonomic tone on the QT interval. Circulation 1982;65:435–439.
38. Laks MM: Long QT Interval Syndrome: a new look at an old electrocardiographic measurement: the power of the computer. Circulation 1990;82: 1539–1541.
39. Jackman WM, Friday KJ, Anderson JL, *et al.*: Long QT syndromes: a critical review, new clinical observations and unified hypothesis. Prog Cardiovasc Dis 1988;31:115–172.
40. Moss AJ, Robinson J: Identification of high-risk population: clinical features of the idiopathic long QT syndrome. Circulation 1992;85:140–144.
41. Gottlieb S, Moss AJ, Hall WJ, *et al.*: Statistical identification of delayed repolarization: Applicability in long QT syndrome (LQTS) population (Abstr). J Am Coll Cardiol 1991;17:241A.
42. Löllgen H, Wollschläger H, Schönrich G, *et al.*: Ventricular arrhythmias and QT_c interval during stress-ECG. Herz 1986;11:303–308.
43. AHA Committee Report: Recommendations for standardization of leads and of specifications for instruments in electrocardiography and vectorcardiography. Circulation 1967;35:583–602.
44. Carruth JE, Silverman ME: Torsade de Pointe: atypical ventricular tachycardia complicating subarachnoid hemorrhage. Chest 1980;78:886–888.
45. Hugenholtz PG: Electrocardiographic changes typical for central nervous system disease after right radical neck dissection. Am Heart J 1976;74:438–440.
46. Meissner FL: Taubstummenheit and taubstunnmenbldung. Leipzig und Heidelberg, 1985;6:119–120.
47. Fraser GR, Froggatt P, James TN: Congenital deafness associated with electrocardiographic abnormalities, fainting attacks and sudden death: A recessive syndrome. Q J Med 1964;33:361–385.
48. Itoh S, Munemura S, Satoh HH: A study of the inheritance pattern of Romano-Ward Syndrome. Clin Pediatr (Phila) 1982;21:20–24.
49. Keating M, Atkinson D, Dunn C, *et al.*: Linkage of a cardiac arrhythmia, the long QT syndrome, and the Harvey ras-1 gene. Science 1991;252:704–706.
50. Schwartz PJ: Autonomic modulation of arrhythmias in patients, In Rosen MR, Janse MJ, Wit AL. (eds): Cardiac Electrophysiology. Futura Publishing Co., Mt. Kisco, NY, 1990:951–966.
51. Schwartz PJ, Locati E: The idiopathic long QT syndrome: pathogenetic mechanisms and therapy. Eur Heart J 1985;6:103–114.
52. Benhorin J, Merri M, Alberti M, *et al.*: Long QT syndrome: new electrocardiographic characteristics. Circulation 1990;82:521–527.
53. Merri M, Benhorin J, Alberti M, *et al.*: Electrocardiographic quantitation of ventricular repolarization. Circulation 1989;80:1301–1308.
54. Rode P, Stajer D, Horvat M, *et al.*: Romano-Ward syndrome: Case report, family study and signal averaged electrocardiogram. Cor Vasa 1190;32:335–342.
55. Coumel P: Early afterdepolarizations and triggered activity in clinical arrhythmias. Rosen MR, Janse MJ et al. Cardiac Electrophysiology: A Textbook, 1990;387–411.
56. Santinelli V, Chiarello M: Heart rate acceleration without changes in the QT interval and severe ventricular tachyarrhythmias: a variant of the long QT syndrome. Int J Cardiol 1983;4:69–71.
57. Schechter E, Freeman CC, Lazzara R: Afterdepolarizations as a mechanism for the long QT syndrome: Electrophysiological studies of a case. J Am Coll Cardiol 1984;3:1556–1561.
58. Garza LA, Vick RL, Nora JJ, *et al.*: Heritable QT prolongation without deafness. Circulation 1970;41:39–48.

59. Milne JR, Ward DE, Suprell RAJ, *et al.*: The long QT syndrome: effects of drugs and left stellate ganglion block. Am Heart J 1982;104:194–198.
60. Edvardsson N, Olsson SB: Induction of delayed repolarization during chronic beta-receptor blockade. Eur Heart J 1985;6:163–169.
61. Kupersmith J, Shiang HS: Electrophysiologic effects of beta drenergic blockade with practolol in canine acute myocardial ischemia. J Pharmacol Exp Ther 1979;207:976–982.
62. Jervell A: The surdo-cardiac syndrome. Heart J 1985;6:97–102.
63. Smirk FH, Ng J: Cardiac ballet repetitions of complex electrocardiographic patterns. Br Heart J 1969;31:426–434.
64. Smith WM, Gallagher JJ: "Les Torsades de Pointes": an unusual ventricular arrhythmia. Ann Intern Med 1980;93:578–584.
65. Zilcher H, Glogar D, Kaindl F: Torsades de pointes: occurrence in myocardial ischemia as a separate entity. Multiform ventricular tachycardia or not? Eur Heart J 1980;1:63–71.
66. Rankin R, Parizel G: Ventricular fibrillo-flutter ("Torsade de Pointe"): an established electrocardiographic and clinical entity. Report of eight cases. Angiology 1977;28:115–117.
67. MacWilliams JA: Some applications of physiology to medicine, II. Ventricular fibrillation and sudden death. Br Med J 1923;2:215–219.
68. Loeb HS, Pietras RJ, Gunnar RM, *et al.*: Paroxysmal ventricular fibrillation in two patients with hypomagnesemia: treatment by transvenous pacing. Circulation 1968;37:210–215.
69. Schwartz SP, Margolies MP, Firenzi A: Transient ventricular fibrillation. V. The effects of oral administration of quinidine sulphate on patients with transient ventricular fibrillation during established auriculo-ventricular dissociation. Am Heart J 1953;45:404–415.
70. Kossmann CE: Torsade de pointes: an addition to the nosography of ventricular tachycardia. Am J Cardiol 1977;42:1054–1056.
71. Sclarovksy S, Strasburg B, Lewin RF, Agmon J: Polymorphous ventricular tachycardia: clinical features and treatment. Am J Cardiol 1979;44:339–344.
72. Soffer J, Dreifus LS, Michelson EL: Polymorphous ventricular tachycardia associated with normal and long Q-T intervals. Am J Cardiol 1982;49:2021–2029.
73. Nguyen PT, Scheinman MM, Seger J: Polymorphous ventricular tachycardia: clinical characterization, therapy, and the QT interval. Circulation 1986;74:340–349.
74. Roden DM: The long QT syndrome and torsades de pointes: basic and clinical aspects. In El-Sherif N, Samet P (eds): Cardiac Pacing and Electrophysiology. WB Saunders, Philadelphia, 1991:265–284.
75. Moss AJ, Schwartz PJ, Crampton RS, *et al.*: The long QT syndrome: a prospective international study. Circulation 1985;71:17–21.
76. Moss AJ, Schwartz PJ, Crampton RS, *et al.*: The long QT syndrome: prospective longitudinal study of 328 families. Circulation 1991;84:1136–1144.
77. Matthews EC Jr, Blount AW Jr, Townsend JL: QT prolongation and ventricular arrhythmias with and without deafness in the same family. Am J Cardiol 1972;29:702–711.
78. Jervell A, Thingstad R, Endsjo TO: The surdocardiac syndrome. Three new cases of congenital deafness with syncopal attacks and QT prolongation in the electrocardiogram. Am Heart J 1966;72:582–593.
79. Weintraub RG, Gow RM, Wilkinson JL: The congenital long QT syndromes in childhood. J Am Coll Cardiol 1990;16:674–680.
80. Singer PA, Crampton RS, Bass NH: Familial QT prolongation syndrome. Convulsive seizure and paroxysmal ventricular fibrillation. Arch Neurol 1974;31:64–66.
81. Gospe SM, Choy M: Hereditary long Q-T syndrome presenting as epilepsy: electroencephalography laboratory diagnosis. Ann Neurol 1989;(25):514–516.
82. Schwartz PJ, Periti M, Malliani A: The long QT syndrome. Am Heart J 1975;84:378–390.
83. Coumel P, Fidelle J, Lucet V, *et al.*: Catecholamine-induced severe ventricular arrhythmias with Adams-Stokes syndrome in children: Report of four cases. Br Heart J 1978 (Suppl);40:28–37.
84. Bhandari AK, Scheinman M: The long QT syndrome. Mod Concepts Cardiovasc Dis 1985;54:45–50.
85. Moss AJ, Schwartz PJ: Delayed repolarization (QT or QTU prolongation) and malignant ventricular arrhythmias. Mod Concepts Cardiovasc Dis 1980;51:85–90.
86. Wellens HJJ, Vermuelen A, Durrer D: Ventricular fibrillation occurring on arousal from sleep by auditory stimuli. Circulation 1972;46:661–665.
87. Schrem SS, Belsky P, Schwartzman D, *et al.*: Cocaine-induced torsades de pointes in a patient with the idiopathic long Q-T syndrome. Am Heart J 1990;120:980–984.
88. Vincent GM: The heart rate of Romano-Ward syndrome patients. Am Heart J 1986;112:61–64.
89. Curtiss EI, Heiber RH, Shaver JA: Autonomic maneuvers in hereditary Q-T interval prolongation (Romano-Ward syndrome). Am Heart J 1978;95:420–428.
90. Kernohan RJ, Froggett P: Atrioventricular dissociation with prolonged QT interval and syncopal attacks in a 10-year-old boy. Br Heart J 1974;36:516–519.
91. Greenspon AJ, Kidwell GA, Barrasse LD, *et al.*: Hereditary long QT syndrome associated with cardiac conduction system disease. PACE 1989; 12:479–485.
92. VanHare GF, Franz MR, Rogé C. *et al.*: Persistent functional atrioventricular block in two patients with prolonged QT intervals: elucidation of the mechanism of block. PACE 1990;13:608–618.
93. Jackman WM, Clark M, Friday KJ, *et al.*: Ventricular tachyarrhythmias in the long Q-T syndromes. Med Clin North Am 1984;65:1079–1109.
94. Shaw TRD: Recurrent ventricular fibrillation associated with normal QT intervals. Q J Med 1981;200:451–462.
95. Rubin SA, Brundage B, Mayer W, *et al.*: Usefulness of Valsalva maneuver and cold pressor test for the evaluation of arrhythmias in the long QT syndrome. Br Heart J 1979;42:490–494.
96. Mitsutake A, Takeshita A, Kuroiwa A, *et al.*: Usefulness of the Valsalva maneuver and cold pressor test for the evaluation of arrhythmias in the long QT syndrome. Br Heart J 1979;42:490–494.
96. Mitsutake A, Takeshita A, Kuroiwa A, *et al.*: Usefulness of the Valsalva maneuver in management of the long QT syndrome. Circulation 1981;63:1029–1035.
97. Benhorin J, Hewitt D, Moss AJ: Relationship between repolarization duration and cycle length during exercise testing in normals and long QT syndrome patients (Abstr). J Am Coll Cardiol 1991;17:60A.
98. Gavrilescu S, Luca C: Right ventricular monophasic action potential in patients with long QT syndrome. Br Heart J 1978;40:1014–1018.
99. Shimizu W, Ohe T, Kurita T, *et al.*: Early afterdepolarizations induced by isoproterenol in patients with congenital long QT syndrome. Circulation 1991;84:1915–1923.
100. Schwartz PJ: Idiopathic long QT syndrome: progress and questions. Am Heart J 1985;109:399–411.
101. Coumel P, Leclercq JF, Lucet V: Possible mechanisms of the arrhythmias in the long QT syndrome. Eur Heart J 1985;6:115–129.
102. Horowitz LN: Greenspan AM, Spielman SR, *et al.*: Torsades de pontes: Electrophysiologic studies in patients without transient pharmacologic or metabolic abnormalities. Circulation 1981;93:1120–1128.
103. Kay GN, Plumb VJ, Arciniegas JG, *et al.*: Torsade de pointes: The long-short initiating sequence and other clinical features: Observations in 32 patients. J Am Coll Cardiol 1983;2:806–817.
104. Roden DM, Woosley RL, Primm RK: Incidence and clinical features of the quinidine-associated long QT syndrome: implications for patient care. Am Heart J 1986;111:1088–1093.
105. Kahn MM, Logan KR, McComb JM, *et al.*: Management of recurrent ventricular tachyarrhythmias associated with QT prolongation. Am J Cardiol 1981;45:1301–1308.
106. Kupersmith J, Hoff P, Guo S: In vitro characteristics of repolarization abnormality—a possible cause of arrhythmias. J Electrocardiol 1986; 19:361–370.

107. Brachmann J, Scherlag BJ, Rosenshtraukh LV, *et al.*: Bradycardia-dependent triggered activity: Relevance to drug-induced multiform ventricular tachycardia. Circulation 1983;68:846–856.
108. Piergies AA, Ruo TI, Jansyn EM, *et al.*: Effect kinetics of N-acetylprocainamide-induced QT interval prolongation. Clin Pharm Ther 1987;107–112.
109. Ejvinsson G, Prinius E: prodromal ventricular premature beats preceded by a diastolic wave. Acta Med Scan 1980;208:445–450.
110. Steinbrecher UP, Fitchett DH: Torsade de pointes: A cause of syncope with atrioventricular block. Arch Intern Med 1980;140:1223–1226.
111. Chow MJ, Piergies AA, Bowsher DJ, *et al.*: Torsade de pointes induced by n-acetylprocainamide. J Am Coll Cardiol 1984;4:621–624.
112. Bender KS, Shematek JP, Leventhal BG, *et al.*: QT interval prolongation associated with anthracycline cardiotoxicity. J Pediatr 1984;105:442.
113. Abinader EG, Shahar J: Possible female preponderance in prenylamine-induced 'torsade de pointes' tachycardia. Cardiol 1983;70:37–40.
114. Mehta D, Warwick GL, Goldberg MJ: QT prolongation after ampicillin anaphylaxis. Br Heart J, 1986;55:308–310.
115. VanderMotten M, Verhaeghe R, DeGeest H: Ventricular arrhythmias and QT-prolongation during therapy with ketanserin: report of a case. Acta Cardiol 1989;44:431–437.
116. Kern MJ, Deligonul U, Serota H, *et al.*: Ventricular arrhythmia due to intracoronary papaverine: analysis of QT intervals and coronary vasodilatory reserve. Cath Cardiovasc Diag 1990;19:229–236.
117. Matsuhashi H, Onodera S, Kawamura Y, *et al.*: Probucol-induced QT prolongation and torsades de pointes. Jpn J Med 1989;28:612–615.
118. Freedman RA, Anderson KP, Green LS, *et al.*: Effect of erythromycin on ventricular arrhythmias and ventricular repolarization in idiopathic long QT syndrome. Am J Cardiol 1987;59:168–169.
119. Aunsholt NA: Prolonged QT interval and hypokalemia caused by haloperidol. Acta Psychiatr Scand 1989;79:411–412.
120. Little RE, Kay GN, Cavender JB, *et al.*: Torsade de pointes and T-U wave alternans associated with arsenic poisoning. PACE 1990;13:164–170.
121. Eiferman C, Chanson P, Cohen A, *et al.*: Torsades de pointes and Q-T prolongation in secondary hypothyroidism. Lancet 1988;1:170–171.
122. Bryer-Ash M, Zehnder J, Angelchik P, *et al.*: Torsades de pointes precipitated by a Chinese herbal remedy. Am J Cardiol 1987;60:1186–1187.
123. Nattel S, Ranger S, Talajic M, *et al.*: Erythromycin-induced long QT syndrome: concordance with quinidine and underlying cellular electrophysiologic mechanism. Am J Med 1990;89:235–238.
124. Webb CL, Dick II M, Rocchini AP, *et al.*: Quinidine syncope in children. J Am Coll Cardiol 1987;9:1031–1037.
125. James MA, Culling W, Jones JV: Polymorphous ventricular tachycardia due to alpha-blockade. Int J Cardiol 1987;14:225–227.
126. McKibbin JK, Pocock WA, Barlow JB, *et al.*: Sotalol hypokalemia, syncope, and torsade de pointes. Br Heart J 1984;51:157–162.
127. Neuvonen PJ, Elonen E, Vuorenmaa T, *et al.*: Prolonged Q-T interval and severe tachyarrhythmias, common features of sotalol intoxication. Eur J Clin Pharmacol 1981;20:85–89.
128. Kennelly BM: Comparison of lidoflazine and quinidine in prophylactic treatment of arrhythmias. Br Heart J 1977;39:540–546.
129. Barbey JT, Thompson KA, Echt DS, *et al.*: Antiarrhythmic activity, electrocardiographic effects and pharmacokinetics of the encainide metabolites O-desmethyl encainide and 3-meth-oxy-O-desmethyl encainide in man. Circulation 1988;77:380–388.
130. Curry P, Fitchett D, Stubbs W, *et al.*: Ventricular arrhythmia and hypokalemia. Lancet 1976;2:231–233.
131. Ludomirsky A, Klein HO, Sarelli P, *et al.*: Q-T prolongation and polymorphous ("torsade de pointes") ventricular arrhythmias associated with organophosphorus insecticide poisoning. Am J Cardiol 1982;49:1654–1658.
132. Herrmann HC, Kaplan LM, Bierer BE: Q-T prolongation and torsades de pointes ventricular tachycardia produced by the tetracyclic antidepressant agent maprotiline. Am J Cardiol 1983;51:904–906.
133. Luomanmaki K, Heikkila J, Hartikainen M: T-wave alternans associated with failure and hypomagnesemia in alcoholic cardiomyopathy. Eur J Cardiol 1975;3:167–170.
134. Strasbuerg B, Sclarvsky S, Erdberg A, *et al.*: Procainamide-induced polymorphous ventricular tachycardia. Am J Cardiol 1981;47:1309–1314.
135. Wald RW, Waxman MB, Coman JM: Torsade de pointes ventricular tachycardia: A complication of disopyramide shared with quinidine. J Electrocardiol 1981;14:301–308.
136. Olshansky B, Martins J, Hunt S: N-acetylprocainamide causing torsade de pointes. Am J Cardiol 1982;50:1439–1441.
137. Rothman MT: Prolonged QT interval, atrioventricular block, and torsade de pointes after antiarrhythmic therapy. Br Med J 1980;280:922–923.
138. Tzivoni D, Keren A, Stern S, *et al.*: disopyramide-induced torsade de pointes. Arch Intern 1981;141:946–947.
139. Leclercq JF, Kural S, Valere PE: Bepridil et torsades de pointes. Arch Mal Coeur 1983;76:341–348.
140. Bronsky D, Dubin A, Waldstein SS, *et al.*: Calcium and the manifestations of hypoparathyroidism. Am J Cardiol 1961;7:823–831.
141. Kerr WJ, Bender WL: Paroxysmal ventricular fibrillation with cardiac recovery in a case in auricular fibrillation and complete heart block while under quinidine sulfate therapy. Heart 1921;9:269–291.
142. Selzer A, Wray HW: Quinidine syncope: paroxysmal ventricular fibrillation occurring during treatment of chronic atrial arrhythmias. Circulation 1964;30:17–26.
143. Roden DM, Hoffman BF: Action potential prolongation and induction of abnormal automaticity by low quinidine concentrations in canine Purkinje fibers. Relationship to potassium and cycle length. Circ Res 1985;56:857–867.
144. Radford MD, Evans DW: Long-term results of DC reversion of atrial fibrillation. Br Heart J 1968;30:91–96.
145. Thomspon KA, Murray JJ, Blair IA, *et al.*: Plasma concentrations of quinidine its major active metabolites, and dihydroquinidine in patients with torsades de pointes. Clin Pharmacol Ther 1988;43:636–642.
146. Shah A, Schwartz H: Mexiletine for treatment of Torsades de Pointes. Am Heart J 1984;107:589–591.
147. Hersch C: Electrocardiographic changes in head injuries. Circulation 1961;23:853–860.
148. Lee YC, Sutton FJ: Concomitant pulses and U wave alternans associated with head trauma. Am J Cardiol 1984;55:851–852.
149. Sen S, Stober T, Burger L, *et al.*: Recurrent torsades de pointes type ventricular tachycardia in intracranial hemorrhage. Intensive Care Med 1984;10:263–264.
150. Hammer WJ, Lussenhop AJ, Weintraub AM: Observations on the electrocardiographic changes associated with subarachnoid hemorrhage with special reference to their genesis. Am J Cardiol 1975;59:427–433.
151. Burch GE, Myers R, Abildskev JA: A new electrocardiographic pattern observed in cerebrovascular accidents. Circulation 1954;9:719–723.
152. Hugenholtz PG: Electrocardiographic abnormalities in cerebral disorders. Report of six cases and review of the literature. Am Heart J 1962;63:451–461.
153. Gallivan GJ, Levine H, Canzonetti AJ: Ischemic electrographic changes after truncal vagotomy. J Am Med Assoc 1970;211:798–801.
154. Chambers JB, Sampson MJ, Springings DC: QT prolongation on the electrocardiogram in diabetic autonomic neuropathy. Diabetic Med 1990;7:105–110.
155. Bennett KR: Torsades de Pointes and mitral valve prolapse. Am J Cardiol 1980;45:715–716.
156. Kramer HM, Kligfield P, Devereux RB, *et al.*: Arrhythmias in mitral valve prolapse, effect of selection bias. Arch Intern Med 1984;144:360–364.
157. Winkle RA, Lopes MG, Goodman DS, *et al.*: Propranolol for patients with mitral valve prolapse. Am Heart J 1970;93:422–429.
158. Levy D, Savage D. Prevalence and clinical features of mitral valve prolapse. Am Heart J 1978;113:1281–1289.
159. Cowan MD, Fye WB: Prevalence of QT_c prolongation in women with mitral valve prolapse. Am J Cardiol 1989;63:133–134.

160. Chambers JB, Ward DE: The QT and QS_2 intervals in patients with mitral leaflet prolapse. Am Heart J 1987;114:355–361.
161. Bekheit SG, Ali AA, Deglin SM, *et al.*: Analysis of QT interval in patients with idiopathic mitral valve prolapse. Chest 1982;81:620–625.
162. Taylor GJ, Crampton RS, Gibson RS, *et al.*: Prolonged QT interval at onset of acute myocardial infarction in predicting early phase ventricular tachycardia. Am Heart J 1981;102:16–24.
163. Wheelan K, Mukharji J, Rude PE, *et al.*: Sudden death and its relation to Q-T interval prolongation after acute myocardial infarction: two-year follow-up. Am J Cardiol 1986;57:749–50.
164. Kramer B, Brill M, Bruhn A, *et al.*: Relationship between the degree of coronary artery disease and of left ventricular function and the duration of the QT-interval in ECG. Eur Heart J 1986;7:14–24.
165. Maron BJ, Clark CE, Goldstein RE, *et al.*: Potential role of QT interval prolongation in sudden infant death syndrome. Circulation 1976;54:423–430.
166. Guntheroth WG: The QT interval and sudden infant death syndrome. Circulation 1982;66:502–504.
167. Arnsdorf MF: The effect of antiarrhythmic drugs on triggered sustained rhythmic activity in cardiac Purkinje fibers. J Pharmacol Exp Ther 1977; 201:689–700.
168. Levine JH, Spear JF, Guarnieri T, *et al.*: Cesium chloride-induced long QT syndrome: demonstration of afterdepolarizations and triggered activity in vivo. Circulation 1985;72:1092–1104.
169. Davidenko JM, Cohen L, Goodrow R, *et al.*: Quinidine-induced action potential prolongation, early afterdepolarizations, and triggered activity in canine Purkinje fibers. Effects of stimulation rate, potassium, and magnesium. Circulation 1989;79:674–686.
170. El-Sherif N, Bekheit SS, Henkin R: quinidine-induced long-QTU interval and torsades de pointes: role of bradycardia-dependent early afterdepolarizations. J Am Coll Cardiol 1989;14:242–247.
171. Bonatti V, Rolli A, Botti G: Recording of monophasic action potential of the right ventricle in the long QT syndrome complicated by severe ventricular arrhythmias. Eur Heart J: 1983;4:168–176.
172. D'Alnocourt CN, Zierhut W, Luderitz B: "Torsades de pointes" tachycardia: re-entry or focal activity? Br Heart J 1982;48:213–216.
173. Bardy GH, Ungerleider RM, Smith WM, *et al.*: A mechanism of torsades de pointes in a canine model. Circulation 1983;67:52–59.
174. Li ZY, Maldonado C, Zee-Cheng C, *et al.*: Conduction of early afterdepolarizations in sheep Purkinje fibers and ventricular muscle. J Electrocardiol 1992;25:119–127.
175. Li ZY, Maldonado C, Zee-Cheng C, *et al.*: Purkinje fiber-papillary muscle interaction in the genesis of triggered activity. Cardiovas Res 26;543:548,1992
176. Kupersmith J, Hoff P: Occurrence and transmission of repolarization abnormalities in vitro. J Am Coll Cardiol 1985;6:152–160.
177. Hiromasa S, Coto H, Li ZY, *et al.*: Dextrorotatory isomer of sotalol: Electrophysiologic effects and interaction with verapamil. Am Heart J 1988;116:1552–1557.
178. Sclarvosky S, Lewin RF, Kracoff O, *et al.*: Amiodarone-induced polymorphous ventricular tachycardia. Am Heart J 1983;105:6–12.
179. Han J, Moe GK: Nonuniform recovery of excitability of ventricular muscle. Circ Res 1964;14:44–60.
180. Zipes DP: The long QT interval syndrome: A rosetta stone for sympathetic related ventricular tachyarrhythmias. Circulation 1991;84:1414–1419.
181. Abildskov JA: Adrenergic effects on the QT interval of the electrocardiogram. Am Heart J 1976;92:210–216.
182. Schwartz PJ, Snebold NG, Borwn AM: Effects of unilateral cardiac sympathetic denervation on the ventricular fibrillation threshold. Am J Cardiol 1976;37:1034–1040.
183. Christiansen JL, Kirby ML: Experimentally induced long QT syndrome in the chick embryo. Ann NY Acad Sci 1990;588:314–322.
184. Janse MJ, Schwartz PJ, Wilms-Schopman F, *et al.*: Effects of unilateral stellate ganglion stimulation and ablation on electrophysiologic changes induced by acute myocardial ischemia in dogs. Circulation 1985;72:585–595.
185. Puddu PE, Jouve R, Langlet F, *et al.*: Prevention of postischemic ventricular fibrillation late after right or left stellate ganglionectomy in dogs. Circulation 1988;77:935–946.
186. Schwartz PJ, Locati EH, Moss AJ, *et al.*: Left cardiac sympathetic denervation in the therapy of congenital long QT syndrome. Circulation 1991;84:503–511.
187. DeAmbroggi LD, Bertoni T, Locati E, *et al.*: Mapping of body surface potentials in patients with idiopathic long QT syndrome. Circulation 1986;74:1334–1345.
188. Till JA, Shinnebourne EA, Pepper J, *et al.*: Complete denervation of the heart in a child with congenital long QT and deafness. Am J Cardiol 1988;62:1319–1321.
189. Eldar M, Griffin JC, Abbott JA, *et al.*: Permanent cardiac pacing in patients with the long QT syndrome. J Am Coll Cardiol 1987;10:600–607.
190. Tzivoni D, Banai S, Schuger C, *et al.*: Treatment of torsade de pointes with magnesium sulfate. Circulation 1988;77:392–397.
191. Ben-David J, Zipes DP: Differential response to right and left stellate stimulation on early afterdepolarizations and ventricular tachycardia in the dog. Circulation 1988;78:1241–1250.
192. Angelakos ET, King MP, Millard RW: Regional distribution of catecholamines in the hearts of various species. Ann NY Acad Sci 1969;156:219–240.
193. Ben-David J, Zipes DP: Alpha adrenoceptor stimulation and blockade modulates cesium-induced early afterdepolarizations and ventricular tachyarrhythmias in dogs. Circulation 1990;82:225–233.
194. Mary-Rabine L, Hordof AJ, Danilo P, *et al.*: Mechanisms for impulse initiation in isolated human atrial fibers. Circ Res 1980;47:267–277.
195. Pellegrino A, Ho SY, Anderson RH, *et al.*: Prolonged QT interval and the cardiac conduction tissues. Am J Cardiol 1986;58:1112–1113.
196. Hoepp HW, Eggeling T, Hombach V: Pharmacologic blockade of the left stellate ganglion using a drug-reservoir-pump system. Chest 1990;97:250–251.
197. Garcia-Rubira JC, Garcia-Aranda VL, Fernandez JMC: Magnesium sulphate for torsade de pointes in a patient with congenital long QT syndrome. Int J Cardiol 1990;27:282–283.
198. Banai S, Schuger C, Benhorin J, *et al.*: Treatment of Torsade de pointes with intravenous magnesium. Am J Cardiol 1989;63:1539–1540.
199. DeSilvey DL, Moss AJ: Primidone in the treatment of the long QT syndrome: QT shortening and ventricular arrhythmia suppression. Ann Intern Med 1980;93:53–54.
200. Wilmer CI, Stein B, Morris DC: Atrioventricular pacemaker placement in Romano-Ward syndrome and recurrent torsades de pointes. Am J Cardiol 1987;59:171–172.
201. Solti E, Szatmary L, Renyi-Vamos F, *et al.*: Pacemaker therapy for the treatment of the long QT syndrome associated with long-lasting bradycardia and ventricular tachycardia. Cor Vasa 1987;29:428–435.
202. Puddu PE, Torresani J: The QT-sensitive cybernetic pacemaker: a new role for an old parameter? PACE 1986;9:108–123.
203. Platia EV, Griffith LSC, Watkins L, *et al.*: Management of the prolonged QT syndrome and recurrent ventricular fibrillation with an implantable automatic cardioverter-defibrillator. Clin Cardiol 1985;8:490–493.
204. Wilton NCT, Hantler CB: Congenital long QT syndrome: Changes in QT interval during anesthesia with thiopental, vecuronium, fentanyl and isoflurane. Anesth Analg 1987;66:357–360.
205. Palkar NV, Crawford MW: Spinal anesthesia in prolonged Q-T interval syndrome (letter). Br J Anesth 1986;58(5):575–576.
206. Ryan H: Anaesthesia for caesarean section in a patient with Jervell, Lange-Nielsen syndrome. Can J Anaesth 1988;35:422–424.
207. Bhandari AK, Shapiro WA, Morady F, *et al.*: Electrophysiologic testing in patients with the long QT syndrome. Circulation 1985;71:63–71.
208. Perticone F, Adinolfi L, Bonaduce D: Efficacy of magnesium sulfate in the treatment of torsade de pointes. Am Heart J 1986;112:847–849.

209. Roden DM: Magnesium treatment of ventricular arrhythmias. Am J Cardiol 1989;63:43G–46G.
210. Balie BS, Inoue H, Kaseda S, *et al*.: Magnesium suppresses early afterdepolarizations and ventricular tachyarrhythmias induced in dogs by cesium. Circulation 1988;77:1395–1402.
211. Kaplinsky E, Yahinl JH, Barzilai J, *et al*.: Quinidine syncope: report of a case successfully treated with lidocaine. Chest 1972;62:764–766.
212. VanderArk CR, Reynolds EW, Kahn DR: Quinidine syncope: a report of successful treatment with bretylium tosylate. J Thorac Cardiovasc Surg 1976;72:464–467.
213. Fauchier JP, Lanfranchi J, Ginies G, *et al*.: 'Syncope par torsades de pointes' au cours d'un traitement par la chloroquine. Etude de l'electrocardiogramme hisien et traitement par le verapamil. Ann Cardiol Angeiol 1974;23:341–346.

11

ANTIARRHYTHMIC DRUGS: GENERAL PRINCIPLES

Joel Kupersmith, M.D., F.A.C.P., F.A.C.C.

This chapter will review important underlying principles in the use of antiarrhythmic drugs. Chapter 12 will discuss the specific agents.

BASIC ELECTROPHYSIOLOGIC EFFECTS OF ANTIARRHYTHMIC DRUGS

In the discussion of basic electrophysiologic (EP) effects, we will build on the knowledge of basic electrophysiology provided in Chapters 1 and 2. Antiarrhythmic drugs are evaluated by several in vitro and in situ models, of which the clinical EP study is one. Much of our fundamental knowledge of antiarrhythmic drugs comes from the intracellular microelectrode study. Generally speaking, microelectrode studies of antiarrhythmic drugs evaluate parameters that are relevant to the two major mechanisms of arrhythmia—reentry and automaticity. This section focuses on relevant EP properties of antiarrhythmic drugs and then how these properties influence reentry and automaticity.

Action Potential Upstroke and Conduction

Conduction of the cardiac impulse is a most important parameter related to antiarrhythmic drugs. Conduction proceeds from cell to cell via the upstroke of action potentials. It is therefore influenced by factors that influence the upstroke as well as the cell to cell connections. The action potential upstroke (Fig. 11.1) is mediated by either an inward movement of Na^+ (atrium, His-Purkinje system, and ventricle) or predominantly Ca^{2+} (sinus and AV (atrioventricular) nodes). So-called "local anesthetic" antiarrhythmic drugs block Na^+ channels while Ca^{2+} channel blockers are involved with the others.

Conduction velocity can be measured directly. In addition, drug effects on the action potential upstroke (Fig. 11.1) are measured. The primary upstroke parameter that is evaluated is V_{max}, i.e., maximum rate of voltage change (1) during the upstroke. In drug studies, V_{max} is used as a somewhat indirect and imperfect measure of inward Na^+ current (I_{Na}). In atrium, His-Purkinje system, and ventricle, drugs with "local anesthetic" properties block inward Na^+ current, in turn, depress V_{max} (2,3) and therefore slow conduction. In human ventricular muscle slowing of conduction then translates into QRS prolongation in the electrocardiogram (ECG).

The membrane responsiveness curve (Fig. 11.2) is a more detailed analysis of V_{max} (2). When membrane potential is reduced (i.e., made more positive), there is partial inactivation of the Na^+ channel, and therefore a slower rate of rise of the action potential upstroke. One can construct curves, plotting the activation voltage (or "takeoff potential"), i.e., the potential at which the upstroke initiates, versus V_{max}. These plots are called "membrane responsiveness curves." Interventions that reduce inward Na^+ current, i.e., local anesthetic agents, shift membrane responsiveness curves so as to lower V_{max} at given membrane potentials (see Fig. 11.2).

Membrane responsiveness type curves are a requisite piece of information for any antiarrhythmic drug and lowered V_{max} at given activation voltages are the measure of local anesthetic properties.

Another more detailed analysis of V_{max} involves the phenomenon of "use dependence" and the "modulated receptor hypothesis" (4–6) (Fig. 11.3). Drug affinity for its receptor, in this case the Na^+ channel, is not uniform during the course of an action potential. The electrical state of the cell membrane influences affinity of drug for the channel. The channel exists in three basic states—resting (resting phase of the action potential), open (the upstroke), and inactive (plateau) (Fig. 11.3). Local anesthetic antiarrhythmic drugs have different rates of association to and/or dissociation from the receptor (the Na^+ channel) in each of these states. Drug affinity is generally higher during open (upstroke) and inactive (plateau) phases and less during the resting phase when dissociation of drug from the Na^+ channel tends to occur. Thus, the drug moves into the channel during the upstroke (Phase 0) and plateau (Phase 2) of the action potential to block inward Na^+ movement and away from the channel in diastole (i.e., during phase 4) (Fig. 11.1 and 11.3). Different drugs have different rates of association and dissociation from receptor (4,5,8). Lidocaine, a Class IB agent, has rapid association and dissociation, while flecainide, a Class IC agent, reacts much

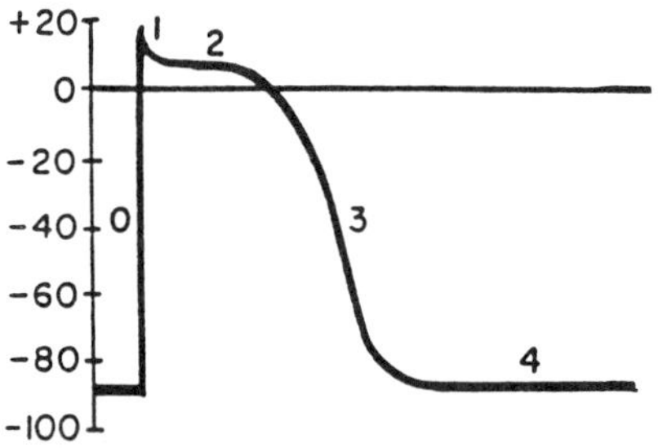

Figure 11.1. Fast response action potential of the type that might be seen in atrium, His-Purkinje system, or ventricle. There are five phases. Phase 0 is the upstroke, Phase 2 the plateau, Phase 3 repolarization, and Phase 4 resting membrane potential. The upstroke (Phase 0) is mediated by rapid inward movement of Na^+ current. The Na^+ channel is considered "open" during phase 0, "inactive" during phase 2, and "resting" during phase 4. Membrane potential during phase 4 is normally about −90. See text for further discussion.

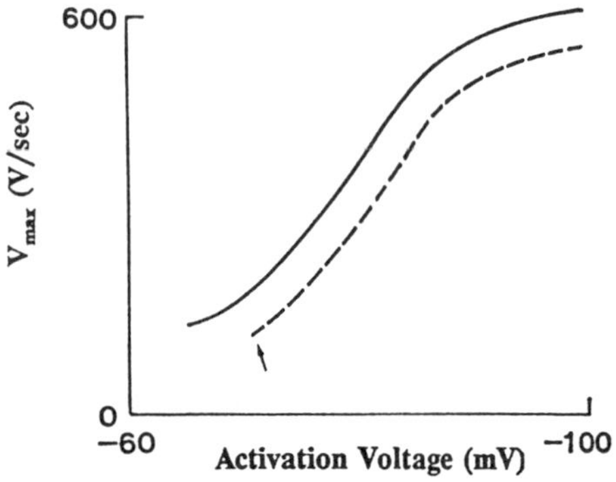

Figure 11.2. Effect of local anesthetic agents on membrane responsiveness curves. *Horizontal axis* is activation voltage and the *vertical axis* maximum rate of rise of the action potential upstroke (V_{max}). *Solid line* shows baseline and dashed line shows local anesthetic effects. Local anesthetic agents lower V_{max} at any given membrane potential. *Arrow* shows minimum activation voltage at which a response can be elicited with drug. This is at a more positive voltage drug than at baseline, another effect of local anesthetic agents. Membrane responsiveness curves are generated by applying progressively premature beats during Phase 3 of the action potential. "Inactivation curves" are similar but generated by using voltage clamp technique (See Chapter 1) and results with certain drugs may be slightly different. mV = millivolts; V/sec = volts/sec.

more slowly. Generally, higher-molecular-weight drugs move slowly (9).

Use-dependent block has particular implications regarding the influence of heart rate on drug effects. During slow rates there is more time in diastole than during fast rates. Thus drugs that move quickly to and from the Na^+ channel have time to completely dissociate during diastole (i.e., phase 4) (Fig. 11.1). However, with fast rates or premature beats, drugs do not have enough time to dissociate from the channel; they then bind to it to a greater degree and their effects are enhanced. The advantage here is more drug activity on the Na^+ channel during tachycardia, when needed. The phenomenon of use dependence has been demonstrated in clinical EP as well as in vitro studies.

Local anesthetic agents may also display another property—

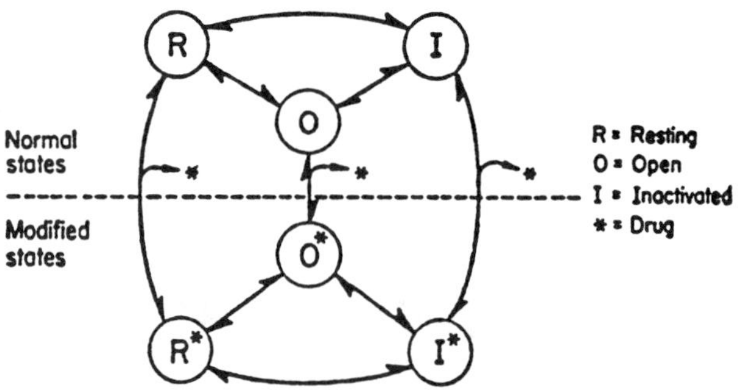

Figure 11.3. Modulated receptor hypothesis. Shown are the Na^+ channel in resting (R), open (O), and inactive (I) forms. The channels are shown in their normal states (R, O, I) and modified states (R* O*, I*) when drug is bound to receptor. Shown are movements between normal and modified states, i.e., binding and unbinding of drug to receptor in the resting, open and inactive phases. Each of these movements has a rate constant. (From Strauss HC: Mechanisms of local anesthetic interaction with the sodium channel. In Rosen MR, Janse MJ, Wit AL (eds): Cardiac Electrophysiology. Mt. Kisco, NY, Futura Publishing Co., 1990:995–1012, with permission.)

injury zone selectivity. That is, they may suppress I_{Na}, reduce V_{max} of the upstroke and slow conduction more in injured than normal tissues (10–12). This property of injury zone selectivity may also be related to use dependence. Drugs with substantial binding to open and inactive channels (e.g., Class IB agents) (4,5) also bind more to the Na^+ channels of injured or ischemic tissue. These tissues have reduced resting membrane potentials and thus channels that are in "partially inactivated" states, even during the "resting" phase. That is, the "resting" membrane potential is more positive and thus closer to plateau levels. Thus there is greater drug affinity for and more binding to the Na^+ channel receptor of these cells than to normal cells. A consequence of this is potentiation of effects in injured tissues where arrhythmias occur (13) (see also Chapter 12).

Other parameters for which drug effects are routinely determined are amplitude and overshoot of the upstroke and excitability (the ability of a stimulus to initiate an action potential). Overall, drugs with local anesthetic effects move membrane responsive curves to lower V_{max} (2), have a variable degree of use dependence (4,5), diminish amplitude, and overshoot of the upstroke, reduce excitability, and slow conduction.

Action Potential Duration and Effective Refractory Period

Effects of antiarrhythmic drugs on action potential duration (APD) and effective refractory period (ERP) are another routine in drug evaluation. APD is usually measured from the time of the upstroke to the time of 50 and 90% of repolarization (so-called "APD_{50}" and "APD_{90}") and many drugs either lengthen or shorten it.

The phenomenon of "reverse use dependence" may occur in relation to APD. Many antiarrhythmic drugs prolong APD. However, many of these drugs (with the notable exception of amiodarone) prolong this parameter *less* at fast rates, a factor that may interfere with antiarrhythmic properties during tachycardia.

The ERP is the time from the upstroke to the earliest stimulus that initiates a propagated response. ERP is substantially but not completely related to APD. It is usually determined using stimuli of two times diastolic threshold.

The ERP/APD ratio has also been utilized as a parameter with possible relevance to antiarrhythmic drug action. If ERP is prolonged relative to APD (increased ERP/APD ratio), then impulses arising toward the end of the action potential, when it is partially refractory, can no longer occur (14). These impulses tend to have slow upstrokes, to conduct slowly, and therefore are more likely to be associated with reentry.

Other Parameters

Measurement of ventricular fibrillation (VF) threshold is a frequently used research technique. It refers to the amount of current necessary to cause VF. Antiarrhythmic drugs generally increase VF threshold but relevance of this parameter to spontaneously occurring VF is still not clear.

Automaticity-related parameters include: (a) rate of depolarization of cells during phase 4 which in turn constitutes the slope (slower slope equals slower rate), (b) threshold of activation of the upstroke (higher threshold means later firing, i.e., activation, and slower rate, and (c) maximum diastolic potential at the end of the action potential (more negative maximum diastolic potential at the onset of phase 4 means that, all other factors being equal, tissue will reach threshold later and the rate will be slower) (15). For example, an intervention that increases maximum diastolic potential and/or reduces the slope of phase 4, and/or makes threshold more positive, will slow automatic firing rate (see Fig. 1.5) (15).

Direct drug effects on ionic currents can be determined using voltage clamp technique in vitro. One can directly determine effects on I_{Na}, I_{Ca}, I_K (involved in APD), and others. Also, effects of drugs on cable properties, which reflect cell-to-cell connections, are important but have not been the subject of as much study as effects on ionic currents.

Normal Versus Abnormal Tissue

One problem in determination of drug effects on normal tissue in vitro is that arrhythmias arise in abnormal tissues in situ where drug effects may differ. As noted above, local anesthetic drugs may have enhanced effects on the upstroke of the action potentials and the conduction velocity in injured tissues. They may also have different effects on APD and ERP (14,16). For this reason, a number of models of abnormal tissues have been used to determine drug effects. These include in situ effects on ischemia or infarcted zones, in vitro effects on infarcted tissue, effects on triggered activity models, and others (13).

Drug Effects on Reentry and Automaticity

The two major mechanisms of arrhythmias are reentry (17) and automaticity. Reentry is shown in Fig. 11.4A. The basis of reentry is one-way block and it occurs because of a primary abnormality of conduction or a longer ERP (i.e., a disparity in refractoriness) in the depressed segment. Figure 11.4B shows

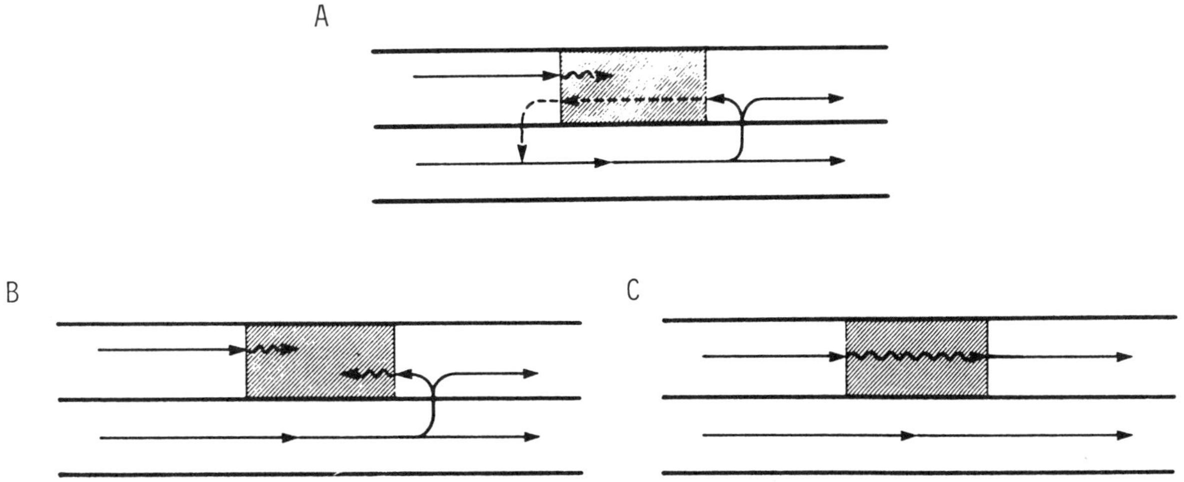

Figure 11.4. Schematic of reentry. **A** shows reentry. There are two contiguous strips of ventricular muscle. The *upper strip* has a depressed area which displays one-way block. An impulse (*arrow*) proceeds into this zone and is blocked in an antegrade direction. A corresponding impulse proceeds in the contiguous strip and then reenters in a retrograde direction through the zone of one-way block to complete a reentrant cycle which may become repetitive to cause a reentrant tachycardia. **B** shows the usual effects of antiarrhythmic drugs, i.e., further depression of conduction and/or prolongation of refractoriness in the depressed segment. Here the impulse again proceeds antegrade slows and is blocked as in **A.** However, in this case, the retrograde impulse is also blocked. **C** shows an more favorable but probably less common effect of antiarrhythmic drugs. Here the impulse, rather than being blocked in an antegrade direction, passes on through making reentry impossible.

what is believed to be the common mechanism for antiarrhythmic drug action. One-way block is converted to two-way block and this may occur via: (a) further depression of conduction, which in turn is related to depression of V_{max} of the upstroke (Fig. 11.2), interference with cable properties, or excitability. Use-dependent block may also be important here as its presence would cause greater depression of the upstroke at faster rates and (b) prolongation of refractoriness. This may occur along with prolongation of APD or there may be a primary effect on ERP and thus an increase in the ERP/APD ratio. In this regard, lidocaine has a primary effect prolonging the ERP, especially in ischemic tissue (10,16). Quinidine, on the other hand, lengthens both APD and ERP, though it still increases the ERP/APD ratio somewhat.

It is clear from these effects that the same factors that are "antiarrhythmic" can at times be "proarrhythmic." For example, slowing of conduction or prolongation of refractoriness could, in one circumstance, abolish reentry but, in other circumstances, facilitate reentry through the same type of reentrant pathway. This paradoxic effect may occur because reentry depends on the relationship between the conduction velocity and refractory periods of two pathways constituting the reentry loop. Slowing of conduction in one pathway may allow sufficient time for the second pathway to recover, thus paradoxically promoting reentry.

Figure 11.4C shows a more unusual circumstance for antiarrhythmic drugs. Here there is no one-way block and impulses pass on through the depressed segment. Drugs may do this in the following ways: (a) by improving conduction in the depressed segment. One way for this to occur is via movement of activation voltage to a more negative level. Reentrant arrhythmias tend to arise in abnormal zones where membrane potential is reduced, i.e., tissue is partly inactivated. An antiarrhythmic drug might move this membrane potential to a more negative level, i.e., move the cell from partial inactivation to complete activation (e.g., from −75 to −90 mV). This would improve activation voltage and move V_{max} to a higher point on the membrane responsiveness curve (Fig. 11.2). Thus conduction would be improved and reentry made impossible. Catecholamines, especially in cardiac arrest situations, and occasionally lidocaine may do this; (b) by decreasing disparity in ERP between abnormal and contiguous normal zones (14,18).

Reentry is induced in the electrophysiology laboratory by programmed stimulation. Here the concept of "trigger" versus "substrate" is also important. This concept is thoroughly discussed in Chapter 2. The substrate is the reentrant pathway. The trigger is either a spontaneous or a stimulated beat that initiates the arrhythmia. An antiarrhythmic drug can influence upstroke, conduction, APD or ERP in the trigger, the substrate or the pathway, from trigger to substrate. This is a point to remember in the EP study where the trigger is an artificially applied stimulus. In the ambient state, the trigger would be a spontaneous premature beat.

Enhanced or abnormal automaticity is the other major mechanism for arrhythmias. This is divided into two main groups—enhanced normal/abnormal automaticity and triggered activity which in turn is related to early and delayed afterdepolarizations (Chapter 2). Antiarrhythmic drugs may reduce the frequency of spontaneous depolarizations and suppress normal or abnormal automaticity by one of the mechanisms described above via actions on a variety of currents, including I_f, the pacemaker current, I_K (potassium current), and T-type inward calcium current (I_{Ca}). Drugs may also suppress both early and delayed afterdepolarizations and triggered activity (see Chapter 2).

PHARMACOKINETICS

Knowledge of drug pharmokinetics (19–21) is vital when using antiarrhythmic agents and especially when performing a clinical EP study.

When a drug is administered orally, there are several steps in its progression into the bloodstream. First, it undergoes disintegration and dissolution, or if in a sustained-release form, it slowly elutes from the binding gel. The drug is then absorbed from the intestine (with a "half-life" of absorption) into the portal circulation which carries it to the liver. It subsequently passes through the liver to the systemic circulation. In the liver, certain drugs, e.g., propranolol and verapamil, undergo extensive "first-pass metabolism." That is, the liver removes and metabolizes them with a high extraction ratio such that a large percent of drug is removed in a single passage (22,23). For example, 60–70% of propranolol is removed.

Figure 11.5 shows a schematic of first pass metabolism (23). Drugs that exhibit first-pass metabolism have certain features: (a) intravenous doses are much lower than oral (for obvious reasons), (b) if metabolites formed by the liver on first pass are pharmacologically active, they play an important role when the drug is used orally and play less of a role in intravenous forms, (c) food improves bioavailability. This occurs because the increased hepatic blood flow that accompanies the ingestion of food causes more rapid drug passage through the liver and thus less time for hepatic metabolism. (d) Diminished cardiac output reduces elimination of these drugs. After a drug reaches the systemic circulation, there is still a high hepatic extraction ratio, i.e., the liver removes drug from the bloodstream as soon as it is delivered. For this reason, the amount of drug eliminated depends essentially on its delivery to the liver or, in other words, on the hepatic blood flow. If blood flow is reduced, there is less drug delivered and therefore, less elimination.

Several concepts are important to understanding antiarrhythmic drug pharmacokinetics. These include the concepts of bioavailability, volume of distribution (V_D), drug clearance, and half-life ($T_{1/2}$). Each of these concepts is discussed in detail below.

Bioavailability refers to the percent of drug that enters the body. It is defined as the area under the curve of serum drug

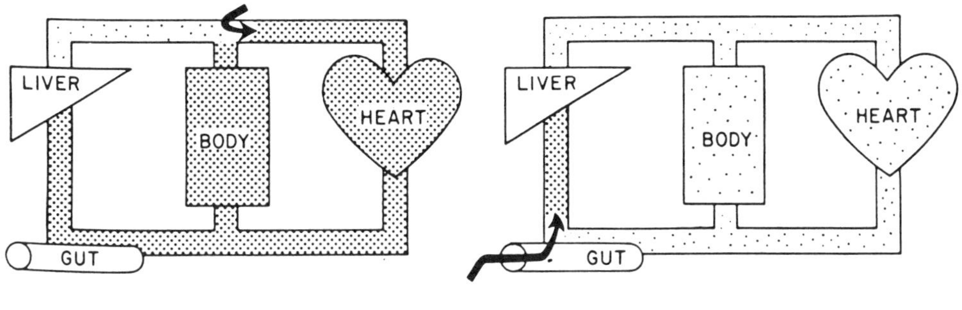

INTRAVENOUS ORAL

Figure 11.5. First-pass metabolism. On the **right** a drug is administered orally. It passes through the gut into the portal circulation and arrives at the liver where most of it is extracted and metabolized leaving a small proportion to enter the body. Bioavailability is low. On the **left** with intravenous administration, the liver is bypassed and much more of the drug enters the body. (From Nies AS, Shand DG: Clinical pharmacology of propranolol. Circulation 1975;52:6–15, by permission of the American Heart Association, Inc.)

level after oral administration divided by the area under the curve after intravenous administration (20) (Fig. 11.6). Bioavailability is influenced by the factors described above—gastrointestinal absorption and hepatic extraction.

When a drug is administered intravenously, it reaches the systemic circulation immediately.

When a drug arrives at the systemic circulation after either oral or intravenous administration it is then distributed throughout the body. The theoretical construct that describes this for most drugs is the two-compartment model (19). In this model, the drug moves from the so-called "central" to the "peripheral" compartment (Fig. 11.7). Each of these compartments is a theoretical entity and not a specific anatomic location. The central compartment is related to the blood volume, extracellular space, and rapidly equilibrating tissues while the peripheral compartment has to do with the more slowly equilibrating peripheral tissues.

Each compartment has a *volume of distribution* (V_D), which is defined on the volume of fluid into which a dose of drug would have to be diluted to give a particular plasma concentration (C_p) (V_D = total drug in body/C_p). The size of the V_D in the peripheral compartment depends on the amount of tissue uptake. It in turn influences the loading dose of the drug. The greater the V_D, the higher the loading dose has to be to fill it. Certain disease states influence V_D. For example, congestive heart failure reduces the V_D of lidocaine (because of diminished peripheral tissue uptake) and therefore loading dose of lidocaine has to be reduced in this state.

Figure 11.8 shows a schematic of drug levels after a single intravenous dose of drug (19). There is a distribution phase, representing movement to tissue, and an elimination phase. Half-life ($T_{1/2}$) (i.e., the time it takes to fall to half of the initial or peak levels) of the distribution phase is called the "alpha half-life" (alpha $T_{1/2}$) and that of the elimination phase the "beta half life." (beta $T_{1/2}$) Lidocaine, for example, has an alpha $T_{1/2}$ of about 8 and a beta $T_{1/2}$ of about 120 min.

Drug clearance (Cl) (like renal clearance) is defined as the volume of blood cleared of drug per unit time (24). Equations relating V_D Cl and beta $T_{1/2}$ are listed in Table 11.1.

Several factors may influence drug clearance. Renal, hepatic, or congestive heart failure have an influence depending on the particular metabolism of the given drug. Another factor, stereospecificity, refers to a preferred clearance of an isomer of a drug. For example, an *l*-form of a drug might be cleared by the liver or kidneys at a greater rate. Since *l* and *d*-isomers may differ in their activity, such preferential elimination might also have implications regarding drug activity. Verapamil is a drug with stereospecific clearance; see the section on verapamil in Chapter 12 (25).

Proper initiation of drug therapy, especially intravenous therapy, involves the concepts of "loading" and "maintenance" doses. Without a loading dose, there is a gradual rise of drug level and a prolonged interval before steady state is reached. It takes 3.3 half-lives to arrive at 90% and 5 half-lives to arrive at 97% of steady state of serum drug level (Fig. 11.9). The purpose of a loading dose or "bolus" is to fill the peripheral compartment and bring it into more rapid equilibration so as to arrive at steady state more quickly.

Figure 11.10 shows drug levels of lidocaine with different methods of administration (26). While loading doses bring drug into equilibrium more quickly, they do not do so immediately. As seen in Figure 11.10B, the loading dose is followed by a dip in drug level and then a slow rise representing the constant rate infusion. During the dip, drug levels may fall below minimum effective concentration (24). This is corrected by use of a second bolus (Fig. 11.10C) which in this case brought drug levels briefly into the toxic range. A more slowly administered loading dose allows for a more consistent and less variable drug level (Figure 11.10D). However, here there is an initial delay in achieving therapeutic levels, a situation that may not be desirable in emergencies.

Similar principles apply when drug is administered orally. However, drug levels with oral administration have an obligatory

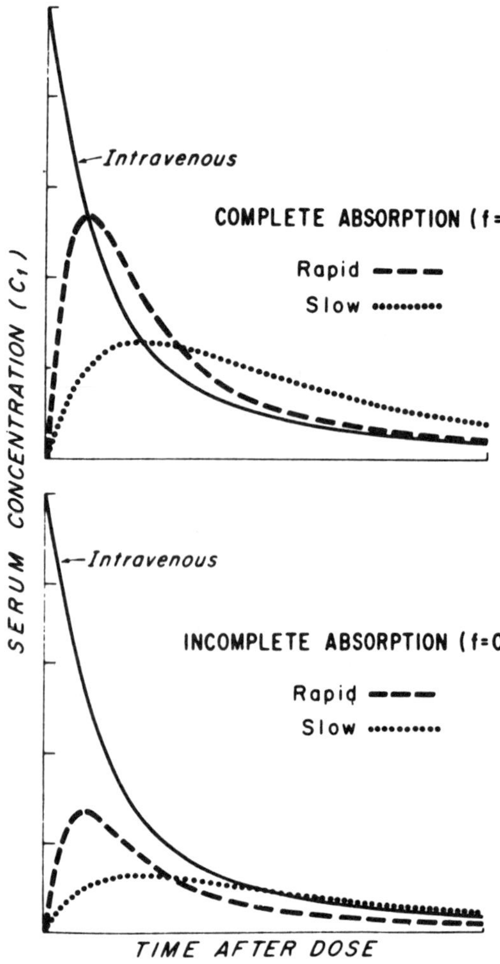

Figure 11.6. Bioavailability curves. Bioavailability (f) is AUC_{po}/AUC_{iv}, i.e., area under the curve of oral/area under the curve of intravenous drug. *Upper curves* show complete absorption of a drug (*f* = 1.0) and *lower curves* 50% absorption (*f* = 0.5). Also shown are rapid (*dashed lines*) and slow (*dotted lines*) absorption. For complete absorption (*f* = 1.0), area under the curve of oral and intravenous drug are the same though the time course of rise and decline of serum concentration of the rapidly and slowly absorbed (e.g. sustained release) drugs are different. For incomplete absorption (*f* = 0.5), area under the curve of oral drug is half that of intravenous drug. (From Greenblatt DJ, Koch-Weser J: Medical intelligence: drug therapy-clinical pharmacokinetics (second of two parts). N Engl J Med 1975:19:964–979, with permission.)

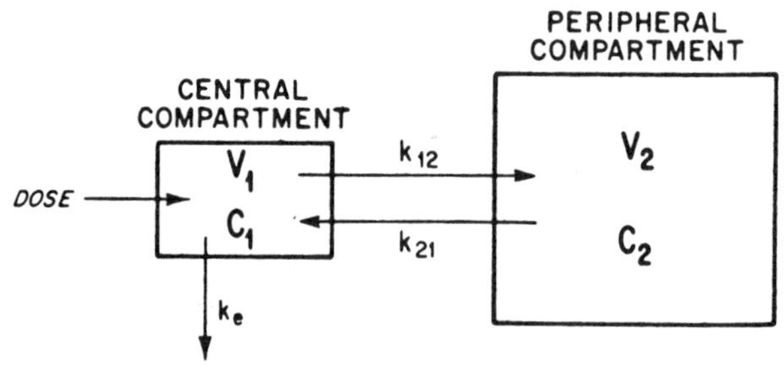

Figure 11.7. Intercompartmental movement of drug. Shown are a two-compartment model with a central and a peripheral compartment. Drug moves into the central compartment after administration of dose. From the central compartment the drug may move into the peripheral compartment or be eliminated (*downward arrow*). Each of these movements has a time constant. K_{12} represents movement from the central to the peripheral compartment while K_{21} represents movement from the peripheral to the central compartment. K_e represents elimination consistent, V_1 and V_2 represent volume of distribution, and C_1 and C_2 concentrations in the central and peripheral compartments, respectively. It is important to remember that these compartments are theoretical constructs and not anatomic structures. The *central compartment* generally has to do with blood volume, extracellular space, and rapidly equilibrating tissue while the *peripheral compartment* has to do with peripheral uptake in the more slowly equilibrating tissue. (From Greenblatt DJ, Koch-Weser J: Medical intelligence: drug therapy-clinical pharmacokinetics (first of two parts). N Engl J Med 1975;14:702–705, with permission.)

peak/trough variation with each dose taken and also depend on the rate of absorption, hepatic extraction, and overall bioavailability.

Once steady state is reached, the timing of the oral doses depends on the desired peak/trough ratio. Figure 11.11 and Table 11.2 show peak/trough ratios at various multiples of a half-life (20). If the drug is given at intervals of every $T_{1/2}$, peak/trough ratio will be 2:1. If it is given at two times $T_{1/2}$ this ratio is 4:1; at intervals of half of a $T_{1/2}$, 1.4:1. For antiarrhythmic drugs which have narrow toxic/therapeutic ratios and the need for minimum effective levels to be maintained at all times, a narrow peak/trough is generally desirable. Drug administration should take this into consideration.

In the blood, drug may be bound to protein. The bound portion is inactive and free drug is responsible for drug activity. Protein binding of drugs is an issue in interpretation of serum levels when elevations in or saturation of binding sites occur (see Chapter 12, sections on lidocaine and disopyramide).

Active metabolites exist for a number of antiarrhythmic drugs. These have antiarrhythmic and toxic properties of their own. While they are similar to the parent compound, active metabolites rarely have precisely the same EP effects, antiarrhythmic spectrum, and toxicity.

Each antiarrhythmic drug has a suggested therapeutic range of drug levels. However, it is important to realize that these ranges are by no means precise. For most drugs, there is considerable overlap and interpatient variation between therapeusis and toxicity at the upper boundary of the therapeutic window and effectiveness and ineffectiveness at the lower boundary (Fig. 11.12). An individual patient can easily be an outlier.

Knowledge of pharmacokinetic parameters permits relatively precise dosing to achieve target serum levels (27). Some relevant dosing formulae are given in Table 11.1. Precise dosing is especially important for antiarrhythmic drugs because of their narrow toxic/therapeutic ratios.

It is also important to remember that both the physician and

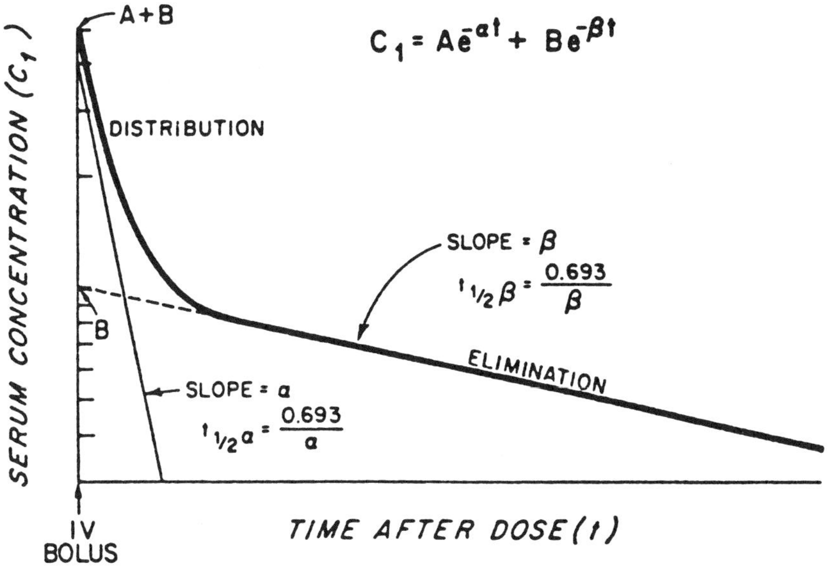

Figure 11.8. Schematic of drug concentration (C_1) (*vertical axis*) on a logarithmic scale versus time (*horizontal axis*) after a single intravenous dose of drug based on a two-compartment model. There is a distribution (alpha) and an elimination (beta) phase of drug decline. Both alpha and beta phases have their own half-lives. (From Greenblatt DJ, Koch-Weser J: Medical intelligence: drug therapy-clinical pharmacokinetics (first of two parts). N Engl J Med 1975;14:702–705, with permission.)

Table 11.1.
Useful Pharmacokinetic Formulas

1. $D_L = V_D \times C_p$ (intravenous)
2. $D_M = Cl \times C_p$ (intravenous)
3. $D_M = \dfrac{C_p \times Cl \times T}{f}$ (oral)
4. $C_p = \dfrac{f \times D_M}{Cl \times T}$
5. $f = \dfrac{AUC_{po}}{AUC_{iv}}$
6. $\beta T_{1/2} = \dfrac{0.693 \times V_D}{Cl}$
7. $Cl = \dfrac{A_D/t}{C_p}$
8. $K_e = \dfrac{0.693}{T_{1/2}}$

Abbreviations: A_D = drug amount; AUC_{po} = area under the curve after oral administration; AUC_{iv} = area under the curve after intravenous administration; C_p = plasma drug concentration; Cl = drug clearance; D_L = loading dose; D_M = maintenance dose; f = bioavailability; K_e = elimination constant; t = time; T = dosing interval; $T_{1/2}$ = half-life; V_D = volume of distribution.

HALF LIVES	1	2	3	4	5	6	7
Accumulation	50%	75%	87.5%	93.8%	96.9%	98.4%	99.2%
Elimination	50%	25%	12.5%	6.2%	3.1%	1.6%	.8%
	1/2	1/4	1/8	1/16	1/32	1/64	1/128

Figure 11.9. Accumulation and elimination of drugs during one to seven half-lives. Shown are percentages of steady-state levels. "Accumulation" shows percentages after initiation of a constant rate infusion and "elimination" after cessation of an infusion that was at steady-state levels. The *bottom line* shows elimination fractions. After one half-life, drug accumulates to 50% of final steady-state levels after two 75%, etc. It takes 3.3 and 5 half-lives to reach 90 and 97% of steady state, respectively. Elimination: after one half-life drug declines to 50% (½) of steady state, after two half-lives to 25%, (¼), etc.

the patient have a responsibility for proper dosing. In life-threatening arrhythmias antiarrhythmic drugs have to be taken consistently. They must be at a certain minimal effective concentration to be protective at all times. Achieving therapeutic concentration of antiarrhythmic drugs assumes that the drug is presented and taken properly. The physician must prescribe them based on clinical, pharmacologic, and EP principles. The patient must take the drug according to the prescribed regimen. Unfortunately, patient compliance can often be a problem, especially with agents that have short half-lives and therefore require frequent administration (28) (Fig. 11.13).

Figure 11.14 shows the problem of missing even one drug dose in the case of procainamide. Note the drug levels, which were within the therapeutic range virtually all the time before the missed dose subsequently fall below minimum effective concentration for the time from the missed to the next dose and a good percentage of time afterward.

CLINICAL EVALUATION OF ARRHYTHMIC DRUG EFFECTIVENESS

Ambulatory Electrocardiogram

The main clinical techniques used in evaluating specific drug effects on arrhythmias are ambulatory electrocardiography and EP testing. The 24- to 72-hr ambulatory ECG or "Holter" monitor is the predominant monitoring technique. Here, arrhythmia is analyzed during a control period of monitoring and then on drug. The technique is widely used but is expensive, a factor that places limits on the number of ambulatory ECGs that can be performed in a given situation and time consuming.

In using ambulatory electrocardiographic monitoring, it is

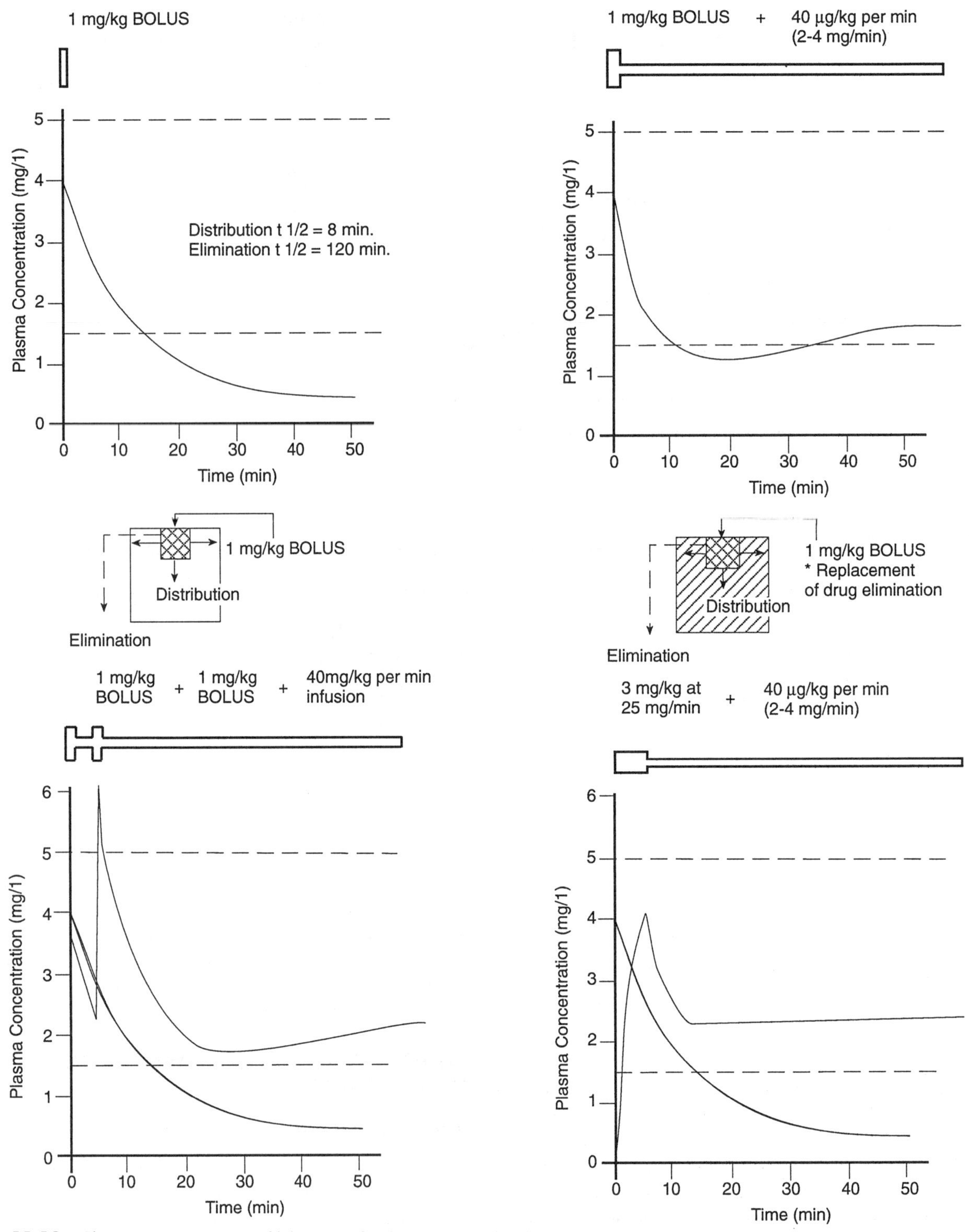

Figure 11.10. Plasma concentrations of lidocaine after four different types of administration. Distribution (α) $T_{1/2}$ of 8 min and elimination (β) $T_{1/2}$ of 120 min are assumed. **A** shows rapid intravenous administration. **B** shows an intravenous loading dose plus a constant rate infusion at 40 µg/kg/min. Note that it takes some time for steady-state drug levels to be reached and there is a dip below minimum effective concentration (*dashed line*) with nadir at about 40 min. **C** shows administration of a second bolus of 1 mg/kg. Here drug levels remain above minimum effective concentration at all times. However, they do not enter into the toxic range briefly, at about 15 min. **D** shows results when loading dose was administered more slowly over 10 min. Drug levels remained in the therapeutic range but attainment of therapeutic levels had some delay. (From Nattel S, Zipes DP: Clinical pharmacology of old and new antiarrhythmic drugs. Cardiovasc Res 1980;11:221–248, with permission.)

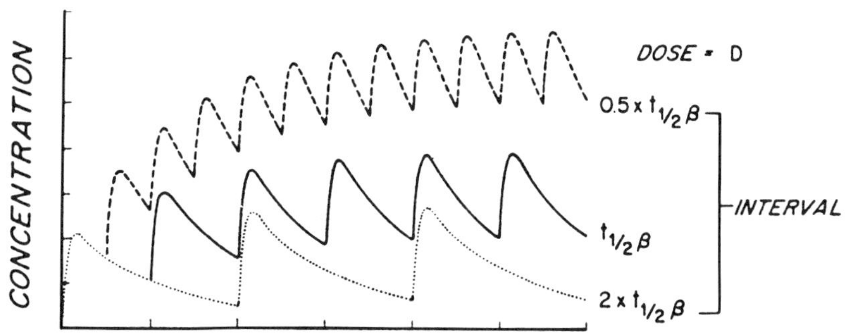

Figure 11.11. Concentration of drug (*vertical axis*) vs. time (*horizontal axis*) when drug given at three different dose intervals. Drug is given at an interval of half a T½ (upper), one T½ (middle), and two T½s (lower). With a more frequent dosing interval peak:trough ratios are much narrower (see Table 11.2). This is a generally desirably effect for antiarrhythmic drugs which require a minimum effective concentration at all times and have narrow toxic/therapeutic ratios. (From Greenblatt DJ, Koch-Weser J: Medical intelligence: drug therapy-clinical pharmacokinetics (second of two parts). N Engl J Med 1975;19:964–979, with permission.)

Table 11.2.
Peak/Trough Ratios

Half-life Multiple	Peak/Trough
1 $T_{1/2}$	2:1
2 $T_{1/2}$	4:1
4 $T_{1/2}$	16:1
0.5 $T_{1/2}$	1.4:1

important to note that there is considerable spontaneous variation in arrhythmia, making drug evaluation more difficult. For example, it was found that the occurrence of spontaneous ventricular premature complexes (VPCs) had a 23% day-to-day, 29% 8-hr, and 48% hourly variation. On the basis of this data, the established guideline for distinguishing drug-induced suppression of VPCs from spontaneous biologic variation is: 83% reduction in VPCs with 24-hr and 65% with 72-hr monitoring periods (29). Other briefer monitoring periods have been tried for specific purposes. (It should, however, be noted that the relevance of VPC suppression to occurrence of more serious arrhythmias is particularly open to question in view of the Cardiac Arrhythmia Suppression Trial) (see below).

Sustained arrhythmias of all types may also display considerable variation. They may or may not appear within a given ambulatory monitoring interval making antiarrhythmic drug evaluation difficult or impossible. In addition, ECG monitoring does not assess the hemodynamic consequences of arrhythmias.

Event monitors may be helpful, particularly when arrhythmias are relatively infrequent. These recordings only detect abnormal rhythms, e.g., tachycardias, and are attached to patients for more prolonged periods. Several types of event recorders are available and these are discussed in Chapter 3. Another commonly used technique is the transtelephonic recorder. This device is carried about by the patient and then applied to the body by means of direct contact electrodes when symptoms occur. Recordings are then transmitted via telephone to an interpretation center. If a serious arrhythmia is detected, the patient's physician or emergency squads are alerted. Also, in evaluation of nonlife-threatening arrhythmias (e.g. atrial fibrillation) this sort of monitoring plus symptom diaries is a useful approach in the evaluation of drug therapy.

Clinical Electrophysiology Testing

An important function of the clinical electrophysiologic (EP) test is to determine effectiveness of antiarrhythmic drugs (see also Chapters 4–8). The test is used not only when drugs are administered alone but also when they are combined with implantable defibrillators (where they are used to reduce the frequency of episodes and avoid excessive defibrillatör discharges) or to evaluate effectiveness of surgical therapy. The clinical EP study involves (a) induction of arrhythmia, (b) repeat testing using an intravenous drug (procainamide and/or lidocaine) as a screen, (c) 3 or more days of oral drug dosing (in the case of amiodarone 2–3 wk), followed by (d) an abbreviated electrophysiologic test to examine drug effects on arrhythmia inducibility. For ventricular arrhythmias most commonly, a Class IA drug is tried first (at one or occasionally more doses), and if not effective, a Class IB or β-adrenergic blocking agent may be added. Serum drug levels are measured at all times of testing. Effectiveness of Type IC drugs or a combination of different classes of drugs may also be tested in specific situations. For Wolff-Parkinson-White syndrome and other supraventricular tachycardias, a wider variety of drugs are employed.

In the example of ventricular tachycardia (VT), drug is considered completely effective if it prevents VT induction. However, some investigators define drug effectiveness of five or less repetitive ventricular complexes after antiarrhythmic drug administration, when VT or VF had been induced at baseline (30–32). A drug is considered partially effective if a more aggressive protocol (including the use of isoproterenol) is required for induction during drug testing or if VT rate is importantly slower or less sustained than at baseline (though how one should properly interpret a "partially effective" EP test is not resolved). Induction of VF has less certain implications in EP testing in general. Figure 11.15 is an example of drug testing for VT.

Sampling of plasma level of drug at the time of testing is important to determine target plasma levels for long-term therapy and also to determine if the effective level at the time of testing is in fact a reasonable target for the future or if it is a level at which toxicity is likely to occur.

For most drugs, effectiveness in EP testing predicts long-term

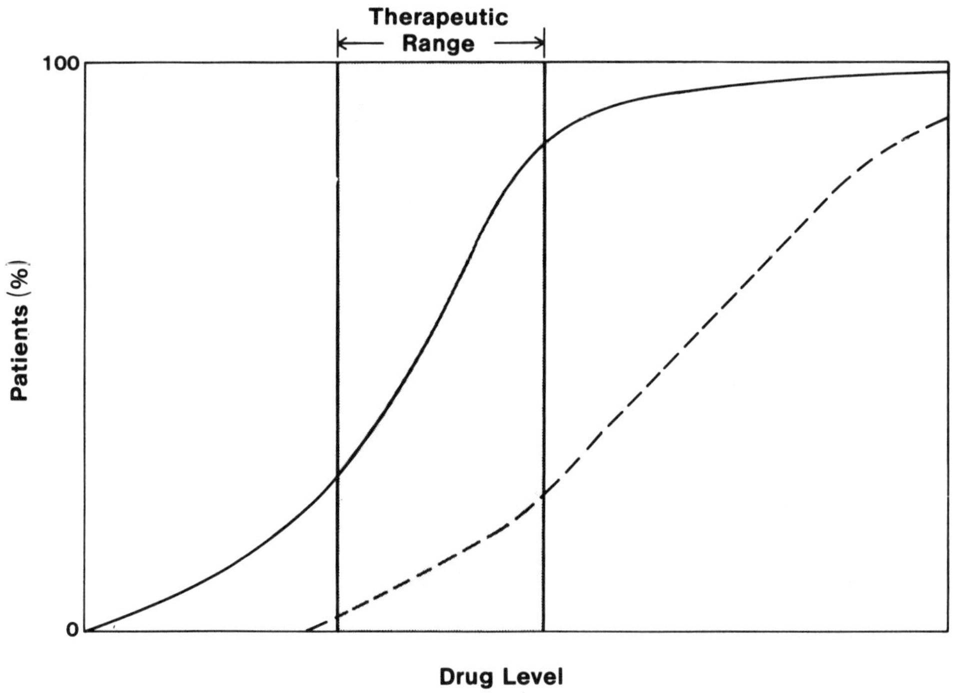

Figure 11.12. Schematic of effectiveness (*solid line*) and toxicity (*dashed line*) in a population of patients. The *horizontal axis* shows drug levels. The *vertical axis* shows the percent of patients with effectiveness or toxicity. The *central area* shows the accepted therapeutic range. As drug levels rise, the percent of patients with both effectiveness and toxicity increases but the therapeutic range does not completely reflect drug properties. Drug will be effective in a certain number of patients below the "therapeutic" range (i.e., below "minimum effective concentration") and other patients require higher levels than the "therapeutic" range for effectiveness. Similarly, a certain percentage of patients have drug toxicity within the "therapeutic" window and there are even occasional patients with toxicity below this window. However, for most patients the therapeutic window reflects both therapeusis and lack of toxicity. These curves are schematic; actual curves would vary with drug as well as with types of population studied.

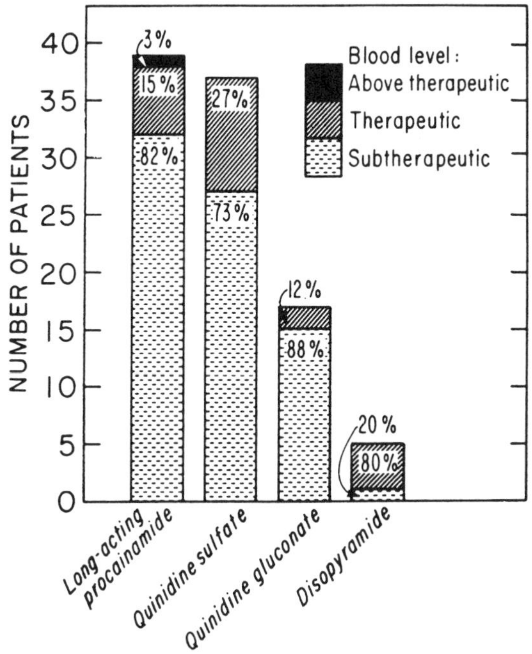

Figure 11.13. Serum drug levels in 100 patients in which therapeutic doses of the antiarrhythmic drugs indicated were prescribed. Drug levels were subtherapeutic in the predominant number indicating poor patient compliance. (From Squire A, Goldman M, Kupersmith J, *et al.*: Chronic antiarrhythmic therapy—a problem of low serum drug levels and patient noncompliance. Am J Med 1984;77:1035–1038, with permission.)

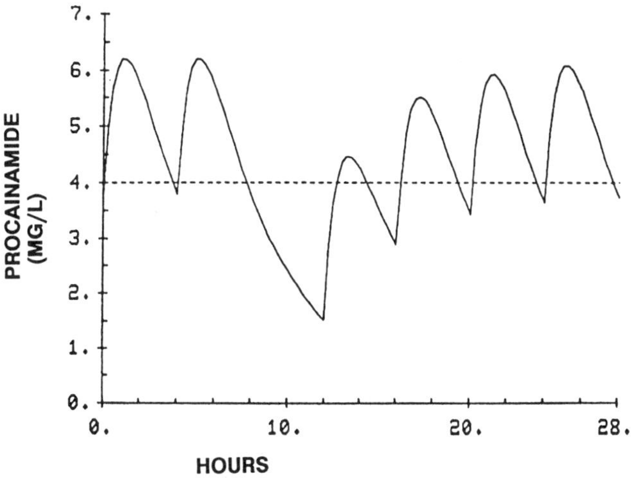

Figure 11.14. Computer simulation of drug levels of procainamide showing effects of one missed dose. Shown are serum levels of procainamide in a 70-kg male given 750 mg/Q4H. The *dashed line* shows the standard minimum effective concentration for procainamide. The early portion of the curve shows steady state during which serum levels are in the therapeutic range for almost the entire 4-hr interval. The patient does not take the third dose at 8 hr and then resumes taking the medication at 12 hr. Drug levels are below minimum effective concentration not only for the time of the missed dose but for several hours afterward until steady state is again achieved. This shows the importance of patient compliance and that even one missed dose results in drug levels that are below minimum effective concentration for many hours.

outcome. Figure 11.16 shows an example of a study in which there was improved survival when antiarrhythmic drugs were effective in EP tests versus when they were not (32). However, mortality was still significant in both groups. Other studies have shown a 1-yr incidence of "arrhythmia" events (including sudden death) of about 10–15% (34,35) in patients with noninducibility at EP testing through some of the studies included arrhythmia surgery as well as strictly drug treated patients (31,35).

Regarding which drug(s) is (are) more likely to be more effective, such data are hard to come by and evaluate. Most investigational electrophysiology laboratories have selected populations with higher proportions of difficult to treat patients. Data on relative (or absolute) effectiveness of various drugs may thus be skewed.

Regarding atrial arrhythmias, EP studies predict drug efficacy in the case of circus movement tachycardias due to Wolff-Parkinson-White and AV nodal reentry (36). There was also some predictability in the case of inducible atrial fibrillation (37) though this is far less certain. A therapeutic response in atrial fibrillation with accessory pathway conduction is predicted by slowing of the ventricular response and prolongation of accessory pathway refractoriness in the electrophysiology laboratory (see also Chapter 9) (38).

It should be remembered that the electrophysiology test is designed for analysis of reentrant and not automatic arrhythmias and also does not detect arrhythmias due to acute ischemia. In addition, the test examines mainly substrate and not trigger. An antiarrhythmic drug could suppress or alter the trigger, an occurrence that might not be detected in EP testing.

Another confounding factor in the evaluation of the EP test for drug response is the autonomic nervous system. The EP test does not assess changes in autonomic tone which, of course, have great relevance to arrhythmias. In recent years a number of methods of autonomic analysis, including tilt testing, Valsalva maneuver and infusion of catacholamines, have been added to the standard EP tests (39–43). Infusion of epinephrine, for example, was found to reverse antiarrhythmic efficacy of quinidine but not amiodarone for ventricular arrhythmias in the EP laboratory (40). Also antiarrhythmic effects of the flecainide in paroxysmal supraventricular tachycardia (PSVT) associated with accessory pathways were reversed by epinephrine in these patients in whom the drug would prove ineffective long-term (43). (See also Chapter 2 for discussion of autonomic influences on reentry.) It is hoped that in the future, autonomic analysis will be elaborated and refined so as to become a routine part of the EP test.

Pharmacokinetics and the Electrophysiologic Study

There are certain considerations related to drug kinetics that must be borne in mind when performing EP drug testing.

1. One generally does not achieve a true study state in a short

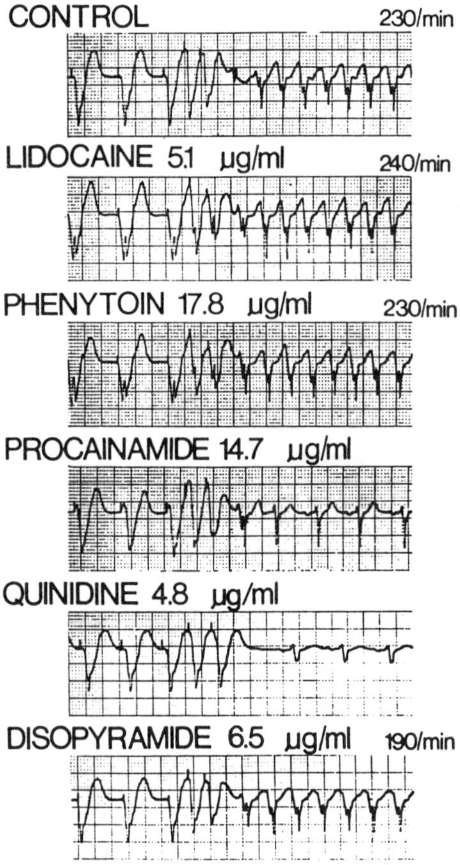

Figure 11.15. Programmed premature stimulation during control and after administration of several antiarrhythmic drugs. Two premature stimuli were applied in each instance. During control, sustained monomorphic ventricular tachycardia at a rate of 230/min was induced. Both quinidine and procainamide prevented induction of tachycardia. Lidocaine and phenytoin had no effect. Disopyramide caused induction of VT at 190 beats/min which would be considered partial effectiveness. Serum levels of drug at the time of induction are also shown. The usual therapeutic ranges of these drugs are in Table 12.3. (From Kastor JA, Horowitz LN, Harken AH, *et al.*: Clinical electrophysiology of ventricular tachycardia. N Engl J Med 1981:304:1004–1020, with permission.)

period of time with intravenous drug. As seen in Figure 11.10, no matter how the infusion is administered, there is variation. This is especially troublesome in terms of drug levels versus pharmacologic effects in the earliest infusion time interval (post–loading dose) when drug level is rapidly changing and tissues are not yet saturated (unless one uses an exponential infusion). It is thus important to wait until the major variation in drug levels have passed and to obtain serum levels at precisely the time of programmed stimulation. For lidocaine as seen in Fig 11.10, this is about 60–90 min; for procainamide, more than 2 hr.

2. The use of intravenous drugs to screen for oral drugs is a common approach. Lidocaine is often administered intravenously as a screen for other Class IB drugs such as tocainide and mexiletine. It is important to remember that these are different drugs with limited cross-responsiveness (44). On the other hand, of interest, Waxman, *et al.* (45) found that if procainamide (15 mg/kg at rate of 50 mg/min) prevents induction of VT, there is an 85% likelihood that a single or combination of Class IA, IB, and IC drugs will be effective. Though it may not be easy to delineate the successful regimen, this particular screen at least permits some insight as to likelihood of success in general with a pharmacologic approach.

3. Active metabolites do not play a role in intravenous drug administration. Clinically important active metabolites generally have longer half-lives and thus take longer to reach steady state than the parent compound (27,46,47a). They are also less prominent after 3 days of oral administration of drug than they would be with more chronic use. This is important for some drugs. The procainamide metabolite *N*-acetyl procainamide (NAPA) is probably the offending agent in torsade de pointes more than the parent compound. (47) This form of toxicity may not be apparent in intravenous or short-term oral use, while it may appear later as NAPA levels rise. Propranolol and verapamil both have active metabolites and extensive first-pass metabolism (22,23). Thus, intravenously administered drug (where only parent compound is important), may act rather differently than orally administered drug. Figure 11.17 shows the example of encainide where two of its active metabolites take considerably longer than the parent compound to arrive at steady state.

4. When more than one intravenous drug is administered in relatively close succession, there will almost surely be additive effects making interpretation of test results more difficult.

5. Certain factors may cause a different response to drug acutely than clinically. These include a heightened adrenergic state during the invasive EP test or alterations in serum K^+ or Mg^{2+} levels.

6. Some drugs have a lag time between peak serum level and peak effect. This effect may be due to delayed tissue uptake or delay in reaching the specific active site in the myocardial cell. Bretylium is an example of this effect (48).

7. Testing of intravenous drug in the EP lab is an "idealized" condition, i.e., drug is evaluated at a specific level during constant rate infusion, the environment is controlled, etc. These idealized conditions are not replicated in the ambulatory patient.

8. For the above several reasons, use of intravenous drug in EP testing can never be considered conclusive. It can only be used as a screen for future testing of oral drug.

9. Half-lives of drug may be prolonged by congestive heart failure, renal failure or hepatic dysfunction. Thus, 3 days of oral drug may not, in certain instances, be sufficient to arrive at steady-state serum levels.

10. There may be some day-to-day variability in the EP test (due to autonomic changes, etc.) creating a problem with oral testing (49). However, this problem may not be as great as one would think, e.g., for monomorphic ventricular tachycardia (50).

11. Amiodarone presents a special problem. Some observers feel that the electrophysiology test is associated with uniquely less reliable predictability of outcome in the case of amiodarone.

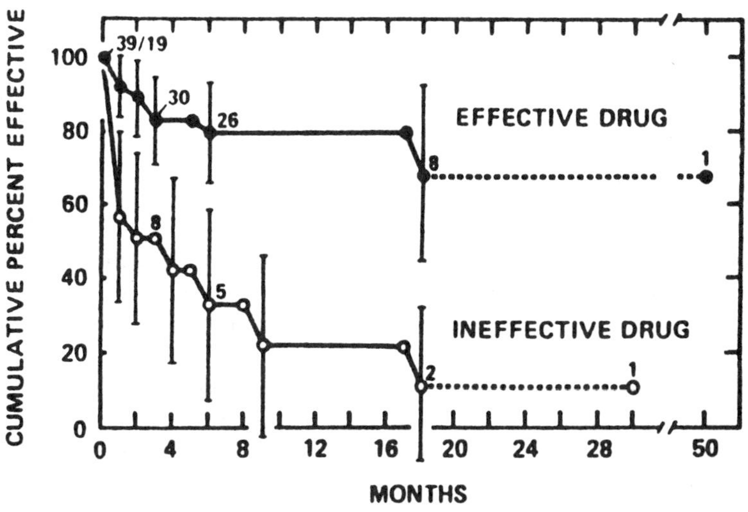

Figure 11.16. Long-term efficacy of antiarrhythmic drugs after electrophysiologic testing. Cumulative percentage effective, i.e., freedom from arrhythmia events, is shown on the *vertical axis*. The *solid circles* represent patients with drug efficacy by EP testing and the *open circles* represent patients with ineffectiveness by EP testing. Patients with a successful EP tests have less recurrences, mainly in the earlier months. Numbers represent numbers of patients in each group at the various follow-up time intervals. It should be noted that this was a nonrandomized study. (From Mason JW, Winkle RA: Accuracy of the ventricular tachycardia-induction study for predicting long-term efficacy and inefficacy of antiarrhythmic drugs. N Engl J Med 1980; 303:1073–1077, with permission.)

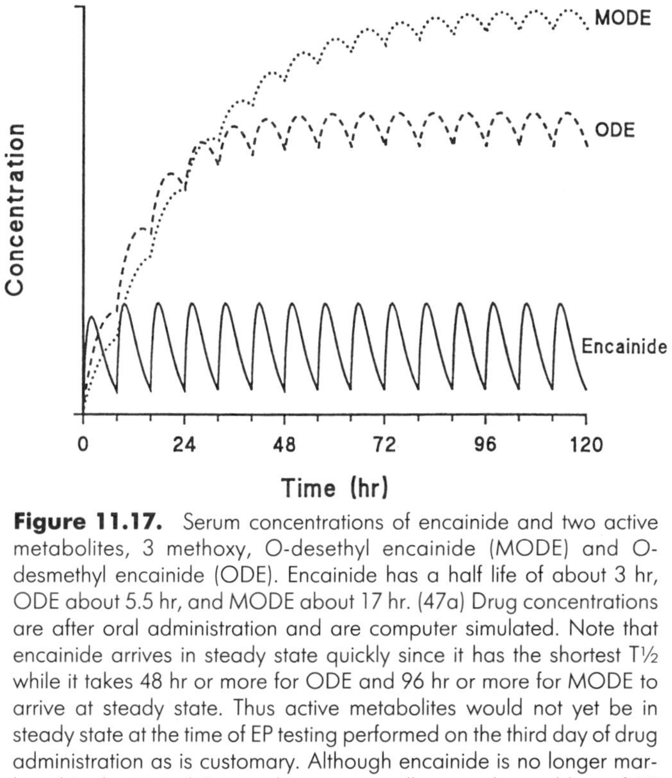

Figure 11.17. Serum concentrations of encainide and two active metabolites, 3 methoxy, O-desethyl encainide (MODE) and O-desmethyl encainide (ODE). Encainide has a half life of about 3 hr, ODE about 5.5 hr, and MODE about 17 hr. (47a) Drug concentrations are after oral administration and are computer simulated. Note that encainide arrives in steady state quickly since it has the shortest T½ while it takes 48 hr or more for ODE and 96 hr or more for MODE to arrive at steady state. Thus active metabolites would not yet be in steady state at the time of EP testing performed on the third day of drug administration as is customary. Although encainide is no longer marketed in the United States, this serves to illustrate the problem of EP studies and active metabolites. (From Roden DM: Clinical pharmacological requisites to ensure the adequacy of antiarrhythmic therapy. In Rosen MR, Janse MJ, With AL (eds): Cardiac Electrophysiology. Mt. Kisco, NY, Futura Publishing Co., 1990:1095–1115, with permission.)

Others feel that a longer waiting time for the drug assessment EP test is needed because of amiodarone's long half-life (1–2 mo rather than 3 days) and that partial EP effectiveness has predictive value for long-term suppression of arrhythmias. This topic will be discussed in more detail in the amiodarone section of Chapter 12.

12. If a patient was already taking antiarrhythmic drugs before the study, at least five half-lives must pass before drug is cleared from the system. At this point, serum level is at 3% of steady state (Fig. 11.9).

13. Frequent use of lidocaine to locally anesthetize tissues may lead to therapeutic serum levels confounding EP test results.

14. Repeated drug testing is expensive. This fact will surely be important not only in determining the overall role of EP drug testing but also in limiting the number of drugs one can test.

DRUG COMBINATIONS

For various reasons antiarrhythmic drug combinations may be useful to achieve certain ends. Proper selection depends on evaluating EP properties, pharmacokinetics, and possible adverse effects. For example, combining two local anesthetic drugs may allow one to achieve therapeusis at a relatively lower level of each drug and thus avoid the bothersome extra cardiac effects of a particular drug (e.g., diarrhea with quinidine or neurologic toxicity with Class IB agents)

There may be an advantage in administering drugs with slow and fast receptor kinetics to achieve a more complete range of properties, i.e., substantial blockade of both open and closed channels with consequent potentiated effect on premature beats and tachycardia (51,52). Also, drugs that prolong APD will as a result maintain membrane potential at inactivated (plateau levels) for more prolonged periods of time. This can potentiate effects of other drugs that have had high affinity for the Na^+ channel in the inactivated state. On the other hand, there may be competition for the Na^+ channel between a weaker and stronger blocking drug. In this instance, the stronger agent will be weakened. If the drug that causes less intense Na^+ blockade has greater affinity to the Na^+ channel, the overall effect of the competition will be less Na^+ blockade. In some instances metabolites of a drug may have such an effect.

Beta blockers may be administered with Class I drugs (53) to obtain a different type of pharmacologic benefit, i.e., antiadrenergic effects, which may be important in certain patients and are difficult to assess by presently used EP techniques. Beta blockers may also counteract the adverse effects of some agents, e.g., mexiletine-induced tremors.

PROARRHYTHMIA

General

Proarrhythmia is an important issue in consideration of "antiarrhythmic" drugs. As indicated above and in Chapter 2, the very properties which convey antiarrhythmic effects, e.g., conduction delay and block, can also increase arrhythmias. In addition, many agents are capable of inducing arrhythmias by causing early or delayed afterdepolarizations. Drugs may also exert proarrhythmic effects in ways that are not primarily EP. They may cause mechanical or hemodynamic depression, alter autonomic function, or promote adverse drug interactions.

Proarrhythmia has been recognized with a number of antiarrhythmic agents. A long-recognized example is VF due to quinidine (54) as well as torsade de pointes in the acquired long QT syndrome (55). More recently, increase in VPCs on ambulatory ECG and proarrhythmic effects on EP testing have been recognized with a wide variety of agents. Specific criteria are, however, somewhat arbitrary.

The following criteria for proarrhythmia have been used in ambulatory ECGs (56): (a) a 4-fold increase in VPCs per hour, (b) a 10-fold increase in repetitive forms (couplets or VT) per hour, (c) first occurrence of sustained VT not present during drug-free control monitoring.

For EP testing in VT/VF, the following criteria have been proposed (57): (a) induction of sustained VT or VF on drug while only nonsustained VT was induced at baseline, (b) development of induced sustained VT, reversible only by cardioversion when arrhythmia was reversible by pacing at baseline, (c) induction of ventricular arrhythmias via a less aggressive mode on drug than at baseline (see Chapter 4), (d) occurrence of spontaneous VT on drug in a patient when induction by programmed stimulation was required at baseline, (e) shorter cycle length of induced VT on drug than at baseline. The degree of shortening is again somewhat arbitrary but more than 20% has been suggested (57,58), (f) lack of inducibility of arrhythmia off drug but inducibility with drug administration. This situation, i.e., drug testing for proarrhythmia, would come up in patient with an episode of VT/VF while taking a drug for lesser arrhythmia such as VPCs or atrial flutter (59).

Criteria for proarrhythmia in supraventricular tachycardia and preexcitation syndromes are less well defined but would presumably follow along similar lines.

Cardiac Arrhythmia Suppression Trial

The question of proarrhythmia and the danger of "antiarrhythmic" drugs was brought to particular public and professional attention by the Cardiac Arrhythmia Suppression Trial (CAST) (60–62). CAST was a post–myocardial infarction sudden death prevention trial. It has long been known that the occurrence of VPCs after myocardial infarction was associated with an increased overall cardiac as well as sudden death mortality (63–65). It was not known, but was a reasonable hypothesis, that suppression of VPCs with antiarrhythmic drugs would prevent sudden death. Previous trials of antiarrhythmic drugs in this setting had been inconclusive except for these showing diminished mortality with nonsympathomimetic beta blockers (66,67). CAST was launched with the hypothesis that reduction of VPCs by antiarrhythmic drugs would result in a diminished incidence of arrhythmic death after myocardial infarction.

CAST examined three drugs, encainide, flecainide, and moricizine, all of which had been found in a pilot trial (the Cardiac Arrhythmia Pilot Study) (68) to suppress VPCs post–myocardial infarction without much in the way of either adverse effects or proarrhythmia on ambulatory ECGs. CAST enrolled post–myocardial infarction patients with six or more VPCs/hr and no runs of VT greater than 120 beats/min or a total of 15 beats (61).

Patients first underwent an open-label VPC suppression dose titration (encainide 35–50 mg t.i.d.; flecainide 100–150 mg b.i.d.; moricizine 200–250 mg t.i.d.). Patients responding to the drug with at least 80% suppression of VPCs and 90% suppression of VT runs were randomized to that particular drug. No patient entered into the study had "proarrhythmia," i.e., increased VPCs by the above definition on ambulatory ECG (60,61).

In 1989, the encainide and flecainide arms of CAST were stopped before completion of enrollment because of the striking results shown in Figure 11.18. Encainide and flecainide had increased mortality/cardiac arrest (60,61). The moricizine limb was stopped in 1991 because of drug ineffectiveness in diminishing mortality.

Reasons for excess mortality with encainide and flecainide are not clear, but adverse interactions with ischemic tissue (i.e., enhanced ischemia-induced conduction delay), depression of myocardial function as well as others have been postulated (60–62). It is of interest that the drugs increased the incidence of mortality due to myocardial infarction with shock and congestive heart failure as well as due to arrhythmia (though it should be noted that classification of mortality into arrhythmic versus nonarrhythmic causes is rather difficult).

CAST has many implications and it will take some time to completely sort them out. The hypothesis that suppression of VPCs of its own will reduce mortality is now disproved. Thus, the value of ambulatory monitoring of VPCs in the evaluation of therapy for more serious arrhythmias in the setting of ischemia is also in question. In addition, previously held concepts about proarrhythmia and how to assess it must be reevaluated. No patient entered in CAST had proarrhythmia, as defined above by an increase in ventricular arrhythmia on ambulatory ECG (see above) (60–62). In addition, adverse consequences in CAST occurred over a wide spectrum of patients, not, as would have been previously thought, only in those with more severe disease factors. CAST included mostly patients with VPCs and not those

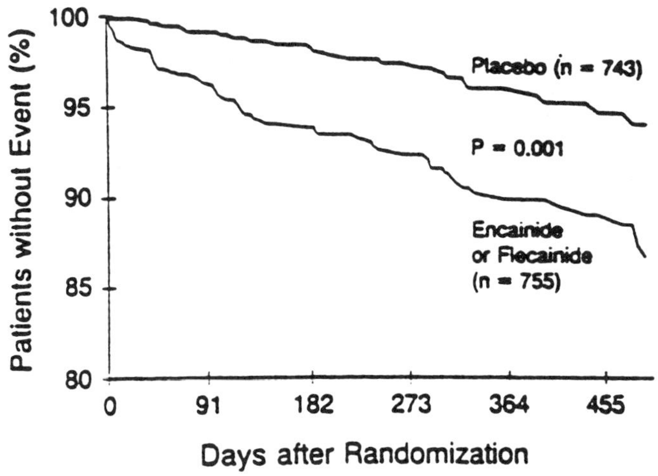

Placebo	743	625	516	412	292	181
Active drug	755	619	507	392	286	186

Figure 11.18. Actuarial probability of freedom from death or cardiac arrest due to arrhythmia in patients receiving encainide/flecainide or placebo in the cardiac arrhythmia suppression trial (CAST). Numbers in the lower section are patients at risk of an event. Numbers of events are less in the placebo than in the encainide/flecainide group. (From Echt DS, Liebson PR, Mitchenn LB, *et al.*: Mortality and morbidity in patients receiving encainide, flecainide, or placebo. N Engl J Med 1991:324:781–788, with permission.)

with more severe arrhythmias (69). Also, increased mortality in CAST occurred independent of ejection fraction, baseline QRS duration, and a number of other factors.

Extrapolation of results to other situations besides myocardial infarction may or may not be appropriate. However, the burden of proof (except in the case of beta blockers) (66,67) is now on any hypothesis stating that a particular antiarrhythmic drug will reduce mortality in a given situation.

A meta-analysis review published since and including the encainide and flecainide data from CAST, examined agents used after myocardial infarction by class (see Chapter 12 for antiarrhythmic drug classification), and found the following. Classes I (local anesthetic) and Class IV agents (Ca^{2+} channel blockers) caused a nonsignificant excess in mortality. When Classes IA, B, and C were examined separately, only Class IC displayed a statistically significant excess. Class III agents were associated with a nonsignificant and Class II (beta blockers) a highly significant reduction in mortality (70).

Meta-analysis reviews of quinidine have found an increased mortality in trials of patients with all but most severe ventricular arrhythmias (71) and in those with paroxysmal atrial fibrillation (72). Results with Class IB agents over a number of trials showed a nonstatistically significant trend in this direction (70,73). These included the International Mexiletine and Placebo Antiarrhythmia Coronary Trial (IMPACT) of patients post–myocardial infarction which on its own had the same nonstatistically significant trend (74).

Meta-analysis reviews such as these have contributed greatly to our understanding of antiarrhythmic drugs. However, it should be noted that meta-analysis involves summation of previous known trials which may have tested various and different hypotheses than the one evaluated by meta-analysis. The previous trials generally but not always (71,72) have involved broad patient categories rather than specific subgroups. Clinicians, on the other hand, may have to face patients in specific subgroups where results may vary from the group as a whole. Also, there may have been negative trials that were not published and not available for inclusion.

Clinical trials now underway with amiodarone (75) and other drugs should help us to assess the proper role of antiarrhythmic therapy. Because of CAST and other findings related to proarrhythmia, it has been suggested that Class I and III drugs be started in hospital.

References

1. Weidmann S: The effect of the cardiac membrane potential on the rapid availability of the sodium-carrying system. J Physiol 1955;127:213–224.
2. Weidmann S: Effects of calcium ions and local anesthetics on electrical properties of Purkinje fibers. J Physiol 1955;129:568–582.
3. Vaughan Williams EM: A classification of antiarrhythmic actions reassessed after a decade of new drugs. J Clin Pharmacol 1984;24:129–147.
4. Hondgehem L, Katzung BG: Test of a model of antiarrhythmic drug action: Effects of quinidine and lidocaine on myocardial conduction. Circulation 1980;61:1217–1224.
5. Hondgehem, LM, Katzung BG: Antiarrhythmic agents: The modulated receptor mechanism of action of sodium and calcium channel-blocking drugs. Annu Rev Pharmacol Toxicol 1984;24:387–423.
6. Hille B: Local anesthetics: hydrophilic and hydrophobic pathways for the drug-receptor reaction. J Gen Physiol 1977;69:497–515.
7. Strauss HC: Mechanisms of local anesthetic interaction with the sodium channel. In Rosen MR, Janse MJ, Wit AL (eds): Cardiac Electrophysiology. Mt. Kisco, NY, Futura Publishing Co., 1990;995–1012.
8. Gintant GA, Hoffman BF, Naylor RE: The influence of molecular form of local anesthetic-type antiarrhythmic agents on reduction of the maximum upstroke velocity of canine cardiac Purkinje fibers. Circ Res 1983;52:735–746.
9. Courtney KR: Interval-dependent effects of small antiarrhythmic drugs on excitability of guinea-pig myocardium. J Mol Cell Cardiol 1980;12:1273–1286.

10. Kupersmith J, Antman EM, Hoffman BF: *In vivo* electrophysiologic effects of lidocaine in canine acute myocardial infarction. Circ Res 1975;36:84–91.
11. Allen JD, Pomerantz J, Wit AL: Actions of lidocaine on transmembrane potentials of subendocardial Purkinje fibers surviving in infarcted canine hearts. Circ Res 1978;43:470–481.
12. Hiromasa S, Li ZY, Coto H, *et al.*: Selective effects of tocainide in canine acute myocardial infarction. Int J Cardiol 1990;27:79–86.
13. Kupersmith J: Antiarrhythmic drugs—changing concepts. Am J Cardiol 1976;38:119–121.
14. Kupersmith J, Shiang H, Litwak RS, *et al.*: Electrophysiological and antiarrhythmic effects of propranolol in canine acute myocardial ischemia. Circ Res 1976;38:302–307.
15. Hoffman BF, Cranefield PF: Electrophysiology of the Heart. McGraw-Hill, New York, 1960.
16. Kupersmith J: Electrophysiologic and antiarrhythmic effects of lidocaine in canine acute myocardial ischemia. Am Heart J 1979;97:320–327.
17. Schmitt OF, Erlanger J: Directional differences in the conduction of the impulse through heart muscle and their possible relation of extrasystolic and fibrillary contractions. Am J Physiol 1928-1929;87:326–347.
18. Han J, Moe GK: Nonuniform recovery of excitability of ventricular muscle. Circ Res 1964;14:44–60.
19. Greenblatt DJ, Koch-Weser J: Medical intelligence: drug therapy-clinical pharmacokinetics (first of two parts). N Engl J Med 1975;14:702–705.
20. Greenblatt DJ, Koch-Weser J: Medical intelligence: drug therapy-clinical pharmacokinetics (second of two parts). N Engl J Med 1975;19:964–979.
21. Scheiner LB, Tozer TN: Clinical Pharmacokinetics: the use of plasma concentrations of drugs. In Melmon KL, Morrelli HF (eds): Clinical Pharmacology. MacMillan, New York, 1978:71–109.
22. Kates RE, Keefe DL, Schwartz J, *et al.*: Verapamil disposition kinetics in chronic atrial fibrillation. Clin Pharmacol Ther 1981;30:44–51.
23. Nies AS, Shand DG: Clinical pharmacology of propranolol. Circulation 1975;52:6–15.
24. Roden DM: Clinical pharmacological requisites to ensure the adequacy of antiarrhythmic therapy. In Rosen MR, Janse MJ, Wit AL (eds): Cardiac Electrophysiology. Mt. Kisco, NY, Futura Publishing Co., 1990;1095–1115.
25. Echizen H. Vogelgesang B, Eichelbaum M: Effects of d, I-verapamil on atrioventricular conduction in relation to its stereoselective first-pass metabolism. Clin Pharmacol Ther 1985;38:71–76.
26. Nattel S, Zipes DP: Clinical pharmacology of old and new antiarrhythmic drugs. Cardiovas Res 1980;11:221–248.
27. Kupersmith J: Monitoring of antiarrhythmic drug levels: values and pitfalls. Ann NY Acad Sci 1984;432:138–154.
28. Squire A, Goldman M, Kupersmith J, *et al.*: Chronic antiarrhythmic therapy—a problem of low serum drug levels and patient noncompliance. Am J Med 1984;77:1035–1038.
29. Morganroth J, Anderson JL, Gentzkow GD: Classification by type of ventricular arrhythmia predicts frequency of adverse cardiac events from flecainide. J Am Coll Cardiol 1986;8:607–615.
30. Mason JW, Winkle RA: Electrode-catheter arrhythmia induction in the selection and assessment of antiarrhythmic drug therapy for recurrent ventricular tachycardia. Circulation 1978;58:971–985.
31. Swerdlow CD, Winkle RA, Mason JW: Determinants of survival in patients with ventricular tachyarrhythmias. N Engl J Med 1983;308:1436–1442.
32. Mason JW, Winkle RA: Accuracy of the ventricular tachycardia-induction study for predicting long-term efficacy and inefficacy of antiarrhythmic drugs. N Engl J Med 1980;303:1073–1077.
33. Kastor JA, Horowitz LN, Harken AH, *et al.*: Clinical electrophysiology of ventricular tachycardia. N Engl J Med 1981;304:1004–1020.
34. Eldar M, Sauve M, Scheinman, M: Electrophysiologic testing and follow-up of patients with aborted sudden death. J Am Coll Cardiol 1987;10:291–296.
35. Wilber JD, Garan H, Kelly E, *et al.*: Out-of-hospital cardiac arrest: role of electrophysiologic testing in the prediction of long-term outcome. N Engl J Med 1988;318:19–24.
36. Bauernfeind RA, Wyndham CRC, Dhingra RC, *et al.*: Serial electrophysiologic testing of multiple drugs in patients with atrioventricular nodal reentrant paroxysmal tachycardia. Circulation 1980;62:1341–1349.
37. Bauerfeind RA, Swiryn SP, Strasberg B, *et al.*: Electrophysiologic drug testing in prophylaxis of sporadic paroxysmal atrial fibrillation: technique, application, and efficacy in severely symptomatic preexcitation patients. Am Heart J 1982;103:941–949.
38. Morady F, Sledge C, Shen E, *et al.*: Electrophysiologic testing in the management of patients with the W-P-W syndrome and atrial fibrillation. Am J Cardiol 1983;51:1623–1628.
39. Brugada P, Facchini M, Wellens HJJ: Effects of isoproterenol and amiodarone and the role of exercise in initiation of circus movement tachycardia in the accessory atrioventricular pathway. Am J Cardiol 1986;57:146–149.
40. Calkins H, Sousa J, El-Atassi R, *et al.*: Reversal of antiarrhythmic drug effects by epinephrine: quinidine versus amiodarone. J Am Coll Cardiol 1992;19:347–352.
41. Jazayeri MR, VanWyhe G, Avitall B, *et al.*: Isoproterenol reversal of antiarrhythmic effects in patients with inducible sustained ventricular tachyarrhythmias. J Am Coll Cardiol 1989;14:705–711.
42. Morady F, Kou WH, Kadish AH, *et al.*: Antagonism of quinidine's electrophysiologic effects by epinephrine in patients with ventricular tachycardia. J Am Coll Cardiol 1988;12:388–394.
43. Cockrell JL, Scheinman MM, Titus C, *et al.*: Safety and efficacy of oral flecainide therapy in patients with atrioventricular reentrant tachycardia. Ann Intern Med 1991;114:189–194.
44. Podrid PJ, Lown B: Tocainide for refractory symptomatic ventricular arrhythmias. Am J Cardiol 1982;49:1279–1286.
45. Waxman HL, Buxton AE, Sadowski LM, *et al.*: The response to procainamide during electrophysiologic study for sustained ventricular tachyarrhythmias predicts the response to other medications. Circulation 1982;67:30–37.
46. Roden DM, Reele SB, Higgins SB, *et al.*: Antiarrhythmic efficacy, pharmacokinetics and safety of N-acetylprocainamide in human subjects: comparison with procainamide. Am J Cardiol 1980;46:463–468.
47. Olshansky B, Martins J, Hunt S: N-acetylprocainamide causing Torsades de Pointes. Am J Cardiol 1982;50:1439–1441.
47a. Barbey JT, Thompson KA, Echt DS, *et al.*: Antiarrhythmic activity, electrocardiographic effects and pharmacokinetics of the encainide metabolites O-desmethyl encainide and 3-methoxy-O-desmethyl encainide in man. Circulation 1988;77:380–391.
48. Anderson JL, Patterson E, Conlon M, *et al.*: Kinetics of antifibrillatory effects of bretylium: correlation with myocardial drug concentrations. Am J Cardiol 1980;46:583–589.
49. Bigger JT Jr, Reiffel JA, Livelli FD Jr, *et al.*: Sensitivity, specificity, and reproducibility of programmed ventricular stimulation. Circulation 73 (Suppl II) 1986;73–78.
50. Horowitz LN, Josephson ME, Farshidi A, *et al.*: Recurrent sustained ventricular tachycardia. 3. Role of the electrophysiologic study in selection of antiarrhythmic regimens. Circulation 1978;58:986–987.
51. Duff HJ, Roden D, Primm RK, *et al.*: Mexiletine in the treatment of resistant ventricular arrhythmias: Enhancement of efficacy and reduction of dose-related side effects by combination with quinidine. Circulation 1983;67:1124.
52. Valois M, Sasyniuk BI: Modification of the frequency- and voltage-dependent effects of quinidine when administered in combination with tocainide in canine Purkinje fibers. Circulation 1987;76(2):427–441.
53. Deedwania PC, Olukotun AY, Kupersmith J, *et al.*: Beta blockers in combination with class I antiarrhythmic agents. Am J Cardiol 1987;60:21D–26D.
54. Selzer A, Wray HW: Quinidine syncope: Paroxysmal ventricular fibrillation occurring during treatment of chronic atrial arrhythmias. Circulation 1964;30:17–23.
55. Roden DM, Woosley RL, Primm RK: Incidence and clinical features of the quinidine-associated long QT syndrome: Implications for patient care. Am Heart J 1986;111:1088–1093.

56. Velebit V, Podrid PJ, Lown B, *et al.*: Aggravation and provocation of ventricular arrhythmias by antiarrhythmic drugs. Circulation 1982;65:886–894.
57. Horowitz L, Greenspan A, Spielman S, *et al.*: Usefulness of electrophysiologic testing in evaluation of amiodarone therapy for sustained ventricular tachyarrhythmias associated with coronary heart disease. Am J Cardiol 1985;55:367–371.
58. Rinkenberger RL, Prystowsky EN, Jackman WM, *et al.*: Drug conversion of nonsustained ventricular tachycardia to sustained ventricular tachycardia during serial electrophysiologic studies: identification of drugs that exacerbate tachycardia and potential mechanisms. Am Heart J 1982;103:177–184.
59. Ruskin JN, McGovern B, Garan H, *et al.*: Antiarrhythmic drugs: A possible cause of out-of-hospital cardiac arrest. N Engl J Med 1983;309:1302–1306.
60. The Cardiac Arrhythmia Suppression Trial (CAST) Investigators: Effect of encainide and flecainide on mortality in a randomized trial of arrhythmia suppression after myocardial infarction. N Engl J Med 1989;321:406–412.
61. Echt DS, Liebson PR, Mitchenn LB, *et al.*: Mortality and morbidity in patients receiving encainide, flecainide, or placebo. N Engl J Med 1991;324:781–788.
62. Bigger JT: The events surrounding the removal of encainide and flecainide from the cardiac arrhythmia suppression trial (CAST) and why CAST is continuing with moricizine. J Am Coll Cardiol 1990;15:243–245.
63. Bigger JT Jr, Fleiss JL, Kleiger R, *et al.*: The relationships among ventricular arrhythmias, left ventricular dysfunction and mortality in the 2 years after myocardial infarction. Circulation 1984;69:250–258.
64. Ruberman W, Weinblatt JE, Goldberg JD, *et al.*: Ventricular premature beats and mortality after myocardial infarction. N Engl J Med 1977;297:750–757.
65. Moss AJ, Davis HT, DeCamilla J, *et al.*: Ventricular ectopic beats and their relation to sudden and non-sudden cardiac death after myocardial infarction. Circulation 1979;60:998–1003.
66. Beta-Blocker Heart Attack Trial Research Group: A randomized trial of propranolol in patients with acute myocardial infarction: I. Mortality results. JAMA 1982;247:1707–1714.
67. The Norwegian Multicenter Study Group. Timolol-induced reduction in mortality and reinfarction in patients surviving acute myocardial infarction. N Engl J Med 1981;304:801–807.
68. Cardiac Arrhythmia Pilot Study (CAPS) Investigators: Effect of encainide, flecainide, imipramine and moricizine on ventricular arrhythmias during the year after acute myocardial infarction: the CAPS. Am J Cardiol 1988;61:501–506.
69. Morganroth J, Anderson JL, Gentzkow GD: Classification by type of ventricular arrhythmia predicts frequency of adverse cardiac events from flecainide. J Am Coll Cardiol 1986;8:607–15.
70. Teo K, Yusuf S, Furberg C: Effect of antiarrhythmic drug therapy on mortality following myocardial infarction. Circulation (Suppl) 1990;82:III–197.
71. Morganroth J, Goin JE: Quinidine-related mortality in the short-to-medium-term treatment of ventricular arrhythmias: a meta-analysis. Circulation 1991;84:1977–1983.
72. Coplen SE, Antman EM, Berlin JA, *et al.*: Efficacy and safety of quinidine therapy for maintenance of sinus rhythm after cardioversion: a meta-analysis of randomized control trials. Circulation 1990;82:1106–1116.
73. Anderson JL: Reassessment of benefit-risk ratio and treatment algorithms for antiarrhythmic therapy after the cardiac arrhythmia suppression trial. J Clin Pharmacol 1990;30:981–989.
74. IMPACT Research Group: International mexiletine and placebo antiarrhythmic coronary trial: I. Report on arrhythmia and other findings. J Am Coll Cardiol 1984;6:1148–1163.
75. The Cascade Study. Cardiac Arrest in Seattle: Conventional versus amiodarone drug evaluation. Am J Cardiol 1991;67:578–584.

12

ANTIARRHYTHMIC DRUGS: SPECIFIC AGENTS

Joel Kupersmith, M.D., F.A.C.P., F.A.C.C.

This chapter deals with the antiarrhythmic agents used in the United States. Before discussing the specifics of the drugs, it is worthwhile to remember the goals of this form of therapy. These goals include: (a) prevention of sudden cardiac or other death, (b) diminution of symptoms, (c) diminution of complications secondary to arrhythmia such as emboli, syncope, and hypotension, (d) suppression of arrhythmia events in patients with implantable defibrillators to prevent excessive firing of the device.

These goals should be in mind when balancing a drug or regimen against risk and cost.

CLASSIFICATION OF ANTIARRHYTHMIC DRUGS

The Vaughan-Williams (1–3) classification of antiarrhythmic drugs with the Harrison (4) modification is now widely accepted for antiarrhythmic drugs (Table 12.1). It is based mainly on electrophysiologic (EP) properties. Drugs are separated into five classes: Class I, the local anesthetic agents with three subclasses, A, B and C; Class II, beta blockers; Class III, drugs that primarily prolong action potential duration (APD), Class IV, Ca^{2+} channel blockers, and Class V, miscellaneous.

This classification has been open to scrutiny in several ways and any classification has imperfections. However, it is still the most useful. It is important to remember that groupings are based on idealized properties of drugs while an individual drug may have characteristics of more than one class. Amiodarone, for example, is considered the prototype Class III drug but it has properties of all classes. Many drugs overlap and few fit perfectly into any category.

Drug effects are also dependent on dose and serum levels. In high and low concentrations, there are bound to be even more overlaps between categories.

In addition, though EP effects within a group or subgroup are very similar, this does not necessarily mean that response to one drug absolutely predicts response to another drug in the same group. Differences in kinetics, local tissue concentration, and a variety of other factors can account for such differences in response in an individual patient. However, in general, there should be a similar response spectrum.

Table 12.1 shows the antiarrhythmic drug classification and Tables 12.2–12.6 give pharmacologic and kinctic information on individual agents.

CLASS I AGENTS

Class I are the local anesthetic agents that block inward Na^+ current, shift membrane responsiveness curves to lower the maximum rate of depolarization (V_{max}) of the action potential upstroke (Fig. 12.1) and slow conduction (5). These effects are in fast response tissue—atrium, His-Purkinje system, and ventricle (2)—where upstroke is inward Na^+ current (I_{Na}). Class I agents also depress automaticity.

Class I agents increase pacemaker thresholds which can at times cause failure to capture. Intravenous isoproterenol is used acutely to restore thresholds. In addition, Class I drugs are negatively inotropic to a variable degree—most prominent with Class IC agents and least with the Class IB agents. The postulated reason for negative inotropic effects is that blockade of inward Na^+ movement leads to diminution of intracellular Na^+, followed by diminution of Na-Ca exchange, and consequent diminution of intracellular Ca^{2+}.

Class I has been divided into IA, IB, and IC subclasses (addition of IC is the "Harrison modification") (4). (Table 12.1). The subdivision is somewhat complicated. While it is clear that drugs in each of these subclasses are distinct in several ways, it is not always clear which feature should be the one used to define the subclass, especially as there are drugs that overlap categories. The Class IA–IC subclassification is based on the degree of I_{Na} block and in particular on the rate kinetics of use dependence of the Na^+ channel (3) (fast, slow, or intermediate—Table 12.1) (see Chapter 11 for discussion of use dependence). There are also differences in effects on APD and effective refractory period ERP among the subclasses (Table 12.1).

CLASS IA AGENTS

General

Class IA drugs have intermediate potency in blocking I_{Na} and use-dependent kinetics that are intermediate in rate of association to and dissociation from the Na^+ channel receptor (i.e., intermediate between Class IB and Class IC agents). Thus, there are some rate-related effects on I_{Na} and in slowing conduction across the physiologic and tachycardic ranges of heart rates (19). In membrane responsiveness curves Class IA agents uniformly lower V_{max} at any given membrane potential (6). (Fig. 12.1A) Class IA drugs prolong APD (due to blockade of one or more K^+ currents) and ERP and increase ERP/APD ratio. The agents slow conduction, prolong QRS duration (less than the Class IC drugs), and prolong both rate-corrected QT interval (QT_c) and JT (the "J" point is the junction of the QRS and ST segment) intervals on the electrocardiogram (ECG) (2,20).

The Class IA agents presently approved for use in the United States are quinidine, procainamide, and disopyramide. These drugs are the most protean of the antiarrhythmics and are of use in a wide variety of atrial and ventricular arrhythmias. They have become first-line drugs for EP testing in ventricular tachycardia/ventricular fibrillation (VT/VF). They are moderately effective against ventricular premature complexes (VPC s) (more than the Class IB drugs, less than the Class ICs) and of use in supraventricular tachycardias, especially these associated with preexcitation. Cardiac adverse effects include the possibility of causing or exacerbating almost any bradycardic or tachycardic arrhythmia, including torsade de pointes and the acquired long QT syndrome (21). Class IA drugs should not be given to patients who have prolonged QT intervals at baseline.

Table 12.1.
Antiarrhythmic Drug Classification

Class I—local anesthetic agents
Class IA—intermediate suppression of I_{Na} and UDB with intermediate rate kinetics[a]
Class IB—modest suppression of I_{Na} and UDB with rapid kinetics[b]
Class IC—considerable suppression of I_{Na} and UDB with slow kinetics[c]
Class II—β-adrenergic blocking agents
Class III—drugs that primarily prolong APD
Class IV—calcium channel blockers
Class V—miscellaneous

Based on Vaughan Williams EM: A classification of antiarrhythmic actions re-assessed after a decade of new drugs. J Clin Pharmacol 1984;24:129–147; Vaughan Williams EM: Classification of the antiarrhythmic action of moricizine. J Clin Pharmacol 1991;31:216–221; Harrison DC: Antiarrhythmic drug classification: New science and practical applications. Am J Cardiol 1985;56:185–187.
[a]Class IA agents prolong APD.
[b]Class IB agents shorten APD.
[c]Class IC agents have no effect on APD.
Abbreviations: APD = action potential duration; UDB = use-dependent block.

Table 12.2.
Electrocardiogram's Clinical Electrophysiologic Effects of Antiarrhythmic Drugs

	Sinus Node		ECG			Conduction		ERP				
	Rate	SNRT	PR	QRS	QT/JT	AH	HV	ATR	AVN	HPS	VENT	AP
Class IA												
Quinidine	– ↑	–	– ↓ ↑	↑	↑ / ↑	– ↓ ↑	– ↑	↑	– ↓ ↑	↑	↑	↑
Procainamide	– ↑	–	– ↓ ↑	↑	↑ / ↑ [a]	– ↓ ↑	– ↑	↑	– ↓ ↑	↑	↑	↑
Disapyramide	– ↑	–	– ↓ ↑	↑	↑ / ↑	– ↓ ↑	– ↑	↑	– ↓	↑	↑	↑
Class IB												
Lidocaine	–	–	–	–	– / –	–	– ↑ [b]	–	–	– ↑	–	– ↑
Mexiletine	–	–	–	–	– / –	–	– ↑ [b]	–	–	– ↑	–	–
Tocainide	– ↓	–	–	–	– ↓ / – ↓	–	– ↑ [b]	–	–	– ↑	–	↑
Class IC												
Flecainide	– ↓	–	↑	↑	– ↑ / –	↑	↑	– ↑	–	↑	↑	↑
Encainide	–	–	↑	↑	– ↑ / –	↑	↑	↑	↑	↑	↑	↑
Propafenone	– ↓	–	↑	↑	– ↑ / –	↑	↑	– ↑	– ↑	–	↑	↑
Moricizine	–	–	↑	↑	– ↑ / –	↑	↑	↑	↑	↑	↑	– ↑
Class III												
Amiodarone	↓	↑	– ↑	– ↑	↑ ↑ / ↑ ↑	↑	– ↑	↑	↑	↑	↑	↑
Bretylium[c]	– ↓		– ↑	–	– ↑ / – ↑	– ↑		– ↑	– ↑	– ↑	– ↑	–
Class IV												
Verapamil	– ↑ ↓	↑	↑	–	– / –	↑	–	–	↑	–	–	–
Class V												
Digoxin	– ↓	↑	↑	–	–	↑	–	↓	↑	–	–	– ↓ ↑
Adenosine	↓		↑	–		↑	–	↓	↑	–	–	– ↓ ↑

[a]*N*-acetyl procainamide is mainly responsible for QT/JT prolongation.
[b]Further prolongation when abnormal at baseline—see text.
[c]Effects may differ in the early catecholamine release phase vs. later.
Abbreviations: AP = accessory pathway; ATR = atrium; AVN = AV nodal; HPS = His-Purkinje system; SNRT = sinus node recovery time; VENT = ventricular.
From Woosley RL: Antiarrhythmic Agents. In Hurst JW, Schlant RC (eds): The Heart. McGraw-Hill, New York, 1990:1682–1711; Beaufils P, Leenhardt A, Denjoy E, *et al.*: Antiarrhythmic drugs in the adult population. In Rosen MR, Janse MJ, Wit AL (eds): Cardiac Electrophysiology. Futura Publishing Co., Mt. Kisco, NY, 1990;1175–1187; Frishman WH, Sonnenblick EH: Calcium channel blockers. In Hirst JW, Schlant RD (eds): The Heart. McGraw-Hill, New York, 1990;1731–1748; Antiarrhythmic drugs. Medical Letter on Drugs and Therapeutics 1991;33:55–60; Marcus FI, Huang SK: Digitalis. In Hurst JW, Schlant RC (eds): The Heart, 7th ed. McGraw-Hill, New York, 1990;1748–1761; Zipes DP: Management of cardiac arrhythmias: Pharmacological, electrical, and surgical techniques. In Braunwald E (ed): Heart Disease. WB Saunders, Philadelphia, 1988; Mann HJ: Moricizine: a new Class I antiarrhythmic. Clin Pharmacol 1990;9:842–852; Squire A, Kupersmith J: Beta adrenergic blocking agents, review and updata. Mt Sinai Med J 1985;52:553–558; Funck-Brentano C, Woosley RL: Current antiarrhythmic agents: clinical pharmacology. In El-Sherif N, Samet P (eds): Cardiac Pacing and Electrophysiology. WB Saunders, Philadelphia, 1991;409–435, with permission.

Table 12.3.
Pharmacology of Antiarrhythmic Drugs

	Time to Peak Level (t_{max}) (po) (hr)	Bioavailability (%)	Volume of Distribution (V_D) (L/kg)	Protein Binding (%)	Beta $T_{1/2}$ (hr)	Therapeutic Levels (mg/L)	Clearance
Class IA							
Quinidine	1.5–3	60–80	2.5	80–90	5–9	2–5	200–400
Procainamide	1 (tab) 2–3 (SR)	80–100	2	15	3–5	4–10	400–700
Disapyramide	1–2	80–90	1.5	20–50[a]	6–8	2–5	90
Class IB							
Lidocaine		35[b]	2	40–70	1.5–2.5	1.5–5	650–850
Mexiletine	2–4	70–90	5.5–9.5	70	8–17	0.5–2	400–700
Tocainide	0.5–2	80–95	1.5–3	50	8–15	3–10	150–200
Class IC							
Encainide	1–2	25–65[c,d]	3.5–6	70	3–4[c]	1–2[d]	200–12,000[c]
Flecainide	2–4	90–95	7–10	40	20	0.2–1.0	200–800
Morcizine	1–2.5	34–45	4–5	95	1.5–2.5		1000–2000
Propafenone	1–3	—[e]	3–4	90	.5–8[c]	0.5–3.0[d]	800–5000[e]
Class III							
Amiodarone	3–5	20–80	20–200	95	30–60[f] days	1–2.5[d]	6500–11,000
Bretylium	—[c]	10–35[a,b]	3–4	Low	8–14	0.5–1.5	1300
Class IV							
Verapamil	1–2	10–35	4–5	90	6–10	0.1–0.3	700–1000
Class V							
Digoxin	1–2	50–80 (tab) 80–100 (cap)	4–8	25	1.1–1.9 days	1.2–2.0	150–250
Adenosine					0.6–10 sec		

(From Woosley RL: Antiarrhythmic Agents. In Hurst JW, Schlant RC (eds): The Heart. McGraw-Hill, New York, 1990:1682–1711; Beaufils P, Leenhardt A, Denjoy E, *et al.* Slama R: Antiarrhythmic drugs in the adult population. In Rosen MR, Janse MJ, Wit AL (eds): Cardiac Electrophysiology. Futura Publishing Co., Mt. Kisco, NY, 1990:1175–1187; Frishman WH, Sonnenblick EH: Calcium channel blockers. In Hirst JW, Schlant RD (eds): The Heart. McGraw-Hill, New York, 1990;1731–1748; Frishman WH, Sonnenblick EH: B-adrenergic blocking drugs. In Hirst JW, Schlant RC (eds): The Heart. McGraw-Hill, New York, 1990;1712–1731; Antiarrhythmic drugs. Medical Letter on Drugs and Therapeutics 1991;33:55–60; Marcus FI, Huang SK: Digitalis. In Hurst JW, Schlant RC (eds): The Heart, 7th ed. McGraw-Hill, New York, 1990;1748–1761; Zipes DP: Management of cardiac arrhythmias: Pharmacological, electrical, and surgical techniques. In Braunwald E (ed): Heart Disease. WB Saunders, Philadelphia, 1988;621–657; Mann HJ: Moricizine: a new Class I antiarrhythmic. Clin Pharmacol 1990;9:842–852; Funck-Brentano C, Woosley RL: Current antiarrhythmic agents: clinical pharmacology. In El-Sherif N, Samet P (eds): Cardiac Pacing and Electrophysiology. WB Saunders, Philadelphia, 1991, 409–435, with permission.)

[a]Protein binding is concentration dependent.
[b]Not available as an oral agent in the United States.
[c]Genetic variation in metabolism (see text).
[d]Active metabolite may play an important role (see text).
[e]Saturable hepatic first-pass metabolism (see text).
[f]Highly variable (see fig. 12.7) (18).
Abbreviations: CAP = capsule; SR = sustained-release form; tab = tablet.

Quinidine

Quinidine is a *d*-isomer of quinine and has been in use since 1917. It is administered in either a sulfate or a more slowly absorbed gluconate form. An intravenous form is rarely used because of hypotension, tinnitus, and other adverse effects.

Quinidine has anticholinergic properties (24) and may thus speed the ventricular response in atrial fibrillation as well as having a slight stimulating effect on sinus rate. The drug can cause hypotension via α-adrenergic blockade (25). It has mild negative inotropic properties but in clinical use these are generally counteracted by afterload reducing effects (25). Active metabolites of quinidine include 3-OH quinidine (22) but they have questionable clinical significance. Dihydroquinidine is an active impurity accounting for 10–20% of drug (23).

Quinidine is used as a first-line drug in the treatment and prevention of atrial fibrillation, in ventricular arrhythmias (VAs) where it is widely used in EP laboratories, and in arrhythmias due to Wolff-Parkinson-White syndrome (WPW). It is also useful but somewhat lower in the therapeutic hierarchy in other supraventricular arrhythmias.

Quinidine can cause polymorphous VT and arrhythmias of this type probably account for quinidine-induced syncope (spontaneous VF) (26) as well as quinidine-induced sudden death. Hypokalemia enhances the likelihood of these arrhythmias and therefore, close attention should be paid to maintain serum K^+ levels above 4.0 mEq/liter in patients taking the drug. Na^+-containing solutions have been used to antagonize severe toxicity. Meta-analysis studies have also suggested an increased mortality in quinidine in patients with paroxysmal atrial fibrillation (27) and with all but the most serious VAs (28). It has been advised that patients beginning quinidine be hospitalized (29).

Quinidine causes elevation of serum digoxin levels (30), worsens neuromuscular blockade in myasthenia gravis (31) and

Table 12.4.
Active Metabolites

	Active Metabolites
Class IA	
Quinidine	3-OH Quinidine; 2′-Oxoquinidinone *O*-Desmethyl Quinidine
Procainamide	*N*-Acetyl procainamide
Disapyramide	*N*-Desisopropyl disopyramide
Class IB	
Lidocaine	Monoethylglycine xylidine Glycine xylidine
Mexiletine	
Tocainide	
Class IC	
Encainide	*O*-Desmethyl (ODE) 3-Methoxy-*O*-desmethyl encainide (MODE) N-Desemythyl encainide (NDE)
Flecainide	
Moricizine	Moricizine sulfoxide Phenothiazine-2-carbamic acid ethyl ester sulfoxide
Propafenone	3-OH Propafenone *N*-de-propyl propafenone
Class III	
Amiodarone	Desethyl amiodarone
Bretylium	
Class IV	
Verapamil	Norverapamil
Class V	
Digoxin	
Adenosine	

(From Woosley RL: Antiarrhythmic Agents. In Hurst JW, Schlant RC (eds): The Heart. McGraw-Hill, New York, 1990:1682–1711; Beaufils P, Leenhardt A, Denjoy E, *et al.*: Antiarrhythmic drugs in the adult population. In Rosen MR, Janse MJ, Wit AL (eds): Cardiac Electrophysiology. Futura Publishing Co., Mt. Kisco, NY, 1990:1175–1187; Frishman WH, Sonnenblick EH: Calcium channel blockers. In Hirst JW, Schlant RD (eds): The Heart. McGraw-Hill, New York, 1990;1731–1748; Antiarrhythmic drugs. Medical Letter on Drugs and Therapeutics 1991;33:55–60; Marcus FI, Huang SK: Digitalis. In Hurst JW, Schlant RC (eds): The Heart, 7th ed. McGraw-Hill, New York, 1990;1748–1761; Zipes DP: Management of cardiac arrhythmias: Pharmacological, electrical, and surgical techniques. In Braunwald E (ed): Heart Disease. WB Saunders, Philadelphia, 1988;621–657; Mann HJ: Moricizine: a new Class I antiarrhythmic. Clin Pharmacol 1990;9:842–852; Funck-Brentano C, Woosley RL: Current antiarrhythmic agents: clinical pharmacology. In El-Sherif N, Samet P (eds): Cardiac Pacing and Electrophysiology. WB Saunders, Philadelphia, 1991, 409–435, with permission.)

potentiates effects of succinyl choline (32). Other adverse effects include gastrointestinal distress, diarrhea (common), tinnitus and other manifestations of cinchonism, hepatitis, fever, hemolytic anemia, thrombocytopenia, and various bradycardic rhythms.

Procainamide

Procainamide, a derivative of procaine, is another early antiarrhythmic drug which has been in use since 1960. The drug is administered intravenously or orally as a conventional tablet, taken every 3–4 hr (Fig. 12.2) or, more commonly in a sustained-release form taken every 6–8 hr.

Procainamide has an active metabolite *N*-acetyl procainamide (NAPA) (also called acecainide) which is a Class III antiarrhythmic (34). The two compounds are different in EP and pharmacologic effects. Procainamide has local anesthetic effects on upstroke and causes some APD prolongation (35) while NAPA has virtually no effect on upstroke but considerably prolongs APD (36). In an individual patient, it is not clear whether procainamide, NAPA, or some combination of both, is responsible for antiarrhythmic effects. However, NAPA, because of its APD-prolonging effects, is more likely responsible for torsade de pointes and similar arrhythmias; for this reason considerable caution is advised when NAPA levels begin to rise above 25–30 μg/L. NAPA does not contribute to procainamide-induced lupus, an important adverse effect (37).

The liver acetylates procainamide to NAPA and both of these are eliminated by the kidney. Both, but especially NAPA, tend to accumulate in renal failure for which dose of drug has to be considerably modified. Also (as is common with metabolites) the parent compound and NAPA interfere with renal elimination of each other. Of interest is the fact that there are fast and slow acetylators of procainamide (37). Slightly over half the population are fast acetylators and they are less likely to have lupus.

Since NAPA has a longer half-life than procainamide (7–8 or more hr vs. 3–4 hr), it tends to be at lower serum levels during earlier phases of administration than later (38). Thus, during EP

Table 12.5.
Dosage of Antiarrhythmic Drugs

	Dosage (IV)			Dosage[a]	
	Loading	Maintenance	Initial	Loading[b] (mg)	Maintenance (mg/day)
Class IA					
Quinidine sulfate	6–10 mg/kg at 0.3–0.5 mg/kg/min[c]		200 mg q6hr	600–1000	800–2400
Procainamide	6–15 mg/kg at 0.2–0.5 mg/kg/min[d]	2–6 mg/min	SR 500 mg q6hr	50–1000	2000–6000 (SR)
Disopyramide	1–2 mg/kg over 15 or 45 min[c]	1 mg/kg/hr[c]	100 mg q6hr		300–800
Class IB					
Lidocaine	—[e]	—[e]			
Mexiletine	500 mg[c]	0.5–1.0 g/day[c]	200 mg q8hr	400–600	400–1200
Tocainide	750 mg[c]		400 mg q8hr	400–600	600–2400
Class IC					
Encainide			25 mg q8hr		75–400
Flecainide	2 mg/kg[c]		100 mg q12hr		200–400
Propafenone	1–2 mg/kg[c]		150 mg q8hr	600–900	300–900
Moricizine			200 mq q8hr		600–900
Class III					
Amiodarone	—[c,e]	—[c,e]	—[e]	—[e]	—[e]
Bretylium	5–30 mg/kg	0.5–2 mg/min			
Class IV					
Verapamil	5–10 mg over 1–2 min × 2 Q30min[f]	0.125 μg/kg/min	80–120 mg		240–1600 SR or tab
Class V					
Digoxin	0.75–1 mg	0.125–0.375 mg/day	0.25–0.50 mg	1–1.5 mg	0.125–0.5 mg/day
Adenosine	6–12 mg × 2 q1–2 min[f]				

(From Scheiner LB, Tozer TN: Clinical Pharmacokinetics. The use of plasma concentrations of drugs. In Melmon KL, Morrelli HF (eds): Clinical Pharmacology. MacMillan, New York, 1978;71–109; Woosley RL: Antiarrhythmic Agents. In Hurst JW, Schlant RC (eds): The Heart. McGraw-Hill, New York, 1990:1682–1711; Beaufils P, Leenhardt A, Denjoy E, *et al.*: Antiarrhythmic drugs in the adult population. In Rosen MR, Janse MJ, Wit AL (eds): Cardiac Electrophysiology. Futura Publishing Co., Mt. Kisco, NY, 1990:1175–1187; Frishman WH, Sonnenblick EH: Calcium channel blockers. In Hirst JW, Schlant RD (eds): The Heart. McGraw-Hill, New York, 1990;1731–1748; Antiarrhythmic drugs. Medical Letter on Drugs and Therapeutics 1991;33:55–60; Marcus FI, Huang SK: Digitalis. In Hurst JW, Schlant RC (eds): The Heart, 7th ed. McGraw-Hill, New York, 1990;1748–1761; Zipes DP: Management of cardiac arrhythmias: Pharmacological, electrical, and surgical techniques. In Braunwald E (ed): Heart Disease. WB Saunders, Philadelphia, 1988;621–657; Mann HJ: Moricizine: a new Class I antiarrhythmic. Clin Pharmacol 1990;9:842–852; Funck-Brentano C, Woosley RL: Current antiarrhythmic agents: clinical pharmacology. In El-Sherif N, Samet P (ed): Cardiac Pacing and Electrophysiology. WB Saunders, Philadelphia, 1991, 409–435, with permission.)

[a]Loading dosages are highly individual and depend on response, observation of toxicity and presence of renal, hepatic or congestive heart failure.
[b]Oral loading must be done with caution and careful observation.
[c]Not Food and Drug Administration (FDA) approved or available for intravenous use in the United States.
[d]Alternative dosing regimen for acute arrhythmias: 100 mg q5min until initial arrhythmia converts, toxicity, or a total dose of 1000 mg is administered.
[e]See text for dosage regimens.
[f]Second dose, only if necessary.
Abbreviations: IV = intravenous; po = oral; SR = sustained release; Tab = tablet.

Table 12.6.
β-Adrenergic Blocking Agents[a]

	B_1 Selectivity	ISA	MSA	Lipid Solubility	Bioavailability (%)	First-Pass Metabolism	Protein Binding (%)	Beta $T_{1/2}$[b] (hr)	Beta Blocking (mg/ml)	Clearance (Cl) (ml/min)	Active Metabolites	Dose (oral) mg/day	Dose (IV)
Acebutolol	+	+	+	Moderate	40	No	25	3–4	0.2–2.0 μg/ml	6–15	Yes	400–1200	
Atenolol	++	–	–	Low	40	No	<5	6–9	0.2–5.0 μg/ml	130	No	50–200	—[c]
Esmolol	++	–	–	Low			55	9 min	0.15–1.0 μg/ml	27,000	No		—[d]
Metoprolol	++	–	–	Moderate	50	No	50	3–4	50–100	1,100	No	100–400	5 mg × 3 q2min
Propranolol	–	–	++	High	20–30	Yes	90–95	3–4	50–100	1,000	Yes	30–240	—[e]
Timolol	–	–	–	Low	75	No	10	4–5	5–10	660	No	20–60	

From Frishman WH, Sonnenblick EH: β-adrenergic blocking drugs. In Hirst JW, Schlant RC (eds): The Heart. McGraw-Hill, New York, 1990;1712–1731; Squire A, Kupersmith J: Beta adrenergic blocking agents, review and update. Mt Sinai Med J 1985;52:553–558.

[a]Only beta blockers FDA approved for arrhythmias or mortality reduction post–myocardial infarction are included.
[b]Effects of beta blockers may last longer than expected from $T_{1/2}$.
[c]5 mg over 5 min, × 2 q10 min, if necessary.
[d]Loading—500 μg over 1 min; maintenance—start 25 μg/kg/min, increase 25–50 μg/kg/min q4min to desired effect, usually at 100–300 μg/min.
[e]1–3 mg may be repeated in 2 min, then wait 4 hr.
Abbreviations: C_p = drug level; ISA = intrinsic sympathomimetic activity; MSA = membrane stabilizing activity; $T_{1/2}$ = half-life.

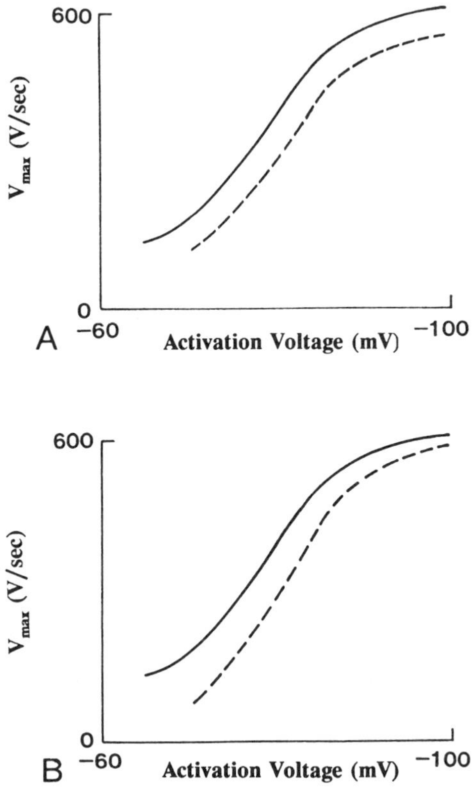

Figure 12.1. Effects of local anesthetic agents on membrane responsiveness curves. Activation voltage vs. V_{max} at baseline (*solid line*) and with drug (*dashed line*) are shown. As membrane potential declines, V_{max} also declines. Local anesthetic agents shift V_{max} curves to the right lowering V_{max} at a given membrane potential. **A** shows a uniform shift to the right i.e., V_{max} is lowered similarly at all membrane potentials. Generally speaking, this represents the effect of Class IC and often IA antiarrhythmic drugs.(6) **B** shows curves in which drug causes little reduction of V_{max} at fully activated voltages (−90 to −100 mV) but greater reductions of V_{max} at "partially inactivated" (i.e., reduced) membrane potentials. This is the type of response associated with Class IB drugs (6) but may also be associated with other agents depending on drug concentration. Note also that in both **A** and **B** the minimum activation voltage (minimum voltage at which an action potential can be initiated) is made less negative, i.e., moved from about −65 to about −70 mV.

testing, which is performed immediately with intravenous administration or after 3 days with oral administration, serum levels of NAPA may be lower than during chronic administration. At later times, accumulation of NAPA may be relevant both to antiarrhythmic properties and toxicity.

It is generally accepted that procainamide levels of 4–10 μg/ml are at least an approximate therapeutic range (with considerable overlap at both ends). Higher levels appear to be necessary for treatment of VT and to prevent induction of VT in EP studies (39). NAPA also plays some role in antiarrhythmic properties and its levels must be taken into consideration. However, as indicated above, it has different EP properties and a somewhat different antiarrhythmic spectrum and this complicates interpretation of serum levels. Thus the commonly used practice of adding levels of parent compound and metabolite do not seem appropriate as these are different drugs.

Like quinidine, procainamide has slight negative inotropic effects which may be compensated by its afterload reducing properties. However, in intravenous use, negative inotropic effects and hypotension become important (40). Procainamide also has vagolytic (somewhat less than quinidine) and mild ganglionic blocking properties (25).

Oral procainamide has a similar antiarrhythmic spectrum as quinidine with effectiveness in atrial fibrillation, paroxysmal supraventricular tachycardia (PSVT) (not first line), WPW arrhythmias, and VAs. Intravenous procainamide is also an important drug and this form may be used to directly convert atrial fibrillation or ventricular tachycardia. A suggested approach has been to administer 100 mg q5min until arrhythmia is converted, hypotension or other toxicity occurs or a total of 1000 mg is given (41) (see Table 12.5 for dosage in other situations). Intravenous procainamide is also frequently used as a screening drug in EP studies and it can predict its own oral effectiveness as well as, to a lesser degree, that of other Class IA drugs. It has been found that if IV procainamide prevents induction of VT, there is an 85% probability that a single or combined Class I drug regimen will be effective (42).

Procainamide has troublesome adverse effects and up to 30–40% of patients may have to have the drug discontinued. The most important of these is the lupus syndrome which occurs in 15–20%. Virtually all patients on procainamide develop antinuclear antibodies against single-, not double-stranded, deoxyribonucleic acid (DNA) but only the clinical lupus syndrome is reason for discontinuing the drug. Procainamide-induced lupus is characterized by fever, arthralgia, arthritis, pericardial effusion, rash, and no renal involvement (43). It responds to withdrawal of drug. Other adverse effects include leukopenia (which seems to be more with the sustained-release form perhaps because of more constant serum levels), psychosis (rare), fever, and similar EP toxicity as other Class IA drugs. Congestive heart failure is not a common complication of oral procainamide but acute congestive heart failure may occur with intravenous administration especially if prolonged.

Disopyramide

Disopyramide is an oral Class IA agent. Its intravenous form is not in use in the United States. The drug is administered in racemic form. Both isomers have about equal local anesthetic properties on action potential upstroke. However, prolongation of APD resides mainly in S−(+)−disopyramide form while anticholinergic and negative inotropic effects are primarily in the R−(−) form (44).

Among the pharmacologic peculiarities of disopyramide is concentration-dependent protein binding. At higher serum levels, there is relatively less bound and more free drug (45) (about 20% vs. 50%), a situation which makes the therapeutic range of total disopyramide levels (free plus bound) less useful. It also

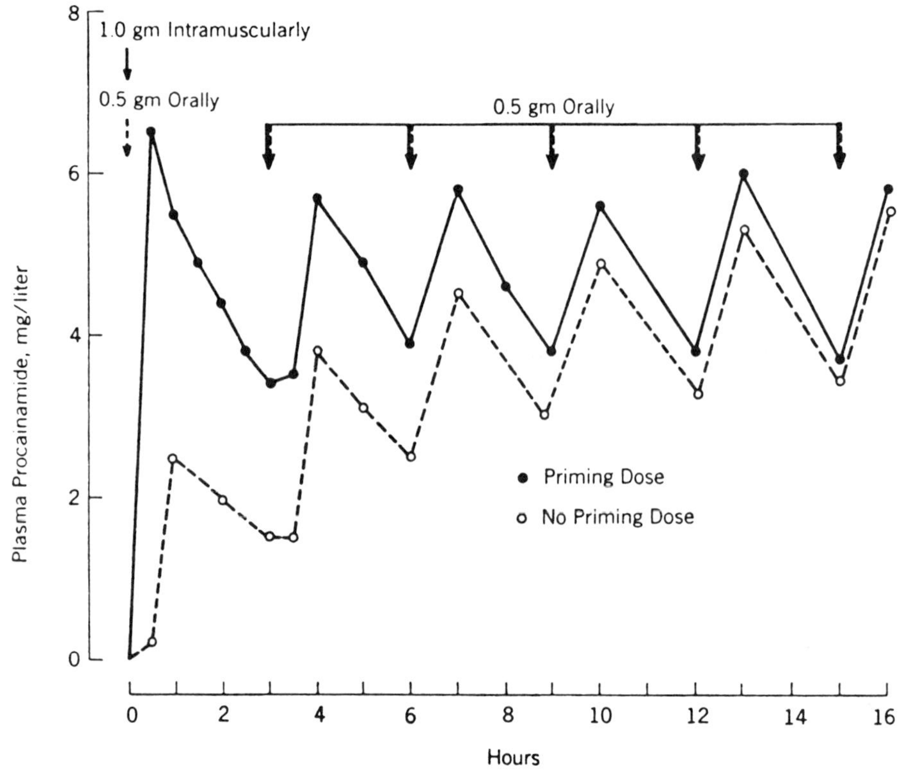

Figure 12.2. Plasma levels of procainamide with oral administration of 0.5 gm q8hr with (*solid lines*) and without (*dashed lines*) a loading (or "priming") intramuscular dose of 1 g. With the loading dose, steady state variation in levels is achieved much more quickly. Curves would differ with sustained-release forms of procainamide which are absorbed more slowly and which are now in common use. Overall value of loading dose, however, would be the same. (From Koch-Weser J, Klein SW: Procainamide dosage schedules, plasma concentrations, and clinical effects. JAMA 1971;215:1454–1460, Copyright, 1971, American Medical Association with permission.)

creates problems in initial drug administration, which must be done with extra caution and without a loading dose, since small changes in dose may lead to great fluctuations in free drug level.

Disopyramide has an active metabolite, *N*-dealkyl disopyramide formed via hepatic transformation. Both disopyramide and *N*-dealkyl disopyramide are eliminated by the kidneys. Interestingly, disopyramide exhibits stereoselective elimination. *d*-disopyramide, unlike the *l*-isomer, is not protein bound and has a higher renal clearance.

Disopyramide is available as a conventional form (administered every 6–8 hr) and a sustained-release form (administered every 8–12 hr). The drug has a similar spectrum of effect on atrial and ventricular arrhythmias as other Class IA agents though it is not as widely used. Compared to other Class IA agents, it has a greater propensity to cause congestive heart failure (special caution is advised in patients with reduced myocardial function) and much more marked anticholinergic effects, a special problem for elderly males with obstructive uropathy and patients with glaucoma.

Hepatic metabolism of disopyramide is enhanced by phenobarbital, rifampicin and phenytoin (46) with accompanying loss of effectiveness.

CLASS IB AGENTS

General

Class IB drugs have very modest effects on I_{Na} (47) and slow conduction in abnormal but not in normal tissue (48–50). They exhibit use dependent block of I_{Na} with fast kinetics of association to and dissociation from the Na^+ channel (19,51,52). For reasons discussed in Chapter 11, this property has several consequences. First, effects at fast rates are considerably enhanced (Fig. 12.3) Thus drug effects are greater during tachycardias than in slower, normal rhythms. Second, drug effects are enhanced in partially inactivated tissue, i.e., injured or otherwise altered tissue in which resting membrane potential is more positive. Drug association to the Na^+ channel is greater at these membrane potentials. This will result in the type of effect on membrane response curves shown in Figure 12.1B (6,53) where drugs have little effect at normal resting membrane potential ($-$ 90 to $-$100 mV) but have greater effect at more positive partially inactivated membrane potentials (e.g., $-$70 to $-$80 mV). Third, drugs exhibit injury zone selectivity. IB agents slow conduction only in ischemic or infarcted tissue (48–50,54) where cardiac cells tend to be at reduced membrane potential, a property that has been demonstrated in human (55) as well as experimental studies (Fig. 12.4). This selectivity allows for greater effects in injured tissues where arrhythmias arise rather than in normal tissues (56).

Class IB agents also have other selective effects. They prolong ERP, both absolutely and relative to APD, and do so to a greater degree in injured tissue (49,50). Lidocaine, the prototype IB, also shortens APD in normal and not in ischemic zones. Since APD is longer in normal than ischemic zones prior to drug, lidocaine serves to make APDs nearly equal and this is probably one of its antiarrhythmic properties (49).

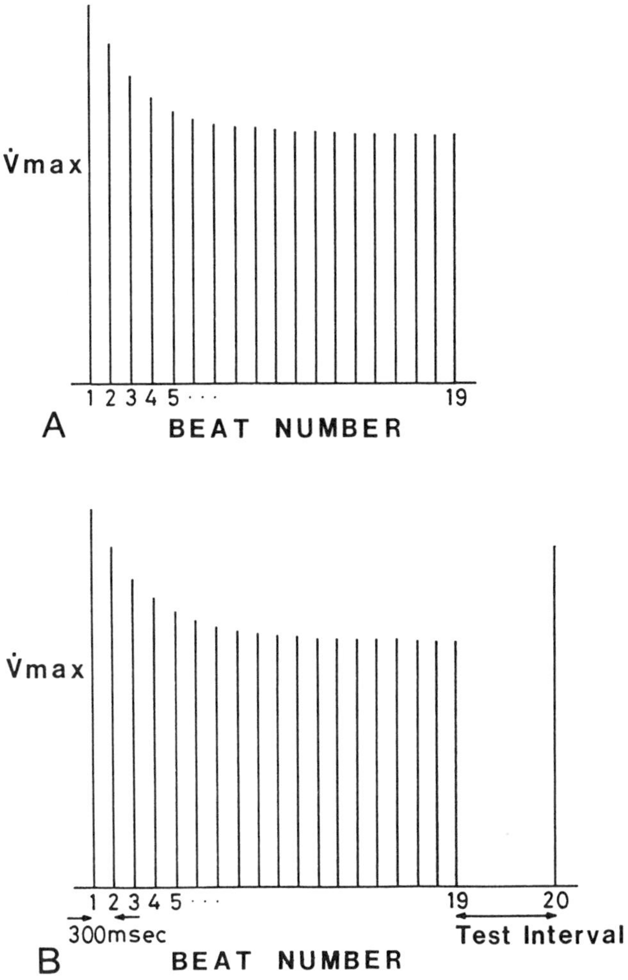

Figure 12.3. V_{max} during and after rapid beating in a sheep Purkinje fiber superfused with tocainide (5 mg/liter). Tocainide displays use dependence with fast kinetics. **A** shows effects of rapid pacing and in **B** an additional stimulus was applied after the rapid pacing sequence (after a "test interval"). Note that V_{max} declined during rapid pacing and reached a steady state after about 10 beats. After cessation of rapid pacing and after the "test interval" in **(B),** there was partial recovery of V_{max}. With a longer postpacing test interval (not shown), V_{max} returned to its baseline level. This experiment simulates what would happen during a spontaneous tachycardia, i.e., drug effect (decline in V_{max}) would be enhanced with the rapid rate. Effects of certain other local anesthetic agents, such as the Class IC drugs, would tend to be more uniform over these rates. (Hiromasa S, Kupersmith J, unpublished observations.)

Clinically, Class IB drugs have no measurable effect on QRS duration or QT_c interval. The agents are effective in ventricular but usually not in supraventricular arrhythmias. They are, however, only modestly effective in suppressing VPCs. Class IB agents are probably not associated with torsade de pointes and have in fact been used to treat this arrhythmia. Negative inotropic effects are almost nonexistent in clinical usage, especially with oral drugs.

Lidocaine

Lidocaine was used for several years as a local anesthetic agent before its first use as an antiarrhythmic in 1950 (57). It is a strictly intravenous Class IB agent which is generally the drug of choice for acute treatment of VAs and in cardiac arrest. Lidocaine is widely used for this purpose in coronary care units, during surgery and other similar acute settings.

Lidocaine exhibits extensive first-pass hepatic metabolism and therefore, cannot be administered orally. The high hepatic extraction ratio also causes metabolism to be heavily dependent upon blood flow. The drug is eliminated more slowly when cardiac output is reduced (Fig. 12.5) (58) (not uncommon in patients needing lidocaine), including by drugs such as propanolol. For this reason maintenance doses of lidocaine must be reduced by about 50% in congestive heart failure because of decreased elimination. In addition, loading dose must be reduced similarly because there is also a decreased volume of distribution of lidocaine in this state.

Lidocaine elimination is reduced after 24 hr of infusion (59), perhaps because of interference via an accumulated dimethyl metabolite. On the other hand, another metabolite which accumulates at times, glycine xylidine, competes with lidocaine for the Na^+ channel and blunts its effects.

Lidocaine is partially bound to α-1-acid glycoprotein, an acute phase reactant which increases an acute myocardial infarction and other acute states. When α-1-acid glycoprotein increases, drug levels rise without a concomitant rise in free (i.e., active) drug, a fact that must be taken into account in evaluating these levels.

The traditional method of lidocaine administration is as follows: (a) loading: 1–2 mg/kg at rate of 20–50 μg/min; (b) constant rate (maintenance) infusion: 1–4 mg/min (or about 20–60 μg/kg/min.).

With this infusion, serum levels may drop below minimum effective concentration at 30–60 min and for this reason various multiple loading dose regimens have been suggested as follows (see also Fig. 11.10 for drug levels with various intravenous regimens of lidocaine):

1. 1–2 mg/kg at rate of 20–50 mg/min (as above) followed by a second bolus of 0.5 mg/kg in 30 min
2. 1 mg/kg followed by up to two doses of 1 mg/kg q5min if initial bolus is ineffective (60)
3. 75 mg followed by 5.33 mg tapering to 2 mg/min over 25 min (exponential) (61)
4. 75 mg followed by 50 mg/min q5min × 3 (in a 75-kg person) (62).

Once steady state is established, an additional small bolus is required if higher levels are needed quickly.

It has been stated that patients who require higher total loading doses of lidocaine for suppression of arrhythmias also require higher maintenance doses (60).

Lidocaine may also administered intramuscularly at a dose of

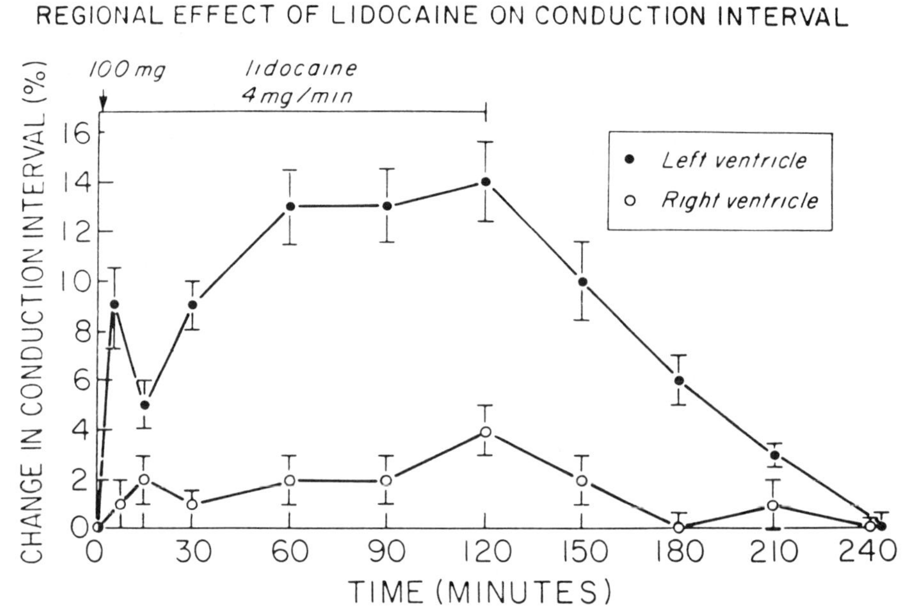

Figure 12.4. Effects of lidocaine on conduction intervals measured at time of coronary artery bypass surgery. Recordings were made in abnormal, chronically infarcted segments of the left ventricle and in normal segments in the right ventricle. Lidocaine was administered as a bolus of 100 mg and a constant rate infusion of 4 mg/min for 120 min. Lidocaine prolonged conduction interval to a much greater degree in the abnormal (chronically infarcted) left than in the normal right ventricle indicating injury zone selectivity. (From Wiener I, Mindich B, Kupersmith J: Regional differences in the effects of lidocaine on intramyocardial conduction in patients with coronary artery disease. Am Heart J 1981;102:53–58, with permission.)

300–400 mg. This has been suggested for outpatient prophylaxis in acute myocardial infarction (63).

Lidocaine is used in VAs and in supraventricular arrhythmias with associated preexcitation. Like all Class IB agents, it is not generally effective in other supraventricular arrhythmias.

Adverse effects of lidocaine include hypotension, congestive heart failure (rare), central nervous system effects such as drowsiness and dysarthria (common), seizures, and sinus node dysfuntion. All are directly related to serum levels. His-Purkinje block may occur in patients with baseline abnormalities because of selective depression in abnormal tissue.

Mexiletine

Mexiletine is a Class IB agent approved for all use in the United States. It is (moderately) effective against VAs and unlike other Class IB agents, is occasionally effective against supraventricular tachycardias. Although it is in the same class as lidocaine, response in an individual patient may or (often) may not be predicted by previous response to lidocaine.

Mexiletine is now more frequently used in combination with other drugs than alone, especially a Class IA agent or a beta blocker (64–67). It is often added to Class IA drugs in EP testing for ventricular arrhythmias and to beta blockers in the treatment of torsade de pointes.

Mexiletine is administered every 6–8 hr. Administration with food is suggested to modulate wide swings in serum levels and therefore reduce adverse effects without diminishing overall bioavailability. The drug is eliminated mainly by the liver (85–90%) (68) and has no known active metabolites (69). Dosage reduction may be necessary in hepatic or cardiac failure. Renal elimination is reduced with increased pH.

The main adverse effects of mexiletine are neurologic—tremor, dizziness, and visual difficulties. These are rather common and often necessitate reduction in dosage or discontinuation of drug. Mexiletine also causes nausea. It can cause severe bradycardia in patients with sick sinus syndrome (70) and presumably by virtue of injury zone selectivity prolongs His-Purkinje intervals and may cause block in patients with baseline abnormalities (71). Overall, however, the drug appears to be relatively safe with little negative inotropic effects or organ toxicity (rare thrombocytopenia) (72–73).

Tocainide

Tocainide was approved in the United States as a Class IB agent for oral use. It has EP and antiarrhythmic effects that are very similar to lidocaine which it resembles in effects more than does mexiletine. However, antiarrhythmic response to one still does not absolutely predict response to the other. It has been said that if lidocaine suppresses a given ventricular arrhythmia on ambulatory ECG, tocainide has a 60% chance of being effective versus 15% when lidocaine was ineffective (74). In addition there is rather limited (53%) concordance of response between mexiletine and tocainide in inducibility of VT/VF (75).

Tocainide has also been used for ventricular arrhythmias, both individually and in combination with Class IA agents and beta blockers. However, more recently its use has been limited by organ toxicities (see below).

Tocainide is administered as a tablet preferably taken with food every 8 hr. It is eliminated by both the liver and kidney and there are no active metabolites. R−(+)− tocainide is pharmacologically active and is eliminated much more rapidly than the S(−) form. Thus, levels of pharmacologically inactive S(−) enantiomers may be four times that of the R(+) from making for a wide and inexact therapeutic window (76). Binding of drug to

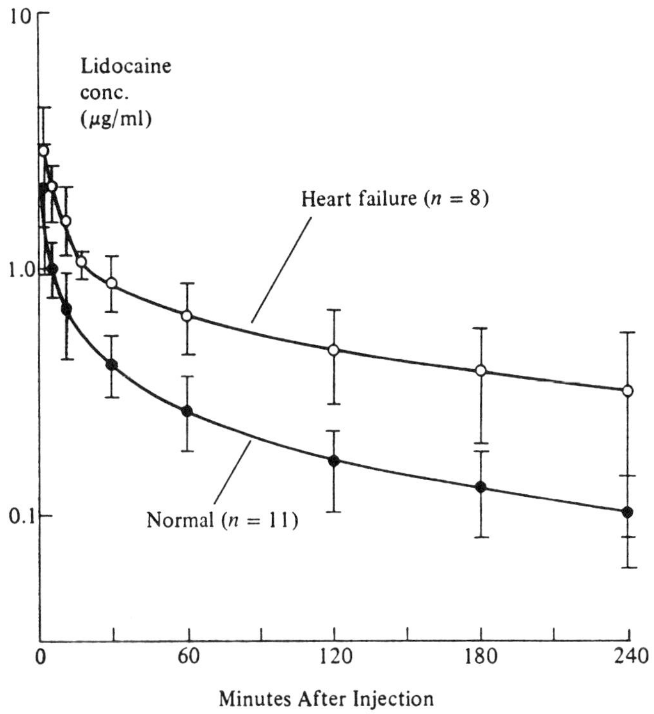

Figure 12.5. Effect of heart failure on drug level decline after administration of intravenous lidocaine. Shown are drug levels after IV lidocaine in normals and patients with heart failure. Heart failure caused a reduced distribution and elimination of the drug and thus much higher drug levels with the same dose. (From Nies AS: Cardiovascular disorders. In Melmon KL, Morrelli HF (eds): Clinical Pharmacology: Basic Principles in Therapeutics. McGraw-Hill, New York, 1972:142–261, with permission.)

plasma proteins is low (about 10%). Dosages should be reduced with hepatic or renal failure.

Tocainide is well tolerated hemodynamically (slight negative inotropic action) and EP adverse effects are similar to mexiletine. However, the drug has been reported to cause thrombocytopenia, interstitial pneumonitis, and agranulocytosis (this with an incidence estimated at 0.18%) (77). These organ toxicities have limited use of the drug. Tocainide also frequently causes dose-related neurologic adverse effects (in 30–50% of patients) leading to diminution of dose or discontinuation. These effects include tremor, visual blurring, paresthesia, and others.

CLASS IC AGENTS

General

Class IC agents profoundly suppress I_{Na} (78) and thus profoundly slow conduction. They exhibit slow kinetics of use-dependent block and thus do not have substantial rate related effects on the Na^+ channel (Table 12.1) (79). Class IC drugs have no effect on APD, ERP, or the ERP/APD ratio.

Class IC agents substantially prolong QRS duration and by virtue of this effect also prolong QT_c but not the JT interval (80). All Class IC agents are negatively inotropic.

IC drugs are effective against a wide variety of atrial and ventricular arrhythmias. They may also be associated with proarrhythmic VT, generally not of the torsade de pointes type. Findings of the Cardiac Arrhythmia Suppression Trial (CAST) (see Chapter 11) have strongly influenced the use of Class IC agents. Flecainide and propafenone are the IC agents in use in the United States. Indecainide was also approved by the Food and Drug Administration (FDA) but has not been marketed and encainide and moricizine were withdrawn from the market in 1991.

Flecainide

Flecainide has an interesting fluoride-containing structure. Like other Class IC agents, it is a potent inhibitor of inward Na^+ current and causes impressive prolongation of QRS duration in the ECG (81). Also like other Class IC agents, it is a potent suppressor of VPCs.

Flecainide is available as a tablet administered every 12 hr. The drug is mainly eliminated by the liver to inactive metabolities and has a relatively long half-life (Table 12.3).

Regarding indications, flecainide is occasionally used in EP studies for VT/VF, but it does not appear to be as effective as Class IA agents which are preferred. It is not recommended for less severe VAs.

Flecainide is now approved for use in supraventricular arrhythmias based on a number of reports showing suppression of arrhythmias (82–86) without undue adverse effects or (in retrospective studies) mortality (87).

Flecainide has been found of use in PSVT, including those with an extra nodal accessory pathway, and atrial fibrillation. The drug increases intervals between PVST attacks from 12 days (placebo) to 55 days and reduces mean heart rates during tachycardia from 178 to 143 beats/min (84). In paroxysmal atrial fibrillation, flecainide increases time intervals between attacks from 6.2 (placebo) to 27.0 days and is associated with complete arrhythmia elimination over 4 mo in 30% of patients (vs. 9% on placebo) (85).

The drug is also effective in about half the patients with supraventricular tachycardia and an extranodal accessory pathway (83). Interestingly, an isoproterenol challenge intensified arrhythmias in most patients in whom flecainide would prove ineffective (83).

Proarrhythmia is an important consideration for flecainide and because of the CAST study, indications and toxicity have been reevaluated (see Chapter 11) (88). As with other drugs, toxicity can occur at any drug level of flecainide including the promulgated therapeutic range (89,90). Rather impressive PR and QRS prolongation have been allowed (up to 180 msec) but at this point, considerable caution is advised, especially if intervals jump by 40 msec or more. With exercise there is further prolongation of QRS duration (91).

Proarrhythmic manifestations include a dangerous, unremitting sinusoidal VT. For this and other cardiac instances of severe flecainide intoxication, intravenous administration of Na^+ containing solutions may be helpful (92). Flecainide considerably raises pacemaker thresholds (93) and may also cause a variety of block forms of intracardiac block. It is negatively inotropic and may worsen congestive heart failure. Central nervous systems complications (dizziness and difficulty in visual accommodation) occur (89) and may be transient.

All of the above complications are in general related to dose/drug level, though they can occur at any drug level. However, most patients, symptomatically at least, tolerate the drug well. Among drug interactions, cimetidine reduces clearance of flecainide (94) and flecainide may increase digoxin and propranolol levels (95).

Encainide

Encainide is similar to flecainide in effects but has more complex pharmacology. It has similar effects on the ECG, EP testing, and arrhythmias (see above) and should be used with the same guidelines and precautions. However, it does appear to have somewhat less, though not absent negative inotropic properties. In 1991 encainide was withdrawn from the U.S. market.

Encainide is converted by the liver into three main metabolites—*O*-desmethyl encainide (ODE), 3-methoxy ODE (MODE), and *N*-desmethyl encainide. All are pharmacologically active but ODE and MODE appear to account for both effects and toxicity in most patients (96,97). ODE slows conduction velocity and prolongs ventricular refractoriness while MODE is similar to encainide but uniquely prolongs APD (96). There are both slow and fast metabolizers of encainide. In the slow metabolizers (a small percentage of the population), the parent compound accounts for most effects (98). The fact that these metabolites are different and are present in different proportions in patients taking encainide may account for differences in effects.

Encainide is administered as a tablet every 8 hr and like flecainide, one should wait at least 3 days before changing dosage.

Encainide has a similar proarrhythmic propensity as flecainide. It is less likely to, but may exacerbate congestive heart failure, and also causes dose-related central nervous system complications (alleviated by taking the drug with food).

Propafenone

Propafenone is a Class IC agent, recently approved by the FDA for use in the United States. It has a number of interesting features including unique pharmacology, a structure similar to propranolol, and partial beta blocking effects. It is effective against VAs but because it is a Class IC agent, concerns have been raised about it in light of the CAST study.

Propafenone has typical Class IC EP effects—blockade of inward I_{Na} with slow use-dependent kinetics and little change (or slight prolongation) of APD. It also has beta blocking properties, very slight Ca^{2+} channel blocking properties, and it suppresses delayed afterdepolarizations. The drug depresses the sinus node and prolongs AH, HV, and QRS intervals. Propafenone is also negatively inotropic due both to local anesthetic and beta blocking properties.

The beta blocking properties of propafenone may be highly relevant to its actions. Previously they were considered unimportant because of a 40:1 propanolol:propafenone potency ratio (99,100). However, a more recent analysis emphasizes, the high serum levels of the drug (making beta blockade important at any ratio) and the fact that potency ratio may be only 4:1 (3).

Since beta blockade diminishes post–myocardial infarction mortality and may also counteract proarrhythmic effects of flecainide (101), these actions may be relevant and separate propofenone from the other Class IC drugs. On the other hand, this notion still awaits clinical confirmation.

Pharmacokinetics of propafenone are complex and mandate close clinical observation of patients on this drug. Propafenone undergoes extensive first-pass metabolism but bioavailability depends on dose. Metabolism of propafenone is saturable, an important issue in drug loading. As dose is increased from 150–300 to 450 mg, bioavailability increases from 5 to 12% to from 40 to 50% (102). Daily doses of 900 mg lead to serum levels that are 10 times those at doses of 300 mg.

Once in the bloodstream, propafenone has a rather variable half-life (depending in part on whether hepatic enzymes have been saturated).

There are additional complexities. Propafenone has active metabolites, 5-OH propafenone and *N*-de-propylpropafenone (103) both of which have similar EP effects as the parent compound and which play an important role in antiarrhythmia. These metabolites have long half-lives and their levels depend on dose, saturation of hepatic enzymes, and time after initiation of therapy (104). It takes about 4–5 days to load a patient with propafenone and, as time goes by, active metabolites rise to higher and higher levels.

Another complexity: about 10% of patients are slow metabolizers and thus have much higher levels of propafenone and lower levels of metabolites (104). Also, in some patients R-(−) propafenone, which has lower beta blocking activity may be cleared more rapidly than S-(+)-propafenone (105).

The above makes for difficulties in evaluating patients, especially during early treatment. During drug loading, there are bound to be highly variable levels of both propafenone and its active metabolites, depending on dose, duration of therapy, and patient phenotype. Pharmacodynamic consequences of this may, however, be somewhat blunted because of the similarities in the EP effect of parent compound and metabolites. Still, one must be very cautious and close monitoring is advised. It is also prudent to delay the drug assessment EP test longer than the 3 days allowed for other antiarrhythmic agents.

Propafenone is used in VAs. Like other Class IC agents, it is highly effective in suppressing VPCs and nonsustained VT and moderately effective in suppressing inducible sustained VT (102,106). The drug is also effective in supraventricular tachycardias (where it clearly should not be a first-line drug), atrial flutter and fibrillation (especially when adrenergic dependent) (107,108) and arrhythmias due to WPW syndrome in which it prolongs the refractory periods of accessory pathways (109), though propafenone is not at this time FDA approved for these uses.

Besides proarrhythmia, other adverse effects of propafenone include conduction abnormalities, myocardial depression (102), various gastrointestinal disturbances, neurologic problems (dizziness is the most common but also change in mental status and rarely seizures) and those related to beta blockade (including exacerbation of asthma).

Among drug interactions, it increases levels of digoxin (110), warfarin (with an accompanying 25% increase in prothrombin time) (111), propranolol (112), and metoprolol. Cimetidine increases its levels (113).

Moricizine (Ethmozin)

Moricizine was originally synthesized in the U.S.S.R. in 1964. It has a phenathiazide-like structure and was later found to have antiarrhythmic properties. It was approved for use in the United States but withdrawn from the market in 1991 after CAST results were released.

Moricizine appears to have properties of all three Class I subclasses. It suppresses I_{Na}, not as greatly as the Class IC drugs but with similar slow kinetics (3) and has no effect on or shortens APD like the Class IB agents (114). The drug modestly prolongs AH, HV, and QRS intervals, has no effect on JT interval, and prolongs QT_c slightly by virtue of its effects on QRS (114). These effects are somewhat more pronounced in patients with baseline abnormalities. Sinus node abnormalities also occur in patients with baseline dysfunction. Moricizine has modest negative inotropic but no vasoactive properties.

Kinetics of moricizine are similar to other phenothiazides. It undergoes extensive first-pass hepatic metabolism with mean bioavailability of about 38% (15). Moricizine has 26 known metabolites (15) (only two with known pharmacologic activity) (Table 12.4), a high volume of distribution, and interestingly, somewhat induces its own clearance after some time.

Half-life of moricizine is short (1 1/2 hr) but duration of action is long (24 hr), suggesting the presence of as yet unidentified active metabolite(s) with long half-life(s). Thus, one should bear in mind caveats expressed earlier regarding active metabolites in early (3-day) EP testing of drugs.

The dose of moricizine is 200–300 mg every 8 hr. One should wait at least 3 days before increasing the dose. The drug is effective against VPCs (115), and nonsustained VT (somewhat more than Class IA drugs and less than other Class IC drugs), has modest effects on sustained VT (75), and there are insufficient data on atrial arrhythmias.

Moricizine has a proarrhythmic spectrum similar to other agents. The drug is generally well tolerated and in the cardiac arrhythmia pilot study, only dizziness occurred more commonly than placebo (115). However, the drug may also have gastrointestinal and other neurologic adverse effects. Exacerbation of congestive heart failure is uncommon but occurs.

CLASS II—β-ADRENERGIC BLOCKING AGENTS

Table 12.6 shows properties of beta blockers that are approved for arrhythmias or post–myocardial infarction prevention of mortality. Beta blockers have slow channel blocking properties. They are useful in atrial arrhythmias where they may convert or prevent arrhythmia, or in the case of atrial flutter and fibrillation, to slow the ventricular response. Beta blockers are only modestly effective in suppressing VAs in the ambulatory ECG and in EP testing, probably due to their anti-adrenergic effects. They are often combined with other drugs in EP testing and their long-term value may be greater than reflected in an individual EP test. These drugs (i.e., these without sympathomimetic activity) are the only group to clearly prevent sudden and other deaths in long-term post–myocardial infarction trials (116,117).

CLASS III AGENTS

General

Class III agents prolong APD as a primary effect (Table 12.1). They do so mainly by effects on one or more K^+ currents (116), though in the case of ibutilide, APD prolongation is via enhancement of window I_{Na}. Almost all Class III drugs, with the notable exception of amiodarone, exhibit reverse use dependence. That is, effects in prolonging APD are less at tachycardic rates, a possible limitation.

Class III drugs considerably prolong QT_c interval and if they are "pure" Class III agents, they have no effect on conduction or QRS duration. Amiodarone is considered the prototype, though it is rather a unique drug. Other newer agents include sematilide, ipazilide, ibutilide, and NAPA. Sotalol has both Class II and III properties. Class III agents are effective against a wide variety of atrial and ventricular arrhythmias and are the subject of considerable investigative effort. They are associated with torsade de pointes, though in the case of amiodarone this is rather unusual.

Amiodarone

Amiodarone was originally developed as an antithyroid and vasodilating antianginal agent. Although classified as a Class III agent and sometimes considered the prototype, it has properties of every class.

Amiodarone's most impressive effect is marked prolongation of APD, perhaps in part due to antithyroid properties (118), and consequently of QT_c and JT interval (Fig. 12.6). Unlike other Class III agents, amiodarone does not display reverse use dependence of APD. That is, amiodarone's effects in prolonging APD are still substantial at tachycardic heart rates, a probable antiarrhythmic advantage.

Amiodarone has Class I properties in depressing inward Na^+ current. It also displays substantial use dependence of I_{Na} (119).

The drug has both beta (120) and Ca^{++} channel blocking properties and blocks muscarinic channels.

Amiodarone has an active metabolite, desethyl amiodarone, which has somewhat greater effects on upstroke and conduction than the parent compound (121).

Which combination of the above factors is responsible for the drug's antiarrhythmic effect is unclear and probably varies among patients and rhythms. For one, there is a synergism between APD prolongation and use dependent block of I_{Na}. During the long plateau, the drug has enhanced affinity to the receptor which then translates into greater Class I type activity. Beta and Ca^{2+} channel blocking effects also play a role at times, especially in atrial arrhythmias. Amiodarone thus has many special properties, which must be borne in mind when evaluating other Class III agents which may be rather different.

Amiodarone prolongs sinus rate AH, HV intervals, and atrial, atrioventricular (AV) nodal, ventricular, and accessory pathway refractoriness, as well as PR, QRS, and QT_c intervals (122) (Fig. 12.6). After acute intravenous administration, however, primarily AV nodal and accessory pathway changes are seen which may be in part due to the solubilizing agent, polysorbate 80 (Tween 80). Oral amiodarone has few hemodynamic effects while the IV form can cause both hypotension and decrease in myocardial contractility, also possibly due in part to the Tween 80. Amiodarone does not appear to influence pacemaker thresholds.

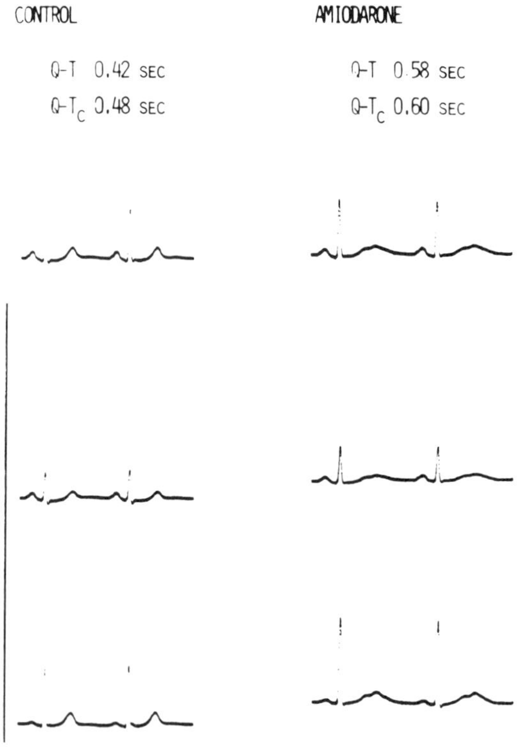

Figure 12.6. Effect of amiodarone on QT interval in a 38-yr-old male with ventricular arrhythmias. Dose of amiodarone was 200 mg/day. Shown are ECG leads I, II, and III.

Both oral and intravenous amiodarone are used clinically, although only the oral form is presently FDA approved for use in the United States. Kinetics of amiodarone are most interesting and highly variable from patient to patient. The drug has a huge volume of distribution and an incredibly long beta half-life of 23–103 days (Fig. 12.7) (123). After intravenous administration, (alpha) half-life is highly variable (5–68 hr) (124). Part of this variability is due to complex drug distribution. The long half-life of amiodarone must be considered when comparing its efficiency to that presumed for other Class III agents. It permits skipped doses and other patient errors without loss of antiarrhythmic effectiveness, an advantage in long-term administration.

After initial administration, the drug rapidly concentrates in the heart and more slowly in the adipose and other tissues. However, it may redistribute out of the heart while still accumulating elsewhere (124). This may account for initial response followed by recurrence of arrhythmia, especially with intravenous use. In chronic therapy, desethyl amiodarone accumulates to levels of up to two times the parent compound (125).

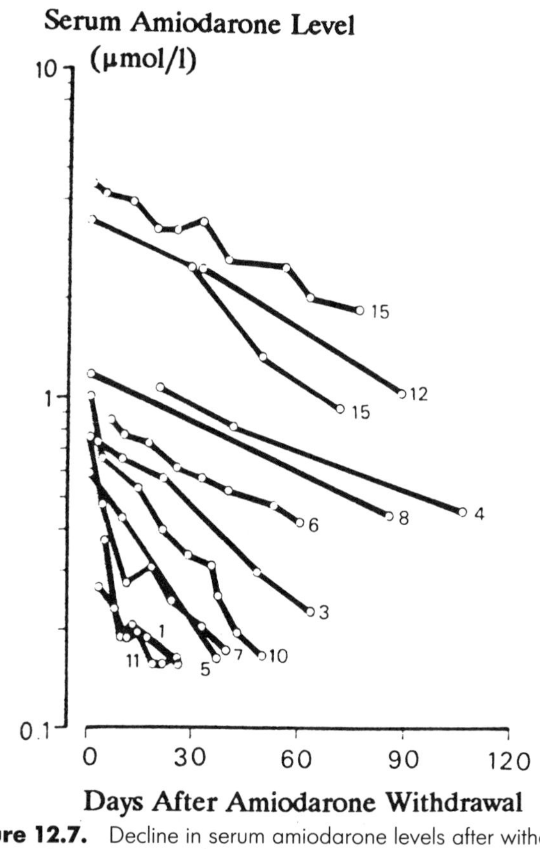

Figure 12.7. Decline in serum amiodarone levels after withdrawal from steady state in 12 evaluations in 11 patients. Numbers referred to patient numbers in the original study. There is a slow but variable decline in amiodarone levels. Mean half-life of amiodarone in these 11 patients was calculated at 41 ± 19 days. (From Staubli M, Bircher J, Gateazzi RL, *et al.*: Serum concentrations of amiodarone during long-term therapy. relation to dose, efficacy, and toxicity. Eur J Clin Pharmacol 1983; 24:485–494, with permission.)

With intravenous use, in spite of the above variability and complexity, one can expect an initial response within a few hours, often within a half-hour. In oral use, with a loading dose, some effectiveness can be expected within a few days. However, it takes weeks for efficacy to fully take hold.

The following dosing regimens of amiodarone have been suggested (14,126):

1. Intravenous: (a) 5–10 mg/kg over 20–30 min followed by 1 g/day for several days. Additional 1–3 mg/kg doses may be given. (b) 2–2.5 mg/min for 12 hr followed by 0.7 mg/min for the next 36 hours.

2. Oral: 800–1600 mg/day for 1–3 wk followed by 800 mg/day for 2–4 wk, followed by 600 mg for 4–8 wk. After this, maintenance of 200–400 mg/day

Because of highly variable kinetics, dosage regimen should be individualized with close attention to ECGs and drug levels.

Oral amiodarone is effective in atrial arrhythmias including PSVT, atrial flutter, and atrial fibrillation but it is not at present FDA approved for this use. It is most effective in arrhythmias related to the WPW syndrome where it causes substantial prolongation of ERP in the accessory pathway. The drug may be effective in WPW even in small doses of less than 200 mg/day. Amiodarone suppresses VPCs for which it is not recommended because of toxicity.

The most common use and only FDA approved use of amiodarone is for serious VAs. Here it is administered alone or in combination with implantable defibrillator or surgical therapy. A number of clinical trials are now underway to fully establish the use of amiodarone versus other drugs or versus defibrillator therapy in VT/VF (127).

Intravenous amiodarone is also effective for VAs and in spite of its usual kinetics has been used for acute therapy including in cardiac arrest situations. It is effective acutely for atrial arrhythmias including especially those associated with preexcitation. Intravenous amiodarone has not yet been approved by the FDA.

Assessment of amiodarone's long-term effectiveness for VT by EP studies is problematic. The test clearly does not predict efficacy to amiodarone as well as it does to other antiarrhythmic agents. It is not known whether this is due to some EP peculiarity, or, perhaps more likely, to the unusual kinetics which makes early evaluation difficult. The drug evaluation EP study should be performed 2 wk after start of therapy using IV plus oral drug loading. But even then, final drug distribution may not have been achieved. In addition, the active metabolite desetheyl amiodarone, which has different EP effects from the parent compound may only come into effect much later.

Data on the predictability of EP studies have been variable. Several investigators have found that many VT patients were inducible after administration of amiodarone yet had an apparently good clinical outcome (127–130) while others have found some usefulness for the test. In one study, negative inducibility of VT post amiodarone was predictive of an 18-month arrhythmia-free interval (though it is likely that some patients in this category will have recurrences) whereas inducibility was associated with a 48% recurrence (131).

Partial effectiveness of amiodarone in EP testing may be a more reliable indicator for the long-term effectiveness of this than of other drugs (131,132). For example, requirement of a more aggressive stimulation protocol for induction and a slower rate of induced VT with amiodarone are probably also associated with less likely recurrence. One study also showed that hemodynamic tolerance of induced VT correlated with later tolerance of spontaneously occurring VT while cardiovascular collapse during the induced arrhythmia correlated with later sudden death (131). Clinical parameters such as degree of prolongation of QT_c interval and recurrence of spontaneous VT during monitoring (132) as well as certain additional EP parameters such as prolongation of ventricular ERP may be helpful but do not, by any means, assure complete predictability.

Amiodarone has impressive toxicity, highly limiting its use (133). Pulmonary toxicity beginning as lipoidal pneumonia and progressing to pulmonary fibrosis is the most feared (134). It is characterized by cough, dyspnea, and (early) fever. Pulmonary function tests show reduced diffusion capacity and gallium scans are positive for inflammation. Incidence is unclear but may be about 10% over 1 yr. Steroids as well as discontinuation of the drug are advised.

Amiodarone commonly causes hepatic enzyme abnormalities, mild elevations of which can be tolerated, and also rarely, hepatic injury. Photosensitivity, slate blue skin discoloration, corneal microdeposits, anorexia, and constipation are common. The drug causes a slight increase in thyroxine (T_4), reverse triiodothyronine (T_3) and thyroid stimulating hormone (TSH), and a slight decrease in T_3. Hyperthyroidism (due to iodine load in sensitive patients) and hypothryoidism (due to inhibition of conversion of T_4 to T_3) occur uncommonly. Chemical diagnosis of hyperthyroidism is difficult to make because the drug distorts thyroid function tests even when it does not have a metabolic effect. However, there may be a more substantial increase in TSH.

Cardiac toxicity includes sinus bradycardia (which may be severe and lethal), rare torsades de pointes (even in spite of its tendency to considerably prolong QT_c intervals; see Chapter 10 for a more complete discussion of this subject), and worsening of congestive heart failure. For better evaluation of possible toxicity, baseline QT_c intervals, thyroid, pulmonary, and liver function tests, chest x-rays and ophthalmologic slit lamp examinations are advised, as well as the usual routine blood tests. Toxicity is more likely at serum levels above 2.5 μg/ml, but one cannot depend on this.

Amiodarone interferes with elimination of warfarin and prothrombin time must be closely watched (135). A jump in values with accompanying bleeding may occur suddenly after 2–4 wk of therapy. Amiodarone also causes increased serum levels of digoxin, quinidine, procainamide, disopyramide, mexiletine, and propafenone (136).

Bretylium

Bretylium usually is put in Class III, though its mechanism of action is unclear. It is used exclusively in intravenous form for arrhythmias. The drug has sympathomimetic effects—it first causes catecholamine discharge with its consequences (including possible proarrhythmia) and then sympathetic depletion. Hypotension due to such depletion is common. Bretylium also has primary effects in prolonging atrial and ventricular APD and ERP (137) (the reason for its placement in Class III) and in reducing ERP disparity between injured and normal tissue (138). However, it is not known which of these properties leads to antiarrhythmia. Bretylium has negative inotropic effects by virtue of sympathetic depletion, but not primarily.

Bretylium is used in acute treatment of VT/VF after lidocaine has failed. It is given as a 5 mg/kg loading dose, quickly in emergencies. Additional loading doses may be given to tolerance with hypotension the limiting feature. In some patients, high doses have been given. Maintenance is 1–4 mg/min. Therapeutic effects occur over a wide range of serum levels (139). It should be noted that there may be a larger lag time between administration and effect than, e.g., with lidocaine or procainamide because of delay in myocardial uptake of drug.

Besides hypotension, the complications include nausea and vomiting. Also, there may be hypertension and proarrhythmia (increased VPCs) in the initial catecholamine-release phase.

Sotalol

Sotalol has been used for many years in Europe and elsewhere for treatment in angina and hypertension but is not, as of this writing FDA approved for use in the United States. Over the years, a number of antiarrhythmic properties have been recognized.

Sotalol is a combined Class II and III drug. *d*-Sotalol has exclusive Class III properties and appears to be an antiarrhythmic drug in its own right (140), though data are limited. The drug's main effect is an increase in APD and ERP which (141) are both counteracted by verapamil in vitro. (142). Sotalol has little or no effect on upstroke in atrium, His-Purkinje tissue, or ventricle (142,143).

Sotalol's beta blocking effects depress automaticity, slow conduction, and prolong refractoriness in the sinus and AV nodes. The drug prolongs AH and QT_c intervals but not HV or QRS (144). In vitro, the drug has milder negatively inotropic properties than other beta blockers. These are due to increased cellular Ca^{2+} uptake due to APD prolongation. However, a decrease in cardiac output may be observed in patients with congestive heart failure (145). Sotalol has few primary vasoactive effects other than from beta blockade.

Sotalol has relatively simple pharmacokinetics (146). It is virtually 100% bioavailable and half-life of 7–18 hr. The drug is not at all bound to serum protein. Since it is eliminated unchanged by the kidneys, dosage reduction must be made in renal failure.

Sotalol is effective against both atrial and ventricular arrhythmias. It suppresses VPCs and is effective against sustained VT in EP testing (147), though more data are needed on this subject. It is useful in PSVT and atrial fibrillation as well as arrhythmias due to WPW (148).

Torsades de pointes, (1.9% in one study (149) and other proarrhythmia (4.3%), are significant considerations with sotalol. Patients need to be monitored carefully for excessive prolongation of QT_c interval, though prolongation is not necessarily greater in patients with torsades de pointes than in the others (149). Close attention to serum K^+ levels (150) are advised and interactions with thiazide diuretics make these drugs risky for coexisting administration. Also, bradycardia due to beta blocking actions of sotalol may predispose to torsade de pointes.

Congestive heart failure may be exacerbated (about 1.5%) (149) and there are other adverse effects related to beta blockade. Overall, however, sotalol is a well-tolerated drug and few patients discontinue it because of adverse effects.

CLASS IV AGENTS—CALCIUM CHANNEL BLOCKERS

General

Ca^{2+} channel blockers are useful in acute treatment of supraventricular tachycardias and to slow the ventricular response in atrial flutter and fibrillation (though they should be used with extreme caution in atrial fibrillation associated with preexcitation syndromes) (see Chapter 9). Class IV drugs are generally not useful in VAs, with the exception of an interesting group of exercise-induced VAs that may be due to delayed afterdepolarizations. Verapamil is the prototype Ca^{2+} channel blocker used for arrhythmia and it alone will be reviewed here. Diltiazem has been approved by the FDA for rate control in atrial flutter-fibrillation. In addition, bepridil has some antiarrhythmic properties while nifedipine and other purine derivatives do not have sufficient electrophysiologic effects for antiarrhythmic use.

Verapamil

Verapamil is a papaverine derivative that blocks slow channels. It therefore slows sinus and AV nodal automaticity and prolongs conduction and refractoriness in the AV node. These effects may be somewhat modulated by enhanced sympathetic activity due to hypotension, especially at lower concentrations.

Verapamil displays first-pass hepatic metabolism. It also displays stereoselectivity of both effect and metabolism. The Ca^{2+} channel blocking properties reside in the *l*-isomer while *d*-verapamil has slight local anesthetic properties that are probably of little clinical significance. *l*-Verapamil is more extensively metabolized by the liver on first pass and thus relatively more *d*-verapamil gets into the blood stream with oral administration. With intravenous administration both *d*- and *l*-verapamil get into the bloodstream equally (151,152). For this reason at a given drug level of verapamil after oral administration there is less *l*-verapamil and thus less effect on sinus and A-V nodes and PR interval than at the same drug level after intravenous administration. Effects of oral versus intravenous administration of verapamil on PR interval are shown in Figure 12.8 (152). This phenomenon may in some part explain why antiarrhythmic effects on PSVT with oral verapamil may be disappointing compared to intravenous effects. Norverapamil, an active metabolite, also plays a greater role with oral administration.

Hemodynamically, verapamil causes hypotension and is negatively inotropic. It also blocks α-2 receptors.

Intravenous verapamil is used to terminate PSVT due to either AV nodal reentry or WPW (153,154). It is also used to slow the ventricular response in atrial flutter and fibrillation, occasionally as a constant rate infusion; it may also convert atrial flutter to fibrillation.

Chronically, verapamil has been used to prevent recurrence of PSVT, for which it is probably less effective than other agents. It is also used either alone or in combination with other agents to slow the ventricular response in atrial flutter and fibrillation.

Several precautions in intravenous use of verapamil should be noted. (a) The drug is risky in VT where it may cause hemodynamic collapse. It should therefore not be given to patients with wide complex tachycardia unless one is certain that the tachycardia is supraventricular, a distinction that can only be made definitively in the EP laboratory. However there is one unusual form of rate/exercise-induced VT, believed due to triggered activity in which verapamil may be useful (155). (b) Verapamil may dangerously accelerate ventricular rate in atrial fibrillation due to WPW through either loss of retrograde concealed conduction in the accessory pathway or sympathetic stimulation (156). (c) Use of verapamil in atrial flutter should be cautious as the drug may not slow ventricular rate but may cause hypotension. (d) VPCs and occasionally VT may occur with administration for PSVT but these tend to be self-limited (157).

Complications of verapamil include hypotension, congestive heart failure, AV nodal block, and sinus node depression acutely. As antidotes, intravenous calcium chloride may reverse hypotension and isoproterenol is used for bradycardic/blocked rhythms. All of the depressant effects are additive to other negatively inotropic and hypotensive agents and particular caution should be exercised in using verapamil with β-adrenergic blockers.

CLASS V AGENTS

Adenosine

Adenosine is approved for intravenous use in the treatment of acute PSVT. Adenosine (as well as adenosine triphosphate which has been tried clinically, and adenosine mono- and di-phosphate) (158) suppresses automaticity and conduction and prolongs refractoriness in the AV node. Clinically, it prolongs AH intervals (159). In the sinus node adenosine has a somewhat lesser effect in suppressing automaticity (160,161) which may be counteracted by reflex tachycardia due to hypotension (162).

Mode of action of adenosine is not yet clear, but there appears to be direct enhancement of K^+ current and indirect suppression of catecholamine-induced Ca^{2+} and pacemaker currents (via inhibition of adenyl cyclase activity and cAMP which in turn prevents intracellular Ca^{2+} overload). Hemodynamically, adenosine is a coronary and peripheral vasodilator and can cause hypotension as well as coronary steal syndrome. It is slightly negatively inotropic.

Adenosine has proven effective in treatment of paroxysmal supraventricular tachycardia with a major advantage in having an extremely short half-life of 1–7 sec (163). It therefore has virtually no important complications and is nearly universally

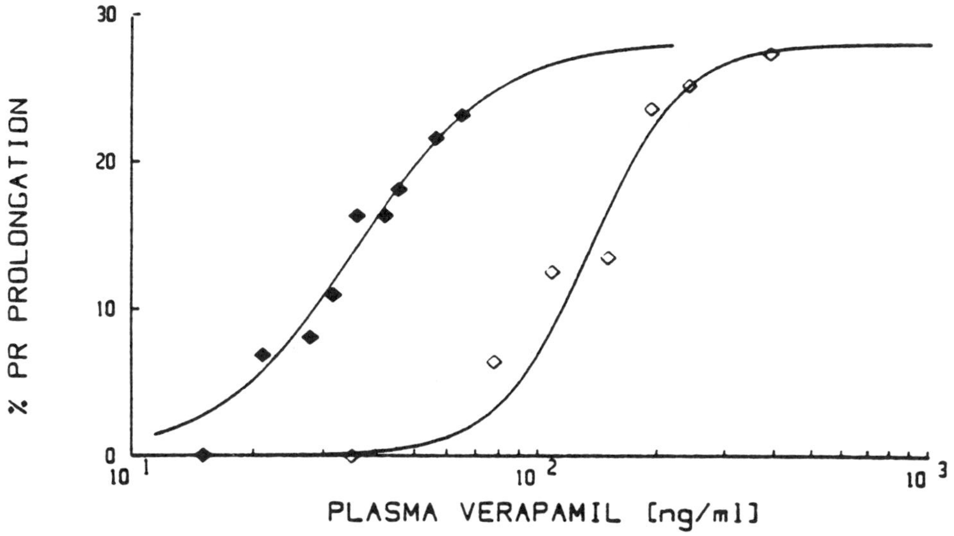

Figure 12.8. Plasma verapamil levels vs. PR prolongation on the ECG after intravenous (*closed squares*) and oral (*open squares*) administration. At the same plasma verapamil levels, effects on PR interval are less after oral administration. This is due to stereospecific hepatic first-pass metabolism as described in text. (From Echizen H, Vogelgesang B, Eichelbaum M: Effects of d,l-verapamil on atrioventricular conduction in relation to its stereoselective first-pass metabolism. Clin Pharmacol Ther 1985;38:71–76, with permission.)

effective. In one study, 12 mg of adenosine terminated 91% of PSVTs (164). The drug is also effective in supraventricular tachycardias due to WPW, AV junctional tachycardia, and a group of exercise-induced ventricular tachycardias that may be due to cyclic adenosine monophosphate (cAMP)-mediated triggered activity (165).

Dose of adenosine is 6–12 mg administered rapidly intravenously. It is less effective when given slowly. Recurrences may occur and this dose can be repeated in 1–2 min. The drug should not be given in atrial flutter/fibrillation or ectopic atrial tachycardia. In WPW, it has occasionally caused atrial fibrillation and atrial flutter. Also, as with verapamil, VPCs may occur following adenosine use in PSVT.

Adenosine is antagonized by quinidine (166), theophylline, and other xanthines (167). Dipyridamole inhibits adenosine uptake and thus may potentiate and prolong its duration of action (167). Atropine does not block its effects.

Digoxin

Extensive reviews of digitalis preparations are available elsewhere and this chapter will focus only on antiarrhythmic essentials in its use (13). Only digoxin which is now the predominant preparation will be discussed. Digoxin's arrhythmia uses are, generally speaking, confined to supraventricular arrhythmia.

Effects of digoxin are both direct and indirect. The drug inhibits Na, K-adenosine triphosphatase (Na, K-ATPase), enhances parasympathetic (168) and diminishes sympathetic activity (169), and is a direct systemic and pulmonary vasoconstrictor (170,171). Electrophysiologic effects are suppression of sinus node automaticity, variable effects on the atrium (mainly but not always shortening of ERP), prolonged conduction and enhanced automaticity in the A-V node, and little effect on His-Purkinje system and ventricular muscle. The drug may also shorten (or at times lengthen) refractory periods in accessory pathways (172–174).

Pharmacokinetics of digoxin have been well studied (175–177). The drug is administered intravenously or orally as a tablet (bioavailability about 50–80% or 60%), an elixir (bioavailability 60–80%) and a capsulated gel-form (greatest bioavailability at 80–100%). The drug has a very large volume distribution and a mean half-life of 36 hr (range 26–44 hr).

Digoxin is mainly eliminated by the kidney and to some degree by the enterohepatic circulation which may be enhanced with renal failure. Half-life in renal failure may be considerably prolonged (178), but hepatitis and congestive heart failure have little influence (179).

About 37% of drug is excreted per day with normal renal function and 14% in anephric patients (179). Volume of distribution of digoxin is also smaller in renal failure so the loading dose must be also reduced (180).

Digoxin was one of the first drugs for which plasma levels were part of routine clinical thinking. Therapeutic plasma levels are approximately 1.2–2.0 mg/ml with exceptions and considerably overlap at both ends of the scale. Many patients do not have digitalis toxicity in higher concentrations.

Digoxin can be used in the acute treatment of PSVT but verapamil and adenosine are now the first-line drugs. Digoxin is, however, a valuable drug in long-term prevention of this arrhythmia and has relatively less adverse effects than other drugs used. Digoxin is used to control ventricular response in atrial flutter and fibrillation (flutter requires a higher dose) (181,182) with verapamil or beta blockers added when it is inadequate. Digoxin is also commonly employed to prevent occurrence of atrial fibrillation or convert it to sinus rhythm though in fact there is data as to its ineffectiveness for this use here (183,184).

Digoxin has been used in ventricular arrhythmias but with little justification. It may be effective in WPW due to its AV blocking properties. However, it may also be risky in this situation because shortened atrial and accessory pathway refractory periods may increase the ventricular rate in atrial fibrillation possibly leading to VF (185,186). Use of digoxin for WPW is not generally recommended for this reason.

Digitalis toxicity has been widely discussed (187,188). Arrhythmias include sinus bradycardia (not usually of pathologic significance unless there was previous disease in the sinus node), AV nodal block, junctional tachycardia, paroxysmal atrial tachycardia with block, VPCs, VT, and VF. Hypocalcemia and hypomagnesemia increase the risk of digitalis toxicity. Delayed afterdepolarizations (see Chapter 2) probably play an important role in the tachycardic arrhythmias.

Digitalis suicidal overdoses generally result in sinus bradycardia and in its last phases hyperkalemia due to poisoning of the Na-K pump (189). Fab fragment treatment (190) and hemoperfusion with XAD-4 (191) have been used in this instance. Since there is an enterohepatic circulation of digoxin, cholestyramine (192) and both oral (193) and hemoperfused (194) charcoal have been used to enhance fecal elimination via binding and reduction of enteral reabsorption. Other drug toxicity include nausea and vomiting, various neurologic symptoms including, at their worst, visual disturbances, gynecomastia, and sexual dysfunction in males.

Phenytoin and lidocaine (for ventricular arrhythmias) and potassium have been used for digitalis-toxic arrhythmias. Potassium is used in ectopic tachycardias but care should be used in the presence of associated intracardiac conduction blocks.

A situation that occasionally arises is the need for electroconversion of atrial arrhythmias in the presence of digoxin. In the presence of digitalis toxicity there are risks of inducing VAs and if electroconversion is absolutely necessary, use of lower energy doses, which may be gradually increased, and lidocaine are helpful.

Drug interactions with digoxin are numerous and are based on interference with absorption, tissue uptake, and elimination. Bile acid binding resins and antacids, kaolin, pectate, and certain antibiotics (erythromycin and tetracycline) decrease absorption (195). Quinidine, verapamil, and amiodarone significantly increase serum levels (196,197) while propofenone, diltiazem, nifedipine, spironolactones, triamterene, and indomethacin cause somewhat lesser increases. While these interactions have been reported to cause digitalis toxicity at times, their overall significance is not as yet clear.

References

1. Vaughan Williams EM: Classification of anti-arrhythmic drugs. In Sandoe E, Flensted-Jansen E, Olesen KH (eds): Symposium on Cardiac Arrhythmias. AB Astra, Soderatalje, Sweden, 1970:449–472.
2. Vaughan Williams EM: A classification of antiarrhythmic actions reassessed after a decade of new drugs. J Clin Pharmacol 1984;24:129–147.
3. Vaughan Williams EM: Classification of the antiarrhythmic action of moricizine. J Clin Pharmacol 1991;31:216–221.
4. Harrison DC: Antiarrhythmic drug classification: new science and practical applications. Am J Cardiol 1985;56:185–187.
5. Mirro MJ, Watanabe AM, Bailey JC: Electrophysiologic effects of the optical isomers of disopyramide and quinidine in the dog: Dependence on stereochemistry. Circ Res 1981;48:867–874.
6. Chen C-M, Gettes LS, Katzung BF: Effect of lidocaine and quinidine on steady-state characteristics and recovery kinetics of (d/V/dt) max in guinea pig ventricular myocardium. Circ Res 1975;37:20–29.
7. Scheiner LB, Tozer TN: Clinical Pharmacokinetics: The use of plasma concentrations of drugs. In Melmon KL, Morrelli HF (eds): Clinical Pharmacology. MacMillan, New York, 1978;71–109.
8. Woosley RL: Antiarrhythmic agents. In Hurst JW, Schlant RC (eds): The Heart. McGraw-Hill, New York, 1990:1682–1711.
9. Beaufils P, Leenhardt A, Denjoy E, *et al.*: Antiarrhythmic drugs in the adult population. In Rosen MR, Janse MJ, Wit AL (eds): Cardiac Electrophysiology. Futura Publishing Co., Mt. Kisco, 1990:1175–1187.
10. Frishman WH, Sonnenblick EH: Calcium channel blockers. In Hirst JW, Schlant RD (eds): The Heart. McGraw-Hill, New York, 1990:1731–1748.
11. Frishman WH, Sonnenblick EH: B-adrenergic blocking drugs. In Hirst JW, Schlant RC (eds): The Heart. McGraw-Hill, New York, 1990:1712–1731.
12. Antiarrhythmic Drugs. Medical Letter on Drugs and Therapeutics 1991;33:55–60.
13. Marcus FI, Huang SK: Digitalis. In Hurst JW, Schlant RC (eds): The Heart, 7th ed. McGraw-Hill, New York, 1990;1748–1761.
14. Zipes DP: Management of cardiac arrhythmias: Pharmacological, electrical, and surgical techniques. In Braunwald E (eds): Heart Disease. WB Saunders, Philadelphia, 1988:621–657.
15. Mann HJ: Moricizine: A new Class I antiarryhthmic. Clin Pharmacol 1990;9:842–852.
16. Squire A, Kupersmith J: Beta adrenergic blocking agents, review and update. Mt Sinai Med J 1985;52:553–558.
17. Funck-Brentano C, Woosley RL: Current antiarrhythmic agents: clinical phramacology. In El-Sherif N, Samet P (eds): Cardiac Pacing and Electrophysiology. WB Saunders, Philadelphia, 1991:409–435.
18. Stäubli M, Bircher J, Galeazzi RL, *et al.*: Serum concentrations of amiodarone during long term therapy. Relation to dose, efficacy and toxicity. Eur J Clin Pharmacol 1983;24:485–494.
19. Hondgehem L, Katzung BG: Test of a model of antiarrhythmic drug action: Effects of quinidine and lidocaine on myocardial conduction. Circulation 1980;61:1217–1224.
20. Kupersmith J, Reder RF, Slater W: New antiarrhythmic drugs. Cardiovasc Rev Rep 1985;6:35–56.
21. Roden DM, Woosley RL, Primm RK: Incidence and clinical features of the quinidine-associated long QT syndrome: implications for patient care. Am Heart J 1986;111:1088–1093.
22. Vozeh S, Oti-Amoako K, Uematsu T, *et al.*: Antiarrhythmic activity of two quinidine metabolites in experimental reperfusion arrhythmia: Relative potency and pharmacodynamic interaction with the parent drug. J Pharmacol Exp Ther 1987;243:297–301.
23. Thompson KA, Blair A, Woosley RL, *et al.*: Comparative in vitro electrophysiology of quinidine, its major metabolites and dihydroxyquinidine. J Pharmacol Exp Ther 1987;241:84–90.
24. Mirro MJ, Manalan AS, Bailey JC, *et al.*: Anticholineric effects of disopyramide and quinidine on guinea pig myocardium: Mediation by direct muscarinic receptor blockade. Circ Res 1980;47:855–858.
25. Schmid PG, Nelson LD, Heistad DD *et al.*: Vascular effects of procainamide in the dog: Predominance of the inhibitory effect on ganglionic transmission. Circ Res 1974;35:948–960.
26. Selzer A, Wray HW: Quinidine syncope: paroxysmal ventricular fibrillation occurring during treatment of chronic atrial arrhythmias. Circulation 1964;30:1031–1034.
27. Coplen SE, Antman EM, Berlin JA, *et al.*: Efficacy and safety of quinidine therapy for maintenance of sinus rhythm after cardioversion: A meta-analysis of randomized control trials. Circulation 1990;82:1106–1116.
28. Morganroth J, Goin JE: Quinidine-related mortality in the short-to-medium-term treatment of ventricular arrhythmias: A meta-analysis. Circulation 1991;84:1977–1983.
29. Weintraub RG, Gow RM, Wilkinson JL: The congenital long QT syndromes in childhood. J Am Coll Cardiol 1990;16:674–680.
30. Leahey EB Jr, Reiffel JA, Giardina EGV, *et al.*: The effect of quinidine and other oral antiarrhythmic drugs on serum digoxin: A prospective study. Ann Intern Med 1980;92:605–608.
31. Kornfeld P, Horowitz SH, Genkins G, *et al.*: Myesthenia gravis unmasked by antiarrhythmic agents. Mt Sinai J Med 1976;43:10–14.
32. Grogono AW: Anesthesia for atrial fibrillation: Effect of quinidine on muscle relaxation. Lancet 1963;2:1039.
33. Koch-Weser J, Klein SW: Procainamide dosage schedules, plasma concentrations, and clinical effects. JAMA 1971;215:1454–1460.
34. Elson J, Strong MJ, Lee W-K *et al.*: Antiarrhythmic potency of N-acetylprocainamide. Clin Pharmacol Ther 1975;17:134–140.
35. Rosen MR, Merker C, Gelband H, *et al.*: Effects of procainamide on the electrophysiologic properties of the canine ventricular conduction system. J Pharmacol Exp Ther 1973;185:438–446.
36. Dangman KH, Hoffman BF: In vivo and in vitro antiarrhythmic and arrhythmogenic effects of N-acetryl procainamide. J Pharmacol Exp Ther 1981;217:851–862.
37. Woosley RL, Drayer DE, Reidenberg MM, *et al.*: Effect of actylator phenotype on the rate at which procainamide induces antinuclear antibodies and the lupus syndrome. N Engl J Med 1978;298:1157–1159.
38. Roden DM, Reele SB, Higgins SB, *et al.*: Antiarrhythmic efficacy, pharmacokinetics and safety of N-acetylprocainamide in human subjects: Comparison with procainamide. Am J Cardiol 1980;46:463–468.
39. Myerburg RJ, Kessler KM, Kiem I, *et al.*: Relationship between plasma levels of procainamide, suppression of premature ventricular complexes and prevention of recurrent ventricular tachycardia. Circulation 1981;64:280–290.
40. Miller RR, Hillard G, Lies JE *et al.*: Hemodynamic effects of procainamide in patients with acute myocardial infarction and comparison with lidocaine. Am J Med 1973;55:161–168.
41. Giardina EGV, Heissenbuttel RH, Bigger JT: Intermittent intravenous procainamide to treat ventricular arrhythmias. Correlation of plasma concentration with effect on arrhythmia, electrocardiogram, and blood pressure. Ann Intern Med 1973;78:183–193.
42. Waxman HL, Buxton AE, Sadowski LM, *et al.*: The response to procainamide during electrophysiologic study for sustained ventricular tachyarrhythmias predicts the response to other medications. Circulation 1982;67:30–37.
43. Blomgren SE, Condemi JJ, Vaughan JH: Procainamide-induced lupus erythematosus-clinical and laboratory observations. Am J Med 1972;52:338–348.

44. Giacomini KM, Cox BM, Blaschke TF: Comparative anticholinergic potencies of R- and S-disopyramide in longitudinal muscle strips from guinea pig ileum. Life Sci 1980;27:1191–1197.
45. Meffin PJ, Robert EW, Winkle RA, *et al.*: The role of concentration-dependent plasma protein binding in disopyramide disposition. J Pharmacokinet Biopharm 1979;7:29–46.
46. Aitio M, Mansury L, Tala E, *et al.*: The effect of enzyme-induction on the metabolism of disopyramide in man. Br J Clin Pharmacol 1981;11:279–285.
47. Singh BN, Vaughan Williams EM: The effect of altering potassium concentration on the action of lidocaine and diphenylhydantoin on rabbit atrial and ventricular muscle. Circ Res 1971;29:286–296.
48. Kupersmith J, Antman EM, Hoffman BF: *In vivo* electrophysiologic effects of lidocaine in canine acute myocardial infarction. Circ Res 1975;36:84.
49. Kupersmith J: Electrophysiologic and antiarrhythmic effects of lidocaine in canine acute myocardial ischemia. Am Heart J 1979;97:320–327.
50. Hiromasa S, Li ZY, Coto H, *et al.*: Selective effects of tocainide in canine acute myocardial infarction. Int J Cardiol 1990;27:79–86.
51. Hille B: Local anesthetics: Hydrophilic and hydrophobic pathways for the drug-receptor reaction. J Gen Physiol 1977;69:497–515.
52. Courtney KR: Interval-dependent effects of small antiarrhythmic drugs on excitability of guinea-pig myocardium. J Mol Cell Cardiol 1980;12:1273–1286.
53. Roden DM: Clinical pharmacological requisites to ensure the adequacy of antiarrhythmic therapy. In Rosen MR, Janse MJ, Wit AL (eds): Cardiac Electrophysiology. Futura Publishing Co., Mt. Kisco, New York, 1990;1095–1115.
54. Allen JD, Pomerantz J, Wit AL: Actions of lidocaine on transmembrane potentials of subendocardial Purkinje fibers surviving in infarcted canine hearts. Circ Res 1978;43:470–481.
55. Weiner I, Mindich B, Kupersmith J: Regional differences in the effects of lidocaine on intramyocardial conduction in patients with coronary artery disease. Am Heart J 1981;102:53–58.
56. Kupersmith J: Antiarrhythmic drugs—changing concepts. Am J Cardiol 1976;38:119–121.
57. Southworth JL, McKusick VA, Pierce EC II, *et al.*: Ventricular fibrillation precipitated by cardiac catheterization. JAMA 1950;143:717–720.
58. Nies, AS: Cardiovascular disorders. In Melmon KL, Morrelli HF (eds): Clinical Pharmacology: Basic principles in Therapeutics. McGraw-Hill, New York, 1972:142–261.
59. LeLorier J, Grenon D, Latour Y, *et al.*: Pharmacokinetics of lidocaine after prolonged intravenous infusions in uncomplicated myocardial infarction. Ann Intern Med 1977;87:700–702.
60. Nattel S, Zipes DP: Clinical pharmacology of old and new antiarrhythmic drugs. Cardiovas Res 1980;11:221–248.
61. Sefaldt RJ, Nattel S, Kreeft JH, *et al.*: Lidocaine therapy with an exponentially declining infusion. Ann Intern Med 1984;101:632–634.
62. Wyman MG, Slaughter RL, Farolino DA, *et al.*: Multiple bolus technique for lidocaine administration in acute ischemic heart disease. II. Treatment of refractory ventricular failure. J Am Coll Cardiol 1983;2:764–769.
63. Koster RW, Dunning AJ: Intramuscular lidocaine for prevention of lethal arrhythmias in the prehospitalization phase of acute myocardial infarction. N Engl J Med 1985;313:1105–1110.
64. Duff HJ, Roden DM, Primm RK, *et al.*: Mexiletine for resistant ventricular tachycardia: Comparison with lidocaine and enhancement of efficacy by combination with quinidine. Am J. Cardiol 1981;47:438–445.
65. Duff HJ, Roden D, Primm RK, *et al.*: Mexiletine in the treatment of resistant ventricular arrhythmias: Enhancement of efficacy and reduction of dose-related side effects by combination with quinidine. Circulation 1983;67: 1124–1128.
66. Leahey EB Jr, Heissenbuttel RH, Giardina EGV, *et al.*: Combined mexiletine and propranolol treatment of refractory ventricular arrhythmia. Br Med J 1980;281:357–358.
67. Greenspan AM, Spielman SR, Webb CR, *et al.*: Efficacy of combination therapy with mexiletine and a type IA agent for inducible ventricular tachyarrhythmias secondary to coronary artery disease. Am J Cardiol 1985;56:277–284.
68. Beckett AH, Chidomere EC: The distribution, metabolism and excretion of mexiletine in man. Postgrad Med J 1977;53(Suppl 1):60.
69. Campbell RWF: Mexiletine. N Engl J Med 1987;316:29–34.
70. Campbell RWF, Dolder MA, Prescott LF, *et al.*: Comparison of procainamide and mexiletine in prevention of ventricular arrhythmias after acute myocardial infarction. Lancet 1975;1:1257–1260.
71. Roos JC, Paalman ACA, Dunning AJ: Electrophysiological effects of mexiletine in man. Br Heart J 1976;38:1262–1271.
72. Fasola GP, D'Osualdo F, dePangher V, *et al.*: Thrombocytopenia and mexiletine. Ann Intern Med 1984;100:162–163.
73. Girmann G, Pees H, Scheurelen PG: Pseudothrombocytopenia and mexiletine. Ann Intern Med 1984;100:767–768.
74. Podrid PJ, Lown B: Tocainide for refractory symptomatic ventricular arrhythmias. Am J Cardiol 1982;49:1279–1286.
75. Hession MJ, Lampert S, Podrid PJ, *et al.*: Ethmozine (moricizine HCI) therapy for complex ventricular arrhythmias. Am J Cardiol 1987;60:59F–66F.
76. Block AJ, Merrill D, Smith ER: Stereoselectivity of tocainide pharmacodynamics in vivo and in vitro. Fed Proc 1986;45:513.
77. Roden DM, Woosley RL: Tocainide. N Engl J Med 1986;315:41–45.
78. Ikeda N, Singh BN, Davis LD, *et al.*: Effects of flecainide on the electrophysiologic properties of isolated canine and rabbit myocardial fibers. J Am Coll Cardiol 1985;5:303–310.
79. Campbell TJ, Vaughn Williams EM: Voltage- and time-dependent depression of maximum rate of depolarization of guinea-pig ventricular action potentials by two new antiarrhythmic drugs, flecainide and lorcainide. Cardiovasc Res 1983;17:251–258.
80 Estes NAM, Garan H, Ruskin JN: Electrophysiologic properties of flecainide acetate. Am J Cardiol 1984;53:26B.
81. Hellestrand KJ, Bexton RS, Nathan AW, *et al.*: Acute electrophysilogical effects of flecainide acetate on cardiac conduction and refractoriness in man. Br Heart J 1982;48:140–148.
82. Pritchett F, Smith WM, Kirsten E: Pharmacokinetics and pharmacodynamic interaction between cimetidine and propafenone. J Clin Pharmacol 1988;28:619–24.
83. Cockrell JL, Scheinman MM, Titus C, *et al.*: Safety and efficacy of oral flecainide therapy in patients with atrioventricular reentrant tachycardia. Ann Intern Med, 1991;114:189–194.
84. Henthorn RW, Waldo AL, Anderson JL, *et al.*: Flecainide acetate prevents recurrence of symptomatic paroxysmal supraventricular tachycardia. Circulation 1991;83:119–125.
85. Anderson JL, Gilbert EM, Alpert BL, *et al.*: Prevention of symptomatic recurrences of paroxysmal atrial fibrillation in patients initially tolerating antiarrhythmic therapy. Circulation 1989;80:1557–1570.
86. Hellestrand KJ, Nathan AW, Bexton RS, *et al.*: Cardiac electrophysiologic effects of flecainide acetate for paroxysmal reentrant junctional tachycardias. Am J Cardiol 1983;51:770–776.
87. Pritchett ELC, Wilkinson WE: Mortality in patients treated with flecainide and encainide for supraventricular arrhythmias. Am J Cardiol 1991;67:976–980.
88. Echt DS, Liebson PR, Mitchenn LB, *et al.*: Mortality and morbidity in patients receiving encainide, flecainide, or placebo. N Engl J Medicine 1991;324:781–788
89. Salerno DM, Granrud G, Sharkey P: Pharmacodynamics and side effects of flecainide acetate. Clin Pharmacol Ther 1986;40:101–107.
90. Winkelman BR, Leinberger H: Life-threatening flecainide toxicity. Ann Intern Med 1987;106:807–814.
91. Ranger S, Talajic M, Lemery R, *et al.*: Amplication of flecainide-induced ventricular conduction slowing with exercise. A potentially significant clinical consequence of use-dependent sodium channel blockade. Circulation 1990;79:1000–1006.
92. Chouty F, Funck-Brentano C, Landau JM, *et al.*: Efficacite de fortes doses

de lactate molaire par voie veineuse lors des intoxications au flecainide. Presse Med 1987;16:808–815.

93. Hellestrand KJ, Burnett PJ, Milne JR, *et al.*: The effect of the antiarrhythmic agent flecainide on acute and chronic pacing thresholds. PACE 1983;6:892.

94. Tjandra Maga TB, van Hecken A, van Melle P, *et al.*: Altered pharmacokinetics of oral flecainide by cimetidine. Br J Clin Pharmacol 1986;22:108.

95. Lewis GP, Holtzman JL: Interaction of flecainide with digoxin and propranolol. Am J Cardiol 1984;52B–55B.

96. Barbey JT, Thompson KA, Echt DS, *et al.*: Antiarrhythmic activity, electrocardiographic effects and pharmacokinetics of the encainide metabolites O-desmethyl encainide and 3-methoxy-O-desmethyl encainide in man. Circulation 1988;77:380–391.

97. Carey EL, Duff HJ, Roden DM *et al.*: Encainide and its metabolites. Comparative effects in man on ventricular arrhythmia and electrocardiographic intervals. J Clin Invest 1984;73:539–549.

98. Wang T, Roden DM, Wolfenden HT, *et al.*: Influence of genetic polymorphism on the metabolites and disposition of encainide in man. J Pharmacol Exp Ther 1984;228:605–611.

99. McLeod AA, Stiles GL, Shand DG: Demonstration of beta andrenoceptor blockade by propafenone hydrochloride: Clinical pharmacologic, radioligand binding and adenylate cyclase activation studies. J Pharmacol Exp Ther 1984;228:461–466.

100. Ledda F, Mantelli L, Manzini S, *et al.*: Electrophysiological and antiarrhythmic properties of propafenone in isolated cardiac preparations. J Cardiovasc Pharmacol 1981;3:1162–1173.

101. Myerburg RJ, Kessler KM, Cox MM, *et al.*: Reversal of proarrhythmic effects of flecainide acetate and encainide hydrochloride by propanolol. Circulation 1989;80:1571–1579.

102. Shen EN, Sung RJ, Morady F, *et al.*: Electrophysiologic and hemodynamic effects of intravenous propafenone in patients with recurrent ventricular tachycardia. J Am Coll Cardiol 1984;3:1291–1297.

103. von Phillipsborn G, Gries J, Hofmann HP, *et al.*: Pharmacological studies of propafenone and its main metabolite 5-hydroxypropafenone. Arzneimittelforsch 1984;34:1489–1497.

104. Siddoway LA, Thompson KA, McAllister CB, *et al.*: Polymorphism of propafenone metabolism and disposition in man: Clinical and pharmacokinetic consequences. Circulation 1987;75:785–791.

105. Kroemer HK, Turgeon J, Parker RA, *et al.*: Flecainide enantiomers: Disposition in human subjects and electrophysiologic actions in vitro. Clin Pharmacol Ther 1989;46:584–590.

106. Brodsky MA, Allen BJ, Abate D, *et al.*: Propafenone therapy for ventricular tachycardia in the setting of congestive heart failure. Am Heart J 1985;110:794–799.

107. Bianconi L, Boccadamo R, Pappalardo A, *et al.*: Effectiveness of intravenous propafenone for conversion of atrial fibrillation and flutter of recent onset. Am J Cardiol 1989;61:335–38.

108. Kerr CR, Klein GJ, Axelson JE, *et al.*: Propafenone for prevention of recurrent atrial fibrillation. Am J Cardiol 1988;61:914–16.

109. Breithardt G, Borgreffe M, Wiebringhaus E, *et al.*: Effect of propafenone in the Wolff-Parkinson-White syndrome: Electrophysiologic findings and long-term follow-up. Am J Cardiol 1984;54:29D–39D.

110. Beltz GG, Matthews J, Doering W, *et al.*: Digoxin antiarrhythmics: Pharmacodynamics and pharmacokinetic studies with quinidine, propafenone, and verapamil. Clin Pharmacol Ther 1982;31:202–203.

111. Kates RE, Yee YG, Kirsten EB: Interaction between warfarin and propafenone in healthy volunteer subjects. Clin Pharmacol Ther 1987;42:305–11.

112. Kowley PR, Kirsten EB, Fu C-HJ, *et al.*: Interaction between propanolol and propafenone in healthy volunteers. J Clin Pharmacol 1989;29:512–517.

113. Pritchett F, Smith WM, Kirsten E: Pharmacokinetics and pharmacodynamic interaction between cimetidine and propafenone. J Clin Pharmacol 1988;28:619–624.

114. Bigger JT Jr: Cardiac electrophysiologic effects of moricizine hydrochloride. Am J Cardiol 1990;65:15D–20D.

115. Cardiac Arrhythmia Pilot Study (CAPS) Investigators: Effect of encainide, flecainide, imprismine and moricizine on ventricular arrhythmias during the year after acute myocardial infarction: The CAPS, Am J Cardiol 1988;61:501–506.

116. Beta-Blocker Heart Attack Trial Research Group: A randomized trial of propranolol in patients with acute myocardial infarction: I. Mortality results. JAMA 1982;247:1707–1714.

117. The Norwegian Multicenter Study Group: Timolol-induced reduction in mortality and reinfarction in patients surviving acute myocardial infarction. N Engl J Med 1981;304:801–807.

118. Yabek S, Kato R, Singh BN: Acute electrophysiologic effects of amiodarone and desethylamiodarone in isolated cardiac muscle. J Cardiovasc Pharmacol 1986;8:197–207.

119. Mason JW, Hodeghem LM, Katzung BG: Block of inactivated sodium channels and of depolarization-induced automaticity in guinea-pig papillary muscle by amiodarone. Circ Res 1984;55:277–285.

120. Charlier R, Delaunois G, Bauthier J: Opposite effects of amiodarone and beta-blocking agents on cardiac functions under adrenergic stimulation. Arzneimittelforschung 1972;22:545–552.

121. Talajic M, DeRoode MR, Nattel S: Comparative electrophysiologic effects of intravenous amiodarone and desethylamiodarone in dogs: Evident for clinically relevant activity of the metabolite. Circulation 1987;75:265–268.

122. Nademanee K, Hendrickson J, Kannan R, *et al.*: Antiarrhythmic efficacy and electrophysiologic actions of amiodarone in patients with life-threatening arrhythmias. Am Heart J 1982;103:950–959.

123. Holt DW, Tucker GT, Jackson PR, *et al.*: Amiodarone pharmacokinetics. Br J Clin Pract (Symp Suppl) 1986;44:109–112.

124. Plomp TA, van Rossum JM, Robles de Medina EO, *et al.*: Pharmacokinetics and body distribution of amiodarone in man. Arzneimittelforschung, 1984;34:513–520.

125. Adams PC, Holt DW, Storey GC, *et al.*: Amiodarone and its desethyl metabolite: Tissue distribution and morphologic changes during long-term therapy. Circulation 1985;72:1064–1075.

126. Wellens HF, Brugada P, Abdollah H, *et al.*: A comparison of the electrophysiological effects of intravenous and oral amiodarone in the same patient. Circulation 1984;69:120–124.

127. The Cascade Study: Cardiac arrest in Seattle: conventional versus amiodarone drug evaluation. Am J Cardiol 1991;67:578–584.

128. Heger J, Prystowsky E, Jackman W, *et al.*: Amiodarone: Clinical efficacy and electrophysiology during long-term therapy for recurrent ventricular tachycardia or ventricular fibrillation. N Engl J Med 1981;305:539–545.

129. Hamera, Finerman W, Peter T, *et al.*: Disparity between the clinical and electrophysiologic effects of amiodarone in the treatment of recurrent ventricular arrhythmias. Am Heart J 1981;102:992–1000.

130. Veltri E, Reid P, Platia E, *et al.*: Results of late programmed electrical stimulation and long-term electrophysiologic effects of amiodarone therapy in patients with refractory ventricular tachycardia. Am J Cardiol 1985;55:375–379.

131. Horowitz LN, Greenspan AM, Spielman SR, *et al.*: Usefulness of electrophysiologic testing in evaluation of amiodarone therapy for sustained ventricular tachyarrhythmias associated with coronary heart disease. Am J Cardiol 1985;55:367–371.

132. Naccarelli GV, Fineberg NS, Zipes DP, *et al.*: Amiodarone: risk factors for recurrence of symptomatic ventricular tachycardia identified at electrophysiologic study. J Am Coll Cardiol 1985;6:814–821.

133. Greene HL, Graham EL, Werner JA, *et al.*: Toxic and therapeutic effects of amiodarone in the treatment of cardiac arrhythmias. J Am Coll Cardiol 1983;2:1114–1128.

134. Sobel SM, Rakita L: Pneumonitis and pulmonary fibrosis associated with amiodarone treatment: A possible complication of a new antiarrhythmic drug. Circulation 1982;65:819–824.

135. Almog S, Shafran N, Halkin H, *et al.*: Mechanism of warfarin potentiation by amiodarone: Dose- and concentration-dependent inhibition of warfarin elimination. Eur J Clin Pharmacol 1985;28:257–261.
136. Marcus FI: Drug interactions with amiodarone. Am Heart J 1983;106:924–930.
137. Bigger JT Jr, Jaffee CC: The effect of bretylium tosylate on the electrophsyiologic properties of ventricular muscle and Purkinje fibers. Am J Cardiol 1971;27:82–92.
138. Cardinal R, Sasyniuk BI: Electrophysiological effects of bretylium tosylate on subendocardial Purkinje fibers from infarcted canine hearts. J Pharmacol Exp Ther 1978;204:159–174.
139. Harrison DC, Meffin PJ, Winkle RA: Clinical pharmacokinetics of antiarrhythmic drugs. Prog Cardio Dis 1977;20:217–242.
140. Somani P, Watson DL: Antiarrhythmic activity of the dextro- and levorotatory isomers of 4-(2-isopropylamino-l-hydroxyethyl) methanesulfonanilide (MJI9999). J Pharmacol Exp Ther 1968;164:317–325.
141. Edvardsson N, Olsson B: Effects of acute and chronic beta-receptor blockade on ventricular repolarization in man. Br Heart J 1981;45:628–636.
142. Hiromasa S, Coto H, Li ZY, *et al.*: Dextrorotatory isomer of sotalol: Electrophysiologic effects and interaction with verapamil. Am Heart J 1988;116:1552–1557.
143. Nademanee K, Feld G, Hendrickson JA, *et al.*: Electrophysiologic and antiarrhythmic effects of sotalol in patients with life-threatening ventricular tachyarrhythmias. Circulation 1985;72:555–564.
144. Creamer JE, Nathan AW, Shennan A, *et al.*: Acute and chronic effects of sotalol and propranolol on ventricular repolarization using constant rate-packing. Am J Cardiol 1986;57:1092–1096.
145. Mahmarian JJ, Verani MS, Pratt CM: Hemodynamic effects of intravenous and oral sotalol. Am J Cardiol 1990;65:28A–34A.
146. Antonaccio MJ, Gomoll A: Pharmacology, pharmacodynamics and pharmacokinetics of sotalol. Am J Cardiol 1990;65:12A–21A.
147. Nademanee K, Singh BN: Effects of sotalol on ventricular tachycardia and fibrillation produced by programmed electrical stimulation: comparison with other antiarrhythmic agents. Am J Cardiol 1990;65:53A–57A.
148. Borggrefe M, Breithart G: Electrophysiologic effect of sotalol in supraventricular tachycardias. Z Kardiol 1985;74:506–511.
149. Soyka LF, Wirtz C, Spangenberg RB: Clinical safety profile of sotalol in patients with arrhythmias. Am J Cardiol 1190;65:74A–81A.
150. McKibbin JK, Pocock WA, Barlow JB, *et al.*: Sotalol, hypokalemia, syncope and Torsade de Pointes. Br Heart J 1984;51:157–162.
151. Eichelbaum B, Birkel P, Grube E, *et al.*: Effects of verapamil on P-R intervals in relation to verapamil plasma levels following single i.v. and oral administration and during chronic treatment. Klin Wochenschr 1980;58:919–925.
152. Echizen H, Vogelgesang B, Eichelbaum M: Effects of d,I-verapamil on atrioventricular conduction in relation to its steroselective first-pass metabolism. Clin Pharmacol Ther 1985;38:71–76.
153. Rinkenberger RL, Prystowsky EN, Heger JJ, *et al.*: Effects of intravenous and chronic oral verapamil administration in patients with supraventricular tachyarrhythmias. Circulation 1980;62:996–1010.
154. Matsuyama E, Konishi T, Okazaki H, *et al.*: Effects of verapamil on accessory pathway properties and induction of circus movement tachycardia in patients with the Wolff-Parkinson-White syndrome. J Cardiovasc Pharmacol 1981;3:11–24.
155. Palileo EV, Ashley WW, Swiryn S, *et al.*: Exercise-provacable right ventricular outflow tract tachycardia. Am Heart J 1982;104:185–193.
156. Gulamhusein S, Ko P, Carruthers SG, *et al.*: Acceleration of the ventricular response during atrial fibrillation in the Wolff-Parkinson-White syndrome after verapamil. Circulation 1982;65:348–354.
157. Winters S, Schweitzer P, Kupersmith J, *et al.*: Verapamil-induced polymorphic ventricular tachycardia. J Am Coll Cardiol 1985;6:257–259.
158. Belardinelli L, Linden J, Berne RM: The cardiac effects of adenosine. Prog Cardiovasc Dis 1989;32:73–97.
159. Clemo HF, Belardinelli L: Effect on adenosine on atrioventricular conduction. I. Site and characterization of adenosine action in the guinea pig atrioventricular node. Circ Res 1986;59:427–436.
160. DiMarco JP, Sellers TD, Berne RM, *et al.*: Adenosine: Electrophysiologic effects and therapeutic use for terminating paroxysmal supraventricular tachycardia. Circulation 1983;68:1254–1263.
161. DiMarco JP, Sellers TD, Lerman BB, *et al.*: Diagnostic and therapeutic use of adenosine in patients with supraventricular tachyarrhythmias. J Am Coll Cardiol 1985;6:417–425.
162. Szentmiklosi AJ, Nemeth M, Szegi J, *et al.*: Effect of adenosine on sinoatrial and ventricular automaticity of the guinea pig. Naynyn Schmiedebergs Arch Pharmacol 1989;311:147–149.
163. Moser GH, Schrader J, Deussen A: Turnover of adenosine in plasma of human and dog blood. Am J Physiol 1989;256:C799–806.
164. Bauernfeind RA, Wyndham CRC, Dhingra RC, *et al.*: Serial electrophysiologic testing of multiple drugs in patients with atrioventricular nodal reentrant paroxysmal tachycardia. Circulation 1980;62:1341–1349.
165. Lerman BB, Belardinelli L, West GA, *et al.*: Adenosine sensitive ventricular tachycardia: evident suggesting cyclic AMP-mediated triggered activity. Circulation 1986;74:270–80.
166. Meszaros J, Kelemen K, Kecskemeti V, *et al.*: Interaction between adenosine and antiarrhythmic agents in atrial mycardium of guinea pig. Arch Int Pharmacodyn Ther 1986;280:84–96.
167. Klabunde RE: Dipyridamole inhibition of adenosine metabolism in human blood. Eur J Pharmacol 1983;93:21–26.
168. Pace DG, Gillis RA: Neuroexcitatory effects of digoxin in the cat. J Pharmacol Exp Ther 1976;199:583–600.
169. Ten Eick RE, Hoffman BF: Chronotropic effect of cardiac glycosides in cats, dogs and rabbits. Circ Res 1969;25:365–378.
170. Hamlin NP, Willerson JT, Garan H, *et al.*: The neurogenic vasoconstrictor effect of digitalis on coronary vascular resistance. J Clin Invest 1974;54:288–296.
171. Mikkelsen E: Effects of digoxin on isolated human pulmonary vessels. Acta Pharmacol Toxicol 1979;45:25–31.
172. Dhingra RC, Amet-Y-Leon F, Wyndham C, *et al.*: The electrophysiological effects of ouabain on sinus node and atrium in man. J Clin Invest 1975;56:555–562.
173. Gomes JAD, Dhatt MS, Akhtar M, *et al.*: Effects of digitalis on ventricular myocardial and His-Purkinje refractoriness and reentry in man. Am J Cardiol 1978;42:931–938.
174. Hayward RP, Hamer J, Taggart P, *et al.*: Observations on the biphasic nature of digitalis electrophysiological actions in the human right atrium. Cardiovasc Res 1983;17:533–541.
175. Reuning RH, Sams RA, Notari RE: Role of pharmacokinetics in drug dosage adjustment. I. Pharmacological effect, kinetics and apparent volume of distribution of digoxin. J Clin Pharmacol 1973;13:127–141.
176. Huffman DH, Manion CV, Azarnoff DL: Inter-subject variation in absorption of digoxin in normal volunteers. J Pharm Sci 1975;64:433–437.
177. Lukas DS: Some aspects of distribution and disposition of digitoxin in man. Ann NY Acad Sci 1971;1979:338–361.
178. Marcus FI, Peterson A, Salel A, *et al.*: The metabolism of tritiated digoxin in renal insufficiency in dogs and man. J Pharmacol Exp Ther 1966;152:372–382.
179. Marcus FI, Kapadia GG: The metabolism of tritiated digoxin in carrhotic patients. Gastroenterology 164;47:517–526.
180. Gault MH, Churchill DN, Kalra J: Loading dose of digoxin in renal failure. Br J Clin Pharmacol 1980;9:593–597.
181. Redfors A: Digoxin dosage and ventricular rate at rest and exercise in patients with atrial fibrillation. Acta Med Scan 1971;190:321.
182. Aberg H, Srom G, Werner I: The effect of digitalis on the heart rate during exercise in patients with atrial fibrillation. Acta Med Scand 1972;191:441–445.
183. Falk RH, Knowlton AA, Bernard SA, *et al.*: Digoxin for converting recent-onset atrial fibrillation to sinus rhythm. Ann Intern Med 1987;106:503–506.

184. Steinbeck G, Doliwa R, Bach P: Cardiac glycosides for paroxysmal atrial fibrillation? Circulation 1985;74:100–102.
185. Wu D, Amat-Y-Leon F, Simpson RJ, *et al.*: Electrophysiological studies with multiple drugs in patients with atrioventricular re-entrant tachycardia utilizing an extranodal pathway. Circulation 1977;56:727–736.
186. Dreiful LS, Hiat R, Watanabe Y, *et al.*: Ventricular fibrillation: A possible mechanism of sudden death in patients with Wolff-Parkinson-White syndrome. Circulation 1971;43:520–527.
187. Smith TW, Antman EM, Friedman PL, *et al.*: Digitalis glycosides: Mechanisms and manifestations of toxicity. Prog Cardiovasc Dis 1984;26:413–458, 495.
188. Rosen MR: Cellular electrophysiology of digitalis toxicity. J Am Coll Cardiol 1985;5:22A–34A.
189. Smith TW, Willerson JT: Suicidal and accidental digoxin ingestion: report of 5 cases with serum digoxin level correlations. Circulation 1971;44: 29.
190. Smith TW, Butler VP Jr, Haber E, *et al.*: Treatment of life threatening digitalis intoxication with digoxin-specific Fab antibody fragments. N Engl J Med 1982;307–1357.
191. Hoy WE, Gibson TP, Rivero AJ, *et al.*: XAD-4 resin hemoperfusion for digitoxic patients with renal failure. Kidney Int 1983;23:79–82.
192. Baciewitz AM, Isaacson ML, Lipscomb GL: Cholestryramine resin in the treatment of digitoxin toxicity. Drug Intell Clin Pharm 1983;17:57–59.
193. Pond S, Jacobs M, Marks J, *et al.*: Treatment of digitoxin overdose with oral activated charcoal. Lancet 1981;2:1177–1178.
194. Gilfrich HJ, Okonek S, Manns M, *et al.*: Digoxin and digitoxin elimination in man by charcoal hemoperfusion. Klin Wochenschr 1978;56: 1179–1183.
195. Brown DD, Juhl RP: Decreased bioavailability of digoxin due to antacids and kaolin-pectin. N Engl J Med 1976;295–1034.
196. Fenster PE, White NW Jr, Hanson CD: Pharmacokinetic evaluation of the digoxin-amiodarone interaction. J Am Coll Cardiol 1985;5:108–112.
197. Lee TH, Smith TW: Serum digoxin concentration and diagnosis of digitalis toxicity: Current concepts. Clin Pharmacokinet 1983;8:279–285.

III

PACING FOR BRADYARRHYTHMIAS

13

CURRENT AND FUTURE LEAD TECHNOLOGY

Frank Callaghan M.S., M.S.E.E., and Mark Christensen B.A.

INTRODUCTION

Permanent pacing leads evolved from a large, unreliable weak link in the pacing system to a focal point of materials design innovation. Often ignored and misunderstood, they remain the most significant component of the pacing system, accounting for a large percentage of the complications associated with pacer systems (1). Knowledge of pacing leads and experience in implanting techniques are imperative for successful results.

It is helpful to begin by understanding the basic terminology being used. Figure 13.1 is a diagram of a typical endocardial pacing lead and describes its essential components.

Currently, a variety of pacing lead types exist which are described by Table 13.1. The components of the chart are organized in a manner similar to the lead diagram in Figure 13.1. Starting at the left of the chart and proceeding to the right via any path, one can describe the lead of choice. In most cases, such a lead may already be commercially available.

Based on this chart, there are 288 possible combinations. At least that many different lead models are available. The following sections will briefly discuss advantages and disadvantages of the possible choices in each area. Implantation techniques will be discussed briefly since it is crucial to achieving good chronic lead performance. Finally, future lead designs will be discussed, particularly those likely to become available in the near future.

ENDOCARDIAL VERSUS EPICARDIAL

The very first permanently implantable pacing lead used in conjunction with an implanted cardiac pacemaker was an epicardial lead, which fractured three days postimplantation. This was the first of many problems encountered in the development of pacing leads.

Limitations of epicardial pacing leads are well known, while their advantages are almost solely limited to the lack of alternative surgical options. High pacing thresholds, chronic exit block, lead fracture, damage to the lead body or connector and poor sensing are some of the complications associated with this approach. As a result, epicardial leads are rarely used today, accounting for less than 4% of all implants. In the adult pacemaker recipient, the epicardial approach is used only in the presence of a prosthetic tricuspid valve or if endocardial access is unattainable.

In the pediatric population, the situation is somewhat different. Pediatric implants for premature and newborn infants are almost exclusively performed using the epicardial approach. The small size of the veins and rapid growth has discouraged many physicians from using endocardial leads. On the other hand, the increasing success in placing endocardial leads in pediatric patients is likely to make the endocardial approach the technique of choice.

Endocardial leads are preferred whenever possible and offer a number of advantages. These are: relatively small lead size, ease of implantation, superior long-term performance, and mechanical reliability. The first endocardial leads to be implanted were large and stiff with large surface area electrodes that remained securely positioned by the most basic of fixation mechanisms—gravity. Placement was analogous to dropping a pencil into a cup. Acute dislodgement was as easy as turning the cup upside down.

Endocardial lead development has concentrated on reducing the lead body and electrode size, increasing the lead flexibility and reducing its mass. Optimization of these attributes is likely to further diminish the trauma to the heart, the venous access and soft tissues.

UNIPOLAR OR BIPOLAR

The term "unipolar" or "bipolar" refers to the number of electrodes on the pacing lead. All electrical systems must form a complete circuit in order to function and are therefore, by definition, bipolar. All unipolar pacing systems use the pacing electrode as the cathode (−) and the metal pacemaker "can" as the anode (+). A bipolar pacing system has a second electrode at the distal end of the lead which acts as the anode. The generic lead in Figure 13.1 is a bipolar pacing lead.

The lead must provide the conduit for cardiac stimulation and

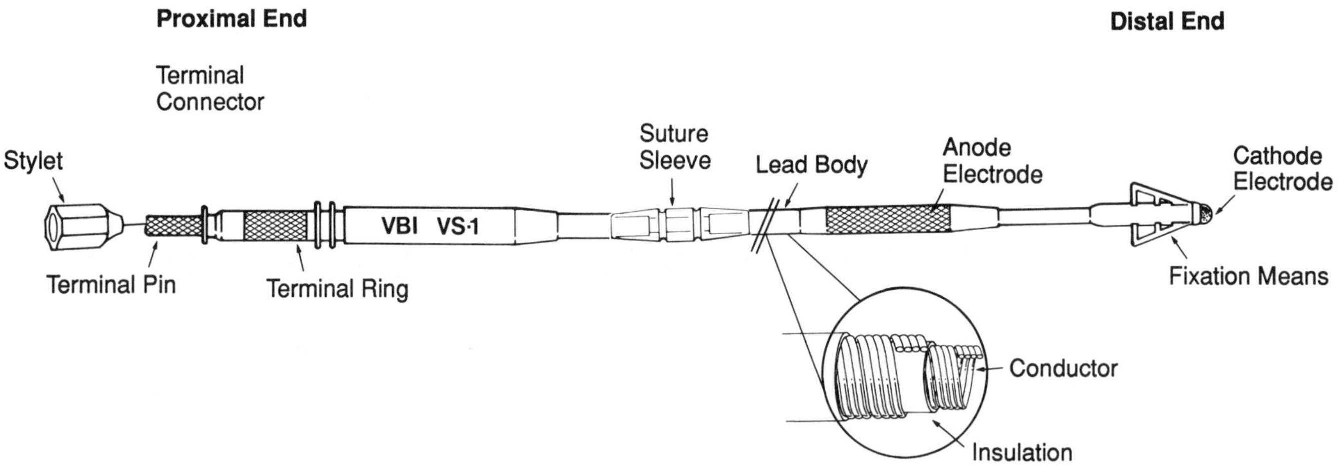

Figure 13.1. Current endocardial pacing leads can be either unipolar or bipolar (bipolar shown), have a small 3.2 mm in-line terminal connector (VS-1/IS-1), coaxial multifilar conductor(s) and porous or microporous, small surface area electrodes.

Table 13.1.
Pacing Lead Design Variables

Position	Polarity	Connector	Insulation	Fixation	Electrode
		VS-1/IS-1 (3.2 mm)		Tined	Polished platinum
Endocardial	Unipolar		Silicone		
		5 mm		Finned	Porous platinum
Epicardial	Bipolar		Polyurethane		
		6 mm		Screw-in	Carbon Drug eluting

for sensing of the intrinsic cardiac activity. Unipolar lead and pacing systems offer the advantage of small size, simplicity, and large signal artifact on the surface electrocardiograms (ECG's), which may be helpful for interpretation of paced rhythms. The large sensing field created by the distance between the tip of the electrode and the pacemaker can however, increase the chance for these systems to inappropriately sense extra-cardiac signals, including muscle activity and electromagnetic interference (EMI) emitted by such devices as automobile alternators, high-voltage power stations, welding equipment, and microwave ovens.

Although sensing using a bipolar lead offers little practical difference in cardiac signal strength compared to a unipolar lead, it is less susceptible to far-field signal detection. Since bipolar leads require that the lead have two electrodes within the heart, and therefore two conductors within the lead body, they have traditionally been somewhat larger and possibly stiffer than unipolar leads (2).

Superiority of bipolar sensing, particularly for dual-chamber pacing systems is now well recognized (3). The number of unipolar leads now being implanted is diminishing. The use of bipolar leads has been further enhanced by the introduction of a large number of programmable unipolar/bipolar pacemaker models (which are only fully utilized if attached to a bipolar lead) and a recent introduction of bipolar leads using a single multifilar coated conductor coil (see Fig. 13.3C.) which make the lead identical in size and flexibility to unipolar leads.

TERMINAL CONNECTORS

The lead terminal connector creates an insulated electrical connection between the pacing lead and the implanted pulse generator. The electrical connection is made through the metal terminals. The terminal pin is electrically continuous with the distal tip electrode of the lead as the cathodal (−) limb of the circuit. If the lead is bipolar there is a second metal terminal ring located distal to the pin which is electrically continuous with the ring electrode for the anodal (+) limb. Silicone rubber is used to electrically isolate these terminals from each other and to create an electrically insulated seal between the lead and the generator.

Lead terminals have undergone progressive downsizing concurrently with implanted devices. The most commonly encountered lead terminal designs are illustrated in Fig. 13.2. The lead connectors labeled VS-1 and IS-1 are the result of physicians' and industry's efforts, in coordination with the International Standards Organization (ISO), to establish a standard for pacemaker and lead connections. They are physically identical and represent the progression of this standardization effort. The standard was at first voluntary (VS-1) and, after it was ratified by the ISO, became an official international standard (IS-1). All

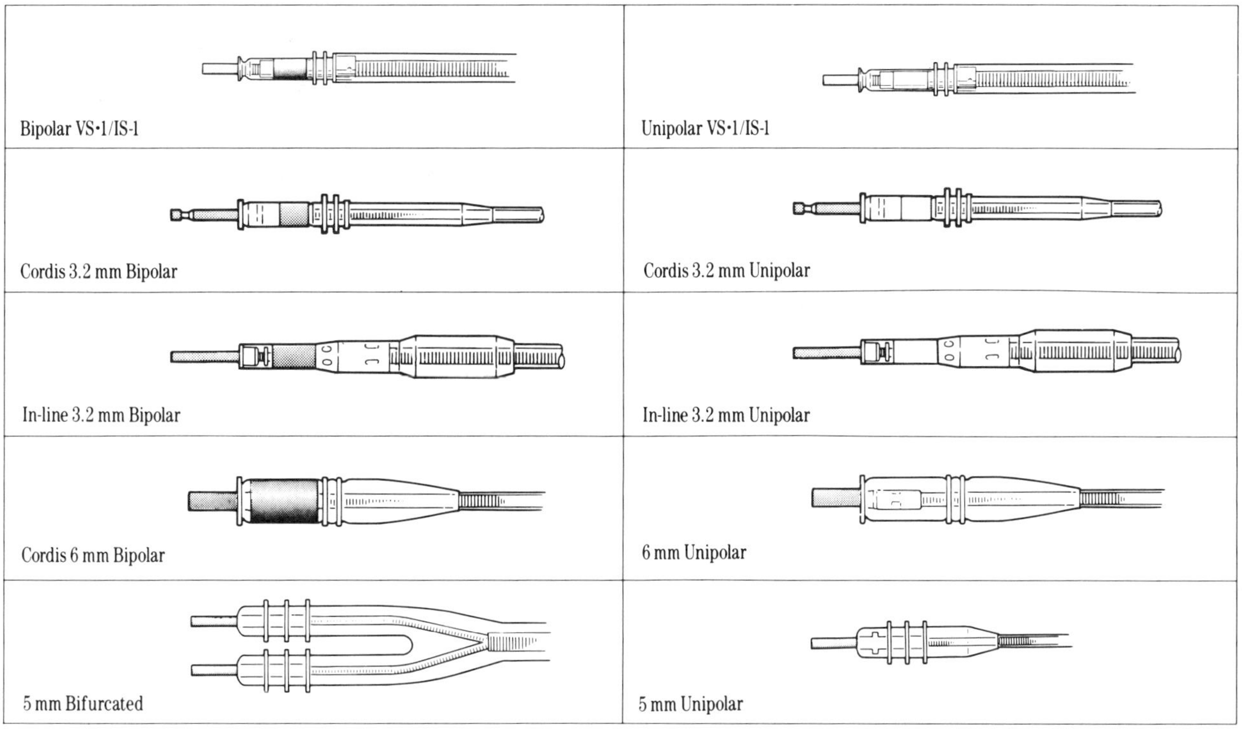

Figure 13.2. Bipolar lead terminals are on the **left,** unipolar on the **right.** The VS-1/IS-1 terminals shown at the top represent the current standard for pacing lead terminals. Older 3.2-, 5-, and 6-mm unipolar and bipolar terminals are frequently encountered during pacemaker replacement.

leads currently implanted should have the designation VS-1 or IS-1.

LEAD BODIES

Lead bodies are made up of the electrical conductor(s) and insulating tubing which electrically isolates each conductor from other conductors and from body fluids. The conductors are multifilar coils of a nickel-cobalt alloy (MP35N). The coil design is used for its flexibility and fatigue resistance. The nickel-cobalt alloy is used for its bioelectric stability, even if totally exposed to body fluids (4). The coil creates an inner lumen (Fig. 13.3A) through which a stiffening stylet wire can be passed to aid in lead placement.

The insulating tubing material has been either silicone or polyurethane. Both materials have proven to have desirable qualities which are not available in the other. Silicone is generally softer, more flexible, and easier to manufacture. Polyurethane is four to six times stronger than silicone and can therefore be made smaller. Two polyurethane leads will slide past each other in the vein with less frictional resistance and polyurethane is more resistant to scalpel injury.

The use of either material beyond its physical capabilities has caused more than one product failure and continues to be an issue which affects long term lead reliability. Additionally, both materials are easily damaged by surgical trauma. Several precautions have become standard for all lead designs and include: (a) use of the anchoring sleeve is absolutely required when suturing the lead to the tissue, (b) care to avoid kinking or pinching of the lead during the implant or in its permanent implant position, (c) if a subclavian introducer is used, avoidance of an insertion site immediately adjacent to the junction of the clavicle and first rib since this location allows the lead to be pulled into the acute angle created by this junction, resulting in chronic pinching of the lead body, and (d) coiling of the lead behind the pacemaker in the pacemaker pocket to help prevent damage to the lead during subsequent pacemaker replacement or revision.

For bipolar leads, addition of a second coil and insulating tube over a unipolar lead body is shown in Figure 13.3B. This coaxial design makes bipolar leads slightly larger and stiffer than their unipolar counterparts. Several manufacturers are now introducing the use of a single multifilar coil conductor of a standard unipolar lead, insulating each individual wire within the coil and creating multiple electrical pathways in a single coil as shown in Figure 13.3C. This process allows bipolar leads to be designed with the same dimensional attributes of the unipolar leads.

FIXATION DEVICES

As leads become more flexible, the incidence of dislodgement increases (5). The three most common fixation designs are

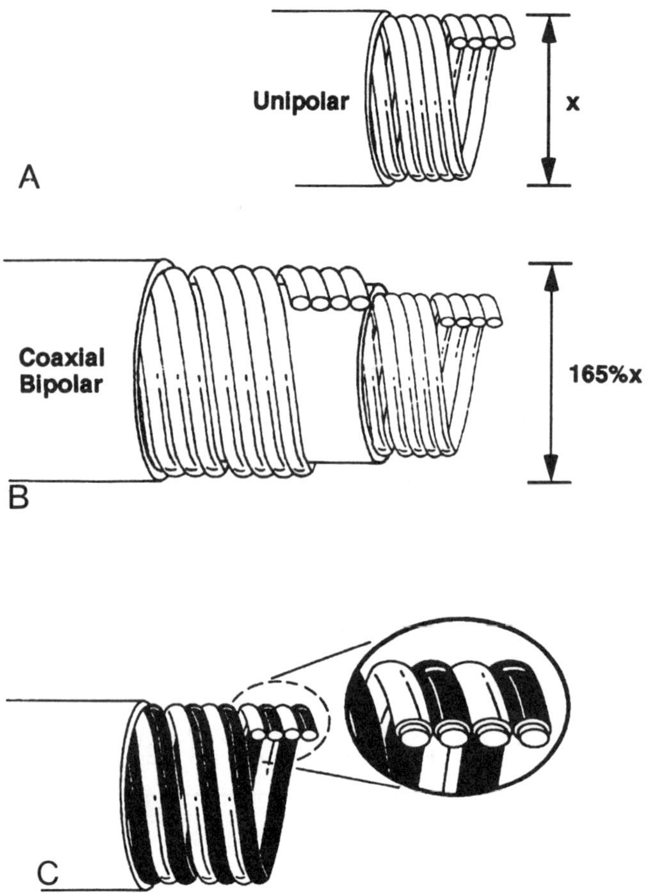

Figure 13.3. Multifilar unipolar (A) and bipolar coaxial (B) lead designs. Lumen created by the coiled wire design allows passage of a stylet which is used to stiffen the lead during implantation. Single, multifilar conductor coils with each individual strand of wire insulated (C) allows for multiple conductive pathways in a single coil. In the illustration, four separate conductive pathways are possible.

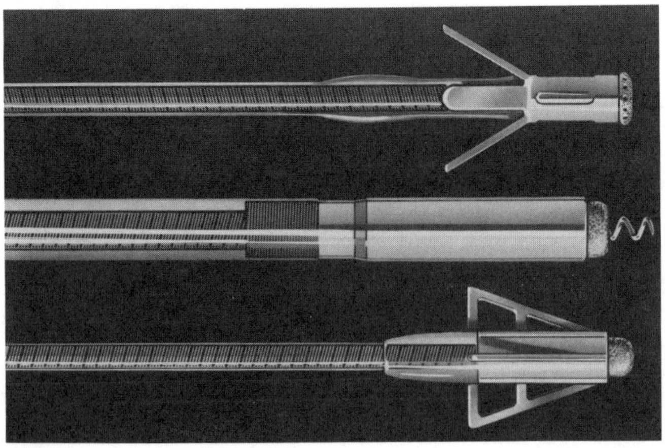

Figure 13.4. Available fixation mechanisms. **Top:** passive fixation flexible tines protruding at an acute angle away from the electrode. **Middle:** active fixation screw-in design. **Bottom:** passive fixation flexible fin design.

illustrated in Figure 13.4. The first of these, proposed by Citron in the mid-1970's, was the use of flexible tines placed immediately adjacent to the distal pacing electrode that would passively entrap themselves within the trabeculae (6). Though greatly modified since its original introduction, this passive fixation tine design is still the most widely implanted. A later variation of the tine, flexible fins, was developed by Cordis Corp. (Miami, FL) and provided an added advantage of lesser susceptibility to being ensnared on the tricuspid valve during the implant. Chronically, however, the fibrotic encapsulation of both types of flexible protrusions, make passive fixation leads virtually impossible to remove (Figure 13.4).

Higher dislodgement rates of passive fixation atrial leads, smooth-walled ventricles, anatomic abnormalities, and chronic removability have prompted many implanters to consider the use of active fixation leads (1). Active fixation leads use a corkscrew-shaped helix to actively affix the lead to the endocardial surface. This helix can be of either a fixed design, requiring a counter-clockwise rotation of the lead as it is being introduced through the vein and then a clockwise rotation to affix it to the heart, or it may be of an extendable/retractable design, allowing the lead to be introduced and anchored more simply and safely. The development of antitachycardia pacemakers and implantable defibrillators requiring bipolar sensing and brady and antitachycardia pacing has further increased the use of active fixation leads.

The advantages of active fixation leads include the following: (a) placement of the lead in various parts of the right atrium and ventricle, (b) greater lead stability, and (c) easier removal chronically.

ELECTRODES

Although electrodes are available in virtually every imaginable size and shape, there are few significant differences in their therapeutic performance. For biocompatibility and electrical performance, electrodes are made of platinum, platinum/iridium alloy, or carbon materials. To reduce the pacemaker battery current drain, electrodes have been downsized from greater than 20 mm^2 to between 6 and 8/mm^2. Surface area reduction increases the current density at the electrode tissue interface and increases the pacing lead impedance. Higher current density, will lower the pacing threshold. Higher impedance will lower the current drain on the battery of the pacemaker with each paced pulse. Recent testing of electrodes with surface areas less than 5 mm^2 indicates that this size reduction may continue (7,8).

The concept of electrode porosity was introduced to increase the microsurface area of the electrode for improved sensing and to reduce the traumatization of endocardium at the electrode/tissue interface (9,10). The addition of porous treatment, particularly microporous coatings, has the added benefit of reducing the electrical polarization after a pacing pulse.

Electrode performance, as measured by low pacing thresholds and chronic stability, has been shown to improve with the timed release of a small amount of steroid adjacent to the electrode (11,12). The addition of steroid eluting leads to the implanters armamentarium of available lead options may further enhance pacing threshold stability over time, allowing for lower programmed pacemaker outputs, minimizing current drain and extending the battery life.

THE LEAD IMPLANT

Perhaps the most critical aspect of implantation of a "pacing system" is the implantation of the pacing lead. Retrospective studies have shown that the procedure can be performed with equal safety in either the operating room or the electrophysiology or cardiac catheterization laboratory (13,14) with minimal complications. The implant procedure typically consists of the following steps: (a) obtaining venous access, (b) positioning the lead(s) into the desired cardiac chamber(s), (c) mapping the sites of the most optimal sensing and pacing, (d) anchoring of the lead(s), (e) pacer pocket preparation, and (f) connection to the pacemaker.

A comprehensive description of the surgical aspects of pacemaker implantation may be found elsewhere (15,16). The primary objective here is to focus on information that may be helpful in optimizing chronic lead performance.

Venous Access

Venous access is generally obtained either via a cephalic cutdown or through a direct subclavian puncture. The external jugular may also be used, but this approach requires tunneling of the lead subcutaneously over the clavicle to the pulse generator implant site. Use of the cephalic reduces the potential that the lead will be placed too medially, at the junction of the clavicle and first rib where it may be compressed. The subclavian introducer technique is simpler, requires less time, and allows insertion of more than one lead through a single-needle puncture (e.g., retained guidewire technique). Also, the subclavian vein more easily accommodates two leads required for dual chamber pacemaker implants.

If the cephalic vein is chosen, access to the vein often can be obtained with a small lateral extension of the pacemaker pocket. If a subclavian approach is used, a similarly small extension can be made medially. In either case, venous access should be approached from deep within this incision. This allows the lead to enter the pacemaker pocket from behind the pacemaker where it is ultimately positioned.

With the cephalic vein cut down, the vein is isolated and temporarily tied off both distally and a loose ligature is placed proximally to the incision site. The incision into the cephalic vein is then made and the lead is passed proximally into the vein. The proximal suture is released to allow the passage of the distal tip of the lead and tightened around the generally smaller diameter lead body to maintain hemostasis.

With the subclavian approach, a single 18-gauge needle puncture allows access to the venous circulation. A flexible guide wire is passed through the needle and the needle is then removed. The guide wire may be viewed using fluoroscopy. The introducer set, which is composed of a dilator and a peel-away introducer sheath, is then placed over the guide wire and introduced into the vein. The dilator and the guide wire are then removed, leaving the peel-away sheath in the subclavian vein through which the lead can then be easily passed. The guide wire may be left in the sheath alongside the lead body when two leads are required. A second introducer may then be advanced over the guide wire, obviating the need for a second venous puncture, with its attendant risks. There are several variations to this approach which are described in the literature (17,18). An uncommon, but helpful secondary use for the guide wire is for temporary emergency unipolar pacing (e.g., asystole, which may occur in some patients during lead placement).

Passage of the lead through the vein and into the heart is aided by the insertion of a stylet through the central lumen of the lead to stiffen its flexible body. By fashioning a curve in the distal portion of the stylet, placement of the lead into the appropriate chamber may be facilitated. It is important to emphasize that during the removal and reinsertion of the stylet, meticulous care should be given not to introduce blood into the central lumen of the lead, since coagulated blood within the lumen may prevent further insertion or removal of the stylet. When two leads are required (atrial and ventricular), the ventricular lead is usually positioned first to allow emergency ventricular pacing during pacemaker implant, if required.

Positioning of the Lead(s)

Advancing the lead through the tricuspid valve and into the right ventricle can be difficult at times. Two methods commonly used are the "forward pass" and the "slack loop" techniques. The forward pass method is usually tried first and is simply an attempt at passing the distal tip straight into the ventricle. With a slightly curved stylet fully inserted into the lead, rotation of the stylet is used to direct the distal tip of the lead through the center of the tricuspid valve as the lead is being advanced. Withdrawing the stylet approximately 3 cm may allow the flexible distal tip of the lead to "flow" through the valve. A potential drawback of this approach is that, if a passive fixation tined lead is being used, it may become entrapped within the tricuspid valve.

In the "slack loop" method, the distal tip of the lead is intentionally positioned against the atrial wall. The stylet is withdrawn 10–15 cm creating a flexible loop in the distal portion of the lead. The loop is advanced through the valve by advancing more lead into the vein. With the looped portion of the lead in the right ventricle, the stylet is slowly advanced back into the lead toward the apex. As the stylet is being advanced, the lead body is simultaneously retracted. This dual motion of advancing the stylet while retracting the lead body causes the distal tip of the lead to pass backward through the valve and into the right ventricle. If resistance is met, caution should be exercised to assure that the stylet does not perforate the lead body.

Atrial leads are available in either passive or active fixation designs (preformed J shaped or as straight active fixation). The preformed J shaped aids positioning the lead in the right atrial appendage. If the lead is of an active fixation straight design, preformed J stylets are provided for the same purpose. A regular straight stylet is placed into the preformed J shaped leads to temporarily straighten the J portion of the lead, allowing for easy passage of the lead through vein and into the atrium. Once in the atrium, the stylet is slowly withdrawn while the lead is rotated, so as to direct the lead tip towards the atrial appendage. The stylet is only withdrawn to the point where it is completely outside the J portion of the lead. Advancing it back into the lead will cause the J to open, permitting lead repositioning. The distal tip is pulled up into the atrial appendage by slowly retracting the lead. Gentle twisting of the lead is helpful during this maneuver. The appropriate flexing of the preformed atrial J design is achieved only if the lead is positioned in the atrial appendage or, if the patient has an amputated appendage, in the high right atrium. If other locations within the atrium are desired, a straight, active fixation lead must be used. The preformed J design in other locations may impede the atrial contraction and/or cause atrial perforation (19).

With an active fixation lead, a straight stylet is used to advance the distal tip into the atrium. The straight stylet is then removed and a performed J stylet is inserted. Positioning can then be achieved as described above. With a straight, active fixation lead, alternative positions within the right atrium are possible. Once the final position is determined, the tip is actively affixed to the atrial wall and the stylet removed.

Mapping for Optimal Pacing and Sensing Thresholds

Whether in the atrium or in the ventricle, it is important to optimize pacing and sensing thresholds. Using a commercially available pacing systems analyzer (PSA), the electrode(s) are maneuvered to a location where QRS or P wave amplitudes and pacing thresholds are optimized. Impedance measurements and slew rates should also be obtained. Generally accepted values for each are listed in Table 13.2 (20). While these are acceptable values, ventricular pacing thresholds of 0.5 V or less and electrogram amplitudes of greater than 8 mV, and, in the atrium, pacing thresholds of 0.8 V or less and atrial electrogram amplitudes greater than 2.5 mV are often obtained. Achieving more optimal values has been associated with a reduced incidence of subsequent pacing or sensing complications. As a general guideline, atrial and ventricular electrogram amplitude should be at least twice the most sensitive programmable setting of the pacemaker generator to be implanted.

With bipolar pacing leads, electrogram amplitudes can be influenced by the position of the bipolar electrodes relative to the vector of the electrical depolarization (3). As illustrated in Figure 13.5, the strongest bipolar signal will be received when the bipolar electrodes are directly in line with the depolarization vector. The pacemaker measures the difference in electrical potential between its cathode (−) and anode (+). As the depolarization wave front passes the cathodal electrode first, the electrical potential of this electrode becomes more positive while the anodal electrode potential remains unchanged (baseline). The difference between these two potentials is "seen" as a positive deflection. As the depolarization wave front passes the anodal electrode, the electrical signal is reversed and is recorded as a negative deflection. If the bipolar electrodes are positioned exactly perpendicular to the depolarization wave, the electrical potential of both electrodes change at exactly the same time as the depolarization wave passes over them and the pacemaker sees no difference between the electrical potentials of the two electrodes. Repositioning of the lead to change the orientation of the electrodes is usually sufficient to correct this potential problem (Fig. 13.5).

Table 13.2.
Acute Threshold Values

Chamber	Signal Amplitude (mV)	Pacing Threshold at 0.5 msec Pulse Width (V)	Lead Impedance (ohms)
Atrium	>1.5	<1.0	>350 <1200
Ventricle	>4.0	<1.0	>400 <1400

Once the final position is determined, pacing thresholds should be measured at several different pulse widths. Graphically plotting this data generates a strength-duration curve (21,22) (Fig. 13.6).

The strength-duration curve plots the relationship between voltage (or current) and pulse width for any pacing lead. It should be noted that the relationship between the voltage and pulse width is asymptotic, therefore a point is reached at which increasing the pulse width does not reduce further the voltage required to stimulate the heart muscle. This is known as the *rheobase* and normally occurs between pulse widths of 1–2 msec. The pulse duration at which the voltage is twice the rheobase is known as the *chronaxie*. Programming the pulse widths to values greater than the rheobase provides little additional safety margin, while greatly increasing the battery current drain.

Anchoring the Lead

Adequate fixation of the distal tip should be checked by applying slight traction and by asking the patient to take a deep breath. The electrode should be stable during inspiration and expiration. Enough slack should be left in the ventricular lead to produce a gentle curve through the atrium and into the ventricle. For atrial leads, a preformed J lead should be positioned in such a way as to allow sufficient flexing but not permit the J shape to open to an angle greater than 60° or completely close against itself. With an active fixation lead, the slack left in the lead should not be too great, so that it would interfere with the tricuspid valve function.

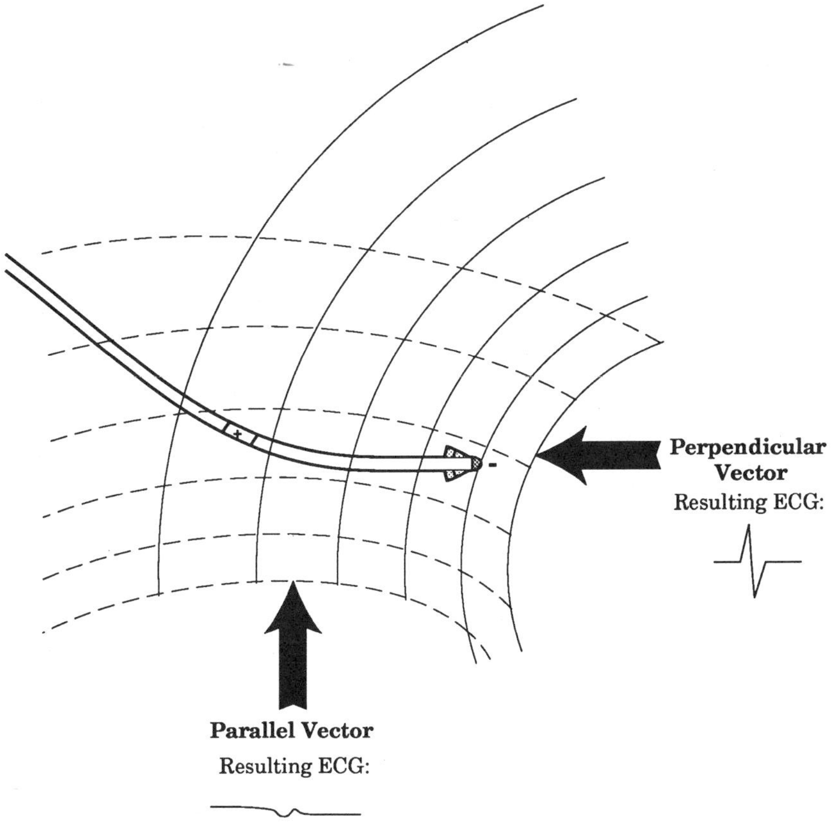

Figure 13.5. The relationship of the electrodes to the vector of the intrinsic depolarization wave can influence the size of the intracardiac signal "seen" by the pacemakers sensing circuit. When the electrodes are perpendicular to the depolarization wave, the signal is strongest, when the electrodes are parallel to the depolarization wave, the signal is minimized.

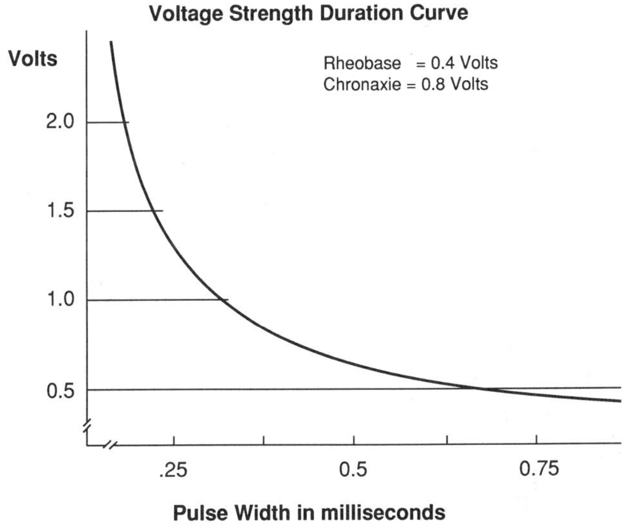

Figure 13.6. A strength duration curve is obtained by plotting the voltage threshold at various stimulation pulse widths. The rheobase is the voltage value at which additional increases in stimulation pulse width will not produce a lower voltage threshold. The chronaxie is the point on the curve that is twice the rheobase.

Proper anchoring of the lead at the point of venous access requires the use of a suture sleeve. Failure to use a suture sleeve can cause permanent lead damage. The suture sleeve is slid into a position immediately adjacent to the point of venous access. A minimum of three nonabsorbable sutures are then tied around the sleeve, proximally and distally, to anchor the suture sleeve to the lead. Additional sutures are then used to secure the suture sleeve to the tissue. It is important that sufficient tension is applied to the sutures to prevent the lead from slipping within the sleeve. At the same time, excessive tightening of the sutures can cause lead damage chronically (23).

Pacemaker Pocket Preparation

It is important that both the incision and the pocket be sized appropriately for the pulse generator. The incision should be only as wide as necessary to allow passage of the generator. The pocket is formed using blunt dissection of the subcutaneous tissue to the muscle fascia. The pacemaker should fit snugly into the pocket. If the pocket is too large and the pacemaker is allowed to move easily within, it could potentially migrate or rotate within the pocket. If the pocket is too tight and the tissue is stretched, the pacemaker may erode through the skin.

Extra care should be taken to assure complete hemostasis, checking deep within the pocket to verify that no bleeding is occurring. All electrocautery should be completed before the pacemaker is inserted, taking care to avoid direct contact with the lead.

Connection of the Lead(s) to the Pacemaker

The pulse generator should be placed over the pocket in the same position as it is to be inserted. The lead(s) should be uncoiled and it should be verified that there are no twists or torquing of the lead body which may put stress on the lead or cause kinking. Chronically, these forces may be transferred to the distal tip and cause a late dislodgement or additional irritation of the endocardium. The lead(s) are then carefully wound, not looped, behind the pulse generator. An alternative to this is to wind the lead directly into the pocket at this time. The location of the exposed portion of the lead's terminal connector pin and ring should be noted and the lead connector inserted into the aperture of the pacemaker. Visual confirmation that the exposed metal portions of the lead terminal are properly aligned within the pacer's terminals is important to ensure proper electrical contact. The set screws are then tightened.

When placing the pacemaker into the pocket care should be taken to keep the leads behind the generator and to avoid kinking of the leads. With a unipolar generator, or one programmable to a unipolar mode, the exposed portion of the generator which is used as the anode will have a large plus sign (+). This exposed portion of the generator should face away from the muscle. Most pacemakers provide a suture hole in the top of the device which may be used to anchor the unit to the fascia. This is helpful in preventing migration, particularly when a larger device is implanted.

Finally, pocket closure is begun deep within the subcutaneous tissue. Three layers of suturing using absorbable suture material, e.g., 3.0 Vycril or similar, should be employed to approximate fascial, dermal, and subepidermal tissue planes. Care should be taken to assure that the lead insulation is not nicked or punctured during this procedure.

ACUTE TO CHRONIC LEAD MATURATION

Pacing thresholds can change significantly as the lead becomes chronically encapsulated within the heart. A graphic representation of the three phases of the maturation process, and the corresponding changes in pacing thresholds, is illustrated in Figure 13.7 (24). At implant, the pacing electrode is positioned directly against the endocardium and the resulting thresholds are optimized. The acute phase begins with micromovement of the electrode against the endocardium causing an inflammation of that region. This inflammation pushes the lead away from its original position and simultaneously a fluid layer forms between the electrode and the healthy myocardial cells. As the electrical current emanates from the electrode, it must pass through this barrier on its way to the cells that are actually being simulated. The effective pacing surface area is enlarged by the thickness of this barrier, causing the current density to decrease. Pacing impedance decreases as the pacing threshold increases. During the later portion of the acute phase, fibrotic encapsulation results in reduced irritation of the endocardium, as the micromovement of the electrode eases. As edema within the tissue dissipates, there is further fibrotic sheath development, with reduction in the distance between the electrode and the healthy myocardial cells. This results in an increase in the current density and impedance, and a decrease in the stimulation threshold. Early fibrotic growth into appropriately sized porous electrodes limits the thickness of this fibrotic layer by reducing the amount of time for micromovement of the electrode (25).

Chronically, if the fibrotic encapsulation sufficiently stabi-

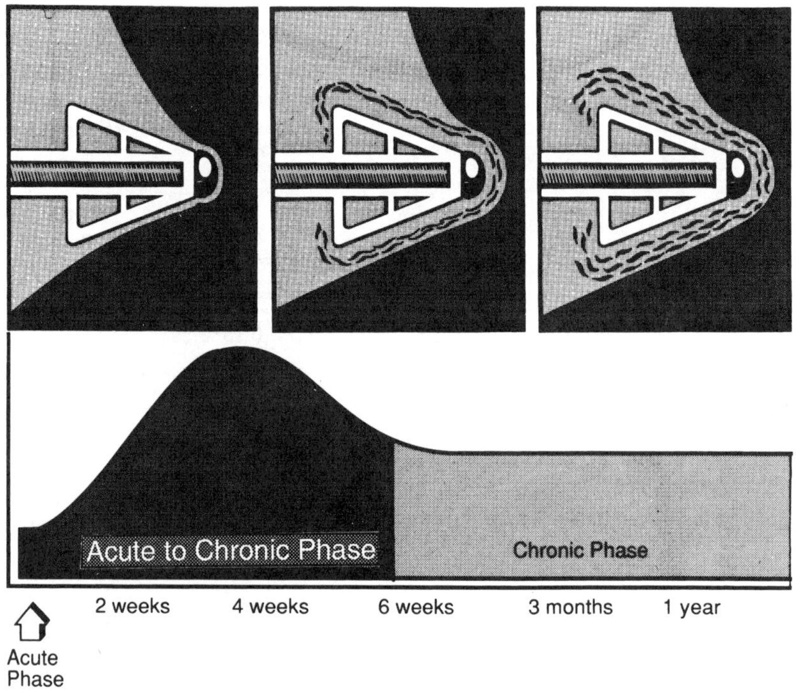

Figure 13.7. Changes in stimulation threshold that occur over time as the electrode becomes chronically encapsulated. Acute phase: direct electrode to tissue contact for optimal thresholds. Acute to chronic phase: micromovement of the electrode against the tissue causes irritation and an inflammatory response, thresholds increase two to three times the acute phase value. Chronic phase: fibrotic encapsulation stabilizes the distal tip and electrode/tissue interface improves, thresholds decrease, however, due to the fibrotic layer, not to the original acute value.

lizes the distal tip of the lead, no additional electrode/tissue interface reactions take place, and the thresholds remain constant. If electrode movement continues, or if there is a pathologic reaction to the presence of the lead, thresholds will continue to increase during the chronic phase and ultimately will cause exit block to occur.

Although the actual mechanism is not completely understood, leads that elute a small amount (less than 1 mg) of the steroid dexamethasone, have had a significant effect in reducing the pacing thresholds during the acute and chronic phases postimplant primarily by reducing the initial inflammatory response of the cardiac tissue adjacent to the electrode (11,12). This development has also been successfully used in patients with previously documented chronic exit block (26,27).

LEAD-RELATED PROBLEMS

Postimplant, lead-related complications may occur in up to 5% of patients. Incidence of lead-related complications decreases with frequency of use and the experience of the implanter (1). In the past, troubleshooting a possible lead problem, other than a gross conductor fracture, was almost impossible. Telemetry and noninvasive measurement tests available in state-of-the-art implantable pulse generators simplifies this diagnostic process significantly. At a minimum, the implanted pacemaker should provide real-time lead impedance data, intracardiac electrograms, and a simple, safe method for measuring pacing thresholds.

As with all surgical procedures, infection is always a potential complication. Good antiseptic technique prevents most infectious complications. If infection occurs, it is almost always necessary to remove the entire system—pacemaker and lead(s) (28,29).

The most common early complications is lead dislodgement. Macro or gross dislodgement of the pacing electrode occurs when the entire distal portion of the lead becomes separated from the original implant site and is found to be free floating within the heart or displaced to another location. The primary indicator is the loss of capture at any programmable output. It is easily confirmed by viewing the lead under fluoroscopy or by conventional radiography. Macrodislodgement can occur with either passive or active leads, and reoperation is required to reposition the leads.

With microdislodgement, the distal portion of the lead remains in the original implant position but the electrode becomes separated from the endocardial wall. Visual confirmation is therefore impossible and the primary indicators are elevated thresholds and/or loss of capture (also indicators for chronic exit block). If microdislodgement results in elevated but still acceptable thresholds, noninvasive programming to a higher output is frequently all that is required. If the threshold continues to increase, it may be due to continued micromovement of the lead tip causing cellular irritation. This is often the case with epicardial or epi/myocardial pacing leads. If loss of capture occurs, repositioning is required. Use of the noninvasive threshold testing at each follow-up is particularly helpful when the threshold increase is sudden, and therefore most likely due to the lead dislodgement. A more gradual increase is commonly associated with micromovement or exit block.

Exit block results in a steady increase in pacing thresholds over time, clue to an exaggerated physiologic reaction of the tissue to the pacing electrode. As with microdislodgement, its primary indicator is the loss of capture. Repositioning the lead however, usually only results in the phenomenon repeating itself. The only proven effective method of dealing with this complication is to use steroid eluting leads. Although the reported incidence of exit block has been relatively high, many reported cases may actually be due to lead dislodgements, with the true exit block occurring uncommonly.

Penetration or perforation of the heart wall by the pacing lead is a rare, but potentially significant complication. There are several methods available to assist in diagnosing these events; however, few if any, will provide a definitive reason for their occurrence. The physiologic condition of the heart and stiffness of the lead, particularly in the distal portion, can both be a factor, as can the force used during lead placement or lead positioning, and the presence of other leads within the heart (2). Fluoroscopy or ultrasound may be used to diagnose this condition. With perforation, a comparison of the intracardiac electrogram to one taken at the time of implant or a previous follow-up visit may also be a reasonable indicator (see also Chapter 18). If the sensed electrogram (P wave or R wave) exhibit changes from the reference intracardiac electrocardiogram (IECG), the electrodes are "seeing" the depolarization vector from an alternate direction. Although rare, cardiac tamponade may occur and the patient should be closely monitored for this complication.

The removal of chronically implanted leads has traditionally proven difficult, and the available techniques remain less than adequate to the need. Due to the lead design, the distal portion of the lead is larger than the lead body. This "golf club" configuration, fibrous encapsulation of the lead body in the vein, and fibrosis of the distal tip makes lead removal difficult at times. As a result, the most common, and still the safest method of dealing with an unused implanted lead is to cut off the terminal connector, securely cap the exposed end, suture it to the fascia, and abandon the lead.

The most common technique for removing a chronically implanted lead is to simply apply continuous traction (28–30). Although this may be successful, particularly with unipolar leads, this is not a recommended technique for newer bipolar leads. The recent development of specialized lead removal kits with a special stylet that "locks" onto the distal electrode, allows the physician to pull on the stylet and not the lead (31). Special dilating sheaths are also available to separate and expand the fibrous sheath away from the lead body. This kit makes chronic lead removal possible. Removals should be performed only in

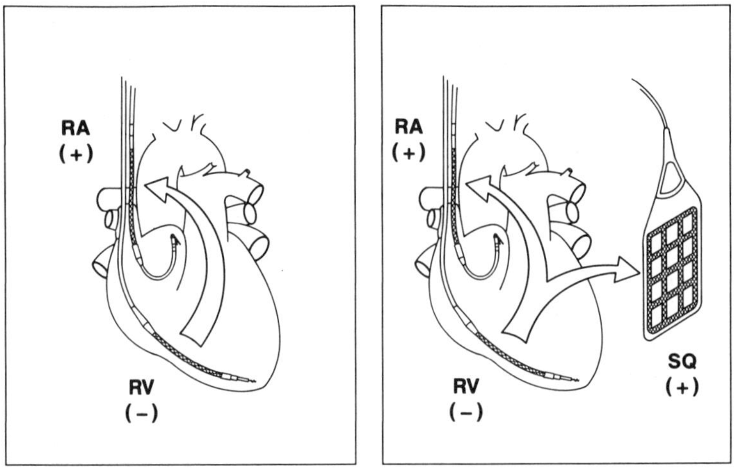

Figure 13.8. High-voltage endocardial leads (Enguard, Telectronics, Englewood, CO.) with large electrode surface areas (*shaded areas*) are positioned in the right ventricle and superior vena cava. A unidirectional shock **(left)** has been found to be effective in a small number of patients. More frequently, the addition of a subcutaneously placed patch electrode is required to deliver a bidirectional shock **(right)**. (Courtesy of Telectronics Inc. Englewood, CO.).

centers which are actively doing this procedure on a regular basis. Surgical removal may be required when these techniques are unsuccessful and lead removal is mandatory, e.g., with lead/generator infection.

FUTURE LEADS

With the increasing use of bipolar pacing systems, future pacing lead designs will aim to eliminate differences in size, stiffness, and "positionability" between unipolar and bipolar models. Given the limitations of existing insulators, the introduction of new materials for this purpose is inevitable. The use of such materials to create a single coated conductor coil to provide both anodal and cathodal current pathways is presently being tested by several manufacturers and is anticipated to eliminate the need for the coaxial lead design (Fig. 13.3C). This same technology may also be used to provide additional current pathways for lead-based sensors. Rate-responsive pacing systems, for example, requiring the use of temperature, pressure, and oxygen saturation sensors mounted on the distal portion of the lead, are all being investigated.

Recent investigations of several atrial synchronous, ventricular pacing (VDD) systems using a single-pass atrioventricular lead with free-floating atrial electrode(s) has proven beneficial for a subgroup of patients with healthy sino-atrial nodes and no significant atrial arrhythmias (32).

The single greatest area of lead development will undoubtedly be associated with implantable cardioverter/defibrillator devices. These devices must sense both bradycardia and tachycardias, provide antitachycardia pacing therapies, deliver high-voltage cardioversion/defibrillation, and possibly be modified to deliver antiarrhythmic drugs. The current practice of using large epicardial patches for high-voltage defibrillation represents the very beginning of lead development in this area. As shown in Figure 13.8, endocardial leads with flexible large surface area electrodes and resembling early dual-chamber pacing leads are already being investigated (33,34). Here, too, lead-based sensors are anticipated.

CONCLUSION

Variety of lead types implanted in the past, present, and future make it almost impossible for any one individual to be the definitive expert in leads. As a result, every major pacemaker manufacturer maintains a product data base and technical staff which is available to assist the physician, nurse, or technician in resolving a wide variety of questions that may arise.

Frequently, data about a particular product become available after the lead has been implanted and the physician may not have the most current information. For this reason it is usually best to start with the lead manufacturer first.

As no one lead is suited for every patient or application, and new leads are continually being introduced, the physician's use of a given lead model will constantly be challenged. It is therefore helpful to develop a method of evaluation that can be used to periodically assess new products as they become available.

As a standard, new lead types to be considered should be bipolar, with competitive pacing and sensing threshold performance, high pacing impedances, and small size. Long-term reliability of lead technology used should be the primary concern and closely monitored. Ease of implantation is also an important factor in assuring a consistent and optimal performance. The more technically challenging the lead is to implant, the less likely it is to be properly positioned. Most importantly, the best leads for a specific physician are the models that consistently work for that physician. This requires that the physician monitor, at a minimum, the threshold performance and complication rates of their individual patient population.

The implantable lead is increasingly being called upon to complement the pulse generator in an effort to provide the most efficient pacing "system" possible. Efforts to standardize the lead to pacer connection should be viewed as providing the physician with the ability to always use the most optimal lead with the most appropriate pulse generator. Defining the "best lead" is an evolutionary process and will change with the clinical evaluation of smaller leads with multiple conductors, multiple electrodes, sensors, high-voltage defibrillation, and drug delivery systems.

References

1. Parsonnet V, Bernstein AD, Lindsay BD: Pacemaker-implantation complication rates: an analysis of contributing factors (Abstract). PACE 1987;10:409.
2. Cameron J, Mond HG, Ciddor G, *et al.*: Stiffness of the distal tip of bipolar pacing leads. PACE 1990;13 (II):1915–1920.
3. Mond HG: Unipolar versus bipolar pacing—poles apart. PACE 1991;14: 1411–1424.
4. Aubert AE: Evaluation of pacemaker lead corrosion. In Aubert AE, Ector H (eds): Pacemaker Leads. Elsevier Science Publishers, Amsterdam, 1985; 411–417.
5. Timmis GC, Helland J, Westveer DC, *et al.*: The evolution of low threshold leads. Clin Prog Pacing Electrophysiol 1983;1:313–334.
6. Gordon S, Timmis GC, Ramos RG, *et al.*: Improved transvenous pacemaker electrode stability. In Macre C. (ed): Proceedings of Sixth World Symposium on Cardiac Pacing. Publishers Pacesymp, Montreal, 1979;31–33.
7. Furman S, Parker B, Escher DJ: Decreasing electrode size and increasing efficiency of cardiac stimulation. J Surg Res 1971;11:105–110.
8. Mond H, Holley L, Hirshorn M: The high impedance dish electrode-clinical experience with a new tined lead. PACE 1982;5:529–534.
9. MacGregor DC, Wilson G, Lixfield W, *et al.*: The porous surface electrode: a new concept in pacemaker leads. J Thorac Cardiovasc Surg 1979;78: 281–291.
10. MacCarter DJ, Lundberg KM, Corstiens JPM: Characteristics of advanced porous and textured surface pacemaker electrodes. PACE 1983;6: 427–435.
11. Timmis GC, Gordon S, Westveer DC, *et al.*: A new steroid-eluting low threshold lead (Abstract). PACE 1983;6:316.
12. Wilson A, Cowling R, Mathivanar R, *et al.*: Drug eluting collar—a new approach to reducing thresholds. PACE 1990;13(II):1876–1878.
13. Parsonnet V, Furman S, Smyth NPD, *et al.*: Optimal resources for implantable cardiac pacemakers. Circulation 1983;68:226A–244A.
14. Miller G, Leman R, Kratz J, *et al.*: Comparison of lead dislodgment and pocket infection after pacemaker implantation in the operating room versus cardiac catheterization laboratory. Am Heart Journal 1988;115:1048–1051.
15. Byrd C: Permanent pacemaker implantation techniques. In Samet P, El-Sherif N (eds): Cardiac Pacing, 2nd ed. Grune & Stratton, New York, 1980;229–253.
16. Holmes DR, Hayes DL, Furman S: Permanent pacemaker implantation. In Holmes DR, Hayes DL, Furman S(eds): A Practice of Cardiac Pacing, 2nd ed. Futura Publishing Co. New York, 1989:239–287.
17. Bognolo DA, Vijayanagar R, Eckstein PF, *et al.*: Two leads in one introducer technique for A-V sequential implantations. PACE 1982;5:217–218.
18. Parsonnet V, Werres R, Atherley T, *et al.*: Transvenous insertion of double sets of permanent electrodes. JAMA 1980;243:62–64.
19. Portnow AS, Greene TO, Mittleman RS, *et al.*: Acute pericarditis resulting from an active fixation screw-in atrial lead (Abstract). PACE 1991;14(II): 731.
20. Love C, Pashkow F: Telectronics paving systems—implant workshop. Educational slide set, 1990. Englewood, CO.
21. Davies JG, Sowton E: Electrical threshold of the human heart. Br Heart J 1966;25:231–239.
22. Irnich W: The chronaxie time and its practical importance. PACE 1980;3:292–301.
23. Pacesetter Systems, Inc.: Technical memorandum no. 17. Pacesetter Systems, Sylmar, CA, 1991.
24. Stokes K, Bornzin G: The electrode-biointerface: stimulation. In Barold SS (ed): Modern Cardiac Pacing. Futura Publishing Co., New York, 1985:33–77.
25. Miller SL, MacGregor DC, Klement P, *et al.* Performance of a Platinum-iridium porous-surface electrode. In Aubert AE, Ector H (eds): Pacemaker Leads. Elsevier Science Publishers, Amsterdam, 1985;337–342.
26. Stokes K, Church T: The elimination of exit block as a pacing complication using a transvenous steroid eluting lead (Abstract). PACE 1987;10:748.
27. King DH, Gillette PC, Shannon C, *et al.*: Steroid-eluting endocardial pacing lead for treatment of exit block. Am Heart J 1983;126:1438–1440.
28. Meyers MR, Parsonnet V, Bernstein AD: Extraction of implanted transvenous pacing leads: a review of a persistent clinical problem. Am Heart J 1991;121(I):881–888.
29. Phibbs B, Marriott HJL: Complications of permanent transvenous pacing. N Engl J Med 1985;312:1428–1432.
30. Madigan NP, Curtis JJ, Sanfelippo JF, *et al.*: Difficulty of extraction of chronically implanted tined ventricular endocardial leads. J Am Coll Cardiol 1984;3:724–731.
31. Byrd CL, Schwartz SJ, Hedin N: Intravascular techniques for extraction of permanent pacemaker leads. J Thorac Cariovasc Surg 1991;101:989–997.
32. Varriale P, Pilla AG, Tekriwal M: Single-lead VDD pacing system. PACE 1990;13:757–766.
33. Schmitt C. Brachmann, J, Saggau W, *et al.*: Early experience with transvenous implantation of pacemaker-defibrillator systems (Abstract). PACE 1991;14(II):717.
34. Saksena S, Ward D, Krol R, *et al.*: Efficacy of braided endocardial defibrillation leads: acute testing and chronic implant (Abstr). PACE 1991;14(II):719.

14

INDICATIONS FOR PERMANENT CARDIAC PACEMAKERS

S. Serge Barold, M.B., B.S., F.R.A.C.P., F.A.C.P., F.A.C.C., F.E.S.C.

The most complete and authoritative guidelines concerning the indications for permanent pacing were originally published in 1984 by a joint committee established by the American College of Cardiology (ACC) and the American Heart Association (AHA) (1). These guidelines were revised in 1991 (2). The document recognizes the fact that indications for permanent pacing in an individual patient may not always be clear-cut, and the guidelines are liberal enough to cover the majority of clinical situations. The ACC/AHA guidelines (1,2) emphasize the indications for pacing and various pacing modes whereas recommendations concerning the optimal pacing mode for the individual patient are limited. For example, the answer to the question: What is the optimal pacing mode for the patient with sick sinus syndrome? is not addressed in detail.

Indications for permanent pacing in the ACC/AHA guidelines have been grouped according to the following classifications (1,2):

- Class I: Conditions for which there is general agreement that permanent pacemakers should be implanted.
- Class II: Conditions for which permanent pacemakers are frequently used but there is a divergence of opinion with respect to the necessity of their insertion.
- Class III: Conditions for which there is general agreement that pacemakers are unnecessary.

In patients being considered for pacemakers, decision making may be influenced by the following additional factors (1,2):

1. Overall physical and mental state of the patient, including the absence of associated diseases that may result in a limited quality or prognosis for life
2. Presence of associated underlying cardiac disease that may be adversely affected by bradycardia
3. Desire of the patient to operate a motor vehicle
4. Remoteness of medical care, including patients who travel widely or live alone who therefore might be unable to seek medical help if serious symptoms arise
5. Necessity for administering medication that may depress escape heart rates or aggravate atrioventricular (AV) block
6. Slowing of the basic escape rates
7. Significant cerebrovascular disease that might result in a stroke if cerebral perfusion were to suddenly decrease
8. Desires of the patient and family

ACQUIRED ATRIOVENTRICULAR BLOCK IN ADULTS (Table 14.1)

The 1991 ACC/AHA guidelines (2) state the following:

> *Atrioventricular block* is classified as first-degree, second-degree, or third-degree (complete) heart block; anatomically, it is defined as supra-His, intra-His, and infra-His. Second-degree heart block may be further classified as type I (progressive prolongation of PR interval before a blocked beat) or type II (no progressive prolongation of PR interval before blocked beats) and is usually associated with a wide QRS complex. *Advanced second degree block* refers to the block of two more consecutive P waves.

According to the definitions codified by the World Health Organization (3) (WHO) and the ACC (4) (both in 1978), Type II second-degree AV block should be defined as the occurrence of a single nonconducted P wave associated with a constant PR interval before and after the blocked impulse, provided there are at least two consecutive conducted P waves (i.e., 3:2 AV block) to determine the behavior of the PR interval (5). 2:1 AV block cannot be classified into Type I or Type II, an important concept clearly emphasized in the 1989 ACC/AHA guidelines for clinical intracardiac electrophysiologic study (6) (EPS). 2:1 AV block is best considered as advanced block as are higher degrees of block such as 3:1, 4:1, etc., according to the definitions promulgated by the WHO and ACC (3,4). Many workers have adopted these definitions (7–9), although the above 1989 ACC/AHA guidelines for EPS (6) mentioned that some experts recommend advanced AV block as an additional category (outside of Type I, Type II, and 2:1 AV block) in which multiple consecutive P waves are blocked but complete AV block is not present.

The 1984 and 1991 ACC/AHA guidelines do not specifically mention 2:1 AV block (1,2). I believe this represents a major

Table 14.1.
ACC/AHA 1991 Guidelines—Indications for Permanent Pacing in Acquired Atrioventricular Block in Adults

Class I

A. Complete heart block, permanent or intermittent, at any anatomic level, associated with any one of the following complications:
   1. Symptomatic bradycardia. In the presence of complete heart block, symptoms must be presumed to be due to heart block unless proved otherwise.
   2. Congestive heart failure
   3. Ectopic rhythms and other medical conditions that require drugs that suppress the automaticity of escape pacemakers and result in symptomatic bradycardia
   4. Documented periods of asystole ≥ 3.0 sec or any escape rate < 40 beats/min in symptom-free patients
   5. Confusional states that clear with temporary pacing
   6. Post-AV junction ablation, myotonic dystrophy

B. Second-degree AV block, permanent or intermittent, regardless of the type or the site of block, with symptomatic bradycardia

C. Atrial fibrillation, atrial flutter, or rare cases of supraventricular tachycardia with complete heart block or advanced AV block, bradycardia, and any of the conditions described under (1A). The bradycardia must be unrelated to digitalis or drugs known to impair AV conduction.

Class II

A. Asymptomatic complete heart block, permanent or intermittent, at any anatomic site, with ventricular rates of 40 beats/min or faster

B. Asymptomatic type II second-degree AV block, permanent or intermittent

C. Asymptomatic type I second-degree AV block at intra-His or infra-His levels

Class III

A. First-degree AV block

B. Asymptomatic type I second-degree AV block at the supra-His (AV node) level

omission that promises to cloud the understanding of AV block and its treatment. It is unclear why the ACC/AHA guidelines chose to define advanced second-degree AV block as block of two or more consecutive P waves. Furthermore, the definition of type II second-degree AV block in the 1984 and 1991 ACC/AHA guidelines lends itself to misinterpretation because the constancy of the PR interval after a blocked impulse is not emphasized (5).

Natural History of First- and Second-Degree Atrioventricular Block

As expected, the prognosis of isolated first-degree AV block is benign (10). In 1981, Strasberg, *et al.* (11) reported on the natural history of 56 patients with second-degree AV block followed for periods of 157–2280 days. These workers concluded that the prognosis was related to the presence or absence of organic heart disease, usually benign without organic heart disease and more malignant with organic heart disease and related to the severity of underlying disease. However, the weakness of the study centers around the group of patients with no disease, because it consisted of only 19 subjects; 7 were trained athletes and 12 were under 35 yrs old, all expected to have an excellent prognosis.

Only one study has addressed the prognosis of asymptomatic patients with type II second-degree AV block (12). Most patients were found eventually to develop symptoms within a relatively short time. These observations form the basis for the current recommendation of permanent pacing in patients with asymptomatic type II second-degree AV block (or type I infranodal block that carries the same prognostic significance as type II AV block).

In 1985, Shaw, *et al.* (13) presented provocative data showing that chronic type I second-degree AV block had a similar prognosis to second-degree type II or advanced AV block in unpaced patients. Shaw, *et al.* (13) followed 214 patients with second-degree AV block (unrelated to acute myocardial infarction) between 1968 and 1982. The patients were divided into three groups: (1) 77 patients with type I second-degree AV block, (2) 86 patients with type II second-degree AV block, (3) 51 patients with 2:1 or 3:1 AV block. Pacemakers were received by 103 patients (33 in group 1, 49 in group 2, and 21 in group 3). The 5-yr survival was similar in the three groups of unpaced patients. The presence or absence of bundle branch block did not appear to influence the prognosis. Group 1 unpaced patients without bundle branch block (BBB) did not fare any better than unpaced patients in group 2, both with or without BBB. In contrast, patients with permanent pacemakers exhibited improved survival and did as well as expected compared to the normal population (13).

Guidelines from the British Pacing and Electrophysiology Group

The recently published document entitled "Recommendations for Pacemaker Prescription for Symptomatic Bradycardia" by the British Pacing and Electrophysiology Group (14) (BPEG) recommends using the 1984 ACC/AHA guidelines except in two areas where the BPEG indicates that pacing should be more widely used as first-line therapy. First, referring to the work of Shaw, *et al.* (13) the BPEG guidelines state that "asymptomatic patients with either Wenckebach or Mobitz II second-degree AV block occurring during much of the day and night would quality for pacemaker implantation as would patients with asymptomatic complete heart block"(14). In this respect, the BPEG also cautions that 'the Wenckebach phenomenon can occur during sleep in normal individuals with high vagal tone and these people do not need to be considered for treatment" (14). Second, the BPEG indicates that carotid sinus syndrome and malignant vasovagal syncope would now qualify as firm indications for pacemaker implantation when appropriate investigation shows a major cardioinhibitory effect (14) and indeed the 1991 ACC/AHA guidelines (2) have addressed this subject with basically the same recommendations (discussed below).

The data of Shaw, *et al.* (13) if confirmed by others would have enormous impact on the utilization of permanent pacemakers. Considering the findings of Shaw, *et al.* (13) and the

ACC/AHA guidelines (2), it seems reasonable at present to recommend permanent pacing in *asymptomatic* patients with Type I, Type II, or advanced second-degree AV block where the block is localized in the His-Purkinje system. Despite the BPEG guidelines, it also seems reasonable at this juncture to continue conservative therapy in asymptomatic patients with type I or advanced second-degree AV nodal block regardless of QRS duration, though such patients should be followed carefully.

PACING AFTER MYOCARDIAL INFARCTION

The requirement for temporary pacing in acute myocardial infarction (MI) does not by itself constitute an indication for permanent pacing. Unlike many other indications, the need for permanent pacing after acute MI does not necessarily depend on the presence of symptoms (2) (Table 14.2).

Inferior Wall Myocardial Infarctions

In patients with inferior MI and AV block with a narrow QRS complex, permanent pacing is very rarely needed (15–20). Atrioventricular block (mostly confined to the AV node) may take as long as 16 days or even 3 wk in exceptional cases to subside with the return of 1:1 AV conduction. Even relatively uncommon intra-Hisian block is almost always reversible and rarely requires permanent pacing.

Tans, *et al.* (17) evaluated 144 patients who developed high-degree (second- and third-degree) AV block during acute inferior MI. The in-hospital mortality was 22%, but all the patients that survived were discharged with 1:1 AV conduction. In the study of Nicod, *et al.* (16) involving 95 patients surviving inferior MI and complete heart block, only one patient required a permanent pacemaker, but the duration of AV block was not stated. Dubois, *et al.* (21) reported their experience with 88 patients with acute inferior MI complicated by second- and third-degree AV block. Sixty-seven patients survived and 45% had third-degree AV block (30 patients). Six of those patients received a permanent pacemaker. Assuming that a permanent pacemaker was implanted only in patients with complete heart block, this constitutes 20% of all the patients with complete heart block in the acute phase. This is not in keeping with the almost invariable return of 1:1 AV conduction, provided one waits for up to 3 wk. Consequently, it would appear that these workers implanted pacemakers probably too early in the course of AV block, and had they waited longer, perhaps fewer or none of the pacemakers might have been necessary. In this respect, Lie and Durrer (22) stated over 10 yr ago that "there is little controversy over the indications for permanent pacing in conduction disturbance following inferior infarctions, since these are always transient and do not have a tendency to recur. Permanent pacing is generally not necessary in this setting." This statement is still true today, although in rare instances AV block can persist for over 3 wk and might require permanent pacing. I do not agree with suggestions from some workers that permanent pacemakers should be implanted when AV block is prolonged so as to facilitate mobilization and rehabilitation, especially if the patient is dependent on temporary pacemakers and requires multiple replacements (23). Most patients with persistent complete heart block during inferior MI may not be truly pacemaker-dependent if one gradually decreases the pacing rate so as to allow the emergence of a spontaneous rhythm, often with an acceptable rate.

Rarely, a patient with preexistent right BBB and left anterior hemiblock presents with an acute inferior MI complicated by left posterior hemiblock and the development of complete heart block in the His-Purkinje system (24). A permanent pacemaker seems justified in such an exceptional situation. Concerning the incidence of type II second-degree AV block, Scheinman and Gonzales (25) wrote in 1980 that "classic type II AV block has not been documented in patients with acute inferior myocardial infarction," and this statement is still true today. The existence of true type II second-degree AV block with a narrow QRS complex remains to be documented in acute MI, particularly inferior MI (26) despite claims to the contrary (27–33).

Table 14.2.
ACC/AHA 1991 Guidelines—Indications for Permanent Pacing After Myocardial Infarction

Class I
- A. Persistent advanced second-degree AV block or complete heart block after acute myocardial infarction with block in the His-Purkinje system (bilateral bundle branch block)
- B. Patients with transient advanced AV block and associated bundle branch block

Class II
- A. Patients with persistent advanced block at the AV node

Class III
- A. Transient AV conduction disturbances in the absence of intraventricular conduction defects
- B. Transient AV block in the presence of isolated left anterior hemiblock
- C. Acquired left anterior hemiblock in the absence of AV block
- D. Patients with persistent first-degree AV block in the presence of bundle branch block not demonstrated previously

Anterior Myocardial Infarction

Permanent pacing is not indicated in patients with acute anterior MI and residual intraventricular conduction disorders without documented transient second- or third-degree AV block because there is no appreciable risk of late development of complete AV block. Measurement of the HV interval does not predict which patients will develop progressive conduction system disease. As a rule, lesions in the bundle branch system once established during acute MI lesions tend to remain constant and generally do not show progressive deterioration with the passage of time (34,35).

Transient Atrioventricular Block in Anterior Myocardial Infarction

Bundle branch block occurs in about 8–13% of patients with acute anterior MI. Patients who develop BBB and transient second- or third-degree AV block during anterior MI have a high in-hospital mortality and are at a high risk of sudden death after hospital discharge. Sudden death usually is due to malignant ventricular tachyarrhythmias and less commonly related to the development of complete AV block with prolonged ventricular asystole (although the latter can occasionally precipitate a ventricular tachyarrhythmia). The use of permanent pacing in patients with transient trifascicular AV block during acute anterior MI is still controversial (19,36–41). In 1978, Roos and Dunning (40) put this problem into clear perspective by pointing out that: (a) about 10% of patients reaching the hospital with acute anterior MI will develop BBB, (b) approximately one-third of these patients will progress to complete heart block, and (c) 80% of patients with transient or permanent complete heart block will die in the hospital. This means that less than 1% of patients admitted with an acute anterior MI will survive the first four weeks to obtain possible benefit from permanent pacing. By analyzing the available literature, Roos and Dunning (40) concluded that there was a trend that late sudden death in patients developing transient AV block might be reduced by permanent pacing. In the same year, the study of Hindman, *et al.* (34) involving a relatively large number of patients, also suggested a reduction in sudden death mortality by implantation of a permanent pacemaker in patients with bundle branch block who developed transient AV block during anterior MI. A 1983 review of the subject pooling patients from the available literature also suggested that permanent pacing might be helpful (19). As emphasized in 1978 by Roos and Dunning (40), the numbers of patients in all the trials have been far too small to make firm conclusions and the situation has not really changed to this day. Thus, permanent pacing, though still controversial, should be considered in those patients who develop transient trifascicular block and eventual return of 1:1 AV conduction with the aim of preventing sudden death from asystole.

Some questions remain unanswered: (a) Is there need for prophylactic permanent pacing in the absence of transient AV block if there is alternating BBB or right BBB and left posterior hemiblock? (23) (b) In patients with residual BBB, because of the high incidence of deaths in the first 6 wks post-MI from ventricular tachyarrhythmias rather than AV block, would a combination of permanent pacing and antiarrhythmic drugs be more appropriate than antiarrhythmic therapy alone?

Comments on the ACC/AHA Guidelines: Indications for Permanent Pacing After Myocardial Infarction

The Class 1A indication in Table 14.2 should include all forms of second-degree AV block rather than only advanced second-degree AV block. With regard to the Class 1B indication in Table 14.2, transient advanced AV block with associated bundle branch block does not necessarily constitute an indication for permanent pacing in some circumstances. For example, a patient with an inferior MI associated with right BBB and AV nodal block (the latter almost always transient) rarely requires permanent pacing.

In the Class IIA indication (Table 14.2), the term "persistent" is not defined and complete AV block should obviously have been included. Permanent pacing is rarely required for second- or third-degree AV nodal block after MI. Furthermore, in the 1984 guidelines "patients with transient advanced AV block and associated bundle branch block" represented a Class II indication (1). The same group was recently promoted to a Class I indication in the 1991 guidelines (2) without any new data (since 1984) to justify the change.

BIFASCICULAR AND TRIFASCICULAR BLOCK (Table 14.3)

Asymptomatic Bundle Branch Block

Eighty percent of patients with BBB have clinical evidence of associated heart disease, and coronary artery disease is found in almost half the patients. Half the deaths are sudden and usually not the result of bradycardia but rather MI or ventricular tachycardia (42). There is a high prevalence of HV prolongation in patients with BBB or bifascicular block and a prolonged HV (<100 msec) interval is generally not predictive of future events such as syncope and death (42). Although the development of AV block is more frequent in patients with HV interval prolongation (1–2%/yr), the incidence is so low that no investigation is indicated in the asymptomatic patient.

Table 14.3.
ACC/AHA 1991 Guidelines: Indications for Permanent Pacing in Bifascicular and Trifascicular Block

Class I
- A. Bifascicular block with intermittent complete heart block associated with symptomatic bradycardia
- B. Bifascicular or trifascicular block with intermittent type II second-degree AV block without symptoms attributable to the heart block

Class II
- A. Bifascicular or trifascicular block with syncope that is not proved to be due to complete heart block, but other possible causes for syncope are not identifiable
- B. Markedly prolonged HV (>100 msec)
- C. Pacing-induced infra-His block

Class III
- A. Fascicular block without AV block or symptoms
- B. Fascicular block with first-degree AV block without symptoms

Infranodal Block Induced by Atrial Pacing and Exercise

Dhingra, *et al.* (43) found that His-Purkinje AV block induced by atrial pacing (generally at a rate faster than 130/min) occurred in only 3–5% of their large number of patients with intraventricular conduction blocks. This response is considered abnormal and correlates with a high incidence of AV block or sudden death and requires a permanent pacemaker. Indeed, in the study of Dhingra, *et al.* (43), 8 of 15 such patients developed AV block over a mean follow-up of 3.4 yrs. This abnormal response to atrial pacing should not be confused with *functional* infranodal block, a rare response during rapid atrial pacing because the effective refractory period of the His-Purkinje system is frequently shorter than the AV nodal functional refractory period (44). Functional His-Purkinje AV block is usually seen with abrupt initiation and random coupling of atrial stimulation to the spontaneous rhythm at the start of atrial pacing. Such functional His-Purkinje block represents a normal response to a lengthening of the preceding cycle length followed by abrupt shortening of the coupling interval, i.e., a form of Ashman phenomenon—long-short H-H sequences (45).

Despite the report of McAnulty, *et al.* (46), it is widely believed that His-Purkinje block induced by atrial pacing, although an insensitive sign of conduction system disease, constitutes a definite indication for permanent pacing (47,48) provided functional infranodal block is ruled out.

Permanent pacing is also recommended in patients with exercise-induced AV block even in the asymptomatic state because recent studies have demonstrated that almost all cases of exercise-induced (or tachycardia-dependent) AV block are due to disease of the His-Purkinje system and associated with a poor prognosis (49–57). Many patients with exercise-induced AV block also demonstrate abnormal tachycardia-dependent infranodal AV block with incremental atrial pacing.

Symptomatic Bundle Branch Block

Three large and well-known prospective studies (46,47,58) focusing only on the HV interval did not indicate whether a permanent pacemaker can reduce the risk of death in patients with symptomatic bifascicular block and a prolonged HV interval. More recent studies have demonstrated the importance of performing a complete electrophysiologic study (EPS) in patients presenting with BBB and syncope (48,59,60). A comprehensive EPS increases the diagnostic yield and offers a rational therapeutic approach not previously available. EPS should include measurement of the HV interval, atrial pacing, programmed ventricular stimulation for the induction of sustained monomorphic ventricular tachycardia (VT), sinus node function tests, ventricular pacing to test for the "fatigue" phenomenon in the His-Purkinje system (61,62), programmed stimulation for supraventricular tachycardia (useful if associated with hypotension), and carotid sinus massage to unmask infranodal Phase 4 bradycardia-dependent block or demonstrate carotid hypersensitivity.

An EPS yields a positive result in about 50% of patients and sustained monomorphic VT constitutes the most common abnormality (in 20–30% of patients subjected to EPS) (48,59,60,63–65). The incidence of VT and therefore the value of EPS is greater in patients with structural heart disease compared with patients who do not have structural heart disease in whom the incidence of VT is low (65–68). A positive EPS is associated with a greater incidence of total and sudden death during follow-up (66–69). A negative or nondiagnostic EPS in patients with BBB and syncope indicates a good prognosis and a higher rate of remission of symptoms and identifies a group of patients at low risk of dying from an arrhythmia (66). Obviously a negative EPS does not exclude transient bradycardia as a cause of syncope and possibly sudden death, although the risk is low (66,67,70) and recurrence of syncope does not correlate with higher mortality or sudden death. A comprehensive EPS can define by a process of exclusion which patients with HV interval prolongation (HV interval > 70 msec) and no other electrophysiologic abnormality might benefit from permanent pacing. A markedly prolonged HV ≥ 100 msec is associated with a higher risk of AV block and clearly requires permanent pacing (47). However, a finding of HV ≥ 100 msec does not guarantee that AV block is the cause of symptoms, and HV < 100 msec and an otherwise negative EPS do not exclude symptomatic AV block. If EPS demonstrates prolongation of the HV interval (≥ 70 msec) and inducible sustained monomorphic VT, a permanent pacemaker and antiarrhythmic drugs can be given in combination (48,59). The role of drug provocation studies to define patients with BBB at risk of developing AV block is unclear and no definite recommendations concerning challenge studies can be made on the basis of present data, particularly because Ajmaline, the most widely used agent, is not available in the United States.

Comments on the ACC/AHA Guidelines: Bifascicular and Trifascicular Block (Table 14.3)

In the 1984 ACC/AHA guidelines (1), "bifascicular and trifascicular block with intermittent Type II second-degree AV block without symptoms" was labeled a Class II indication. Surprisingly, in the 1991 ACC/AHA guidelines (2) the identical condition described in terms of "bifascicular or trifascicular block with intermittent Type II second-degree AV block without symptoms attributable to the heart block" was promoted to a Class I indication. Yet the same 1991 ACC/AHA guidelines (2) in the section acquired AV block in adults (Table 14.1) state that "asymptomatic Type II second-degree AV block, permanent or intermittent" constitutes a Class II indication for permanent pacing. Because Type II second-degree AV block is associated with bifascicular or trifascicular block in at least 2/3 of the cases (71), this 1991 Class II recommendation in the section on acquired AV block in adults, does not agree with the 1991 Class I indication of the same condition in a different section on bifascicular and trifascicular block. This important discrepancy should be corrected by stating that asymptomatic Type II AV block is a Class I indication for permanent pacing. Furthermore, Indication 1B in the 1991 guidelines should be extended to patients with advanced second degree AV block (2:1, 3:1, etc.).

SICK SINUS SYNDROME

Sick sinus syndrome (SSS) (Table 14.4) is the most common indication for cardiac pacing in the United States, accounting for 40–55% of the pacemaker population. SSS constitutes a spectrum of abnormalities including sinus arrest or block, severe sinus bradycardia, alternating bradycardia-tachycardia (bradycardia-tachycardia syndrome) with normal sinus rate, or bradycardia between the attacks. Characteristically at the termination of supraventricular tachycardia there is overdrive suppression with long periods of sinus arrest or asystole. In the bradycardia-tachycardia syndrome, drugs alone may worsen the bradycardia and symptomatic patients are usually best managed by a combination of pacemaker and antiarrhyhmic drugs. As a rule, a pacemaker should only be implanted if there is a documented relationship between bradycardia and symptoms, which may be difficult to establish in elderly patients with vague symptoms. The treatment of patients with SSS should be directed toward control of symptoms and amelioration of organ dysfunction secondary to poor perfusion, e.g., congestive heart failure with sinus bradycardia. When bradycardia is secondary to drug therapy, e.g., beta blocker or antiarrhythmic agent, without any acceptable alternative, a pacemaker may be used to counteract the consequences of successful pharmacologic therapy. If one is in doubt about the need for pacing, it is usually safe to wait because arrhythmias associated with SSS rarely if ever result in sudden cardiac death. Permanent pacing is not indicated when there is transient bradycardia due to an increase in vagal tone, acute myocardial infarction, or secondary to drug therapy that may be discontinued or the dose lowered.

Table 14.4.
ACC/AHA 1991 Guidelines—Indications for Permanent Pacing in Sinus Node Dysfunction

Class I
A. Sinus node dysfunction with documented symptomatic bradycardia. In some patients this occurs as a consequence of long-term (essential) drug therapy of a type and dose for which there are no acceptable alternatives.

Class II
A. Sinus node dysfunction, occurring spontaneously or as a result of necessary drug therapy, with heart rates <40 beats/min when a clear association between significant symptoms consistent with bradycardia and the actual presence of bradycardia has not been documented

Class III
A. Sinus node dysfunction in asymptomatic patients, including those in whom substantial sinus bradycardia (heart rate <40 beats/min) is a consequence of long-term drug treatment
B. Sinus node dysfunction in patients in whom symptoms suggestive of bradycardia are clearly documented not to be associated with a slow heart rate

The prognosis of SSS is generally poor because most patients have structural heart disease. Single-lead ventricular pacing (VVI) prevents symptoms due to bradycardia but does not reduce the overall mortality. Recent data suggest that atrial pacing improves the quality and duration of life and may prevent or facilitate the treatment of supraventricular arrhythmias, an important consideration because half of SSS patients exhibit some form of supraventricular tachycardia, usually atrial fibrillation (as discussed in another chapter).

The role of prophylactic pacing in asymptomatic patients with electrocardiographic evidence of SSS has not been established. Asymptomatic patients should be followed closely, and drugs that depress sinus node function should be avoided. Pauses up to 2 sec are often quite harmless. Indeed, during sleep the sinus rate may fall to as low as 30/min with pauses up to 2.8 sec in the normal situation. Although many authorities agree that spontaneous sinus pauses are abnormal if they exceed 3 sec without intervening escape, the role of permanent pacing in these patients has not been established although some workers feel that such a pause justifies permanent pacemaker insertion in an asymptomatic patient (72,73).

CONGENITAL ATRIOVENTRICULAR BLOCK

The indications for pacing in children are discussed in detail in the ACC/AHA guidelines (1,2). With regard to congenital AV block, at present permanent pacing in *asymptomatic* patients is recommended in the following situations (74,75): (a) mean daytime junctional rate of less than 50/min, (b) poor response of ventricular rate on exercise, (c) sudden prolongation of RR interval due to high-degree AV block during sleep, (d) cardiomegaly, (e) depressed left ventricular function detected echocardiographically, (f) electrocardiographic evidence of atrial enlargement, (g) pacing should be strongly considered in the presence of a prolonged QRS complex (or block below the His bundle) or prolongation of the corrected QT interval, or frequent multiformic or repetitive ventricular ectopy.

CAROTID SINUS SYNDROME AND NEURALLY MEDIATED (VASOVAGAL) SYNCOPE (Table 14.5)

Carotid Sinus Syndrome

In the carotid sinus syndrome, patients with dominant cardioinhibitory reflex response (slowing of sinus rate and/or prolongation of AV conduction with AV block) benefit from permanent pacing. Single-lead atrial pacing (AAI mode) is contraindicated because it offers no protection against reflex AV block which may occur in up to 70% of patients with carotid sinus syndrome (76,77). In patients with cardioinhibitory and vasodepressor type of carotid sinus syndrome, pacing prevents syncope due to ventricular asystole or bradycardia, but not neurologic symptoms

Table 14.5.
ACC/AHA 1991 Guidelines—Indications for Permanent Pacing in Hypersensitive Carotid Sinus and Neurovascular Syndromes

Class I

A. Recurrent syncope associated with clear spontaneous events provoked by carotid sinus stimulation; minimal carotid sinus pressure induces asystole of >3 sec duration in the absence of any medication that depresses the sinus node or AV conduction

Class II

A. Recurrent syncope without clear, provocative events and with a hypersensitive cardioinhibitory response
B. Syncope with associated bradycardia reproduced by a head-up tilt with or without isoproterenol or other forms of provocative maneuvers and in which a temporary pacemaker and a second provocative test can establish the likely benefits of a permanent pacemaker

Class III

A. A hyperactive cardioinhibitory response to carotid sinus stimulation in the absence of symptoms
B. Vague symptoms, such as dizziness or lightheadedness, or both, with a hyperactive cardioinhibitory response to carotid sinus stimulation
C. Recurrent syncope, lightheadedness, or dizziness in the absence of a cardioinhibitory response

due to reflex hypotension. Some workers have reported good results with VVI pacing in carefully selected patients with an isolated cardioinhibitory component of carotid sinus syndrome (78–80) while others have observed poor tolerance and persistent symptoms with VVI pacing (76,77,81–83). Patients with a large vasodepressor response are especially at risk of episodic hypotension following VVI pacing. In patients with mixed cardioinhibitory and vasodepressor form of carotid sinus syndrome, VVI pacing is contraindicated and a dual-chamber device should be used. In predominant vasodepressor syncope, even dual-chamber pacing may not abolish symptoms. Most workers now recommend dual-chamber pacing with the DDI mode, preferably with hysteresis (77,79,82–87).

Neurally Mediated Syncope

Neurally mediated syncope refers to tilt induced (malignant) vasovagal syncope (88,89). Many patients with this syndrome develop profound bradycardia, and there is always a major component of vasodilatation in contradistinction to some forms of carotid sinus syndromes. Symptomatic relief by temporary pacing during tilt table testing shows promise as a predictive test for symptomatic control via implanted dual-chamber pacemakers with hysteresis (90,91). Kenny, *et al.* (92) first reported in 1986 the benefit of dual-chamber pacemakers in neurally mediated syncope, but permanent pacing for this condition is still controversial (93). However, Morgan, *et al.* (94) recently reported the beneficial effects of dual-chamber pacing for the treatment of cardioinhibitory malignant vasovagal syndrome in a large group of patients and found that symptoms were abolished or considerably ameliorated in 92% of patients who received mostly DDI pacemakers with hysteresis.

CARDIOMYOPATHY

Several recent studies suggest that dual-chamber pacing may be effective therapy for the treatment of hypertrophic obstructive cardiomyopathy (HOCM) resistant to pharmacologic therapy (95–100). These studies (in patients not requiring a pacemaker for the treatment of bradycardia) have demonstrated that in most patients DDD pacing with a *short* AV interval (AV = 50–150 msec and often less than 100 msec) causes significant long-term improvement in exercise capacity and reduction of symptoms (angina and dyspnea) in association with diminution of the left ventricular outflow tract gradient. Recently, Hochleitner *et al.* (101) also reported the beneficial effects of DDD pacing (short AV interval of 100 msec) in the treatment of end-stage idiopathic dilated cardiomyopathy in 16 patients without AV block in whom conventional drug therapy had failed. There was striking improvement in such symptoms as severe dyspnea at rest and pulmonary edema, as well as significant decrease in the New York Heart Association Class. DDD pacing actually increased left ventricular ejection fraction, reduced left atrial and right atrial size, and reduced the cardiothoracic ratio. The short AV interval appears to reduce mitral regurgitation and improve left ventricular filling (102,103).

References

1. Frye RL, Collins JJ, DeSanctis RW, *et al.*: Guidelines for permanent cardiac pacemaker implantation, May 1984. A report of the Joint American College of Cardiology/American Heart Association task force on assessment of cardiovascular procedures (Subcommittee on pacemaker implantation). J Am Coll Cardiol 1988;11:1882.
2. Dreifus LS, Gillette PC, Fisch C, *et al.*: Guidelines for Implantation of Cardiac Pacemakers and Antiarrhythmia Devices. A report of the American College of Cardiology/American Heart Association Task Force on Assessment of Diagnostic and Therapeutic Cardiovascular Procedures (Committee on Pacemaker Implantation). J Am Coll Cardiol 1991;18:1.
3. WHO/ISC Task Force. Definition of terms related to cardiac rhythm. Am Heart J 1978;95:796.
4. Surawicz B, Uhley H, Borun R, *et al.*: Optimal electrocardiography, Tenth Bethesda Conference Co-sponsored by the American College of Cardiology and the Health Resources Administration of the Department of Health, Education and Welfare Task Force. I. Standardization of terminology and interpretation. Am J Cardiol 1978;41:130.
5. Barold SS, Friedberg HD: Second degree atrioventricular block. A matter of definition. Am J Cardiol 1974;33:311.
6. Zipes DP, Gettes LS, Akhtar M, *et al.*: Guidelines for Clinical Intracardiac Electrophysiologic Studies. A report of the American College of Cardiology/American Heart Association Task Force on assessment of diagnostic and therapeutic cardiovascular procedures (subcommittee to assess clinical intracardiac electrophysiologic studies). J Am Coll Cardiol 1989;14:1827.
7. Puech P, Wainwright RJ: Clinical electrophysiology of atrioventricular block. Cardiol Clin 1983;1:209.
8. Ward DE, Camm AJ: Clinical Electrophysiology of the Heart. Edward Arnold, London, 1987.
9. Homey CJ: Atrioventricular block. In Eagle KA, Haber E, DeSanctis RW, *et*

al. (eds): The Practice of Cardiology, 2nd ed., Little, Brown, Boston, 1989: 267.
10. Mymin D, Mathewson FAL, Tate RB, *et al.*: The natural history of primary first-degree atrioventricular heart block. N Engl J Med 1986;315:1183.
11. Strasberg B, Amat-Y-Leon F, Dhingra RC, *et al.*: Natural history of chronic second-degree atrioventricular nodal block. Circulation 1981;63:1043.
12. Dhingra RC, Denes P, Wu D, *et al.*: The significance of second degree atrioventricular block and bundle branch block. Observations regarding site and type of block, Circulation 1974;49:638.
13. Shaw DB, Kerwick CA, Veale D, *et al.*: Survival in second degree atrioventricular block. Br Heart J 1985;53:587.
14. Clarke M, Sutton R, Ward D, *et al.*: Recommendations for pacemaker prescription for symptomatic bradycardia. Br Heart J 1991;66:185.
15. Gupta PK, Lichstein E, Chadda KD: Heart block complicating acute inferior wall myocardial infarction. Chest 1976;69:599.
16. Nicod P, Gilpin E, Dittrich H, *et al.*: Long-term outcome in patients with inferior myocardial infarction and complete atrioventricular block. J Am Coll Cardiol 1988;12:589.
17. Tans AC, Lie KI, Durrer D: Clinical setting and prognostic significance of high degree antrioventricular block in acute inferior wall myocardial infarction: a study of 144 patients. Am Heart J 1980;99:4.
18. Kaul U, Haran VH, Malhotra A, *et al.*: Significance of advanced atrioventricular block in acute inferior wall myocardial infarction. A study based on ventricular function and Holter monitoring. Int J Cardiol 1986;11:187.
19. Codini MA: Conduction disturbances in acute myocardial infarction. The use of pacemaker therapy. Clin Prog Pacing Electrophysiol 1983;1:142.
20. Constans R, Marco J, Berthoumieu H, *et al.*: Devenir des infarctus du myocarde compliqués en phase aigue de troubles de la conduction. Arch Mal Coeur 1979;72:957.
21. Dubois C, Piérard LA, Smeets JP, *et al.*: Long term prognostic significance of atrioventricular block in inferior acute myocardial infarction. Eur Heart J 1989;10:816.
22. Lie KI, Durrer D: Indications for temporary and permanent pacing in ischemic conduction disturbances. In Samet P, El-Sherif N (eds): Cardiac Pacing, 2nd ed., Grune & Stratton, New York, 1980:459.
23. Rosenfeld LE: Bradyarrhythmias, abnormalities of conduction, and indications for pacing in acute myocardial infarction. Cardiol Clin 1988;6:49.
24. Sobrino JA, delRio A, Maté L, *et al.*: Anterograde and retrograde bradycardic block in the His-Purkinje system. Finding in a patient with acute myocardial infarction. Chest 1978;73:109.
25. Scheinman MM, Gonzalez RP: Fascicular block and acute myocardial infarction. JAMA 1980;244:2646.
26. Barold SS: Narrow QRS-Mobitz type II second degree AV block in acute myocardial infarction. True or false? Am J Cardiol 1991;68:1291.
27. Haft JI: Clinical implications of atrioventricular and intraventricular conduction abnormalties. II. Acute myocardial infarction. Cardiovasc Clin 1977;8:65.
28. Schamroth L: The Disorders of Cardiac Rhythms. 2nd ed. Blackwell Scientific Publications, St. Louis, 1980.
29. Silber EN: Heart Disease, 2nd ed., Macmillan, New York, 1987.
30. Lamas GA, Muller JE, Turi ZG, *et al.*: A simplified method to predict occurrence of complete heart block during acute myocardial infarction, Am J Cardiol 1986;57:1213.
31. Hayes DL: Indications for permanent pacing. In Furman S, Hayes DL, Holmes DR (eds): A Practice of Cardiac Pacing, 2nd ed. Futura Publishing Co., Mt. Kisco, NY, 1989:3.
32. Silver MD, Goldschlager N: Temporary transvenous cardiac pacing in the critical care setting, Chest 1988;93:607.
33. Alpert JS: Conduction disturbances: Temporary and permanent pacing in patients with acute myocardial infarction. In Gersh B, Rahimtoola SH (eds): Acute Myocardial Infarction, Elsevier, New York, 1991: 249.
34. Hindman MC, Wagner GS, Jaro M, *et al.*: The clinical significance of bundle branch block. 2. Indications for temporary and permanent pacemaker insertion, Circulation 1978;58:639.
35. Nauer R, Lie KI, Liem KL, *et al.*: Long term prognosis in patients with bundle branch block complicating acute anteroseptal infarction. Br. Heart J 1984;52:408.
36. Edhag O, Berfeldt L, Edvardsson N, *et al.*: Pacemaker dependence in patients with bifascicular block during acute anterior myocardial infarction. Br Heart J 1984;52:408.
37. Klein RC, Vera Z, Mason DT: Intraventricular conduction defects in acute myocardial infarction: Incidence, prognosis, and therapy. Am Heart J 1984;108:1007.
38. Murphy E, DeMots H, McAnulty J, *et al.*: Prophylactic permanent pacemakers for transient heart block during myocardial infarction? Results of a prospective study. Am J Cardiol 1982;49:952.
39. Talwar KK, Kalra GS, Dogra B, *et al.*: Prophylactic permanent pacemaker implantation in patients with anterior wall myocardial infarction complicated by bundle branch block and transient AV block. A prospective long term study. Indian Heart J 1987;39:22.
40. Roos JC, Dunning AJ: Bundle branch block, Eur J Cardiol 1978;6:403.
41. Grigg L, Pitt A, Kertes P, *et al.*: The role of permanent pacing after anterior myocardial infarction complicated by transient atrioventricular block. Aust NZ J Med 1988;18:685.
42. Barold SS, Falkoff MD, Ong LS, *et al.*: Atrioventricular block: New insights In Barold SS, Mugica J (eds): New Perspectives in Cardiac Pacing, 2. Futura Publishing Co., Mt. Kisco, NY, 1991:23.
43. Dhingra RC, Wyndham C, Bauerfeind R, *et al.*: Significance of block distal to the His bundle induced by atrial pacing in patients with chronic bifascicular block. Circulation 1979;60:1455.
44. Damato AN, Varghese PJ, Caracta AR, *et al.*: Functional 2:1 AV block within the His-Purkinje system. Simulation of type II second-degree AV block. Circulation 1973;47:534.
45. Young ML, Gelband H, Castellanos A: Rapid atrial pacing-induced infra-His conduction block in children. Am Heart J 1985;110:652.
46. McAnulty JH, Rahimtoola SH, Murphy E, *et al.*: Natural history of "high-risk" bundle branch block. Final report of prospective study. N Engl J Med 1982;307:137.
47. Scheinman MM, Peters RW, Morady F, *et al.*: Electrophysiologic studies in patients with bundle branch block. PACE 1983;6:1157.
48. Click RL, Gersh BJ, Sugrue DD, *et al.*: Role of invasive electrophysiologic testing in patients with symptomatic bundle branch block. Am J Cardiol 1987;59:817.
49. Bakst A, Goldberg B. Schamroth L: Significance of exercise induced second degree AV block. Br Heart J 1975;37:984.
50. Kalusche D, Roskamm H: Tachycardia-dependent second degree AV block in a patient with right bundle branch block. J Electrocardiol 1987;20:169.
51. Woelfel AK, Simpson RJ, Gettes LS, *et al.*: Exercise induced distal atrioventricular block. J Am Coll Cardiol 1983;2:578.
52. Freeman G, Hwang MH, Danoviz J, *et al.*: Exercise induced "Mobitz type II" second degree AV block in a patient with chronic bifascicular block (right bundle branch block and left anterior hemiblock). J Electrocardiol 1984;17:409.
53. Peller OG, Moses JW, Kligfield P: Exercise-induced atrioventricular block: Report of three cases. Am Heart J 1988;115:1315.
54. Donzeau JP, Dechandol AM, Bergeal A, *et al.*: Blocs auriculo-ventriculaires survenant à l'effort: considerations générales à propos de 14 cas. Coeur 1985;15:513.
55. Petrač D, Gjurović J, Vukosavić D, *et al.*: Clinical significance and natural history of exercise-induced atrioventricular block. In Belhassen B, Feldman S, Copperman Y (eds): Cardiac Pacing and Electrophysiology, Proceedings of the VIIIth World Symposium on Cardiac Pacing and Electrophysiology. R&L Creative Communications, Jerusalem, Israel, 1987:265.
56. Paillard F, Mabo P, BenSlimane A, *et al.*: Les blocs auriculoventriculaire desmasqués à l'épreuve d'effort. Ann Cardiol Angeiol 1990;39:55.
57. Chokshi SK, Sarmiento J, Nazari J, *et al.*: Exercise-provoked distal atrioventricular block. Am J Cardiol 1990;66:114.
58. Dhingra RC, Palileo E, Strasberg B, *et al.*: Significance of the HV interval

in 517 patients with chronic bifascicular block. Circulation 1981;64: 1265.

59. Morady F, Higgins J, Peters RW, *et al.*: Electrophysiologic testing in bundle branch block and unexplained syncope. Am J Cardiol 1984;54:587.
60. Kaul U, Dev V, Narula J, *et al.*: Evaluation of patients with bundle branch block and "unexplained" syncope. A study based on comprehensive electrophysiologic testing and ajmaline stress. PACE 1988;11:289.
61. DiLorenzo DR, Sellers D: Fatigue of the His-Purkinje system during routine electrophysiologic studies. PACE 1988;11:263.
62. Takahashi N, Gilmour RF, Zipes DP: Overdrive suppression of conduction in the canine His-Purkinje system after occlusion of the anterior septal artery. Circulation 1984;70:495.
63. Wellens HJJ, Brugada P, Stevenson WG: Programmed electrical stimulation. Its role in the management of ventricular arrhythmias in coronary artery disease. Prog Cardiovasc Dis 1986;29:165.
64. Ezri M, Lerman BB, Marchlinski FE, *et al.*: Electrophysiologic evaluation of syncope in patients with bifascicular block. Am Heart J 1983;106:693.
65. Krol RB, Morady F, Flaker GC, *et al.*: Electrophysiologic testing in patients with unexplained syncope. Clinical and noninvasive predictors of outcome. J Am Coll Cardiol 1987;10:358.
66. Denes P, Uretz E, Ezri MD, *et al.*: Clinical predictors of electrophysiologic findings in patients with syncope of unknown etiology. Arch Intern Med 1988;148:1922.
67. Doherty JV, Penbrook-Rogers D, Grogan EW, *et al.*: Electrophysiologic evaluation and follow-up characteristics of patients with recurrent unexplained syncope and presyncope. Am J Cardiol 1985;55:703.
68. DiMarco JP. Electrophysiologic studies in patients with unexplained syncope. Circulation 1987;75 (Suppl III):140.
69. Bass EB, Elson JJ, Fogoros RN, *et al.*: Long-term prognosis of patients undergoing electrophysiologic studies for syncope of unknown origin. Am J Cardiol 1988;62:1186.
70. Fujimura O, Yee R, Klein GR, *et al.*: The diagnostic sensitivity of electrophysiologic testing in patients with syncope caused by transient bradycardia. N Engl J Med 1989;321:1703.
71. Narula OS: Clinical concepts of spontaneous and induced atrioventricular block. In Mandel WJ (ed): Cardiac Arrhythmias. Their Mechanisms, Diagnosis, and Management, 2nd ed., JB Lippincott, Philadelphia, 1987:321.
72. Ector H, Rolies L, DeGeest H: Dynamic electrocardiography and ventricular pauses of 3 seconds and more: etiology and therapeutic implications. PACE 1983;6:548.
73. Hilgard J, Ezri MD, Denes P: Significance of ventricular pauses of three seconds or more detected on twenty-four Holter recordings. Am J Cardiol 1985;55:1005.
74. Dewey RC, Capeless MA, Levy AM: Use of ambulatory electrocardiographic monitoring to identify high-risk patients with congenital complete heart block. N Engl J Med 1987;316:835.
75. Sholler GF, Walsh EP: Congenital complete heart block in patients without anatomic cardiac defects. Am Heart J 1989;118:1193.
76. Strasberg B, Sagie A, Erdman S, *et al.*: Carotid sinus hypersensitivity and the carotid sinus syndrome. Prog Cardiovasc Dis 1989;5:379.
77. Morley CA, Sutton R: Carotid sinus syndrome. Int J Cardiol 1984;6:287.
78. Stryjer D, Friedensohn A, Schlesinger Z: Ventricular pacing as the preferable mode for long-term pacing in patients with carotid sinus syncope of the cardioinhibitory type. PACE 1986;9:705.
79. Menozzi C, Brignole M, Pagani P, *et al.*: Assessment of VVI diagnostic pacing mode in patients with cardioinhibitory carotid sinus syndrome. PACE 1988;11:1641.
80. Brignole M, Menozzi C, Lolli G: Validation of a method for choice of pacing in carotid sinus syndrome with or without sinus bradycardia. PACE 1991;14:196.
81. Torresani J, Ebagosti A, Aubran M, *et al.*: Carotid sinus syndrome. Single or dual pacing. In Perez Gomez R (ed): Cardiac Pacing; Electrophysiology. Tachyarrhythmias. Edition Grouz, Madrid, 1985:243.
82. Madigan NP, Flaker GC, Curtis JJ, *et al.*: Carotid sinus hypersensitivity. Beneficial effects of dual chamber pacing. Am J Cardiol 1984;53: 1034.
83. Morley CA, Perrins EJ, Grant P, *et al.*: Carotid sinus syndrome treated by pacing. Analysis of persistent symptoms and role of atrioventricular sequential pacing. Br Heart J 1982;47:411.
84. Ahmed R, Guneri S, Ingram A, *et al.*: Double blind comparison of DDI, DDI with rate hysteresis, VVI, and VVI with rate hysteresis in symptom control in carotid sinus syndrome. PACE 1991;(Part II):623.
85. Sutton R, Ingram A, Clarke M: DDI pacing in the treatment of sick sinus, carotid sinus, and vasovagal syndromes. PACE 1988;11:827.
86. Griebenow R, Kramer L, Bartels S: Therapeutic decisions in carotid sinus syndrome. PACE 1991;14 (Part II):692.
87. Morley CA, Perrins EJ, Chan SL, *et al.*: The role of rate hysteresis pacing in the hypersensitive carotid sinus syndrome. PACE 1983;6:1224.
88. Milstein S, Reyes WJ, Benditt DG: Upright body tilt for evaluation of patients with recurrent unexplained syncope. PACE 1989;12:117.
89. Milstein S, Buetikofer J, Lesser J, *et al.*: Cardiac asystole: a manifestation of neurally mediated hypotension-bradycardia. J Am Coll Cardiol 1989;14:1626.
90. Fitzpatrick A, Theodorakis G, Ahmed R, *et al.*: Dual chamber pacing aborts vasovagal syncope induced by head-up 60° tilt. PACE 1991;13:13.
91. McGuinn P, Moore S, Edel T, *et al.*: Temporary dual chamber pacing during tilt table testing for vasovagal syncope. A predictor of therapeutic success, PACE 1991;14 (Part II):734.
92. Kenny RA, Ingram A, Bayliss J, *et al.*: Head-up tilt: a useful test for investigating unexplained syncope. Lancet 1986;1:1352.
93. Sra J, Dhala A, Shen HY, *et al.*: Efficacy of atrioventricular pacing in preventing hypotension in patients with significant bradycardia or asystole during head up tilt table. Circulation 1991;84 (Suppl. II):II-234.
94. Morgan JM, Amer AS, Ingram A, *et al.*: Diagnosis and treatment of vasovagal syndrome, PACE 1991;14 (Part II):667.
95. McDonald KM, Maurer B: Permanent pacing as treatment for hypertrophic cardiomyopathy. Am J Cardiol 1991;68:108.
96. Erwin J, McWilliams E, Gearty G, *et al.*: Haemodynamic assessment of dual chamber pacing in hypertrophic cardiomyopathy using radionuclide ventriculography. Br Heart J 1986;55:507.
97. McDonald K, McWilliams E, O'Keeffe B, *et al.*: Functional assessment of patients treated with permanent dual chamber pacing as a primary treatment for hypertrophic caridomyopathy. Eur Heart J 1988;9:893.
98. Ovadia M, Clynne C, Tripodi D, *et al.*: Dual chamber permanent pacing is an alternative to surgery in hypertrophic cardiomyopathy with severe left ventricular outflow obstruction. Circulation 1990;82:III-333.
99. Kappenberger L, Jeanrenaud X, Vogt P, *et al.*: Pacemaker treatment of hypertrophic obstructive cardiomyopathy (HOCM). Acute and longterm efficacy. PACE 1991;14 (Part II):668.
100. Fananapazir L, Cannon RO, Tripodi D, *et al.*: Dual chamber pacing is an alternative to cardiac surgery in hypertrophic patients with symptoms refractory to medical therapy. Circulation 1991;84 (Suppl II):II-326.
101. Hochleitner M, Hörtnagl H, Ng CK, *et al.*: Usefulness of physiologic dual chamber pacing in drug-resistant idiopathic dilated cardiomyopathy. Am J Cardiol 1990;66:198.
102. Kataoza H: Hemodynamic effect of physiological dual chamber pacing in a patient with end-stage dilated cardiomyopathy: a case report. PACE 1991;14:1330.
103. Iskandrian A: Pacemaker therapy in congestive heart failure. Am J Cardiol 1990;66:223.

15

SINGLE- AND DUAL-CHAMBER PACEMAKERS: ELECTROPHYSIOLOGY, PACING MODES AND MULTIPROGRAMMABILITY

S. Serge Barold, M.B., B.S., F.R.A.C.P., F.A.C.P., F.A.C.C., F.E.S.C.

A *pacemaker* is a battery-operated device that delivers electrical stimuli to the heart. The *lead* is the component of the pacing system that connects the pulse generator to the heart. There are two types of pacemaker leads: (a) unipolar with only one electrode (cathode) in the heart. The other electrode (anode) is situated on the pacemaker can; (b) bipolar with two electrodes in the heart (the tip is usually the cathode). All leads serve as two-way conductors for (a) delivery of the electrical impulse to the heart and (b) detection of spontaneous electrical activity from the heart (electrogram, i.e, intracardiac electrocardiogram (ECG)) and transmission of the sensed signal to the pacemaker.

The first pacemaker was implanted in 1958, and over 30 yr later cardiac pacing continues its spectacular and accelerated growth as a high-tech specialty (1, 2). Few fields in medicine have evolved so rapidly. In the United States there are now more than 500,000 patients living with implanted pacemakers. In the last few years, major advances in pacemaker technology (3–6) have fostered a large array of pulse generators with a variety of functions that must be understood if these devices are to be used wisely (7, 8). Selection of the optimum pacing device or mode for the individual patient requires knowledge of pacemaker technology, cardiac electrophysiology, and hemodynamics. In the nineties, the aim of permanent antibradycardia pacing should be to (a) restore normal or near normal hemodynamics at rest and exercise rather than simply the prevention of symptoms due to bradycardia and (b) change favorably the natural history of the condition requiring pacing, especially reduction of certain atrial tachyarrhythmias and their thromboembolic complications related to atrial dysfunction. Selection of the optimal device or pacing mode for the individual patient requires knowledge of the pacemaker code (9) and the operational characteristics of a relatively large number of single- and dual-chamber pacing modes (Table 15.1).

POWER SOURCES

The lithium-iodine battery is the gold standard of pacemaker power sources (10) and remains the only type of lithium battery left, though other obsolete types will remain in service for years, e.g., lithium cupric sulfide. The lithium-iodine battery has a high energy density (energy content/volume), low internal losses caused by self-discharge, a long shelf life, and can be hermetically sealed to prevent ingress of body fluids. The lithium-iodine cell develops a progressive rise in internal impedance that causes a fairly linear drop in cell voltage translated by circuit design into a gradual decline of the pacing rate that reflects the status of the battery. A lithium-iodine battery will retain a satisfactory voltage for 90% of its life. The longevity of the lithium-iodine battery is directly proportional to the useful battery capacity (expressed as ampere-hours (A-hr)) and inversely proportional to the continuous current drain from the battery or circuit (expressed in μA). The life of the battery (years) = capacity/drain. In a single chamber pacemaker with a circuit current drain (not to be confused with the current output in mA. delivered to the lead) of 20 μA (used for pacing and also for internal "housekeeping," i.e., basic functions such as sensing) and a capacity of 2 A-hr, longevity = $2 \times 10^6/20 \times 365$ (days of the yr) $\times$ 24 (hr/day) = 11.42 yr. For single-chamber pulse generators, the expected life should be between 7 and 12 yr and for a DDD pulse generator from 4 to 8 yr depending on programmed parameters, periods of inhibition, etc.

PACEMAKER IMPLANTATION

The Inter-Society Commission for Heart Disease Resources (American Heart Association) has published the optimal resources for implantable cardiac pacemakers (11). In the early days, pacemakers were all implanted epicardially, a route now

Table 15.1.
The NASPE/BPEG Generic Pacemaker Code

Position	I	II	III	IV	V
Category	Chamber(s) Paced	Chamber(s) Sensed	Response to sensing	Programmability, rate modulation	Antitachyarrhythmia function(s)
	0 = none	0 = none	0 = none	0 = none	0 = none
	A = atrium	A = atrium	T = triggered	P = simple programmable	P = pacing (antitachyarrhythmia)
	V = ventricle	V = ventricle	I = inhibited	M = Multiprogrammable	S = shock
	D = dual (A + V)	D = dual (A + V)	D = dual (T + I)	C = communicating	D = dual (P + S)
				R = rate modulation	
Manufacturer's designation only	S = single (A or V)	S = single (A or V)			

Abbreviations: BPEG = British Pacing and Electrophysiology Group; NASPE = North American Society of Pacing and Electrophysiology.

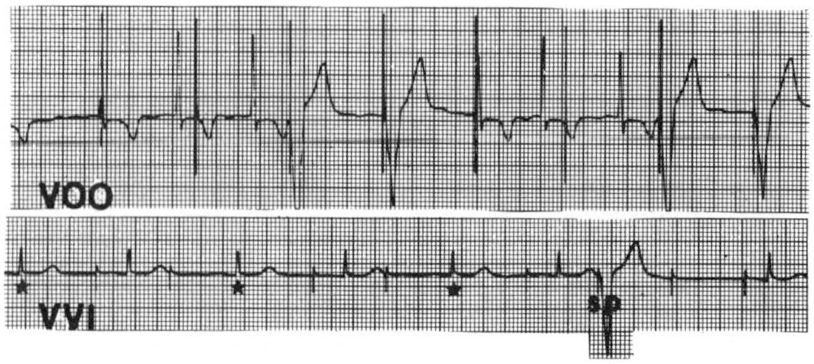

Figure 15.1. Top: VOO pacing. The pacemaker competes with the spontaneous rhythm. Pacemaker stimuli capture the ventricle only beyond the myocardial refractory period. **Bottom:** Supernormal phase. The recording shows a ventricular demand (VVI) pacemaker with ineffectual pacemaker stimuli. The high pacing threshold was close to the output of the pulse generator. The third last stimulus captures the ventricle in the supernormal phase when the excitability threshold attains its lowest value. Spontaneous QRS complexes falling within the pacemaker refractory period (350 msec after the stimulus), are not sensed; those beyond the pacemaker refractory period are sensed and recycle the pacemaker. (Reproduced with permission from Barold SS, Zipes DP: Cardiac pacemakers and antiarrhythmic devices. In Braunwald E (ed): Heart Disease, a Textbook of Cardiovascular Medicine. WB Saunders, Philadelphia, 1991:726.)

utilized in rare cases if there is no venous access, in certain pediatric patients, or in patients undergoing open heart surgery. Virtually all pacemakers are implanted transvenously under local anesthesia using either the cephalic vein exposed by cutdown or blind percutaneous puncture of the subclavian vein. Pacing leads and implantation techniques are discussed elsewhere in this book (Chapter 13).

PACEMAKER CODE

Pacemakers are categorized according to the site of pacing electrodes and the mode of pacing (9) (Table 15.1). The letters in the identification code are few and easy to remember: V = ventricle, A = atrium, D = double (A and V), I = inhibited, T = triggered, and 0 = none. The first position denotes the chamber(s) paced. The second position indicates the chamber(s) sensed. The third position describes the response to sensing, if any, with "I" response indicating an inhibited response (output suppressed by a sensed signal), "T" indicating a triggered response (output discharged by a sensed signal, either P or QRS), and "D" indicating both inhibited and triggered functions. Both I and T responses reset the timing circuit. In the third position, "0" indicates that the pulse generator is not influenced by cardiac events because it does not sense. Therefore, when the third position is zero, the second one must always be zero, and vice versa. Occasionally the letter "S" is used in the first and second positions to indicate that a single-chamber unit is suitable for either atrial or ventricular pacing, depending on how its parameters are programmed. For most pacemakers, the first three positions contain all the information of practical importance. The fourth and fifth positions describe additional functions, but the letters are infrequently stated in practice except for "R" which indicates a rate-adaptive, sensor-driven pulse generator.

OPERATIONAL CHARACTERISTICS OF SINGLE-CHAMBER PACEMAKERS

Asynchronous AOO and VOO Modes

In the AOO and VOO modes, pacemaker stimuli are generated at a fixed rate with no relationship to the spontaneous rhythm. During VOO pacing, stimuli will capture the ventricles only when they fall outside the ventricular refractory period following spontaneous beats (Fig. 15.1). Ventricular fibrillation induced by a pacemaker stimulus falling in the ventricular vulnerable period is extremely rare (12,13) outside of circumstances such as myocardial ischemia or infarction, electrolyte abnormalities, or autonomic imbalance. VOO pacemakers were popular in the early days of pacing because of electronic simplicity and they worked remarkably well in preventing symptoms of bradycardia. Dedicated VOO or other asynchronous pacemakers (that cannot sense) are now obsolete. However, asynchronous modes are often used temporarily during pacemaker testing when a special magnet is applied over the device. The asynchronous mode can occasionally be used for competitive pacing in the treatment of reentrant tachycardias. Rarely a multiprogrammable pacemaker is permanently programmed to the asynchronous mode to prevent undesirable oversensing.

VVI Mode

In the early 1970s, sensing circuits were added to ventricular pacemakers to allow stimulation only on demand when the sensing circuit detects no underlying ventricular activity (Fig. 15.2). The pacemaker senses the *intracardiac* ventricular depolarization or electrogram, i.e., the potential difference between the two electrodes (anode and cathode) also utilized for pacing. A VVI pacemaker programmed to a predetermined rate of 70/min will pace with a cycle length of 857 msec whenever the spontaneous rate falls below 70/min or the RR interval lengthens beyond 857 msec. The timing cycle (or internal clock) of a VVI pulse generator begins with either a sensed or paced ventricular event. The initial portion of the cycle consists of a refractory period (usually 200–350 msec) during which the pulse generator is insensitive to any signals. The refractory period prevents the pulse generator from sensing its own stimulus, the paced or spontaneous QRS complex, T waves, and the decaying residual voltage (polarization or afterpotential) at the electrode-myocardial interface due to an electrochemical process (14–16). Beyond the pacemaker refractory period, a sensed event inhibits and resets the pacemaker so that its timing clock returns to the baseline: a new pacing cycle is initiated and the output circuit remains inhibited for a period equal to the programmed pacemaker (or lower rate) interval (Fig. 15.2). If no signal is sensed, the timing cycle ends with the delivery of a ventricular stimulus and a new cycle is started. The sensing function prevents competition between pacemaker and intrinsic rhythm and conserves battery capacity.

AAI Mode

AAI pacing may be used for patients with sick sinus syndrome and intact atrioventricular (AV) conduction. The AAI mode is identical to the VVI mode except that it paces the atrium and senses atrial electrical activity. AAI pacemakers differ from VVI ones in two respects: (a) they need a greater sensitivity because the atrial electrogram is considerably smaller than the ventricular one, (b) the pacemaker refractory period should be longer (≥400 msec) to prevent sensing of the "far-field" ventricular electrogram (registered by the atrial lead) that may cause inappropriate inhibition of the pacemaker (17) (Fig. 15.3).

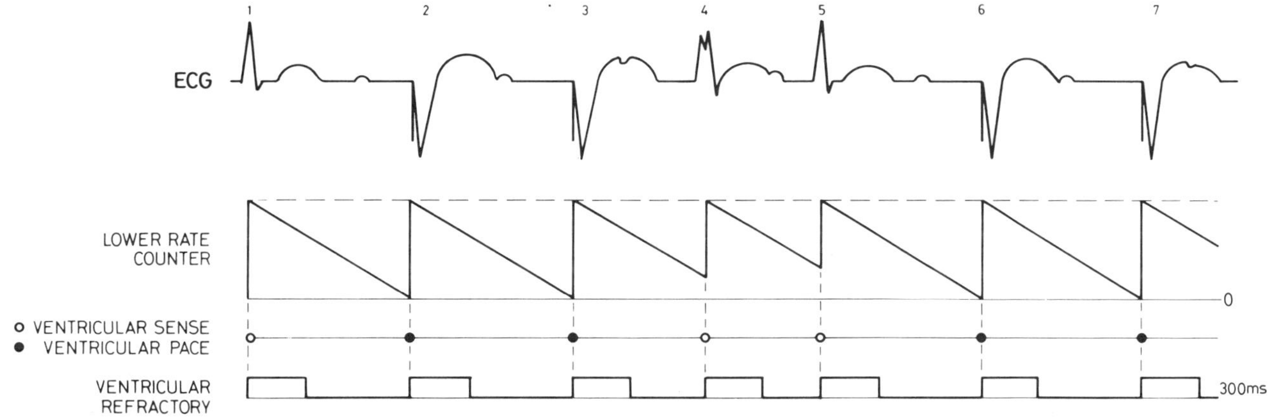

Figure 15.2. Diagrammatic representation of the VVI mode of pacing (rate = 80 ppm). The QRS marked 1 is sensed. Beats 2 and 3 are paced complexes. A ventricular extrasystole (4) and a normal QRS (5) are then sensed. The sixth and seventh beats are paced. The pacemaker ventricular refractory period (300 msec) is shown by a *rectangle*. Complexes 4 and 5 reset and start the lower rate counter before the zero level has been reached, i.e., before completion of the escape or automatic interval. The pacemaker emits its stimulus only from the zero level. (Reproduced with permission from Lindemans PW: Diagrammatic representation of pacemaker function in Barold SS (ed): Modern Cardiac Pacing. Mt. Kisco, NY, Futura Publishing Co., 1985:323.)

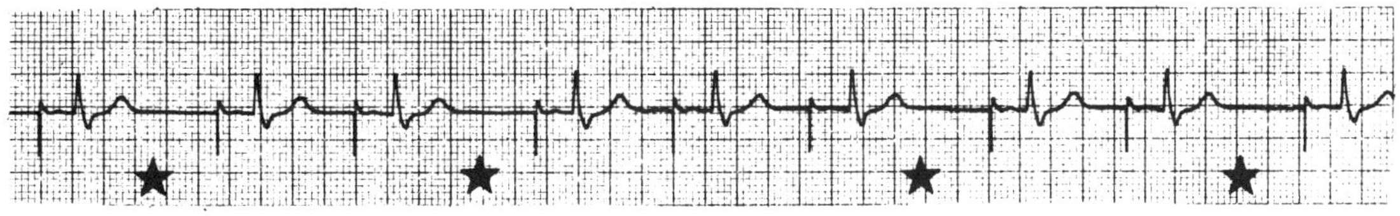

Figure 15.3. AAI pacemaker, rate = 70/min (automatic interval = 857 msec) and refractory period = 250 msec. There is intermittent prolongation of the interstimulus interval because the atrial lead senses the far-field QRS complex just beyond the 250 msec pacemaker refractory period. When the refractory period was programmed to 400 msec the irregularity disappeared with restoration of regular atrial pacing at a rate of 70/min. (Reproduced with permission from Barold SS, Zipes DP: Cardiac pacemakers and antiarrhythmic devices. In Braunwald E (ed): Heart Disease, a Textbook of Cardiovascular Medicine. WB Saunders, Philadelphia, 1992:726.)

VVT Mode

In the VVT mode, a sensed ventricular event causes immediate release or triggering of a pacemaker stimulus. The VVT mode therefore requires three timing intervals: lower rate interval, upper rate interval, and refractory period (RP). In many simple VVT designs, the pacemaker RP determines the maximal pacing rate according to the formula: upper rate (ppm) = 60/RP (sec). On sensing a QRS complex, a VVT pacemaker discharges its stimulus during the absolute refractory period of the ventricular myocardium (Fig. 15.4, bottom strip). Such ineffectual stimulation wastes battery capacity and distorts the ECG. As in the VVI mode, if no QRS is sensed during the lower rate interval (LRI), the pacemaker delivers its impulse at the completion of the LRI. Dedicated single-mode VVT (AAT) pulse generators are now obsolete, but in the early days of pacing they constituted important systems because they prevented prolonged pacemaker inhibition (exhibited by unsophisticated VVI pacing systems) secondary to detection of extraneous or electromagnetic interference. The triggered VVT mode therefore ensures stimulation (i.e., prevents inhibition) whenever the pulse generator senses signals other than the QRS complex.

The triggered function is generally available in contemporary single- and dual-chamber pacemakers as a programmable mode for either temporary or permanent use. In the temporary VVT (AAT) mode, the capability of triggering an implanted pacemaker by the application of chest wall stimuli (generating signals for sensing) from an external pacemaker (Fig. 15.5) provides a way of performing noninvasive electrophysiologic studies or terminating reentrant tachycardias by appropriately timed stimuli or burst pacing (18–20). The temporary VVT or AAT mode may also delineate the presence and exact time of sensing by "marking" the sensed signal with a stimulus, a function useful in the diagnosis of oversensing spurious signals (invisible on the surface electrocardiogram) generated by a fractured or defective lead (17). Rarely, the VVT (AAT) mode is used to prevent inhibition of a unipolar pulse generator by myopotentials (musculoskeletal electrical activity originating near the anodal electrode on the pacemaker case) when programming of sensitivity cannot correct the problem without compromising QRS (or P) sensing (15). In the VVT mode, a unipolar pulse generator will increase its pacing rate on sensing myopotentials, a better tradeoff than ventricular inhibition.

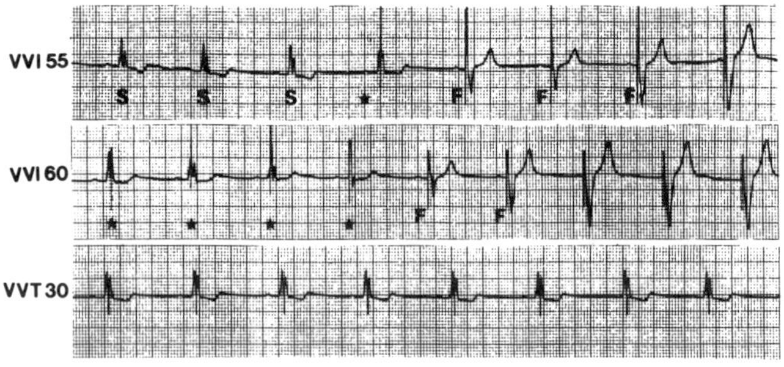

Figure 15.4. Top: VVI pacemaker at a rate of 55/min. The first three beats are sensed, and the fourth beat (star) is a pseudofusion beat (i.e, superimposition of a pacemaker stimulus on the surface QRS complex because the *intracardiac* ventricular electrogram registered by the pacing lead has not yet developed sufficient amplitude to inhibit the pacemaker output). The fifth, sixth, and seventh complexes are ventricular fusion beats (F). **Middle:** VVI pacemaker at a rate of 60/min. The first three beats (*stars*) are pseudofusion beats. The fourth beat (*star*) appears to be a pseudofusion beat because the initial QRS vector occurs just before the stimulus. Note that in beat 4 the T wave is identical to that of the previous beats, suggesting that depolarization was also identical. The fifth and sixth complexes are fusion beats (F) while the last three beats are pure ventricular paced beats. **Bottom:** Same patient as above. The pacemaker was programmed to the VVT mode, rate = 30/min. The pacemaker emits a stimulus immediately on sensing each QRS complex. Thus a stimulus marks the precise time of sensing in the VVT mode. This may be correlated with the pseudofusion beats in the middle tracing where the first pseudofusion beat is deformed by a stimulus just before the R wave returns to the baseline, i.e., just before sensing would have occurred as determined from the VVT mode in the lower tracing. (Reproduced with permission from Barold SS, Zipes DP: Cardiac Pacemakers and Antiarrhythmic Devices. In Braunwald E (ed): Heart Disease, A Textbook of Cardiovascular Medicine. WB Saunders, Philadelphia, 1992:726.)

SINGLE-CHAMBER PACEMAKERS: INTERVALS AND RATES

There are several basic intervals or rates in single-chamber pacemakers. The *automatic interval* is the period between two

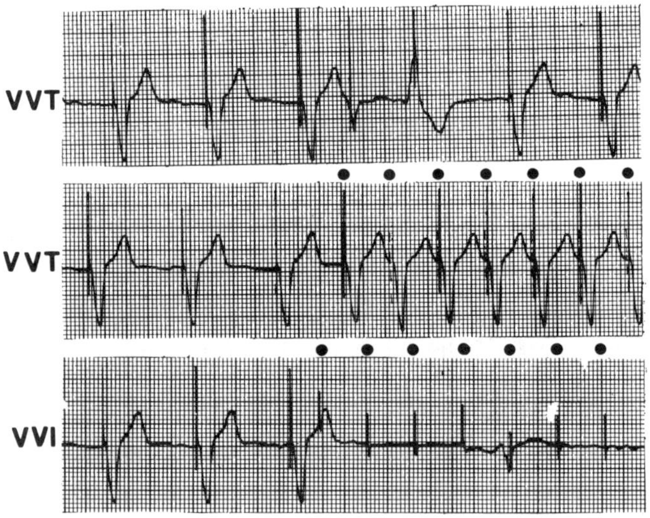

Figure 15.5. VVI pacemaker programmed to the VVT mode, rate = 70/min. **Top:** there are two sensed ventricular extrasystoles, both deformed by ventricular stimuli. **Middle:** VVT mode. Chest wall stimulation (*solid black circles*) delivered from an external pacemaker (to electrodes on the chest) provides signals detected by the implanted VVT pacemaker which therefore discharges its stimuli in synchrony with the sensed signals. This leads to an increase in the rate of ventricular pacing equal to the rate of chest wall stimulation. **Bottom:** Same patient. The pacemaker was reprogrammed back to the VVI mode, rate = 70/min. Chest wall stimulation at the same rate and amplitude as in the **middle tracing** now causes inhibition with the emergence of a slow spontaneous rhythm.

consecutive stimuli during continuous pacing and corresponds to the programmed freerunning or lower rate. The *escape interval* is measured in the electrocardiogram for the sake of simplicity from the onset of the sensed QRS complex (or other signal) to the succeeding pacemaker stimulus. In the case of a VVI pulse generator, sensing ventricular activity, the exact time when the ventricular electrogram activates the sensing circuit (when the timing clock returns to the baseline as in Fig. 15.2) and initiates a new (electronic) escape interval cannot be determined precisely from the surface electrocardiogram (21). Consequently, in pacemakers with identical automatic and "electronic" escape intervals, the escape interval determined from the surface ECG must of necessity be slightly longer than the automatic interval by a value ranging from a few milliseconds to almost the entire duration of the QRS complex depending on the temporal relationship of the intracardiac electrogram and the surface electrocardiogram. Application of a special magnet over a pulse generator closes a magnetic reed switch that inactivates the sensing function with conversion to the asynchronous mode (22). The *magnet rate* (interval) varies according to the manufacturer and is generally faster (shorter interval) than the programmed rate so as to override the spontaneous rhythm. The magnet interval is often used for assessment of battery status, lengthening with impending battery depletion. The *interference rate* is the rate (often equal to the lower rate) at which a pulse generator will revert automatically in the presence of continually sensed extraneous interference.

Rate-Adaptive Pacemakers

In the VVIR (AAIR) mode the lower rate interval is variable and changes according to the activity of the sensor (that monitors activity in terms of body vibration, minute ventilation volume, temperature, etc.) designed to increase the pacing rate with effort. At any given time, the duration of the lower rate interval can either be its basic programmed value or the constantly changing sensor-controlled lower rate interval, whichever is shorter (Fig. 15.6). The shortest sensor-driven lower rate interval is equal to the programmed sensor-driven upper rate interval (URI).

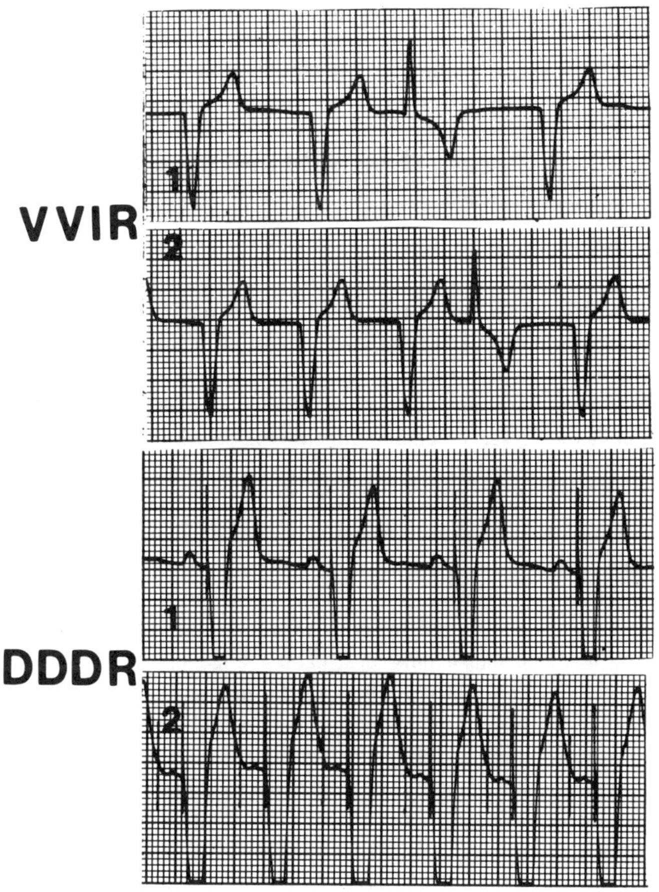

Figure 15.6. Response of rate-adaptive VVIR and DDDR pacemakers to exercise. **Top:** VVIR. The tiny bipolar stimuli cannot be discerned. **Panel 1** shows pacing at the programmed lower rate interval (LRI) = 857 msec (corresponding to a rate of 70/min). The third beat is a ventricular extrasystole sensed by the pacemaker. The escape interval is essentially equal to the automatic interval. **Panel 2** shows the response on exercise when the ventricular rate increases to about 88/min (sensor-driven interval = 680 msec) so that the sensed ventricular extrasystole now recycles the pacemaker with an escape interval of about 680 msec. **Bottom panels:** DDDR. **Panel 1** shows DDD pacing with sensing of P waves (LRI = 1000 msec). In **panel 2** during exercise the AV sequential pacing rate increases to 107/min (cycle length 560 msec). (Reproduced with permission from Barold SS, Falkoff MD, Ong LS, *et al.*, Cardiac Pacing in the Nineties. Technologic, hemodynamic and electrophysiologic considerations in the selection of the optimal mode of pacing. In Rackley CE (ed): Challenges in Cardiology I. Futura Publishing Co., Mt. Kisco, NY, 1992:39.)

Hysteresis

When the escape interval is significantly longer than the automatic interval, the pacemaker is said to operate in the hysteresis mode (23). The purpose of hysteresis is to maintain sinus rhythm (i.e., AV synchrony) for as long as possible at a spontaneous rate lower (e.g., 50/min) than the automatic rate of the pacemaker (e.g., 70/min). Thus, when the spontaneous rate drops below 50/min, the pacemaker will take over at a pacing rate of 70/min. The pacemaker will then continue to pace at a rate of 70/min until the spontaneous rate exceeds the automatic rate, i.e., when the spontaneous QRS complex occurs within the 857-msec automatic interval. In some advanced systems, the device lengthens one or more pacing cycles automatically after a given number of paced cycles at the programmed duration to allow the return of the slower spontaneous rhythm. Hysteresis is a frequent source of confusion in electrocardiographic interpretation of pacemaker function. Although hysteresis is available as a programmable option in many contemporary pacemakers, it is probably used infrequently because its advantages are more theoretical than real and it may predispose to undesirable arrhythmias (24, 25). Indeed, hysteresis appears to have no advantage over simply decreasing the pacing rate in those patients with symptoms due to loss of AV synchrony (26). However, when pacing is required for carotid sinus syndrome or malignant vasovagal syndrome (neurally mediated syncope), a dual-chamber pulse generator with deep hysteresis is generally recommended (7).

Fusion and Pseudofusion Beats

Ventricular fusion beats occur when the ventricles are depolarized simultaneously by spontaneous and pacemaker-induced activity. A ventricular fusion beat is often narrower than a pure paced beat and can exhibit various morphologies depending on the relative contribution of the two foci to ventricular depolarization (Fig. 15.4). Ventricular fusion can mimic lack of capture if it produces an isoelectric complex in a single electrocardiographic lead. In this situation the presence of a T wave (repolarization) indicates that preceding depolarization has taken place while ventricular depolarization should be obvious in other leads.

Pseudofusion beats consist of the superimposition of an ineffectual pacemaker stimulus on the surface QRS complex originating from a single focus and represent a normal manifestation of VVI pacing (21,27) (Fig. 15.4). A substantial portion of the *surface* QRS complex can be inscribed before *intracardiac* electrical activity or the electrogram monitored by the pacing lead generates the required voltage or signal to inhibit the output circuit of a VVI pacemaker (Fig. 15.7). Therefore a normally functioning VVI pacemaker according to its programmed timing mechanism can deliver its impulse within a spontaneous surface QRS complex (mimicking undersensing) before the pulse generator has the opportunity to sense the "delayed" *intracardiac* signal or electrogram at the right ventricular apex. In a pseudofusion beat, the pacemaker stimulus falls within the absolute refractory period of the myocardium (Fig. 15.4). In the presence of normal ventricular sensing, striking examples of ventricular pseudofusion beats with pacemaker stimuli released late within the surface QRS complex can occur in right bundle branch block, left ventricular extrasystoles, and deranged intraventricular conduction because of delayed arrival of activation at the sensing electrode(s) at the right ventricular apex (28). Whenever pseudofusion beats are observed, true sensing failure must be excluded with long electrocardiographic recordings. Pacemaker stimuli falling clearly beyond the surface QRS complex indicate undersensing. Fusion and pseudofusion atrial beats may also occur with atrial pacing, but are more difficult to recognize in view of the smaller size of the P wave in the ECG.

PACEMAKER ELECTROPHYSIOLOGY

The pacing threshold is the minimal amount of "electrical activity" required to pace the heart (29–34). Determination of pacing threshold is crucial to ensure consistent pacing and optimize pacemaker longevity, an important consideration with complex pacemakers with special functions such as rate modulation that increase current drain from the battery. The most important factor in determining battery longevity is battery current drain measured in microamperes or the rate at which charge (current × time) is drained from the battery. The current drain required to provide the output parameters (including rate) can be controlled by programming. On the other hand, the current drain of the "static" circuit (for "housekeeping") cannot be controlled except by the pacemaker manufacturer.

Pacing Threshold and Strength Duration Curve

The pacing threshold may be determined in terms of (a) voltage (V), (b) current (mA), (c) energy (microjoules (μJ)), (d) charge (microcoulombs (μC)), and (e) pulse width (milliseconds (msec)) at a fixed voltage or current. The voltage and current waveforms of the testing device must be identical to those of the implantable device and specified if they are different (29,35–38). In practice, the pacing threshold is determined in terms of voltage (at a fixed pulse width) or pulse width (at a fixed voltage). Determination of pacing threshold in terms of energy expressed in microjoules (although popular in Europe) is not recommended because it is affected by too many factors (36).

The output of most implantable pulse generators is often considered in terms of a constant voltage source, a misnomer because only the leading edge of the voltage pulse remains constant regardless of the impedance (resistance) (39). Such a waveform should be called a voltage-limited (capacitor-coupled) output. The acute or chronic pacing threshold at the time of implantation or replacement should be determined in terms of volts at a given pulse width duration (with a device that delivers a waveform identical to that of the implantable pulse generator) (29,30,33,35,38). If only one measurement is made at the time

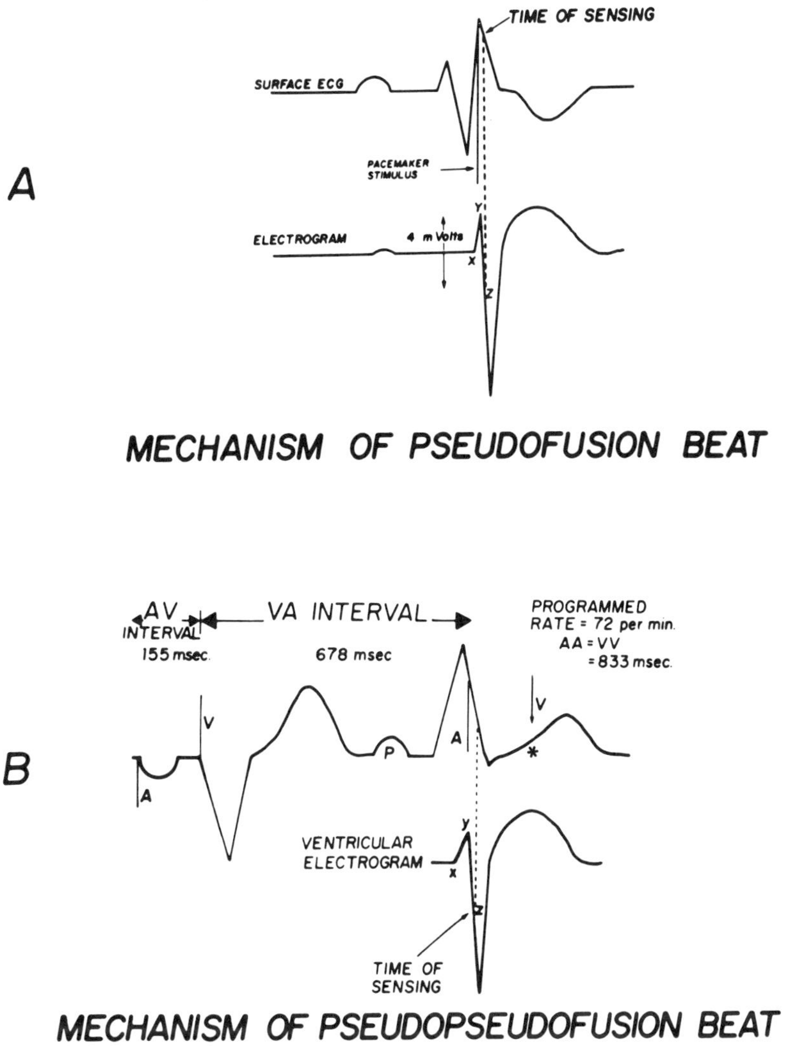

Figure 15.7. A, Diagrammatic representation of the mechanism of pseudofusion. The surface electrocardiogram and ventricular electrogram are recorded simultaneously. The electrogram generates the necessary intracardiac voltage to inhibit the pacemaker (yz, assumed at 4 mV) at a point corresponding with the descending limb of the surface QRS complex in its second half (at *dotted line*). Consequently it is possible for a pacemaker stimulus to occur at the apex of the R just before the *dotted line* (or point of sensing) because the ventricular electrogram has not yet generated the required voltage to inhibit the pulse generator. **B,** Diagrammatic representation of the mechanism of pseudopseudo-fusion. Assume a DVI pulse generator with an AV interval of 155 msec and an atrial escape (pacemaker VA) interval of 678 msec. The atrial channel cannot sense in the DVI mode. The first beat shows atrial and ventricular capture by the atrial and ventricular stimuli. The relatively early occurrence of a spontaneous P wave and the ensuing conducted QRS complex allows the atrial stimulus to fall within the surface QRS complex according to the programmed atrial escape interval of 678 msec. The ventricular electrogram generates the necessary voltage for sensing (yz) relatively late in relation to the surface QRS complex (corresponding to the *dotted line*). Consequently the pulse generator delivers its atrial stimulus within the surface QRS complex (before the point of sensing at the *dotted line*) according to its programmed VA interval because the electrogram has not yet generated sufficient intracardiac voltage to suppress the pulse generator. In a DVI or (DDD) pulse generator release of the atrial stimulus initiates a short ventricular refractory period (known as the blanking period) to prevent the ventricular channel from sensing the atrial stimulus as crosstalk). If a substantial portion of the ventricular electrogram falls within the ventricular blanking period, the ventricular channel will not sense the QRS complex, leading the pacemaker to deliver its ventricular stimulus on the ascending limb of the T wave at the completion of the programmed AV delay (*asterisk*). This mechanism may be called pseudopseudofusion (98–100) beat because two chambers are involved. It is the atrial stimulus that falls within the QRS complex in contrast to a pseudofusion mechanism where only one chamber is involved. The same mechanism can occur during DDD pacing with ventricular extrasystoles or atrial undersensing. (In ventricular pseudofusion the ventricular stimulus deforms the QRS complex.) (Reproduced with permission from Barold SS, Falkoff MD, Ong LS, *et al.*: Electrocardiographic analysis of normal and abnormal pacemaker function. In Dreifus LS (ed): Pacemaker therapy. Cardiovas Clin 1983;14(2):97.)

of implantation, the pulse width of the external testing device should be 0.5–0.6 msec. To measure the acute threshold at the time of implantation, the external pulse generator is set at 5 V and pulse width = 0.5–0.6 msec (usually the nominal parameters of an implantable device). The pacing rate is increased until regular pacing is achieved. The voltage is then gradually decreased until loss of capture occurs. When the output of the pulse generator is near the pacing threshold, capture may occur only when stimuli fall in the supranormal phase of excitability (Fig. 15.1). The lowest voltage causing consistent capture outside the myocardial refractory period determines the stimulation threshold. The relationship of voltage and pulse width at threshold is not linear and is represented by the strength-duration curve (Fig. 15.8). A shorter pulse width requires a higher voltage to attain pacing threshold. The strength duration curve is steep with a short pulse width and becomes essentially flat at a pulse width greater than 2 msec (rheobase) (34,40–42).

Acute Pacing Threshold

The acute ventricular pacing threshold at the time of implantation should be ≤0.8V at 0.5 msec and the *acute* atrial pacing threshold ≤1.5 V at 0.5 msec. Lower values are often obtained. The acute pacing threshold should be measured during quiet and deep respiration and during coughing to evaluate stability. A high initial pacing threshold value requires lead repositioning. All effort should be made to obtain a threshold as low as possible at implantation because its initial value may ultimately determine the threshold at maturity and hence the voltage and pulse width required for long-term pacing. Initial data with screw-in

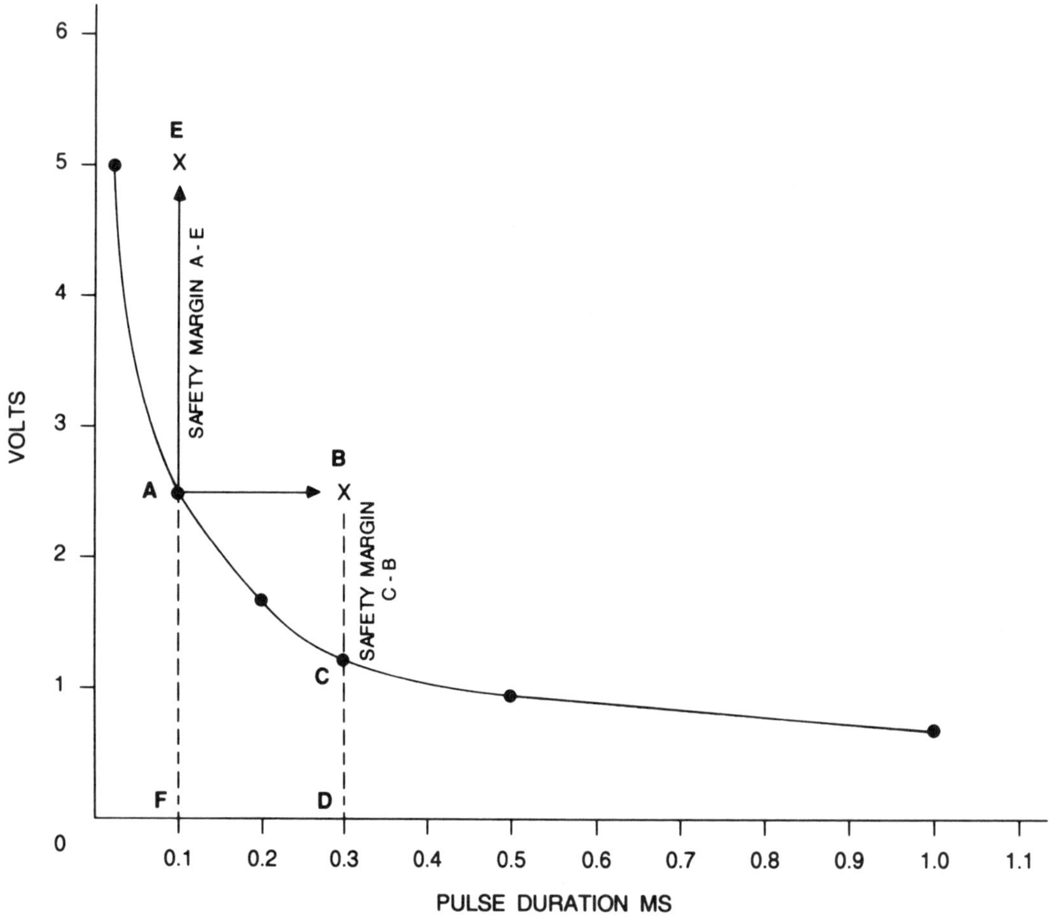

Figure 15.8. Strength-duration curve relating voltage and pulse width at the pacing threshold. Values above the curve pace the heart while values below the curve fail to capture. The threshold for pacing at *point A* is 2.5 V at a pulse width of 0.1 msec. Consequently, starting from the threshold at *point A*, the output voltage of the pulse generator could be doubled to 5 V while keeping the pulse width constant at 0.1 msec, i.e., going to *point E*. This would provide a safety margin EA/AF × 100 = 100%, or a safety factor of 2, i.e., E − F/A − F = 2. Alternatively the output voltage might be left at 2.5 V. and the pulse width increased to 0.3 msec to *point B*. This yields a safety margin slightly exceeding 100% or a safety factor yielding a value slightly more than 2. The second option requires less current drain from the battery and improves battery longevity more than the first option of 5 V. at 0.1 msec. (Reproduced with permission from Barold SS, Zipes DP: Cardiac pacemakers and antiarrhythmic devices. In Braunwald E (ed): Heart Disease, A Textbook of Cardiovascular Medicine. WB Saunders, Philadelphia, 1992:726.)

leads may reveal a rather high pacing threshold due to acute trauma. In this situation, repeat measurement of the pacing threshold after 10–15 min often show a substantial reduction (43). After implantation the output of the pulse generator is usually left at 5 V, 0.5 msec or longer for the first 8 wk.

Factors Influencing Pacing Threshold

The pacing threshold rises shortly after implantation because edema and inflammation separate the tip from the myocardium. Most of the threshold increase appears to result from the formation of nonexcitable fibrous tissue around the electrode, increasing the effective size of the "virtual" electrode at the interface with the myocardium. The threshold with most leads reaches its maximum value 10–20 days after implantation (peaking) and stabilizes to about two to four times the acute value at 1–2 months (31–34). Small electrodes have lower initial thresholds and a greater proportionate rise during the initial reaction, but their chronic threshold is lower than that of larger electrodes. Occasionally threshold evolution takes longer than the classic response and rarely the threshold continues to rise gradually with ultimate failure to capture (44,45). If there is no lead displacement, this abnormality is often called exit block, now a relatively rare complication with contemporary pacing leads.

Steroid eluting leads have a reservoir within the electrode tip that elutes a trace of dexamethasone directly at the electrode-tissue interface (no systemic effect occurs). An anti-inflammatory action reduces the local tissue reaction and the thickness of the fibrous capsule surrounding the tip electrode (46). Steroid eluting leads are associated with low initial and chronic pacing thresholds and characteristically avoid the initial postoperative peaking of thresholds seen with other electrodes (34,47–50). Steroid eluting leads also avoid the occasional unpredictable rise of thresholds seen with other good performance leads and have virtually eliminated "exit block" (50–52). Like conventional porous leads, they are associated with low polarization and therefore also possess good sensing characteristics (47,48).

The pacing threshold is also influenced by a variety of drugs, physiologic and clinical conditions (33,34,53,54). The threshold is decreased by exercise, sympathomimetics, and glucocorticoids. The threshold is increased by eating, sleeping, insulin, ischemia, hypothyroidism, hyperkalemia, mineralcorticoids, and certain antiarrhythmic agents (55–58). Pacemaker failure may occur with the administration therapeutic doses of a Type 1C antiarrhythmic drug (especially flecainide), toxic levels of Type 1A antiarrhythmic agents, and hyperkalemia (59–63). A high threshold may be treated temporarily with an Isoproterenol infusion or systemic steroids until the underlying condition is corrected (53,54,64).

Chronic Thresholds and Safety Margin

Eight weeks after implantation, the threshold has attained its chronic value in most cases. Then the output voltage and pulse width should be programmed to maintain consistent capture with an adequate margin of safety and maximal conservation of battery longevity.

The safety margin for capture is the amount by which voltage output of the pulse generator exceeds the threshold voltage at a given pulse duration. The safety margin can be determined noninvasively by appropriate programming. In the early days of pacing, it was established that the safety margin for chronic lead systems with a stable threshold should be about three times the threshold value in terms of energy (microjoules) to allow for physiologic fluctuations (65). An energy safety factor of 3 corresponds to a factor of 1.75 in terms of voltage, i.e., the output voltage should be at the minimum of 1.75 × chronic threshold voltage at the same pulse width (29,33). In practice, a voltage safety margin of two (or 100%) is often used. Voltage safety margin = output voltage/threshold voltage = 2:1, i.e., the output voltage of the pulse generator should be double the chronic voltage threshold at the same pulse width. An output voltage higher than 5 V should not be used routinely for long-term pacing because it leads to reduced pulse generator efficiency and longevity.

No data are available to back up the assumption that patients need a 100% voltage safety margin with contemporary pacing leads. Data on circadian variations of pacing threshold based on work done in the 1960s are probably irrelevant to modern pacing. Furthermore, many of these old measurements were made with constant-current devices and polished electrodes (mostly myocardial) that are no longer used today.

Threshold Determination: Variable Pulse Width with Fixed Voltage Output

When the pulse width "threshold" is measured, one actually determines the pulse width on the strength duration curve where the pacing threshold is the output voltage of the pacemaker. Let us assume a threshold of 5 V (nonprogrammable fixed voltage output) at a pulse width of 0.1 msec. When the output voltage cannot be changed (fixed at 5 V), the actual voltage threshold provided by the strength duration curve at a pulse width of 0.2 msec is unknown and could be smaller or greater than 2.5 V depending on the configuration of the curve. Thus with 5-V pulse generator, doubling the pulse width from 0.1 (threshold) to 0.2 msec may not necessarily yield a voltage safety margin of 2 or 100% despite the steepness of the strength duration curve for short pulse widths. Consequently, in the case of a pacemaker with a nonprogrammable voltage output, the pulse width should not be adjusted to double its duration at threshold, e.g., when the threshold was equivalent to 5 V. Rather, the pulse width should be increased to three times its value at "threshold" to allow for an adequate voltage safety margin of 2 or 100% provided the pulse width at "threshold" ≤0.2 msec, an accurate assumption based on the configuration of the strength duration curve. With a pulse width at threshold ≥0.3 msec, tripling the pulse width at a fixed voltage output may not provide a voltage safety margin of 2 because of the less steep and eventually almost straight configuration of the strength duration curve at longer pulse widths. The relatively flat configuration of the voltage strength duration curve from 0.5 to 1.5 msec indicates an increase in the pulse width in this range (keeping the voltage constant) will certainly not provide an adequate voltage safety margin of 2. Therefore, at a given voltage, if the pacing threshold requires a pulse width ≥0.4–0.5 msec, a voltage safety margin of 1.75–2 cannot be obtained by keeping the voltage constant and programming pulse width alone to any value.

Threshold Determination: Programmable Voltage and Pulse Width

Older pulse generators used rather inefficient voltage doublers to convert battery voltage to "full output." The lithium-iodine cell delivers about 2.7 V and a 2.5 V output was more efficient than 5.0 V. With today's doublers and dividers substantially more efficient, the optimal output voltage is no longer important at voltages other than 2.5–2.7 V in terms of wasting battery capacity, though voltage greater than 5–5.4 V should not be used unless there is a high threshold problem. The pulse generator should be programmed to minimize current drain from the battery as long as the (voltage) safety margin is maintained and in most cases reduction of pacer voltage will give the best decrease in current drain.

The voltage threshold may be determined by lowering the output voltage at a given pulse width. Alternatively, the threshold may be determined by programming the voltage to a fixed value, e.g., 2.5 V, and then lowering the pulse width, as already discussed. With a threshold of 2.5 V/0.1 msec, the pulse generator could be programmed either to 2.5 V/0.3 msec, or 5 V/0.1 msec, to provide a voltage safety factor of at least 2. In terms of output energy (which correlates with battery current drain), multiplying the voltage output by 2 (keeping the pulse width constant) is equivalent to multiplying the pulse width by 4 (keeping the voltage constant). Therefore an output of 2.5 V at 0.3 msec should be used because of reduced battery current drain compared to an output of 5 V/0.1 msec. Similarly, with a threshold of 2.5 V/0.2 msec, the output should be programmed to 2.5 V/0.6 msec. However a threshold of 2.5 V/0.3 msec requires an output of 5 V/0.3 msec for a safety factor of 2 because of the configuration of the strengthduration curve. With relatively high chronic thresholds greater than 3–3.5 V at a pulse width of 0.5 msec, the output voltage of the pulse generator should exceed 5 V. In this situation, a new lead or a pulse generator programmable to a high voltage (7.5–10 V) should be used.

Contemporary steroid eluting leads may produce exceedingly low pacing thresholds, e.g., <1.25 V at 0.05 msec. The question arises as to whether an output of 2.5 V, 0.05 msec pulse width is acceptable. By assuming that the patient's threshold changes throughout the day, it means that the strength duration curve also shifts up and down throughout the day. Although the overall slope of the curve may not change substantially, it is theoretically possible that the 0.05 msec value may shift significantly if it is on the vertical leg of the curve. Until solid data become available concerning the safety of pacing at pulse widths ≤0.1 msec, it appears more prudent to pace near the knee of the curve and pulse width of 0.2–0.3 msec are acceptable. The longevity of an ideal SSI pulse generator with a 4.0 μA circuit and a deliverable 0.5 A-hr lithium-iodine power source, on a 500 ohm lead at 72 ppm is as follows: (a) at 2.5 V/0.05 msec—13.3 yr, (b) at 2.5 V/0.2 msec—11 yr, a difference of 17%. An equivalent DDD device would produce 6.9 yr at 2.5 V/0.05 msec (both channels) and 6.2 yr at 2.5 V/0.2 msec (both channels), a difference of 10%.

Evaluation of Lead Integrity and Pacing Impedance

The pacing impedance (resistance) is determined by measuring the delivered current to the lead according to Ohm's law. Lead impedance normally ranges between 250 and 1000 ohms when determined at a nominal output of 5 V. An external testing device or implanted pulse generator (by telemetry) measures impedance in a variety of ways: at the leading edge, at the specific point during delivery of the pacemaker impulse (e.g., midpoint) or as an average value from leading to trailing edge. However, for practical purposes the value of lead impedance does not differ substantially according to the way it is measured (30).

The integrity of new and old leads may be evaluated by determining lead impedance either directly at operation or by telemetry (29,39,66). With the passage of time, the lead impedance normally remains constant or falls slightly, and the chronic value does not differ significantly from the original value (66). A high voltage threshold due to lead displacement or an excessive tissue reaction around the electrode (exit block) is associated with a normal lead impedance. With a lead fracture both the voltage threshold and lead impedance will be high (greater than 1000 ohms). With an insulation defect, the voltage threshold may be low or normal and the lead impedance will be low (less than 250 Ohms) (29,30,39).

Sensing

A pacemaker senses the potential difference between the two electrodes (anode and cathode) used for pacing. A bipolar system senses the potential difference between the two electrodes in the heart and requires recording of a bipolar electrogram to determine the characteristics of the signal available for sensing. For a unipolar system (one electrode in the heart and the other on the pacemaker can), the unipolar electrogram from the tip electrode (cathode) closely resembles the available electrogram for sensing, because the anodal contribution from the pacemaker plate is generally negligible.

The amplitude and slew rate (dV/dt) of the electrogram must exceed the sensitivity of the pulse generator to ensure reliable sensing (37,56,67–70). The ventricular signal often measures

6–15 mV, a range that exceeds the nominal sensitivity (2–3 mV) of a pulse generator (21,68). The atrial electrogram is smaller and should measure at least 2 mV. A signal with a gradual slope (lower slew rate) is more difficult to sense than a sharp upstroke signal (71,72). If the amplitude of the signal is large enough, the slew rate will always be sufficient and there is no need to measure it. Determination of slew rate is most useful when a signal is low or borderline (3–5 mV for ventricular signals). An inadequate electrographic signal may or may not be associated with a low pacing threshold and requires repositioning of the lead. Rarely, unipolar and bipolar ventricular electrograms are too small for sensing at the highest pacemaker sensitivity because of chronic ischemia or cardiomyopathy; in this situation a bipolar pulse generator programmable to a high sensitivity should be used.

On a long-term basis, the amplitude of the intracardiac QRS signal diminishes slightly (66,67), but the slew rate may diminish further (about 40%) (67). These changes are usually of no clinical importance for ventricular sensing, but could be important in the case of smaller atrial signals, though recent studies with contemporary leads have documented the functional stability of the atrial signal on a chronic basis.

Unipolar or Bipolar Pacing and Sensing?

New lead technology and design have eliminated the previous advantages of unipolar leads over bipolar leads. Long-term follow-up has shown no significant difference in the pacing and sensing characteristics of bipolar and unipolar systems (73–77). Bipolar leads by virtue of a greater signals-to-noise ratio allow the use of higher sensitivities, especially useful for atrial pacing (71,72). Bipolar systems are less sensitive to extraneous interference (especially skeletal myopotentials) and avoid muscle stimulation occasionally seen at the anodal site of unipolar pulse generators in the absence of malfunction. Bipolar leads are also associated with less frequent crosstalk (atrial stimulus sensed by ventricular lead) in dual chamber pacing systems (76). Consequently unipolar systems will probably become obsolete except for replacement of existing unipolar pacemakers (78).

OPERATIONAL CHARACTERISTICS OF A SIMPLE DDD PULSE GENERATOR

The DDD mode of pacing (with pacing and sensing in both chambers) is no longer considered the "universal" mode because the pacing rate does not increase appropriately on exercise in patients with atrial chronotropic incompetence. Furthermore, P-synchronous pacing (sensing in the atrium and pacing in the ventricle) is impossible in patients with chronic atrial fibrillation or a paralyzed or nonexcitable atrium. These limitations led to the development of rate-adaptive pacemakers (also known as rate-modulated, rate-responsive, or sensor-driven) to provide an increase in the pacing rate on exercise independent of atrial activity (discussed below).

Ventricular Channel (Lower Rate Interval and Ventricular Refractory Period)

As in a standard VVI pacemaker, the ventricular channel of a DDD device requires two basic timing cycles. First, LRI (corresponding to the programmed lower rate). In most dual-chamber pacemakers lower rate timing is ventricular-based (V-V timing) in that the lower rate interval is controlled and initiated only by a paced or sensed ventricular event (79). In this situation, the lower rate interval is the longest interval from a paced or sensed ventricular event to the succeeding ventricular stimulus (without any intervening atrial or ventricular sensed events). Second, pacemaker ventricular refractory period (traditionally defined as the period during which the pulse generator is insensitive to incoming signals (16)). Yet many contemporary pulse generators can sense during part of the refractory period and use such signals to initiate or reset certain timing cycles with the exception of the inviolable LRI (80).

VVI Pacing with an Atrial Channel (AV Interval and Upper Rate Interval)

The addition of an atrial channel to a VVI system (the latter supplying the LRI and ventricular refractory period) creates a simple DDD pulse generator (9). Two new intervals are required: an AV interval (the electronic analogue of the PR interval) and an upper rate interval (the speed limit) to control the response of the ventricular channel to sensed atrial activity. The AV interval is initiated either by an atrial pacing or sensed event. If the pulse generator does not detect ventricular activity during the AV interval, it will emit a ventricular stimulus at the end of the programmed AV delay.

If the upper rate interval of a DDD pacemaker is 500 msec (upper rate = 120/min), a P wave occurring earlier than 500 msec from the previous atrial event will not be followed by a ventricular stimulus. Such an arrangement allows atrial sensing with 1:1 AV synchrony between the lower and upper rate intervals. In such a simple DDD pulse generator with only four intervals, the URI is equal to the refractory period of the atrial channel (or total atrial refractory period) as discussed later (Fig. 15.9).

The atrial escape (pacemaker VA) interval is a *derived* timing interval obtained by subtracting the programmed AV delay from the lower rate interval. In a pacemaker with ventricular-based (V-V) lower rate timing, the atrial escape (pacemaker VA) interval always remains constant and starts with a sensed or paced ventricular event and terminates (in the absence of sensed atrial or ventricular activity) with the release of an atrial stimulus (80–82).

Influence of Events of One Chamber on the Other

The functions of the two channels of a DDD pacemaker are intimately linked and an event detected by one channel gener-

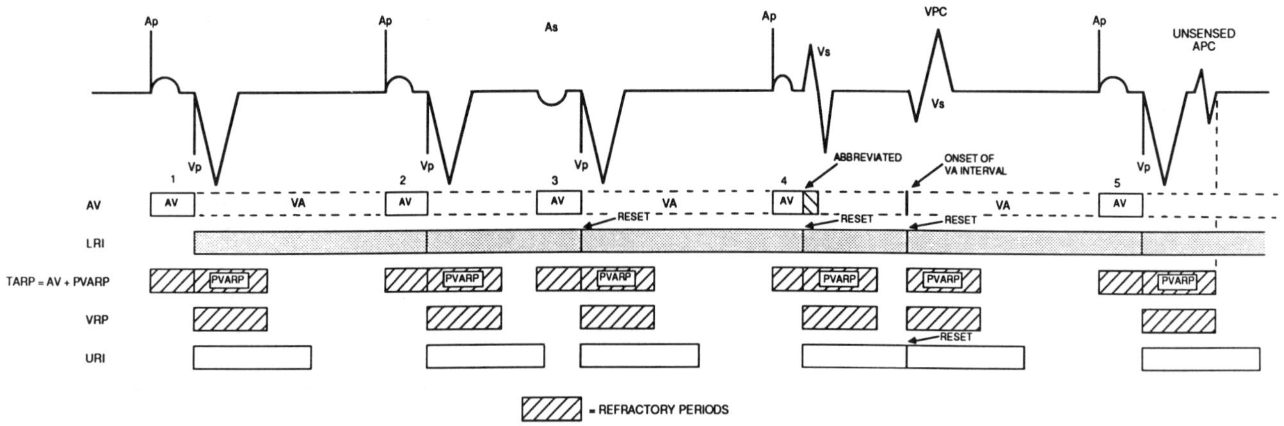

Figure 15.9. Diagram showing the function of a simple DDD pacemaker with only four basic intervals. Ap = atrial paced beat, As = atrial sensed event, Vp = ventricular paced beat, Vs = ventricular sensed event. The four fundamental intervals are: LRI = lower rate interval; VRP = ventricular refractory period; AV = atrioventricular delay; PVARP = postventricular atrial refractory period. The two derived intervals are: atrial escape (pacemaker VA) interval = LRI − AV, and total atrial refractory period (TARP) = AV + PVARP. Reset refers to the termination and reinitiation of a timing cycle before it has timed out to its completion according to its programmed duration. Premature termination of the programmed AV delay by Vs is indicated by its abbreviation. The upper rate interval (URI) is equal to TARP. As (third beat) initiates an AV interval terminating with Vp; As also aborts the atrial escape interval initiated by the second Vp. The third Vp resets the LRI and starts the PVARP, VRP, and URI. The fourth beat consists of Ap which terminates the atrial escape interval initiated by the third Vp, followed by a sensed conducted QRS (Vs). The AV interval is therefore abbreviated. Vs initiates the atrial escape interval, LRI, PVARP, VRP, and URI. The fifth beat is a ventricular extrasystole (VPC) that initiates an atrial escape interval, PVARP, VRP, and resets the LRI and URI. The last beat is followed by an unsensed atrial extrasystole because it occurs within the PVARP. (Reproduced with permission from Barold SS, Zipes DP: Cardiac pacemakers and antiarrhythmic devices. In Braunwald E (ed): Heart Disease, a Textbook of Cardiovascular Medicine. WB Saunders, Philadelphia, 1992:726.)

ally influences the other (80–82). A sensed atrial event alters pacemaker response in two ways: (a) it triggers a ventricular stimulus after the completion of the programmed AV interval, provided the ventricular channel senses no signal during the AV interval, and (b) it inhibits the release of the atrial stimulus expected at the completion of the atrial escape (pacemaker VA) interval because there is no need for atrial stimulation. Thus the atrial channel functions simultaneously in the triggered mode by delivering ventricular stimulation (it triggers a ventricular output after a sensed P wave) and in the inhibited mode by preventing competitive release of an atrial stimulus when a P wave is sensed, i.e., the atrial escape interval does not time out in its entirety. When the ventricular channel senses a signal, both atrial and ventricular channels are inhibited simultaneously. A sensed ventricular event inhibits release of the atrial stimulus (the atrial escape interval does not time out) and initiates new atrial escape and lower rate intervals.

If a sensed ventricular event occurs during the AV interval, there is obviously no need for a ventricular stimulus at the completion of the programmed AV interval. The AV interval is therefore terminated (i.e., abbreviated) and the pacemaker initiates new atrial escape (pacemaker VA) and lower rate intervals. The ventricular channel of a DDD pulse generator functions in the inhibited mode under all circumstances. The code DD TI/I was originally proposed for the DDD mode because the atrial channel functions both in the triggered and inhibited modes, while the ventricular channel is restricted to the inhibited mode. This designation, although correct, was considered unwieldy and was eventually replaced by the simpler but less descriptive DDD mode requiring that the last position be labeled D (double) if both T and I responses occur, regardless of other considerations.

Refractory Periods

In a DDD pulse generator, an atrial sensed or paced event initiates the AV interval and atrial refractory period. The atrial channel of a DDD pulse generator must remain refractory during the entire AV interval to prevent initiation of a new AV interval while one is already in progress (83). Thus, the first part of the atrial refractory period lasts for the duration of the AV interval in the form of Ap-Vs, Ap-Vp, As-Vp, As-Vs (Ap = atrial paced event, As = atrial sensed event, Vp = ventricular paced event, Vs = ventricular sensed event). The AV interval terminates with a ventricular event (Vp or Vs) which immediately restarts (or continues) the atrial refractory period. The part of the atrial refractory period initiated by a ventricular event is called the postventricular atrial refractory period (PVARP). The PVARP is designed to prevent the atrial channel from sensing a variety of signals such as retrograde P waves related to retrograde VA condition, very early atrial extrasystoles, and farfield ventricular signals registered in the atrial electrogram (84,85). The total atrial refractory period is equal to the sum of the AV delay and the PVARP.

In a DDD pulse generator, does a paced or sensed event in one channel initiate a refractory period in both atrial and ventricular channels to ensure that a given paced or sensed event in one

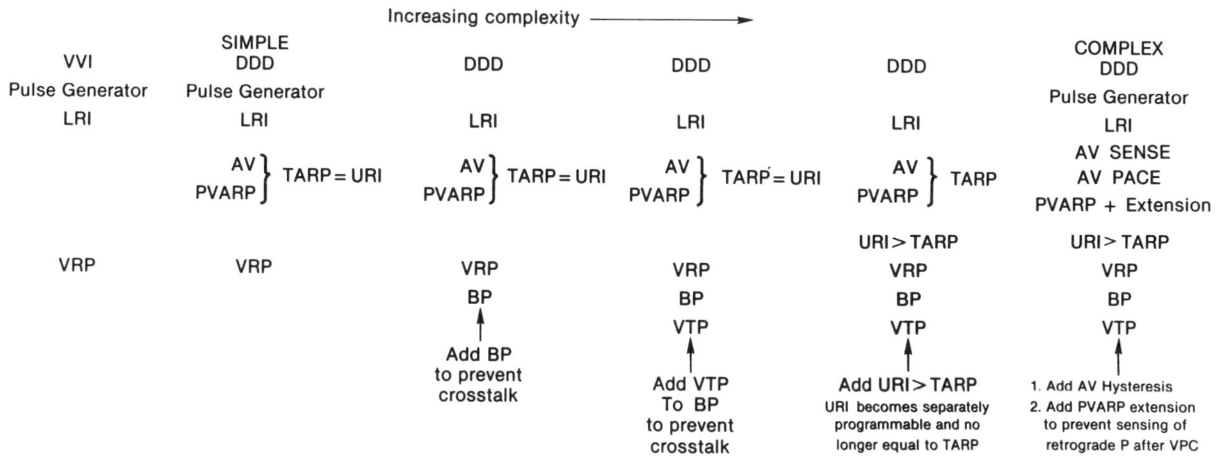

Figure 15.10. The progressive addition of new timing cycles to a simple DDD pacemaker (**left**) creates a more complex device (**right**) (see text for details). Abbreviations as in Figure 15.9. AV pace = AV interval initiated by Ap; AV sense = AV interval initiated by As; BP = blanking period; VTP = ventricular triggering period or ventricular safety pacing period. (Reproduced with permission from Barold SS, Falkoff MD, Ong LS, *et al.*: Timing cycles of DDD pacemakers. In Barold SS, Mugica J (eds): New Perspectives in Cardiac Pacing. Futura Publishing Co., Mt. Kisco, NY, 1988:69.)

(electrical) chamber or channel does not interfere with the function of the other? Four possible events may be considered, i.e., Ap, As, Vs, and Vp. (a) Vs or Vp initiates the ventricular refractory period and the PVARP simultaneously. (b) Ap initiates the AV interval and the atrial refractory period and simultaneously initiates a short ventricular refractory period (ventricular blanking period) to avoid sensing of the atrial stimulus by the ventricular channel (interference known as crosstalk) (80,86,87). (c) As is the only one of the four possible events (As, Ap, Vs, Vp) that generates a refractory period only in the atrial channel. No ventricular refractory period is needed after As because it cannot be ordinarily sensed by the ventricular electrode and therefore cannot directly disturb the function of the ventricular channel.

Control of Upper Rate Interval in a Simple DDD Device

In a simple DDD pulse generator (without a separately programmable URI), URI = total atrial refractory period (TARP). The TARP (AV delay + PVARP) and upper rate interval are interrelated according to the formula: upper rate (ppm) = 60,000/TARP in msec or 60/TARP in sec. When the TARP is selected at 400 msec, the pulse generator will sense atrial signals (P waves) 400 msec or longer apart up to a repetition rate of 150 per minute. An atrial signal occurring earlier than 400 msec (the URI) from the previous atrial event will fall in the atrial refractory period and will not be sensed (80,82,83).

Basic and Derived Timing Cycles of DDD Pulse Generators

Although the upper rate interval was previously considered a basic timing cycle, it is preferable at this stage to use the PVARP as a fundamental interval and relegate the URI and TARP to derived functions. At this point in the discussion, a simple DDD pulse generator has been built with only four basic intervals: LRI, AV interval, ventricular refractory period, and PVARP, and three derived intervals: atrial escape interval, TARP (AV delay + PVARP), and URI (the last two being equal). Theoretically a DDD pulse generator equipped with these timing cycles should function well, provided the ventricular channel does not sense the atrial stimulus (crosstalk) (86,87). Prevention of crosstalk is mandatory and requires the addition of a fifth fundamental timing interval in the form of a brief ventricular refractory (blanking) period starting with the release of the atrial stimulus. Indeed, a DDD device with only these five basic intervals was successfully used clinically in early DDD pulse generators manufactured by Cordis. Further refinements related to crosstalk and the upper rate response created the need for two other basic intervals, the ventricular safety pacing (VSP) period (to complement the ventricular blanking period in dealing with crosstalk) and a URI programmable independently of the TARP for an upper rate response smoother than the sudden mechanism provided only by the TARP (80–83,88,89) (Figs. 15.10 and 15.11).

Crosstalk Intervals

Crosstalk with self-inhibition refers to the inappropriate detection of the atrial stimulus by the ventricular channel. In patients without an underlying ventricular rhythm, inhibition of the ventricular channel by crosstalk could be catastrophic (Fig. 15.12).

VENTRICULAR BLANKING PERIOD

The prevention of crosstalk requires a basic timing cycle called the ventricular blanking period that consists of a brief absolute

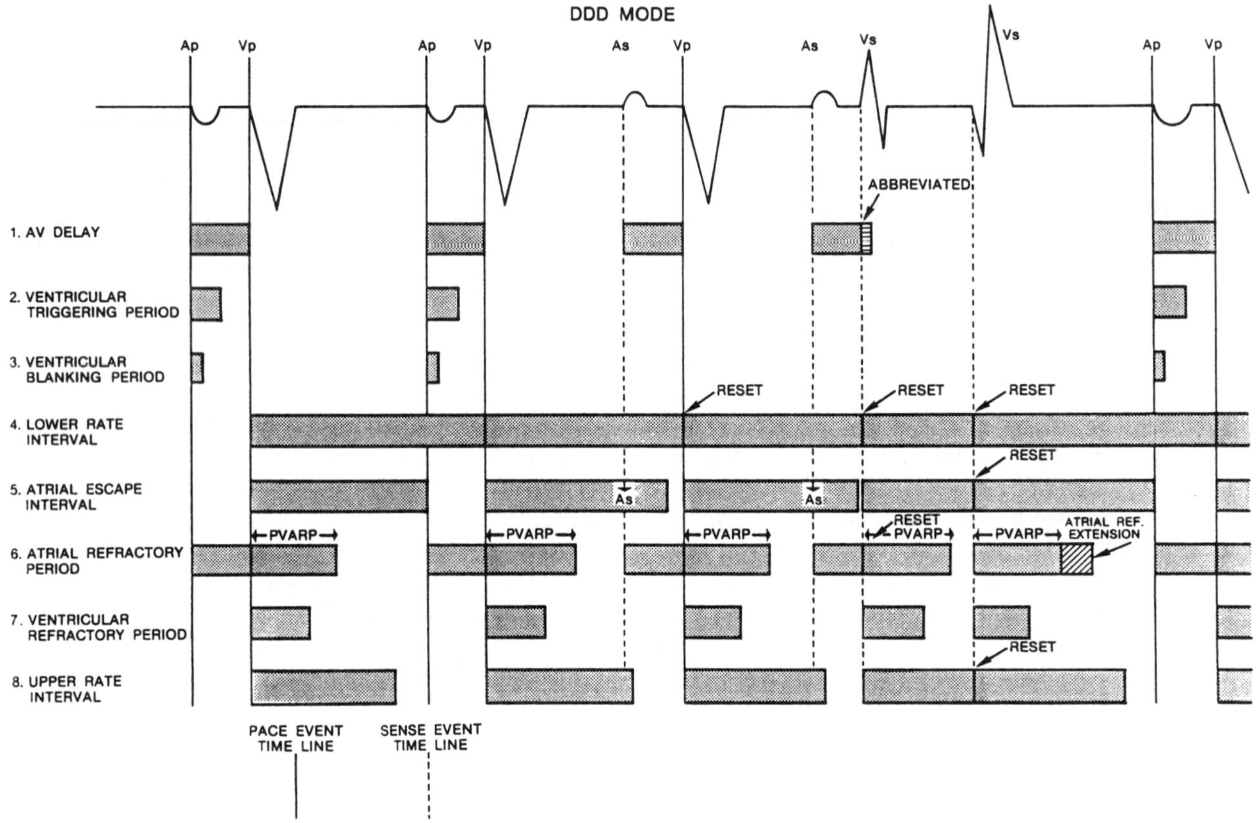

Figure 15.11. DDD mode. Diagrammatic representation of timing cycles. REF = refractory, ventricular triggering period = ventricular safety pacing period. The second Vs event is a sensed ventricular extrasystole. The fourth AV interval initiated by As is abbreviated because Vs occurs before the AV interval has been timed out. The PVARP generated by the ventricular extrasystole is automatically extended by the atrial refractory period extension. This design is based on the concept that most episodes of endless loop tachycardia (pacemaker macroreentrant tachycardia due to repetitive sensing of retrograde atrial depolarization) are initiated by a ventricular extrasystole with retrograde ventriculoatrial conduction (see Figure 15.34). Whenever possible, the AV interval and atrial escape (pacemaker VA) interval are depicted in their entirety for the sake of clarity. The *arrow* pointing down within the atrial escape (pacemaker VA) interval indicates that As has taken place. As inhibits the release of the atrial stimulus expected at the completion of the atrial escape interval. The abbreviations and format used in this illustration are the same for Figures 15.18, 15.20–22 and 15.25. (Reproduced with permission from Barold SS, Falkoff MD, Ong LS, *et al.*: All dual-chamber pacemakers function in the DDD mode. Am Heart J 1988;115:1353.)

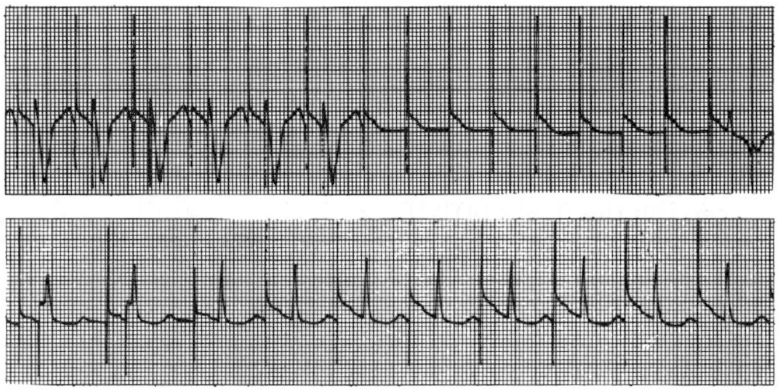

Figure 15.12. Crosstalk during DDD pacing without a ventricular safety pacing mechanism. **Top strip:** The lower rate was increased to test for crosstalk. LRI = 580 msec, AV = 170 msec. During crosstalk, the interval between atrial stimuli on the right becomes shorter than the LRI because the ventricular channel initiates a new atrial escape interval on sensing the atrial stimulus. Crosstalk therefore causes an increase in the atrial pacing rate faster than the freerunning (**lower**) AV sequential rate on the **left.** Continual crosstalk causes prolonged ventricular asystole. **Bottom strip:** Crosstalk with AV conduction. LRI = 857 msec, AV interval = 200 msec. Crosstalk occurs with the third atrial stimulus and produces characteristic prolongation of the interval between the atrial stimulus and the succeeding conducted QRS complex to a value longer than the programmed AV interval. The rate of atrial pacing increases because the sensed atrial stimulus by the ventricular channel initiates a new atrial escape interval just beyond the termination of the ventricular *blanking period.* Consequently the interval between two consecutive atrial stimuli becomes equal to the atrial escape interval of 657 msec (857 − 200) plus the duration of the ventricular blanking period (50 msec) providing a total of about 700 msec. (Reproduced with permission from Barold SS, Zipes DP: Cardiac Pacemakers and Antiarrhythmic Devices. In Braunwald E (ed): Heart Disease, A Text- book of Cardiovascular Medicine. WB Saunders, Philadelphia, 1992:726.)

ventricular refractory period starting coincidentally with release of the atrial stimulus (Fig. 15.11). The duration of the ventricular blanking period varies from 10 to 60 msec according to the manufacturer and is programmable in some pulse generators (87). Some devices adjust the duration of the blanking period automatically according to the programmed atrial output and ventricular sensitivity. There is no need for ventricular blanking after atrial sensing. The reverse of crosstalk, sensing of a ventricular stimulus or QRS complex by the atrial channel, is also prevented by appropriate blanking of the atrial channel provided automatically by the PVARP.

VENTRICULAR SAFETY PACING

In many dual-chamber pulse generators the AV interval initiated by an atrial stimulus contains an additional safety mechanism to prevent the potentially serious consequences of crosstalk. The AV delay initiated by an atrial stimulus is divided into two parts. The first part is called the ventricular safety pacing (VSP) period (also known as the nonphysiologic AV delay or ventricular triggering period) (87,90). During the VSP period, a signal (crosstalk, QRS, etc.) sensed by the ventricular channel does not inhibit the pulse generator. Rather the signal initiates or triggers a ventricular stimulus delivered prematurely only at the completion of the VSP period, producing a characteristic abbreviation of the paced AV interval (Figs. 15.13 and 15.14). In this way, when a QRS complex is sensed during the VSP period, the early triggered ventricular stimulus is supposed to fall harmlessly during the absolute refractory period of the myocardium because of the abbreviated AV interval (91) (Fig. 15.14).

The VSP period usually encompasses the first 100–110 msec of the AV interval and is programmable in some devices. Although the duration of the VSP is generally described as beginning from the atrial stimulus, obviously ventricular sensing cannot occur until termination of the initial ventricular blanking period. A sensed ventricular signal beyond the VSP period in the second part of the AV interval inhibits rather than triggers the ventricular output. Pulse generators without a VSP period generally require a relatively long ventricular blanking period to prevent crosstalk. A long ventricular blanking period (being an absolute refractory period) therefore predisposes to undersensing by the ventricular channel (Fig. 15.15). Consequently VSP provides a "backup" mechanism to deal with crosstalk and allows the use of relatively short ventricular blanking periods to optimize ventricular sensing. Figure 15.16 shows further refinements of the VSP response of contemporary dual chamber pacemakers.

Upper Rate Response

NO SEPARATELY PROGRAMMABLE UPPER RATE INTERVAL

In a DDD pacemaker without a separately programmable upper rate interval (URI), the TARP (AV delay + PVARP) is equal to the (ventricular) URI and provides a simple way of controlling the paced ventricular response to a fast atrial rate. The TARP defines the fastest atrial rate associated with 1:1 AV pacemaker response (80,82–84). An atrial rate faster than the programmed upper rate causes 2:1, 3:1, etc., fixed-ratio pacemaker AV block (*n*:1 block where *n* is a whole number). The AV interval (As-Vp) always remains fixed and equal to the programmed value (Fig. 15.17).

SEPARATELY PROGRAMMED UPPER RATE INTERVAL

A pacemaker Wenckebach (or pseudo-Wenckebach according to some authors) upper rate response during DDD pacing can occur only if the URI is longer than the TARP (67,81,82,84,88–90,92–95) (Fig. 15.18). During the Wenckebach upper rate response, if w is equal to the increment of the AV interval per cycle, w = URI − (P-P interval). If W is equal to the maximum increment of the AV (As-Vp) interval (W) = URI − TARP. Thus the AV interval will vary from the basic value of As-Vp (as programmed) to a value equal to (As-Vp) + (URI − TARP). For example, if URI = 600 msec, AV = 200 msec, PVARP = 200 msec, and PP interval = 550 msec, the increment per cycle w

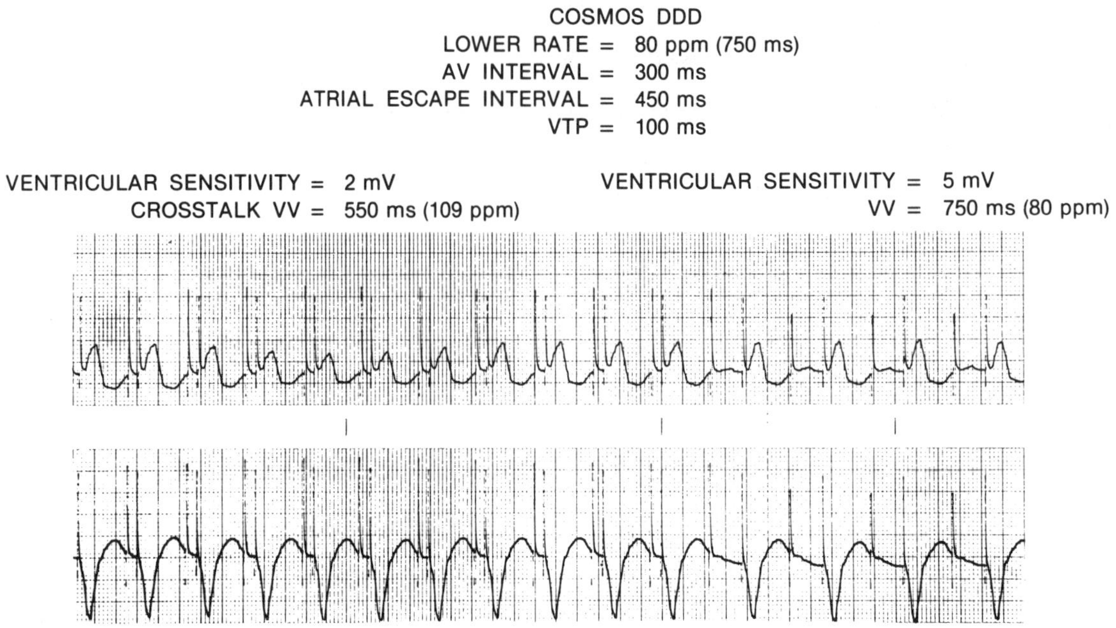

Figure 15.13. Cosmos I Intermedics unipolar DDD pulse generator with ventricular safety pacing mechanism (VTP = ventricular triggering period) showing on the **left** crosstalk characterized by abbreviation of the AV interval to 100 msec. The lower rate interval is controlled by ventricular events. Consequently the atrial escape interval remains constant at 450 msec. The interval between two consecutive ventricular stimuli (Vp − Vp) therefore shortens from 750 to 450 + 100 = 550 msec, increasing the AV sequential pacing rate from 80 to 109/min during continual crosstalk. On the right, crosstalk disappears when the ventricular sensitivity is reduced from 2 to 5 mV (less sensitive setting).

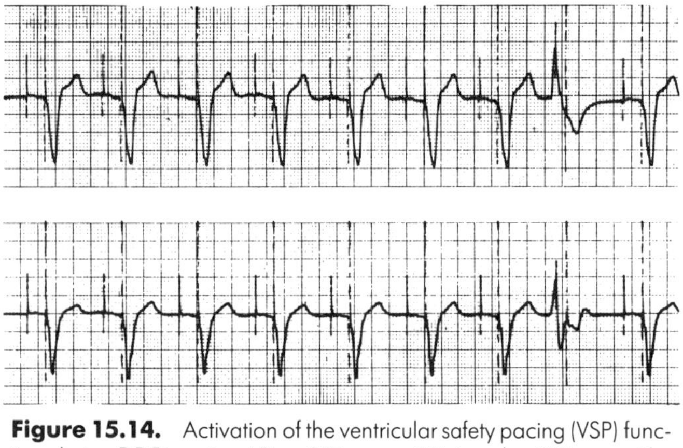

Figure 15.14. Activation of the ventricular safety pacing (VSP) function during DDD pacing. LRI = 857 msec, AV interval = 200 msec. The second last QRS complex is a ventricular extrasystole sensed by the ventricular channel during the VSP period whereupon the pulse generator triggers a ventricular stimulus at the termination of the VSP period, producing characteristic abbreviation of the AV interval (100 msec). An atrial stimulus falls within the QRS complex because the ventricular electrogram at that point has not yet generated sufficient voltage to inhibit the pulse generator, in effect producing a pseudofusion beat. A pseudofusion beat in this situation has been called a pseudopseudofusion beat because an atrial and not a ventricular stimulus falls within the QRS complex (98–100). (See Fig. 15.7.)

= URI − (P-P interval) = 50 msec. The maximum increment of the AV interval, W = URI − TARP = 600 − 400 = 200 msec (Fig. 15.19). The pacemaker will respond to an atrial rate faster than 100 ppm and less than 150 ppm with a Wenckebach upper rate response. The Wenckebach ratio can be calculated for the aforementioned parameters according to the formula of Higano and Hayes (96) as follows: n = W/w = 4. If N is the next integer above n, N = 5, Wenckebach ratio = $N + 1/N$ = 6/5. Thus, with this situation, a DDD pulse generator will exhibit 6:5 Wenckebach pacemaker AV block. The duration of the pause terminating the Wenckebach cycle can also be calculated by another formula published by Higano and Hayes (96) by knowing the atrial rate (P-P interval), TARP, and URI. In the above example, when the P-P interval becomes shorter than TARP, i.e., less than 400 msec (corresponding to an atrial rate faster than 150 ppm), the Wenckebach upper rate response gives way to fixed ratio 2:1 pacemaker AV block.

Upper Rate Interval Shorter than Total Atrial Refractory Period

When the URI is programmed to a shorter value than the TARP (despite the fact that the programmer and the pulse generator may seem to have accepted the command), the pacemaker obviously cannot exhibit Wenckebach pacemaker AV block. The actual URI will be the longer of the two intervals (TARP vs. programmed URI).

Upper Rate Interval Equal to the Total Atrial Refractory Period

If a separately programmable URI is equal to the TARP, a Wenckebach upper rate response cannot occur and the pulse

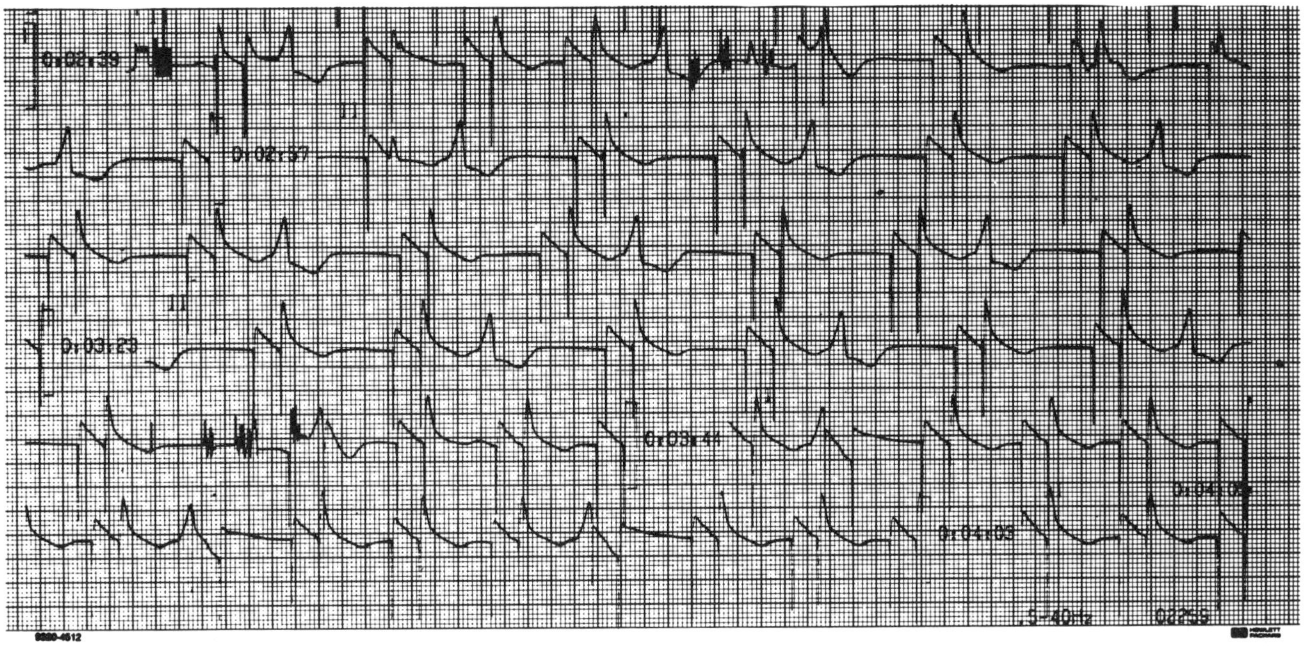

Figure 15.15. Ventricular undersensing due to blanking period. The electrocardiogram shows a normally functioning Cordis Gemini DDD pulse generator programmed to a relatively slow lower rate. There are frequent ventricular extrasystoles with a varying coupling interval. The ventricular extrasystoles are all sensed by the pulse generator. At the beginning of the fifth strip, the pacemaker was reprogrammed to a faster lower rate. Atrial stimuli now fall within the QRS complexes of the ventricular extrasystoles because of "late sensing" of these beats by the ventricular channel (pseudopseudofusion beats) (98–100) (see Fig. 15.7). The ventricular channel does not sense the ventricular extrasystole because their ventricular electrogram falls within the ventricular blanking period (39–47 msec). The pulse generator therefore emits a ventricular stimulus on the apex of the T wave at the completion of the full AV interval of 250 msec. (Reproduced with permission from Barold SS, Ong LS, Falkoff MD, *et al.*: Crosstalk or self-inhibition in dual-chambered pacemakers. In Barold SS (ed): Modern Cardiac Pacing. Futura Publishing Co., Mt. Kisco, NY, 1985:615.)

generator will respond to fast atrial rates with only fixed ratio pacemaker AV block.

UPPER RATE INTERVAL LONGER THAN TOTAL ATRIAL REFRACTORY PERIOD

When URI > TARP, the upper rate response of a DDD pulse generator depends on the duration of three variables: TARP, URI, and P-P intervals (corresponding to the atrial rate) and three situations may be considered.

1. P-P interval > URI. The pulse generator maintains 1:1 AV synchrony because the atrial rate is slower than the programmed upper rate.
2. P-P interval < URI. When the P-P interval becomes shorter than the URI but remains longer than the TARP, i.e., URI > PP interval > TARP, the pulse generator responds with Wenckebach pacemaker AV block.
3. P-P interval < TARP. When the P-P interval is shorter than TARP (and therefore also shorter than URI), a Wenckebach upper rate response cannot occur and the upper rate response consists of only fixed-ratio pacemaker AV block regardless of the duration of the separately programmable URI (Fig. 15.20).

Therefore, when the URI > TARP, a progressive increase in the atrial rate (shortening of the P-P interval) causes first pacemaker Wenckebach upper rate response (when TARP < P-P < URI). When P-P < TARP, the upper rate response switches from pacemaker Wenckebach AV block to 2:1 fixed-ratio pacemaker AV block.

DURATION OF AV INTERVAL AND UPPER RATE

The AV interval initiated by As (As-Vp) (and not the one initiated by Ap) determines the point where fixed-ratio pacemaker AV block occurs, i.e., when P-P interval < TARP, i.e., (As-Vp) + PVARP. In many pacemakers, As-Vp can be programmed to a shorter value than Ap-Vp, thereby shortening the TARP during atrial sensing. In some pulse generators, the TARP can shorten further on exercise by one of three mechanisms (84). (a) The As-Vp decreases with an increase of the sensed atrial rate and/or sensor activity (adaptive AV interval). PVARP shortens on exercise (adaptive PVARP). (b) Both As-Vp interval and PVARP shorten on exercise.

In terms of the upper rate response, abbreviation of the AV interval initiated by atrial sensing (As-Vp < Ap-Vp) provides important advantages over the situation where As-Vp = Ap-Vp: (a) shorter TARP duration (As-Vp + PVARP) so that fixed-ratio

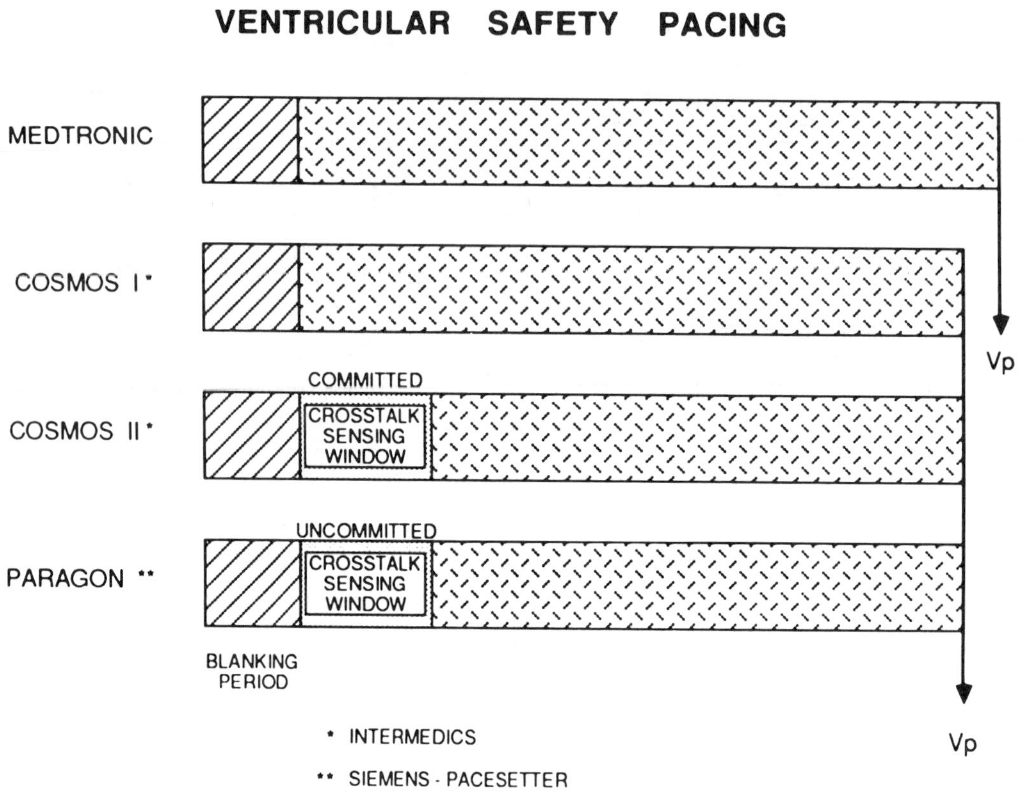

Figure 15.16. Behavior of the ventricular safety pacing (VSP) mechanism of DDD pacemakers. The VSP period actually begins at the completion of the ventricular blanking period, but its total duration is generally expressed as starting from the atrial stimulus with the onset of the ventricular blanking period. Medtronic dual-chamber pulse generators possess a VSP period of 110 msec while other pulse generators have a VSP period with a nominal value of 100 msec. Medtronic and Intermedics Cosmos I pulse generators: a signal sensed anywhere during the VSP period (beyond the blanking period) by the ventricular channel of these pulse generators triggers an obligatory (committed) ventricular stimulus at the termination of the VSP period. In the Intermedics Cosmos II DDD pulse generator, the VSP period contains an initial crosstalk sensing window. When the ventricular channel senses a signal during the crosstalk window, the pulse generator triggers a committed ventricular stimulus at the termination of the VSP period regardless of any other sensed ventricular events sensed during the VSP period beyond the crosstalk sensing window. In contrast, an isolated ventricular signal sensed in the VSP beyond the crosstalk sensing window inhibits the ventricular output. In the Pacesetter Siemens Paragon DDD and Synchrony DDDR pulse generators, the crosstalk sensing window functions as in the Cosmos II pulse generator. A signal sensed by the ventricular channel during the crosstalk sensing window triggers a ventricular stimulus at the termination of the VSP period. In contrast to the Cosmos II pulse generator, the ventricular output triggered by sensing in the VSP is uncommitted. Thus another ventricular event sensed in the VSP (beyond the crosstalk sensing window) will inhibit the triggered ventricular response initiated by ventricular sensing within the crosstalk sensing window.

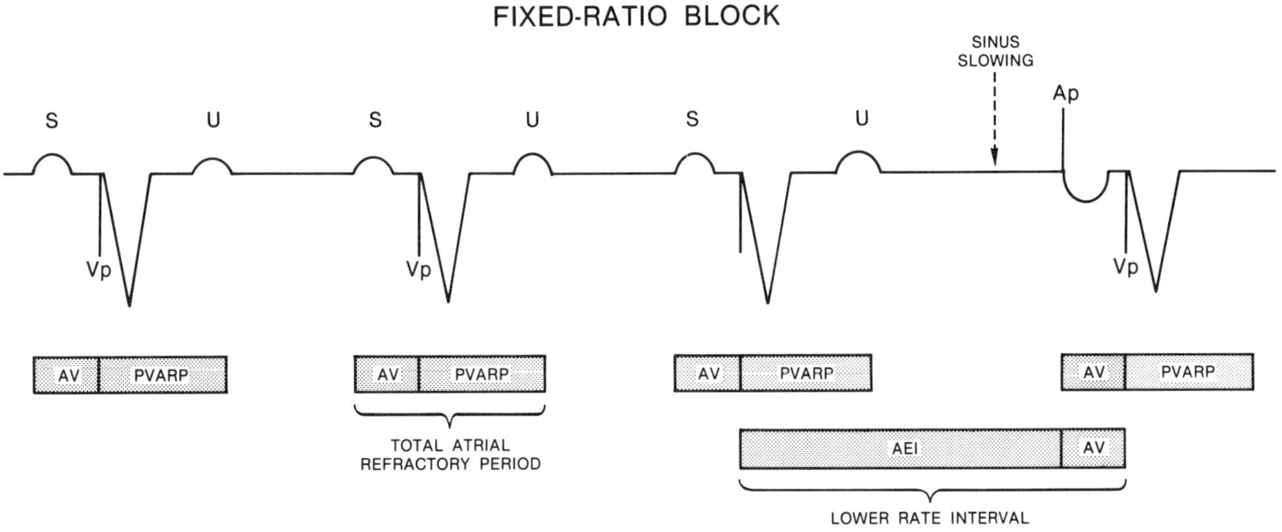

Figure 15.17. Diagrammatic representation of pacemaker fixed-ratio AV block. The TARP (AV + PVARP) controls the URI. Every second P wave is unsensed because it falls within the PVARP (2:1 block). When sinus slowing occurs on the right, the pacemaker functions according to the programmed LRI, thereby delivering an atrial stimulus that terminates the pause. AEI = atrial escape interval; Ap = atrial pace event; S = sensed P wave; U = unsensed P wave; Vp = ventricular pace event. (Reproduced with permission from Barold SS, Falkoff MD, Ong LS, *et al.*: Electrocardiography of contemporary DDD pacemakers. A. Basic concepts, upper rate response, retrograde ventriculoatrial conduction, and differential diagnosis of pacemaker tachycardia. In Saksena S, Goldschlager N (eds): Electrical Therapy for Cardiac Arrhythmias, Pacing, Antitachycardia Devices, Catheter Ablation. WB Saunders, Philadelphia, 1990:225.)

pacemaker AV block begins at a faster sensed atrial rate when P-P interval < TARP; (b) with the separately programmable URI remaining constant, a shorter TARP widens the range of atrial rates associated with pacemaker Wenckebach AV block, i.e, the Wenckebach upper rate response begins at the same atrial rate, but fixed-ratio pacemaker AV block begins at a faster atrial rate; (c) a shorter TARP allows programming of a shorter (separately programmable) URI (keeping URI > TARP) with preservation of the Wenckebach pacemaker AV block response at faster atrial rates.

TYPES OF DUAL-CHAMBER PACEMAKERS

The function and timing intervals of the various modes of dual chamber pacing are best understood by focusing first on the DDD mode. Simpler pacing modes are then derived by the removal of "building blocks" from the DDD mode and equalizing certain timing intervals (92). A DDD pacemaker may have to be downgraded to a simpler mode for the treatment of certain complications. In contrast, a DDDR pacemaker consists of a DDD system with the addition of a non-P-wave sensor to provide an increase in the pacing rate in patients with abnormal sinus node function on exercise.

DVI Mode

Dedicated permanent DVI pacemakers (but not the DVI mode) are now obsolete. The DVI mode may be considered as the DDD mode with the PVARP extending through the entire atrial escape interval (101). Thus, in the DVI mode the TARP in effect lasts through the entire LRI because during the AV interval the atrial channel of a DDD pacemaker always remains refractory. The URI cannot exist because a DVI pacemaker cannot sense atrial activity. Therefore, in the DVI mode the LRI, TARP, and URI are all equal. Asynchronous atrial pacing may precipitate atrial fibrillation (97).

In the uncommitted DVI mode (Fig. 15.21) the ventricular channel can sense through the entire duration of the AV interval (no ventricular blanking period) while in the partially committed DVI mode the ventricular channel can sense only during part of the AV interval beyond the initial ventricular blanking period (98–100). In contrast, a committed DVI pacemaker may be regarded as having a ventricular blanking period that encompasses the entire AV interval, rendering crosstalk impossible (98–100). In the committed DVI mode, AV sequential stimulation therefore occurs in an all-or-none fashion, i.e., no stimuli occur during inhibition and two sequential stimuli always occur during pacing because the ventricular channel cannot sense during the AV interval (Vp is committed after Ap).

VDD Mode

The VDD mode functions like the DDD mode except that the atrial output is turned off (Fig. 15.22). Failure to deliver an atrial stimulus precludes initiation of crosstalk intervals (ventricular blanking and safety pacing periods) (92). As far as the timing cycles are concerned, the omitted atrial stimulus begins an implied AV interval during which the atrial channel must be refractory as in the DDD mode. This behavior explains why in most contemporary designs a P wave occurring during the im-

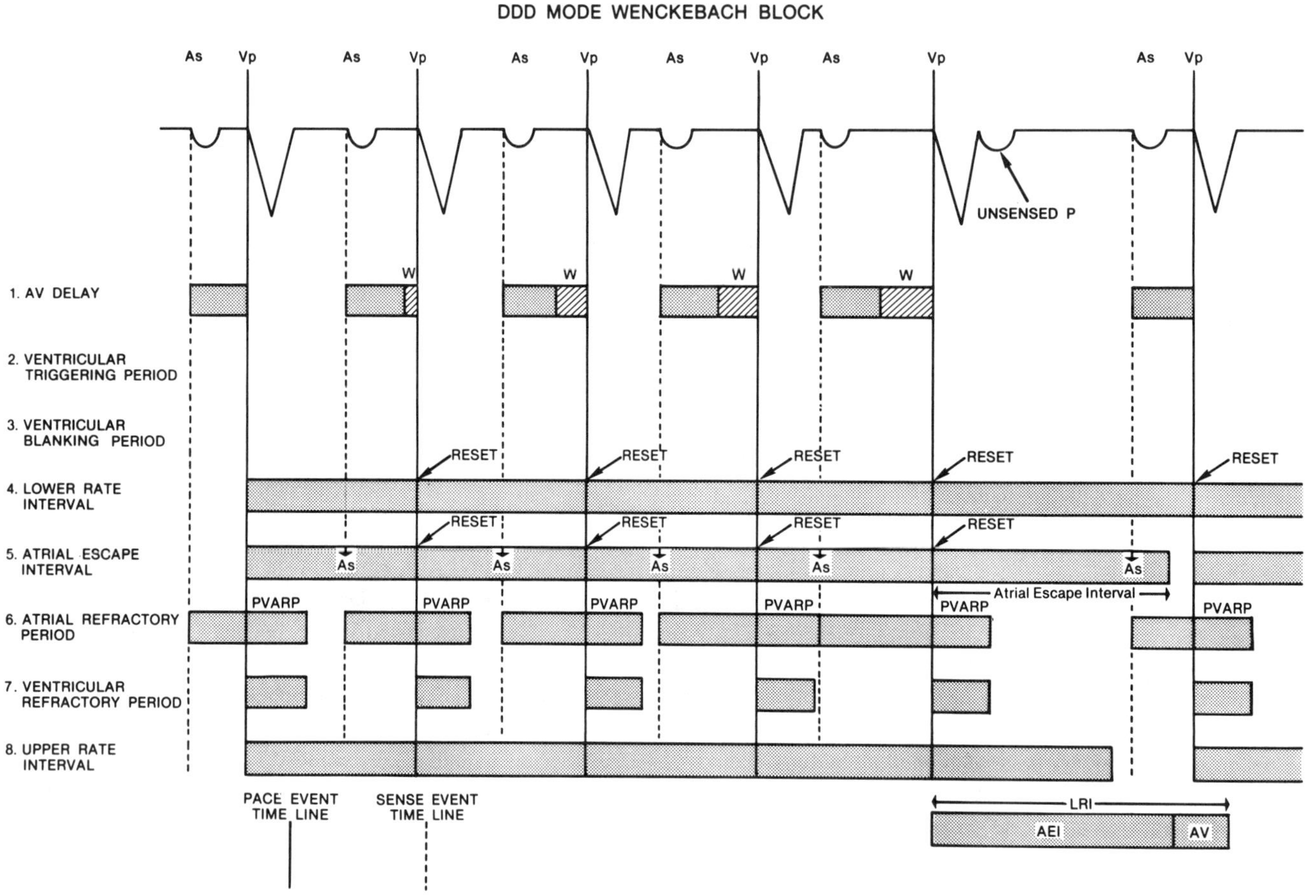

Figure 15.18. DDD mode. Upper rate response with pacemaker Wenckebach AV block. AEI = atrial escape interval. The URI is longer than the programmed TARP. The PP interval (As-As) is shorter than the URI, but longer than the programmed TARP. The As-Vp interval lengthens by a varying period (W) to conform to the URI. During the Wenckebach response, the pacemaker synchronizes Vp to As, and because the pacemaker cannot violate its (ventricular) URI, Vp can be released only at the completion of the URI. The AV delay (As-Vp) becomes progressively longer as the ventricular channel waits to deliver its Vp until the URI has timed out. The maximum prolongation of the AV interval represents the difference between the URI and the TARP. The As-Vp interval lengthens as long as the As-As interval (P-P) is longer than the TARP. The sixth P wave falls within the PVARP and is unsensed and not followed by Vp. A pause occurs and the cycle restarts. In the first four pacing cycles, the intervals between ventricular stimuli (Vp-Vp) are constant and equal to the URI interval. When the P-P interval becomes shorter than the programmed TARP, Wenckebach pacemaker AV block cannot occur and fixed-ratio pacemaker AV block (e.g., 2:1) supervenes. (Reproduced with permission from Barold SS, Falkoff MD, Ong LS, *et al.*: All dual-chamber pacemakers function in the DDD mode. Am Heart J 1988;115:1353.)

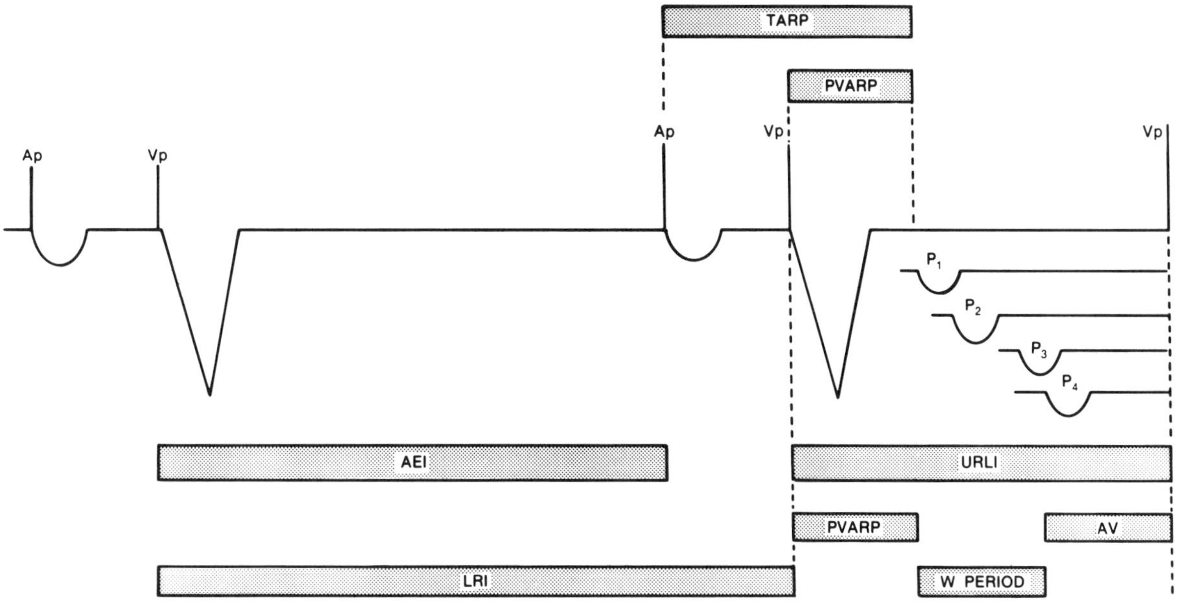

Figure 15.19. Diagrammatic representation of the mechanism of AV interval prolongation in a pulse generator with a separately programmable TARP and upper rate limit interval (URLI). The maximum AV extension, or waiting, period (W) = URLI – (AV + PVARP) = URLI – TARP. A P wave (P_1) occurring immediately after the termination of the PVARP exhibits the longest AV interval, i.e., AV + W. A P wave just beyond the W period (P_4) initiates an AV interval equal to the programmed value. P waves occurring during the W period (P_2 and P_3) exhibit varying degrees of AV prolongation to conform to the URLI depicted as the shortest interval between two consecutive ventricular paced beats. AEI = atrial escape interval; LRI = lower rate interval; Ap = atrial paced beat; Vp = ventricular paced beat. (Reproduced with permission from Barold SS, Falkoff MD, Ong LS, *et al.*: Electrocardiography of contemporary DDD pacemakers. A. Basic concepts, upper rate response, retrograde ventriculoatrial conduction, and differential diagnosis of pacemaker tachycardias. In Saksena S, Goldschlager N (eds): Electrical Therapy for Cardiac Arrhythmias, Pacing, Antitachycardia Devices, Catheter Ablation. WB Saunders, Philadelphia, 1990:225.)

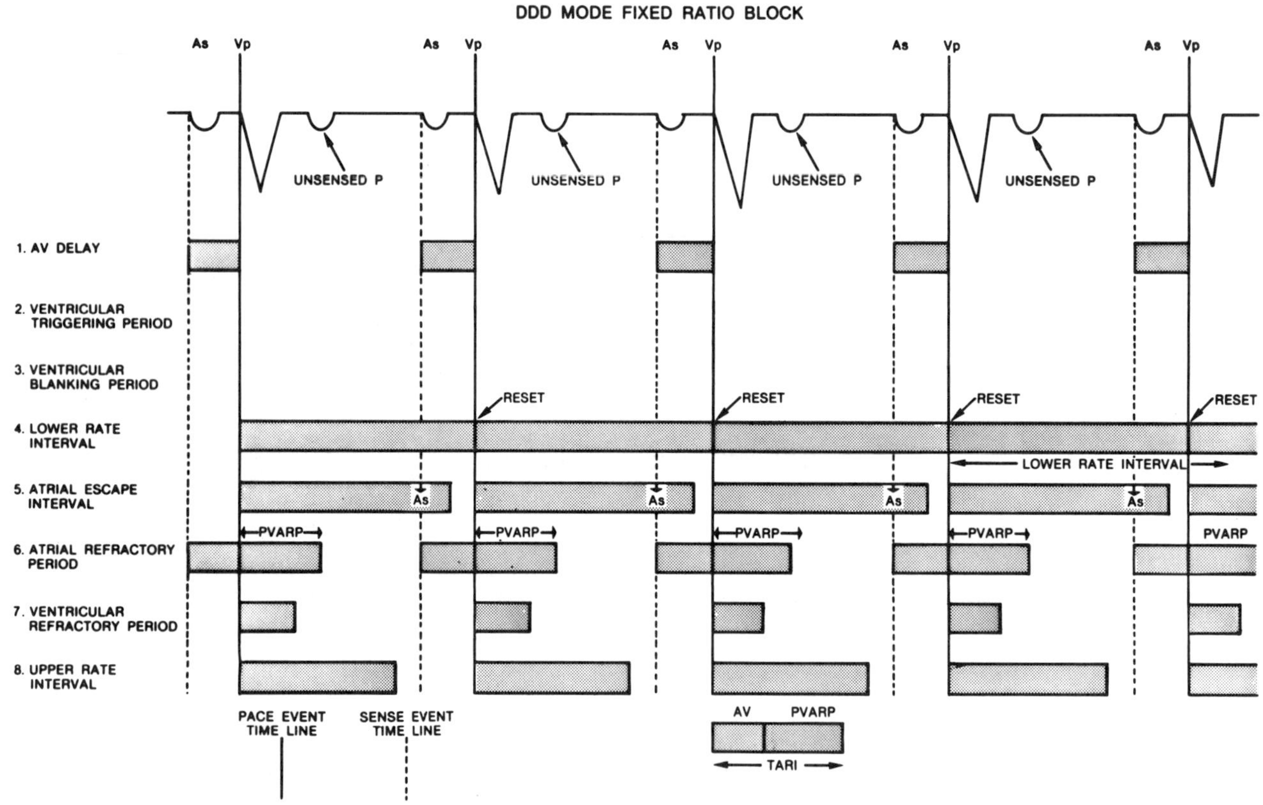

Figure 15.20. DDD mode. **Top:** upper rate response with fixed ratio pacemaker AV block. The URI is longer than the TARP (AV + PVARP) and the PP interval (As-As) is shorter than the TARP. Thus, a Wenckebach upper rate response cannot occur. Every second P wave falls within the PVARP and is unsensed. The AV interval remains constant. (Reproduced with permission from Barold SS: Management of patients with dual chamber pulse generators: central role of pacemaker atrial refractory period, Learning Center Highlights (Heart House, American College of Cardiology) 1990;5(4):8.)

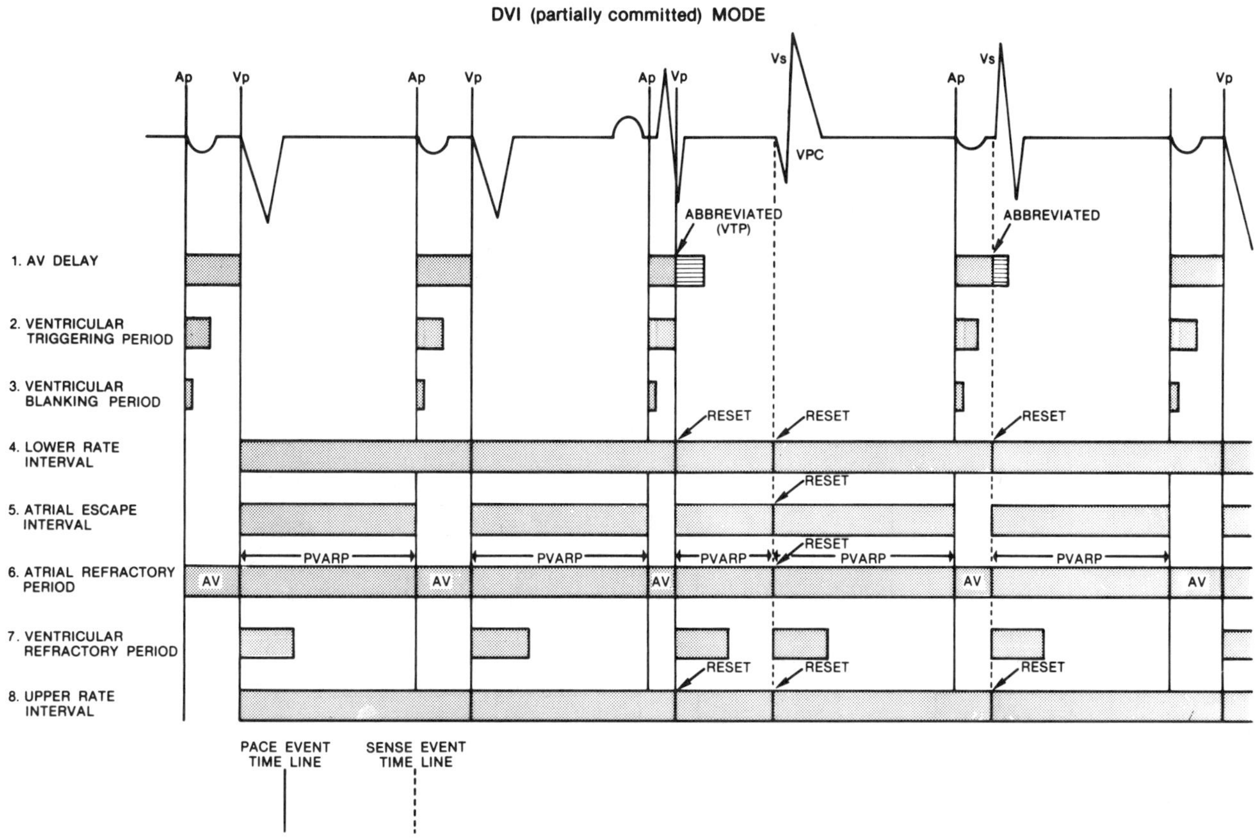

Figure 15.21. DVI mode (partially committed). The PVARP, LRI, and URI are all equal. Atrial pacing is asynchronous. The AV interval is longer than the VSP (triggering) period and the latter is in turn longer than the ventricular blanking period (VBP). The third P wave is unsensed because the atrial channel functions asynchronously. The first spontaneous QRS complex (between the third Ap and the third Vp) is sensed within the VSP period (or VTP) so that the ventricular channel delivers Vp at the completion of the VSP period. Therefore, the third AV interval (Ap-Vp) is abbreviated by premature delivery of Vp. The fourth Ap initiates an AV interval that is terminated prematurely because Vs occurs before the AV interval has timed out; premature emission of Vp does not occur because Vs is sensed beyond the VSP period. The fourth beat is a ventricular extrasystole (VPC) sensed by the ventricular channel. In an uncommitted DVI device, the VBP and VTP are absent. In a committed DVI device, the VBP is equal to the AV interval. (Reproduced with permission from Barold SS, Falkoff MD, Ong LS, *et al.*: All dual chamber pacemakers function in the DDD mode. Am Heart J 1988;115:1353.)

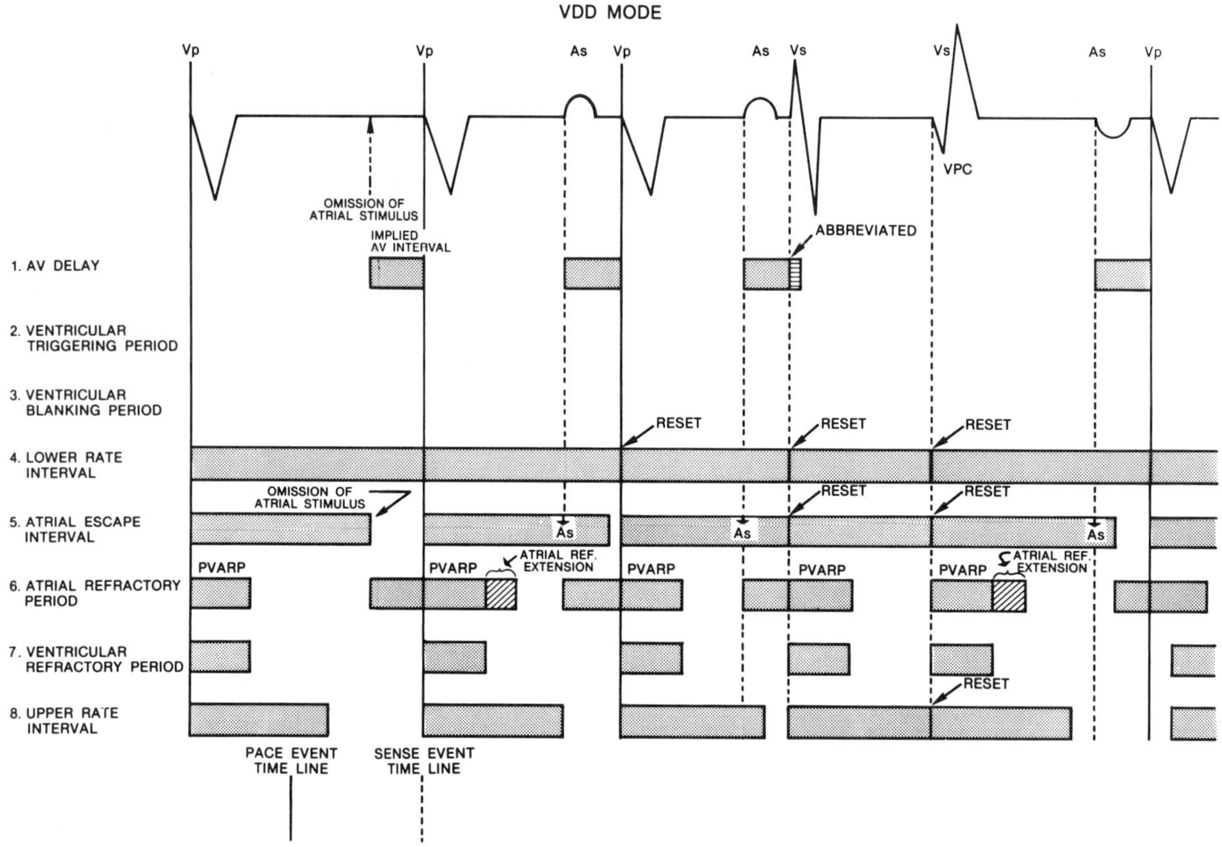

Figure 15.22. VDD mode. In the DDD mode, an atrial stimulus is released at the completion of the atrial escape interval whenever no As occurs within the atrial escape interval. In the VDD mode (equivalent to the DDD mode without an atrial output), the atrial stimulus is omitted. Nevertheless, the pulse generator initiates an implied AV interval with the same characteristics as in the DDD mode. In the first Vp-Vp cycle, the pacemaker extends its PVARP automatically as after a sensed ventricular extrasystole (Fig. 15.11) because Vp terminating the implied AV interval is not preceded by Ap or As. No ventricular blanking and VSP (triggering) periods are needed because there are no atrial stimuli in the VDD mode. With the omission of Ap at the end of the implied AV interval and the absence of As, the pulse generator effectively paces in the VVI mode at the programmed DDD lower rate interval (first cycle). (Reproduced with permission from Barold SS, Falkoff MD, Ong LS, *et al.*: All dual chamber pacemakers function in the DDD mode. Am Heart J 1988;115:1353.)

plied AV interval (after an aborted atrial stimulus) cannot initiate a new AV interval. However, in some DDD pulse generators programmed to the VDD mode a P wave during the implied AV interval can be sensed and actually reinitiate an entirely new AV interval so that the Vs-Vp or Vp-Vp interval becomes longer (maximum extension equal to As-Vp interval) than the programmed (ventricular-based) LRI, producing a form of hysteresis. In the absence of sensed atrial activity, the VDD mode will continue to pace effectively in the VVI mode (at the LRI of the DDD mode) because the VDD mode preserves all the other timing cycles of the DDD mode despite the missing atrial output.

DDI Mode

The DDI mode has been described as an improved DVI mode or in terms of a hybrid of the DVI and DDD modes (101). In the DDI mode, atrial sensing occurs beyond the PVARP as in the DDD mode. Atrial sensing inhibits release of the atrial stimulus at the end of the atrial escape interval. Despite atrial sensing, a DDI pacemaker cannot increase its ventricular pacing rate in response to a faster atrial rate (unlike the DDD mode) and ventricular pacing always occurs at the programmed lower rate (Fig. 15.23). This response is sometimes described as inability to track the atrial rate. Constancy of the paced ventricular rate in the DDI mode requires a ventricular-based lower rate timing (V-V timing) after a paced ventricular event. With this arrangement, the DDI mode can be considered as the DDD mode with identical upper and lower intervals (92,102). In this way, an atrial sensed event (As) initiates an AV interval that terminates (as in the DDD mode) only at the completion of the URI (identical to the LRI in the DDI mode). The DDI mode is useful in patients with the sick sinus syndrome and paroxysmal atrial tachyarrhythmias (103) (Fig. 15.24). The DDI mode provides atrial pacing and AV synchrony (in the absence of atrial tachyarrhythmias), with the potential of preventing atrial tachyarrhythmias by overdrive suppression (103). During the episodes of atrial tachyarrhythmias, the DDI pacemaker simply paces the ventricle at the constant programmed lower rate. In the DDI mode, sensing of a retrograde P wave outside the PVARP may cause VA synchrony that tends to perpetuate itself (like endless loop tachycardia—discussed below) and may lead to the pacemaker syndrome (104) (Fig. 15.25).

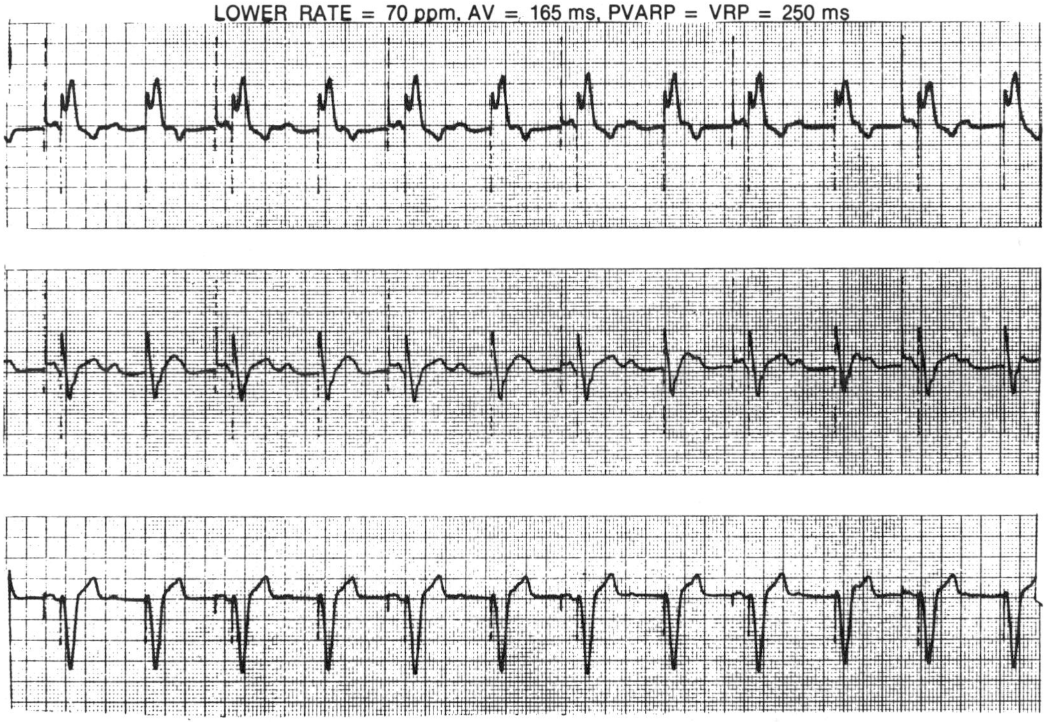

Figure 15.23. DDI mode. With V-V lower rate timing, the DDI mode is equivalent to the DDD mode with LRI = URI. However, the URI (equal to LRI) is longer than the programmed TARP (AV + PVARP). As in the DDD mode, P waves outside the 250-msec PVARP are sensed and initiate an AV interval (i.e., atrial stimulus is inhibited). With atrial sensing the As-Vp interval lengthens by a varying period to conform to the URI (equal to the LRI). As in the DDD mode (Fig. 15.18), the maximum prolongation of the AV interval during Wenckebach pacemaker AV block represents the difference between the URI and the programmed TARP. When the P wave is unsensed during the PVARP, the pulse generator emits an atrial stimulus at the end of its programmed atrial escape interval. (Reproduced with permission from Barold SS, Falkoff MD, Ong LS, *et al.*: Electrocardiography of contemporary DDD pacemakers. A. Basic concepts, upper rate response, retrograde ventriculoatrial conduction, and differential diagnosis of pacemaker tachycardias. In Saksena S, Goldschlager N (eds): Electrical Therapy for Cardiac Arrhythmias, Pacing, Antitachycardia Devices, Catheter Ablation. WB Saunders, Philadelphia, 1990:225.)

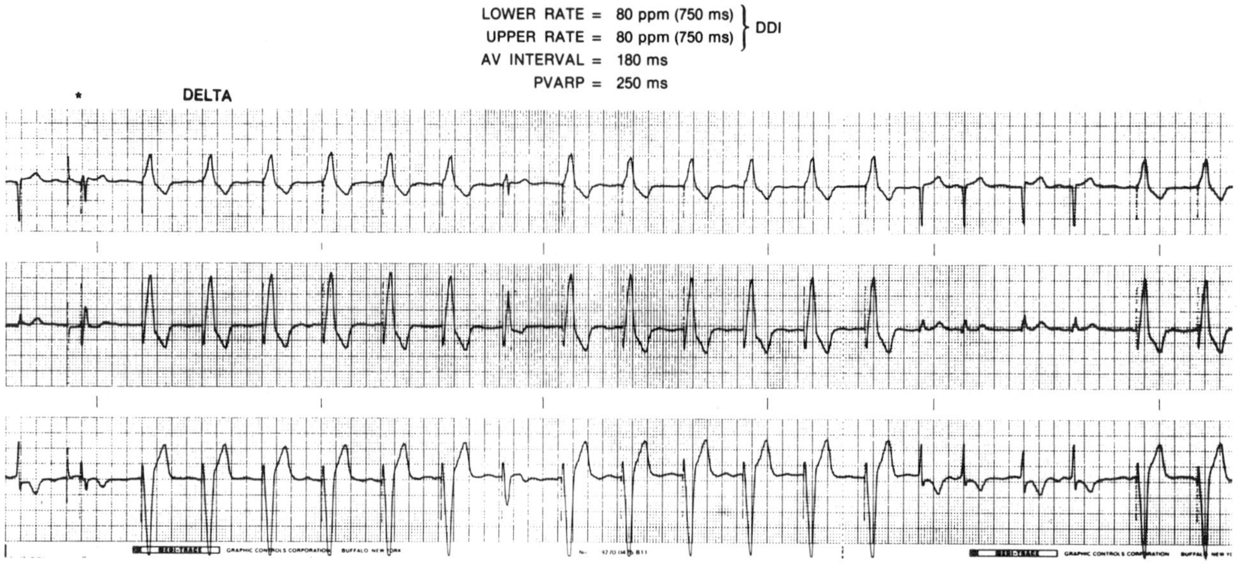

Figure 15.24. DDI mode in CPI Delta DDD pacemaker with V-V lower rate timing. Although the pulse generator was left programmed to the DDD mode, it functions as in the DDI mode because the upper rate was programmed to a value equal to the lower rate (80 ppm). The underlying rhythm is atrial fibrillation. Barring the first beat, the DDI mode resembles VVI pacing at 80 ppm with normal ventricular pacing and sensing. The presence of atrial and ventricular stimuli in relation to the first beat provides the only clue that the pulse generator functions in the DDI mode. The atrial fibrillatory waves generate sufficient voltage to inhibit the atrial channel continually except on the left before the first QRS complex. Three ECG leads were recorded simultaneously. (Reproduced with permission from Barold SS, Falkoff MD, Ong LS, *et al.*: Timing cycles of DDD pacemakers. In Barold SS, Mugica J (eds): New Perspectives in Cardiac Pacing. Futura Publishing Co., Mt. Kisco, NY, 1988:69.)

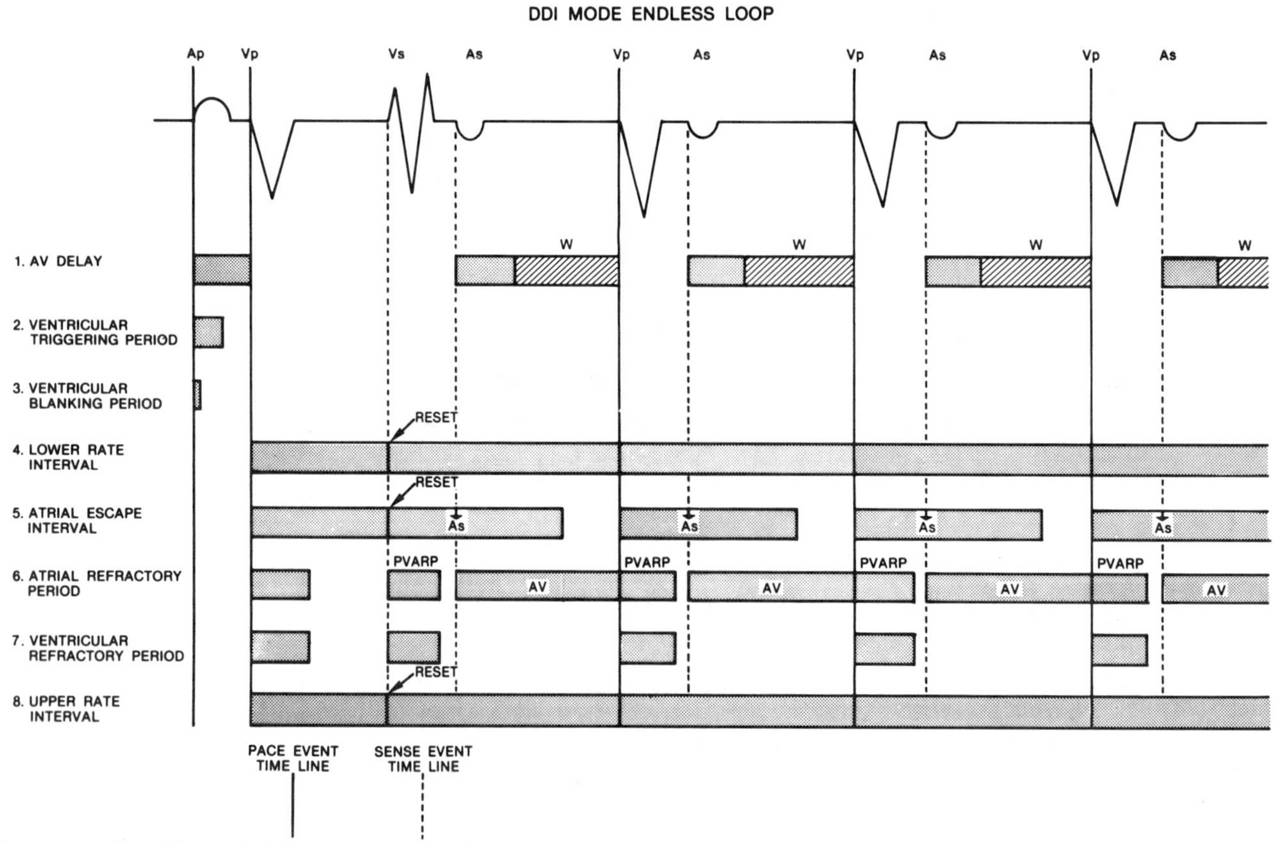

Figure 15.25. DDI mode (V-V lower rate timing). Repetitive reentrant VA synchrony. This mechanism is identical to that of endless loop tachycardia (Fig. 15.34), but no tachycardia occurs in the DDI mode because URI = LRI. A sensed ventricular extrasystole (Vs) generates retrograde ventriculoatrial conduction (As). The pacemaker senses As and initiates an extended AV interval lengthened by W to conform to the upper rate interval (Vp-Vp), also equal to the lower rate interval. (Reproduced with permission from Barold SS, Falkoff MD, Ong LS, *et al.*: All dual chamber pacemakers function in the DDD mode. Am Heart J 1988;115:1353.)

VENTRICULAR-BASED LOWER RATE TIMING OF DUAL-CHAMBER PACEMAKERS

Behavior of Single Cycles

The behavior of DDD pacemakers with V-V lower rate timing may be simplified by examining a single cycle at a time. The DDD mode incorporates three simple modes—DVI, AAI, and VDD. In any one pacemaker cycle, any of these three modes may be seen to start with a ventricular paced or sensed event (Fig. 15.26). The descriptive mode for a single pacemaker cycle is determined only by the way the cycle terminates with a ventricular event. When there are no pacemaker stimuli, the pacemaker is in the inhibited mode (81).

VVI (VOO) MODE

If there is a single ventricular stimulus, the pacemaker may also be functioning in the VVI or VOO mode rather than the VDD mode. Automatic conversion of a DDD pulse generator to the VVI (or VOO) mode may occur as a result of sensing extraneous interference or secondary to battery depletion, the reset mode (VVI or VOO) being an elective replacement indicator. In the DDI mode (with V-V lower rate timing so that the LRI = URI), when rapid atrial activity continually inhibits the atrial channel, the ECG becomes identical to that of the VVI mode.

DDT MODE

A DDD pulse generator may be considered to work in the DDT mode during VSP because a signal sensed by the ventricular channel during the VSP period (or crosstalk sensing window) forces the delivery of a triggered ventricular stimulus at the end of the VSP period with abbreviation of the paced AV interval.

Rate Fluctuation Due to Ventricular Inhibition During Programmed AV Delay

During DVI, DDI, and DDD pacing with V-V lower rate timing, when AV conduction is relatively normal, atrial capture (Ap) may give rise to a normally conducted QRS complex that may in turn inhibit the ventricular channel (Vs). In this situation, the QRS complex must occur before the completion of the programmed interval (Ap-Vp). Because the sensed QRS complex also starts a new LRI and atrial escape interval, this situation may lead to a fluctuation of the atrial pacing rate (faster than the lower rate for ventricular pacing) on a beat-to-beat basis or produce an atrial pacing rate faster than the programmed lower (ventricular) rate (105–107) (Fig. 15.27).

In pulse generators with V-V lower rate timing, increase in the atrial rate due to ventricular inhibition is more pronounced at faster basic pacing rates, an important consideration in the design of rate-adaptive (DDDR) pulse generators (Fig. 15.27B). Rate-adaptive shortening of the AV interval of DDDR pacemakers can effectively narrow or eliminate the difference between the faster atrial pacing rate (due to ventricular inhibition) and the

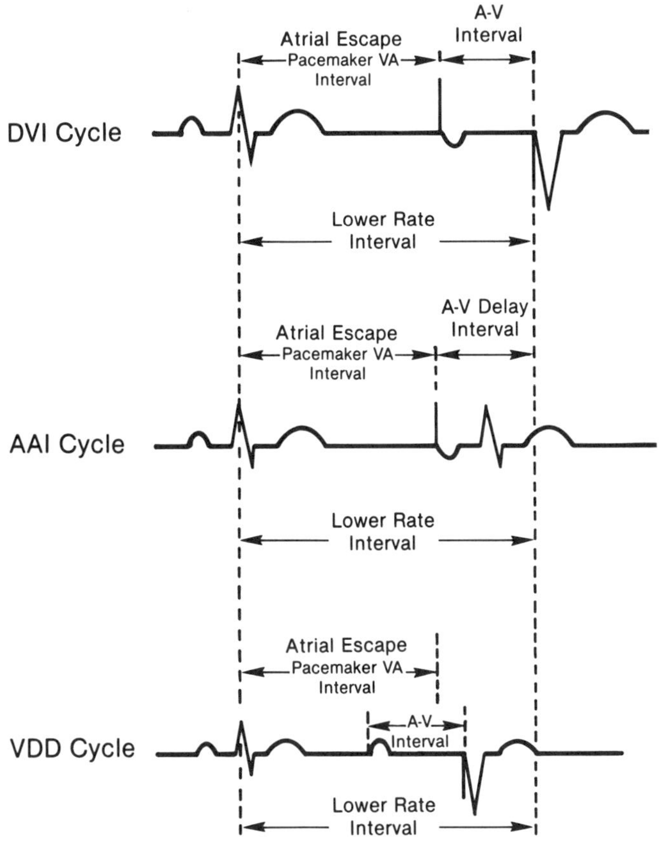

Figure 15.26. Behavior of a DDD pacemaker with V-V lower rate timing based on examination of a single cycle at a time in a continuous electrocardiogram. The DDD mode incorporates the essentials of three simpler modes: DVI, AAI, and VDD. In any one pacemaker cycle, starting with either a sensed or a paced ventricular event (Vs or Vp), one of these three modes may be seen. The descriptive mode for a single pacemaker cycle is determined only by the way the cycle terminates. (a) DVI mode if there are two stimuli. The DVI mode occurs with a slow atrial rate and abnormal AV conduction. (In this context, the DVI mode refers to a partially committed system.) (b) AAI mode. If there is only an atrial stimulus, the pacemaker functions in the AAI mode. The AAI mode occurs if the atrial rate is slow, with intact AV conduction. (c) VDD mode. If there is only a ventricular stimulus, the pacemaker functions in the VDD mode. The VDD mode occurs with a normal atrial rate, but abnormal AV conduction. If there are no stimuli, the pacemaker is fully inhibited and the mode for a given cycle cannot be determined. Thus, if there are no stimuli the pacemaker could be operating in any one of its three modes for any given cycle (AAI, VDD, or DVI). In this situation the RR interval (Vs-Vs) is shorter than the lower rate interval and the PR interval is shorter than the programmed AV interval. However, inhibition does not always mean that the pulse generator senses both ventricular and atrial signals. Thus, during total inhibition a DDD pulse generator may actually be working continuously in the DVI mode with atrial undersensing (if the atrial signal is too small to be sensed), if the RR interval is shorter than the atrial escape interval. (Reproduced with permission from Barold SS, Falkoff MD, Ong LS, *et al.*: Electrocardiography of contemporary DDD pacemakers. A. Basic concepts, upper rate response, retrograde ventriculoatrial conduction, and differential diagnosis of pacemaker tachycardias. In Saksena S, Goldschlager N (eds): Electrical Therapy for Cardiac Arrhythmias, Pacing, Antitachycardia Devices, Catheter Ablation. WB Saunders, Philadelphia, 1990:225.)

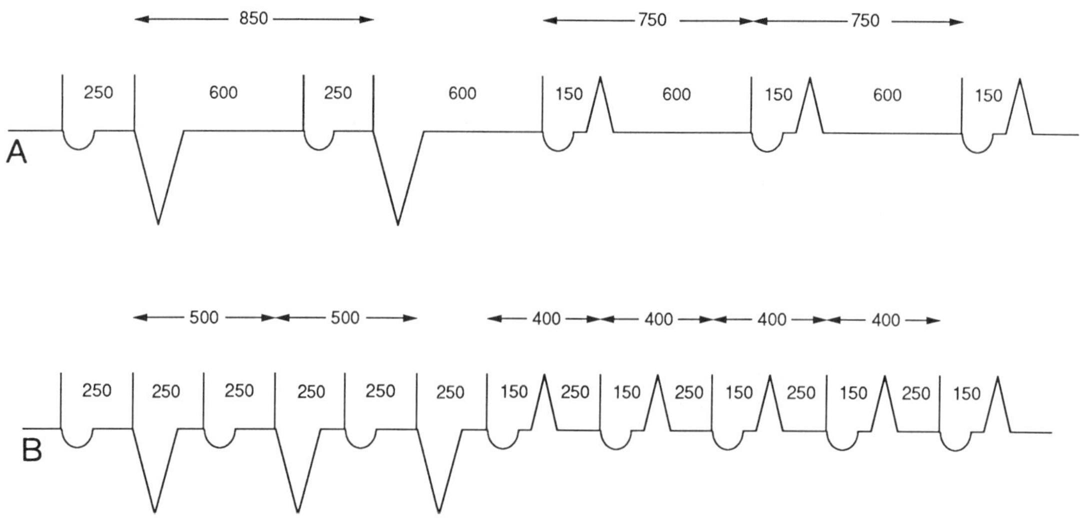

Figure 15.27. Diagrammatic representation of the function of a DDDR pacemaker with V-V LRT showing the effect of ventricular inhibition. **A,** DDD mode: LRI = 850 msec, AV = 250 msec, AEI = 600 msec. On the **right,** when Ap is followed by a conducted QRS complex, the PR (Ap-Vs) interval shortens to 150 msec, but the AEI remains constant at 600 msec. Therefore the Ap-Ap interval decreases to 750 msec, i.e., the atrial pacing rate increases from 70 to 80 ppm. **B,** DDDR mode: the programmed maximum sensor-driven rate is 120 ppm (500 msec). The AV interval remains at 250 msec so that the AEI shortens to 250 msec. On the **right,** when Ap is followed by a conducted QRS complex, the PR (Ap-Vs) interval shortens to 150 msec, but the AEI remains constant at 250 msec. Therefore, the Ap-Ap interval decreases to 400 msec, i.e., the atrial pacing rate increases from 120 to 150 ppm. (Reproduced with permission from Barold SS, Falkoff MD, Ong LS, *et al.*: A-A and V-V lower rate timing of DDD and DDDR pulse generators. In Barold SS, Mugica J (eds): New Perspectives in Cardiac Pacing. 2. Futura Publishing Co., Mt. Kisco, NY, 1991:203.)

programmed maximum rate (106), i.e, upper ventricular rate (Fig. 15.28).

Rate Fluctuation Due to Ventricular Safety Pacing

In pulse generator with V-V timing and a VSP mechanism, activation of VSP (by ventricular sensing of signals such as crosstalk) causes an increase in the atrial pacing rate due to abbreviation of the Ap-Vp interval with the atrial escape interval (Vp-Ap) remaining constant (Fig. 15.13).

TYPES OF LOWER RATE TIMING MECHANISMS OF DUAL-CHAMBER PACEMAKERS

Despite the well-established performance of dual-chamber pacemakers with V-V lower rate timing, recently some pacemaker manufacturers introduced dual-chamber pulse generators with atrial-based lower rate timing (A-A timing), designed to avoid cycle-to-cycle fluctuations or beat-to-beat oscillations. With an atrial-based timing system, the LRI is controlled by atrial rather than ventricular events. In A-A lower rate timing, the LRI is the longest Ap-Ap or As-Ap interval (without an intervening atrial sensed event). Other designs of lower rate control include a variety of hybrids with either A-A or V-V timing according to circumstances (105,106). The definition of the atrial escape interval starting from Vp or Vs to the succeeding Ap (without an intervening atrial sensed event) remains the same for all types of lower rate timing.

V-V and A-A Responses

For descriptive purposes, the behavior of a *single* pacemaker cycle initiated by any combination of atrial and ventricular events (As-Vs, As-Vp, Ap-Vs, Ap-Vp, or isolated VS) can be considered in terms of one of two mechanisms: (a) V-V response in which a ventricular paced or sensed event determines the duration of the succeeding pacing cycle. Vp or Vs initiates a *constant* atrial escape interval (Vs-Vp or Vp-Ap) equal to its basic value in the freerunning mode. If Ap terminating the atrial escape interval is followed by Vp, the Vs-Ap-Vp or Vp-Ap-Vp intervals will be constant and equal to the programmed LRI. (b) A-A response in which an atrial paced or sensed event determines the duration of the succeeding pacing cycle. As or Ap initiates a constant LRI (As-Ap or Ap-Ap) disregarding any Vs or Vp following As or Ap at the beginning of the pacing cycle (Figs. 15.29–15.31). Consequently the atrial escape interval adapts its duration (longer, shorter, or unchanged) to maintain a constant Ap-Ap or As-Ap relationship equal to the atrial-based LRI. During ventricular safety pacing, an atrial-based DDD pulse generator (in contrast to a ventricular-based system) maintains the programmed lower rate (interval) constant: the AV interval shortens and the atrial escape interval lengthens so that the sum of these two intervals is equal to the atrial-based lower rate interval (Fig. 15.29). In hybrid designs, the pulse generator functions either with a V-V or A-A mechanism according to circumstances.

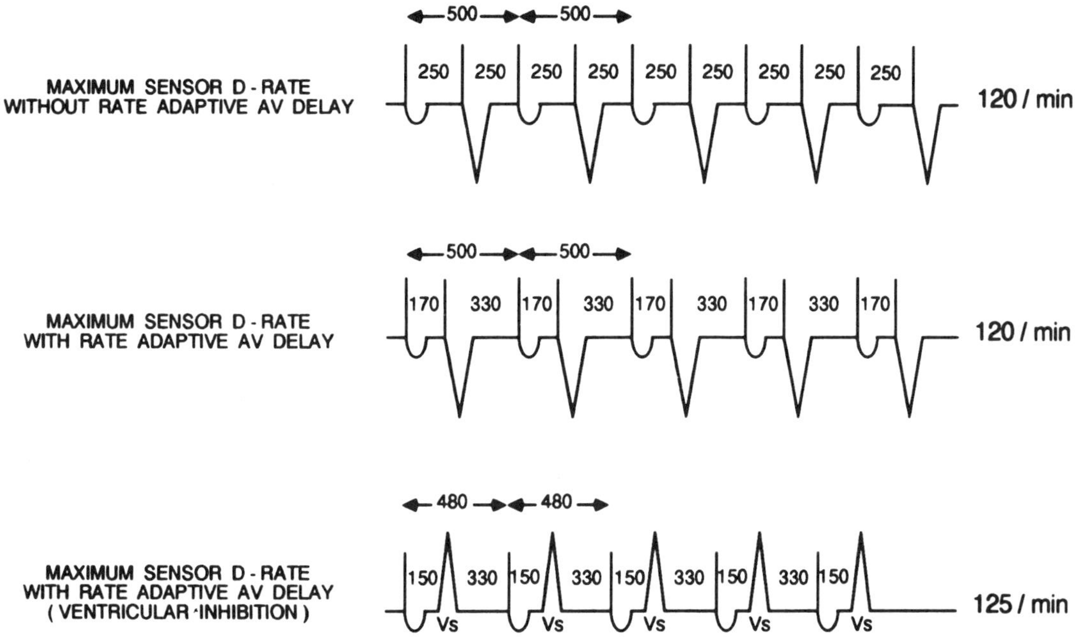

Figure 15.28. Diagrammatic representation of the function of a DDDR pacemaker with V-V LRT showing the effect of a rate-adaptive AV delay that shortens on exercise. The maximum sensor-driven rate is 120 ppm (500 msec). The basic AV interval is 250 msec. **Top:** maximum sensor-driven rate without rate adaptive AV delay. **Middle:** maximum sensor-driven rate with rate-adaptive AV delay. Note that the AV delay has shortened from 250 to 170 msec, and the sensor-driven escape interval has lengthened from 250 msec (**top**) to 330 msec. **Bottom:** The maximum sensor-driven rate is 120 ppm (500 msec). The AV interval shortens to 150 msec because a conducted QRS complex (Vs) is sensed before termination of the rate-adaptive AV interval. As in the **middle example,** the atrial escape interval remains at 330 msec, so that the atrial pacing rate increases to only 125/min (compare with the atrial pacing rate of 150/minute in Fig. 15.27 (Part B)).

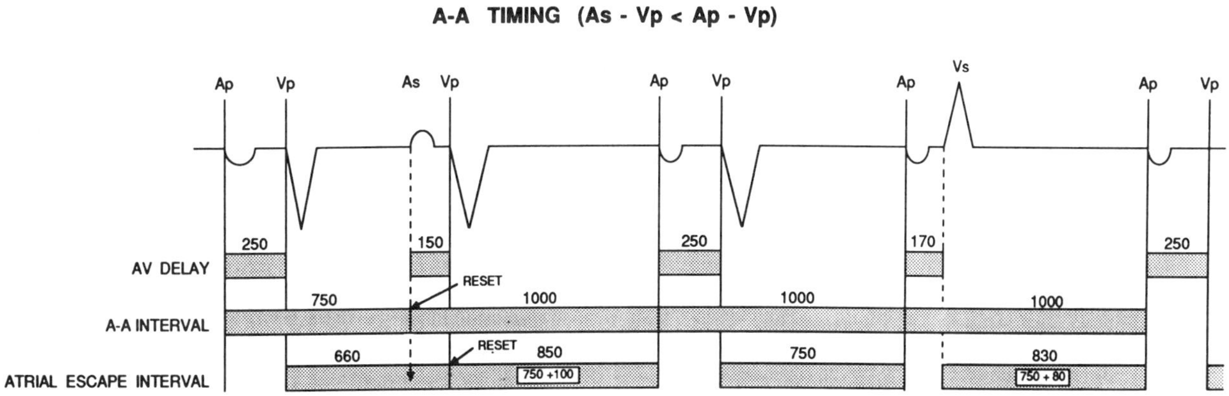

Figure 15.29. Diagrammatic representation of the timing cycles of the Intermedics Cosmos II DDD pulse generator with A-A lower rate timing showing the effect of differential AV delays. LRI = 1000 msec, basic atrial escape interval (AEI) = 750 msec during freerunning AV sequential pacing, As-Vp = 150 msec, and Ap-Vp = 250 msec. The second Vp terminates the As-Vp interval = 150 msec, and initiates an AEI of 750 + (250 − 150) = 850 msec to maintain constancy of the A-A or Ap-Ap interval. On the **right,** the third Ap initiates an Ap-Vs interval = 170 msec. The corresponding escape interval becomes 750 + (250 − 170) = 830 msec to maintain constancy of the A-A or Ap-Ap interval. (Reproduced with permission from Barold SS, Falkoff MD, Ong LS, *et al.*: A-A and V-V lower rate timing of DDD and DDDR pulse generators. In New Perspectives in Cardiac Pacing. 2. Futura Publishing Co., Mt. Kisco, NY, 1991:203.)

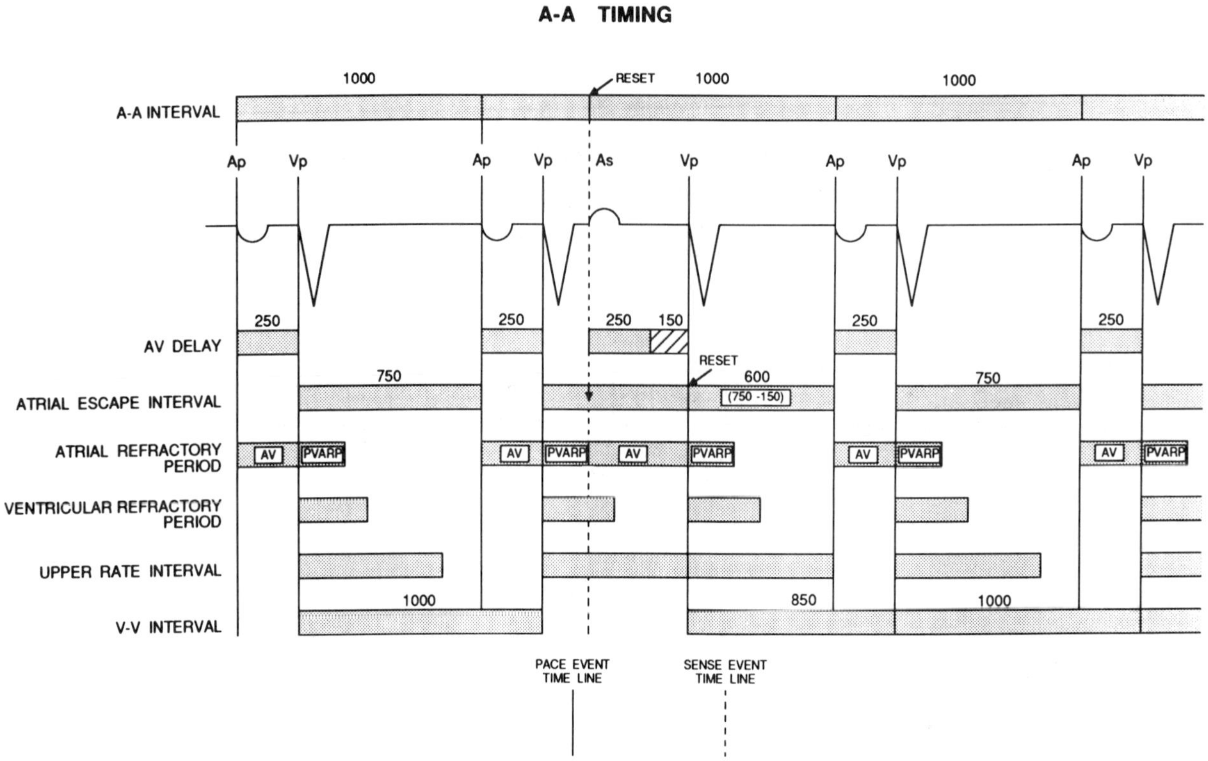

Figure 15.30. Diagrammatic representation of the timing cycles of the Intermedics Cosmos II DDD pulse generator with A-A lower rate timing showing the effect of an early atrial sensed event. LRI = 1000 msec, basic AEI = 750 msec during freerunning AV sequential pacing. An atrial extrasystole (As) initiates an AV interval of 400 msec (As-Vp) to conform to the ventricular URI. Therefore, the pulse generator emits Vp at the completion of the URI. Vp initiates an AEI of 750 + (250 − 400) = 750 − 150 = 600 msec. The A-A interval remains constant at 1000 msec. (Reproduced with permission from Barold SS, Falkoff MD, Ong LS, *et al.*: A-A and V-V lower rate timing of DDD and DDDR pulse generators. In New Perspectives in Cardiac Pacing. 2. Futura Publishing Co., Mt. Kisco, NY, 1991:203.)

TIMING CYCLES OF DDDR PACEMAKERS

Lower Rate Interval

In the DDDR mode (as in the VVIR mode), the LRI is variable and varies as the sensor-driven rate varies (Fig. 15.6). At any given time the duration of the LRI can be either the programmed LRI or the constantly changing sensor-driven LRI, whichever is shorter. The shortest sensor-driven LRI is equal to the programmed sensor-driven URI.

Upper Rate Response

Control of the upper rate involves (a) only two intervals (TARP and P-P intervals) with a simple DDD pacemaker, (b) three intervals (TARP, P-P interval, and URI) with a more complex DDD pacemaker with a separately programmable URI > TARP, and (c) four intervals (TARP, P-P interval, atrial-driven URI, and sensor-driven URI) in DDDR devices (108–112).

Control of the LRI by either an A-A or V-V response should not be confused with behavior of the upper rate response. Atrial-based lower rate timing does not mean that the URI is also atrial based (113). Regardless of the mechanism of lower rate timing, the URI is always a *ventricular* interval initiated by a ventricular paced or sensed event.

The atrial-driven URI refers to the shortest Vs-Vp or Vp-Vp where the second Vp is triggered by a sensed atrial event. The second Vp can only be released at the completion of ventricular URI initiated by the preceding Vs or Vp. The sensor-driven URI (DDDR pacing) refers to the shortest Vs-Vp or Vp-Vp, where the second Vp is controlled by sensor activity. The second Vp can only be released at the completion of the sensor-driven ventricular URI initiated by a preceding Vs or Vp.

The relationship between the sensor-driven URI and atrial-driven URI may take one of three forms: (a) sensor-driven URI > atrial-driven URI, i.e., the sensor-driven upper rate is slower than the atrial-driven upper rate (this response is not useful clinically and should not be used) (110), (b) sensor-driven URI = atrial-driven URI (common upper rates), and (c) sensor-driven URI < atrial-driven URI, i.e, sensor-driven upper rate faster than the atrial-driven upper rate (112,114–116), an arrangement useful to avoid tracking of fast atrial rates in patients with the bradycardia-tachycardia syndrome and atrial chronotropic incompetence.

MULTIPROGRAMMABILITY

A programmable pulse generator may be defined as a device capable of non-invasive adjustment of its function in such a way

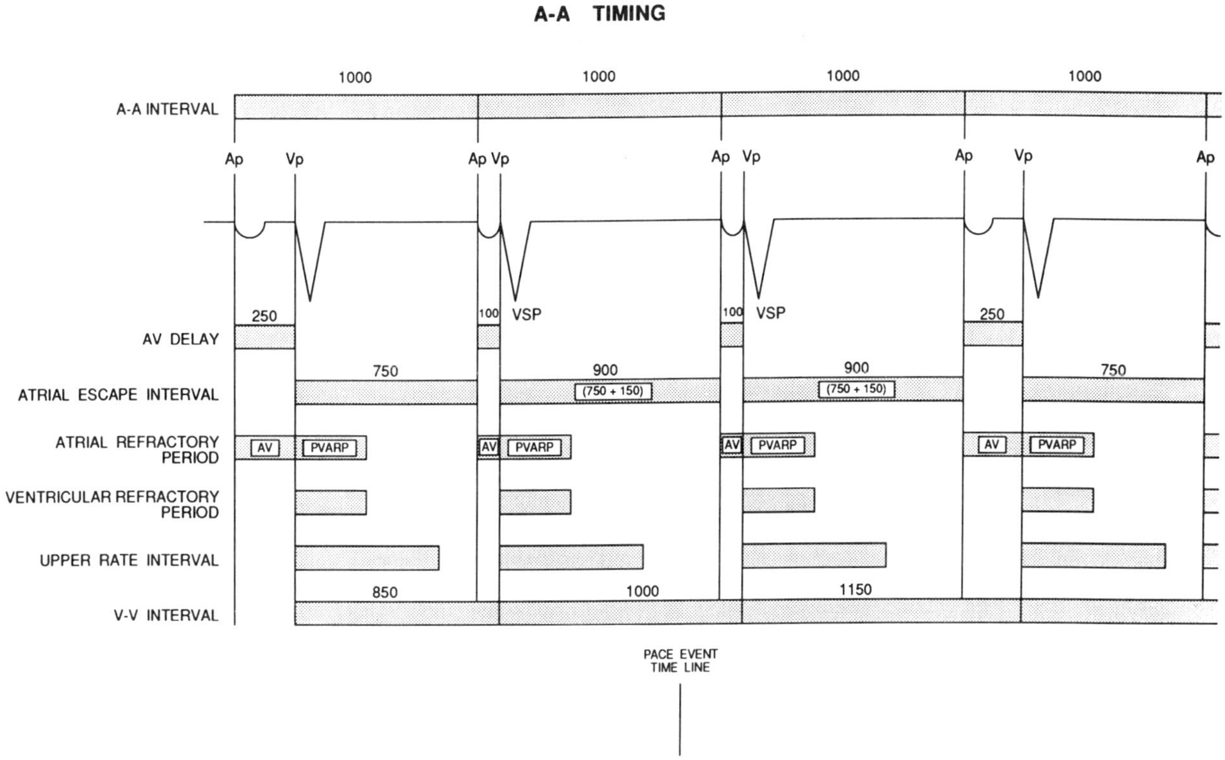

Figure 15.31. Diagrammatic representation of timing cycles of the Cosmos II DDD Pulse generator with A-A lower rate timing. LRI = 1000 msec, basic AEI = 750 msec during freerunning AV sequential pacing. Crosstalk induces ventricular safety pacing (VSP) with abbreviation of the Ap-Vp interval to 100 msec. The Ap-Ap interval remains constant so that the AEI lengthens to 750 + (250 − 100) = 900 msec. During VSP, the pacing rate of a pulse generator with A-A lower rate timing remains constant in contrast to an increase in the pacing rate in a DDD pulse generator with V-V lower rate timing. At the termination of crosstalk, the Vp-Vp interval lengthens to 1150 msec > atrial LRI. (Reproduced with permission from Barold SS, Falkoff MD, Ong LS, *et al.*: A-A and V-V lower rate timing of DDD and DDDR pulse generators. In New Perspectives in Cardiac Pacing. 2. Futura Publishing Co., Mt. Kisco, NY, 1991:203.)

that the change persists indefinitely until the device is reprogrammed again. An appropriate pacemaker "prescription" may thus be "written" by the physician. The available technology is reliable and cost effective. The various communicating mechanisms from programmer to pacemaker and back to the programmer differ somewhat in rapidity and efficiency according to the manufacturer, but they function quite well with rare untoward events. The program change should always be confirmed by telemetry to reduce the likelihood of error. Programmability is mandatory in modern pacemaker practice because it reduces the incidence of secondary interventions and increases pulse generator longevity by optimizing pacemaker output (17,117,121). Yet, programmability after pacemaker implantation still remains underutilized by many practitioners. Multiprogrammability offers the following advantages: (a) Optimal pacing system for a specific clinical situation. Like chronic pharmacologic therapy requiring dose adjustment according to changing circumstances, pacemaker parameters appropriate at the time of implantation may cease to be adequate in the future and may need modification. (b) Diagnosis. Multiprogrammable pulse generators have greatly simplified troubleshooting of many pacemaker problems. (c) Treatment of pacemaker complications. The capability of altering pacemaker characteristics may make operative revision unnecessary in a significant number of patients (17,44,74,121–130).

For single-chamber pacing, the three most important programmable parameters are rate, output (voltage and pulse width) and sensitivity (120,125,126) (Table 15.2). Other parameters such as refractory period, hysteresis, mode, and polarity are also desirable in certain clinical circumstances (Table 15.2). Extensive programmability is essential for dual-chamber pacing.

Output

Situations where output programmability is beneficial include: (a) follow-up of chronic pacing threshold, (b) temporary increase in threshold: the ability to increase output may be useful in dealing with an early disproportionate rise in threshold several days after implantation or a temporary change of the threshold related to a variety of circumstances. (c) Decreasing output is important to conserve battery life and increase longevity of the pulse generator. For most patients the nominal output delivered by the pacemaker is excessive and wasteful. Most patients can be paced at an output substantially lower than nominal settings after the pacing threshold has stabilized several weeks after

Table 15.2.
Multiprogrammability

Rate	Increase	(a) To optimize cardiac output, (b) to overdrive or terminate tachyarrhythmias, (c) to adapt pediatric needs, (d) to test AV conduction with AAI pacemakers, (e) to confirm atrial capture during AAI pacing by observing concomitant change in ventricular rate
	Decrease	(a) To assess underlying rhythm and dependency status, (b) to adjust rate below angina threshold, (c) to allow emergence of normal sinus rhythm and preservation of atrial transport, (d) to test sensing function.
Output	Increase	To adapt to pacing threshold.
	Decrease	(a) To test threshold for pacing, (b) to conserve battery longevity according to threshold for pacing, (c) to reduce extracardiac stimulation (pectoral muscle, diaphragm), (d) to assess underlying rhythm and dependency status.
Sensitivity	Increase (reduction of numeric value)	To sense low electrographic signals (P and QRS)
	Decrease (increase of numerical value)	(a) To test sensing threshold, (b) to avoid T wave or afterpotential sensing (VVI pacing), (c) to avoid sensing extracardiac signals, e.g., myopotentials
Refractory period	Increase	To minimize QRS sensing (AAI pacing), (b) to minimize T wave or afterpotential sensing (VVI pacing)
	Decrease	(a) To maximize QRS sensing (VVI pacing), (b) to detect early premature ventricular complexes
Hysteresis		To delay onset of ventricular pacing to preserve atrial transport function
Polarity	Conversion to unipolar mode	(a) To amplify the signal for sensing in the presence of a low bipolar electrogram, (b) to compensate temporarily for lead fracture in the other electrode
	Conversion to bipolar mode	(a) To decrease electromagnetic or myopotential interference, (b) to evaluate oversensing, (c) to eliminate extracardiac anodal stimulation
Mode	VVT/AAT	(a) To perform noninvasive electrophysiologic study and to terminate reentrant tachycardias (chest wall stimulation with external pacemaker), (b) to prevent inhibition of unipolar pacemaker by extracardiac interference, (c) to evaluate oversensing by "marking" sensed signals
	VOO/AOO	To prevent inhibition of pacemaker by interference when triggered mode is not available or undesirable

Reproduced with permission from Barold SS, Zipes DP: Cardiac Pacemakers and Antiarrhythmic Devices. In Braunwald E (ed); Heart Disease, A Textbook of Cardiovascular Medicine. WB Saunders, Philadelphia, 1992:726.

implantation. (d) Subthreshold stimulation. Programming the output to subthreshold levels (or using a low rate) permits study of the underlying rhythm, the natural history of conduction disorders, etc. (e) Suppression of accessory stimulation: reduction of voltage rather than pulse width often minimizes or eliminates muscle stimulation at the anodal site of normally functioning unipolar pacemakers (in the absence of insulation leak) and undesirable diaphragmatic pacing (right diaphragmatic pacing by stimulation of the right phrenic nerve by an atrial lead and left diaphragmatic pacing by a ventricular lead). (f) High output capability: increasing the voltage output to 7.5–10 V may prevent reoperation in the occasional patient with a high threshold problem (131). Advances in lead technology (e.g., steroid-eluting low threshold leads) may ultimately make the use of high-output voltage virtually obsolete.

Sensitivity

Sensing threshold or sensitivity is a measure of the minimal potential difference required between the terminals of a pulse generator to suppress its output. The numeric value of sensitivity is extremely complex, but may be expressed simply in terms of an arbitrary signal. Test signals have not been standardized and because of their dissimilarity with the natural electrogram, they should be considered only as crude estimates of in vivo sensitivity (29). The higher the numeric value of sensitivity, the less sensitive a pacemaker becomes. Programmability of sensitivity is important because the ideal electrode for sensing does not exist. The sensing threshold is determined by programming the pacing rate lower than the intrinsic rate while sensitivity is gradually reduced (corresponding to a higher numeric value in mV) until failure to sense is observed. The sensitivity threshold is the largest possible numeric value associated with regular sensing (e.g., 8 mV) during deep respiration. As a rule, sensitivity should be programmed to a numeric value of at least half (e.g., 4 mV) the threshold value (e.g., 8 mV). Oversensing of the T wave and/or the afterpotential is easily corrected with a decrease in sensitivity (i.e, increase in the numerical value) and/or prolongation of the refractory period (15,132). Oversensing of myopotentials by a unipolar pacemaker requires reduction of sensitivity, but if it results in undersensing of the QRS, programming to the VVT (AAT) mode may be required (15,78).

MULTIPROGRAMMABILITY IN DDD PACING

Output voltage, pulse width, sensitivity, and refractory period must be individually programmable in each chamber. The PVARP plays a central role in dual-chamber function and must be programmable, particularly to prevent endless loop tachycardia (pacemaker-mediated tachycardia) related to repetitive sensing of retrograde P waves (discussed below—see Figs. 15.32–34). The AV delay, the upper rate, and the lower rate (intervals) must be programmable. A Wenckebach upper rate response cannot be programmed as such but may be obtained by programming a separate URI > TARP. Programmability of the ventricular blanking period (and rarely the duration of the VSP period) may be desirable in the prevention of crosstalk (123).

Atrioventricular Interval

The AV interval should be programmable to obtain maximum hemodynamic advantage. A relatively long AV interval may allow spontaneous AV conduction, providing better left ventricular function and conservation of battery life. A number of DDD pacemakers possess identical AV intervals after atrial pacing and sensing. The pacemaker senses on the right side of the heart. Yet, the timing relationships of atrial and ventricular mechanical activity on the left side of the heart determine hemodynamic performance. Thus, constancy of the programmed AV interval may be associated with markedly different effective PR intervals during atrial pacing (As-Vp) opposed to atrial sensing (As-Vp). In the presence of delayed left atrial activation following right atrial pacing, the programmed AV interval may not provide adequate time for effective left atrial systole before left ventricular systole and in extreme cases left atrial systole may actually begin after the onset of left ventricular systole (133). Alt, *et al*. (134) indicated that as a general rule prolongation of the AV interval after atrial pacing by 50 msec may produce basically the same effective AV interval as that initiated by atrial sensing.

In some DDD pulse generators the AV interval initiated by As may be programmed to a shorter value than that initiated by Ap. Some pulse generators possess algorithms that produce progressive shortening of the AV interval on exercise as in the normal heart (adaptive AV delay). Doppler echocardiography may be useful in "fine-tuning" and individualizing the hemodynamic response to pacing. The optimum AV interval may vary considerably from patient to patient and depends on many factors includ-

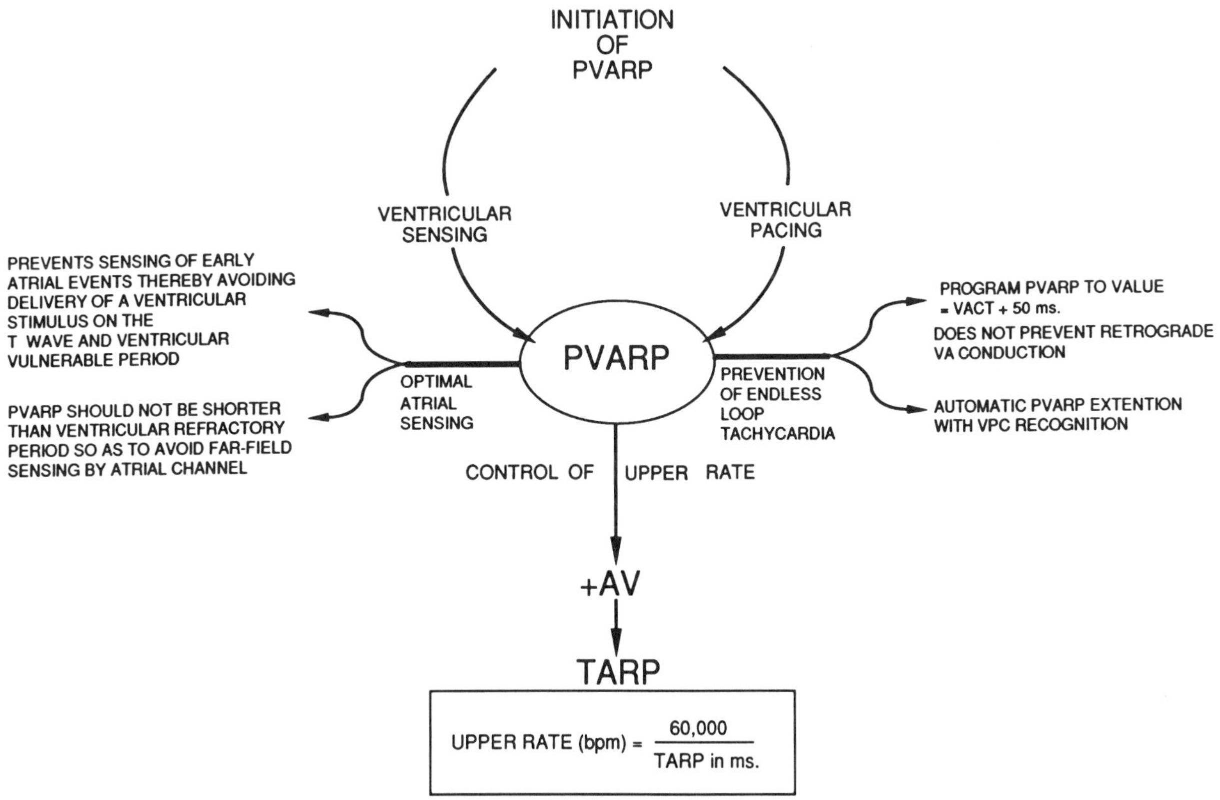

Figure 15.32. Central role of the post-ventricular atrial refractory period in dual chamber pacing (see text for details). (Reproduced with permission from Barold SS: Management of patients with dual chamber pulse generators: central role of the pacemaker atrial refractory period. Learning Center Highlights, Heart House, American College of Cardiology 1990;5(4):8.)

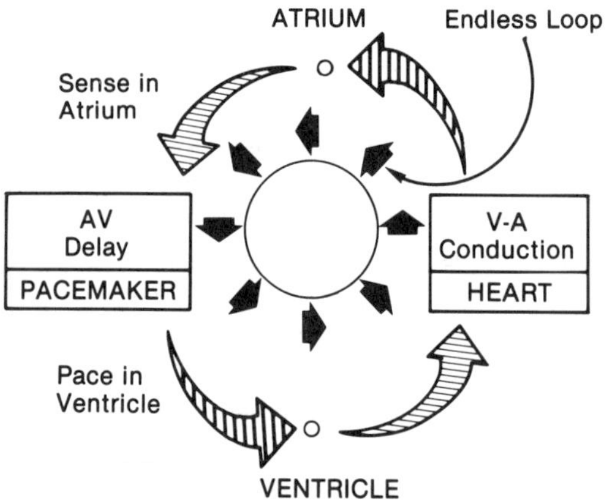

Figure 15.33. Diagrammatic representation of the mechanism of endless loop tachycardia. When the atrial channel senses a retrograde P wave, a ventricular pacing stimulus is issued at the completion of the programmed AV interval. The pulse generator itself provides the anterograde limb of the macroreentrant loop because it functions as an artificial AV junction. Retrograde VA conduction following ventricular pacing provides the retrograde limb of the reentrant loop. The pulse generator again senses the retrograde P, and the process perpetuates itself. Termination of endless loop tachycardia can be accomplished by disrupting either the anterograde limb (by eliminating atrial sensing) or the retrograde limb (by eliminating retrograde VA conduction). (Reproduced with permission from Barold SS, Falkoff MD, Ong LS, *et al.*: Pacemaker endless loop tachycardia: termination by simple techniques other than magnet application. Am J Med 1988;85:817.)

ing left ventricular compliance, left ventricular filling pressure, atrial contractility, mitral valve function, and heart rate and as a rule cannot be predicted in an individual patient (135,136).

Upper Rate Response

The value of the programmed upper rate of a DDD pulse generator depends on the patient's activity, age, left ventricular function, presence of retrograde VA conduction, coronary artery disease, and atrial tachyarrhythmias. The maximal rate of a DDD pacemaker can be defined by either the duration of the TARP (causing fixed-ratio pacemaker AV block such as 2:1, 3:1, etc.) or a separate upper rate timing circuit causing Wenckebach-like AV block (6:5, 5:4, etc.) (81,82,88,93,94). The advantages of other types of upper rate response such as rate-smoothing are unclear and their use should be individualized (88). Holter recording and exercise testing can be useful in tailoring the upper rate response to the needs of the patient.

Pacing Mode

A DDD pulse generator should be programmable at a minimum to the DVI, AAI (or AOO), and VVI modes. With separate programmability to the AAI (or AOO) and VVI modes, the function of each chamber (pacing and sensing) of a DDD pulse generator can be tested individually. Conversion to the AAI or AOO mode provides the fastest and most efficient way of testing for atrial capture (in the absence of AV block with slow spontaneous ventricular rate). (a) VVI mode. Permanent atrial fibrillation necessitates programming to the VVI mode. (b) DDI mode. Frequent paroxysmal supraventricular tachyarrhythmias may require programming to the DDI mode in which the paced ventricular rate remains fixed at the programmed lower rate regardless of the atrial rate. (c) VDD mode. In patients with relatively normal atrial chronotropic function, the VDD mode may be useful in the presence of (a) nonfunctioning atrial lead with high pacing threshold, (b) atrial lead displacement with bothersome right phrenic nerve stimulation, (c) anodal stimulation in a unipolar pulse generator related only to the function of the atrial channel. If the VDD mode is not available, its equivalent in the DDD mode requires turning off the atrial output or programming it to its lowest value for subthreshold atrial stimulation.

Over 90% of contemporary DDD pulse generators with a programmable PVARP should remain in the DDD mode. Permanent mode change to a lesser mode during DDD pacing may arise from: (a) technical causes: problematic atrial pacing or sensing, accessory muscle stimulation or myopotential interference, (b) pathophysiologic causes: sustained atrial arrhythmias, often atrial flutter/fibrillation, constitute the commonest cause of downgrading the pacing mode.

REPETITIVE REENTRANT AND NONREENTRANT VENTRICULOATRIAL SYNCHRONY IN DUAL-CHAMBER PACING

Endless loop tachycardia (sometimes called pacemaker-mediated tachycardia) is a well-known complication of DDD (DDDR, VDD) pacing and represents a form of ventriculoatrial (VA) synchrony (81,89,137,138) or the reverse of atrioventricular (AV) synchrony. Any circumstance causing AV dissociation with separation of the P wave away from the QRS complex coupled with the capability of retrograde VA conduction may initiate endless loop tachycardia (Figs. 15.33 and 15.34). The most common initiating mechanism is a ventricular extrasystole with retrograde VA conduction. Other initiating mechanisms include loss of atrial capture, myopotential sensing by the atrial channel of unipolar devices, undersensing of sinus P waves (sometimes associated with preserved sensing of retrograde P waves), an excessively long AV interval, and application and removal of the pacemaker magnet.

The atrial channel of the pacemaker can sense retrograde atrial activation only when it falls beyond the refractory period (for sensing) of the atrial channel, i.e., the PVARP initiated by a sensed or paced ventricular event. The rate of endless loop tachycardia is often equal to the programmed upper rate of the DDD pacemaker. In the presence of a long retrograde VA conduction time, endless loop tachycardia may occur at a rate slower than the programmed upper rate (Fig. 15.35). The following terminology best describes the mechanism of endless loop tachycardia: repetitive reentrant pacemaker VA synchrony, reentrant VA pacemaker tachycardia, or antidromic reentrant

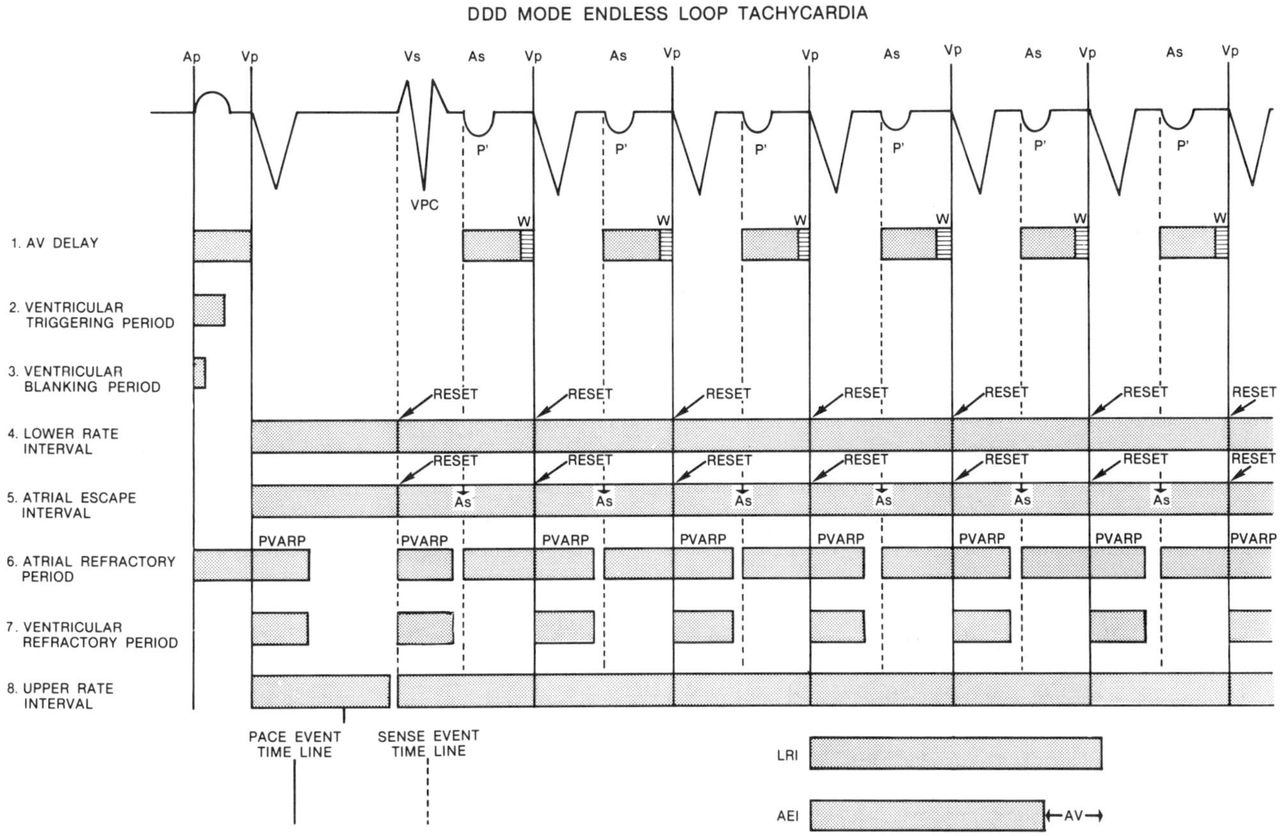

Figure 15.34. DDD mode. Endless loop tachycardia initiated by a ventricular extrasystole (VPC, second beat) with retrograde ventriculoatrial (VA) conduction (As). The atrial channel senses the retrograde P wave (P′) and a ventricular pacing stimulus (Vp) is issued after extension of the AV interval to conform to the URI. Vp generates another retrograde P wave, again sensed by the pulse generator, and the process perpetuates itself. The pulse generator itself provides the antegrade limb of the macroreentrant loop because it functions as an artificial AV junction. Retrograde VA conduction following ventricular pacing provides the retrograde limb of the reentrant loop. The cycle length of the endless loop tachycardia is equal to the URI. The cycle length of an endless loop tachycardia may occasionally be longer than the URI if retrograde VA conduction is prolonged. (Fig. 15.35). (Reproduced with permission from Barold SS, Falkoff MD, Ong LS, *et al.*: All dual chamber pacemakers function in the DDD mode. Am Heart J 1988;115:1353.)

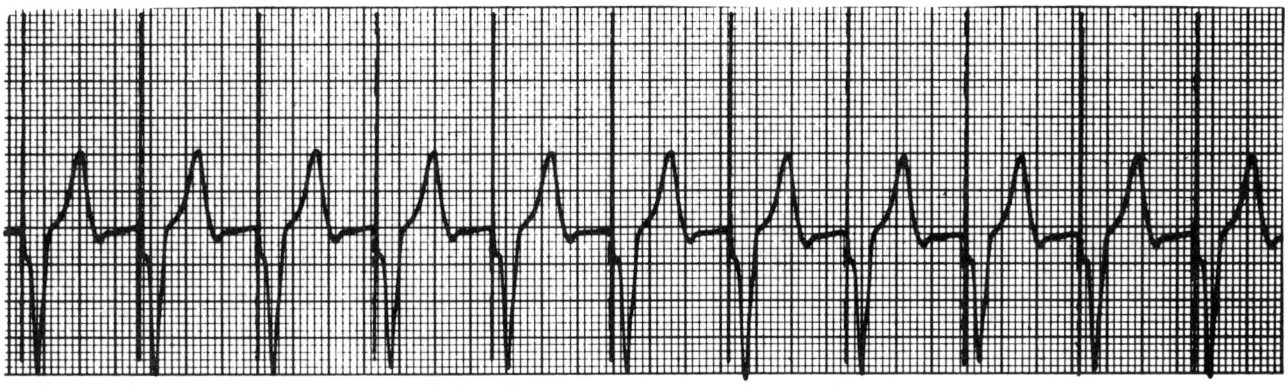

Figure 15.35. Endless loop tachycardia at a rate of 90/min, slower than the programmed upper rate of 100/min. This slower rate permits calculation of the retrograde VA conduction time because the AV interval is not prolonged to conform to the supremacy of the URI. Therefore, the VA conduction time is equal to the cycle length of the tachycardia (650 msec) minus the AV delay (250 msec), i.e., approximately 400 msec (Reproduced with permission from Barold SS, Falkoff MD, Ong LS, *et al.*: Function and electrocardiography of DDD pacemakers. In Barold SS (ed): Modern Cardiac Pacing. Futura Publishing Co., Mt. Kisco, NY, 1985:645.)

dual-chamber pacemaker tachycardia (the pacemaker acting as an electronic accessory pathway).

Endless loop tachycardia may terminate spontaneously because of VA conduction block either from a fatigue phenomenon in the conduction system or the occurrence of a ventricular extrasystole sufficiently premature to cause retrograde VA conduction block (139). Elimination of atrial sensing terminates endless loop tachycardia by affecting the anterograde limb of the reentrant process (Fig. 15.33) in a variety of circumstances: (a) magnet application when the pulse generator converts to the DOO or VOO mode. Rarely the tachycardia recurs upon magnet removal, (b) PVARP prolongation, (c) decrease in atrial sensitivity, (d) programming to a nonatrial tracking mode such as the DVI or VVI mode.

Disruption of the retrograde limb of the reentrant process can also terminate endless loop tachycardia by one of two mechanisms. First, a direct effect on VA conduction with carotid sinus massage or the administration of drugs such as Verapamil or beta blockers (140,141). Second, uncoupling of VA synchrony at (a) any ventricular sensed event unaccompanied by retrograde VA conduction block, e.g., sufficiently premature ventricular extrasystole with retrograde VA conduction block, myopotential (in unipolar pulse generators) or chest wall stimulation (142), and (b) omission of a single ventricular stimulus as in the automatic tachycardia terminating algorithm of some DDD pacemakers (143) (Fig. 15.36). Uncoupling of VA synchrony allows restoration of AV synchrony by promoting either a paced or sensed atrial event.

Approximately 70–80% of patients with sick sinus syndrome and 35% of patients with AV block exhibit retrograde VA conduction (144). Consequently, over 50% of patients receiving dual-chamber pacemakers are susceptible to endless loop tachycardia. The VA conduction time ranges from 100 to 400 msec, rarely longer, and is influenced by autonomic factors, drugs, etc. (144–147). Only a minority of patients (5%) with no VA conduction at the time of implantation subsequently develop

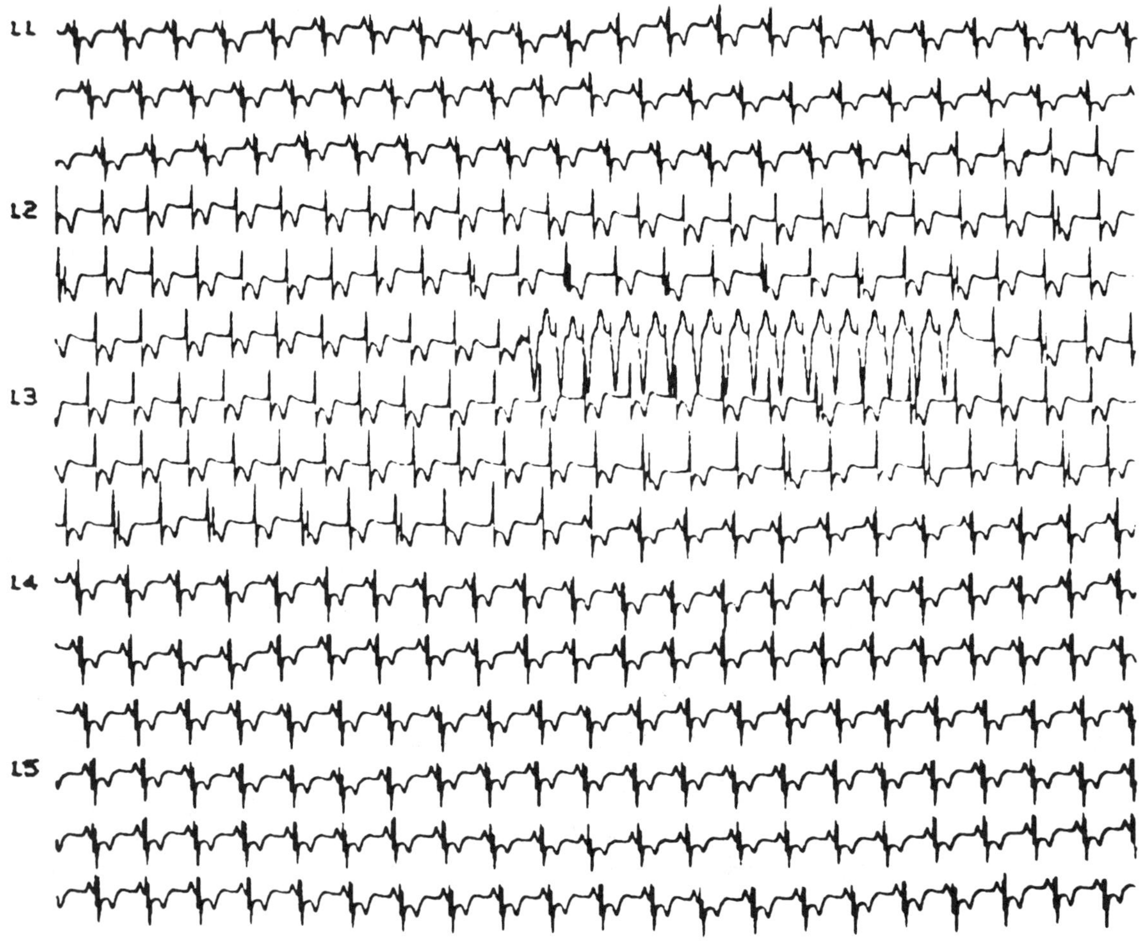

Figure 15.36. Tachycardia terminating algorithm of the Intermedics Cosmos I DDD pulse generator. Endless loop tachycardia is initiated by an AV junctional rhythm and retrograde VA conduction. After 15 consecutive ventricular paced cycles at the upper interval, the pacemaker automatically inhibits the delivery of a single ventricular stimulus, whereupon uncoupling of ventricular and atrial activity terminates the endless loop tachycardia. (Reproduced with permission from Barold SS, Falkoff MD, Ong LS, *et al.*: Function and electrocardiography of DDD pacemakers. In Barold SS (ed): Modern Cardiac Pacing. Futura Publishing Co., Mt. Kisco, NY, 1985:645.)

VA conduction (148,149). With appropriate programming of sophisticated contemporary pulse generators, endless loop tachycardia can be prevented in virtually all cases (150–152), but the problem cannot be considered eradicated because its management may prevent optimum programming of a number of pacemaker indices. These compromises themselves may sometimes lead to new pacemaker problems.

EVALUATION OF RETROGRADE VA CONDUCTION AND PROPENSITY FOR ENDLESS LOOP TACHYCARDIA

Although the presence and duration of retrograde VA conduction can be determined in the VVI mode or even automatically by telemetry to the programmer of advanced pacemakers (153), the propensity for endless loop tachycardia is best tested by programming the pulse generator to the DDD mode as follows: (a) lower rate faster than the spontaneous rate, (b) highest atrial sensitivity, (c) shortest PVARP, (d) lowest possible atrial output (pulse width and voltage) to produce subthreshold atrial stimulation (81,154). An ineffectual atrial stimulus preceding a paced ventricular beat favors retrograde VA conduction by separating the P wave from the QRS complex. Endless loop tachycardia occurs if retrograde VA conduction is sustained and the retrograde P wave falls beyond the PVARP (Figs. 15.37 and 15.38). Alternatively, a pulse generator may be programmed to the VDD mode with the above parameters, the VDD mode being equivalent to the DDD mode with zero atrial output. However, the VDD mode is not universally available as a programmable option. Furthermore, in the presence of a relatively fast sinus rate, programming to the VDD mode with a lower rate faster than the sinus rate makes evaluation difficult. Occasionally in the DDD mode the threshold for atrial pacing is so low that subthreshold atrial stimulation cannot be achieved by programming the lowest

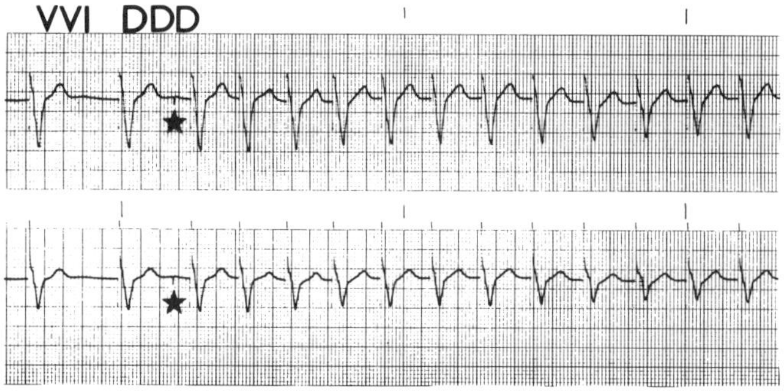

Figure 15.37. Subthreshold atrial stimulation in the DDD mode leading to sustained endless loop tachycardia in a patient with a Cosmos (Intermedics) DDD pulse generator. The threshold for ventricular pacing was tested in the VVI mode (first two paced beats). Then the pacemaker was programmed to the DDD mode: lower rate = 80 ppm, upper rate interval = 120 ppm (500 msec), AV delay = 180 msec, PVARP = 170 msec, atrial output = 2.7 V at 0.03 msec. The first atrial stimulus does not capture the atrium. The subsequent ventricular paced beat causes retrograde VA conduction and initiates endless loop tachycardia at a rate of 120/min (cycle length = 500 msec) with gradual slowing to a cycle length of 540–560 msec (on **right**) because of slowing of VA conduction. Consequently the tachycardia terminating algorithm (Fig. 15.36) is not activated, and the tachycardia continued indefinitely at a cycle length of 540–560 msec.

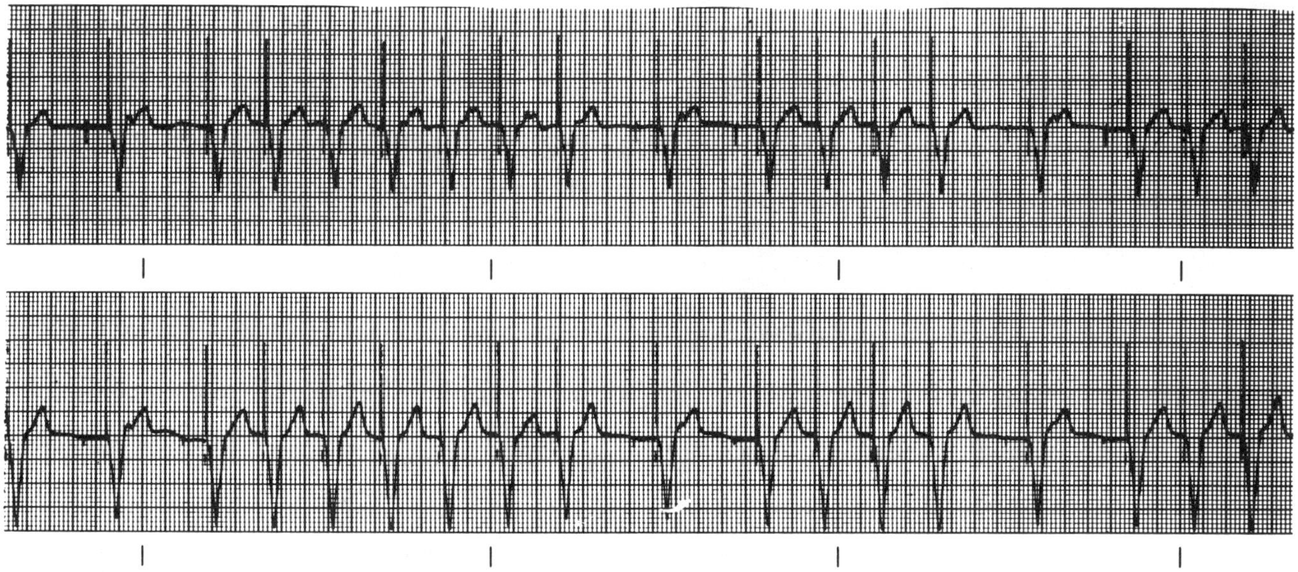

Figure 15.38. Subthreshold atrial stimulation in the DDD mode leading to unsustained endless loop tachycardia in a patient with a Cosmos (Intermedics) DDD pulse generator (two-lead electrocardiogram). The programmed parameters were as follows: LRI = 880 msec, URI = 480 msec, PVARP = 200 msec, and AV interval = 180 msec. The retrograde VA conduction time is just over 200 msec, so that the retrograde P wave is sensed by the atrial channel, thereby initiating runs of nonsustained endless loop tachycardia. (Reproduced with permission from Barold SS, Falkoff MD, Ong LS, *et al.*: Function and electrocardiography of DDD pacemakers. In Barold SS (ed): Modern Cardiac Pacing. Futura Publishing Co., Mt. Kisco, NY, 1985:645.)

atrial output. In these situations, chest wall stimulation (with an external pacemaker providing signals sensed selectively by the atrial channel) will easily precipitate endless loop tachycardia in susceptible individuals by separating the P wave from the paced QRS complex (142,155,156) (Fig. 15.39). Other techniques such as application and withdrawal of the magnet, isometric muscle exercise (with unipolar devices), maximum prolongation of the AV interval, treadmill exercise, and chest thumping (to produce ventricular extrasystoles) are inconsistently effective and not recommended (142,154).

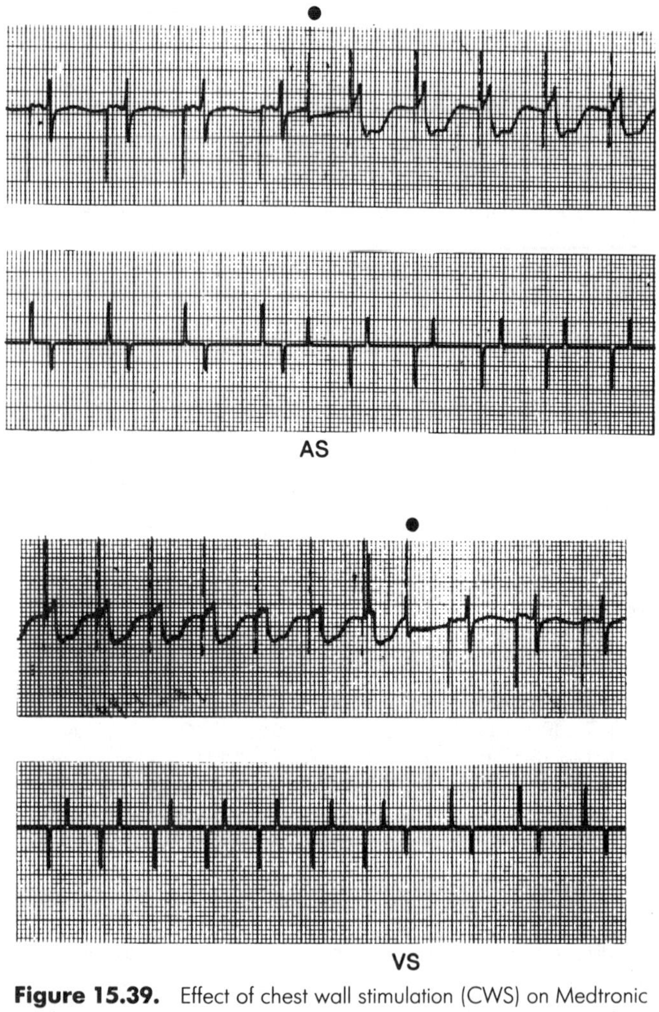

Figure 15.39. Effect of chest wall stimulation (CWS) on Medtronic Symbios 7005 unipolar DDD pulse generator. Real-time event markers are shown below the electrocardiogram. **Top:** CWS (*solid black circle*) sensed only by the atrial channel initiates endless loop tachycardia. **Bottom:** Endless loop tachycardia terminated by the second CWS (*solid black circle*) sensed by the ventricular channel. The first CWS falls within the refractory period of the ventricular channel. The markers depicting sensed events are smaller than those related to paced events. As = atrial sensed event; Vs = ventricular sensed event. (Reproduced with permission from Barold SS, Falkoff MD, Ong LS, *al.*: Electrocardiography of DDD pacemakers. B. Multiprogrammability, follow-up, and troubleshooting. In Saksena S, Goldschlager N (eds): Electrical Therapy for Cardiac Arrhythmias, Pacing, Antitachycardia Devices, Catheter Ablation. WB Saunders, Philadelphia, 1990:242.)

PREVENTION OF ENDLESS LOOP TACHYCARDIA

The maneuvers to initiate endless loop tachycardia are repeated until appropriate programming of the pacemaker prevents induction of tachycardia. In general, the PVARP should be programmed at 50–75 msec beyond the duration of the retrograde VA conduction time determined noninvasively (157). A PVARP of 300 msec offers protection against endless loop tachycardia in most patients with retrograde VA conduction. Programmability of the PVARP constitutes presently the most effective way of preventing endless loop tachycardia. A long PVARP lengthens the total atrial refractory period and therefore limits the upper rate of the pacemaker (83). Other measures to prevent endless loop tachycardia include (a) shorter AV interval; (b) differential discrimination of the larger antegrade P wave from the smaller retrograde atrial depolarization, a potential option in ¾ of patients (80,81,158,159); (c) activation of a special mechanism after a sensed ventricular event (outside the AV delay) that the pacemaker interprets as a ventricular extrasystole: synchronous atrial stimulation (by preempting retrograde atrial depolarization) or automatic extension of the PVARP for one cycle to ensure containment of retrograde atrial depolarization (160,161).

The availability of a programmable PVARP has virtually eliminated endless loop tachycardia with second- and third-generation DDD pulse generators (151,152) but it does not guarantee total prevention because VA conduction may be variable (145,162,163). The experience with contemporary DDD devices stands in sharp contrast to the frequent occurrence of endless loop tachycardia with first generation pulse generators equipped with a short, nonprogrammable PVARP. A contemporary DDD pacemaker should rarely if ever be downgraded to a simpler mode, e.g., DVI or VVI, to prevent endless loop tachycardia (164–166).

AUTOMATIC TERMINATION AND PREVENTION OF ENDLESS LOOP TACHYCARDIA

Some pulse generators can terminate endless loop tachycardia automatically almost as soon as it starts with diagnostic algorithms using rate recognition (143,167,168) or AV interval modulation regardless of the rate (169) (automatic shortening of a single AV interval by advancing ventricular activation may occasionally terminate tachycardia by causing retrograde VA conduction block (169)). A pacemaker can reliably terminate endless loop tachycardia automatically either by omitting a single ventricular stimulus (143) (uncoupling of VA synchrony) or by substantial PVARP prolongation for one cycle (167–169). Obviously algorithms for the detection of endless loop tachycardia should not be based solely on the programmed upper rate because some tachycardias are slower than the upper rate in the presence of relatively prolonged VA conduction. Furthermore, the pulse generator should recognize the nature of tachycardia because pacing at the upper rate obviously does not discriminate endless loop tachycardia from tracking of a normal atrial rhythm.

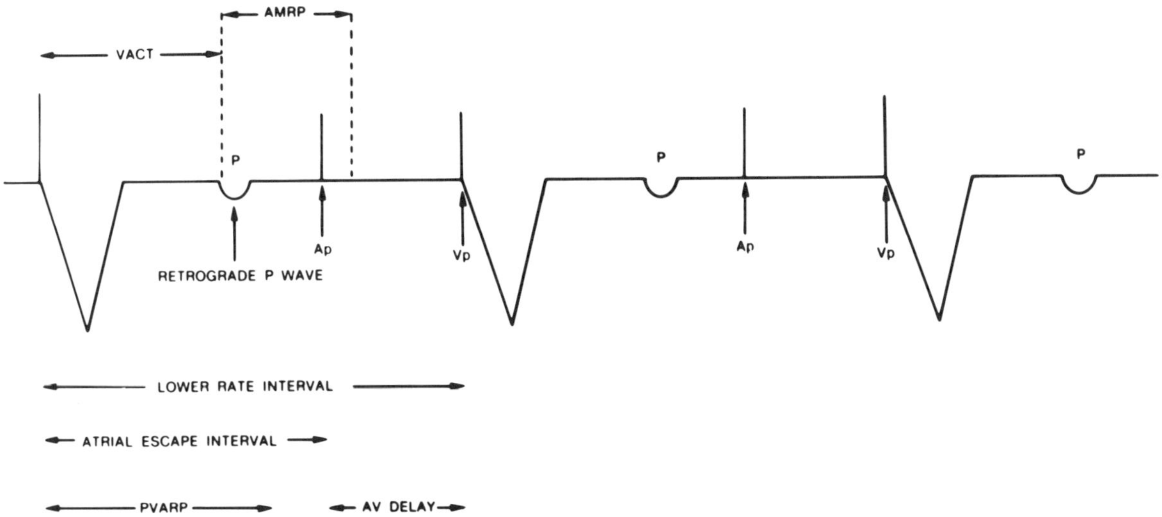

Figure 15.40. Diagrammatic representation of AV desynchronization arrhythmia. There is relatively slow retrograde VA conduction. The first ventricular paced beat causes retrograde VA conduction. The retrograde P wave (P′) is unsensed either because it falls within the PVARP (or because the magnet causes asynchronous DOO pacing). At the completion of the AEI, the pacemaker delivers an atrial stimulus (Ap) falling too close to the preceding retrograde P wave and therefore still within the atrial myocardial refractory period (AMRP) engendered by the preceding retrograde atrial depolarization. Ap is therefore ineffectual. Barring any perturbations, this process becomes self-perpetuating. VACT = retrograde VA conduction time; Vp = ventricular stimulus. (Reproduced with permission from Barold SS, Falkoff MD, Ong LS, *et al.*: Magnet unresponsive pacemaker endless loop tachycardia. Am Heart J 1988;116:726.)

REPETITIVE NONREENTRANT VENTRICULOATRIAL SYNCHRONY

Ventriculoatrial synchrony may occur without endless loop tachycardia when a paced ventricular beat engenders an *unsensed* retrograde P wave usually falling within the PVARP of a DDD pacemaker. Under certain circumstances this form of VA synchrony may become self-perpetuating because the pacemaker continually delivers an ineffectual atrial stimulus during the atrial myocardial refractory period generated by the preceding retrograde atrial depolarization (170–173) (Figs. 15.40 and 15.41). This form of VA synchrony has been called "AV desynchronization arrhythmia" (AVDA), repetitive nonreentrant VA synchrony, or VA synchrony nonreentrant arrhythmia.

During AVDA the pacemaker provides an anterograde pathway (atrial stimulus followed by ventricular stimulus) while the condition system provides a retrograde pathway back to the atrium. In contrast to endless loop tachycardia, the potential reentrant circuit does not close because the pacemaker does not sense the retrograde P wave. The process repeats itself with each cardiac cycle and release of the ventricular stimulus does not depend on the timing of the retrograde P wave. A retrograde P wave beyond the PVARP but unsensed because of its low amplitude or low sensitivity of the atrial channel may also initiate AVDA. Both endless loop tachycardia and AVDA depend on retrograde VA conduction and are physiologically similar. Both share similar initiating and terminating mechanisms and under certain circumstances one arrhythmia may convert spontaneously to the other (174). Occasionally during endless loop tachycardia, magnet application over the pulse generator causes AVDA (with preservation of repetitive retrograde VA conduction) and reinitiation of endless loop tachycardia on magnet removal, producing a magnet-unresponsive ELT.

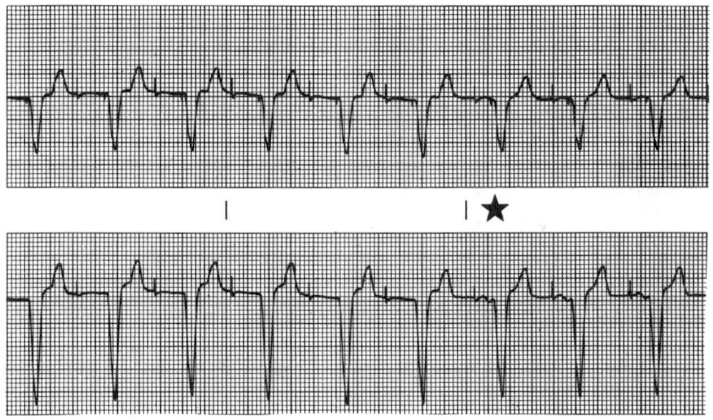

Figure 15.41. AV desynchronization arrhythmia during DDD pacing. On the **left,** ventricular pacing causes retrograde VA conduction. The retrograde P wave falls in the PVARP and is therefore unsensed. The subsequent atrial stimulus (delivered at the completion of the atrial escape interval) is ineffectual because it falls within the atrial myocardial refractory period generated by the preceding retrograde atrial depolarization. Shortening of the AV interval (*star*), keeping the lower rate interval constant, displaces the atrial stimulus away from the preceding P wave and restores AV synchrony by producing atrial capture beyond the atrial myocardial refractory period.

When sustained, AVDA may cause the pacemaker syndrome during normal function of a DDD pulse generator (175). AVDA should not be an important problem with conventional DDD pulse generators because the duration of the atrial escape (pacemaker VA) interval can be easily controlled. However, DDDR pulse generator can induce AVDA on exercise when the sensor-driven increase in pacing rate shortens the atrial escape (pacemaker VA) interval.

References

1. Parsonnet V: Cardiac pacing as a subspecialty. Am J Cardiol 1987;59:989.
2. Harthorne JW, Parsonnet VP: Task Force VI: training in cardiac pacing-Bethesda Conference. J Am Coll Cardiol 1986;7:1213.
3. Furman S. The fourth decade of cardiac pacing. In Barold SS, Mugica J (eds): New Perspectives in Cardiac Pacing. Futura Publishing Co., Mt. Kisco, NY, 1988:429.
4. Brinker JA: Pursuing the perfect pacemaker. Mayo Clin Proc 1989;64:587.
5. Parsonnet V, Bernstein AD: Transvenous pacing: a seminal transition from the research laboratory. Ann Thorac Surg 1989;48:738.
6. Parsonnet V, Bernstein AD: Pacing in perspective: concepts and controversies. Circulation 1986;73:1087.
7. Clarke M, Sutton R, Ward D, *et al.*: Recommendations for pacemaker prescription for symptomatic bradycardia. Report of a working party of the British Pacing and Electrophysiology Group. Br Heart J 1991;66:185.
8. Luceri RM, Myerburg RJ: Indications for and management of cardiac pacemakers. Disease of the month 1985;31:1.
9. Bernstein AD, Camm AJ, Fletcher R, *et al.*: The NASPE/PBEG generic pacemaker code for antibradyarrhythmia and adaptive-rate pacing and antitachy-arrhythmia devices. PACE 1987;10:794.
10. Lillehei RC, Romero LH, Beckman CB, *et al.*: A new solid-state, long-life, lithium-powered pulse generator. Ann Thorac Surg 1974;18:479.
11. Parsonnet V, Furman S, Smyth NPD, *et al.*: Optimal resources for implantable cardiac pacemakers. Report on Inter-society Commission for Heart Disease Resources. Circulation 1983;68:226a.
12. Bilitch M, Cosby RS, Cafferky EA: Ventricular fibrillation and competitive pacing. N Engl J Med 1967;276:598.
13. Tommaso C, Belic N, Brandfonbrener B: Asynchronous ventricular pacing: A rare cause of ventricular tachycardia. PACE 1982;5:561.
14. Barold SS, Carroll M: "Double reset" of demand pacemakers. Am Heart J 1972;84:276.
15. Barold SS, Falkoff MD, Ong LS, *et al.*: Oversensing by single-chamber pacemakers. Mechanisms, diagnostics, and treatment. Cardiol Clin 1987;3:565.
16. Barold SS: Clinical significance of pacemaker refractory periods. Am J Cardiol 1971;28:237.
17. Barold S, Mugica J, Falkoff MD, *et al.*: Multiprogrammability in cardiac pacing. In Barold SS (ed): Modern Cardiac Pacing. Futura Publishing Co., Mt. Kisco, NY, 1985:377.
18. Barold SS, Falkoff MD, Ong LS, *et al.*: Cardiac pacing for the treatment of tachycardia. In Barold SS (ed): Modern Cardiac Pacing. Futura Publishing Co., Mt. Kisco, NY, 1985:693.
19. Barold SS, Falkoff MD, Ong LS, *et al.*: Termination of ventricular tachycardia by chest wall stimulation during DDD pacing. Am J Med 1988;84:549.
20. Barold SS: Clinical uses of chest wall stimulation in patients with DDD pulse generators. Intelligence Reports in Cardiac Pacing and Electrophysiology 1988;7:2.
21. Barold SS, Gaidula JJ: Evaluatin of normal and abnormal sensing functions of demand pacemakers. Am J Cardiol 1971;28:201.
22. Driller J, Barold SS, Parsonnet V: Normal and abnormal function of the pacemaker magnetic switch. J Electrocardiol 1973;6:1.
23. Friedberg HD, Barold SS: On hysteresis in pacing. J Electrocardiol 1973;6:1.
24. Rosenqvist M, Vallin HO, Edhag KO: Rate hysteresis pacing: how valuable is it? A comparison of the stimulation rates of 70 and 50 beats per minute and rate hysteresis in patients with sinus node disease. PACE 1984;7:332.
25. Thompson ME, Shaver JA: Undesirable cardiac arrhythmias associated with rate hysteresis pacemakers. Am J Cardiol 1976;38:685.
26. Hollins WJ, Leman RB, Kratz JM, *et al.*: Limitations of the long-term clinical application of rate hysteresis. PACE 1987;10:302.
27. Spritzer RC, Donoso E, Gadboys HI, *et al.*: Arrhythmias induced by pacemaking on demand. Am Heart J 1969;77:619.
28. Vera Z, Mason DT, Awan NA, *et al.*: Lack of sensing by demand pacemakers due to intraventricular conduction defects. Circulation 1975;51:815.
29. Barold SS, Ong LS, Heinle RA: Stimulation and sensing thresholds for cardiac pacing. Electrophysiologic and technical aspects. Prog Cardiovasc Dis 1981;24:1.
30. Angello DA: Principles of electrical testing for analysis of ventricular endocardial pacing leads. Prog Cardiovasc Dis 1984;27:57.
31. Furman S, Hurzeler P, Mehra R. Cardiac pacing and pacemakers. IV threshold of cardiac stimulation. Am Heart J 1977;94:115.
32. Furman S. Basic concepts. In Furman S, Hayes DL, Holmes DR (eds): A Practice of Cardiac Pacing, 2nd ed. Futura Publishing Co., Mt. Kisco, NY, 1989:23.
33. Stokes K, Bornzin G: The electrode-biointerface: stimulation. In Barold SS (ed): Modern Cardiac Pacing. Futura Publishing Co., Mt. Kisco, NY, 1985:33.
34. Timmis GC. The electrobiology and engineering of pacemaker leads. In Saksena S, Goldschlager N (eds): Electrical Therapy for Cardiac Arrhythmias. Pacing. Antitachycardia Devices. Catheter Ablation. WB Saunders, Philadelphia, 1990:35.
35. Preston TA, Barold SS: Problems in the measurement of threshold for cardiac pacing. Am J Cardiol 1977;40:658.
36. Ector H, Witters E, Aubert A, *et al.*: Measurement of pacing threshold. PACE 1985;8:66.
37. Ohm OJ, Breivik K, Hammer EA, *et al.*: Intraoperative electrical measurements during pacemaker implantation. Clin Prog Pacing Electrophysiol 1984;2:1
38. Greenspan AM. Electrophysiology of pacing. In Hakki AH (ed): Ideal Cardiac Pacing. WB Saunders, Philadelphia, 1984:29.
39. Barold SS, Winner JA: Techniques and significance of threshold measurement for cardiac pacing. Relationship to output circuit of cardiac pacemakers. Chest 1976;70:760.
40. Irnich W: The chronaxie time and its practical importance. PACE 1980;3:292.
41. Irnich W: The electrode myocardial interface. Clin Prog Electrophysiol Pacing 1985;3:338.
42. Hynes JK, Holes DR Jr, Meredith J, *et al.*: An evaluation of long-term stimulation thresholds by measurement of chronic strength duration curves. PACE 1981;4:376.
43. deBuitleir M, Kou WH, Schmaltz S, *et al.*: Acute changes in pacing threshold and R- and P wave amplitude during pacemaker implantation. Am J Cardiol 1990;65:999.
44. Furman S, Pannizo F: Output programmability and reduction of secondary intervention after pacemaker implantation. J Thorac Cardiovasc Surg 1981;81:713.
45. Luceri RM, Furman S, Hurzeler P, *et al.*: Threshold behavior of electrodes in long-term ventricular pacing. Am J Cardiol 1977;40:184.
46. Radovsky AS, VanVleet JF: Effects of dexamethasone elution on tissue reaction around stimulating electrodes of endocardial pacing leads in dogs. Am Heart J 1989;117:1288.
47. Mond H, Stokes K, Helland J, *et al.*: The porous titanium steroid eluting electrode: A double blind study assessing the stimulation threshold effects of steroid. PACE 1988;11:214.
48. Pirzada FA, Moschitto LJ, Diorio D: Clinical experience with steroid-eluting unipolar electrodes. PACE 1988;11:1739.
49. Klein HH, Steinberger J, Knake W: Stimulation characteristics of a steroid-eluting electrode compared with three conventional electrodes. PACE 1990;13:134.

50. Mond H, Stokes K: The electrode-tissue interface. The revolutionary role of steroid elution. PACE 1992;15:95.
51. Jones BR, Midei MG, Brinker JA: Does the long term performance of the target tip electrode justify reducing a pacemaker's nominal output? PACE 1986;9:299.
52. Stokes K, Church T: The elimination of exit block as a pacing complication using transvenous steroid eluting lead. PACE 1987;10:748.
53. Dohrmann ML, Goldschlager N: Myocardial stimulation threshold in patients with cardiac pacemakers: effect of physiologic variables, pharmacologic agents, and lead electrodes. Cardiol Clin 1985;3:527.
54. Barold SS. Effect of drugs on pacing thresholds. In Antonioli GI, Aubert AE, Ector H (eds): Proceedings of the Second International Symposium on Pacing Leads. Elsevier Science Publishers, Amsterdam, 1991:73.
55. Schlesinger Z, Rosenberg T, Stryjer D, *et al.*: Exit block in myxedema treated effectively by thyroid hormone therapy. PACE 1980;3:737.
56. Basu D, Chatterjee K. Unusually high pacemaker threshold in severe myxedema, decrease with thyroid hormone therapy. Chest 1976;70:677.
57. Bashour TT: Spectrum of ventricular pacemaker exit block owing to hyperkalemia. Am J Cardiol 1986;57:337.
58. Barold SS, Falkoff MD, Ong LS, *et al.*: Hyperkalemia-induced failure of atrial capture during dual chamber cardiac pacing. J Am Coll Cardiol 1987;10:467.
59. Hellestrand KF, Burnett PJ, Milne JR, *et al.*: Effect of the antiarrhythmic agent flecainide acetate on acute and chronic pacing thresholds. PACE 1983;6:892.
60. Montefoschi N, Boccadamo R: Propafenone induced acute variation of chronic pacing threshold. A case report. PACE 1990;13:480.
61. Gay RJ, Brown DF: Pacemaker failure due to procainamide toxicity. Am J Cardiol 1974;34:728.
62. Salel AP, Seagren SC, Pool PE: Effects of encainide in the function of implanted pacemakers. PACE 1989;12:1439.
63. O'Reilly MV, Murnaghan DP, Williams MB: Transvenous pacemaker failure induced by hyperkalemia. JAMA 1974;228:336.
64. Nagamoto Y, Ogawa T, Kumagae H, *et al.*: Pacing failure due to markedly increased stimulation threshold 2 years after implantation: successful management with oral prednisolone. A case report. PACE 1989;12:1034.
65. Preston TA, Fletcher RD, Lucchesi BR, *et al.*: Changes in myocardial threshold. Physiologic and pharmacologic factors in patients with implanted pacemakers. Am Heart J 1967;174:235.
66. Platia EV, Brinker JA: Time course of transvenous pacemaker stimulation impedance, capture threshold and electrogram amplitude. PACE 1986;1:620.
67. Furman S: Sensing and timing the cardiac electrogram. In Furman S, Hayes DL, Holmes DR (eds): A Practice of Cardiac Pacing, 2nd ed., Futura Publishing Co., Mt. Kisco, NY, 1989:79.
68. Bornzin G, Stokes K: The electrode-biointerface: sensing. In Barold SS (ed): Modern Cardiac Pacing. Futura Publishing Co., Mt. Kisco, NY, 1985:79.
69. Irnich W: Intracardiac electrograms and sensing test signals: electrophysiological physical and technical considerations. PACE 1985;8:870.
70. Furman S, Hurzeler P, DeCaprio V: The ventricular endocardial electrogram and pacemaker sensing. J Thorac Cardiovasc Surg 1977;73:258.
71. Bagwell P, Pannizzo F, Furman S: Unipolar and bipolar right atrial appendage electrodes: comparison of sensing characteristics. Med Instrum 1985;19:132.
72. Griffin JC: Sensing characteristics of the right atrial appendage electrode. PACE 1983;6:22.
73. DeCaprio V, Hurzeler P, Furman S: A comparison of unipolar and bipolar electrograms for cardiac pacemaker sensing. Circulation 1977;56:750.
74. Hauser RG, Edwards LM, Stafford JL: Bipolar and unipolar sensing: basic concepts and clinical applications. In Barold SS (ed): Modern Cardiac Pacing. Futura Publishing Co., Mt. Kisco, NY, 1985:137.
75. Nielsen AP, Cashion WR, Spencer WH, *et al.*: Long-term assessment of unipolar and bipolar stimulation and sensing thresholds using a lead configuration programmable pacemaker. J Am Coll Cardiol 1985;5:1198.
76. Mond H. Unipolar versus bipolar pacing—poles apart. PACE 1991;14:1411.
77. Breivik K, Ohm O, Engedal H: Long-term comparison of unipolar and bipolar pacing and sensing, using a new multiprogrammable pacemaker system. PACE 1983;6:592.
78. Barold SS, Falkoff MD, Ong LS: Interference in cardiac pacemakers: endogenous sources. In El-Sherif N, Samet P (eds): Cardiac Pacing and Electrophysiology, 3rd ed., WB Saunders, Philadelphia, 1991:634.
79. Barold SS, Falkoff MD, Ong LS, *et al.*: Arrhythmias caused by dual-chambered pacing. In Steinbach K (ed): Proceedings of the 7th World Symposium on Cardiac Pacing. Steinkopff Verlag, Darmstadt, 1983: 505.
80. Barold SS, Falkoff MD, Ong LS, *et al.*: Timing cycles of DDD pacemakers. In Barold SS, Mugica J (eds): New Perspectives in Cardiac Pacing. Futura Publishing Co., Mt. Kisco, NY, 1988:69.
81. Barold SS, Falkoff MD, Ong LS, *et al.*: Electrocardiography of contemporary DDD pacemakers. A. Basic concepts, upper rate response, retrograde ventriculoatrial conduction and differential diagnosis of pacemaker tachycardias. In Saksena S, Goldschlager N (eds): Electric Therapy for Cardiac Arrhythmias. Pacing, Antitachycardia Devices, Catheter Ablation. WB Saunders, Philadelphia, 1990:225.
82. Barold SS, Falkoff MD, Ong LS, *et al.*: Function and electrocardiography of DDD pacemakers. In Barold SS (ed): Modern Cardiac Pacing, Futura Publishing Co., Mt. Kisco, NY, 1985:645.
83. Furman S: Comprehension of pacemaker cycles. In Furman S, Hayes DL, Holmes DR (eds): A Practice of Cardiac Pacing, 2nd ed. Futura Publishing Co., Mt. Kisco, NY, 1989:115.
84. Barold SS: Management of patients with dual chamber pacemakers: central role of the pacemaker atrial refractory period, Learning Center Highlights (Heart House). Am Coll Cardiol 1990;5(4):8.
85. Levine PA: Post ventricular atrial refractory periods and pacemaker mediated tachycardias. Clin Prog Pacing. Electrophysiol 1983;1:394.
86. Furman S, Reicher-Reiss H, Escher DJW: Atrio-ventricular sequential pacing and pacemakers. Chest 1973;63:783.
87. Barold SS, Ong LS, Falkoff MD, *et al.*: Crosstalk or self-inhibition in dual-chamber pacemakers. In Barold SS (ed): Modern Cardiac Pacing. Futura Publishing Co., Mt. Kisco, NY, 1985:615.
88. Barold SS, Falkoff MD, Ong LS, *et al.*: Upper rate response of DDD pacemakers. In Barold SS, Mugica J (eds): New Perspectives in Cardiac Pacing. Futura Publishing Co., Mt. Kisco, NY, 1988:121.
89. Furman S, Gross J: Dual chamber pacing and pacemakers. Curr Prob Cardiol 1990;15:119.
90. Levine PA: Normal and abnormal rhythm associated with dual-chamber pacemakers. Cardiol Clin 1985;3:595.
91. Barold SS, Belott PH: Behavior of the ventricular triggering period of DDD pacemakers. PACE 1987;10:1237.
92. Barold SS, Falkoff MD, Ong LS, *et al.*: All dual-chamber pacemakers function in the DDD mode. Am Heart J 1988;115:1353.
93. Furman S: Dual-chamber pacemakers. Upper rate behavior. PACE 1985;8:197.
94. Luceri RM, Castellanos A, Zaman L, *et al.*: The arrhythmia of dual chamber cardiac pacemakers and their management. Ann Intern Med 1983;99:354.
95. Stoobrandt R, Willems R, Holvoet G, *et al.*: Prediction of Wenckebach behavior and block response in DDD pacemakers. PACE 1986;9:1040.
96. Higano ST, Hayes DL: Quantitative analysis of Wenckebach behavior in DDD pacemakers. PACE 1990;13:1456.
97. Furman S, Cooper A: Atrial fibrillation during AV sequential pacing. PACE 1982;5:133.
98. Barold SS, Falkoff MD, Ong LS, *et al.*: Characterization of pacemaker arrhythmias due to normally functioning AV demand (DVI) pulse generators. PACE 1980;3:712.

99. Barold SS, Falkoff MD, Ong LS, *et al.*: Function and electrocardiography of DVI pacing systems. In Barold SS (ed): Modern Cardiac Pacing. Futura Publishing Co., Mt. Kisco, NY, 1985:625.
100. Barold SS, Falkoff MD, Ong LS, *et al.*: Interpretation of electrocardiograms produced by a new unipolar multiprogrammable "committed" AV sequential (DVI) pulse generator. PACE 1981;4:692.
101. Floro J, Castellanet M, Florio J, *et al.*: DDI: a new mode for cardiac pacing. Clin Prog Pacing Electrophysiol 1984;2:255.
102. Barold SS: The DDI mode of cardiac pacing. PACE 1987;10:480.
103. Sutton R, Ingram A, Kenny RA, *et al.*: Clinical experience of DDI pacing. In Belhassen B, Feldman S, Copperman Y (eds): Cardiac Pacing and Electrophysiology. Proceedings of the VIIIth World Symposium on Cardiac Pacing and Electrophysiology, Jerusalem. R&L Creative Communications Ltd., Jerusalem, 1987:161.
104. Cunningham TM: Pacemaker syndrome due to retrograde conduction in a DDI pacemaker. Am Heart J 1988;115:478.
105. Barold SS: Electrocardiography of rate-adaptive dual chamber (DDDR) pacemakers. 1. Lower rate behavior. In Alt E, Barold SS, Stangl K (eds): Rate Adaptive Pacing. Springer-Verlag, New York (in press).
106. Barold SS, Falkoff MD, Ong LS, *et al.*: A-A and V-V lower rate timing of DDD and DDDR pulse generators. In Barold SS, Mugica J (eds): New Perspectives in Cardiac Pacing. 2. Futura Publishing Co., Mt. Kisco, NY, 1991:203.
107. Markowitz T, Prest-Berg K, Betzold R, *et al.*: Clinical implications of dual chamber responsive rate pacing. In Belhassen B, Feldman S, Copperman Y (eds): Cardiac Pacing and Electrophysiology, Proceedings of the VIIIth World Symposium on Cardiac Pacing and Electrophysiology. Keterpress Enterprises, Jerusalem, 1987:165.
108. Levine PA, Hayes DL, Wilkoff BL, *et al.*: Electrocardiography of rate-modulated pacemaker rhythms. Siemens-Pacesetter, Inc., Sylmar, CA, 1990.
109. Ritter PH: La stimulation DDDR définitive: aspects techniques. Stimucoeur 1990;18:29.
110. Hayes D, Higano ST: DDDR pacing. Follow-up and complications. In Barold SS, Mugica J (eds): New Perspectives in Cardiac Pacing. 2. Futura Publishing Co., Mt. Kisco, NY, 1991:473.
111. Hayes DL, Higano ST, Eisinger G: Electrocardiographic manifestations of a dual-chamber, rate-modulated (DDDR) pacemaker. PACE 1989;12:555.
112. Higano ST, Hayes DL, Eisinger G: Sensor-driven rate smoothing in a DDDR pacemaker. PACE 1989;12:922.
113. Barold SS: Electrocardiography or rate-adaptive dual chamber (DDDR) pacemakers. 2. Upper rate behavior. In Alt E, Barold SS, Stangl K (eds): Rate Adaptive Pacing. Springer-Verlag, New York, (in press).
114. Higano SR, Hayes DL, Eiseinger G: Advantage of discrepant upper rate limits in a DDDR pacemaker. Mayo Clin Proc 1989;64:932.
115. Hanich RF, Midei MG, McElroy BP, *et al.*: Circumvention of maximum tracking limitations with a rate-modulated dual chamber pacemaker. PACE 1989;12:392.
116. Higano ST, Hayes DL: P wave tracking above the maximum tracking rate in a DDDR pacemaker. PACE 1989;12:1044.
117. Levine PA, Belott PH, Bilitch M, *et al.*: Recommendations of the NASPE Policy Conference on Pacemaker Programmability and Follow-up. PACE 1983;6:1221.
118. Levine PA: Proceedings of the policy conference of the North American Society of Pacing and Electrophysiology on programmability and pacemaker follow-up programs. Clin Prog Pacing Electrophysiol 1984;2:145.
119. Pless P, Simonsen E, Arnsbo P, *et al.*: Superiority of multiprogrammable to nonprogrammable VVI pacing. A comparative study with special reference to management of pacing systems malfunction. PACE 1986;9:739.
120. Hayes DL, Osborn MJ: Pacing. A. Antibradycardia devices. In Guiliani ER, Fuster V, Gersh BJ, *et al.*: (eds), Cardiology Fundamentals and Practice, 2nd ed. Mosby Year Book, St. Louis, 1991:1014.
121. Mugica J, Birkui P: Multiprogrammability of modern cardiac pacemakers. In El-Sherif N, Samet P (eds): Cardiac Pacing and Electrophysiology. WB Saunders, Philadelphia, 1991:505.
122. Furman S: Pacemaker programmability. Contemp Surg 1982;20:35.
123. Barold SS, Falkoff MD, Ong LS, *et al.*: Electrocardiography of DDD pacemakers. B. Multiprogrammability, follow-up, and troubleshooting. In Saksena S, Goldschlager N (eds): Electrical Therapy for Cardiac Arrhythmias. Pacing, Antitachycardia Devices, Catheter Ablation. WB Saunders, Philadelphia, 1990:242.
124. Billhardt RA, Rosenbush SW, Hauser RG: Successful management of pacing system malfunctions without surgery. The role of programmable pulse generators. PACE 1982;5:675.
125. Hauser RG: Programmability. A clinical approach. Cardiol Clin 1985;3:539.
126. Hayes DL. Programmability. In Furman S, Hayes DL, Holmes DR (eds): A Practice of Cardiac Pacing, 2nd ed. Futura Publishing Co., Mt. Kisco, NY, 1989:563.
127. Mond H: The Cardiac Pacemaker. Grune & Stratton, New York, 1983:37.
128. Barold SS, Falkoff MD, Ong LS, *et al.*: The third decade of cardiac pacing. Multiprogrammable pulse generators. Br Heart J 1981;45:357.
129. O'Keefe JH Jr, Hayes DL, Holmes DR Jr, *et al.*: Importance and long-term utility of a multiprogrammable pulse generator. Mayo Clin Proc 1984;59:239.
130. Harthorne JW: Programmable pacemakers: technical features and clinical applications. Cardiovasc Clin 1983;14:135.
131. Smyth NPD, Sager D, Keshishian JM: A programmable pulse generator with high output option. PACE 1981;4:566.
132. Hauser RG, Susmano A: Afterpotential oversensing by a programmable pulse generator. PACE 1981;4:391.
133. Wish M, Fletcher RD, Gottdiener JS, *et al.*: Importance of left atrial timing in the programming of dual chamber pacemakers. Am J Cardiol 1987;60:566.
134. Alt EU, VonBibra H, Blömer H: Different benefit AV intervals with sensed and paced atrial events. J Electrophysiol 1987;1:250.
135. Pearson AC, Janosik DL, Redd RM, *et al.*: Hemodynamic benefit of atrioventricular synchrony. Prediction from baseline Doppler-echocardiographic variables. J Am Coll Cardiol 1989;13:1613.
136. Janosik DL, Pearson AC, Buckingham TA, *et al.*: The hemodynamic effect of differential atrioventricular delay intervals for sensed and paced atrial events during physiologic pacing. J Am Coll Cardiol 1989;14:499.
137. Furman S, Fisher JD: Endless loop tachycardia in an AV universal (DDD) pacemaker. PACE 1982;5:476.
138. Tolentino AO, Javier RP, Byrd C, *et al.*: Paced-induced tachycardia associated with an atrial synchronous ventricular inhibited (ASVIP) pulse generator. PACE 1982;5:251.
139. Ausubel K, Gabry MD, Klementowicz PT, *et al.*: Pacemaker-mediated endless loop tachycardia at rates below the upper rate limit. Am J Cardiol 1988;61:465.
140. Friart A: Termination of magnet-unresponsive pacemaker endless loop tachycardia by carotid sinus massage. Am J Med 1989;87:1.
141. Perrins EJ, Morley CA, Dixy J, *et al.*: The pharmacologic blockade of retrograde atrioventricular conduction in paced patients. PACE 1983;6:A-112.
142. Barold SS, Falkoff MD, Ong LS, *et al.*: Pacemaker endless loop tachycardia. Termination by simple techniques other than magnet application. Am J Med 1988;85:817.
143. Fontaine JW, Maloney JD, Castle LW, *et al.*: Noninvasive assessment of ventriculoatrial conduction and early experience with the tachycardia termination algorithm in pacemaker-mediated tachycardia. PACE 1986;9:212.
144. Hayes DL, Furman S: Atrioventricular and ventriculo-atrial conduction times in patients undergoing pacemaker implant. PACE 1983;6:38.
145. Cazeau S, Daubert C, Mabo P, *et al.*: Dynamic electrophysiology of ventriculoatrial conduction. Implications for DDD and DDDR pacing. PACE 1990;13:1649.

146. Akhtar M, Gilbert C, Mahmud R, *et al*.: Pacemaker-mediated tachycardia. Underlying mechanism, relationship to ventriculoatrial conduction, characteristics and management. Clin Prog Pacing Electrophysiol 1985;3:90.
147. Westveer DC, Stewart JR, Goodfleish R, *et al*.: Prevalence and significance of ventriculoatrial conduction. PACE 1984;7:784.
148. Rubin JW, Frank MJ, Boineau JP, *et al*.: Current physiologic pacemakers: A serious problem with a new device. Am J Cardiol 1983;52:88.
149. VanMechelen RV, Ruiter J, Vanderkerchkhove Y, *et al*.: Prevalence of retrograde conduction in heart block after DDD pacemaker implantation. Am J Cardiol 1986;57:797.
150. Calfee RV: Pacemaker-mediated tachycardia: engineering solution. In Barold SS, Mugica J (eds): New Perspectives in Cardiac Pacing. Futura Publishing Co., Mt. Kisco, NY, 1988:357.
151. Hayes DL, Holmes DR, Vliestra RA, *et al*.: Changing experience with dual chamber (DDD) pacemakers. J Am Coll Cardiol 1984;4:556.
152. Hayes DL: Endless loop tachycardia. The problem has been solved. In Barold SS, Mugica J (eds): New Perspectives in Cardiac Pacing. Futura Publishing Co., Mt. Kisco, NY, 1988:375.
153. Mugica J, Barold SS, Ripart A: The smart pacemaker. In Barold SS, Mugica J (eds): New Perspectives in Cardiac Pacing. 2. Futura Publishing Co., Mt. Kisco, NY, 1991:545.
154. DenDulk K, Lindemans FW, Wellens HJJ. Noninvasive evaluation of pacemaker circus movement tachycardia. Am J Cardiol 1984;53:537.
155. Littleford P, Curry RC Jr, Schwartz KM, *et al*.: Pacemaker mediated tachycardia: a rapid bedside technique for induction and observation. Am J Cardiol 1983;52:287.
156. Greenspon AJ, Greenberg RM: Noninvasive evaluation of retrograde conduction times to avoid pacemaker-mediated tachycardia. J Am Coll Cardiol 1985;5:1403.
157. DenDulk K, Lindemans FW, Wellens HJJ: Management of pacemaker circus movement tachycardia. PACE 1984;7:346.
158. Klementowicz PT, Furman S: Selective atrial sensing in dual chamber pacemakers eliminates endless loop tachycardia. J Am Coll Cardiol 1986;7:590.
159. Bernheim C, Markewitz A, Kemkes BM: Can reprogramming of atrial sensitivity avoid an endless loop tachycardia? PACE 1986;9:293.
160. DenDulk K, Wellens HJJ: Failure of the post ventricular premature beat DVI mode of preventing pacemaker circus movement tachycardia. Am J Cardiol 1984;34:1371.
161. DenDulk K, Lindeman FW, Wellens HJJ: Merits of various antipacemaker circus movement tachycardia features. PACE 1986;9:1055.
162. Harriman RJ, Pasquariello JL, Gomes JAC, *et al*.: Autonomic dependence of ventriculoatrial conduction. Am J Cardiol 1985;56:285.
163. Klementowicz P, Ausubel K, Furman S: The dynamic nature of ventriculoatrial conduction. PACE 1986;9:1050.
164. Markewitz A, Hemmer W, Weinhold C: Complications in dual chamber pacing. A six year experience. PACE 1986;9 (Part II):1014.
165. Byrd CL, Schwartz SJ, Gonzales M, *et al*.: DDD pacemakers maximize hemodynamic benefits and minimize complications for most patients. PACE 1988;11 (Part II):1911.
166. Jordaens L, Robbens E, VanWassenhove E, *et al*.: Incidence of arrhythmias after atrial or dual-chamber pacemaker implantation. Eur Heart J 1989;10:102.
167. Goldschlager N: Advances in avoidance and termination of pacemaker-mediated tachycardia. In Barold SS, Mugica J (eds): New Perspectives in Cardiac Pacing. Futura Publishing Co., Mt. Kisco, NY, 1991:459.
168. Duncan JL, Clark MF: Prevention and termination of pacemaker-mediated tachycardia in a new DDD pacing system (Siemens-Pacesetter Model 2010T), PACE 1988;11:1679.
169. Nitzsche R, Gueunoun M, Lamaison D, *et al*.: Endless loop tachycardia: description and first clinical results of a new fully automatic protection algorithm. PACE 1990;13(Part II):1711.
170. Barold SS: Repetitive reentrant and non-reentrant ventriculoatrial synchrony in dual chamber pacing. Clin Cardiol 1991;14:754.
171. Barold SS, Falkoff MD, Ong LS, *et al*.: AV desynchronization arrhythmia during DDD pacing. In Belhassen S, Feldman S, Copperman Y (eds): Cardiac Pacing and Electrophysiology: Proceedings of the VIIIth World Syndrome on Cardiac Pacing and Electrophysiology, Jerusalem. Keterpress Enterprises, Jerusalem, Israel, 1987:177.
172. Barold SS: Repetitive non-reentrant ventriculoatrial synchrony in dual chamber pacing. In Santini M, Pistolese M, Alliegro A (eds): Progress in Clinical Pacing, 1990. Excerpta Medica, Amsterdam, 1990:451.
173. Barold SS, Falkoff MD, Ong LS, *et al*.: Magnet unresponsive pacemaker endless loop tachycardia. Am Heart J 1988;116:726.
174. Ausubel K, Furman S: The pacemaker syndrome. Ann Intern Med 1985;103:420.
175. Chief WW, Foster E, Phillips B, *et al*.: Pacemaker syndrome in a patient with DDD pacemaker for long QT syndrome. PACE 1991;14:1209.

16

HEMODYNAMICS OF CARDIAC PACING AND RATE-ADAPTIVE PACEMAKERS

S. Serge Barold, M.B., B.S., F.R.A.C.P., F.A.C.P., F.A.C.C., F.E.S.C.

HEMODYNAMICS OF CARDIAC PACING

Normally, cardiac output increases about 350% during maximal exercise; the largest component (accounting for about 300%) is provided by an increase in heart rate, whereas increased stroke volume makes only a modest contribution (about 50%). With advancing age, the relative contributions change so that at age 70, increased heart rate provides approximately two-thirds of the total increase in cardiac output with maximal exercise. At normal activity levels, many patients tolerate the loss of atrioventricular (AV) synchrony associated with fixed-frequency VVI pacing; however, effort tolerance is limited, as augmentation of cardiac output depends solely on increases in stroke volume. Such increases probably are due to a greater preload and enhanced contractility during VVI pacing (1,2). This creates particular difficulty for patients with severe left ventricular (LV) dysfunction who cannot increase their stroke volume and who ordinarily depend on rate augmentation for improved hemodynamic performance during exercise.

Atrioventricular Synchrony

The relative contribution of atrial systole to cardiac output depends on heart rate, LV systolic and diastolic function, LV filling pressure, presence of valvular disease, left atrial size, contractility, and compliance, retrograde ventriculoatrial (VA) conduction, and the timing between atrial and ventricular systole (3). In a normal heart, AV synchrony at rest contributes about 20–30% of the cardiac output (4). Many but not all studies have demonstrated that this benefit persists in the upright position. Labovitz, *et al*. (5) demonstrated that patients with normal left atrial size were most likely to benefit from AV synchrony, but this could not be confirmed by Lau and Camm (6). Greenberg, *et al*. (7) found that in a small number of patients the benefits of atrial transport were inversely related to LV filling pressure. Indeed, atrial systole may contribute little to the resting cardiac output in some congestive heart failure (CHF) patients who have high LV filling pressures associated with their dilated left ventricles (represented by the flat portion of the Frank-Starling LV function curve (7)). But others have shown that patients with significantly elevated pulmonary capillary wedge pressures (PCWP) and symptomatic left ventricular failure derive substantial benefit from AV synchrony (8,9). Reiter and Hindman (10) demonstrated the great variability in hemodynamic improvement with AV synchrony in individual patients even when mean PCWP exceeded 20 mm Hg. Even in patients with identical wedge pressures, the benefit of AV synchrony varied and did not correlate with ejection fraction (EF), cardiothoracic ratio (10) or a number of other indices, a finding recently confirmed by Mukharji, *et al*. (8). Lavovitz, *et al*. (5) also found that neither LV size nor echocardiographically determined LV function correlated with the fall in stroke volume that was seen with a loss of AV synchrony.

The mean PCWP rises both in normal individuals and in patients with severe CHF when pacing is switched from the atrial to the ventricular mode. Ventricular pacing is often poorly tolerated in patients with heart failure or severe systolic LV dysfunction (11). Indeed, symptoms of heart failure in patients with bradycardia are rarely improved by the increase in heart rate alone that is provided by VVI pacing.

Patients with a high LV filling pressure unresponsive to the restoration of AV synchrony should not be denied atrial or AV sequential pacing, as they may again become responsive to the benefits of atrial transport if medical therapy improves LV performance. Even when maintenance of AV synchrony provides little or no hemodynamic benefit from atrial transport, AV synchrony is important because it prevents VA conduction, which may further increase systemic and pulmonary venous pressure and aggravate CHF. Permanent dual-chamber pacing should therefore be considered in all CHF patients, if the atrium can be paced.

The atrial contribution to ventricular filling is very important in patients with diastolic LV dysfunction (i.e., decreased compliance with normal LV systolic function) where it provides 30–40% of the end-diastolic volume and cardiac output at rest. Loss of AV synchrony in these patients leads to marked reduction in cardiac output and serious hemodynamic consequences.

The optimal AV delay at rest depends on whether a P wave is paced or sensed, so that the use of differential AV delay intervals, or hysteresis (shorter delays following an atrial sensed event) results in an increase in cardiac output at rest (3,12,13). It is difficult to predict the optimal AV delay in any given patient (1,3,12,14–17). Therefore, optimal duration of the AV delay should be individualized at rest by evaluating the stroke volume or cardiac output with Doppler echocardiography, especially in patients with CHF and diastolic LV dysfunction (12).

Atrioventricular Synchrony on Exercise

The contribution of AV synchrony on exercise is difficult to quantitate. Recent studies have demonstrated better exercise performance with DDDR as opposed to VVIR pacing in patients with atrial chronotropic incompetence (18–22). Yet, earlier studies suggested that the hemodynamic benefit of correctly synchronized atrial activity may be negligible at relatively high levels of exercise when the cardiac output is controlled mostly by the increased ventricular rate (23–27). The lack of benefit of AV synchrony on exercise in these studies may reflect different methodologies and levels of exercise, as well as different patient populations with normal LV function. Favorable results with recent investigations suggest that AV synchrony further improves cardiac function and efficiency and may be important at lesser levels of exercise, particularly in patients with borderline heart failure, LV dysfunction, or decreased LV compliance (18–20). The PR interval normally shortens on exercise, but the beneficial effect of pacemakers with rate-dependent automatic shortening of the AV delay on exercise is as yet unclear (28–34).

Rate Responsiveness

Many studies have shown that during exercise, an increase in the pacing rate provided by VVIR, VDD, DDD, or DDDR modes increases the cardiac output, achieved work, and duration of exercise more than does fixed-frequency VVI pacing in patients with normal or impaired LV function (6,20,35–45). In addition to superior hemodynamic effects, there is an increase in maximum 0_2 consumption, a reduction in AV 0_2 difference, and an increase in subjective well-being. The acute hemodynamic advantage is retained on a long-term basis. Moreover, by 6–12 mo after implantation, rate-adaptive pacemakers may further augment LV function, reduce heart size, and improve exercise performance compared to results in the immediate postoperative period (36,43,46–49).

When atrial chronotropic incompetence precludes an increase in the sinus rate on exercise, VVIR pacing (which provides a rate increase only) may improve exercise tolerance more than does DDD pacing (which, in this setting, provides only AV synchrony) (50). On the other hand, exercise performance in the DDD mode is superior to that in the VVIR mode in patients with AV block and normal chronotropic function (51,52). In some patients with intact VA conduction and without a clinical pacemaker syndrome at rest, hemodynamics on exercise may not improve in the VVIR mode because the beneficial effects of an increase in heart rate may be negated by the unfavorable hemodynamic effect of retrograde VA conduction.

Valvular Regurgitation

During ventricular pacing, dissociated ventricular systole when the AV valves are in the open position may cause varying degrees of valvular regurgitation contributing to a decrease in stroke volume (48,53). Atrioventricular valvular insufficiency is not related to altered ventricular depolarization. Rarely mitral (or tricuspid) regurgitation can be severe and precipitate congestive heart failure (54).

Abnormal Ventricular Depolarization

Disordered depolarization from ventricular pacing results in an altered contraction pattern that decreases LV performance at rest and during exercise (55–57). Alterations in intraventricular conduction may impair left ventricular systolic and diastolic functions due to asynchronous contraction and relaxation (58). Although these abnormalities may not cause serious deterioration of LV performance in patients with normal LV function, in the diseased heart they may significantly impair function and may contribute to the ultimate development of heart failure (58). Consequently the AV interval of DDD pacemakers should be programmed to promote spontaneous AV conduction provided the duration of the programmed pacemaker AV interval is not excessive. The potential advantage of a shorter AV interval in patients with LV dysfunction may at times be reduced or canceled by the negative impact of pacing-induced abnormal depolarization and asynchronous LV systole.

PACEMAKER SYNDROME

The adverse consequences of ventricular pacing were first recognized by Mitsui, *et al.* (59). Various degrees of intolerance to ventricular pacing may occur. Ausubel and Furman defined the pacemaker syndrome as a clinical complex of "signs and symptoms related to the adverse hemodynamic and electrophysiologic consequences of ventricular pacing" (60,61) in the presence of a normally functioning implanted ventricular pacemaker. Under certain circumstances, intolerance to atrial or dual-chamber pacing may also cause unfavorable hemodynamics identical to those seen in the pacemaker syndrome during single-chamber ventricular pacing. For this reason, Schüller and Brandt (62) recently suggested that the pacemaker syndrome should be redefined more broadly as follows: "The pacemaker syndrome refers to symptoms and signs present in the pacemaker patient which are caused by inadequate timing of atrial and ventricular contractions."

Incidence

The pacemaker syndrome is more commonly related to retrograde VA conduction than to the random timing of atrial and ventricular activity. About 40–50% of patients requiring permanent pacing exhibit retrograde VA conduction (63,64) and its presence is a major determinant of the risk of developing the pacemaker syndrome (65). Most reports suggest that with ventricular pacing only 15–20% of patients with preserved VA conduction develop symptoms suggestive of the pacemaker syndrome, with about half exhibiting its full-blown form (66).

The true incidence of pacemaker syndrome with single-lead ventricular pacing may be higher than realized, as most patients with dual-chamber pulse generators prefer the DDD (VDD) to the VVI mode; only a small number have no preference. In that respect, Heldman, *et al.* (67) recently studied the incidence of the pacemaker syndrome in 40 patients with dual-chamber pacemakers (30 with DDD and 10 with DDI). Eighty-three percent of their patients experienced moderate-to-severe symptoms and 42% of these patients were unable to tolerate VVI pacing for one week. In the same study, 18% of the patients reported no discernible benefit from dual-chamber pacing compared with VVI pacing. Rediker, *et al.* (68) also studied 19 patients with DDD pacemakers in a blinded randomized study comparing VVI versus DDD pacing and found that 63% of the patients preferred DDD pacing and none preferred VVI pacing. Other studies (40,69,70) indicated that on withdrawal of the DDD mode by programming to the VVI mode, a majority of the patients noticed a deterioration in their general condition (including occasional sleep disturbances that disappeared when the DDD mode was restored) (40). In some cases, patients have described a subjective improvement in their feelings of well-being or quality of life with DDD(R) pacing compared with those with the VVI(R) mode, despite lack of objective improvement in functional exercise capacity (71). Not all patients with demonstrable adverse hemodynamic effects of ventricular pacing are actually symptomatic. However, "asymptomatic" patients often feel better when their VVI pacemakers are upgraded to a DDD system, suggesting the existence of a "subclinical" pacemaker syndrome (72).

Clinical Manifestations

The prominent symptoms of the pacemaker syndrome mostly result from reduced cardiac output and hypotension. However, many patients have subtle manifestations. Ventricular pacing may cause substantial hypotension (sometimes postural), especially in the first few seconds of ventricular pacing after switching from normal sinus rhythm. Syncope or near-syncope may result from a reduction in cerebral blood flow. Patients may also experience dyspnea, limited exercise capacity, CHF (73), beat-to-beat variations in cardiac response (reflecting changes from spontaneous to pacemaker beats), cough, a lump in the throat, unpleasant pulsations in the neck or chest, the sensation of pressure or fullness in the chest, neck or head, headaches (74), chest pain, apprehension, or fatigue or malaise (65). Rarely, cardiovascular collapse may occur (75). Confusion or changes in mentation have also been observed. Obviously not all features may be present in any individual patient. The definition and description of the pacemaker syndrome advanced in the 1984 and 1991 American College of Cardiology/American Heart Association (ACC/AHA) Guidelines for Implanted Cardiac Pacemakers and Antiarrhythmia Devices (76,77) (Table 16.1) seems too restrictive in view of the protean manifestations of the syndrome and recent observations that its clinical expression may be subtle. The pacemaker syndrome occurs typically in patients with intermittent VVI pacing because alternating periods of normal sinus rhythm and ventricular pacing produce cyclic variations in blood pressure, cardiac output, and peripheral resistance. Mild symptoms may be ignored or attributed to other causes by the physician. The diagnosis is supported by comparing the blood pressure during AV synchrony with that during VA synchrony, as well as by reproducing symptoms during ventricular pacing. Occasionally invasive hemodynamic measurements during right heart catheterization may be necessary to make the diagnosis of the pacemaker syndrome.

Pathophysiology

The loss of AV synchrony per se does not play the key role in the genesis of the pacemaker syndrome. Hemodynamic compromise is more complex, because retrograde VA conduction causes a "negative atrial kick" with more profound hemodynamic disadvantage than that from simple loss of AV synchrony (78). Atrial contraction against closed mitral and tricuspid AV valves causes systemic and pulmonary venous regurgitation and congestion (cannon A waves) and increases in PCWP regardless of LV ejection fraction (9), sometimes leading to the development of CHF in previously compensated patients (61,62,79). Mitral and tricuspid regurgitation may occur because VA synchrony prevents closure of the AV valves prior to ventricular systole, though in most patients with the pacemaker syndrome, valvular

Table 16.1.
Definition of Pacemaker Syndrome 1984 and 1991 ACC/AHA Guidelines

The pacemaker syndrome was first defined as lightheadedness or syncope related to long periods of AV synchrony that occurred at times during ventricular-inhibited (VVI) or VOO pacing. The definition is now expanded to include (1) episodic weakness or syncope associated with alternating AV synchrony and asynchrony; (2) inadequate cardiac output associated with continued absence of AV synchrony or with fixed asynchrony (persistent VA conduction); and (3) patient awareness of beat to beat variations in cardiac contractile sequence, often as a result of (a) cannon A waves, (b) V waves transmitted to the atria or pulmonary veins, and (c) bundle branch block patterns of ventricular contraction with a paced beat.

Reproduced from Frye RL, Collins JJ, DeSanctis RW, *et al.*: Guidelines for permanent cardiac pacemaker implantation, May, 1984. A report of the Joint American College of Cardiology/American Heart Association task force on assessment of cardiovascular procedures (subcommittee on pacemaker implantation). J Am Coll Cardiol 1984;11:1882, with permission.

regurgitation probably plays a relatively small role in the genesis of the hemodynamic derangement. In addition to the marked reduction in cardiac output, retrograde VA conduction leads to atrial distension and activation of stretch receptors that produce a reflex vasodepressor effect that tends to decrease peripheral resistance. The presence of atrial cannon waves during ventricular pacing appears to be the fundamental basis for the development of the pacemaker syndrome (78). Erlebacher, *et al.* (78) showed that patients with left atrial cannon waves during ventricular pacing increased their total peripheral resistance by considerably (about one-quarter) less than those without cannon waves. In patients with the pacemaker syndrome and absent retrograde VA conduction, hemodynamic studies have demonstrated venous cannon waves that are probably the most important single factor responsible for the hemodynamic derangement (78). Patients with VA conduction but no left atrial cannon waves do not seem at risk of developing pacemaker-induced hypotension. Indeed, atrial fibrillation with ventricular pacing does not produce the pacemaker syndrome, but on restoration of sinus rhythm, VVI pacing can then precipitate the pacemaker syndrome (80).

In most cases of pacemaker syndrome, the increase in the peripheral resistance is inappropriately low for the degree of hypotension (secondary to the low cardiac output), indicating that the compensatory mechanisms that ordinarily increase the peripheral resistance are attenuated (78,81–83). The circulatory response and fall in blood pressure may be modified by position, different degrees of neurohumoral activation, volume depletion, poor LV function, drugs, status of the atrium, and actual VA conduction time. Some cases of pacemaker syndrome with profound hypotension may exhibit a net reduction in peripheral resistance (78). During cardiac pacing the level of atrial natriuretic peptide (ANP) rises during unfavorable hemodynamic circumstances at rest or during exercise, and correlates with left atrial pressure (29,84–88). The changes in the peripheral resistance seen in the pacemaker syndrome may be mediated in part by ANP, but the precise role of ANP in the genesis of the pacemaker syndrome remains unclear. The elevation of ANP level may be secondary to the pacemaker syndrome and may simply act as a marker. Nevertheless, determination of ANP level could be used as a test for the adverse hemodynamic consequences of ventricular stimulation (i.e., for the diagnosis of the pacemaker syndrome).

Prevention and Treatment

The pacemaker syndrome is a preventable condition and should be considered a complication of the past. It cannot occur with the correct type of pacemaker functioning correctly and appropriately programmed. Once established, it may be eliminated by restoring AV synchrony either with atrial pacing (if AV conduction is normal) or dual-chamber pacing with an appropriate AV delay (89). No single parameter can identify individuals who will develop the pacemaker syndrome. However, at the time of pacemaker implantation, a decrease of 20 mm Hg or more in blood pressure with ventricular pacing suggests a high likelihood for development of the pacemaker syndrome, and a dual-chamber pacemaker should then be implanted.

RATE-ADAPTIVE PACEMAKERS

The normally functioning sinus node is the ideal sensor of heart rate. Sinus node function is frequently abnormal in patients requiring pacemakers. Atrial chronotropic incompetence is an important concept that remains poorly defined. The most commonly accepted definition is the inability to develop a heart rate greater than 70% of the maximum heart rate predicted for a given level of metabolic demand. The inability to reach a heart rate of 100/min. on exercise also provides a practical definition. About one-third or more of patients with sick sinus syndrome exhibit varying degrees of atrial chronotropic incompetence. Atrial chronotropic incompetence may be characterized by treadmill stress testing, Holter recordings, and monitoring during walking or ordinary activities. In patients with atrial chronotropic incompetence, the hemodynamic benefits of rate variability may be provided by the activity of a biologic parameter (independent of sinus node function) that varies in parallel with the need for a greater cardiac output and sets the required pacing rate at any given moment. A DDD pulse generator is the prime and best example of a rate-adaptive device using atrial activity as a sensor. It should not be surprising that artificial sensors are inferior to the sinus node in mimicking the heart rate response during standardized activity.

Atrial-independent rate-responsive system may be called rate-modulated, rate-adaptive, or sensor-driven systems and are designated by the letter *R* in the fourth position of the pacemaker code, e.g., VVIR is a rate-adaptive ventricular demand pacemaker and DDDR is a rate-adaptive DDD device. The magnitude of the sensor-driven response and its rate of change are programmable. The ideal sensor should be stable, reliable long-term, easy to implant, program and troubleshoot. It should also respond in direct proportion to metabolic demand (proportionality), use a standard lead, be energy efficient, autoprogrammable, respond quickly, and deceleration should be gradual at the end of exercise.

The first rate-adaptive pacemaker was implanted in Europe in 1981 and determined the change in the endocardial QT interval (from stimulus to maximum downslope of the evoked T wave) based on the principle that the QT interval shortens on physical exercise due to the release of catecholamines. The QT interval also shortens with an increase in the heart rate. QT interval shortening on exercise increases the pacing rate and the increase in pacing rate itself shortens the QT interval, but this problem has been corrected by appropriate software dealing with the QT/rate relationship. The QT interval shortens during physical or emotional stress even if the heart rate is kept constant. The QT system provides a stable, rugged sensor using a standard pacemaker lead (90,91). Its disadvantages include a relatively slow reaction time, nonsustained rate changes, some difficulty in ensuring reliable T wave sensing, and problems in obtaining optimum adjustments in patients with congestive heart failure. The QT system is affected by drugs, ischemia, and electrolyte imbalance. Excessive adrenergic tone may cause a QT pulse generator to pace at the upper limit in the setting of an acute myocardial infarction, creating an undesirable response (92,93). Many of these disadvantages have limited the popularity of this system even though many of the problems have recently been overcome. The QT pacemaker is not currently available in the United States.

At least 10 sensor-based systems are either in clinical use or investigation (Table 16.2). Only those utilizing a standard lead have achieved extensive clinical use. Sensors may be classified according to the way they fit into the pacing system, i.e., (a) activity: may be incorporated in the pacemaker can or within the electronics, (b) QT interval, stroke volume, respiratory rate, or minute ventilation volume can be detected with a standard electrode, (c) central blood temperature, intracardiac pressure, and central venous oxygen saturation require a special sensor inside the vascular system. Pacemakers with sensors using standard leads are ideal for pacemaker replacement.

Currently approved rate-adaptive pulse generators (1992) by the Food and Drug Administration in the United States utilize one of three sensors to modulate the pacing rate: activity, temperature, and minute ventilation (94). This chapter focuses only on devices available for general use in the United States.

ACTIVITY

The most commonly used rate-adaptive systems employ a piezoelectric crystal for detecting mechanical foces of vibrations (body movement, but not myopotentials). Deformation or compression of a quartz crystal generates a tiny electrostatic voltage proportional to the applied stress. The frequency (and in some systems also the amplitude) of the vibration signal is eventually translated into an appropriate pacing rate that increases in proportion to the detected vibration. The response depends on the nature of the forces affecting the piezoelectric crystal and the way the pacemaker processes the sensor signal. The piezoelectric crystal is bonded to the inner surface of the pacemaker can and no special lead is required (Fig. 16.1). There is no metabolic or hemodynamic feedback, and the sensor is regarded as nonphysiologic because it does not respond to an increased metabolic demand unrelated to exercise such as emotional stimuli (42,95). Indeed, response to emotional stimuli may not be clinically important and may actually be a disadvantage in some patients. The sensor is unaffected by drugs or disease. Although the "occurrence" of activity is more important than the "strength" of activity (96), this limitation and other idiosyncrasies of piezoelectric-driven, rate-adaptive systems do not detract substantially from their impressive clinical performance. Activity rate-adaptive single-chamber pacemakers quickly became the largest selling pacemakers in the world because they are simple and work well in practice in contradistinction to the theoretical advantages of a host of other more sophisticated and specific sensor systems.

The activity system is hermetically sealed, simple, reliable, stable, uses a standard lead (any electrode—unipolar or bipolar, atrial and/or ventricular, transvenous, or epicardial) and exhibits a fast response to brief periods of exercise. Its main advantage is related to the precise detection and rapid response at the onset

Table 16.2.
Sensors Incorporated into Rate-Adaptive Pacemakers

Activity[a]
Respiration
Respiratory rate[b]
Minute ventilation volume[a]
Temperature
Ventricular repolarization: QT interval[a]
Ventricular depolarization gradient[a]
Myocardial contractility
Stroke volume and rate of change of stroke volume (dV/dt)[a]
Rate of change of right ventricular pressure (dP/dt)
Preejection interval[a]
Oxygen saturation
Central venous pH

[a]Used with conventional electrodes.
[b]Needs auxilliary lead.

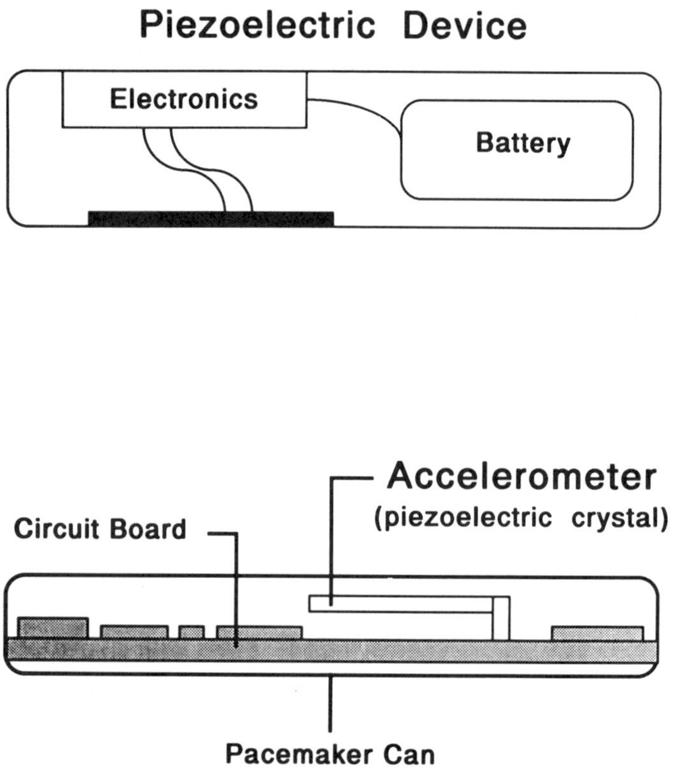

Figure 16.1. Top: Pacemaker cross-section showing location of piezoelectric sensor (*in black*) bonded to the inside surface of the pacemaker can. The sensor responds to vibrations sensed through tissue contact. **Bottom:** Pacemaker cross-section showing location of accelerometer mounted on the electronic circuitry. (Courtesy of Intermedics).

and end of exercise, important characteristics in older patients who do not perform much exercise and do so primarily in short bursts of physical work such as walking or climbing stairs. Programming requires adjustment of activity threshold and slope to provide a certain rate with a given level of activity (Figs. 16.2 and 16.3). The rapid response (97,98) contrasts sharply with other sensor-driven systems that exhibit a delayed response at the onset of exercise and reach a maximum rate after the end of exercise, making them less desirable for the elderly. However the plateau response of activity rate-adaptive pacemakers after the initial increase in rate represents a disadvantage. At the end of the exercise, when vibration stops because there is no feedback, an arbitrary setting controls the decay curve and in early models there was an excessively fast rate drop after exercise. Several programmable decay responses are now available, but without feedback, decay times are necessarily either too long or too short (Fig. 16.4). The pacing rate depends on the type of activity and does not correlate well with the level of exertion or the amount of work, i.e., body vibration is not proportional to the level of energy expenditure.

An activity rate-adaptive pulse generator does not respond to isometric exercise such as hand grip or Valsalva maneuver, weightlifting, postural changes (little or no rate change on standing), and to changes in catecholamines (97,98). Walking at a faster speed on the treadmill will increase the pacing rate. However, the rate will not increase with a steeper incline, keeping the speed constant, because the steeper incline (at the same speed) requires similar body movements and the number of steps remains the same at each speed, i.e., the input or number of counts generated by the piezoelectric crystal reflects the number of steps (96,98) (Fig. 16.5). Consequently, jogging in place achieves a high pacing rate. Bicycle riding employs leg motion rather than body vibration. For this reason, bicycle exercise testing is inappropriate to determine optimal settings of the pacemaker and its rate response because it produces inadequate vibrations from physical activity (99,100). Although the Sensolog (Siemens, Solna, Sweden) (Fig. 16.6) pacemaker possesses the same limitations as the Medtronic Activitrax units (Medtronic, Inc., Minneapolis, MN), it responds better during bicycling because of a different algorithm that integrates vibration waves rather than simply counting peaks of activity (100). Webb, *et al.* (101) reported an inadequate rate response of the Medtronic Activitrax during swimming (breast stroke, back stroke, and freestyle) when the pulse generator was programmed to produce an increase in rate by approximately 30 beats/min. in response to walking.

An activity-driven pulse generator provides a lesser rate response when walking up stairs compared to going down stairs, the opposite of normal physiology (97,102–104) and as a rule the rate increase on walking up stairs is inadequate compared to the normal sinus node response. An activity system is more responsive to lower extremity than upper extremity exercise, yet pacemakers implanted in the abdominal wall or subclavian region do not exhibit significant differences in rate response (101). Simple arm movements such as combing hair or brushing teeth have little effect on the activity pacing rate. Activity pacing produces an appropriate response with bedmaking or washing dishes, and an exaggerated response in rate during tasks involving rapid movement such as scrubbing. Movement of the arm on the side of the implanted activity sensor produces a greater response than movement of the contralateral arm (94). An excessive rate response occurs in response to suitcase lifting by the arm on the side of the pacemaker.

An activity sensor with a piezoelectric crystal is sensitive to

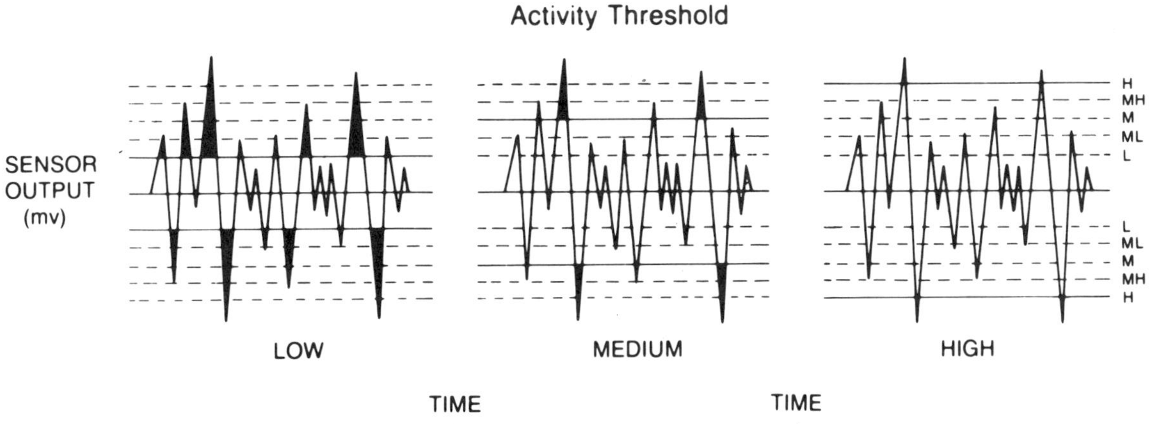

Figure 16.2. Activity threshold response of the Medtronic Legend activity rate-adaptive (VVIR) pulse generator. Sensor deflections due to activity must exceed the programmed threshold before the resultant signal is processed. Five activity threshold settings are available (low, medium/low, medium, medium/high, and high). Signal processing of the piezoelectric signal, counts only the number of times the signal crosses a threshold. (Other systems measure both frequency and the average amplitude of the signal to determine energy content.) A low threshold is exceeded easily and requires minimal activity, while a high threshold requires more vigorous activity before the sensor signals exceed the threshold. Choosing a low threshold causes the device to respond even to minor body movement, whereas a high threshold produces a response only to more intense body movement. (Courtesy of Medtronic, Inc.)

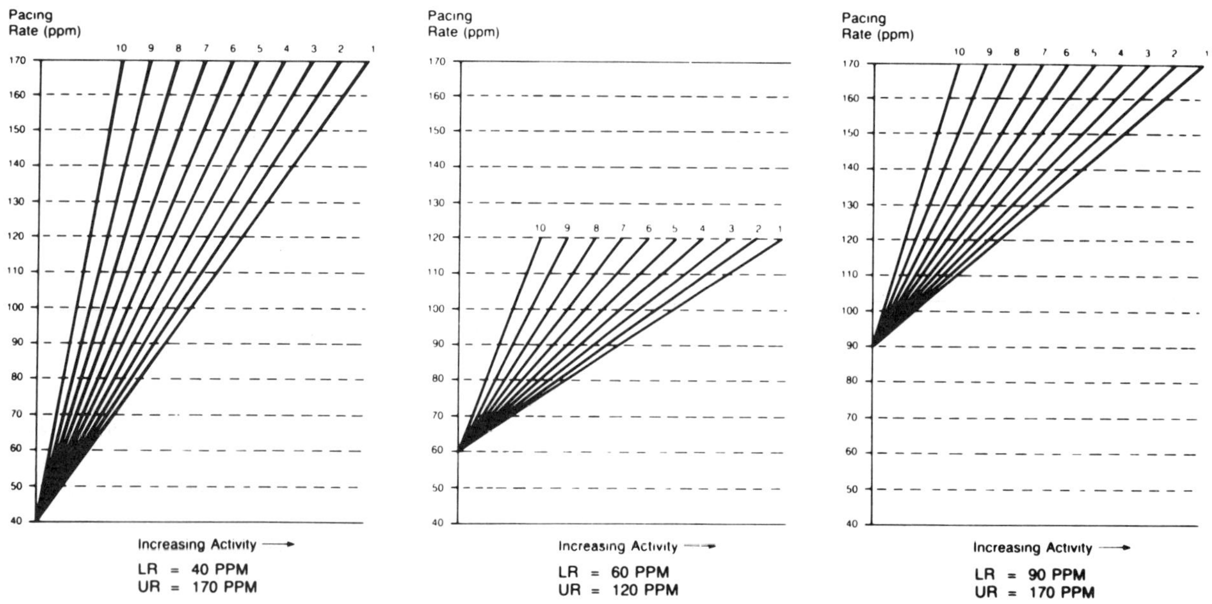

Figure 16.3. Typical slope or linear rate response of the Medtronic Legend activity rate-adaptive (VVIR) pulse generator. The programmed rate response setting establishes the relationship of the pacing rate to the detected physical activity. The number of detected deflections per second, occurring above the programmed activity threshold (Fig. 16.2), and the programmed rate response setting determine the pacing rate. The rate response has 10 settings. The most responsive setting (10) permits the greatest incremental rate change (ppm) in response to detected physical (body) activity. The least responsive setting (1) allows the smallest incremental rate change in response to detected body activity. All the rate response curves intersect and start at the programmed lower rate setting, no matter which setting is selected. The maximum pacing rate attained may be limited either by the detected level of body activity or the programmed upper rate. The sensor-derived pacing rate begins as the programmed lower rate and may reach the programmed upper rate at any rate response setting. If the level of activity stabilizes, the sensor-derived pacing rate will also stabilize and maintain a steady-state response until the activity level changes. (Courtesy of Medtronic, Inc.)

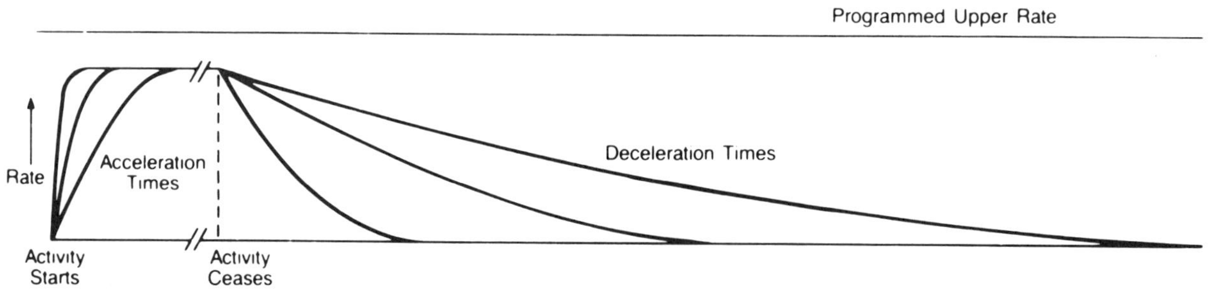

Figure 16.4. Acceleration and deceleration times of the Medtronic Legend activity rate-adaptive (VVIR) pulse generator. The figure illustrates a situation in which the pacemaker reaches a steady state below the programmed upper rate. Response time: when a change in the level of physical (body) activity is detected, the pacing rate will change—up or down, as the case may be. The rapidity of this change is affected by the programmed response time. The setting selected should mimic the acceleration or deceleration times observed in the normal heart. Acceleration time (0.25, 0.5, or 1 min) is the time needed to achieve 90% of the difference between the start of (or increase in) sensor-derived pacing and the maximum achievable pacing rate (due to programmed upper rate or steady-state pacing below the programmed upper rate according to sensor activity). The additional rate increase tapers smoothly to the final elevated rate. The nominal value of programmable acceleration is ½ min. Deceleration Time (2.5, 5, or 10 min) is the time required to achieve 90% of the difference between the maximum (or steady-state) sensor-derived pacing and the programmed Lower (or a lower steady-state) rate. The nominal 2½ min deceleration setting is appropriate for most patients. Note that the pacing rate begins to fall as soon as activity ceases. (Courtesy of Medtronic, Inc.)

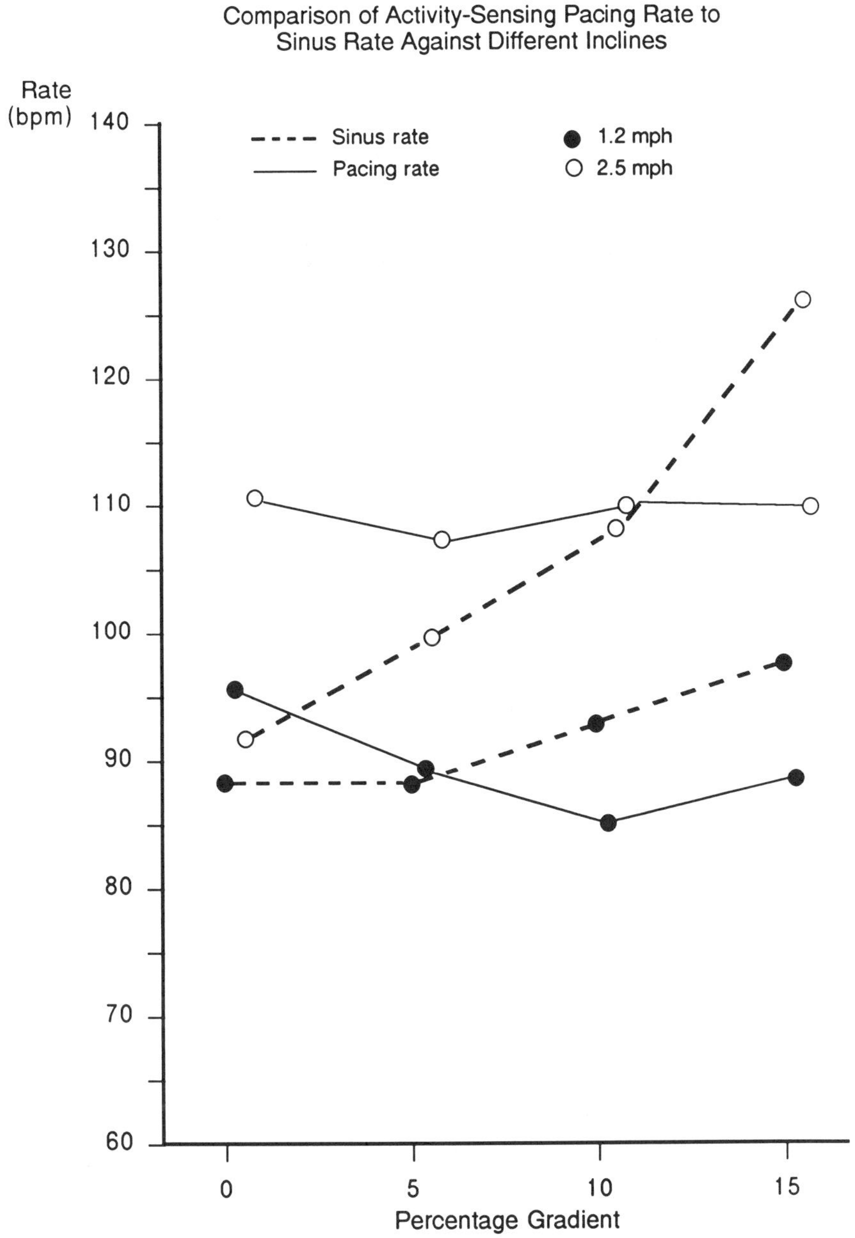

Figure 16.5. Changes in sinus rate without appropriate changes in pacing rate of activity rate-adaptive VVIR pulse generator to different inclines on the treadmill. An external Medtronic Activitrax pacemaker (Model 8403) was attached to the chest wall of normal subjects. The maximum sinus and activity sensing pacing rate responses were determined in six volunteers in treadmill exercises with different inclines at speeds of 1.2 and 2.5 mph. At each speed, four different exercise tests each lasting 3 min were performed (0%, 5%, 10%, and 15% gradient). At 1.2 mph, the sinus and pacing rates were similar at all gradients. At 2.5 mph, statistically significant differences were found at 0% gradient when the pacing rate was faster than the sinus rate, and at 15%, when sinus rate was faster than the pacing rate because the pulse generator failed to increase its rate appropriately. These observations illustrate a higher pacemaker rate response to walking at a faster speed, but not to an increase in slope (gradient) of the treadmill because at each given speed the number of steps used in walking up different slopes remained constant. (Reproduced with permission from Lau CP, Mehta D, Toff W, *et al.*: Limitations of rate response of an activity-sensing rate responsive pacemaker to different forms of activity. PACE 1988;11:141.)

pressure on the pulse generator resulting in an increase in the pacing rate, often seen with application of the programmer over the pulse generator (105). Some patients develop inappropriate increase in the pacing rate at night when sleeping on the chest or turning in bed, as well as when driving a car with seatbelt over the pacemaker site.

Tapping lightly over an activity (piezoelectric) rate-adaptive pacemaker may cause significant increase in the pacing rate that may be useful in certain circumstances. (a) Termination of reentrant supraventricular and ventricular tachycardia. This maneuver is effective only when tachycardia is relatively slow (106). (b) Performance of a thallium stress test by increasing the pacing rate not provided by programming the maximum lower rate. (c) The rate response can sometimes be used beneficially by patients in anticipation of an increase in cardiac output required with certain activities known to produce an inadequate increase in the pacing rate.

Under general anesthesia, vigorous surgical manipulation may cause a substantial increase in pacing rate, but this is unimportant because of its brief duration (107). The muscular twitches produced by suxamethonium and the myoclonus resulting from the intravenous administration of anesthetic agents are unlikely to induce an increase in heart rate (107). Postoperative shivering may cause persistent pacemaker tachycardia (107). In

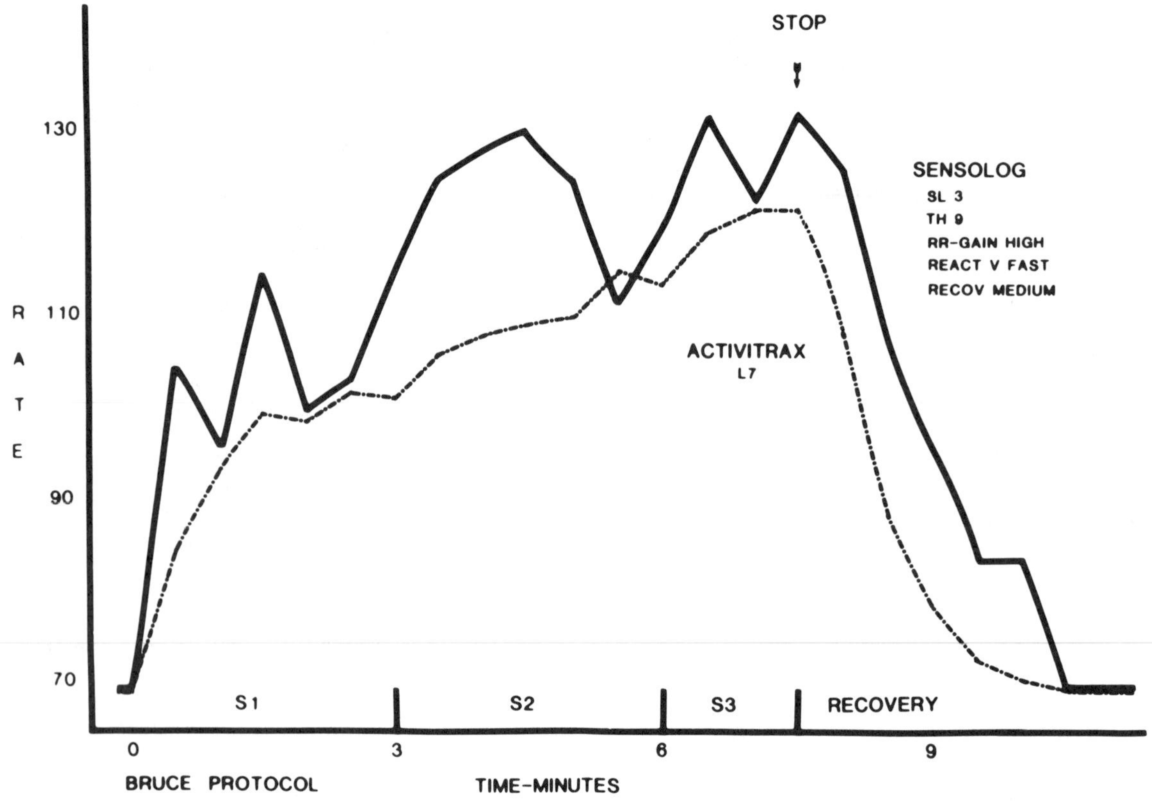

Figure 16.6. Comparison of pacing rate responses of implanted Siemens Sensolog VVIR pulse generator and external Medtronic Activitrax VVIR pulse generator during a Bruce protocol treadmill exercise test. The external Activitrax pacemaker was attached to the skin in the pectoral region. The upper rate of both systems was set at 150/min. There is very little difference between the two activity rate-adaptive systems. Both exhibited dramatic rise in pacing rate at the start of exercise. (Reproduced with permission from Mond HG, Kertes PJ: Rate-responsive cardiac pacing. Telectronics and Cordis Pacing Systems, Englewood, CO, 1988.)

this respect, Mond and Kertes reported a case of anxiety-provoked shivering that resulted in a pacing rate of 120/min (108). Epileptic seizures and myotonic jerking with chorea can also increase the pacing rate (109).

Deep implantation, as in the retromammary area in females, may decrease the response to exercise. As a rule, evaluation of an activity rate-adaptive pacemaker to exercise should be performed about a month after implantation because fluid in the pacemaker pocket may dampen vibrations and rate response. If programmed too early, there may be an excessive rate response several weeks later, after absorption of fluid in the pacemaker pocket (110). Occasionally a unipolar pulse generator implanted in the retromammary position or one that flips in the pacemaker pocket may cause local muscle stimulation and create a self-perpetuating mechanism or sensor-mediated pacemaker tachycardia (111,112) (discussed later).

Environmental interference such as riding on horseback, in a car in rough terrain, train, small engine aircraft, helicopter, hovercraft, motorcycle, the use of drills, and very loud rock music (large amplifier and ultra low frequencies near 20 Hz) may cause an increase in the pacing rate that is rarely of clinical significance (113–116). When bicycling on a paved road, the condition of the road influences the rate response and may provide a better pacing rate compared to the inadequate rate response during stationary bicycle ergometry. Dental drilling represents an important cause of vibrational interference transmitted through the patient with an increase in the rate of activity rate-adaptive pacemakers (99,117). In an effort to eliminate false responses due to environmental vibrations and mechanical noise, activity-driven pacemakers are now being designed with an accelerometer (a modified piezoelectric crystal) that reacts primarily to unidirectional forces of acceleration in the anterior-posterior plane (discussed below).

IMPROVEMENTS IN ACTIVITY RATE-ADAPTIVE PACING

Numerous studies have demonstrated the significant limitations of can-bonded piezoelectric sensor-based pacemakers: excessively rapid increases in the pacing rate at the onset of exercise, unnecessary rate increase at rest, susceptibility to external sources of vibration and localized pressure on the pacemaker can, and a lack of proportionality to different types and levels of exertion. Can-bonded piezoelectric sensors must maintain direct contact with body tissue in order to sense the vibrations or pressure waves produced during physical activity. These pressure waves emanate most frequently from contact of the patient's feet on a hard surface (as in walking or running) and are transmitted throughout the musculoskeletal system. Motion in any direction can cause pressure waves that deflect the can so that sensing with can-bonded piezoelectric systems is omnidirectional, i.e., anything that causes deformity or vibration of the can produces an output from the crystal.

To overcome some of the above limitations, some manufacturers have replaced the can-bonded piezoelectric sensor with an accelerometer which itself contains a piezoelectric crystal (Fig. 16.1). The piezoelectric crystal is mounted on the circuit board and is not can-bonded. The accelerometer responds to changes in motion of the pulse generator (not deflections of the can) and is, therefore, less dependent on vibration. Acceleration forces due to body motion are strongest in the anterior-posterior and superior-inferior plane and weakest in the lateral plane (118). The only stable plane of motion is from logo to nonlogo side or anterior-posterior because the pacemaker is most commonly implanted parallel to the chest wall. The sensor mechanism is principally unidirectional because it detects anterior-posterior acceleration forces. Attempts at processing the acceleration signal have produced a better correspondence with normal sinus rhythm (119–121). Frequencies between 0.5 and 3 Hz are most typical of body motion, and the accelerometer is designed to be most sensitive to this region (122). In contrast, can-bonded piezoelectric sensors are typically most sensitive to frequencies in the 5–7 Hz range, beyond the frequencies normally associated with human motion and therefore more likely to mistakenly interpret environmental vibration as body motion. An accelerometer seems to provide a high discrimination to various work loads, i.e., walking up stairs compared to down stairs, and lower susceptibility to environmental noise (123).

The performance of motion sensors will continue to improve as signal processing techniques are modified to eliminate many of the unwanted effects of a nonmetabolic sensor such as false responses due to environmental vibration and mechanical noise. Preliminary results with accelerometer systems has shown strong correlation between the pacing heart rate and intrinsic heart rate, indicating that an accelerometer-based pacing system will provide adaptive rate response specific to incremental exercise on the treadmill not seen with can-bonded piezoelectric crystals (123–126). The target frequency of the motion sensor systems that causes the maximum pacing rate has gradually decreased. While the Medtronic Activitrax had its greatest sensitivity to frequencies around 7 Hz, and the Pacesetter Sensalog systems around the 4–5 Hz range, the Intermedics Relay and Dash systems perform in the 2–3 Hz range. The lower frequency range is more typical of human motion (122).

MINUTE VENTILATION VOLUME

The Meta MV Telectronics system determines the minute ventilation volume (total volume × respiratory rate) by measuring the transthoracic impedance (a measure of the total opposition to current flow) with the injection of a small current (1 mA for 15 μs every 50 msec) between the pacemaker can and the proximal electrode of a standard bipolar lead (Fig. 16.7). Measurement of the transthoracic impedance is performed between the tip electrode and the pulse generator can every 50 msec. This impedance pulse is less than 10% of the threshold required for ventricular capture. Nevertheless, the additional current required for sensor function may reduce the life span of the pulse generator. The minute ventilation system can function either in the atrium or ventricle, but cannot use unipolar or epicardial leads.

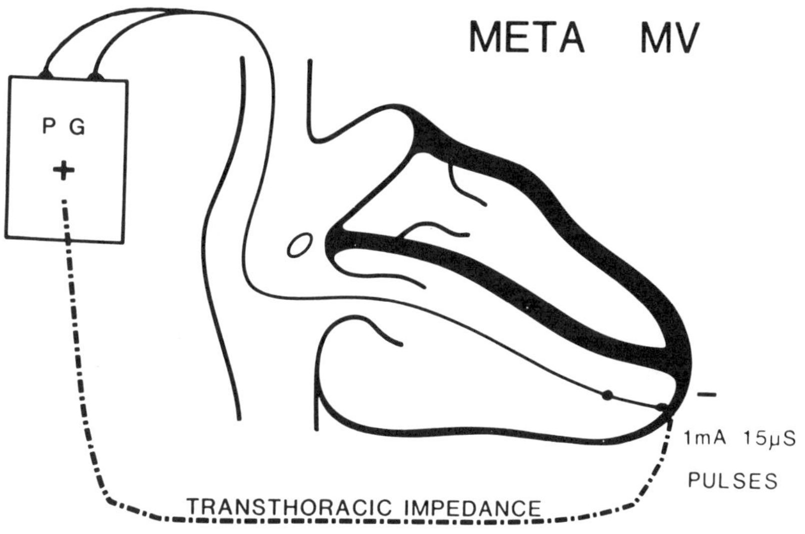

Figure 16.7. Diagram of the Telectronics Meta MV (minute ventilation) transthoracic impedance measurement system. A standard bipolar lead lies at the apex of the right ventricle. Low-energy pulses are generated at the ring electrode. Measurement of transthoracic impedance occurs between the tip electrode and the pulse generator casing. (Reproduced with permission from Mond HG, Kertes PJ. Rate-responsive pacing. Telectronics and Cordis Pacing Systems, Englewood, CO, 1988.)

The correlation with sinus rate is better with minute ventilation volume than respiratory rate alone. The transthoracic impedance increases with inspiration (because air has a higher resistivity than body tissue) and decreases with expiration, and the amplitude varies according to the tidal volume. The impedance can then be used to determine the respiratory rate and tidal volume to yield the minute ventilation volume that is translated into an increase in heart rate (Fig. 16.8). The pulse generator ignores impedance changes related to stroke volume by appropriate rate filtering. The sensor is not affected by drugs other than those that affect respiration. Signals used for impedance measurement can be seen on an electrocardiogram and can interfere with transtelephonic pacemaker monitoring (109).

The first minute ventilation volume was implanted in 1987 and so far no problems with sensor reliability have been reported (127–129). The system is highly physiologic because minute ventilation volume (and its corresponding pacing rate) bears a high correlation with metabolic demand or work load (Fig. 16.9). Actually minute ventilation volume more closely parallels CO_2 production than O_2 consumption (130). The system provides a stable and proportional upper rate with prolonged exercise. The system works well in practice, and occasionally the reaction to the onset of exercise may be delayed and the rate may be too fast after the end of exercise. Future improved algorithms will improve the response at the onset and termination of exercise.

Programming requires a treadmill stress test. Apart from the upper and lower rates, only one other parameter, the rate-responsive factor or slope requires programming and its value is calculated by the pulse generator, producing a suggested optimal slope (displayed by telemetry) based on the patient response. The treadmill exercise test is performed in the VVI mode, and the suggested slope is determined at each level of exercise. Programming the suggested slope will cause the pulse generator to reach its maximum rate at that level of minute ventilation.

Hyperventilation, coughing (131), and tachypnea from a chest infection or congestive heart failure can increase the pacing rate (132). The device is probably contraindicated in patients with chronic obstructive pulmonary disease. Swinging the arm on the side of the pulse generator and rotating shoulder movements cause displacement of the pacemaker in its pocket and a rate increase secondary to artifactual changes in impedance. The effect of shoulder movement is more marked on the ipsilateral side (133). The maximum increase in pacing rate

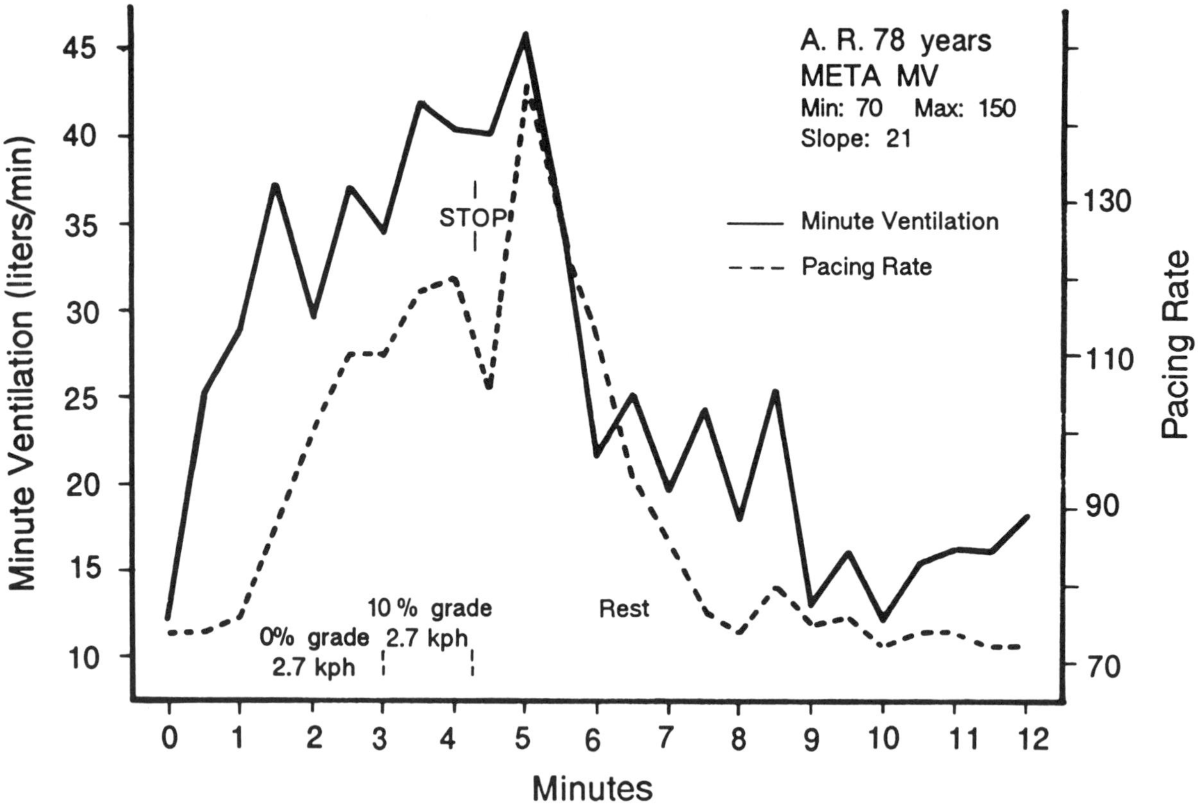

Figure 16.8. Exercise test (modified Bruce protocol) demonstrating the close correlation between measured minute ventilation and pacing rate during exercise and recovery in a patient with an implanted Telectronic Meta MV (minute ventilation) VVIR rate adaptive system. At the end of exercise the patient continued to hyperventilate and the pacing rate rose to the upper rate limit. There was then a physiologic fall in both minute ventilation and pacing rate. Tidal volume and respiratory rate were measured using a Fleisch head pneumotach with air flow converted to volume using a respiratory integrator. (Reproduced with permission from Mond H, Strathmore N, Kertes P, *et al.*: Rate responsive pacing using a minute ventilation sensor. PACE 1988;11:1866.)

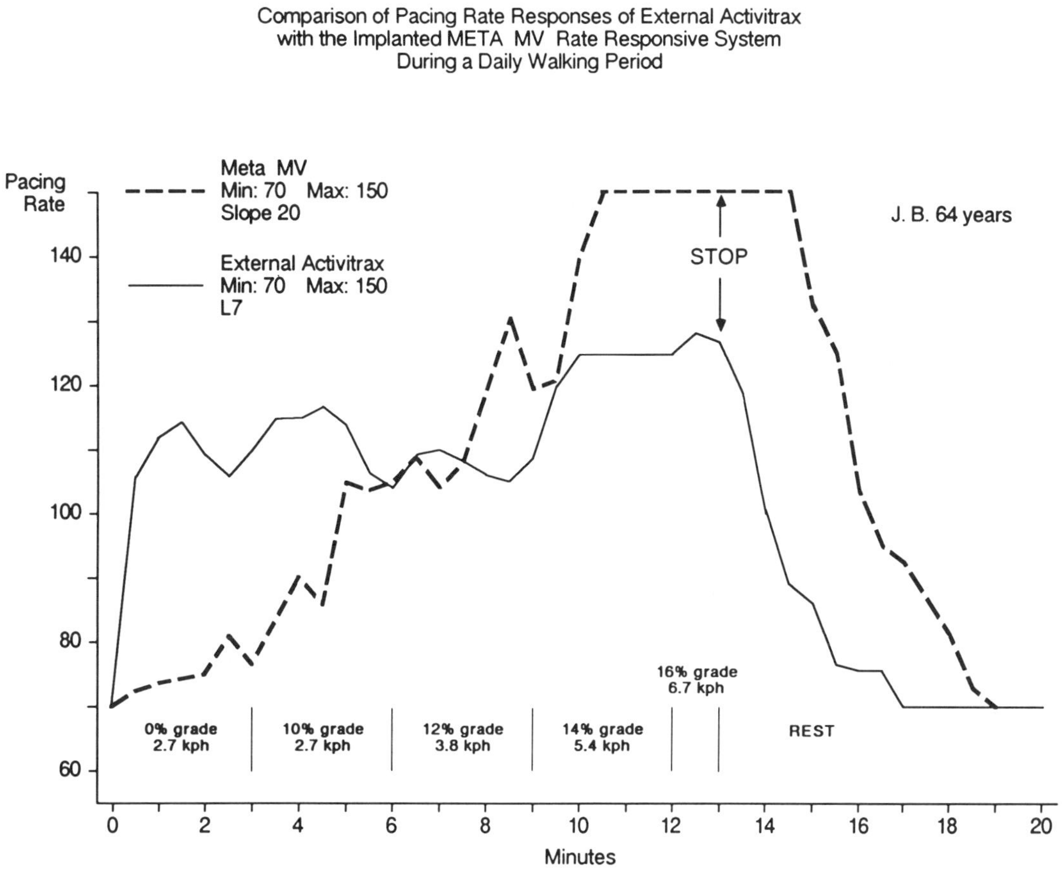

Figure 16.9. Graphs comparing the pacing rate response of an external Medtronic Activitrax activity rate-adaptive (VVIR) pacemaker with an implanted Telectronics META MV (minute ventilation) rate adaptive VVIR system in the same patient at the same time, using a modified Bruce protocol. (During the first 3 min no gradient was introduced. A standard Bruce protocol was then performed.) The activity pulse VVIR generator was tightly strapped to the chest wall, and settings of low activity threshold and rate response of 7 were programmed. These settings correspond to the widely used implanted settings of medium activity threshold and rate response of 7. There was a marked difference between the two rate adaptive pacing systems. At the start of exercise, the Activitrax pacemaker increased its rate to near 120/min within the first min despite the lower work load because it responds to vibrations and not work load. With increasing work load, the rate of the Activitrax pacemaker actually fell before it reached another peak of about 130/min, far below the set upper rate of 150 beats/min. On cessation of exercise, the rate response fell to the low rate within the first minute. In contrast, the minute ventilation rate adaptive VVIR pacemaker increased its pacing rate according to the physiologic work load and was able to reach the upper rate limit of 150 beats/min at peak exercise. The maximum rate response is maintained following cessation of exercise for about 2 minutes before a rapid return to the programmed minimum rate. (Reproduced with permission from Mond H, Strathmore N, Kertes P, *et al.*: Rate responsive pacing using a minute ventilation sensor, PACE 1988;11:1866.)

occurs with swinging of the arms at 30 cycles/min even during breath holding (131,133). Theoretically one could take advantage of this response to overcome the sluggish rate response at the onset of exercise. The response of the minute ventilation volume pacemaker is attenuated by talking continuously during exercise, but this is clinically irrelevant (131,132). Electrocautery changes the impedance between the electrode tip and the pulse generator and can cause an increase in the pacing rate to its upper limit (134). Artificial respiration may also disturb the operation of the pulse generator. The pacemaker can occasionally sense its own impedance measurement pulse with reversion to the asynchronous interference mode (loss of rate-adaptive function), but this form of interference can be prevented by improved design, proper programming, and using only recommended leads to match the device (135). Cheyne-Stokes respiration can also cause an increase in the pacing rate (136). During general anesthesia, an increase in ventilation can produce a substantial increase in the pacing rate that may cause hypotension (137). When the respiratory rate exceeds 50–60 breaths/min, the rate-adaptive function is deactivated and a paradoxic fall in the pacing rate occurs. The device should be avoided in patients susceptible to hyperventilation, particularly in children with high respiratory rates on exercise.

TEMPERATURE

An increase in metabolic rate produces heat that is transported in the blood and can be detected in the right ventricle with a small thermistor (capable of detecting temperature change with an accuracy of 1/100° C) totally incorporated into the pacing lead. Clinical experience with such a system has so far been fairly satisfactory (138).

Temperature sensing rate-adaptive systems have two basic limitations. First, incorporation of a thermistor into the lead itself complicates construction of a reliable system and problems have occurred with signal detection. The special lead consumes additional energy, its long-term stability has not yet been established, and acceptability of the system has been disappointing. Such a pacemaker cannot be used for replacement of a non-rate-adaptive unit. The use of temperature sensing at the atrial level is still under investigation, but the temperature response may be affected by inadequate venous mixing (139). Second, the design must deal with the dip in temperature at the onset of exercise (Fig. 16.10). A small decrease in blood temperature occurs at the onset of exercise as the cooler blood returns from the extremities. This temperature dip can delay the rate response of a temperature based system up to several minutes. However, several designs compensate for this dip by increasing the pacing rate to an interim level when a dip is detected. A paradoxic effect is found in some patients with CHF due to a temperature profile characterized by a very gradual and prolonged dip that sometimes cannot be detected by pacemaker, thereby causing a drop in the paced rate during early exercise. Zegelman, *et al.* (140) have demonstrated a dip in only 57% of their patients, while Fearnot *et al.* (141) found a dip in 91% of their patients (> 0.1°C) at the beginning of exercise. The initiation of exercise in a subject recovering from previous exercise may not produce a dip in temperature. The absence of a dip removes an important early trigger mechanism for accelerating the rate response (140). In anticipation of exercise, temperature can increase secondary to psychologic influences (140,145). Thus, nervousness before exercise can increase the pacing rate and when exercise is then performed, the faster starting pacing rate prevents a dip response because the algorithm provides no dip response beyond a certain pacing rate (140,141).

Temperature accurately reflects O_2 consumption in the middle or late stage of exercise. Central venous temperature is an excellent correlate of metabolic demand at high work loads, but it rises slowly at low work loads. Thus the system is stable and provides a proportional upper rate response to prolonged exertion. Temperature changes during mild exercise (such as walking) are often small, usually not exceeding those at rest. Thus, pacemaker rate response may be too slow (latency) and inadequate at low levels of exercise with brief everyday activities (94). A delayed response causes an increase in rate when activity has already ended (94). A short exercise time may produce a dip, but no temperature above the baseline to the end of the exercise, especially in patients with CHF (141). Increase in heat dissipation during exercise (e.g., swimming) may blunt the rate response (141). Heat dissipation mechanisms after the end of exercise are often impaired in patients with heart failure. A slow rise in central venous body temperature as a result of fever,

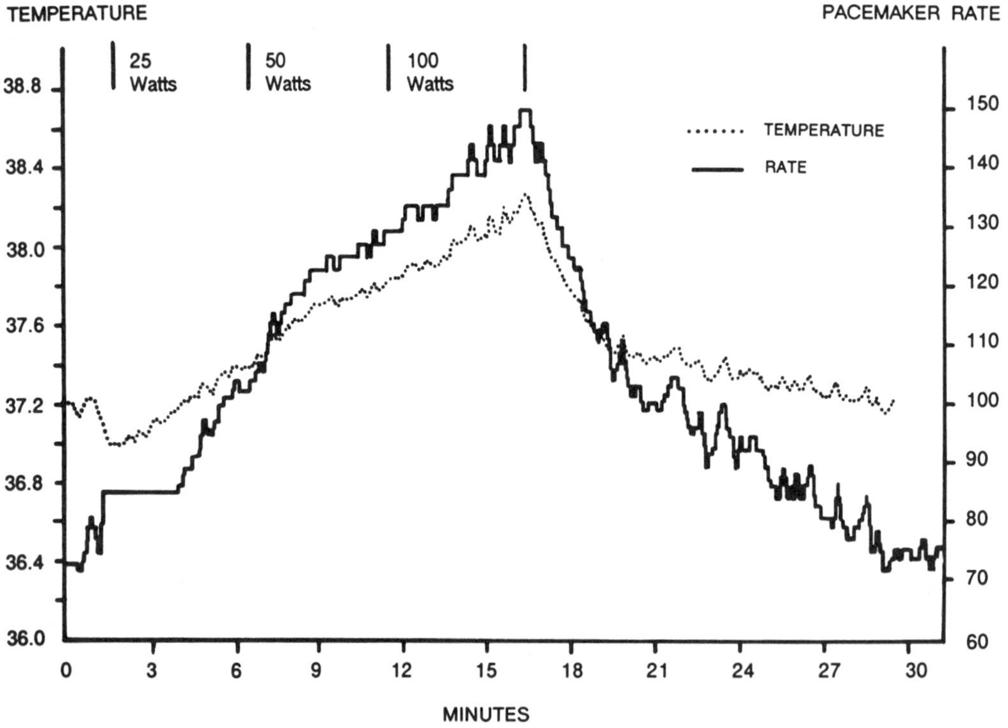

Figure 16.10. Response of an Intermedics Nova MR temperature-based rate-adaptive (VVIR) pulse generator to exercise. The increase in the pacing rate corresponds with the increase in central venous temperature. Note the temperature dip at the beginning of exercise. (Courtesy of Intermedics, Inc.)

emotion, or environmental factors (e.g., high external temperature) generally does not cause a large rate increase because the rate of temperature change is slower than that due to exercise. If they do, the pulse generator will eventually return to the lower rate setting, disregarding the increased temperature. Some algorithms will purposely increase the pacing rate by approximately 12 ppm/°C in an effort to mimic the normal mammallian heart rate response to fever. Likewise, normal hot baths and hot or cold drinks have little effect on temperature-based systems. However, prolonged full-body immersion in a hot tub (> 100°F) could cause a more rapid increase in body temperature and result in an exercise-type rate increase. Hot tubs ≥ 100° F. are therefore contraindicated in patients with temperature responsive pacemakers. Finally, a pulse generator must compensate for circadian temperature fluctuations that may be considerably larger than the changes induced by exercise.

SENSOR COMBINATIONS

New generation pulse generators will utilize two, three, or even more sensors to overcome the drawbacks of each one used alone. Such systems will require increased capability for data storage, processing, and presentation (142). Data will be cross-checked and such a system will take advantage of the physiologically more specific response that one sensor may be capable of providing under certain circumstances (143). With present technology a standard bipolar pacing lead allows the detection of stroke volume, preejection period, minute ventilation volume, QT interval, evoked QRS (depolarization gradient), and activity. Some sensors such as activity react quickly and while nonspecific are more suitable to determine the onset of exercise. An activity sensor could therefore be combined with another more physiologic but slower reacting sensor. The following combinations of sensors could be used: (a) activity and temperature, (b) activity and QT interval, (c) activity and minute ventilation volume, (d) minute ventilation volume and stroke volume, (e) depolarization gradient and minute ventilation volume. Furthermore, the QT sensor is best suited for the detection of increased catecholamines during emotional changes.

Pulse generators with several sensors will be more complex to troubleshoot, their sizes will increase, and the higher current drain will reduce longevity. It is questionable whether a patient will be able to perceive the benefit of a multisensor device when compared to a single sensor device with a refined algorithm and parameters optimally programmed. In the future, physicians may use a light pen on a sensitive screen to outline the desired rate response and the data could then be incorporated automatically into the pacing algorithm (143). True non-invasive hemodynamic data will be obtainable via a stroke-volume signal (impedance related) which multiplified by the heart rate will provide a continuous display of the cardiac output (143,144). Such data will enable optimization of parameters including the AV interval of DDD and DDDR pulse generators at rest and on exercise.

SMART RATE ADAPTIVE PACEMAKERS

Many available DDD and DDDR pacemakers cannot reliably differentiate a physiologic increase in atrial rate with exercise or emotion from an inappropriately high atrial rate due to endless loop tachycardia, myopotential oversensing by the atrial channel, paroxysmal atrial tachycardia, etc. A DDDR pacemaker receives signals from two sources: the atrium provides the P wave, and the independent sensor provides information concerning the need to increase the pacing rate according to changing activity. A smart DDDR pacemaker can differentiate physiologic from nonphysiologic rate variations in the passive sensor mode with the pulse generator itself not necessarily functioning in the rate-adaptive mode. Data from these two inputs can be used to determine whether a high atrial rate is appropriate or not, thereby providing a relatively easy way for the pulse generator to make the diagnosis of abnormal sinus bradycardia on exercise, physiologic and pathologic atrial tachycardia (Table 16.3). If the sensor input is below the level reflecting exercise, the pulse generator can first increase its postventricular atrial refractory period for one or two cycles to terminate endless loop tachycardia immediately. If tachycardia persists, the pulse generator could then identify it as a supraventricular tachycardia other than endless loop tachycardia, whereupon it might switch temporarily its pacing mode and/or rate automatically to avoid atrial tracking and therefore rapid ventricular pacing. The previous parameters could then be automatically restored when the sensed atrial rate falls below a certain level.

Table 16.3.
Interactions of Atrial and Sensor Activity During DDDR Pacing

Atrial rate	Slow	Slow	Fast	Fast
Sensor rate	Slow	Fast	Slow	Fast
Pacemaker interpretation	Sinus bradycardia	Pathologic bradycardia	Pathologic tachycardia	Sinus tachycardia
Pacemaker response	Pace or sense according to lower rate interval	Pace	Automatic conversion to VVIR, VVI, PVARP extension or other responses according to diagnosis or design	Nil

Reproduced with permission from Mugica J, Barold SS, Ripart A. The smart pacemaker. In New Perspectives in Cardiac Pacing. 2. Futura Publishing Co., NY, 1991:545.
PVARP—postventricular atrial refractory period.

PROGRAMMABILITY OF RATE-ADAPTIVE PACEMAKERS

Careful programming of rate-adaptive pacemakers is necessary to ensure that the patient obtains full benefit from the devices. Rate-adaptive pacemaker function in elderly patients should be evaluated at low exercise loads to correspond with their activities of daily living and not with maximum exercise which obviously represents an artificial situation. The procedure is time-consuming and must be adapted to the particular sensor and patient (98,145–147). Protocols include: (a) Casual walk. Program the pulse generator so that after a casual walk of 2–3 min, a rate increase of 10–25 beats/min to a rate of about 90 beats/min is obtained. (b) Fast walk or climbing stairs. Aim for an increment of 20–45 beats/min (rate 100–120 beats/min). (c) Three-minute walk (148). Pacer-derived histograms may be extremely useful to assess rate response (149) (Fig. 16.11). To assist programming, some pulse generators in the passive mode (non-rate-adaptive mode) can derive rate histograms with the expected rate distribution that would have occurred had sensor activity been programmed (149). Too rapid acceleration and deceleration should be avoided and these parameters are now programmable in some contemporary pulse generators. (d) A treadmill exercise stress test may be useful in determining the atrial rate, atrial chronotropic incompetence, arrhythmias, and evaluation of AV conduction at high rates during exercise. (e) A Holter recording during a patient's ordinary activities permits fine-tuning of the rate response.

A new system was recently developed by Intermedics, Inc., capable of storing the sensor-indicated rate or actual rate during a 15-min period of exercise (150,151). These data can be communicated to the programmer which can then display rate profiles for all possible rate-response settings, e.g., 1 to 10, showing the physician what the pacing rate would have been at each setting based on the patient's actual sensor data. These data can be collected even if the patient's intrinsic rate overrides the sensor-driven rate during the exercise. Thus a single exercise test may be sufficient to optimize the rate response setting for a particular patient.

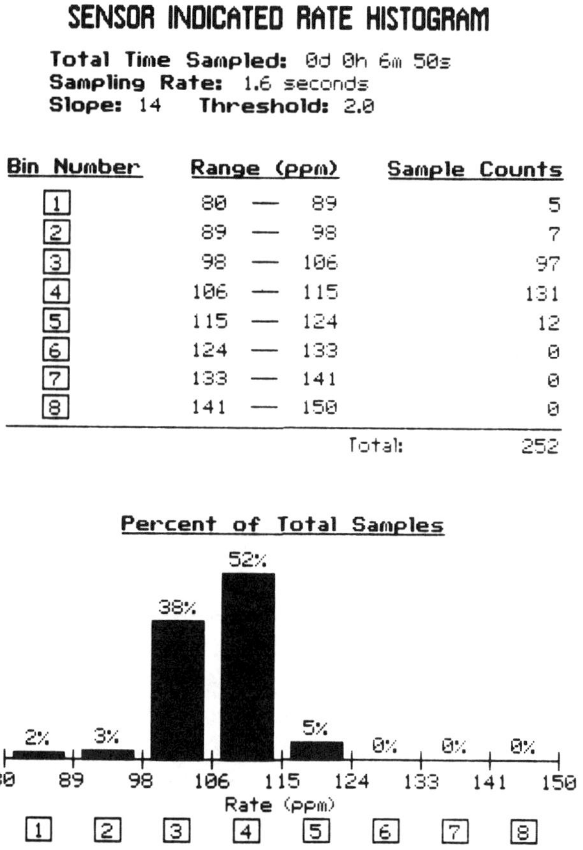

Figure 16.11. Example of telemetered sensor-indicated rate histogram after a brisk walk in a patient with a Pacesetter-Siemens DDDR (Synchrony) pacemaker implanted for the sick sinus (bradycardia-tachycardia) syndrome and atrial chronotropic incompetence. Bin 4 included 131 sample counts or 52% of the total sample providing an average increase in heart rate of about 30 ppm during brisk walking. This desired response was obtained after two other brisk walks at different rate-adaptive settings yielded an unsatisfactory rate increase.

INAPPROPRIATE PROGRAMMING AND SENSOR IDIOSYNCRASY

Inappropriate programming may cause excessive and rapid increase in the pacing rate with activity leading to unpleasant palpitations and other untoward effects. Overprogramming of rate response is generally not acceptable to patients who often request a change in programming (152) in contrast to underprogramming. As already discussed, rate-adaptive pacemakers are subject to idiosyncrasies related to the type of sensor (109). For example, in minute ventilation–driven pacemakers, hyperventilation with general anesthesia may cause pacemaker tachycardia and hypotension that may be misinterpreted as inadequate anesthesia. Consequently during anesthesia these pulse generators should be programmed to the VVI mode or the magnet applied in the VVIR mode to disarm the sensor and prevent inappropriate increases in the pacing rate.

SENSOR FEEDBACK TACHYCARDIA

Occasionally an activity unipolar pulse generator flips over in the pacemaker pocket and causes local muscle stimulation which in turn increases the pacing rate, thereby creating a self-perpetuating mechanism or sensor-mediated tachycardia (positive feedback loop). Lau has called this phenomenon sensor feedback tachycardia (153). However, local muscle stimulation from the anodal plate of a normally functioning unipolar activity driven pacing system is not uniformly associated with an increase in the pacing rate. An activity rate-adaptive pacemaker implanted in the left retromammary position with possible displacement over the apex of the heart carries the risk of an inappropriate rate response by mechanical stimulation of the heart itself (111). Similarly, diaphragmatic pacing by a ventricular lead can cause an increase in temperature which in turn increases the heart rate in a self-perpetuating mechanism (154).

PROBLEMS RELATED TO UNDERLYING PATHOLOGY

Inappropriate upper rate programming may precipitate angina in patients with coronary artery disease (109). Some patients with cardiomyopathy or CHF may not tolerate high VVIR pacing rates and may develop worsening heart failure, hypotension, and syncope (11).

INDUCTION OF VENTRICULAR TACHYCARDIA

The induction of sustained or unsustained ventricular tachycardia by an increase in the ventricular pacing rate is probably an infrequent but important complication of rate adaptive pacing and should be considered in patients with palpitations or unexplained dizziness, particularly in those with a history of previous ventricular tachycardia (109,155). Interestingly, DDDR and DDD pacemakers can actually be used to prevent ventricular tachycardia (possibly working best with a relatively short AV interval) with the DDDR mode probably more useful than the DDD mode for exercise-induced ventricular tachycardia (156–159).

RATE-DEPENDENT OVERDRIVE SUPPRESSION

Schmidinger, *et al.* emphasized that rate-dependent depression of subsidiary ventricular impulse formation can occur with sudden cessation of ventricular pacing (160,161). Thus, sudden inhibition of a pulse generator during fast ventricular stimulation may produce a longer period of asystole compared to similar circumstances during relatively slow pacing. The full extent of overdrive suppression and impulse inhibition may not occur if tested after a long duration of pacing at lower rates or after a short period of pacing at faster rates. For this reason Schmidinger, *et al.* have recommended that pacemaker testing should be performed for at least 60 sec at each pacing level (followed by abrupt cessation of pacing) to determine the risk of overdrive suppression at a particular level of sensor activity or pacing rate (161).

RESPONSE OF RATE-ADAPTIVE PULSE GENERATORS TO INTERFERENCE

Endogenous Sources

As a rule, the consequences of myopotential oversensing in unipolar rate-adaptive pacemakers is similar to that seen with non-rate-adaptive devices (129,162,163). The consequences of myopotential oversensing during exercise can be more dramatic during rapid ventricular pacing in patients with rate-adaptive devices compared to patients with non-rate-adaptive devices. The sudden slowing of the paced rate on exercise in patients with rate-adaptive devices caused by inhibition (with possibly a greater degree of overdrive suppression) or conversion to the slower interference mode can produce serious hemodynamic consequences.

Exogenous Sources

Many sources of interference have been described with standard non-rate adaptive pulse generator (164). As yet, relatively little literature exists concerning interference specifically related to sensor function in the rate-adaptive mode. Electrocautery can increase the pacing rate of a minute ventilation volume pulse generator to its upper rate as already stated. Lithotripsy rarely affects the sensor function rate-responsive pacemakers. Pulse generators with piezoelectric crystals can be affected if the pulse generator is implanted near the extracorporeal shockwave lithotripsy field. Mechanical energy from the lithotripter shock propagates through the tissue, fluid, and bones in the form of pressure waves picked up by the piezoelectric crystal, and the pacemaker may increase its rate. Therefore, it is recommended that the pacemaker be programmed to the VVI nonactivity mode during the procedure and the pacemaker distance from the focal point should be greater than 6 in. Patients with VVIR pulse generators implanted in the abdomen should probably not undergo lithotripsy because the procedure may shatter the crystal in the proximity of the focal point (165,166).

ADVERSE HEMODYNAMIC CONSEQUENCES OF RATE-ADAPTIVE PACING

VVIR-Induced Pacemaker Syndrome

Implantation of a VVIR pacemaker does not protect the patient against the development of the pacemaker syndrome at rest and/or during exercise (167–169). The behavior of retrograde VA conduction on exercise has not been studied in detail and it appears that it cannot be predicted individually (170). Indeed, the pacemaker syndrome may occur on exercise during VVIR pacing in the following circumstances: (a) VA conduction during continuous pacing at rest may persist on exercise (171,172). (b) Development of atrial chronotropic incompetence after a given level of exercise with the spontaneous sinus rhythm giving way to ventricular pacing and therefore retrograde VA conduction only on exercise and not at rest during normal sinus rhythm. (c) Because VA conduction is dynamic, exercise may occasionally induce retrograde VA conduction when it is absent at rest (170). Improved and restored VA conduction on exercise under the influence of catecholamines and other factors may cause an exercise-induced VVIR pacemaker syndrome. Alternatively, a pacemaker syndrome at rest may actually disappear on exercise if an increase in the ventricular pacing rate blocks VA conduction (64,173).

Delayed Left Atrial Systole

A DDDR pacemaker can be programmed to shorten the AV interval (atrial paced-ventricular paced) on exercise automatically according to sensor input. However, when exercise produces little or no associated improvement in latency or interatrial conduction, an adequate AV interval (atrial paced-ventricular paced) at rest may paradoxically become inappropriate on exercise (because of rate-adaptive shortening) and create an exercise-induced pacemaker syndrome if left atrial systole then begins after the onset of left ventricular systole (13,174–176).

DDI and DDIR Modes

The DDI and DDIR modes are useful in some patients with paroxysmal supraventricular tachyarrhythmias, but may cause the pacemaker syndrome if not used appropriately (177). In patients with complete AV block, the DDI mode can produce long periods of AV dissociation that mimic VVI pacing (release of atrial stimuli are inhibited by the sensed P waves) and may not be tolerated in some patients, i.e., pacemaker syndrome. An identical arrangement may occur in the DDIR mode on exercise when the sinus rate exceeds the sensor-driven ventricular pacing rate, a situation that may precipitate the pacemaker syndrome on exercise.

Repetitive Nonreentrant Ventriculoatrial Synchrony

In repetitive nonreentrant VA synchrony during DDD pacing, VA synchrony may occur without endless loop tachycardia (pacemaker-mediated tachycardia) when a paced ventricular beat engenders an *unsensed* retrograde P wave falling within the postventricular atrial refractory period of the pacemaker. Under certain circumstances the process can be self-perpetuating if the pacemaker continually delivers an *ineffectual* atrial stimulus during the atrial *myocardial* refractory period generated by the preceding retrograde atrial depolarization. This form of VA synchrony has been called "AV desynchronization arrhythmia" (AVDA), repetitive nonreentrant VA synchrony, or nonreentrant VA synchrony arrhythmia (178,179). A long AV interval and/or a relatively fast lower rate (or sensor-driven rate with DDDR pacing) favor the development of AVDA. When sustained, AVDA may cause unfavorable hemodynamics similar to the pacemaker syndrome (180). AVDA should not be an important problem with conventional DDD pacemakers because the duration of the atrial escape and AV interval can be easily controlled. However, DDDR pulse generators may induce AVDA on exercise because the sensor-driven pacing rate increases with resultant abbreviation of the atrial escape interval. Conceivably with DDDR pacing, on exercise a ventricular extrasystole could precipitate AVDA, thereby negating the benefit of AV synchrony and producing a VVIR-like pacemaker syndrome.

Single-Chamber Rate-Adaptive Atrial Pacing

In atrial pacing, a marked delay between the atrial pacemaker stimulus and the onset of ventricular systole may produce atrial systole against closed AV valves and a hemodynamic situation identical to retrograde VA conduction. This form of pacemaker syndrome is unlikely to occur with the pacing rates ordinarily used in the AAI mode. However, VA synchrony may occur in the AAIR mode when the atrial pacing rate is increased. When patients are carefully selected for AAIR pacing, the PR interval should shorten (or infrequently remain constant) during exercise (181,182) as the heart rate increases, in contrast to atrial pacing at rest which causes AV conduction delay at faster rates. A fast sensor response in the AAIR mode with an increase in the atrial rate disproportionate to the degree of exercise can lengthen the PR interval before the expected catecholamine surge induces shortening or improvement of AV conduction. The AAIR mode therefore poses the risk of "overstimulation" with rates above exercise requirement that may lead to undesirable paradoxical prolongation of the PR interval. This response usually occurs in patients taking drugs that depress AV conduction (181). The long PR interval places the atrial paced beat too close to the previous QRS complex, resulting in an exercise-induced pacemaker syndrome with atrial contraction against closed AV valve (183–187).

OVERSENSING OF POLARIZATION VOLTAGE AND CROSSTALK

During standard VVI pacing, a larger output (voltage and pulse width) and/or high sensitivity increases susceptibility of afterpotential oversensing (188). When the ventricular pacing rate increases, the polarization voltage at the myocardial-electrode interface (afterpotential) can grow substantially because the shorter pacing cycles provide less time for its dissipation between pacemaker stimuli (189). Indeed, during VVIR pacing, oversensing of the afterpotential is not uncommon at fast pacing rates with the pulse generator programmed to high output and high sensitivity, particularly in the presence of a short pacemaker absolute refractory period that allows detection of a signal relatively close to the preceding stimulus.

In a dual-chamber pacemaker (except for VDD and VAT modes), the atrial stimulus generates a small ventricular signal that must be superimposed on any residual afterpotential at the ventricular electrode-myocardial interface. Although a pulse generator may not be able to sense an enhanced afterpotential or the atrial stimulus individually, a relatively large ventricular afterpotential (associated with a fast pacing rate) can set the stage for crosstalk (even in bipolar systems) if the ventricular channel actually sees a large summation signal consisting of the afterpotential and a superimposed relatively small signal related to the atrial stimulus. Contributions from circuit noise may also play a part in crosstalk and may be design dependent so that data obtained with a particular pulse generator cannot be extrapolated to others (190,191). Unipolar DDDR systems are more likely to exhibit crosstalk at faster pacing rates. Testing for crosstalk in unipolar and bipolar DDDR pulse generators for the worst case situation should be considered in patients with pulse generators programmed to high output, high ventricular sensitivity, and a high upper rate, particularly in unipolar devices.

References

1. Iwase M, Sotobata I, Yokota M, *et al.*: Evaluation of pulsed Doppler echocardiography of the atrial contribution to left ventricular filling in patients with DDD pacemakers. Am J Cardiol 1986;58:104.

2. Pehrsson SK, Astrom H, Bone D: Left ventricular volumes with ventricular inhibited and atrial triggered ventricular pacing. Acta Med Scand 1983; 214:305.
3. Janosik DL, Pearson AC, Buckingham TA, *et al.*: The hemodynamic benefit of differential atrioventricular delay intervals for sensed and paced atrial events during physiologic pacing. J Am Coll Cardiol 1989;14:499.
4. Goldreyer BN: Physiologic pacing: The role of AV synchrony. PACE 1982; 5:613.
5. Labovitz AJ, Williams GA, Redd RM, *et al.*: Noninvasive assessment of pacemaker hemodynamics by Doppler echocardiography. Importance of left atrial size. J Am Coll Cardiol 1985;6:196.
6. Lau CP, Camm AJ: Role of left ventricular function and Doppler-derived variables in predicting hemodynamic benefits of rate-responsive pacing. Am J Cardiol 1988;62:906.
7. Greenberg B, Chaterjee K, Parmley WW, *et al.*: The influence of left ventricular filling pressure on atrial contribution to cardiac output. Am Heart J 1979;98:742.
8. Mukharji J, Rehr RB, Hastillo A, *et al.*: Comparison of atrial contribution to cardiac hemodynamics in patients with normal and severely compromised cardiac function. Clin Cardiol 1990;13:639.
9. DiCarlo LA, Morady F, Krol RB, *et al.*: The hemodynamic effects of ventricular pacing with and without atrioventricular synchrony in patients with normal and diminished left ventricular function. Am Heart J 1987; 114:746.
10. Reiter MJ, Hindman MC: Hemodynamic effects of acute atrioventricular pacing in patients with left ventricular dysfunction. Am J Cardiol 1982; 49:687.
11. Moreira LFP, Costa R, Stolf NAG, *et al.*: Pacing rate increase as cause of syncope in a patient with a severe cardiomyopathy. PACE 1989;12:1027.
12. Pearson AC, Janosik DL, Redd RM, *et al.*: Hemodynamic benefit of atrioventricular synchrony: prediction from baseline Doppler-echocardiographic variables. J Am Coll Cardiol 1989;13:1613.
13. Wish M, Fletcher RD, Gottdiener JS, *et al.*: Importance of left atrial timing in the programming of dual-chamber pacemakers. Am J Cardiol 1987; 60:566.
14. Ronaszeki A, Ector H, Denef B, *et al.*: Effect of short atrioventricular delay on cardiac output. PACE 1990;13 (Part II):1728.
15. Haskell RJ, French WJ: Optimum AV interval in dual chamber pacemakers. PACE 1986;9:670.
16. Lascault G, Bigonzi F, Frank R, *et al.*: Non-invasive study of dual chamber pacing by pulsed Doppler. Prediction of the haemodynamic response by echocardiographic measurements. Eur Heart J 1989;10:525.
17. Rockey R, Quinones MA, Zoghbi WA, *et al.*: Influence of left atrial systolic emptying on left ventricular early filling dynamics by Doppler in patients with sequential atrioventricular pacemakers. Am J Cardiol 1988;62:968.
18. Jutzy RV, Florio J, Isaeff DM, *et al.*: Comparative evaluation of rate modulated dual chamber versus single chamber rate adaptive pacing. PACE 1990;13:1838.
19. Algona P Jr, Batey R, Sweesey M, *et al.*: Improved exercise tolerance with dual chamber versus single chamber rate adaptive pacing. PACE 1990; 13:532.
20. Landzberg JS, Franklin JO, Mahawar SK, *et al.*: Benefits of physiologic atrioventricular synchronization for pacing with an exercise rate response. Am J Cardiol 1990;66:193.
21. Higano S, Hayes DL: Investigation of a new activity sensing rate-responsive dual chamber pacemaker. J Am Coll Cardiol 1989;13:112A.
22. Brinker J, Jutzy R, Hayes D, *et al.*: Initial clinical experience with a dual chamber rate modulated pacemaker. J Am Coll Cardiol 1989;13:112A.
23. Ausubel K, Steingart RM, Shimshi M, *et al.*: Maintenance of exercise stroke volume during ventricular versus atrial synchronous pacing. Role of contractility. Circulation 1985;72:1037.
24. Karlof I: Haemodynamic effect of atrial triggered versus fixed rate pacing, at rest and during exercise in complete heart block. Acta Med Scand 1975; 197:195.
25. Kristensson B, Arnman K, Smedgard P, *et al.*: The haemodynamic importance of atrioventricular synchrony and rate increase at rest and during exercise. Eur Heart J 1985;6:773.
26. Fananapazir L, Bennett DH, Monks PH: Atrial synchronized pacing: contribution of the chronotropic response to improved exercise performance. PACE 1983;6:601.
27. Rydén L, Karlsson O, Kristensson BE: The importance of different atrioventricular intervals to improved exercise performance for exercise capacity. PACE 1988;11:1051.
28. Ritter P, Daubert C, Mabo P, *et al.*: Haemodynamic benefit of a rate-adapted AV delay in dual chamber pacing. Eur Heart J 1989;10:637.
29. Theodorakis G, Kremastinos D, Markianos M, *et al.*: C-AMP and ANP levels in VVI and DDD pacing with different AV delays during daily activity and exercise. PACE 1990;13:1773.
30. Igawa O, Tomokuni A, Saitoh M, *et al.*: Sympathetic nervous system response to dynamic exercise in complete AV block patients treated with AV synchronous pacing with fixed AV delay or with auto-AV delay. PACE 1990; 13:1766.
31. Reed M, Haennel RG, Black WR, *et al.*: Effect of rate-adapting atrioventricular delay on stroke volume and cardiac output during atrial synchronous pacing. Can J Cardiol 1990;6:445.
32. Kutalek SP, Harper GR, Ochetta E, *et al.*: Rate adaptive AV delay improves cardiopulmonary performance in patients with complete heart block. PACE 1991; 14 (Part II):644.
33. Vogt P, Goy JJ, Fromer M, *et al.*: Hemodynamic benefit of atrioventricular delay shortening in DDDR pacing. PACE 1991;14 (Part II):621.
34. Sulke N, Chambers J, Sowton E: The effects of different AV delay programming in DDDR paced patients with out of hospital activity. PACE 1991;14 (Part II):650.
35. Wirtzfeld A, Schmidt G, Himmler FC, *et al.*: Physiological pacing: present status and future developments. PACE 1987;10:41.
36. Perrins EJ, Morley CA, Chan SL, *et al.*: Randomized controlled trial of physiological and ventricular pacing. Br Heart J 1983;50:112.
37. Iwase M, Hatano K, Saito F, *et al.*: Evaluation by exercise Doppler echocardiography of maintenance of cardiac output during ventricular pacing with or without chronotropic response. Am J Cardiol 1989;63:934.
38. Rossi P, Rognoni G, Occhetta E, *et al.*: Respiration-dependent ventricular pacing compared with fixed ventricular and atrial-ventricular synchronous pacing: Aerobic and hemodynamic variables. J Am Coll Cardiol 1985; 6:646.
39. Benditt D, Mianulli M, Fetter J, *et al.*: Single-chamber cardiac pacing with activity initiated chronotropic response: evaluation by cardiopulmonary exercise testing. Circulation 1987;75:184.
40. Fromer J, Kappenberger L, Bobotai I: Subjective and objective response to single versus dual chamber pacing. J Electrophysiol 1987;1:343.
41. Beyersdorf F, Kreuzer J, Happ J, *et al.*: Increase in cardiac output with rate-responsive pacemaker. Ann Thorac Surg 1986;42:201.
42. Benditt DG, Milstein S, Buetikofer J, *et al.*: Sensor-triggered rate-variable cardiac pacing: current technologies and clinical implications. Ann Inter Med 1987;107:714.
43. Kruse I, Arnman K, Conradson TB, *et al.*: A comparison of the acute and long term hemodynamic effects of ventricular inhibited and atrial synchronous ventricular inhibited pacing. Circulation 1982;65:846.
44. Nordlander R, Hedman A, Pehrsson SK: Rate responsive pacing and exercise capacity—a comment. PACE 1989;12:749.
45. Buckingham TA, Woodruff RC, Pennington DG, *et al.*: Effect of ventricular function on the exercise hemodynamics of variable rate pacing. J Am Coll Cardiol 1988;11:1269.
46. Sedney MI, Weijers E, VanderWall EE, *et al.*: Short-term and long-term changes of left ventricular volumes during rate-adaptive and single-rate pacing, PACE 1989;12:1863.
47. Adamec R, Righetti A, Pasquier J: One-year assessment of cardiac parameters in patients with physical activity rate dependent pacemaker. PACE 1987;10:630.

48. Faerestrand S, Ohm OJ: A time-related study by Doppler and M-mode echocardiography of hemodynamics, heart size, and AV valvular function during activity-sensing rate-responsive ventricular pacing. PACE 1987; 10:507.
49. Mugica J, Henry L, Attuel P, *et al.*: Long-term improvement of patient behavior with rate modulated pacemakers. PACE 1990;13:1205.
50. Batey R, Sweesy M, Scala G, *et al.*: Comparison of low rate dual chamber pacing to activity responsive rate variable ventricular pacing. PACE 1990; 13:646.
51. Lau CP, Wong CK, Leung WH, *et al.*: Superior cardiac hemodynamics of atrioventricular synchrony over rate responsive pacing at submaximal exercise: observations in activity sensing DDDR pacemakers. PACE 1990;13 (Part II):1832.
52. Mehta D, Gilmour S, Ward DE, *et al.*: Optimal atrioventricular delay at rest and during exercise in patients with dual chamber pacemakers: A noninvasive assessment by continuous wave Doppler. Br Heart J 1989;61:161.
53. Faerstrand S, Ohm OJ: A time-related study of the hemodynamic benefit of atrioventricular synchronous pacing evaluated by Doppler echocardiography, PACE 1985;8:838.
54. Edhag O, Fagrell B, Lagergren H: Deleterious effects of cardiac pacing with mitral insufficiency. Acta Med Scand 1977;202:331.
55. Rosenqvist M, Isaaz K, Botvinick EH, *et al.*: Relative importance of activation sequence compared to atrioventricular synchrony in left ventricular function. Am J Cardiol 1991;67:148.
56. Bedotto JB, Grayburn PA, Black WH, *et al.*: Alterations in left ventricular relaxation during atrioventricular pacing in humans. J Am Coll Cardiol 1990;15:658.
57. Harper GR, Pina IL, Kutalek SP: Intrinsic conduction maximizes cardiopulmonary performance in patients with dual chamber pacemakers. PACE 1991;14:1787.
58. Tanabe A, Mohri T, Ohga M, *et al.*: The effect of pacing-induced left bundle branch block on left ventricular systolic and diastolic performance. Jpn Heart J 1990;31:309.
59. Mitsui T, Hori M, Suma K, *et al.*: The "pacemaker syndrome." In Jacobs SE (ed): Proceedings of the Eighth Annual International Conference of Mechanical and Biologic Engineering. Association for the Advancement of Medical Instrumentation, Chicago 1969:29.
60. Furman S, Gross J: Dual-chamber pacing and pacemakers. Curr Prob Cardiol 1990;15:123.
61. Ausubel K, Furman S: The pacemaker syndrome. Ann Intern Med 1985; 103:420.
62. Schüller H, Brandt J: The pacemaker syndrome: old and new causes. Clin Cardiol 1991;14:336.
63. Furman S: Atrioventricular and ventriculoatrial conduction. In Furman S. Hayes DL, Holmes DR (eds): A Practice of Cardiac Pacing. Futura Publishing Co., Mt. Kisco, NY, 1986:56.
64. Byrd CL, Scala G, Schwartz SJ: Retrograde conduction and rate responsive pacemakers. PACE 1987;10:1208.
65. Nishimura RA, Gersh BJ, Vliestra RE, *et al.*: Hemodynamic and symptomatic consequences of ventricular pacing. PACE 1982;5:903.
66. Cohen SI, Frank HA: Preservation of active atrial transport: an important clinical consideration in cardiac pacing. Chest 1982;81:51.
67. Heldman D, Mulvihill D, Nguyen H, *et al.*: True incidence of pacemaker syndrome. PACE 1990;13 (Part II):1742.
68. Rediker DE, Eagle KA, Homma S, *et al.*: Clinical and hemodynamic comparison of VVI versus DDD pacing in patients with DDD pacemakers. Am J Cardiol 1988;61:323.
69. Kristensson BE, Arnman K, Smedgard P, *et al.*: Physiological versus fixed rate ventricular pacing. A double-blind cross-over study. PACE 1985;8:73.
70. Dateling F, Obel IWP: Clinical comparison of VVI, VVIR, and DDD pacemakers in the symptomatic relief of bradyarrhythmias. PACE 1989; 12:1278.
71. Sulke N, Dritsas A, Chambers J, *et al.*: A randomized crossover study of four rate responsive pacing modes. PACE 1990;13:534.
72. Sulke N, Dritsas A, Bostock J, *et al.*: "Subclinical" pacemaker syndrome; a randomized study of asymptomatic patients with VVI pacemakers upgraded to dual chamber devices. PACE 1991;14 (Part II):668.
73. Parsonnet V, Myers M, Perry GY: Paradoxical paroxysmal nocturnal congestive heart failure as a severe manifestation of the pacemaker syndrome. Am J Cardiol 1990;65:683.
74. Das G: Pacemaker headaches. PACE 1984;7:802.
75. Haas JM, Strait GB: Pacemaker induced cardiovascular failure: hemodynamics and angiographic observations. Am J Cardiol 1977;33:295.
76. Frye RL, Collins JJ, DeSanctis RW, *et al.*: Guidelines for permanent cardiac pacemaker implantation, May, 1984. A report of the Joint American College of Cardiology/American Heart Association task force on assessment of cardiovascular procedures (subcommittee on pacemaker implantation). J Am Coll Cardiol 1984;11:1882.
77. Dreifus LS, Gillette PC, Fisch C, *et al.*: Guidelines for implantation of cardiac pacemakers and antiarrhythmia devices. A report of the American College of Cardiology/American Heart Association task force on assessment of diagnostic and therapeutic cardiovascular procedures (committee on pacemaker implantation). J Am Coll Cardiol 1991;18:1.
78. Erlebacher JA, Danner RL, Stelzer PE: Hypotension with ventricular pacing. An atrial vasodepressor reflex in human beings. J Am Coll Cardiol 1984;4:550.
79. Naito M, Dreifus LS, David D, *et al.*: Reevaluation of the role of atrial systole to cardiac hemodynamics for pulmonary venous congestion during abnormal atrioventricular sequencing. Am Heart J 1983;105:295.
80. McCormick DJ, Shuck JW, Ansinelli RA: Intermittent pacemaker syndrome: revision of VVI pacemaker to a new cardiac pacing mode for tachy-brady syndrome. PACE 1987;10:372.
81. Ellenbogen KA, Thames MD, Mohanty PK: New insights into pacemaker syndrome gained from hemodynamic humoral and vascular responses during ventriculoatrial pacing. Am J Cardiol 1990;65:53.
82. Alicandri C, Fouad FM, Tarazi RC, *et al.*: Three cases of hypotension and syncope with ventricular pacing: possible role of atrial reflexes. Am J Cardiol 1978;42:137.
83. Witte J, Bondke H, Müller S: The pacemaker syndrome: A hemodynamic complication of ventricular pacing. Cor Vasa 1988;30:393.
84. Noll B, Krappe J, Goke B, *et al.*: Influence of pacing mode and rate on peripheral levels of atrial natriuretic peptide (ANP). PACE 1989;12:1763.
85. Baratto MT, Berti S, Clerico A, *et al.*: Atrial natruiretic peptide during different pacing modes in a comparison with hemodynamic changes. PACE 1990;13:432.
86. Stangl K, Weil J, Laule L, *et al.*: Influence of AV synchrony on the plasma levels of atrial natriuretic peptide (ANP) in patients with total AV block. PACE 1988;11:1176.
87. Nakoka H, Kitahara Y, Imataka K, *et al.*: Atrial natriuretic peptide with artificial pacemakers. Am J Cardiol 1987;60:384.
88. Ellenbogen KA, Kapadia K, Walsh M, *et al.*: Increase in plasma atrial natriuretic factor during ventriculoatrial pacing. Am J Cardiol 1989;64:236.
89. Nashimura RA, Gersh BJ, Holmes DR Jr, *et al.*: Outcome of dual-chamber pacing for the pacemaker syndrome. Mayo Clin Proc 1983;58:452.
90. Rickards AF, Norman J: Relation between QT interval and heart rate. New design of physiologically adaptive cardiac pacemakers. Br Heart J 1981; 45:56.
91. Boute W, Gebhardt U, Begemann MJS: Introduction of an automatic QT interval driven rate responsive pacemaker. PACE 1988;11:1804.
92. Edelstam C, Hedman A, Nordlander R, *et al.*: QT sensing rate responsive pacing and myocardial infarction. PACE 1989;12:502.
93. Robbens EJ, Clement DL, Jordaens LJ: QT-related rate-responsive pacing during acute myocardial infarction. PACE 1988;11:339.
94. Furman S: Rate-modulated pacing. Circulation 1990;82:1081.
95. Ward D, Garratt C: Rate-responsive pacing and sensors. In Saksena S, Goldschlager N (eds): Electrical Therapy for Cardiac Arrhythmias, Pacing, Antitachycardia Devices, Catheter Ablation. WB Saunders, Philadelphia, 1990:343.

96. Lau CP, Mehta D, Toff WD. Limitations of rate response of an activity-sensing rate-responsive pacemaker to different forms of activity. PACE 1988;11:141.
97. Lau CP, Butrous GS, Ward DE, *et al.*: Comparative assessment of exercise performance of six different rate adaptive right ventricular cardiac pacemakers. Am J Cardiol 1989;63:833.
98. McAllister HF, Soberman J, Klementowicz P, *et al.*: Treadmill assessment of an activity-modulated pacemaker. The importance of individual programming. PACE 1989;12:486.
99. Zegelman M, Kreuzer J, Rahn R, *et al.*: Body activity directed pacing. Activitrax versus Sensolog. PACE 1989;12:1574.
100. Lau CP, Tse WS, Camm AJ: Clinical experience with Sensolog 703. A new activity sensing rate responsive pacemaker. PACE 1988;11:1444.
101. Webb SC, Lewis LM, Morris-Thurgood JA, *et al.*: Can activity sensing rate responsive pacemakers match the normal heart rate requirements of recreational swimming. PACE 1988;11:514.
102. Soberman J, McAllister H, Klementowicz P, *et al.*: Paradoxical responses in activity-sensing pacemakers. PACE 1988;11:855.
103. Sulke AN, Pipilis A, Henderson RA, *et al.*: Comparison of the normal sinus node with seven types of rate responsive pacemakers during everyday activity. Br Heart J 1990;64:25.
104. Lau CP, Wong CK, Leung WH, *et al.*: A comparative evaluation of a minute ventilation sensing and activity sensing adaptive-rate pacemaker during daily activities. PACE 1989;12:1514.
105. Wilkoff BL, Denise D, Shimokochi MS, *et al.*: Pacing rate increase due to application of steady external pressure on an activity sensing pacemaker. PACE 1987;10:423.
106. DenDulk K, Brugada P, Wellens HJJ: Tachycardia termination with a rate responsive pacemaker. Am J Cardiol 1987;59:1424.
107. Andersen C, Madsen GM: Rate-responsive pacemakers and anesthesia. A consideration of possible implications. Anesthesia 1990;45:472.
108. Mond HG, Kertes PJ: Rate responsive cardiac pacing. Telectronics and Cordis Pacing Systems, Englewood, CO, 1988.
109. Maloney JD, Vaneiro G, Pashkow FJ: Single chamber rate modulated pacing, AAIR-VVIR. Follow-up and complications. In Barold SS, Mugica J (eds): New Perspectives in Cardiac Pacing. 2. Futura Publishing Co., Mt. Kisco, NY, 1991:429.
110. Bana G, Piatti L, Locatelli V: Sensor related PM syndrome in patients with VVIR PM. RBM 1990;12:23.
111. Ahmed R, Gibbs S, Ingram A, *et al.*: Pacemaker mediated tachycardia in the left retromammary implantation of VVIR (activity) pacemakers. PACE 1990;13:1189.
112. Lau CP, Tai YT, Fong PC, *et al.*: Pacemaker mediated tachycardias in single chamber rate responsive pacing. PACE 1990;13:1573.
113. Toff WD, Leeks C, Joy M, *et al.*: The effect of aircraft vibration on the function of an activity sensing pacemaker. Br Heart J 1987;57:573.
114. Toff WD, Leeks C, Bennett JG, *et al.*: Function of the Activitrax rate-responsive pacemaker during travel by air. PACE 1987;10 (Part II):753.
115. Gordon RS, O'Dell KB, Low RB, *et al.*: Activity sensing permanent internal pacemaker dysfunction during helicopter aeromedical transport. Ann Emerg Med 1990;19:1260.
116. Stangl K. Wirtzfeld A, Lochschmidt O, *et al.*: Physical movement sensitive pacing comparison of two activity-triggered pacing systems. PACE 1989; 12:102.
117. Rahn R, Zegelman M, Kreuzer J: The influence of dental treatment on the Activitrax. PACE 1988;11:499.
118. Alt E, Matula M, Theres H, *et al.*: The basis for activity controlled rate variable cardiac pacemakers: an analysis of mechanical forces on the human body induced by exercise and environment. PACE 1988;12: 1667.
119. Mahaux V, Waleffe A, Mathus E, *et al.*: Preliminary results with a new rate modulated pacemaker sensitive to low frequency vibration and acceleration force. PACE 1990;13:1202.
120. Silvermint EH, Salo RW, Meyerson SC, *et al.*: Distinctive characteristics of Excel VR rate-adaptive pacemaker with an innovative activity sensor. PACE 1990;13:1210.
121. Hage HJ, Niederlag W: A new concept of data processing for activity controlled rate responsive pacing. PACE 1991;13:1196.
122. Lau CP, Stott JRR, Toff WD, *et al.*: Selective vibration sensing: a new concept for activity-sensing rate-responsive pacing. PACE 1988;11:1299.
123. Matula M, Alt E, Heinz M, *et al.*: Rate adaptive pacing: Comparison between Activitrax, Sensolog, and Relay a new activity based system sensitive to low frequency acceleration. PACE 1990;13:1203.
124. Millerhagen J, Bacharach D, Kelly J, *et al.*: An accelerometer based adaptive rate pacemaker, PACE 1991;14 (Part II):699.
125. Millerhagen J, Bacharach D, Street G, *et al.*: A comparison study of two activity pacemakers: An accelerometer versus piezoelectric crystal device. PACE 1991;14 (Part II):665.
126. Erdelitsch-Reiser E, Langenfeld H, Kochsiek K: An acceleration sensor. A new concept in "activity"-controlled pacemaker (Abstr). Eur Heart J 1991; 12 (Suppl):415.
127. Jordaens L, Berghmans L, VanWassenhove E, *et al.*: Behavior of a respiratory driven pacemaker and direct respiratory measurements. PACE 1989;12:1600.
128. Mond H, Strathmore N, Kertes P, *et al.*: Rate-responsive pacing using a minute ventilation sensor. PACE 1988;11:1866.
129. Lau CP, Antoniuou A, Ward DE, *et al.*: Initial clinical experience with a minute-ventilation sensing rate modulated pacemaker: Improvement in exercise capacity and symptomatology. PACE 1988;11:1815.
130. Kay GN, Bubien RS, Epstein AE, *et al.*: Rate-modulated cardiac pacing based on transthoracic measurements of minute ventilation. Correlation with exercise gas exchange. J Am Coll Cardiol 1989;14:1283.
131. Lau CP, Ward DE, Camm AJ: Single chamber cardiac pacing with two forms of respiration controlled rate responsive pacemakers. Chest 1989; 95:352.
132. Lau C, Antoniou A, Ward DE, *et al.*: Reliability of minute ventilation as a parameter for rate responsive pacing. PACE 1989;12:321.
133. Seeger W, Kleinert M: An unexpected rate response of a minute ventilation dependent pacemakers. PACE 1989;12:1707.
134. VanHamel NM, Hamerlijnek RPHM, Pronk KJ, *et al.*: Upper limit ventricular stimulation in respiratory rate responsive pacing due to electrocautery. PACE 1989: 12:1720.
135. Wilson JH, Lattner S: Apparent undersensing due to oversensing of low amplitude pulses in a thoracic impedance-sensing rate-responsive pacemaker. PACE 1988;11:1479.
136. Scanu P, Guilleman D, Groiller G, *et al.*: Inappropriate rate response of the minute ventilation rate responsive pacemakers in a patient with Cheyne-Stokes dyspnea. PACE 1989;12:1963.
137. Madsen GM, Andersen C: Pacemaker-induced tachycardia during general anesthesia. A case report. Br J Anaesth 1989;63:300.
138. Alt E, Heinz M, Theres H, *et al.*: Function and selection of sensors for optimum rate-modulated pacing. In Barold SS, Mugica J (eds): New Perspectives in Cardiac Pacing. 2. Futura Publishing Co., Mt. Kisco, NY, 1991:163.
139. Lau CP, Camm AJ: Rate-responsive pacing. Technical and clinical aspects. In El Sherif N, Samet P (eds): Cardiac Pacing and Electrophysiology. 3rd ed. WB Saunders, Philadelphia, 1991:524.
140. Zegelman M, Winter VJ, Alt E, *et al.*: Effect of different body-exercise modes on the rate response of the temperature-controlled pacemaker, NOVA MR. Thorac Cardiovasc Surg 1990;38:181.
141. Fearnot NE, Smith HJ, Sellers D, *et al.*: Evaluation of the temperature response to exercise testing in patients with single chamber, rate adaptive pacemakers: A multicenter study. PACE 1989;12:1806.
142. Schaldach M. Present state and future trends in electrical stimulation. Med Prog Technol 1987;13:85.
143. Senden PJ, Landman MAJ, VanRooyen H, *et al.*: Sensor cross-checking in a dual sensor pacemaker during exercise and activity sensing artefacts. PACE 1990;13:1209.

144. Geddes LA: The next generation pacemaker. PACE 1990;13:131.
145. denDulk K, Bouwels L, Lindemans F, *et al.*: The Activitrax rate responsive pacemaker system. Am J Cardiol 1988;61:107.
146. Benditt DG, Mianulli M, Fetter J, *et al.*: An office-based exercise protocol for predicting chronotropic response of activity-triggered rate-variable pacemakers. Am J Cardiol 1989;64:27.
147. Hayes DL, VanFeldt L, Higano ST: Standardized informal exercise testing for programming rate adaptive pacemakers. PACE 1991;14 (Part II):1772.
148. Kappenberger L, Monnier P, Passeraul E, *et al.*: Three minute walk-test for adjustment of rate response parameters. PACE 1990;13:1200.
149. Hayes DL, Higano ST, Eisinger G: Utility of rate histograms in programming and follow-up of a DDDR pacemaker. Mayo Clin Proc 1989;64:495.
150. Sanders RS, Brunner U: Use of pacemaker diagnostic data to optimize DDDR pacing. PACE 1990;13:1209.
151. Drumm GW: Rate profile for determination of appropriate aggressiveness of rate adaptation. PACE 1990;13:1193.
152. Sulke N, Dritsas A, Chambers J, *et al.*: Is accurate rate response programming necessary? PACE 1990;13:1031.
153. Lau CP: Sensors and pacemaker mediated tachycardias. PACE 1991; 14:495.
154. Volosin KJ, O'Connor WH, Fabiszewski R, *et al.*: Pacemaker-mediated tachycardia from a single chamber temperature sensitive pacemaker. PACE 1989;12:311.
155. Scanu P, Dorey H, Guilleman D, *et al.*: Tachycardies ventriculaires déclenchées par un stimulateur ventriculaire à fréquence asservie. Stimucoeur 1989;17:158.
156. Adornato E, Pennisi V, Pangallo A: DDD-R pacemaker in the prevention of ventricular tachycardia. A report on one case. RBM 1990;12:84.
157. Adornato E, Pennisi V, Pangallo A: Dual chamber PM in the prevention of ventricular tachycardia—long term follow-up. RBM 1990;12:84.
158. Nicolai P, Blache E: Chronic cardiac pacing. A new therapy for severe ventricular arrhythmias? RBM 1990;12:84.
159. Sartieaux A, Bohyn P, Deperon R, *et al.*: Dual chamber pacing in the treatment of recurrent ventricular tachycardia. RBM 1990;12:85.
160. Schmidinger H, Probst P, Weber H, *et al.*: Rate dependent depression of subsidiary ventricular impulse formation. Cause of Strokes-Adams attack in a patient with rate modulated pacing. PACE 1988;11:1095.
161. Schmidinger H, Probst P, Schneider B, *et al.*: Determinants of subsidiary ventricular pacemaker suppression in man. PACE 1991;14:833.
162. Lau CP, Camm AJ, Ward DE: A severe case of myopotential interference in a patient with a respiratory-dependent rate modulated pacemaker. Int J Cardiol 1987;17:98.
163. Lau CP, Linker NJ, Butrous GS, *et al.*: Myopotential interference in unipolar rate responsive pacemakers. PACE 1989;12:1324.
164. Barold SS, Falkoff MD, Ong LS, *et al.*: Interference in cardiac pacemakers. Exogenous sources. In El-Sherif N, Samet P (eds): Cardiac Pacing and Electrophysiology, 3rd ed. WB Saunders, Philadelphia, 1991:608.
165. Cooper D, Wilkoff B, Masterson M, *et al.*: Effects of extracorporeal shock wave lithotripsy on cardiac pacemakers and its safety in patients with implanted cardiac pacemakers. PACE 1988;11:1607.
166. Fetter J, Patterson D, Aram G, *et al.*: Effects of extracorporeal shock wave lithotripsy on single chamber rate response and dual chamber pacemakers. PACE 1989;12:1494.
167. Wish M, Cohen A, Swartz J, *et al.*: Pacemaker syndrome due to a rate responsive ventricular pacemaker. J Electrophysiol 1988;2:504.
168. Liebert HP, O'Donoghue S, Tullner WF, *et al.*: Pacemaker syndrome in activity-responsive VVI pacing. Am J Cardiol 1989;64:124.
169. Baig MW, Perrins EJ: The hemodynamics of cardiac pacing. Clinical and physiological aspects. Prog Cardiovasc Dis 1991;33:283.
170. Cazeau S, Daubert C, Mabo P, *et al.*: Dynamic electrophysiology of ventriculoatrial conduction. Implications for DDD and DDDR pacing, PACE 1990;13 (Part I):1646.
171. White M, Gessman L, Morse D, *et al.*: Effects of exercise on retrograde conduction during activity sensing rate-adaptive pacing, PACE 1987; 10:424.
172. Fujiki A, Tani M, Mizumaki K, *et al.*: Pacemaker syndrome evaluated by cardiopulmonary exercise testing. PACE 1990;13:1236.
173. Klementowicz P, Ausubel K, Furman S: The dynamic nature of ventriculoatrial conduction, PACE 1986;9 (Part II):1050.
174. Wish M, Gottdiener J, Fletcher R, *et al.*: Use of M mode electrocardiograms for determination of optimal left atrial timing in patients with dual chamber pacemakers. PACE 1986;9:290.
175. Torresani J, Ebagosti A, Allard-Latour G: Pacemaker syndrome with DDD pacing, PACE 1984;7 (Part II):1148.
176. Chirife R, Ortega DF, Salazar AI: Nonphysiologic left heart AV intervals as a result of DDD and AAI "physiological" pacing. PACE 1991;14 (Part II):1752.
177. Cunningham TM: Pacemaker syndrome due to retrograde conduction in a DDI pacemaker. Am Heart J 1988;15:478.
178. Barold SS, Falkoff MD, Ong LS, *et al.*: AV desynchronization arrhythmia during DDD pacing. In Belhassen B, Feldman S, Copperman Y (eds): Cardiac Pacing and Electrophysiology, Proceedings of the VIIIth World Symposium on Cardiac Pacing and Electrophysiology. Jerusalem, Keterpress Enterprises, 1987:117.
179. Barold SS, Falkoff MD, Ong LS, *et al.*: Magnet unresponsive pacemaker endless loop tachycardia, Am Heart J 1988;116:726.
180. Chien WW, Foster E, Phillips B, *et al.*: Pacemaker syndrome in a patient with DDD pacemaker for long QT syndrome. PACE 1991;14:1209.
181. Brandt J, Fahraeus T, Ogawa T, *et al.*: Practical aspects of rate-adaptive atrial (AAIR) pacing. Clinical experiences in 44 patients. PACE 1991; 14:1258.
182. Edelstam C, Nordlander R, Wallgren E, *et al.*: AAIR pacing and exercise. What happens to AV conduction? PACE 1990;13:1193.
183. Clarke M, Allen A: Rate responsive atrial pacing resulting in pacemaker syndrome. PACE 1987;10:1209.
184. Pouillot C, Mabo C, LeLong B: Bénéfices et limites de la stimulation monochambre atriale à fréquence asservie, Arch Mal Coeur 1990; 83:1833.
185. denDulk K, Lindemans FW, Brugada P, *et al.*: Pacemaker syndrome with AAI rate variable pacing. Importance of atrioventricular conduction properties, medication and pacemaker programmability, PACE 1988;11: 1226.
186. Daubert C, Mabo P, Pouillot C, *et al.*: Atrial chronotropic incompetence. Implications for DDDR pacing, In Barold SS, Mugica J (eds): New Perspectives in Cardiac Pacing. 2. Futura Publishing Co., Mt. Kisco, NY, 1991:251.
187. Ruiter J, Burgersdijk C, Zeeders M, *et al.*: Atrial Activitrax pacing. The atrioventricular interval during exercise. PACE 1987;10:1226.
188. Barold SS, Falkoff MD, Ong LS, *et al.*: Differential diagnosis of pacemaker pauses. In Barold SS (ed): Modern Cardiac Pacing, Futura Publishing Co., Mt. Kisco, NY, 1985:587.
189. Barold SS, Roehrich DR, Falkoff MD, *et al.*: Sources of error in the determination of output voltage of pulse generators by pacemaker system analyzers. PACE 1980;3:585.
190. Byrd CL, Schwartz SJ, Gonzales M, *et al.*: Rate responsive pacemakers and crosstalk. PACE 1988;11 (June Suppl.):798.
191. Combs WJ, Reynolds DW, Sharma AD, *et al.*: Crosstalk in bipolar pacemakers. PACE 1989;12:1613.

17

PACEMAKER SELECTION FOR THE INDIVIDUAL PATIENT

S. Serge Barold, M.B., B.S., F.R.A.C.P., F.A.C.P., F.A.C.C., F.E.S.C.

Implantation of a VVI pulse generator in every patient requiring pacing is obviously inappropriate (1). In this regard, the British Pacing and Electrophysiology Group recently developed a position paper entitled "Recommendations for Pacemaker Prescription for Symptomatic Bradycardia" indicating that a basic VVI system for everyone irrespective of need, symptoms, or electrocardiographic findings is clearly inappropriate (1). The British Pacing and Electrophysiology Group also enunciated four general principles for the selection of the various modes of cardiac pacing (1) (Table 17.1) with the recommendation that "the atrium should be paced/sensed unless contraindicated." On the other hand, for clinical and economic reasons, dual-chamber pulse generators, especially DDDR systems, should not be used indiscriminately (2). Despite the advantages of atrial pacing, about 70–80% of all new pacemaker implantations worldwide consist of VVI or VVIR devices (3).

In the last few years, many important retrospective and nonrandomized studies focusing mostly on the sick sinus syndrome have demonstrated convincingly that atrial pacing (single-lead atrial or dual-chamber pacing) improves the quality and duration of life when compared to single-lead ventricular pacing. These studies indicate that single-chamber ventricular pacing in the sick sinus syndrome when compared to atrial or dual-chamber pacing causes a greater incidence of (a) pacemaker syndrome, (b) chronic atrial fibrillation, embolization, and stroke, (c) increase in the cardiothoracic ratio and left atrial size, (d) congestive heart failure, and (e) mortality (4–7). Preliminary evidence suggests that atrial pacing may also prevent attacks of paroxysmal atrial fibrillation in the bradycardia-tachycardia syndrome other than the type associated with vagally induced atrial fibrillation in which atrial pacing alone is often effective (8–14). The hemodynamic and electrophysiologic advantages of atrial pacing form the basis of the recommendation by the British Pacing and Electrophysiology Group that "the atrium should be paced/sensed unless contraindicated"(1).

DISADVANTAGES OF SINGLE-LEAD VENTRICULAR PACING

Pacemaker Syndrome and Retrograde Ventriculoatrial Conduction

The mechanism, incidence, and treatment of the pacemaker syndrome are described in Chapter 16. Irrespective of the pacemaker syndrome, retrograde ventriculoatrial (VA) conduction during single-lead ventricular pacing favors the development of atrial arrhythmias and thromboembolic complications (3,15,16). For this reason alone, some workers feel that single-lead VVI pacing is contraindicated in sick sinus syndrome patients with retrograde VA conduction (15,16).

Chronic Atrial Fibrillation

A prior history of supraventricular tachyarrhythmias appears to be the major determinant of postimplant atrial tachyarrhythmias in patients receiving VVI, DDD, or DDDR pulse generators (17–19). Many workers evaluating the antiarrhythmic benefits of atrial pacing in the sick sinus syndrome failed to analyze the prognostic significance of preexistent paroxysmal supraventricular tachyarrhythmias. When all sick sinus syndrome patients are considered as a group (regardless of preexistent paroxysmal supraventricular tachyarrhythmias), the development of chronic atrial fibrillation is significantly higher with VVI pacing than with AAI (DDD, DDI) pacing (6,20–26).

Fewer workers have focused their investigations on the specific group of sick sinus syndrome patients with a history of prior paroxysmal supraventricular tachyarrhythmias (11,18,27–29). A higher incidence of chronic atrial fibrillation was found in all but one (29) of such studies in the VVI group compared to the group with atrial or dual chamber pacing (the study of Feuer, *et al*. (17) did not separate patients with AV block from sick sinus syndrome).

Table 17.1.
General Principles of Pacemaker Choice. British Pacing and Electrophysiology Group

1. The ventricle should be paced if there is actual or threatened atrioventricular block.
2. The atrium should be paced/sensed unless contraindicated.
3. Rate response is not essential if patient is inactive or has a normal chronotropic response.
4. Rate hysteresis may be valuable if the bradycardia is intermittent.

Reproduced with permission from Clarke M, Sutton R, Ward D, *et al.*: Recommendations for Pacemaker Prescription for Symptomatic Bradycardia. Report of a working party for the British Packing and Electrophysiology Group. Br Heart J 1991;66:185.

Six studies have evaluated specifically the effect of pacing mode on the incidence of chronic atrial fibrillation in sick sinus syndrome patients without preexistent paroxysmal supraventricular tachyarrhythmias (27–32). Three of these studies (30–32) showed a significant decrease in the incidence of chronic atrial fibrillation with atrial or AV sequential pacing compared to the VVI mode, one showed no significant difference (27), and finally in two reports no patients without previous paroxysmal supraventricular tachyarrhythmias developed chronic atrial fibrillation in either the VVI or AAI/DDD modes (28,29).

Congestive Heart Failure

Alpert, *et al.* (33,34) investigated the influence of pacing mode and congestive heart failure (at the time of pacemaker implantation) on long-term survival (one study concentrated on high-degree AV block and the other on sick sinus syndrome) (33,34). In either the AV block or sick sinus syndrome group without congestive heart failure the mortality did not differ significantly when VVI was compared to dual-chamber pacing. On the other hand, in either the AV block or sick sinus syndrome group with congestive heart failure, dual-chamber pacing improved survival significantly compared to VVI pacing. Edelstam, *et al.* (35) also analyzed the survival of patients with AV block treated with VDD and VVI pacemakers and found a higher mortality in the VVI group compared to the VDD group only in the patients that presented with congestive heart failure at the time of pacemaker implantation.

Rosenqvist, *et al.* (27) evaluated the development of congestive heart failure *after* pacemaker implantation for sick sinus syndrome and found a higher incidence with VVI than AAI pacing, as did Stangl, *et al.* (29). However, two other groups (the two studies of Sasaki, *et al.* (6,28) are counted as one) reported no significant difference in sick sinus syndrome patients between VVI versus AAI pacing with regard to the development of congestive heart failure after pacemaker implantation (6,22).

Stroke

Six studies have demonstrated a higher incidence of stroke in sick sinus syndrome patients equipped with VVI pacemakers compared to AAI/DDD devices (6,11,20,22,23,36) with only three studies showing no significant difference (24,29,30). An additional study by Rosenqvist, *et al.* (27) comparing VVI to AAI pacing showed a significant increase in stroke only in sick sinus syndrome patients with paroxysmal supraventricular tachyarrhythmias before pacemaker implantation.

Mortality

Ventricular pacing does not favorably influence mortality in sick sinus syndrome patients (37) and there is no evidence that VVIR versus VVI pacing improves survival. Five studies (6,23,27,36,38) (in addition to those of Alpert, *et al.* (33,34) and Edelstam, *et al.* (35) in patients with preexistent congestive heart failure) have demonstrated a significant reduction in mortality in sick sinus syndrome patients with AAI/DDD pacemakers compared to those with VVI devices. Stangl, *et al.* (29) found in the sick sinus syndrome no difference in the overall mortality of the VVI group versus AAI group, but the mortality was higher in patients with VVI pacemakers if they had either coronary artery disease or no underlying heart disease. In contrast, three other studies of sick sinus syndrome patients have shown no significant difference in mortality comparing VVI pacing with AAI/DDD pacing (22,24,30). Pacemaker rate response to exercise is a highly unlikely protective mechanism increasing survival because fixed-frequency atrial pacing was utilized in most of the studies showing decreased mortality.

PACEMAKER SELECTION: GENERAL CONSIDERATIONS

The 1991 American College of Cardiology/American Heart Association (ACC/AHA) Guidelines for Implantation of Cardiac Pacemakers and Antiarrhythmia Devices (39) recommend VVI pacing as a Class I choice (Table 17.2) for "any symptomatic bradycardia, but particularly when there is no evidence of pacemaker syndrome due to loss of atrial contribution or negative atrial kick (a replacement pacemaker)". Symptomatic bradycardia in the *absence* of retrograde VA conduction is classified as a Class II choice for VVI pacing (Table 17.2). The 1991 ACC/AHA guidelines do not specifically state that the VVI mode is contraindicated in patients with either the sick sinus syndrome and/or retrograde VA conduction as advocated by the British Pacing and Electrophysiology Group and others (1,40–42), though they do indicate that "VVIR pacemakers are particularly contraindicated in the presence of retrograde VA conduction" (Table 17.2). Many workers believe that the last statement also applies to VVI pacing. Furthermore, the 1991 ACC/AHA guidelines do not specifically indicate that single lead atrial (if AV conduction is normal) and dual-chamber pacemakers should be used in patients with retrograde VA conduction. The ACC/AHA guidelines for the selection of the DDD mode are outlined in Table 17.3.

A recent editorial in the *Lancet* entitled "Pacemakers—Practice and Paradox" (43) compared the 1991 (July) ACC/AHA guidelines for antibradycardia pacing (39) with those promul-

Table 17.2.
ACC/AHA Guidelines for Device Selection—VVI Mode

Class I: Conditions for which there is general agreement that such a mode of pacing is appropriate.
- A. Any symptomatic bradyarrhythmia but particularly when there is:
  1. No significant atrial hemodynamic contribution (persistent or paroxysmal atrial flutter/fibrillation, giant atria)
  2. No evidence of pacemaker syndrome due to loss of atrial contribution or negative atrial kick (a replacement pacemaker)

Class II: Conditions for which a given mode of pacing may be used but there is a divergence of opinion with respect to the necessity of that mode of pacing.
- A. Symptomatic bradycardia where pacing simplicity is a prime concern in cases of:
  1. Senility (for life-sustaining purposes only)
  2. Terminal disease
  3. Domicile remote from a follow-up center
  4. Absent retrograde ventriculoatrial (VA) conduction

Class III: Conditions for which there is general agreement that such a mode of pacing is inappropriate.
- A. Known pacemaker syndrome or symptoms produced by temporary ventricular pacing at the time of initial pacemaker implantation
- B. The need for maximum atrial contribution because of
  1. Congestive heart failure
  2. Special need for rate response

VVIR: As in Class I and II but with chronotropic incompetence and anticipated moderate to high level of physical activity. VVIR pacemakers are particularly contraindicated in the presence of retrograde VA conduction or when angina pectoris or congestive heart failure is aggravated by fast rates.

Reproduced with permission from Dreifus LS, Fisch C, Griffin JC, *et al.*: Guidelines for implantation of cardiac pacemakers and antiarrhythmia devices. A report of the American College of Cardiology/American Heart Association Task Force on Assessment of Diagnostic and Therapeutic Procedures (Committee on Pacemaker Implantation). J Am Coll Cardiol 1991;18:1.

Table 17.3.
ACC/AHA Guidelines for Device Selection—DDD Mode[a]

Class I
- A. Requirement for AV synchrony over a wide range of rates such as
  1. The active or young patient with atrial rates responsive to clinical need.
  2. Significant hemodynamic need
  3. Pacemaker syndrome during previous pacemaker experience or a reduction in systolic blood pressure > 20 mm Hg during ventricular pacing at the time of pacemaker implantation (with or without evidence of VA conduction).

Class II
- A. Complete heart block or sick sinus syndrome and stable atrial rates
- B. When simultaneous control of atrial and ventricular rates can be shown to inhibit tachyarrhythmias or when the pacemaker can be adjusted to a mode designed to interrupt the arrhythmia.

Class III
- A. Frequent or persistent supraventricular tachyarrhythmias, including atrial fibrillation or flutter[b]
- B. Inadequate intracavitary atrial complexes
- C. Angina pectoris aggravated by rapid heart rates

DDDR: This mode is indicated in patients with chronotropic incompetence who have an anticipated moderate or high level of activity and in whom there is a stable atrial rhythm. It is particularly applicable in those patients who have persistent VA conduction.

Reproduced with permission from Dreifus LS, Fisch C, Griffin JC, *et al.*: Guidelines for implantation of cardiac pacemakers and antiarrhythmia devices: a report of the American College of Cardiology/American Heart Association Task Force on Assessment of Diagnostic and Therapeutic Procedures (Committee on Pacemaker Implantation). J Am Coll Cardiol 1991;18:1.

[a]Class I, II, and III as in Table 17.2.

[b]The guidelines also state that (1) the DDI mode is useful in patients requiring dual-chamber pacing who have frequent but not constant supraventricular arrhythmias; (2) the DDIR mode is a particularly useful mode in chronotropic incompetence when a moderate to high level of activity is anticipated and when there are fairly frequent atrial arrhythmias or in those individuals who need dual-chamber pacing intermittently.

gated by the British Pacing and Electrophysiology Group (1) (August 1991). The editorial stated:

> The main differences in devices are in the site and number of cardiac leads and the presence or absence of facilities for rate adaptation. The ACC/AHA report itemizes the various pacing systems and modes and recommends the forms of bradycardia for which each would be suitable, using a three-pronged classification, class 1 being the first choice. The British report cuts the cake the other way, listing the principal causes of bradycardia and recommending "optimal," "alternative," and "inappropriate" pacing modes. Both reports encourage the widespread use of dual chamber pacing systems. This emphasis is especially noticeable in the British recommendations, although the difference may be partly attributable to presentation.

Interestingly, as early as 1984 a task force from the North American Society of Cardiac Pacing and Electrophysiology (NASPE) suggested that DDD pulse generators are indicated in 60–80% of all implants (44). However, in 1991 in the United States where single-lead atrial pacing is hardly ever used, only one-third or less of the patients requiring pacemakers presently received dual-chamber (DDD/DDDR) devices (45).

In patients with complete AV block (normal atrial chronotropic function) and without congestive heart failure, DDD and VVIR pacing both provide almost the same degree of enhanced exercise performance, but a substantial number of patients are intolerant of VVIR pacing at *rest*. In patients with atrial chronotropic incompetence unable to increase the sinus rate on exercise, VVIR pacing (providing rate increase only) can improve exercise tolerance more than DDD pacing (providing only AV synchrony (46). If presented with a choice between VVIR and DDD pacing, maintenance of AV synchrony at rest is more important than rate-responsiveness on exercise when considered in terms of quality of life (47) because most pacemaker patients spend their lives predominantly at rest and the heart rate is near basal state for most of 24 hr when symptoms due to pacemaker syndrome with VVI or VVIR pacing are most likely to occur. Recent studies of patients with atrial chronotropic incompetence and DDDR pulse generators suggest a better hemodynamic performance and patient preference in the DDDR mode compared to the VVIR mode (48–52).

The continuing controversy concerning the basically unimportant contribution of AV synchrony to the cardiac output on *exercise* (as opposed to the increase in heart rate) (53–58) should not detract from the well-established and significant hemodynamic and electrophysiologic benefits of atrial pacing and maintenance of AV synchrony at *rest*, as already discussed. VVI and VVIR pacing, by ignoring the atrium contribute to morbidity and mortality, especially in the sick sinus syndrome. Although VVIR units are being recommended by some workers as essentially equivalent to dual chamber systems, this is clearly illogical (39,59,60). Indeed there is no evidence that a VVIR pacemaker improves survival versus a standard VVI device.

The complications of dual-chamber pacemaker implantation (need for reintervention incidence of lead displacement, infection, etc.) do not differ significantly from VVI pacemaker implantation (61). Improved pacemaker design has virtually eliminated many previous problems with dual-chamber pacing such as endless loop tachycardia, crosstalk, and tracking of rapid atrial rates due to atrial tachyarrhythmias (Table 17.4). In the nineties, inability to reliably implant atrial leads or appropriately program a dual-chamber pulse generator should not be an indication for a VVIR device.

SINGLE-CHAMBER ATRIAL PACING

In the United States, perhaps 1% or less of patients requiring pacing receive a single chamber atrial pacemaker. AAI and AAIR pacemakers are underutilized despite the wealth of information showing their superiority over VVI (VVIR) pacing in the sick sinus syndrome (40,62,63). Previous problems with atrial pacing such as instability of the leads, poor lead characteristics, and limited device programmability have been resolved. The pacing and sensing performance of atrial leads compares favorably with that of ventricular leads (40,64) and atrial lead dislodgement is relatively rare (40). Atrial undersensing can often be corrected by programming a higher sensitivity (40,64). In this respect, bipolar atrial leads (insensitive to myopotential oversensing) permit the use of a high atrial sensitivity to optimize atrial sensing (Table 17.5).

The only problem with AAI (AAIR) pacing is the risk of AV block. The development of second- or third-degree AV block in carefully selected patients for AAI (AAIR) pacing is very low with an annual incidence of 1.2% and its occurrence is rarely if ever catastrophic and often related to drug therapy (62,63). AAI or AAIR pacing can be used in patients with the sick sinus syndrome (40) if (a) atrial pacing to rates 120–140 beats/min is associated with 1:1 AV conduction with the realization that this is an arbitrary value. The Wenckebach point (the slowest atrial rate where Type I second-degree AV block develops) may occur at a higher atrial rate when the patient is standing during normal life than when lying during a pacing test. (b) PR interval < 0.24 sec at rest. (c) HV interval < 75 msec and/or absence of bundle branch block according to some workers (40). With careful selection of patients, AAI or AAIR pacing could be used safely in probably half the patients with sick sinus syndrome. Preimplantation stress testing or Holter recordings may be useful in determining the presence of atrial chronotropic incompetence. About 40% of patients who are candidates for atrial pulse generators may require rate adaptive devices (AAIR) because of poor atrial chronotropic response (65). AAIR pacing increases effort capacity compared to AAI pacing (65–68).

The spike-Q interval may be longer in the supine position than when standing. The spike-Q interval may be long when the P-QRS interval is appropriate if there is intraatrial conduction delay, a situation that does not constitute a contraindication to

Table 17.4.
Potential Obstacles to Dual-Chamber Pacing[a]

Problem	Mechanism	Elimination
Crosstalk	Sensing of atrial stimulus by ventricular electrode causing self-inhibition	Use of bipolar systems. Appropriate programming of atrial output, ventricular sensitivity, and duration of ventricular blanking period.
Endless loop tachycardia	Sensing of retrograde P waves by atrial channel leads to a self-perpetuating reentrant pacemaker tachycardia (VpAsVpAs)	Appropriate programming of post-ventricular atrial refractory period. Use of appropriate atrial sensitivity to eliminate sensing of retrograde P waves with preservation of sinus P wave sensing. Use of smart pacemakers to prevent or terminate endless loop tachycardia as soon as it is initiated.
Tracking of nonphysiologic atrial rates	Paroxysmal supraventricular tachyarrhythmias. P or f waves sensed by atrial channel lead to rapid ventricular pacing rate.	DDI (DDIR) mode. Use of rapid automatic switching of pacing mode and/or rate during supraventricular tachyarrhythmias. The fallback mechanism or rate change may be gradual in some pulse generators.
Myopotential oversensing with unipolar systems only.	Sensing of myopotentials by atrial channel triggers rapid ventricular pacing rates	Use of bipolar leads. Contemporary bipolar leads have eliminated previous advantages of unipolar leads.

[a]See Chapter 15.

Table 17.5.
Single-Lead Pacing

Characteristics	VVI (VVIR)	AAI (AAIR)
Simplicity	+ + +	+ + +
Cost effectiveness	+ + +	+ + +
Physiologic	+ (VVIR)	+ + +
Lead dislodgement	Rare	Rare
Reliability of long-term pacing	+ + +	+ + +
Reliability of long-term sensing	+ + +	+ +
Morbidity	±	±
Retrograde ventriculoatrial conduction	+ + +	−
Pacemaker syndrome	+ + +	−
Incidence of		
Congestive heart failure	+ + +	+
Chronic atrial fibrillation	+ + +	+
Stroke	+ + +	+
Mortality	+ + +	+

Reproduced with permission from Barold SS, Falkoff MD, Ong LS, *et al.*: Cardiac pacing in the nineties: technologic, hemodynamic and electrophysiologic considerations in the selection of the optimal mode of pacing. In Rackley CE (ed): Challenges in Cardiology, Futura Publishing Co., Mt. Kisco, NY, 1992:39.

AAI or AAIR pacing. On exercise, the spike-Q interval is significantly shorter than what is seen at rest, probably due to autonomic changes that generally occur during exercise (if the patient is not on drugs) (67).

Despite the favorable experience with AAI and recently with AAIR pacing in sick sinus syndrome patients without AV block (40,62,63,65–72), some workers believe that DDDR devices, although more complex and expensive, provide a greater flexibility for changing conditions and should be used either routinely in the sick sinus syndrome or at least in patients with bradycardia-tachycardia syndrome who will require drug therapy that affects AV conduction and sinus node function (42,73,74). Indeed, if supraventricular tachyarrhythmias become troublesome (or permanent), a DDDR pulse generator can then be programmed to the DDI (DDIR) or VVI (VVIR) mode. Alternatively, a DDD (DDDR) pacemaker could be programmed to the AAI (AAIR) mode with the option of using the dual-chamber mode according to need (42). Some workers advocate implantation of both atrial and ventricular leads in patients with normal AV conduction, but only a single-chamber atrial pulse generator with the option of implanting a dual-chamber device in the future if necessary (41).

SINGLE-LEAD DUAL-CHAMBER PACING

The British Pacing and Electrophysiology Group (1) stated that the indications for the VDD mode are similar to the DDD mode, but with the distinct disadvantage of increasing the chance of pacemaker syndrome at lower atrial rates. Recent satisfactory experience with single-lead VDD pacing suggests that such a dedicated VDD (or VDD/VVIR) system may provide a simpler and less expensive pacing system than the DDD mode for patients with AV block and normal atrial chronotropic function (75–83) and could possibly be used in approximately one-third of patients requiring permanent pacing.

The only difference between the DDD and VDD modes is the behavior of the programmable lower rate during sinus bradycardia: a DDD pacemaker paces the atrium while a VDD device shifts to the VVI mode. Thus when the sinus rate drops below the lower rate, VVI pacing can cause the pacemaker syndrome, particularly in young and active patients that have significant sinus bradycardia at rest (84). Such patients are rare and should receive a dual chamber pacemaker capable of atrial pacing. I believe that a dedicated VDD device is safe and effective in patients with AV block, normal atrial chronotropic function, and retrograde VA conduction, provided a Holter recording confirms the absence of significant sinus bradycardia, especially during waking hours. To guarantee absence of VVI pacing (with associated retrograde VA conduction), the lower rate of the VDD pulse generator can be programmed to a value below the slowest sinus rate. Yet the 1991 ACC/AHA guidelines (39) state retrograde VA conduction as a contraindication (Class III choice) to VDD pacing, while the DDI, DDIR, DDD, and DDDR modes are acceptable in the presence of retrograde VA conduction (Table 17.3). The concern about implanting a VDD device in patients with normal atrial chronotropic function and retrograde VA conduction is probably unwarranted.

SINGLE-LEAD VENTRICULAR PACING: ARE THE VVI AND VVIR PACING MODES CONTRAINDICATED IN THE SICK SINUS SYNDROME?

Special considerations in the sick sinus syndrome include the common potential for retrograde VA conduction and the frequent incidence of paroxysmal supraventricular tachyarrhythmias with their long-term complications. Some workers and the recent report of the British Pacing and Electrophysiology Group have stated categorically that the VVI and VVIR mode are contraindicated in all sick sinus syndrome patients (1,40–42). The British Pacing and Electrophysiology Group has also indicated that atrial fibrillation/flutter (or electrically unresponsive atria) with AV block or slow ventricular response constitutes the only indication for the VVI and VVIR pacing modes (1). In contrast, the 1991 ACC/AHA guidelines are generally more liberal with regard to indications for VVI and VVIR pacing (39) (Table 17.2), but they do emphasize that VVIR pacemakers are contraindicated in patients with retrograde VA conduction, a recommendation echoed by Parsonnet and Bernstein (85).

The British Pacing and Electrophysiology Group also emphasized that "the presence of atrial activity other than chronic or frequently repetitive atrial flutter or fibrillation generally requires an atrial pacemaker electrode. Paroxysmal atrial arrhythmias are not a contraindication to atrial pacing or sensing as atrial pacing may stabilize the atrial rhythm: in others concomitant drug therapy may be beneficial" (1). Thus paroxysmal supraventricular tachycardia previously considered a contraindication to dual-chamber pacing in the sick sinus syndrome now constitutes an important indication for atrial or dual-chamber pacing.

Although I believe that single-chamber ventricular pacing should be avoided in most patients with the sick sinus syndrome (especially those with paroxysmal atrial tachyarrhythmias), there is still a place for single-lead ventricular pacing (in the absence of atrial fibrillation) in some patients with rate episodes of bradycardia (providing a safety net or backup pacing) or in asymptomatic patients requiring replacement of a depleted VVI pacemaker. Single-lead ventricular pacing may also be appropriate in patients who are incapacitated and inactive as well as those with other medical problems associated with a short life expectancy.

DDDR MODE

Because DDDR pacing employs a sensor, it can provide rate responsive pacing in patients with atrial chronotropic incompetence and AV block (86,87). In patients with atrial chronotropic incompetence, DDDR pacing is clearly superior to the DDD mode. Previous studies that minimized the importance of AV synchrony during exercise were generated mostly from populations of patients with AV block and normal left ventricular function (88). Since left ventricular function may be variable in pacemaker recipients, it should not be surprising that recent work has shown that DDD pacing is superior to VVIR pacing in patients with AV block and normal atrial chronotropic function (89,90) while patients with atrial chronotropic incompetence perform better in the DDDR mode compared with the VVIR mode (48–52).

There is concern that DDDR pacing may induce new atrial arrhythmias whenever an unsensed P wave within the postventricular atrial refractory period is closely followed by a sensor-initiated atrial stimulus delivered during the atrial vulnerable period (91). However, preliminary clinical experience suggests that DDDR pacing does not result in a significant increase in atrial arrhythmias (92). A prior history of paroxysmal supraventricular tachyarrhythmias appears to be the major determinant of atrial arrhythmias after implantation of a DDDR pacemaker (17–19).

PACING IN PATIENTS WITH PAROXYSMAL SUPRAVENTRICULAR TACHYARRHYTHMIAS

During supraventricular tachyarrhythmias, conventional or specially designed DDD or DDDR pulse generators can limit the paced ventricular rate by a variety of mechanisms (93) that include (1) using the DDI (DDIR) mode which senses atrial activity but always maintains the paced ventricular rate at the programmed lower rate (or sensor-driven rate in the case of the DDIR mode) (94,95), (2) automatic switching of pacing mode and/or reduction of the pacing rate. Such a response can be either gradual or abrupt with a fallback mechanism to a lower pacing rate with or without a change in the pacing mode (93,96–99). One-to-one AV synchrony returns when the spontaneous atrial rate drops below the programmed upper rate of the pacemaker.

Preliminary data suggest that rate-adaptive AAIR and DDDR modes may be more efficacious in preventing atrial arrhythmias than their non-rate-adaptive counterparts (100,101). If paroxysmal atrial tachyarrhythmias recur after pacemaker implantation, the atrial pacing rate should be increased to 80/min (73). If rate

Table 17.6.
Characteristics of Commonly Used Pacing Modes

Characteristics	VVI	VVIR	AAI	AAIR	DDD	DDI	DDDR	DDIR
Simplicity	+++	+++	++	++	+	+	−	−
AV synchrony	−	−	+	+	+	+[a]	+	+[a]
Potential for pacemaker syndrome	+	+	−	−	−	−	−	−
Normal ventricular activation	−	−	+	+	−[b]	−[b]	−[b]	−[b]
Propensity for endless loop tachycardia	−	−	−	−	+	+[c]	+	+[c]
Tracking of supraventricular tachyarrhythmias	−	−	−	−	+	−[d]	+	−[d]
Contraindicated with AV block	−	−	+	+	−	−	−	−
Increase of pacing rates on exercise in patients with atrial chronotropic incompetence	−	++	−	++	−[e]	−	++	++
Cost	±	+	±	+	++	++	+++	+++

Reproduced with permission from Barold SS, Falkoff MD, Ong LS, *et. al.*: Cardiac pacing in the nineties: technologic, hemodynamic and electrophysiologic considerations in the selection of the optimal mode of pacing. In Rackley CE (ed): Challenges in Cardiology. Futura Publishing Co., Mt. Kisco, NY, 1992:39.

[a]In the DDI mode, if normal sinus rhythm is faster than the programmed lower rate, and in the DDIR if normal sinus rhythm is faster than the sensor-driven rate, AV dissociation is frequent and physiology is largely that of AV dissociation.

[b]Unless AV delay is prolonged to allow for normal anterograde conduction.

[c]Endless loop without tachycardia at the lower rate (DDI) or at the sensor-driven rate (DDIR).

[d]Equivalent to no atrial tracking because ventricular pacing rate remains constant at programmed lower rate (DDI) or sensor-driven rate (DDIR).

[e]Ventricular pacing rate does not increase if sinus rate does not increase on exercise.

manipulation is unsuccessful, antiarrhythmic drug therapy is indicated because poor arrhythmia control predisposes to systemic embolism. Atrial tachyarrhythmias seem to respond better to antiarrhythmic agents in patients with atrial and dual chamber pacemakers (6,102) than in those with single-lead ventricular devices. Long-term anticoagulants should be administered in patients with refractory paroxysmal atrial fibrillation, but the efficacy of warfarin vs. aspirin is presently unknown in this setting (73).

CONCLUSION

In the nineties with presently available technology, the aim of permanent antibradycardia pacing should be (a) restoration of normal or near-normal hemodynamics at rest and on exercise and (b) to change favorably the natural history of the condition requiring pacing, especially reduction of certain atrial tachyarrhythmias and their thromboembolic complications related to atrial dysfunction. In selecting the optimal pacemaker for the individual patient, the physician should always remember the importance of atrial pacing and should resist decisions based on economic constraints that might not serve the patient's best interests (64). Table 17.6 outlines the characteristics of commonly used pacing modes, and Table 17.7 indicates the recommended pacing modes by the British Pacing and Electrophysiology Group (1).

When deciding the type of pacemaker to be selected, three basic questions should be asked and a single algorithm followed (74) (Fig. 17.1). The majority of patients with electrically responsive atria should be considered for either single-chamber atrial or dual-chamber pacing (AAI, AAIR, VDD, DDD, or DDDR). The first question should therefore be "What is the status of the atrium and can it be paced and/or sensed?"; it is the most important one because it focuses on the hemodynamic and electrophysiologic advantages of atrial pacing (1). The first question is then followed by two others: "Is there evidence of latent or overt AV block?" (need for a ventricular lead), and "Is there atrial chronotropic incompetence?" (need for a rate-adaptive pulse generator) (74).

Table 17.7.
Pacemaker Modes Recommended by the British Cardiac Pacing and Electrophysiology Group[a]

Diagnosis	Optimal	Alternative	Inappropriate
SND	AAIR	AAI	VVI VDD
AVB	DDD	VDD	AAI DDI
SND and AVB	DDDR DDIR	DDD DDI	AAI VVI
Chronic AF with AVB	VVIR	VVI	AAI DDD VDD
CSS	DDI	DDD VVI[b]	AAI VDD
MVVS	DDI	DDD	AAI VVI[c] VDD

Reproduced with permission from Clarke M, Sutton R, Ward D, *et al.*: Recommendations for Pacemaker Prescription for Symptomatic Bradycardia. Report of a working party for the British Pacing and Electrophysiology Group. Br Heart J 1991;66:185.

[a]The optimal mode of pacing should be considered for most patients. The alternative mode should be regarded as being less satisfactory, but acceptable in some groups of patients, e.g., those who are disabled by another disease, those with intermittent symptoms, or those who have a short life expectancy because of another disease. When a patient with, for example, a previous hemiplegia or with terminal neoplasia has atrioventricular block, VVI may suffice to reduce symptoms.

[b]If VVI is ever chosen for the management of carotid sinus syndrome, rate hysteresis is recommended (103). Patient selection should follow the guidelines suggested by Brignole, *et al* (104).

[c]See refs. 105, 106.

Abbreviations: AVB = atrioventricular block; AF = atrial fibrillation or flutter; CSS = carotid sinus syndrome; MVVS = malignant vasovagal syndrome; SND = sinoatrial node disease.

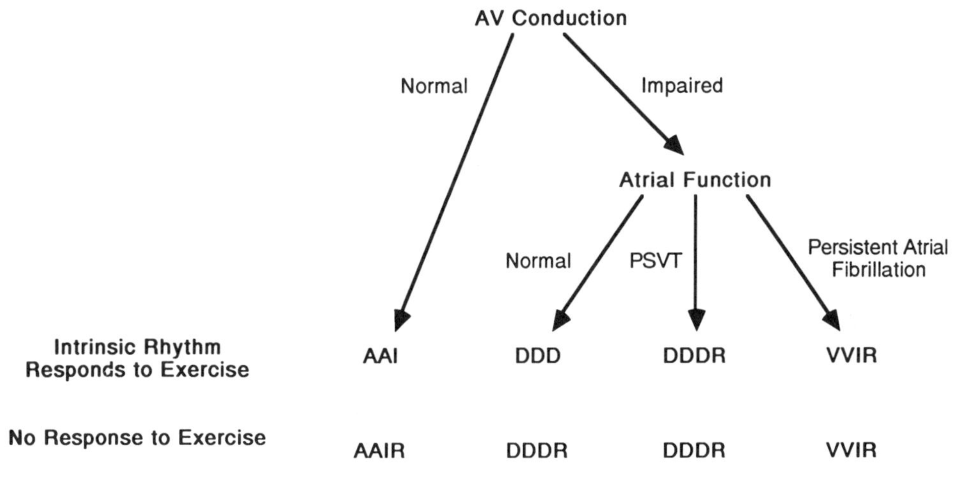

Figure 17.1. Algorithm for determining the optimal pacemaker mode for an individual patient. A DDDR should be considered in patients with the bradycardia-tachycardia syndrome with intrinsic or drug-induced AV conduction delay to provide greater flexibility because (a) drug therapy of supraventricular tachyarrhythmias may further depress the atrial chronotropic response on exercise, and (b) troublesome paroxysmal atrial tachyarrhythmias may necessitate programming to the DDIR mode. PSVT = paroxysmal supraventricular arrhythmias of all types including atrial fibrillation. (Reproduced from Griffin JC: The optimal pacing mode for the individual patient. The role of DDDR. In Barold SS, Mugica J (eds): New Perspectives in Cardiac Pacing. 2. Futura Publishing Co., Mt. Kisco, NY, 1991:325, with permission.)

Other important questions should be addressed: (a) What is the best pacing mode for the patient for his or her level of activity or left ventricular function? (b) What is the best pacing mode in special situations? Patients with angina pectoris generally tolerate DDD, DDDR, or VVIR modes better than the VVI mode, provided the upper rate is not excessively high. The increased MVO_2 related to rate increase on exercise by rate responsive pacemakers is counterbalanced by the increase in MVO_2 during fixed frequency VVI pacing, probably secondary to enhanced contractility and wall tension (107–114). Patients with carotid sinus syndrome, (excluding those with only a vasodepressor component) and neurally mediated syncope (demonstrable by tilt table testing) that require pacing obtain maximal benefit with the DDI mode and hysteresis (103,105,106). (c) What is affordable? (d) What is the simplest system that will optimize hemodynamics? (e) Does the patient have paroxysmal supraventricular tachyarrhythmias? What type of pacemaker response is required to avoid tracking of rapid unphysiologic atrial rates? (98,99) (f) What is the natural history of the condition for which pacing is being used, and what is the impact of present and future drug therapy? (74) Although DDDR pacemakers are complex and expensive, they provide greater flexibility of the pacing mode for changing conditions (115). If cost ever becomes immaterial, only two types of pulse generators will be used in the future, i.e., sensor-driven single-chamber and sensor-driven dual-chamber pacemakers (with appropriate connector to accept a single lead for VDD pacing). All pacemakers will possess extensive programmability of pacing modes and sensor activity. As costs decrease, virtually all patients will receive rate-adaptive pulse generators and the sensor (or combination of sensors) will be just one of the many programmable functions.

References

1. Clarke M, Sutton R, Ward D, *et al*. Recommendations for Pacemaker Prescription for Symptomatic Bradycardia. Report of a working party for the British Pacing and Electrophysiology Group. Br Heart J 1991;66:185.
2. Morgan JM, Joseph SP, Bahri AK, *et al*.: Choosing the pacemaker. A rational approach to the use of modern pacemaker technology. Eur Heart J 1989;11:753.
3. Camm AJ, Katritsis D. Ventricular pacing in sick sinus: a risky business?, PACE 1990;13:695.
4. Ausubel K, Furman S: The pacemaker syndrome. Ann Intern Med 1985; 103:420.
5. Rosenqvist M: Atrial pacing for sick sinus syndrome. Clin Cardiol 1990; 13:43.
6. Sasaki Y, Furihata A, Suyama K, *et al*.: Comparison between ventricular inhibited pacing and physiologic pacing in sick sinus syndrome. Am J Cardiol 1991;67:772.
7. Kubica J, Stolarczyk L, Krzyminska E, *et al*.: Left atrial size and wall motion in patients with permanent ventricular and atrial pacing. PACE 1990;13 (Part II):1737.
8. Mabo P, Denjoy I, Leclerq JF, *et al*.: Comparative efficacy of permanent atrial pacing in vagal atrial arrhythmias and in bradycardia-tachycardia syndrome. PACE 1989;12 (Part II):1236.
9. Attuel P, Pellerin D, Mugica J, *et al*.: DDD pacing: An effective treatment modality for recurrent atrial arrhythmias. PACE 1988;11:1647.
10. Mitsuoka T, Kenny RA, Yeung TA, *et al*.: Benefits of dual chamber pacing in sick sinus syndrome. Br Heart J 1988;60:338.
11. Kosakai Y, Ohe T, Kamakura S, *et al*.: Long term follow-up of incidence of embolism in sick sinus syndrome after pacing. PACE 1991;14 (Part II):690.
12. Hayes DL, Neubauer SA: Incidence of atrial fibrillation after DDD pacing. RBM 1990;12:36.
13. Barr E, Hummel J, Hanich R, *et al*.: VVIR pacing causes more arrhythmias and adverse symptoms than DDDR pacing. RBM 1990;12:57.
14. Galley D, Elharrar C, Ammor M, *et al*.: Is chronic atrial pacing protective against atrial fibrillation, RBM 1990;12:92.
15. Ebagosti A, Gueunoun M, Saadjian A, *et al*.: Long-term follow-up of patients treated with VVI pacing and sequential pacing with special reference to VA retrograde conduction. PACE 1988;11:1929.
16. Curzi GF, Mocchegiani R, Ciampani N, *et al*.: Thromboembolism during VVI permanent pacing. In Pérez-Gómez F (ed): Cardiac Pacing. Electrophysiology. Tachyarrhythmias. Editorial, Grouz, Madrid, 1985:1203.
17. Feuer JM, Shandling AH, Messenger JC, *et al*.: Influence of cardiac pacing mode on the long-term development of atrial fibrillation. Am J Cardiol 1989; 54:1376.
18. Benditt DG, Mianulli M, Buetikofer J, *et al*.: Prior arrhythmia history is the major determinant of post-implant atrial tachyarrhythmias in DDDR pacemaker patients. RBM 1990;12:95.
19. Gross J, Moser S, Benedek ZM, *et al*.: Clinical predictors and natural history of atrial fibrillation in patients with DDD pacemakers. PACE 1990;13 (Part II):1828.
20. Sutton R, Kenny RA: The natural history of sick sinus syndrome. PACE 1986;9:1110.
21. Markewitz A, Schad N, Hemmer W, *et al*.: What is the most appropriate stimulation mode in patients with sinus node dysfunction. PACE 1986;9 (Part II):1115.
22. Zanini R, Facchinetti AI, Gallo G, *et al*.: Morbidity and mortality of patients with sinus node disease. Comparative effects of atrial and ventricular pacing. PACE 1990;13 (Part II):2076.
23. Santini M, Alexidou G, Ansalone G, *et al*.: Relation of prognosis in sick sinus syndrome to age, conduction defect and modes of permanent cardiac pacing. Am J Cardiol 1990;65:729.
24. Biaconi L, Boccadamo R, DiFlorio A, *et al*.: Atrial versus ventricular stimulation in sick sinus syndrome. Effect on morbidity and mortality, PACE 1989;12:1236.
25. Grimm W, Langenfeld H, Maisch T, *et al*.: Symptoms, cardiovascular risk profile and spontaneous ECG in paced patients. A 5 year follow-up study. RBM 1990;12:93.
26. VanErckelens F, Sigmund M, Lambertz H, *et al*.: Atrial fibrillation in different pacing modes. J Am Coll Cardiol 1991(Abstr.);17:272.
27. Rosenqvist M, Brandt J, Schüller H: Long-term pacing in sinus node disease: Effects of stimulation mode on cardiovascular morbidity and mortality. Am Heart J 1988;116:16.
28. Sasaki Y, Shimotori M, Akahane K, *et al*.: Long-term follow-up of patients with sick sinus syndrome. A comparison of clinical aspects among unpaced ventricular-inhibited paced and physiologically paced groups. PACE 1988; 11:1575.
29. Stangl K, Seitz K, Wirtzfeld A, *et al*.: Differences between atrial single chamber pacing (AAI) and ventricular single chamber pacing (VVI) with respect to prognosis and antiarrhythmic effect in patients with sick sinus syndrome. PACE 1990;13 (Part II):2080.
30. Sethi KK, Bajaj V, Mohan JC, *et al*.: Comparison of atrial and VVI pacing modes in symptomatic sinus node dysfunction without associated tachyarrhythmias. Indian Heart J 1990;42:143.
31. Jutila C, Klein R, Shivley B: Deleterious long-term effects of single chamber as compared to dual chamber pacing. Circulation 1990;32 (Suppl III):111.
32. Hesselton AB, Parsonnet V, Perry G: Progression to atrial fibrillation from the DDD, DVI, and VVI pacing modes. PACE 1990;13:564.
33. Alpert MA, Curtis JJ, Sanfelippo JF, *et al*.: Comparative survival after permanent ventricular and dual chamber pacing for patients with chronic

high degree atrioventricular block with and without preexisting congestive heart failure. J Am Coll Cardiol 1986;7:925.
34. Alpert MA, Curtis JJ, Sanfelippo JF, *et al.*: Comparative survival following permanent ventricular and dual chamber pacing for patients with chronic symptomatic sinus node dysfunction with and without heart failure. Am Heart J 1987;113:958.
35. Edelstam C, Gullberg B, Nordlander R, *et al.*: Effects of atrial synchronous pacing on survival in patients with high degree AV block and congestive heart failure. J Am Coll Cardiol 1991;17:289A.
36. Nürnberg M, Frohner K, Podczeck A, *et al.*: Is VVI pacing more dangerous than A-V sequential pacing in patients with sick sinus node syndrome? PACE 1991;14 (Part II):674.
37. Shaw DB, Holman RR, Gowers JI: Survival in sinoatrial disorder (sick sinus syndrome). Br Med J 1980;280:139.
38. Witte J, v.Knorre GH, Volkmann HJ, *et al.*: Survival rate in patients with sick sinus syndrome in AAI/DDD vs. VVI pacing. PACE 1991;14 (Part II):680.
39. Dreifus LS, Fisch C, Griffin JC, *et al.*: Guidelines for implantation of cardiac pacemakers and antiarrhythmia devices. A report of the American College of Cardiology/American Heart Association Task Force on Assessment of Diagnostic and Therapeutic Procedures (Committee on Pacemaker Implantation). J Am Coll Cardiol 1991;18:1.
40. Santini M, Ansalone G, Cacciatore G, *et al.*: Status of single chamber atrial pacing. In Barold SS, Mugica J (eds): New Perspectives in Cardiac Pacing. 2. Futura Publishing Company, Mt. Kisco, NY, 1991:273.
41. Sutton R, Bourgeois I: Pacemaker selection. In Sutton R, Bourgeois I, (eds): The Foundations of Cardiac Pacing: Part I. An Illustrated Practical Guide to Basic Pacing. Futura Publishing Company, Mt. Kisco, NY, 1991:149.
42. Dodinot B: Stimulation cardiaque à fréquence asservie. Ann Cardiol Angeilol 1990;39:597.
43. Pacemakers—practice and paradox. Lancet 1991;338:1178.
44. Parsonnet V, Escher DJ, Furman S, *et al.*: Indications for dual-chamber pacing. PACE 1984;7:318.
45. Parsonnet V, Bernstein AD: The 1989 world survey of cardiac pacing. PACE 1991;14:2073.
46. Batey R, Sweesy MW, Scala G, *et al.*: Comparison of low rate dual chamber pacing to activity responsive rate variable ventricular pacing. PACE 1990; 13:646.
47. Menozzi C, Brignole M, Moracchini PV, *et al.*: Inpatient comparison between chronic VVIR and DDD pacing in patients affected by high degree AV block without heart failure. PACE 1990;13 (Part II):1816.
48. Jutzy RV, Florio J, Isaeff DM, *et al.*: Comparative evaluation of rate modulated dual chamber and VVIR pacing. PACE 1990;13 (Part II):1838.
49. Algona P Jr, Batey R, Sweesy M, *et al.*: Improved exercise tolerance with dual chamber versus single chamber rate adaptive pacing. PACE 1990; 13:532.
50. Lanzberg JS, Franklin JO, Mahawar SK, *et al.*: Benefits of physiologic atrioventricular synchronization for pacing with an exercise rate response. Am J Cardiol 1990;66:193.
51. Higano S, Hayes DL: Investigation of a new activity sensing rate-responsive dual chamber pacemaker. Am Coll Cardiol 1989 (abstr.).;13:112.
52. Brinker J, Jutzy R, Hayes D, *et al.*: Initial clinical experience with a dual chamber rate modulated pacemaker. J Am Coll Cardiol 1989 (Abstr.);13: 112A.
53. Ausubel K, Steingart AM, Shimshi M, *et al.*: Maintenance of exercise stroke volume during ventricular versus atrial synchronous pacing. Role of contractility. Circulation 1985;72:1037.
54. Karlof I: Haemodynamic effect of atrial triggered versus fixed rate pacing, at rest and during exercise, in complete heart block. Acta Med Scand 1975; 197:195.
55. Kristensson BE, Arnman K, Rydén L: The haemodynamic importance of atrioventricular synchrony and rate increase at rest and during exercise. Eur Heart J 1985;6:773.
56. Fananapazir L, Bennett DH, Monks PH: Atrial synchronized pacing contribution to the chronotropic response to improved exercise performance. PACE 1983;6:601.
57. Rydén L, Karlsson O, Kristensson BE: The importance of different atrioventricular intervals to improved exercise performance for exercise capacity. PACE 1988;11:1051.
58. Oldroyd KG, Rae AP, Carter R, *et al.*: Double blind crossover comparison of the effects of dual chamber pacing (DDD) and ventricular rate adaptive (VVIR) pacing on neuroendocrine variables, exercise performance, and symptoms in complete heart block. Br Heart J 1991;65:188.
59. Tyers GF: Current status of sensor-modulated rate adaptive cardiac pacing, J Am Coll Cardiol 1990;15:412.
60. Harthorne JW, Strathmore NR: DDD versus VVIR pacing. Physiologic option versus convenient excuse. In Barold SS, Mugica J (eds): New Perspectives in Cardiac Pacing. 2. Futura Publishing Company, Mt. Kisco, NY, 1991:313.
61. Mueller X, Sadeghi H, Kappenberger L: Complications after single versus dual chamber pacemaker implantation. PACE 1990;13:711.
62. Rydén L: Atrial inhibited pacing: an underused mode of cardiac stimulation. PACE 1988;11:1375.
63. Rosenqvist M, Obel IWP: Atrial pacing and the risk for AV block: is there a time for change in attitude? PACE 1989;12:97.
64. Byrd CL, Schwartz SJ, Gonzales M, *et al.*: DDD pacemakers maximize hemodynamic benefits and minimize complications for most patients. PACE 1988;11:1911.
65. Kallryd A, Kruse I, Rydén L: Atrial-inhibited pacing in the sick sinus syndrome: clinical value and the demand for rate responsiveness. PACE 1989;12:954.
66. Rosenqvist M, Aren C, Kristensson BE, *et al.*: Atrial rate-responsive pacing in sinus node disease. Eur Heart J 1990;11:537.
67. Brandt J, Fahraeus T, Schüller H: Rate-adaptive atrial pacing (AAIR): clinical aspects. In Barold SS, Mugica J (eds): New Perspectives in Cardiac Pacing. 2, Futura Publishing Co., Mt. Kisco, NY, 1991:303.
68. Hatano K, Kato R, Hayashi H, *et al.*: Usefulness of rate responsive atrial pacing in patients with sick sinus syndrome. PACE 1989;12:16.
69. Daubert C, Mabo P, Pouillot C, *et al.*: Incompétence chronotrope: consequences pratiques en stimulation cardiaque définitive. Stimucoeur 1989; 17:76.
70. Rognoni G, Bolognese L, Aina F, *et al.*: Respiratory dependent atrial pacing management of sinus node disease. PACE 1988;11:1853.
71. Meurice G, Lemmens JC: Intéret ryhtmologique de la stimulation à fréquence asservie en mode AAI. Stimucoeur 1988;16:111.
72. Pouillot CH, Mabo PH, Delong B, *et al.*: Bénéfices et limites de la stimulation mono-chambre atriale à fréquence asservie. Arch Mal Coeur 1990;83:1833.
73. Sutton R: Pacing in atrial arrhythmias. PACE 1990;13:1823.
74. Griffin JC: The optimal pacing mode for the individual patient: the role of DDDR. In Barold SS, Mugica J (eds): New Perspectives in Cardiac Pacing. 2, Futura Publishing Co., Mt. Kisco, NY, 1991:325.
75. Curzio G and the Multicenter Study Group: a multicenter evaluation of a single-pass lead VDD pacing system. PACE 1991;14:434.
76. Cornacchia D, Fabbri M, Maresta A, *et al.*: Clinical evaluation of VDD pacing with a unipolar single-pass lead. PACE 1989;12:604.
77. Longo E, Catrini V: Experience and implantation techniques with a new single-pass lead VDD pacing system. PACE 1990;13:927.
78. Varriale P, Pilla AG, Tekriwal M: Single-lead VDD pacing system. PACE 1990;13:757.
79. Antonioli GE, Barbieri D, Marzaloni M, *et al.*: VDD single-lead versus VVI-RR. In Santini M, Pistolese M, Alliegro A (eds): Progress in Clinical Pacing. Excerpta Medica, Amsterdam, 1988:39.
80. Antonioli GE, Ansani L, Barbieri I, *et al.*: Long term experience with the original single-lead for VDD pacing. History and development. PACE 1991; 14 (Part II):693.
81. Furman S, Gross J, Andrews C, *et al.*: Single pass lead atrial synchronous pacing, PACE 1991;14 (Part II):693.

82. Crick JCP: European multicenter prospective follow-up study of 1002 implants of a single lead VDD pacing system. PACE 1991;14 (Part II):1742.
83. Katritsis D, Camm AJ: Single-lead VDD pacing: excellence or expedience? Clin Cardiol 1991;14:917.
84. Levine PA, Seltzer JP, Pirzada FA: The "pacemaker syndrome" in a properly functioning physiologic pacing system. PACE 1983;6:279.
85. Parsonnet V, Bernstein AD: Adaptive rate pacing. In Braunwald E (ed): Heart Disease Update. WB Saunders, Philadelphia, 1989:97.
86. Lemen RB, White JK, Kratz JM, *et al.*: The potential utility of sensor-driven pacing in DDD pacemakers. Am Heart J 1989;118:919.
87. Kappenberger L: DDDR pacing, experiences, comparisons. PACE 1989; 12:1276.
88. Griffin JC: VVIR or DDDR: does it matter? Clin Cardiol 1991;14:257.
89. Lau CP, Wong CK, Leung WH, *et al.*: Superior cardiac hemodynamics of atrioventricular synchrony over rate responsive pacing at submaximal exercise: observations in activity sensing DDDR pacemakers. PACE 1990; 13 (Part II):1832.
90. Mehta D, Gilmour S, Ward DE, *et al.*: Optimal atrioventricular delay at rest and during exercise in patients with dual chamber pacemakers: a non-invasive assessment by continuous wave Doppler. Br Heart J 1989;61:161.
91. Feuer JM, Shandling AH, Ellestad MH: Sensor-modulated dual chamber cardiac pacing: too much of a good thing too fast? PACE 1990;13:816.
92. Spencer WH, Markowitz T, Algona P. Rate augmentation and atrial arrhythmias in DDDR pacing. PACE 1990;13 (Part II):1847.
93. Barold SS. Automatic switching of pacing mode, Cardiostimolazione 1991; 9:121.
94. Floro J, Castellanet M, Florio J, *et al.*: DDI: A new mode for cardiac pacing. Clin Prog Pacing Electrophysiol 1984;2:255.
95. Barold SS. The DDI mode of cardiac pacing. PACE 1987;9:480.
96. Mugica J, Barold SS, Ripart A: The smart pacemaker. In Barold SS, Mugica J (eds): New Perspectives in Cardiac Pacing. 2. Futura Publishing Co., Mt. Kisco, NY, 1991:545.
97. Barold SS, Falkoff MD, Ong LS, *et al.*: Upper rate response. In Barold SS, Mugica J (eds): New Perspectives in Cardiac Pacing. Futura Publishing Co., Mt. Kisco, NY, 1988:121.
98. VanWyhe G, Sra J, Rovang K, *et al.*: Maintenance of atrioventricular sequence after His bundle ablation for paroxysmal supraventricular rhythm disorders: a unique use of the fallback mode in dual chamber pacemakers. PACE 1991;14:410.
99. Vaneiro G, Patel S, Ching E, *et al.*: Early clinical experience with a minute ventilation sensor DDDR pacemaker. PACE 1991;14 (Part II):1815.
100. Kato R, Terasawa T, Gotoh T, *et al.*: Antiarrhythmic efficacy of atrial demand (AAI) and rate-responsive atrial pacing. In Santini M, Pistolese M, Alliegro A (eds): Progress in Clinical Pacing. Excerpta Medica, Amsterdam, 1988:15.
101. Bellocci F, Nobile A, Spampinato A, *et al.*: Antiarrhythmic effects of DDD rate responsive pacing. PACE 1991;14 (Part II):622.
102. Barnay C, Coste A, Quittet F, *et al.*: Stimulation auriculaire permanente exclusive. Expérience clinique à propos de 65 observations avec un recul de 1 à 5 ans. Arch Mal Coeur 1986;79:1710.
103. Sutton R, Clarke M, Ingram AM: DDI pacing in the treatment of sick sinus, carotid sinus and vasovagal syndrome. PACE 1988;11:827.
104. Brignole M, Menozzi C, Lolli G, *et al.*: When is DDD pacing necessary and when is VVI pacing sufficient in carotid sinus syndrome? PACE 1989;12 (Part II):1169.
105. Fitzpatrick AP, Travill CM, Lolli G, *et al.*: Recurrent symptoms after ventricular pacing in unexplained syncope. PACE 1990;13:619.
106. Fitzpatrick A, Theodorakis R, Ahmed R, *et al.*: Dual chamber pacing aborts vasovagal syncope induced by head-up 60° tilt. PACE 1991; 14:13.
107. Baller D, Wolpers HG, Zipfel J, *et al.*: Comparison of the effects of right ventricular apex and atrioventricular sequencing pacing on myocardial oxygen consumption and cardiac efficiency: a laboratory investigation. PACE 1988;11:394.
108. DeCock CC, Panis JHC, VanEenige MJ, *et al.*: Efficacy and safety of rate responsive pacing in patients with coronary artery disease and angina pectoris. PACE 1989;12:1405.
109. Nordlander R, Pehrsson SK, Aström H, *et al.*: Myocardial demands of atrial-triggered versus fixed rate ventricular pacing in patients with complete heart block, PACE 1987;10:1154.
110. Kenny RA, Ingram A, Mitsuoka T, *et al.*: Optimal pacing mode for patients with angina pectoris. Br Heart J 1986;56:463.
111. Kristensson BE, Arnman K, Rydén L: Atrial synchronous ventricular pacing in ischemic heart disease. Eur Heart J 1983;4:668.
112. Fananapazir L, Srinivas V, Bennett DH; Comparison of resting hemodynamic indices and exercise performance during atrial synchronized and asynchronous ventricular pacing. PACE 1983;6:202.
113. DeCock CC, Visser FC, Lourens HJ, *et al.*: Permanent rate-responsive pacing after myocardial infarction: effects on exercise performance and exercise induced ischemia. RBM 1990;12:26.
114. DeCock CC, Visser FC, Stokkel L, *et al.*: Rate-responsive pacing in patients after myocardial infarction and angina pectoris. PACE 1990; 13:1192.
115. Gwinn N, Leman R, Zile M, *et al.*: Pacemaker patients become chronotropic incompetent with time. PACE 1990;13:535.

18

COMPLICATIONS AND FOLLOW-UP OF CARDIAC PACEMAKERS

S. Serge Barold, M.B., B.S., F.R.A.C.P., F.A.C.P., F.A.C.C., F.E.S.C.

Three major groups of complications are associated with pacemaker implantation: (a) acute complications at the time of implantation such as pneumothorax (discussed in Chapter 26), (b) complications of lead placement and pocket formation, and (c) electrical complications or pacemaker malfunction.

COMPLICATIONS OF LEAD PLACEMENT AND POCKET FORMATION

Early complications include loss of pacing and sensing with or without evidence of lead displacement. Dislodgement of ventricular leads should be less than 2% and atrial leads less than 5%. Ventricular perforation is rare with contemporary leads and occurs most often with stiff temporary leads while atrial perforation is even rarer. With perforation, the ventricular pacing lead usually lies more commonly in the pericardial space over the left ventricle than across the ventricular septum (1,2). Ventricular perforation can be asymptomatic or cause intermittent or complete failure to pace and/or diaphragmatic pacing. Ventricular perforation can also cause intercostal muscle stimulation. A friction rub may be audible. If the ventricular lead has migrated toward the left ventricle, the electrocardiogram (ECG) may show ventricular paced beats with a right bundle branch block (RBBB) depolarization pattern in lead V1. The chest x-ray may show displacement of the pacing lead close to the border of the apical cardiac shadow or even beyond it (Fig. 18.1). Two-dimensional echocardiography may be diagnostic in localizing the tip of the lead (1,3). Cardiac tamponade is rare and occurs usually at the time of lead insertion and rarely after the first 24 hr. Thus, after 24 hr the ventricular lead may be simply withdrawn safely and repositioned, though patients should still be carefully observed for the rare development of late cardiac tamponade (4). At this juncture the safety of withdrawing and repositioning an atrial lead in the case of atrial perforation (5) has not been established.

Thromboembolic Complications

Venous thrombosis can occur anywhere along the course of the lead and cause partial or complete occlusion of the axillary, subclavian, innominate veins or the superior vena cava (6). Serial venography has demonstrated that thrombosis can occur early (days) or late (months or years) after pacemaker implantation. The incidence and severity of thrombosis appears unrelated to the site of venous access and a higher incidence with multiple leads has not been established. Clinically manifest pulmonary embolization is extremely rare, but a recent study indicated that early asymptomatic pulmonary embolization occurs in 15% of patients after new pacemaker implantation (7,8).

Although the incidence of symptomatic venous thrombosis is quite low, contrast venography is abnormal in 30–45% of all pacemaker patients. About 10–20% of all pacemaker patients demonstrate total occlusion of the subclavian vein (6,9–14). Yet, symptomatic obstruction occurs in only 1–3% of patients, probably because the gradual formation of thrombus promotes development of collateral channels. Early after implantation, acute thrombosis of the subclavian/axillary veins before the development of collateral venous circulation can cause edema, pain, cyanotic discoloration of the arm, and prominent veins. In all cases of symptomatic thrombosis, infection must be ruled out with blood cultures. Treatment consists of heparin or thrombolytic therapy (if not too soon after implantation). Long-term therapy with coumadin is controversial, but aspirin is probably worthwhile.

Thrombosis of the superior vena cava is rare (0.3–0.4%) and can occur from 1 mo to 15 yr after implantation (14–17). In some cases, the superior vena cava syndrome is due to fibrotic stenosis, a situation where removal of the lead (or leads) followed by balloon angioplasty of the innominate or superior vena cava facilitates lead revision (by providing a channel for access) and eliminates symptoms (18). Superior vena cava obstruction can

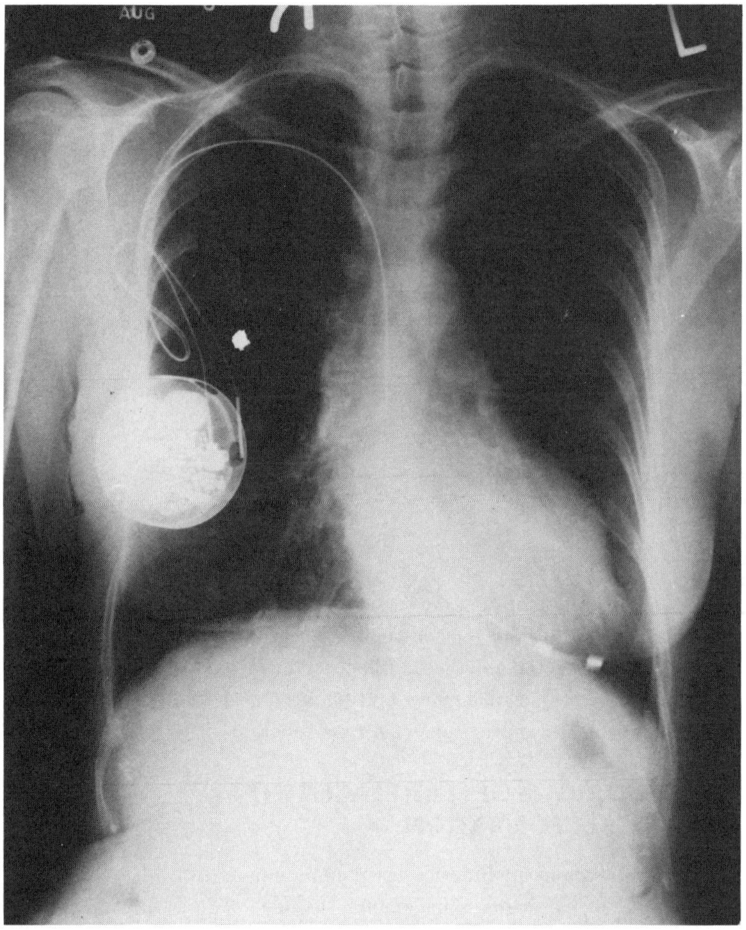

Figure 18.1. Chest x-ray showing right ventricular perforation by bipolar pacing lead. The patient presented with persistent diaphragmatic stimulation; yet pacing and sensing were normal. Note that the tip of the catheter extends to the edge of the cardiac shadow, an appearance suggestive of perforation.

be treated with thrombolytic therapy if recent (1–3 wk) or surgery (14,15,17,19–23). The risk of intracranial bleeding with thrombolytic therapy is increased because of cerebral venous hypertension (15).

The development of a large right atrial thrombus around a pacemaker lead is rare, but carries a high mortality (8,24,25). Such a thrombus may cause right ventricular inflow obstruction or recurrent pulmonary emboli. Right atrial thrombi may occasionally become infected, producing endocarditis (26). Treatment of a large right atrial thrombus includes heparin, thrombolytic therapy (unless it occurs early after implantation), and surgery (8,24,25,27,28).

A pacing catheter inadvertently positioned in the left ventricle may cause serious systemic thromboembolic complications (29) and should be removed even in asymptomatic patients.

Erosion

Erosion usually occurs because of suboptimal implantation technique. Very thin patients pose a greater risk, but erosion has become rare with the use of relatively small pulse generators. Trauma or overexposure to sun predispose to erosion. Erosion without infection can be treated conservatively by moving the pulse generator to a different site, adjacent to the original pocket. To avoid erosion in very thin patients, the pulse generator should be implanted in a retropectoral site.

Infection

Early and late infections are rare and should be less than 1% with proper surgical techniques. Acute infection within a few weeks of implantation is usually caused by *Staphylococcus aureus* and is accompanied with pus formation (30,31) while late infections are more indolent and usually caused by less virulent *Staphylococcus epidermitis* (30,31). Superficial infection (stitch abscess) without pocket infection can be treated conservatively. For skin erosion without obvious infection, the creation of a new pocket away from the eroded site may salvage the system in about half the cases. However, attempts to reposition an obviously eroded pulse generator with an infected pocket are complicated by a very high incidence of recurrence. With obvious pocket infection, long-term therapy with only antibiotics may suppress the clinical manifestations of infection, sometimes for prolonged periods, but is almost never curative (32). Pocket infection, endocarditis, or septicemia require removal of all the hardware and systemic antibiotics (33–42). With obvious infection, partial removal of the lead by simply cutting it virtually guarantees an unsuccessful outcome with significant morbidity and mortality (43) except in rare circumstances when *S. epidermitis* infection does not involve the intravascular portion of the lead (44). Nonsurgical lead extraction by newly developed complex techniques can avoid open heart surgery in most patients, but these procedures should not be undertaken lightly, because even in skilled hands they are associated with a small incidence of hemothorax, cardiac tamponade, pulmonary embolization, and death (45–51). In this respect, retained (abandoned) leads for electrode complications free of infection are not associated with a higher incidence of infection and should generally be left in place (43,44).

Accessory Muscle Stimulation

Accessory muscle stimulation can occur at several sites: (a) Diaphragm. Contraction of the left diaphragm synchronous with a pacemaker stimulus can occur with or without lead perforation of the right ventricle. Late appearance of diaphramatic stimulation suggests an insulation break (52). Contraction of the right diaphragm is due to phrenic nerve stimulation from a malpositioned right atrial electrode. (b) Left intercostal stimulation is invariably due to lead perforation. (c) Deltopectoral muscle twitching. At this site, muscle stimulation can be due to (i) an insulation break causing a current leak from the extravascular portion of the lead (rarely from the pulse generator), (ii) a unipolar pacemaker that has flipped over in a large pocket so that the anodal plate faces skeletal muscle, (iii) a normally functioning and positioned unipolar pacing system without any insulation leak, i.e., the indifferent (anodal) plate of the pulse generator faces the skin. Decreasing the voltage output with preservation of an adequate safety margin for cardiac pacing generally minimizes or eliminates accessory muscle stimulation (53). Decreasing pulse width alone is usually ineffective. Deltopectoral muscle twitching with a bipolar system always indicates an insulation problem.

Tricuspid Valve Abnormalities

A pacing lead across the tricuspid orifice causes little or no valvular dysfunction (54). Hemodynamically significant lesions of the tricuspid valve are rare. Lead puncture of the tricuspid valve (55) and severe avulsion (56) are rare, and require valvuloplasty or valve replacement when hemodynamically significant. Lead-induced tricuspid stenosis sometimes related to chronic endocarditis is also very rare (36,57).

Twiddler's Syndrome

In the twiddler's syndrome, the patient repeatedly turns the implanted pulse generator under the skin, but often denies it. The lead (including those with an active fixation mechanism) retracts from the heart to the right atrium and superior vena cava and becomes twisted into knots (58–63). The chest x-ray shows characteristic twisting of the lead on itself. Twiddler's syndrome occurs more commonly when the pocket is too large for the pulse generator. Intertwinement of the pacing lead may result in pacemaker failure, degradation of insulation, and lead fracture (64).

PACEMAKER FOLLOW-UP

A well-organized pacemaker follow-up clinic is essential for the long-term management of pacemaker patients (52,53,65–77). The most important causes of pacemaker reoperations involve battery failure (at the elective replacement time), lead malfunctions, and pocket complications (53,78). Persistent symptoms, particularly recurrent syncope, may pose difficult problems (79–82). Pacemaker malfunction should not be a major cause of syncope with proper indications for implantation and appropriate pacemaker programming.

Despite the reliability of modern pacemakers, a follow-up program is important because complications are not uncommon and pacemaker failure is ultimately inevitable (53,78,83–86). Lithium-powered pacemakers exhibit a very predictable failure mode. Good follow-up should provide improved pacemaker longevity by appropriate programming and identification of impending pacemaker failure (including battery depletion) (86) before it occurs except for sudden wire fractures or rare unpredictable electronic component malfunction. The frequency and type of follow-up depends on the projected battery life, type, mode, and programming of pulse generators, stability of pacing and sensing, the need for programming changes, underlying rhythm (pacemaker dependency), travel logistics, and the use of alternative methods of follow-up such as the telephone.

Transtelephonic Monitoring

Transtelephonic pacemaker monitoring is the simplest method of pacemaker follow-up and its main function is to detect changes in the rate as an indirect reflection of battery depletion (87–92). Transtelephonic monitoring should complement and not replace comprehensive follow-up and is generally used to document satisfactory pacing function between visits. The Medicare guidelines for transtelephonic monitoring effective since October 1984, are based on pacemaker longevity (77). Transtelephonic monitoring is usually performed every 2–3 mo until the first indication of battery depletion when it should be performed once a month. The ECG is recorded with and without magnet placement. Freerunning and magnet rates (intervals) and pulse width are measured. In dual-chamber pacemakers, rate and pulse width are measured in both channels, as well as the atrioventricular interval. Complex ECGs from DDD pulse generators transmitted transtelephonically are often uninterpretable. As a rule, transtelephonic follow-up does not allow programming or transmission of telemetry data.

Follow-up Visits

When the patient is discharged after implantation, the pulse generator is programmed to optimize function during the expected physiologic changes in the early phase, e.g., output 5 V at 0.5 msec atrial and/or ventricular channel. The patient should then be seen about 2 wk after implantation when the operative site is also inspected for hematoma, infection, etc. The pacing system is then evaluated 2 mo after implantation when pacing and sensing thresholds have stabilized and definitive programming can be performed for long-term function in virtually all patients. Follow-up in the clinic should be done every 6–12 mo for single-chamber and every 3–6 mo for dual-chamber pacemakers (Table 18.1). These visits should be supplemented by periodic transtelephonic pacemaker monitoring. More frequent follow-up may become necessary when impending battery depletion is suspected. Detection and correction of pacemaker malfunction by programming plays a central role in pacemaker follow-up (53,74,86). Programming allows optimal adjustment of pacemaker parameters according to the patient's need (93,94).

Pacemaker follow-up requires equipment such as a three-channel ECG machine, magnet, digital counter for interval measurement, programmers from many manufacturers (no universal programmer exists), temporary pacemaker together with chest electrodes for chest wall stimulation (to inhibit the ventricular channel of a VVI or dual-chamber pacemaker or trigger a DDD pacemaker by selective sensing of chest wall stimulation by the atrial channel) (95,96), echocardiography, Holter recorders, and facilities for cardiopulmonary resuscitation. Accurate record keeping and documentation are essential (Table 1), preferably with computerized system (53,97–100). The physician must be familiar with the "emergency backup" program or "panic button" program available in all programmers (101) designed to provide immediate parameters at the nominal setting for pacemaker-dependent patients. Two programmers for each given family of pulse generators must be available in case of programmer malfunction.

Telemetry

Telemetry is an indispensible feature of all sophisticated pulse generators (102). Transmitted data include: (a) programmed data: a display of programmed settings, e.g., mode, rate, voltage, sensitivity, refractory period, etc. These data merely represent a memory dump and indicate how the pacemaker was instructed and therefore how it is supposed to perform (Fig. 18.2A); (b) real-time or measured data: a display of information actually measured by the pacemaker on how it is operating at the time of interrogation, i.e., self-analysis (Fig. 18.2B). Measured data fall into two groups (102): first, output circuit: pulse amplitude (volts), pulse width (msec). current (mA), pulse energy, pulse charge, and lead impedance for the determination of lead integrity. A low lead impedance (< 250 ohms) suggests a problem

Table 18.1.
Medicare Frequency Guidelines for Pacemaker Follow-up (office or clinic visits)

Single-chamber pacemakers	
First 6 months: twice	
Thereafter: once every 12 months	
Dual-chamber pacemakers	
First 6 months: twice	
Thereafter: every 6 months	

PROGRAMMED PARAMETERS

	INITIAL	PRESENT	
Mode	DDD	DDD	
Rate	70	70	ppm
A-V Delay	200	200	msec
Max Track	110	110	ppm
Vent. Pulse Config.	BIPOLAR	BIPOLAR	
V. Pulse Width	.2	.2	msec
V. Pulse Amplitude	3.0	3.0	Volts
V. Sense Config.	BIPOLAR	BIPOLAR	
V. Sensitivity	2.0	2.0	mVolts
V. Refractory	250	250	msec
Atr. Pulse Config.	BIPOLAR	BIPOLAR	
A. Pulse Width	.2	.2	msec
A. Pulse Amplitude	3.0	3.0	Volts
A. Sense Config.	BIPOLAR	BIPOLAR	
A. Sensitivity	.50	.50	mVolts
A. Refractory	300	300	msec
Blanking	38	38	msec
V. Safety Option	ENABLE	ENABLE	
PVC Options	+PVARP ON PVC	+PVARP ON PVC	
PMT Options	OFF	OFF	
Rate Resp. A-V Delay	DISABLE	DISABLE	
Magnet	TEMPORARY OFF	TEMPORARY OFF	

A

MEASURED DATA

Pacer Rate	70.5	ppm
Ventricular:		
Pulse Amplitude	2.9	Volts
Pulse Current	5.6	mAmperes
Pulse Energy	3	μJoules
Pulse Charge	1	μCoulombs
Lead Impedance	520	Ohms
Atrial:		
Pulse Amplitude	2.9	Volts
Pulse Current	7.6	mAmperes
Pulse Energy	4	μJoules
Pulse Charge	1	μCoulombs
Lead Impedance	379	Ohms
Battery Data: (W.G. 8402 - NOM. 1.2 AHR)		
Voltage	2.80	Volts
Current	12	μAmperes
Impedance	< 1	KOhms

B

Figure 18.2. A, Programmer printout of programmed parameters from the memory of a DDD pulse generator. **B,** Programmer printout of measured (real-time) data transmitted by telemetry from a DDD pulse generator. Note that the output current delivered to the heart in mA. differs from the battery current drain in μA needed to maintain the function of the electronic circuitry.

with lead insulation, while a high impedance (> 1000 ohms) indicates lead fracture, loose set screw, etc. Second, Battery parameters: battery voltage and battery impedance for the diagnosis of impending battery depletion, and average current drain (μA) from the battery (Fig. 18.2B). Battery longevity is directly related to the current required by the circuit—current drain (μA), not to be confused with the current (mA) provided by the output pulse to the heart. Reduction in battery voltage and a major increase in battery impedance in conjunction with slowing of the free-running and/or magnet rate are valuable in confirming the approaching or actual elective replacement time. (c) Diagnostic data: a record of the interaction between pulse generator and patient over an extended period of time serves as a mini-Holter providing cumulative totals of sensed and paced events, etc. (103–106) (Fig. 18.3). (d) Sensor function of rate-adaptive pacemakers: some devices can store recorded sensor generated rates in the form of histograms that may facilitate programming of rate-adaptive parameters. (e) Event markers and transmission of electrograms (107–110): the recording of event markers (for pacing and sensing) recorded simultaneously with the ECG permits real-time evaluation of the pacing system and facilitates interpretation of complex dual chamber pacing rhythms and troubleshooting (Fig. 18.4). Although the actual sensed signal or successful capture cannot be identified by event markers, they do indicate how the pacemaker interprets a specific paced or sensed event and provide precise representation of timing intervals. The telemetered endocardial electrogram is generally less useful than event markers, but may demonstrate the nature of a malfunction caused by lead displacement or fracture, undersensing due to a poor signal, or signals associated with oversensing (111–113), especially when the nature of the signal cannot be determined from the ECG. The telemetered atrial electrogram or

EVENT HISTOGRAM

Total Time Sampled: 0d 0h 27m 6s
Sampling Rate: EVERY EVENT

Mode ———— **DDDR**
Sensor ———— **ON**
Rate ———— **60 ppm**
Max Track ———— **110 ppm**
Maximum Sensor Rate ———— **120 ppm**
A-V Delay ———— **175 msec**
Rate Resp. A-V Delay ———— **ENABLE**

Note: The above values were obtained when the histogram was interrogated.

Rate ppm	Event Counts PV	PR	AV	AR	PVE
0-60	0	0	868	199	0
61-67	0	0	8	371	0
68-75	1	0	0	0	28
76-85	0	0	0	0	6
86-100	0	0	0	0	8
101-119	0	0	0	0	0
120-149	0	0	0	0	0
> 149	0	0	0	0	0
Total:	1	0	876	570	42

Total Event Count: 1,489

Percent Paced in Atrium ———— **97%**
Percent Paced in Ventricle ———— **59%**
Total Time at Max Track Rate ———— **0d 0h 0m 0s**

Percent of Total Time

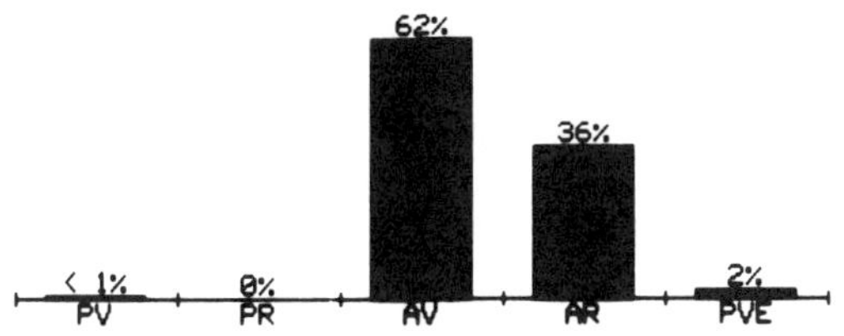

Figure 18.3. Event histogram printout from Pacesetter Synchrony DDDR pacemaker after a brisk walk in a patient with the sick sinus syndrome and atrial chronotropic incompetence. The rate parameters are shown on top. A = atrial paced event; AR = atrial stimulus followed by conducted QRS; AV = atrial stimulus followed by ventricular stimulus; P = atrial sensed event; R = ventricular sensed event; V = ventricular paced event; PR = spontaneous rhythm; PV = P wave synchronous pacing; PVE = premature ventricular event, i.e., extrasystole not preceded by P. The data display the percentage of time pacing occurs in the atrium and ventricle to permit more appropriate programming of the pacemaker. The *printout* shows a summary of the rate distribution of the various pacing rates, i.e., each pacing state complex is placed in the appropriate state bin but also within a rate bin, and the *bar histogram* shows the cumulative percentages of pacing in each of the five pacing states. In this patient the data indicate poor atrial response to exercise and inappropriate pacemaker rate on exercise due to incorrect programming of the sensor parameters.

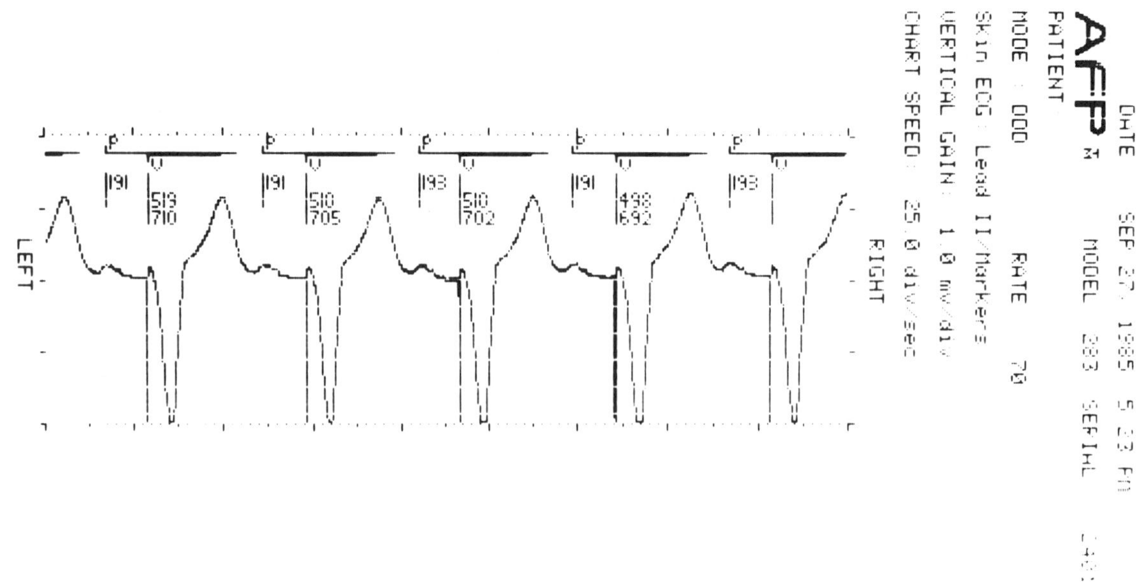

Figure 18.4. Simultaneous recording of telemetered event markers and ECG identify the sensed P wave (P = atrial sensed event) and the ventricular stimulus V. (Other symbols not seen in this recording include A = atrial sensed event and R = ventricular sensed event.) The system displays the duration of various intervals: AV = 191–193 msec, VP intervals = 498–519 msec, and V-V intervals = 692–710 msec. The *horizontal bar* on top of the recording depicts the duration of the atrial refractory period (starting with P and extending beyond V) and the bar underneath depicts the ventricular refractory period (starting with V). In this example, the postventricular atrial refractory period (PVARP) starting at V is longer than the ventricular refractory period (starting at V). Note that the atrial channel remains refractory during the AV interval (PV).

event markers can also easily document the existence of retrograde ventriculoatrial (VA) conduction and its precise duration (Figs. 18.5 and 18.6).

Holter Recordings

Holter monitoring is useful in the investigation of unexplained symptoms such as syncope, dizziness, and palpitations (72,79,114–121). In routine Holter recordings, the commonest abnormalities consist of lack of atrial sensing and myopotential inhibition of the ventricular channel (and/or triggering of synchronized ventricular stimuli if selective atrial oversensing occurs in dual chamber systems). As a rule, the Holter most often demonstrates previously asymptomatic or unsuspected malfunction. In 20–30% of symptomatic patients, supraventricular or ventricular tachycardia unrelated to the pacing is documented. A normal Holter during symptoms excludes a cardiac etiology (72). During a paced rhythm, the atrial stimulus (mostly in unipolar systems) causes a large deflection that often interferes with the depolarization waveform so that atrial capture cannot be determined (72). The interpretation of Holter recordings in patients with DDD pulse generators may be difficult or impossible because of various pauses, apparent shortening of intervals, and missing or concealed pacemaker stimuli. A dual-chamber Holter recording with a special channel to enhance the pacemaker stimulus is extremely useful (116,121,122) (Figs. 18.7 and 18.8). However, such a system may occasionally generate electrostatic discharges that produce deflections resembling pacemaker stimuli, arising from a loose electrode, crushed tape, or a dirty recording head. Some systems can also interpret spontaneous events as being pacemaker outputs creating spurious pacemaker stimuli (Fig. 18.9). A malfunctioning Holter system should not be misinterpreted as pacemaker malfunction (123,124).

The 12-Lead Electrocardiogram During Transvenous Ventricular Pacing

Digital recorders distort the pacemaker stimulus so that it may become larger and show striking changes in amplitude and polarity (125). Digital recorders can miss some of the pacemaker stimuli because of sampling characteristics. Some more advanced digital systems sense all the pacemaker stimuli and process them into a standard-size ECG deflection. However, artifacts can also be misinterpreted by such ECG machines and displayed as pacemaker stimuli, leading to confusion (52). Diagnostic evaluation of the pacemaker stimulus in the ECG is only possible with analog writing systems. Unipolar pacemakers yield a large stimulus in analog machines, but bipolar pacemakers provide small stimuli that can be easily missed when the pacemaker output is low. With an analog recorder, the vector of the pacemaker stimulus in the frontal plane correlates with lead position, while an obvious change from small bipolar stimuli to large ones suggests an insulation defect forming a bipolar-

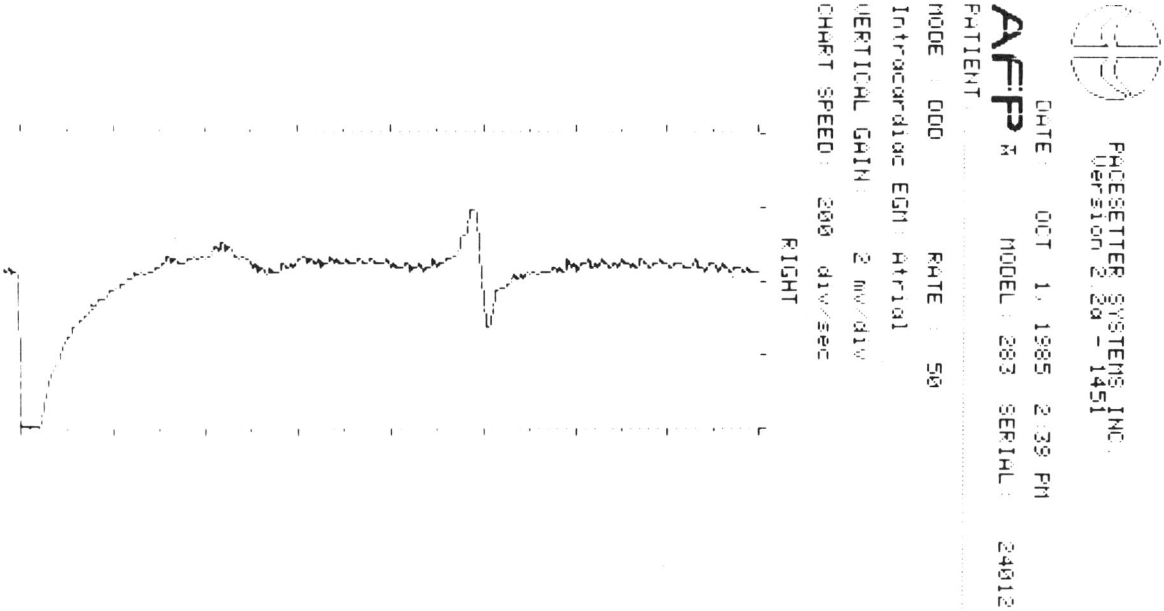

Figure 18.5. Telemetry of atrial electrogram in a patient with a 283 AFP Pacesetter pulse generator showing retrograde ventriculoatrial (VA) conduction following a paced ventricular beat (seen on the **left** of the recording). The atrial output was below the atrial capture threshold. The retrograde P wave is in the middle of the recording. The retrograde VA conduction time is approximately 240 msec from the ventricular stimulus to the onset of the first sharp deflection of the atrial electrogram. (Reproduced with permission from Barold SS, Falkoff MD, Ong LS, *et al.*: Electrocardiography of contemporary DDD pacemakers. A. Basic concepts, upper rate response, retrograde ventriculoatrial conduction and differential diagnosis of pacemaker tachycardias. In Saksena S, Goldschlager N (eds): Electrical Therapy for Cardiac Arrhythmias. Pacing, Antitachycardia Devices, Catheter Ablation. WB Saunders, Philadelphia, 1990:225.)

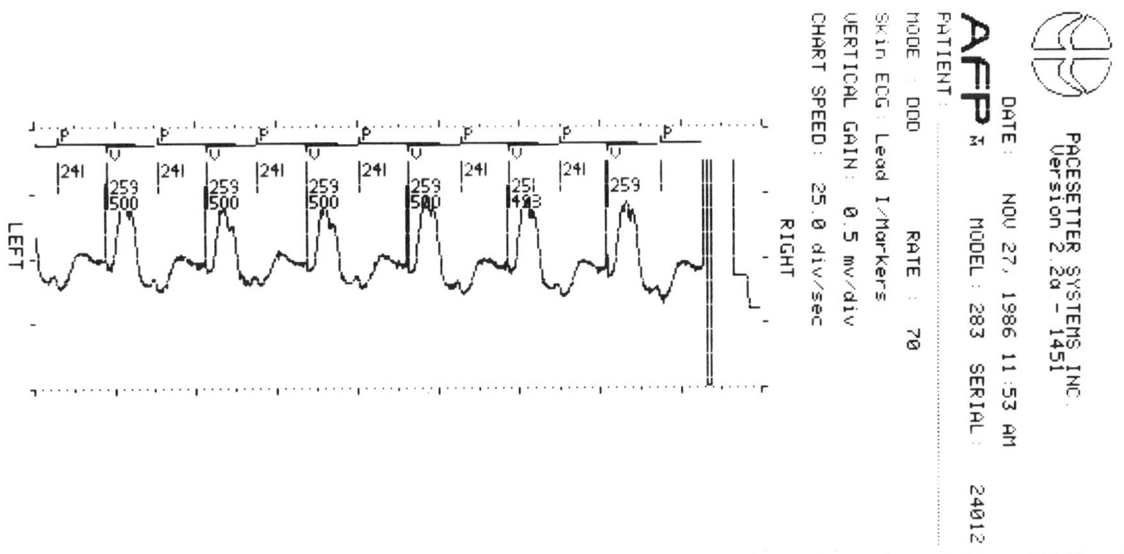

Figure 18.6. Simultaneous recording of telemetered event markers and ECG showing endless loop tachycardia and duration of retrograde ventriculoatrial conduction. P = atrial sensed event; V = ventricular stimulus. The PVARP was deliberately shortened to induce retrograde VA conduction (*upper horizontal bar*—PVARP is shorter than ventricular refractory period shown as horizontal bar beneath the atrial bar). The retrograde VA conduction time measures 251–259 msec.

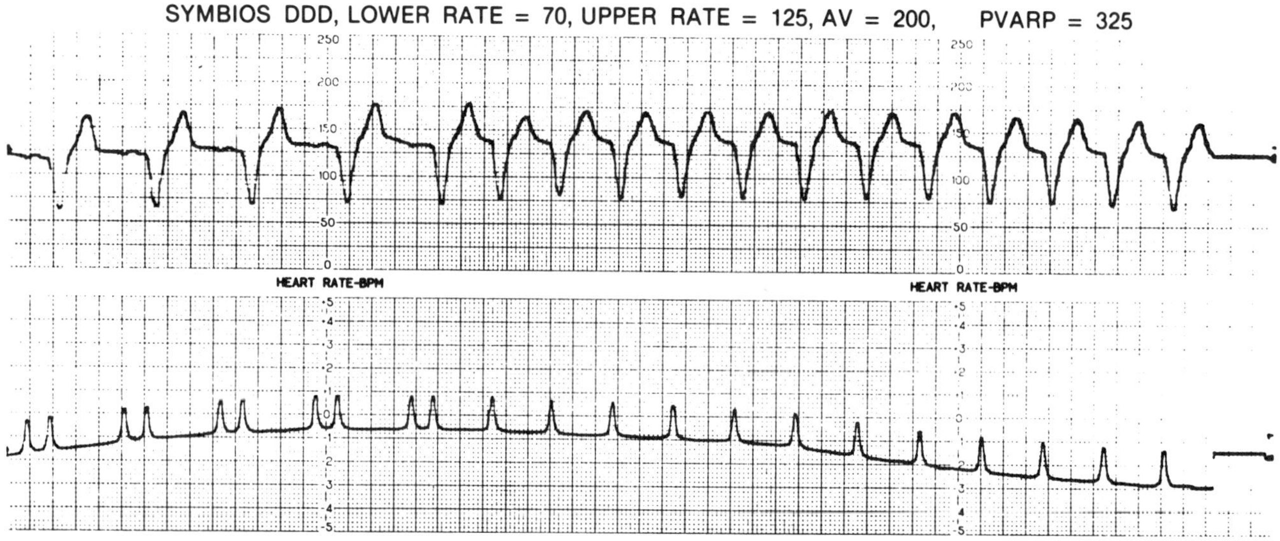

Figure 18.7. Holter recording showing "spontaneous" endless loop tachycardia in a patient with a Medtronic bipolar DDD pulse generator. The *lower channel* depicts the pacemaker stimuli. The initiating mechanism cannot be determined from the surface ECG, but myopotential triggering can be excluded with certainty because no interference could be demonstrated at high atrial sensitivities. Far-field atrial sensing of a ventricular signal is highly unlikely with a relatively long PVARP of 325 msec. The tachycardia was probably initiated by an atrial extrasystole. (Reproduced with permission from Barold SS, Falkoff MD, Ong LS, *et al.*: Electrocardiography of contemporary DDD pacemakers. A. Basic concepts, upper rate response, retrograde ventriculoatrial conduction and differential diagnosis of pacemaker tachycardias. In Saksena S, Goldschlager N (eds): Electrical Therapy for Cardiac Arrhythmias, Pacing, Antitachycardia Devices, Catheter Ablation. WB Saunders, Philadelphia, 1990:225.)

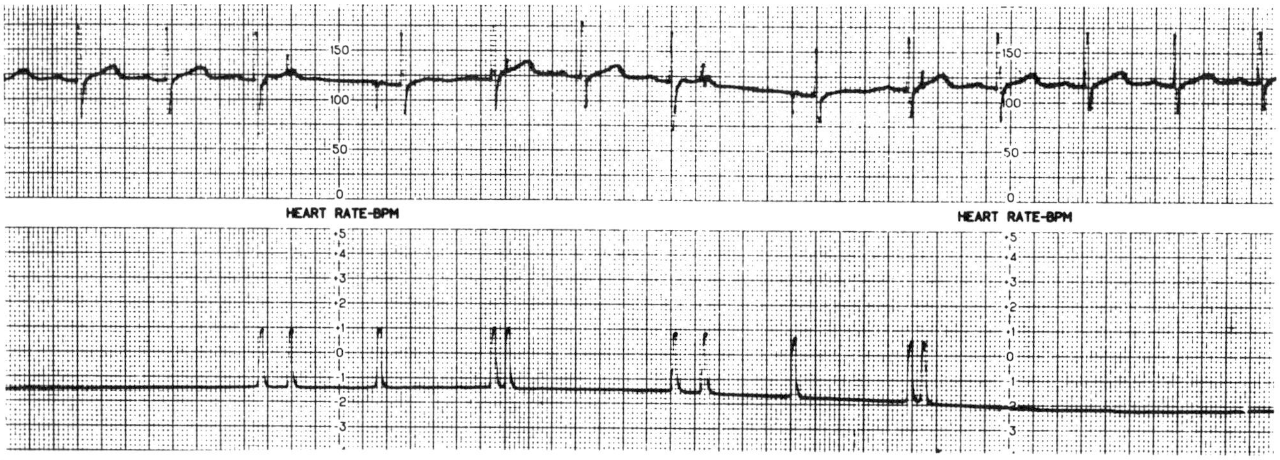

Figure 18.8. Holter recording (with pacemaker channel at **bottom**) in a patient with a DDD pacemaker. There is intermittent atrial undersensing. The invisible pacemaker stimuli on the ECG are clearly delineated by the pacemaker channel at the **bottom.** The abbreviated AV intervals represent ventricular sensing during the ventricular safety pacing period. (Reproduced with permission from Barold SS, Falkoff MD, Ong LS, *et al.*: Electrocardiography of contemporary DDD pacemakers. B. Multiprogrammability, follow-up, and troubleshooting. In Saksena S, Goldschlager N (eds): Electrical Therapy for Cardiac Arrhythmias, Pacing, Antitachycardia Devices, Catheter Ablation, WB Saunders, Philadelphia, 1990:265.)

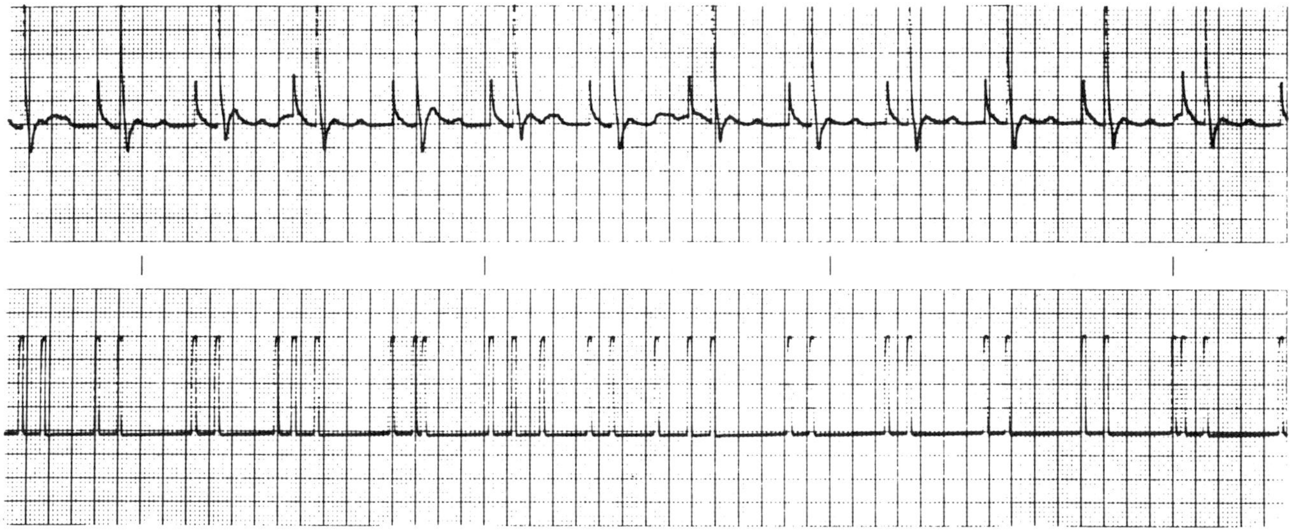

Figure 18.9. Holter recording (with pacemaker channel at bottom) in a patient with a DDD pacemaker, showing multiple artifacts in the pacemaker channel that could be misinterpreted as additional pacemaker stimuli either preceding the atrial stimuli or following the ventricular stimuli.

unipolar system (125) (Fig. 18.10). Obvious attenuation of analog recorded unipolar stimuli during held respiration suggests an increase in lead impedance due to a fracture or loose connection even if capture is preserved (126).

Stimulation of the left ventricle (LV) produces late activation of the right ventricle (RV) and therefore a RBBB pattern of depolarization (127). Conversely, RV pacing produces a left bundle branch block (LBBB) pattern of depolarization. During uncomplicated transvenous RV apical pacing, paced beats usually exhibit a typical LBBB pattern in leads 1 and aVL, but leads V_5 and V_6 sometimes do not show the characteristic LBBB pattern because the main electrical forces point away from the horizontal level where V_5 and V_6 are recorded, thereby producing deep S waves or QS complexes. The mean electrical axis of the paced QRS complex in the frontal plane is oriented superiorly and generally to the left because the sequence of activation travels from apex to base, away from the inferior leads. Occasionally during RV apical pacing the mean frontal plane axis points to the right superior quadrant with resultant negative deflections in leads 1, 2, 3, and aVF, and to a variable degree in aVL. As the pacing electrode moves toward the right ventricular outflow tract, activation travels simultaneously to the base superiorly and the apex inferiorly, and the mean frontal plane electrical axis of the paced QRS complex shifts accordingly and becomes less negative and the axis may point to the right lower quadrant (Fig. 18.11). Right ventricular outflow tract stimulation immediately below the pulmonary valve causes right axis deviation of the QRS complex in the frontal plane because most of the activation travels from base to apex, but the LBBB pattern in the left precordial lead persists, i.e., the rS pattern in leads 1 and aVL does not represent an RBBB pattern because lead V1 displays a predominately negative complex. During pacing from any site in the RV, the left precordial leads display R, Rs, rS, or QS complexes, but never (initial) q waves (i.e., no qR or qRS complexes).

NORMAL Q WAVES IN LEADS 1 AND aVL

During RV outflow tract pacing (in the absence of myocardial infarction), paced beats not uncommonly exhibit a qR, QR, or Qr configuration in leads 1 and aVL when the inferior leads show a dominant R wave. In this situation, as already indicated the precordial leads do not exhibit Qr, qR, or QR complexes. Occasionally with slight displacement of the catheter away from the RV apex, the characteristic negative complexes in leads 2, 3, and aVF persist while leads 1 and aVL show a qR complex (127) (Fig. 18.12). This qR pattern should not be interpreted as representing an St-qR pattern (St refers to pacemaker stimulus) diagnostic of anteroseptal myocardial infarction (128). Rarely, uncomplicated right apical pacing causes a qR complex in lead 1 but not in aVL (127).

SIGNIFICANCE OF A DOMINANT R WAVE OF PACED VENTRICULAR BEATS IN LEAD V1 DURING TRANSVENOUS PACING

The presence of a dominant R wave in V1 during ventricular pacing has been called an "RBBB pattern of depolarization." This terminology is misleading because many cases do not represent late RV activation. The causes of a dominant R wave in V1 include (127,129–131): (a) ventricular fusion with spontaneous beats conducted with RBBB, (b) paced beat in the relative refractory period of the heart, (c) LV endocardial stimulation (132), (d) catheter in the coronary sinus or middle cardiac vein activating the LV epicardial surface (Fig. 18.13), (e) a change of electrically induced ventricular depolarization from LBBB to RBBB strongly suggests catheter perforation of the RV or perfo-

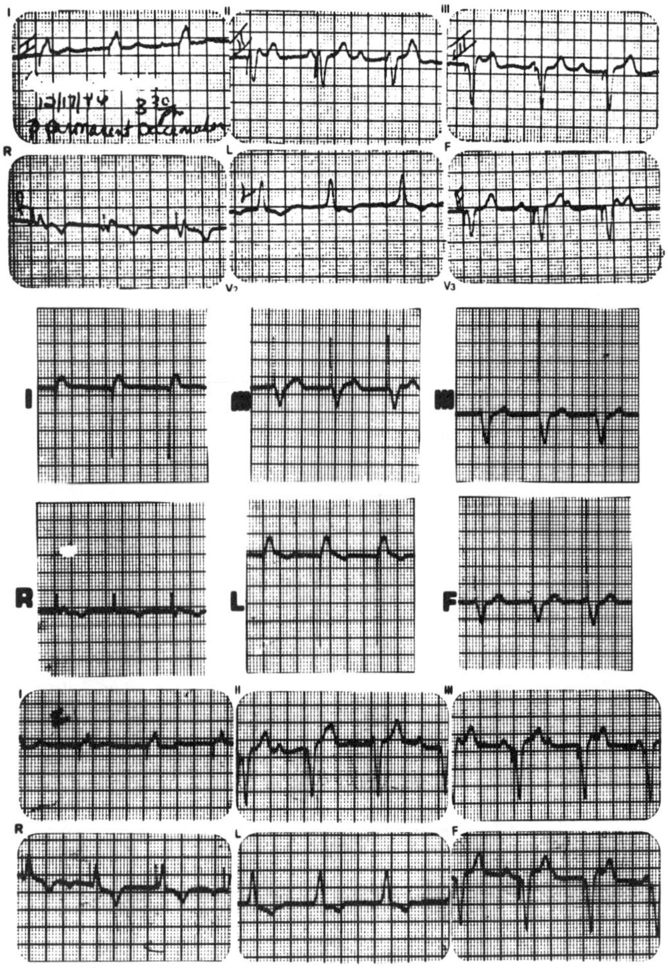

Figure 18.10. Alteration of bipolar pacing stimulus due to defective insulation demonstrated by analog ECGs. **Top:** Frontal plane leads recorded 1 hr after implantation of a permanent transvenous bipolar pacing system. **Middle:** standard leads recorded (at half-standardization) 24 hr after implantation. Note the change in the vector of the pacemaker stimulus from −120° to approximately +120° and a considerable increase in amplitude. At operation it was found that the surgeon had forgotten to insert the seal caps over the set screws holding the leads in place. There was obvious exposure of both leads to body fluids. After insertion of seal caps, the bottom ECG was recorded with restoration of bipolar pacing. Interestingly, in this situation the electrocardiographic abnormalities of an insulation leak took several hours to develop, probably because some time was required for the body fluids to make appropriate electrical contact with the pacemaker connections. (Reproduced with permission from Barold SS, *et al.*: Electrocardiographic diagnosis of pacemaker malfunction. In Wellens HJJ, Kulbertus HE (eds): What's New in Electrocardiography. The Hague, Martinus Nijhoff, 1981:236.)

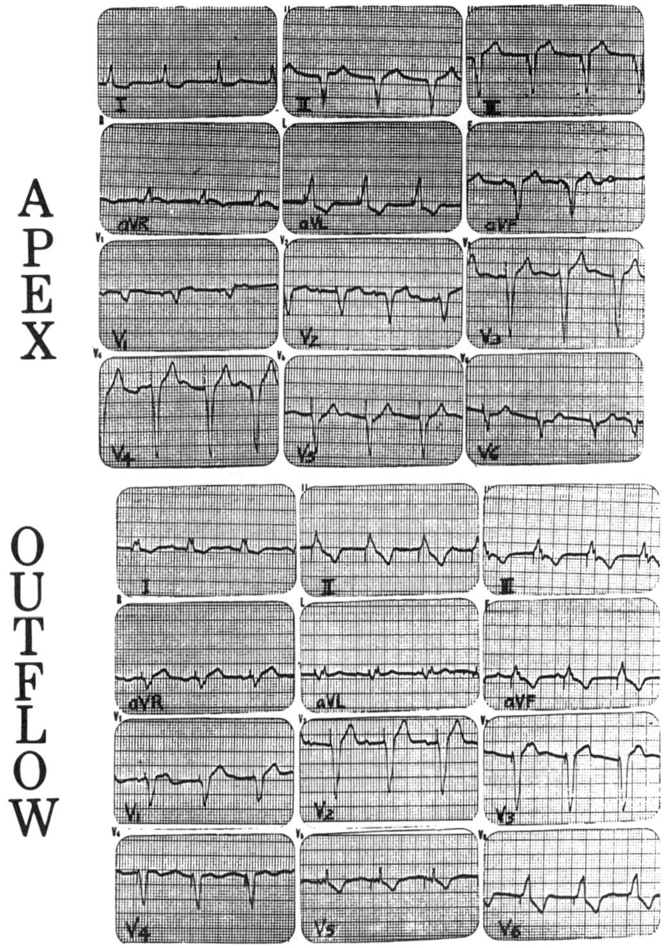

Figure 18.11. Twelve-lead ECG during right ventricular endocardial pacing from the apex and outflow tract respectively. See text for details. (Reproduced with permission from Barold SS, Falkoff MD, Ong LS, *et al.*: Electrocardiographic analysis of normal and abnormal pacemaker function. In Dreifus LS, (ed): Pacemaker Therapy, Cardiovascular clinics. FA Davis, Philadelphia, 1983:97.)

ration of the ventricular septum with LV stimulation, (f) uncomplicated RV stimulation: a dominant R wave in the right precordial leads may occasionally occur during uncomplicated transvenous RV apical stimulation in approximately 10% of cases (127,130). The position of leads V_1 and V_2 should be carefully checked because a dominant R wave may also be recorded during uncomplicated pacing at the level of the third intercostal space and not the fourth (127,130) (Fig. 18.14). When the positivity is mostly confined to lead V1, particularly if the total voltage of the R wave is relatively small, the catheter is almost certainly in the RV if V_1 and V_2 are negative when recorded at the level of the fifth intercostal space (127).

Left ventricular stimulation from the inflow tract or near the AV groove produces paced beats with RBBB and right axis deviation in the frontal plane, while stimulation from the LV apex (e.g., catheter passing from right to left atrium via a patent foramen ovale) produces ventricular depolarization with RBBB and left axis or superior axis deviation in the frontal plane (131). When the lead is in the venous system, the recording of right axis deviation with an RBBB pattern suggests a catheter site near the AV groove, i.e., in the coronary sinus. As a rule, in the presence of an RBBB configuration, the axis in the frontal plane cannot determine the precise site of pacing—left ventricle versus coronary venous system.

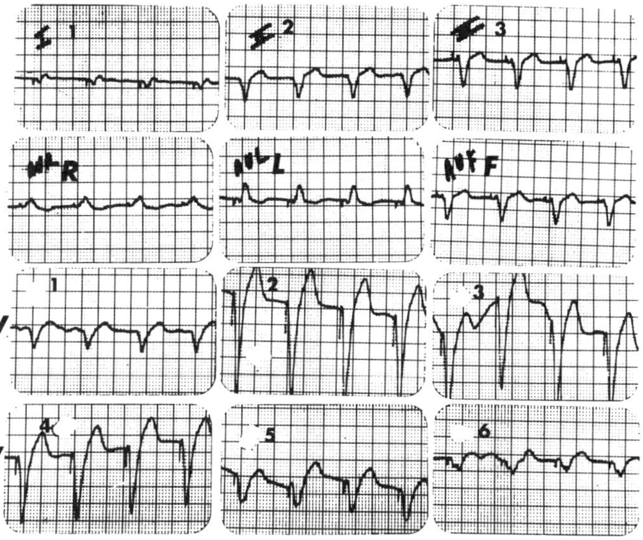

Figure 18.12. Twelve-lead ECG of a patient with a permanent transvenous pacemaker originally positioned at the right ventricular apex. Slight displacement toward the right ventricular outflow tract produced new qR complexes in leads 1 and aVL; yet leads 2, 3, and aVF retained the characteristic negative complexes. The patient did not have coronary artery disease and there was no evidence of an anteroseptal myocardial infarction.

VanGelder, *et al.* (133) reported changes in the ECG during bipolar pacing in over half the patients when the pulse generator was programmed to a very high output. The changes involved the mean frontal plane axis, QRS, and T waves. VanGelder, *et al.* (133) postulated that at a low output setting, ventricular depolarization originates from the distal electrode while at a high output setting, ventricular depolarization emanates from both distal and proximal electrodes (due to the anodal contribution) (134). The electrocardiographic differences between high and low output stimulation are slight and therefore do not invalidate the use of the paced ECG to determine the site of pacing and presence of myocardial infarction.

Diagnosis of Myocardial Infarction During Transvenous Ventricular Pacing

Because of the QRS complex during RV pacing resembles that of spontaneous LBBB (except for the initial forces), the diagnosis of myocardial infarction (MI) can often be made during ventricular pacing by applying the criteria used in complete LBBB (128,131,135). (a) St-qR pattern: An extensive anteroseptal MI may cause an (initial) q in leads 1, aVL, V_5 and V_6, producing an St-qR pattern, (Fig. 18.15) not to be confused with a QS pattern

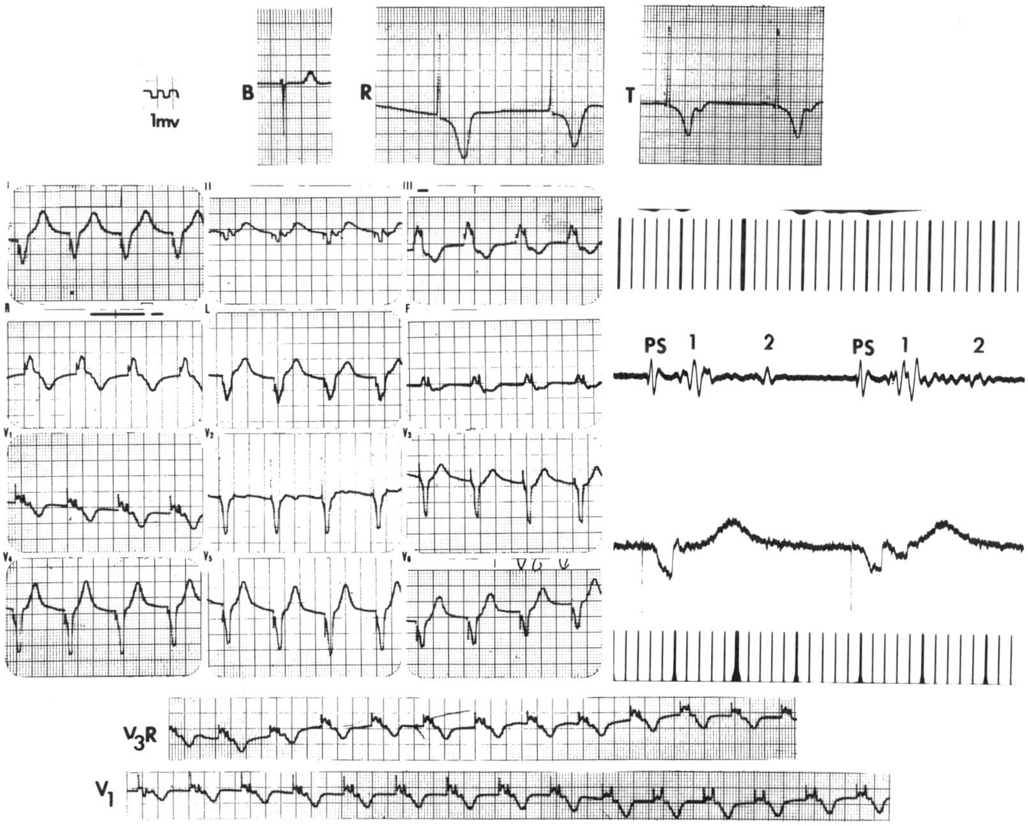

Figure 18.13. Twelve-lead ECG during transvenous ventricular pacing showing a right bundle branch block pattern in V_1 and V_3R (with a dominant R wave) due to right ventricular perforation by pacing lead lying in the pericardium. The previous ECG had shown a left bundle branch block pattern of activation during ventricular pacing. The unipolar electrograms on **top** (B = bipolar, R = ring, T = tip) with a dominant R deflection during spontaneous rhythm suggest an extracardiac lead position. On the **right,** a phonocardiogram shows a pacemaker sound (PS) due to activation of intercostal muscles typical of perforation.

which is normal (St = stimulus) (128,135). The St-qR sign restricted to leads 1 and aVL is not specific for MI (127). The sensitivity of the St-qR sign is low, but its specificity approaches 100% because it is never seen in V_5 and V_6 during uncomplicated RV pacing. A QR or Qr complex in leads 2, 3, and AVF is also diagnostic of an inferior MI (135). Large unipolar stimuli may mask an initial Q wave. (b) Cabrera's sign: An anterior MI can cause late notching of the ascending limb of the QRS complex (≥ 0.03 sec and superior to the lower one-fourth of the S wave) in the left precordial leads (135) (Fig. 18.15). During ventricular pacing, the development of Cabrera's sign requires an extensive anterior MI and can occur together with the St-qR sign. The sensitivity of Cabrera's sign is also low, but its specificity is very high. Ventricular fusion beats must always be excluded in the presence of the St-qR pattern or Cabrera's sign. (c) ST-T wave abnormalities: during RV apical pacing, the inferior and anterior leads (V_1–V_3) often record secondary ST elevation. ST segment depression may occur as a normal finding in leads 1, aVF, V_5 and V_6. Relatively stable ST-T wave changes resembling primary abnormalities may occasionally occur during uncomplicated RV pacing. Discordant or so-called primary T waves are of no diagnostic value. Sequential electrocardiograms are often needed to determine the significance of the ST-T wave abnormalities. Acute MI causes ST-T wave abnormalities more commonly than the St-qR pattern or Cabrera's sign. Useful patterns include (a) pronounced primary ST elevation (same direction as QRS) diagnostic of MI (or severe ischemia). When less obvious, the diagnosis becomes fairly certain only when the polarity of the T wave is opposite to that of the ST segment elevation. Giant ST elevation in leads with a negative QRS complex (Fig. 18.16) also indicates MI or severe ischemia. (b) ST depression concordant with the QRS complex may occasionally occur in V_3–V_6 during uncomplicated RV pacing and rarely in leads V_1 and V_2. Consequently, obvious ST segment depression in leads V_1 and V_2 should be considered abnormal and indicative of anterior or inferior wall MI (or ischemia). Inhibition of a VVI pacemaker by chest wall stimulation or by reduction of the rate or output may allow the emergence of the spontaneous

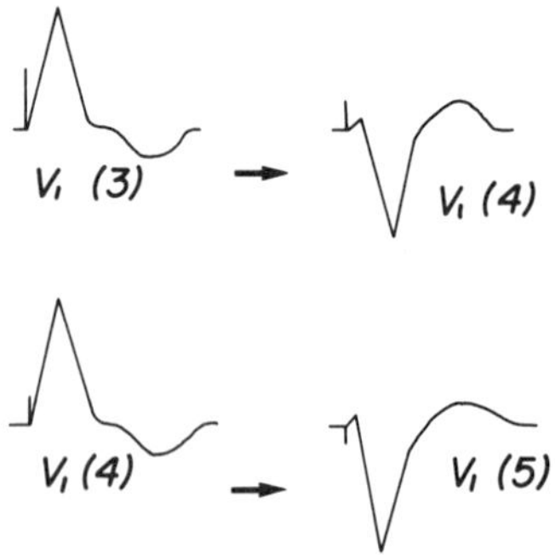

Figure 18.14. Significance of dominant R wave of paced ventricular beats in lead V_1 during uncomplicated transvenous right ventricular pacing. **Top:** A dominant R wave can sometimes be recorded when lead V_1 is recorded one intercostal space (3) too high, but not when lead V_1 is recorded from the correct site (fourth intercostal space). **Bottom:** Lead V_1 shows a dominant R wave when recorded in the fourth intercostal space. In this situation, during uncomplicated right ventricular apical pacing, lead V_1 and V_2 recorded on intercostal space lower (fifth) will show negative complexes.

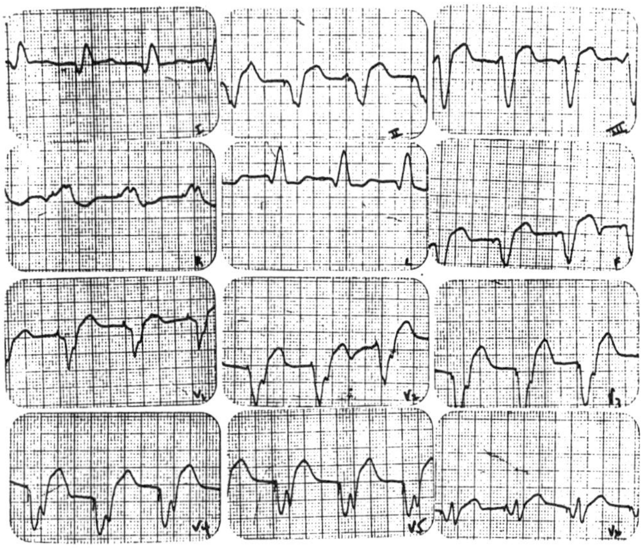

Figure 18.15. Twelve-lead ECG during bipolar ventricular pacing in a patient with extensive anteroseptal myocardial infarction. Leads 1, aVL, and V6 display an St-qR complex best seen in V_6. There is also notching of the S wave (Cabrera's sign) from V_1 to V_5. (Reproduced with permission from Barold SS, *et al.*: Normal and abnormal patterns of ventricular depolarization. In Barold SS, Falkoff MD, Ong LS, *et al.*: (eds): Modern Cardiac Pacing. Futura Publishing Co., Mt. Kisco, NY, 1985:545.)

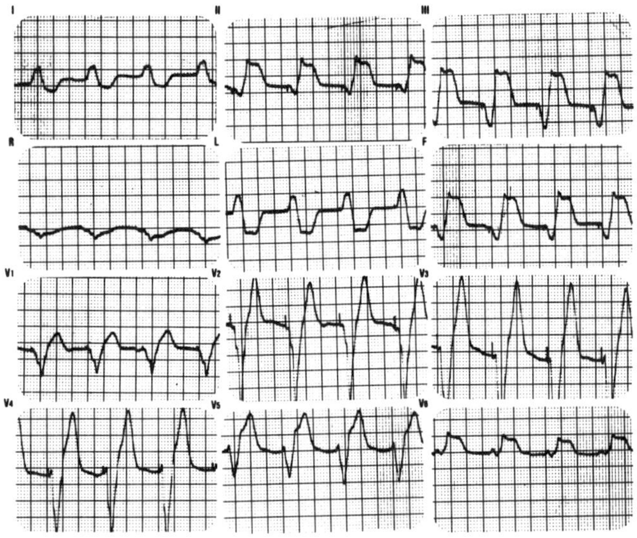

Figure 18.16. Obvious ST elevation in leads 2, 3, aVF, and V_6 during ventricular pacing consistent with acute inferolateral myocardial infarction. (Reproduced with permission from Barold SS, Falkoff MD, Ong LS, *et al.*: Normal and abnormal patterns of ventricular depolarization. In Barold SS (ed): Modern Cardiac Pacing. Futura Publishing Co., Mt. Kisco, NY, 1985:545.)

rhythm and reveal diagnostic Q waves. Repolarization abnormalities may be related to pacing per se and may produce prominent ST-T wave changes that should not be interpreted as representing ischemia or subendocardial infarction (135).

SYSTEMATIC EVALUATION OF PACEMAKER FUNCTION

Various aspects of pacemaker function should be evaluated systematically (Table 18.2). With dual-chamber pacemakers, function of the atrial and ventricular channels are evaluated sequentially.

1. A 12-lead ECG is obtained with and without magnet application. The magnet response varies according to the manufacturers but virtually always occurs in the asynchronous mode. Various intervals (lower rate interval, pulse width, AV interval) are measured with an electronic counter and recorded. Photoanalysis of the pacemaker waveform is now rarely used. If telemetry is available, the pulse generator is interrogated to document initial pacemaker parameters, lead and battery data (Fig. 18.2A and B).

2. Underlying rhythm. The underlying rhythm is determined by programming to the VVI mode and by gradually reducing the rate, sometimes to as low as 30/min, to encourage emergence of the underlying spontaneous rhythm. Most patients tolerate such a slow rate of pacing.

3. Elective replacement indicators. In most pulse generators, when the battery voltage reaches a critical level it will activate the elective replacement indicator (ERI), often in the form of a slower pacing rate. The rate change may be gradual or stepwise (sudden) and in freerunning and/or magnet mode. The ERI of some DDD pulse generators consists of reversion to the

Table 18.2.
Data Required in Pacemaker Chart

Patient Data
Patient's name, age, address, phone number
Pacemaker data
Date(s) of implant(s)
Model and serial number of pacemaker lead(s)
Model and serial number of pacemaker generator
Data from implant
Indication
Pacing threshold(s)
Sensing threshold(s)
Intracardiac electrograms
Lead impedance(s)
Presence of retrograde ventriculoatrial (VA) conduction
Presence of diaphragmatic or accessory muscle stimulation at 5- and 10-V output
Technical specifications
Pacemaker behavior in the magnet mode
Record of elective replacement indicator: magnet and/or freerunning rate, mode change, telemetered battery data (impedance and voltage)
Data from pacemaker clinic
Programmed parameters from time of implant and most recent changes
12-lead ECG and long rhythm strips showing pacing and inhibition of pacing (if possible) to determine underlying rhythm (by programming very low rate or with chest wall stimulation)
12-lead ECG on application of the magnet
Rhythm strip of magnet mode for at least 1 min
Electronic rate intervals and pulse widths freerunning and upon application of the magnet before programming
Interrogation and printout of telemetry, e.g., memory or programmed, and real-time data
Systematic evaluation of pacing system
Atrial and/or ventricular pacing and sensing thresholds
Retrograde ventriculoatrial conduction and propensity to endless loop tachycardia
Crosstalk
Myopotential interference (record best way of reproducing abnormality)
Printouts showing pacemaker function when a parameter is programmed
Evaluation of sensor function with exercise protocols. Histograms or other data to demonstrate heart rate response in the rate-adaptive mode. Efficacy of rate-adaptive parameters.
Final telemetry printout at end of pacemaker evaluation and date. Check that any changes in parameters are intentional by comparing the final parameters with those obtained at the time of initial pacemaker interrogation.[a] Any discrepancy must be justified in the record.
Ancillary data
Symptoms and potential pacemaker problems, e.g., accessory muscle stimulation
ECG with event marker recorders and telemetered electrogram
Intolerance of VOO pacing on application of magnet

[a]In one system, an arrow points to the initial parameter if it differs from the final programmed value.

VVI or VOO mode, VVIR to the VVI mode, or DDDR to the VVI mode (136–139). The behavior of the pulse generator at the elective replacement time should be documented in the chart soon after pacemaker implantation.

4. Ventricular pacing. Ventricular pacing is documented in the VVI mode from the ECG and after application of the magnet over the pulse generator. The pacing rate is programmed faster than the intrinsic rate. Carotid sinus massage is not recommended to slow the intrinsic ventricular rate. Determination of the pacing threshold requires programming voltage and/or pulse width until capture is lost. Appropriate capture should be tested with deep respiration in the supine or other positions and also with gentle movement or traction of the pulse generator in the pocket to expose a lead fracture or loose connection with electrical abnormalities.

The ventricular pacing threshold can also be evaluated in the DDD mode by programming a short AV interval to ensure ventricular pacing before termination of the spontaneous PR interval in the presence of AV conduction. During AV sequential pacing, a QRS that follows a ventricular stimulus may be (a) a pure ventricular paced beat, (b) ventricular fusion beat, (c) pseudofusion beat where the initial vector of the spontaneous QRS complex is not seen clearly, (d) spontaneous QRS complex preceded by an ineffectual ventricular stimulus where the constant delay from the ventricular stimulus to the QRS should not be interpreted as latency with successful ventricular capture.

5. Ventricular sensing. Confirmation of normal ventricular sensing requires reduction of the pacing rate to allow emergence of any existing intrinsic ventricular rhythm. The ventricular sensing threshold is obtained by gradually decreasing ventricular sensitivity until sensing failure occurs (discussed in greater detail in the section on atrial sensing). In DDD pacing, with ventricular pseudofusion beats (ventricular stimulus falling within the spontaneous QRS complex) and normal ventricular sensing, the ventricular stimulus will disappear with an increase in the AV interval. A ventricular stimulus falling beyond the QRS complex represents ventricular undersensing.

6. Atrial pacing. The overshoot of the atrial stimulus in unipolar pulse generators renders the diagnosis of successful atrial depolarization difficult (140–143). A 12-lead ECG recorded at double standardization (occasionally magnified four times) can be invaluable in bringing out a paced P wave and/or tiny bipolar stimuli. Lack of atrial capture can be due to underlying atrial fibrillation.

(a) In the presence of relatively intact AV conduction, reprogramming to the AAI or AOO mode confirms atrial capture by demonstrating a consistent relationship (at several pacing rates) of the atrial stimulus to a succeeding spontaneous QRS complex (Fig. 18.17). In patients with AV block, a gradual reduction of the ventricular rate in the VVI mode to 30/min if tolerated, often leads to ventricular escape at a modest rate, thereby allowing the use of the AAI or AOO mode to evaluate atrial capture (Fig. 18.18). In this way, AAI pacing can be accomplished in most pacemaker-dependent patients.

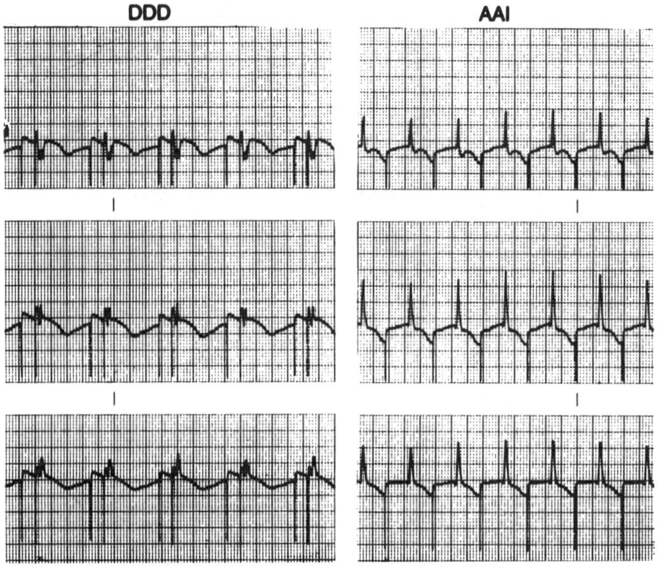

Figure 18.17. DDD pulse generator. On the **left,** during DDD pacing it is impossible to determine successful atrial capture. On the **right,** by reprogramming to the AAI mode at various pacing rates, there is a corresponding increase in the ventricular rate (conducted QRS complex) so that atrial capture can be inferred. (Reproduced with permission from Barold SS, Nanda NC, Ong LS, *et al.*: Determination of successful atrial capture during unipolar dual-chambered pacing. In Barold SS (ed): Modern Cardiac Pacing. Futura Publishing Co., Mt. Kisco, NY, 1985:677.)

(b) A paced P wave may be difficult to discern if the AV interval is short. Occasionally with latency (delay from the atrial stimulus in the onset of visible atrial depolarization) or considerable delay in interatrial conduction, atrial depolarization may be invisible to the presence of a relatively short AV interval, e.g., 150 msec. A relatively late paced P wave can be unmasked by programming a longer AV delay to 250–300 ms.

(c) With dual-chamber pacemakers, atrial capture may be inferred if the paced QRS morphology changes when the AV interval is shortened or lengthened, because with AV conduction either an increased or decreased degree of ventricular fusion will occur from the normally conducted impulse and pacemaker-induced depolarization.

(d) In patients with a relatively fast sinus rhythm, conversion to the DVI mode provides the easiest way to test for atrial capture (Fig. 18.19). A low pacing rate provides competitive atrial pacing so that pacemaker stimuli beyond the atrial myocardial refractory period will demonstrate atrial capture.

(e) In patients with retrograde VA conduction, subthreshold atrial stimulation leads to retrograde VA conduction (142). Identification of a retrograde P wave in the ST segment implies lack of atrial capture by the preceding atrial stimulus (Fig. 18.20). Retrograde P waves invisible on the surface ECG can be documented by telemetry of event markers and/or the atrial electrogram. The disappearance of retrograde P waves with an increase in atrial output (voltage and/or pulse width) indicates successful atrial capture.

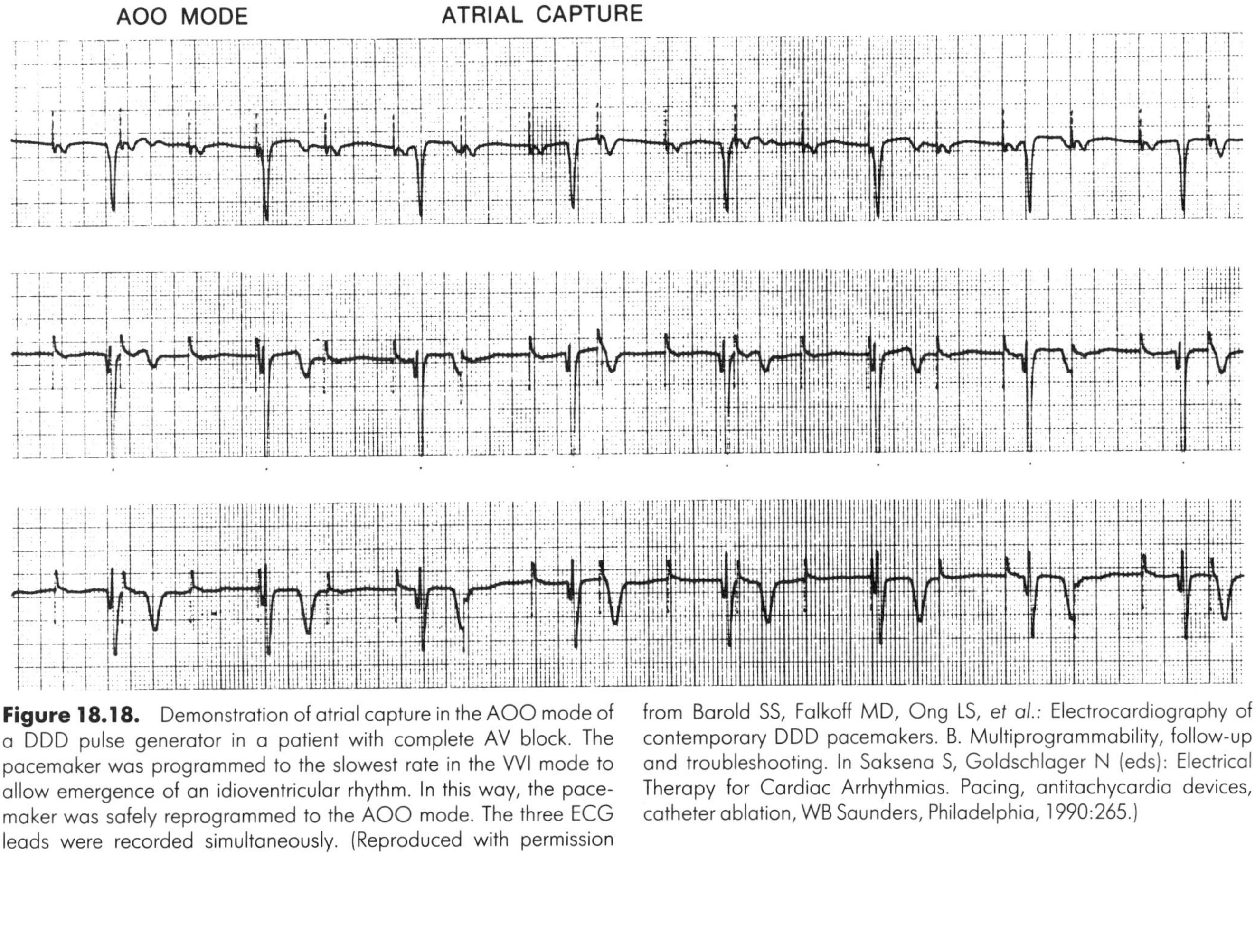

Figure 18.18. Demonstration of atrial capture in the AOO mode of a DDD pulse generator in a patient with complete AV block. The pacemaker was programmed to the slowest rate in the VVI mode to allow emergence of an idioventricular rhythm. In this way, the pacemaker was safely reprogrammed to the AOO mode. The three ECG leads were recorded simultaneously. (Reproduced with permission from Barold SS, Falkoff MD, Ong LS, *et al.*: Electrocardiography of contemporary DDD pacemakers. B. Multiprogrammability, follow-up and troubleshooting. In Saksena S, Goldschlager N (eds): Electrical Therapy for Cardiac Arrhythmias. Pacing, antitachycardia devices, catheter ablation, WB Saunders, Philadelphia, 1990:265.)

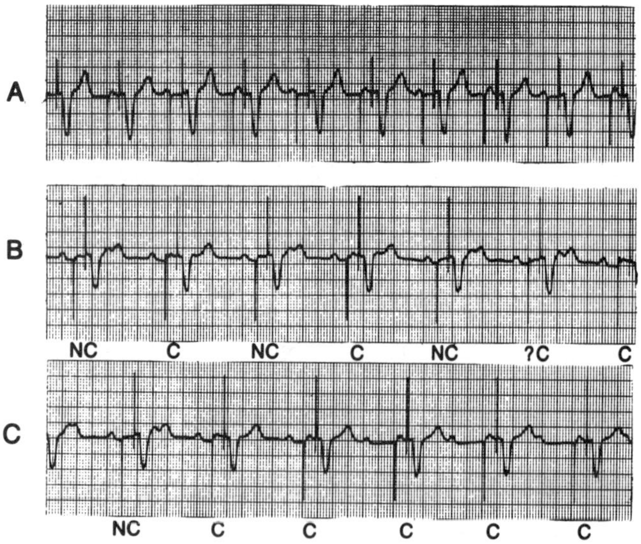

Figure 18.19. **Top:** DVI pacing with relatively fast spontaneous sinus rhythm, makes determination of atrial capture difficult. By programming a dual chamber pulse generator to the DVI mode at a low rate (**B** and **C**), the interplay between the slower paced DVI rhythm and spontaneous atrial depolarization allows the atrial stimulus to depolarize the atrium outside the atrial myocardial refractory period and confirm atrial capture. C = atrial capture outside the atrial myocardial refractory period; NC = noncapture in the atrial myocardial refractory period. (Reproduced with permission from Barold SS, Nanda NC, Ong LS, *et al.*: Determination of successful atrial capture during unipolar dual-chambered pacing. In Barold SS (ed): Modern Cardiac Pacing. Futura Publishing Co., Mt. Kisco, NY, 1985:677.)

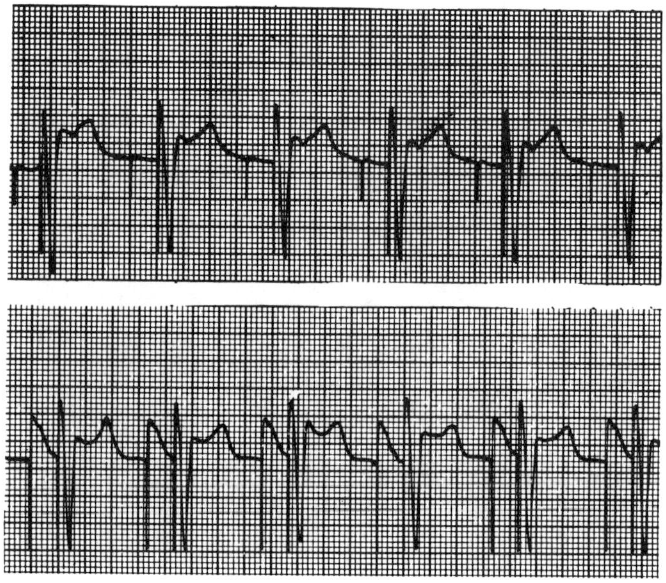

Figure 18.20. DDD pulse generator. **Top:** the atrial stimulus does not give rise to visible atrial depolarization. The presence of notching on the ST segment suggests the presence of retrograde VA conduction indicating lack of atrial capture by the preceding atrial stimulus. **Bottom:** when the atrial output was increased, retrograde VA conduction disappeared, implying that there was appropriate atrial capture despite the absence of a clearly visible P wave. (Reproduced with permission from Barold SS, Nanda NC, Ong LS, *et al.*: Determination of successful atrial capture during unipolar dual-chambered pacing. In Barold SS (ed): Modern Cardiac Pacing. Futura Publishing Co., Mt. Kisco, NY, 1985:677.)

(f) The telemetered electrogram does not allow confirmation of atrial capture because the output of the pulse generator saturates the telemetry amplifier. Event markers merely confirm that the pulse generator has released a stimulus, but they cannot indicate successful capture. In bipolar systems with programmable output configuration, unipolar pacing from the tip electrode and telemetry of the electrogram from the proximal electrode can demonstrate atrial capture. This maneuver can be reversed by pacing from the proximal electrode and recording from the tip electrode (144). Low unipolar pacing thresholds from the tip and ring electrodes indicate a low bipolar pacing threshold.

(g) In difficult cases, echocardiography is preferable to esophageal electrocardiography. Atrial capture may be inferred from a properly timed A wave in the mitral valve echocardiogram and doppler recordings during dual chamber pacing and its disappearance during VVI pacing. In addition, the subcostal four-chamber view easily identifies the right atrium and appropriate M-mode recording of right atrial motion represents a marker of atrial activity (142).

7. Atrial sensing. To evaluate atrial sensing, reduce the lower rate of the pulse generator below that of spontaneous atrial activity, and then shorten the AV delay to 50–100 msec to guarantee that any P wave sensed will be coupled to a ventricular stimulus. A semiquantitative assessment of the atrial signal can be obtained by sequentially changing atrial sensitivity from the lowest numeric value (or most sensitive) to the highest numeric value (or least sensitive) until the P wave is undersensed. The sensing threshold is the lowest sensitivity (highest numerical value) associated with consistent atrial sensing (Fig. 18.21). Atrial sensitivity should be programmed to approximately double (or half the numeric value) the atrial sensing threshold. For

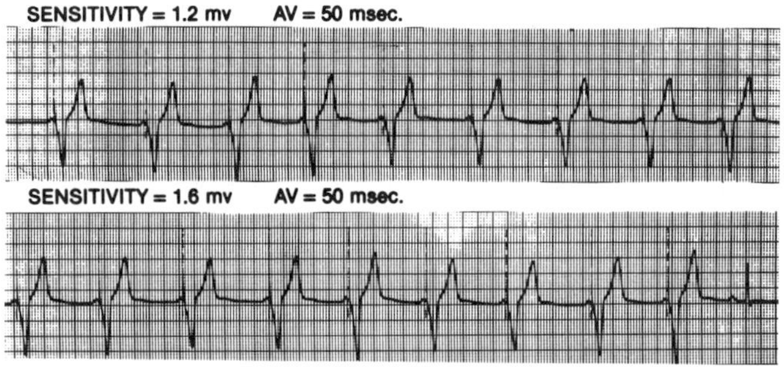

Figure 18.21. Semiquantitative assessment of atrial signal by programmability of sensitivity and short AV interval. **Top:** with an atrial sensitivity of 1.2 mV., all the P waves are tracked. **Bottom:** with an atrial sensitivity of 1.6 mV., there is failure to sense the last P wave. (Reproduced with permission from Barold SS, Falkoff MD, Ong LS, *et al.*: Electrocardiography of contemporary DDD pacemakers. B. Multiprogrammability, follow-up and troubleshooting. In Saksena S, Goldschlager N (eds): Electrical Therapy for Cardiac Arrhythmias. Pacing, Antitachycardia Devices, Catheter Ablation. WB Saunders, Philadelphia, 1990:265.)

example, as in Figure 18.21, if 1:1 sensing occurs at 1.2 mV sensitivity and intermittently at 1.6 mV sensitivity, the final sensitivity should be programmed at 0.6 mV (so-called bracketing). In unipolar devices, atrial sensitivity should also be adjusted to avoid oversensing myopotential interference.

P wave undersensing may be due to causes other than a low electrographic signal, e.g., P wave falling in the postventricular atrial refractory period (145) (Fig. 18.22). If there are no stimuli, one cannot assume that a DDD pacemaker functions in the inhibited mode with sensing of both P waves and QRS complexes. Indeed, if the RR interval is shorter than the atrial escape interval, P wave undersensing can be masked (Fig. 10.23). Telemetry with event markers records sensing of a signal by the atrial channel (and its exact timing) and facilitates the diagnosis of atrial undersensing though markers cannot specifically identify a P wave. Precise confirmation of P wave sensing requires simultaneous recording of the ECG and the telemetered atrial electrogram. Ideally the ECG, event markers, and electrogram should be recorded simultaneously.

8. Special circumstances. In patients with dual-chamber

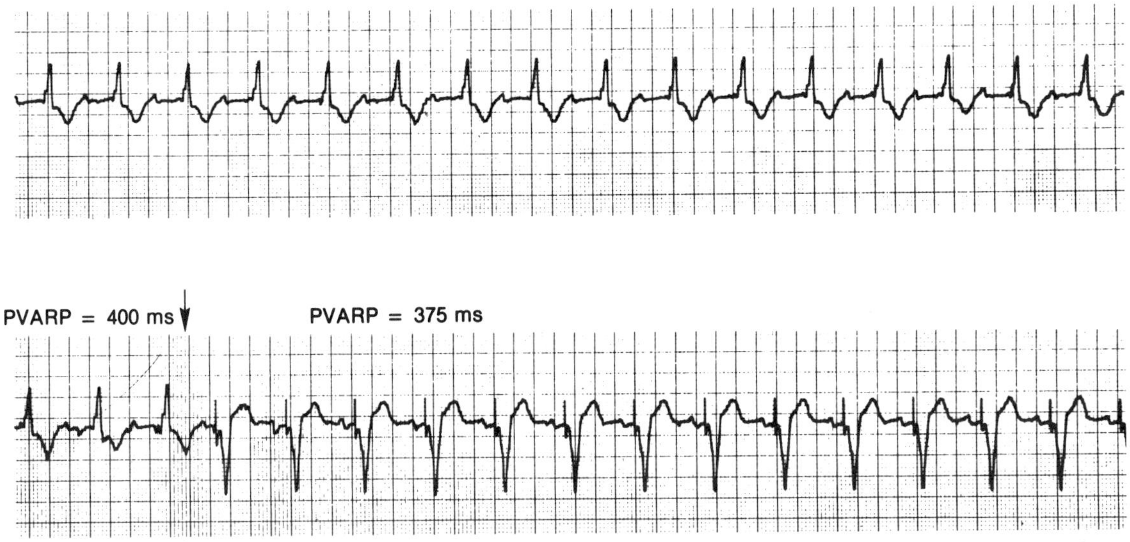

Figure 18.22. DDD pacing (lower rate 70 ppm, upper rate 135 ppm, AV interval 150 msec, PVARP 400 msec, ventricular refractory period 250 msec. Lack of P wave tracking (sensing) due to long PVARP (400 msec). The sinus rate is about 85/min and there is first-degree AV block. The P waves fall within the PVARP initiated by the preceding QRS complex. Shortening the PVARP to 375 msec (**bottom**) restores 1:1 atrial tracking with the programmed AV interval (150 msec). (Reproduced with permission from Barold SS, Falkoff, MD, Ong LS, *et al.*: Timing cycles of DDD pacemakers. In Barold SS, Mugica J (eds): New Perspectives in Cardiac Pacing. Futura Publishing Co., Mt. Kisco, NY, 1988:69.)

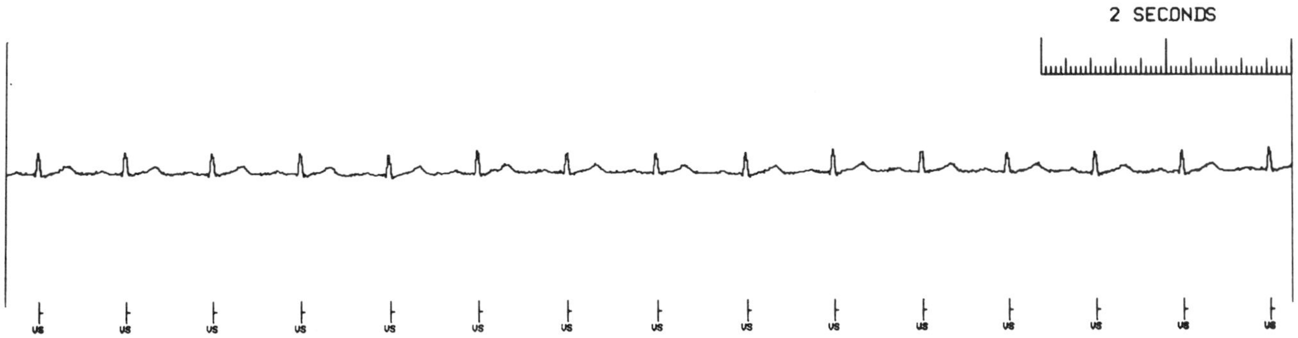

Figure 18.23. Surface ECG recorded simultaneously with marker channel showing that inhibition of DDD pulse generator does not necessarily imply normal atrial and ventricular sensing. The marker channel indicates that P waves are unsensed, but this is masked on the surface ECG. The interval between two consecutive QRS complexes is less than the atrial escape (or pacemaker VA) interval. Consequently the atrial escape interval is aborted when the pacemaker senses the QRS complex. P-wave undersensing is therefore masked. VS = ventricular sensed event. (Reproduced with permission from Barold SS, Falkoff MD, Ong LS, *et al.*: Electrocardiography of contemporary DDD pacemakers. B. Multiprogrammability, follow-up and troubleshooting. In Saksena S, Goldschlager N (eds): Electrical Therapy for Cardiac Arrhythmias. PACING, Antitachycardia Devices, Catheter Ablation. WB Saunders, Philadelphia, 1990:265.)

pacemakers, the propensity to endless loop tachycardia and crosstalk should be evaluated routinely. These situations as well as programming of the AV delay and the sensor response of rate-adaptive pacemakers are discussed elsewhere in this book (Chapters 15 and 16).

PACEMAKER MALFUNCTION

Loss of Capture by Visible Pacemaker Stimuli

The causes of loss of capture by visible pacemaker stimuli are listed in Table 18.3. Many of the abnormalities due to changes in the electrode-tissue interface can be overcome by noninvasive reprogramming or correcting any reversible metabolic or drug-related abnormalities. A temporary acute rise in the pacing threshold with loss of capture can occasionally be controlled with a course of steroid therapy, e.g., prednisone, 60 mg/day. If there is no fall in threshold in 4–6 days, the steroid should be discontinued and the lead repositioned. In some cases of chronic progressive increases in pacing threshold (so-called exit block), lead replacement is required.

Pacing Failure Without Pacemaker Stimuli

Absence of stimuli is usually due to pulse generator failure (battery or component, the latter being rare) or an open circuit with no current flow usually due to a broken electrode with intact insulation (Table 18.4). In the case of an open circuit, event marker telemetry can clearly demonstrate that the emitted stimuli do not reach the heart.

Abnormal Firing of Pacemaker Stimuli

A change in the pacing rate or erratic pacing should not be attributed to malfunction of the pulse generator (Table 18.5). Electronic malfunction is rare and often the diagnosis is one of exclusion. A constantly changing spike-to-spike interval during pacing is often due to an oversensing and/or electrode problem. Runaway pacemakers with rapid life-threatening stimulation are now rare, but no pacemaker should be considered immune to runaway behavior despite manufacturers' claim to the contrary (148,149) (Fig. 18.24). At rapid rates, stimulation is either ineffectual or intermittent. Rapid ventricular pacing may simulate spontaneous ventricular tachycardia if small stimuli are not identifiable. Rapid ventricular pacing rates must be differentiated from functional runaways of DDD pulse generators as in atrial fibrillation. True pacemaker runaway in any form requires immediate disconnection and removal of the pacemaker.

Undersensing

The most common cause of undersensing is a low amplitude electrogram delivered to a normally functioning pulse generator system. Lead dislodgement is the most likely cause of undersensing soon after implantation, and often correctable by reprogramming sensitivity. Occasionally the bipolar electrogram may be too small for sensing despite large unipolar electrograms from

Table 18.3.
Loss of Capture by Visible Pacemaker Stimuli

Electrode–tissue interface: (a) Early displacement or unstable position of pacing leads (most common cause) and late displacement in twiddler's syndrome, (b) perforation, (c) malposition into coronary sinus, middle cardiac vein, (d) elevated threshold (acute or chronic), (e) inapparent displacement (exit block), (f) subcutaneous emphysema with loss of anodal contact of unipolar pacemaker (146), (g) myocardial infarction, ischemia, or fibrosis, (h) hypothyroidism, (i) transient or chronic elevation of pacing threshold after defibrillation or cardioversion, (j) electrolyte abnormalities, e.g., hyperkalemia, severe acidosis, (k) drug toxicity, e.g., Type 1A antiarrhythmic agents or effect, e.g., Type 1C antiarrhythmic agents (flecainide, encainide, and propafenone)

Electrode: fracture and insulation leak

Pulse Generator: (a) Normally functioning pulse generator: inappropriate programming of output parameters, (b) spontaneous pacemaker failure due to battery exhaustion or component failure, (c) component failure from iatrogenic causes: defibrillation and therapeutic radiation.

Table 18.4.
Pacing Failure Without Pacemaker Stimuli

1. Normal situation—100% inhibition of pulse generator when the intrinsic rate is faster than the preset pacemaker rate
2. Normal function with programmed hysteresis: escape interval is longer than automatic interval
3. Pseudomalfunction—overlooking tiny bipolar pacemaker stimuli in the ECG
4. Lead fracture, loose connection, or set screw problem
5. Pulse generator: (a) battery depletion, (b) component failure, (c) sticky magnet reed switch (application of magnet produces no effect), (d) poor anodal contact: air in pacemaker pocket (subcutaneous emphysema) (147)
6. Extreme electromagnet interference
7. Oversensing (signal originating from outside or inside the pulse generator)

Table 18.5.
Problems Related to Stimulus Release

Normal Function of Pulse Generator
(a) Low programmed rate, (b) application of the magnet, (c) inaccurate speed of ECG machine drive, (d) apparent malfunction in special function pulse generator, e.g., hysteresis or triggered mode (AAT, VVT), (e) reversion to interference rate (in response to electromagnetic or other signals) with either a faster or a slower rate than the spontaneous freerunning or magnet rate.

Abnormal Function
(a) Battery failure (slowing of rate), (b) runaway pacemaker: spontaneous or consequent to therapeutic radiation or electric cautery, (c) component failure, e.g., erratic delivery of pacemaker stimuli: spontaneous or consequent to therapeutic radiation, (d) change of mode after defibrillation, electrocautery: DDD to VVI reset (no damage to pacemaker), (e) phantom reprogramming, misprogramming, etc., (f) oversensing.

the tip and proximal electrodes of a bipolar lead (150); the treatment consists of invasive or, if feasible, noninvasive unipolarization of the system (Fig. 18.25). Occasionally a VVI pacemaker senses the supraventricular QRS complex normally, but does not detect some ventricular extrasystoles because their electrogram is smaller, a situation not always correctable by reprogramming sensitivity. An adequate ventricular signal may become suboptimal after myocardial infarction, the development of bundle branch block, or with the passage of time. Lead maturation causes a small reduction in signal amplitude, but a significant drop in the slew rate (dV/dt) that may lead to undersensing, especially if the initial signal was relatively small (151). Undersensing due to electronic component failure is rare. An abnormal (jammed) magnet reed switch (that releases the asynchronous mode on magnet removal), inappropriate programming of sensitivity or refractory period may all cause undersensing. Asynchronous pacing also occurs as a protective response to continually sensed interference. Functional undersensing secondary to normal pacemaker function occurs when a QRS complex falls in the pacemaker ventricular refractory period or the ventricular blanking period (the latter is designed to prevent crosstalk in dual chamber pacemakers). Oversensing of an extraneous signal (by the initiation of a new pacemaker refractory period) can lead to undersensing of the succeeding QRS complex if the ventricular electrogram falls within the pacemaker refractory period initiated by the preceding undesirable sensed event (153) (Fig. 18.26B). Finally, ventricular pseudofusion beats should not be misinterpreted as undersensing.

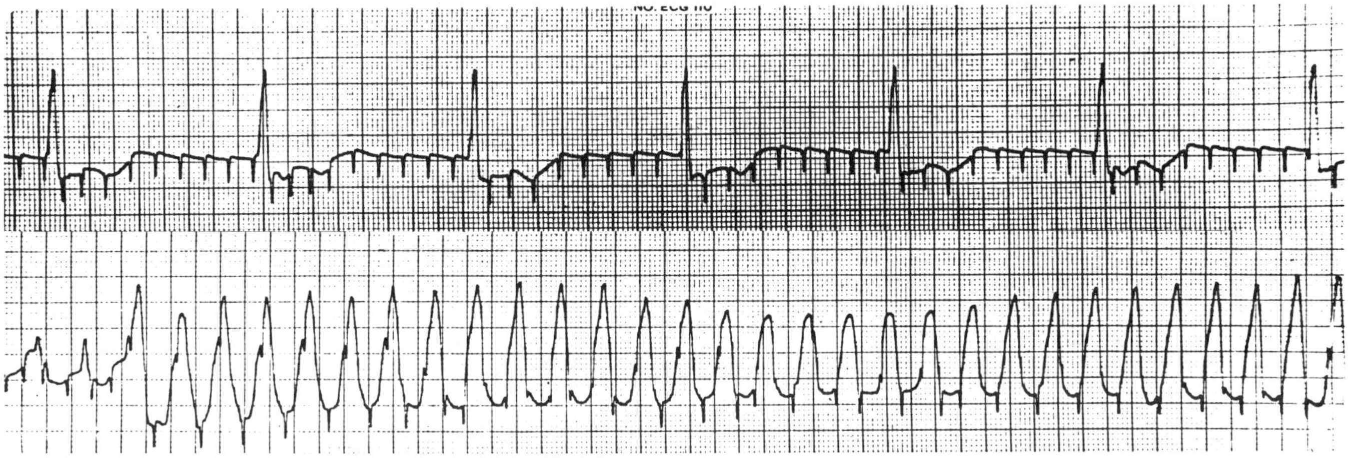

Figure 18.24. Runaway pacemaker. **Top:** the pacemaker rate is 300 beats/min and there is no capture. The patient's heart rate is 35 beats/min. **Bottom:** in the same patient, the pacemaker is now capturing at a rate of 166 beats/min. (Reproduced with permission from Smyth NPD, Millette ML: Complications of pacemaker implantation, In Barold SS (ed): Modern Cardiac Pacing. Futura Publishing Co., Mt. Kisco, NY, 1985:257.)

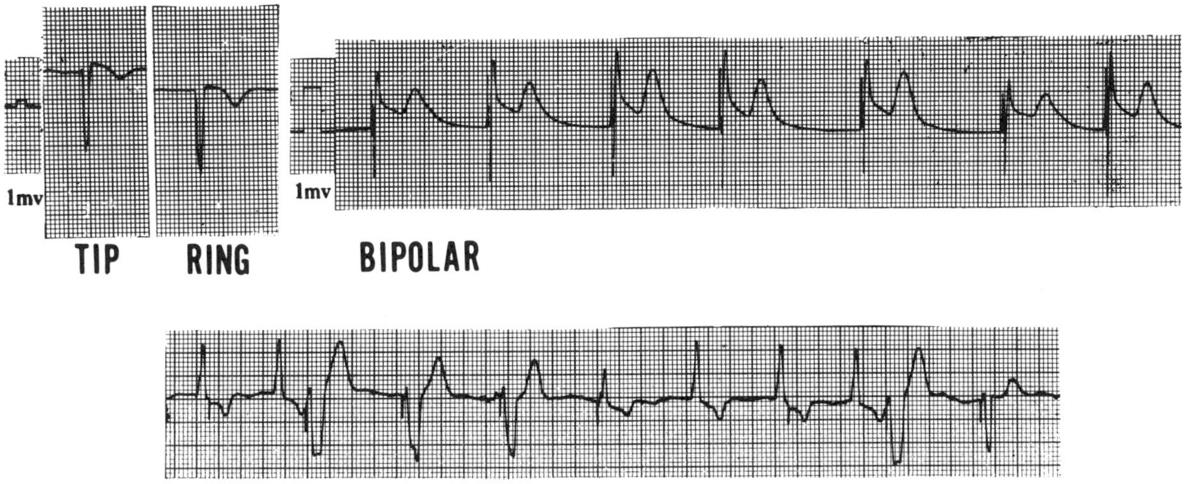

Figure 18.25. Bipolar VVI pacing with intermittent undersensing. Although the unipolar electrograms from the tip and ring electrodes are considerably larger than the programmed 2 mV sensitivity, the bipolar electrogram is much smaller and fluctuates with respiration, the lowest amplitude being slightly less than 2 mV. Conversion to a unipolar system with the tip as the negative pole restored normal sensing.

Insulation or wire fracture defects can also attenuate the effective electrogram detected by the pulse generator and cause undersensing (111,152). Hyperkalemia, toxic effects of antiarrhythmic drugs, and cardioversion-defibrillation can also lead to transient undersensing.

A substantial number of cases of atrial undersensing occurring in the first few days resolve spontaneously. Random rather than sustained loss of atrial sensing is not uncommon in Holter recordings, but rarely of important clinical significance. Atrial sensing may be influenced by changes in body position, respiration (Fig. 18.27), congestive heart failure, and exercise, the latter decreasing the amplitude of the atrial electrogram (154–158). Atrial sensing should be evaluated with deep respiration, lying, sitting, standing, and exercise if necessary.

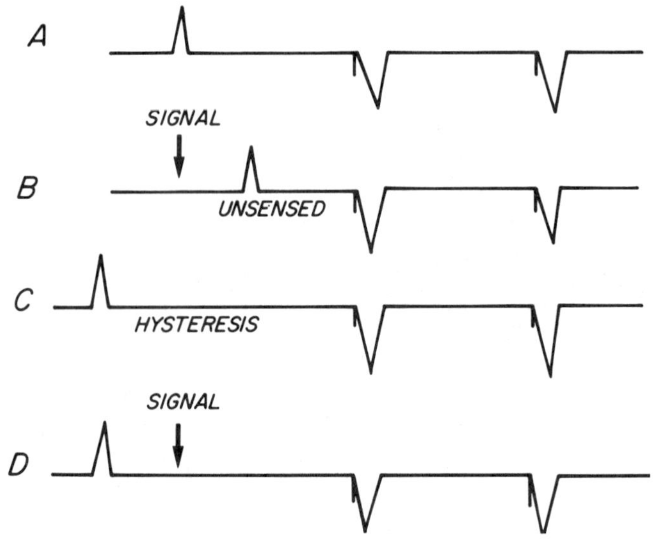

Figure 18.26. Relationship of escape interval (from sensed signal to the succeeding pacemaker stimulus) to automatic interval (corresponding with programmed pacemaker rate). **A,** Pacemaker with equal automatic and escape intervals. **B,** An inapparent signal (such as a false signal from an intermittent wire fracture) invisible on the surface electrocardiogram generates another pacemaker refractory period upon sensing. An ensuing QRS complex falling within the pacemaker refractory period will therefore be unsensed. **C,** Hysteresis: Programmable characteristic of pulse generators in which the escape interval is significantly longer than the automatic interval. **D,** Oversensing of a signal beyond the QRS complex may resemble the normal function of a pulse generator with hysteresis. (Reproduced with permission from Barold SS, Falkoff MD, Ong LS, *et al.*: Electrocardiographic diagnosis of pacemaker malfunction. In Wellens HJJ, Kulbertus HE (eds): What's New in Electrocardiography. The Hague, Martinus Nijhoff Publishers, 1981:236.)

Oversensing

Oversensing during VVI pacing causes pauses during VVI pacing and is a common clinical problem. A pause is defined as failure of delivery of a pacemaker stimulus at the anticipated time according to the programmed escape interval or automatic interval (159,160). Hysteresis should not be interpreted as oversensing (Fig. 18.26) With dual-chamber systems, oversensing should be evaluated sequentially by programming to single-chamber pacing, i.e., VVI and AAI modes. The following discussion focuses primarily on single lead ventricular pacing, but the same concepts apply to single-lead atrial and dual-chamber pacemakers. The diagnosis of oversensing can be easily confirmed by conversion to the asynchronous mode by application of the magnet over the pacemaker, a maneuver that eliminates arrhythmias specially related to the sensing mechanism. Unwanted signals causing oversensing may arise from several sources.

PHYSIOLOGIC VOLTAGES

P wave oversensing during VVI pacing is rare and occurs only with displacement of the lead toward the right ventricular inflow tract and a pacemaker programmed to a high sensitivity. Asystole can occur if the sinus rate exceeds the preset rate of the pacemaker (161) (Fig. 18.28). Emergency treatment consists of magnet application or programming to the VOO or VVT mode. T wave oversensing is rare, and often represents the detection of a summation voltage from the afterpotential of a paced beat and the generated T wave correctable by reprogramming the sensitivity and/or refractory period. The diagnosis of T wave sensing should always be one of exclusion. An acute increase in T wave voltage soon after implantation (related to current of injury at the electrode site) may cause oversensing, with the afterpotential as a necessary but passive bystander to achieve a combined voltage exceeding the sensitivity of the pulse generator. Such a transient abnormality is often of no clinical importance (162) and disappears permanently with regression of the current of injury. Similarly, any process that affects intracardiac T wave voltage

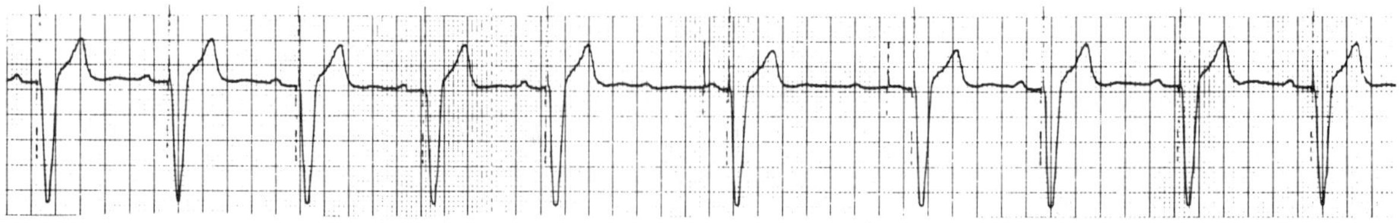

Figure 18.27. Intermittent failure of atrial sensing by a DDD pulse generator unraveled by deep inspiration. (Reproduced with permission from Barold SS, Falkoff MD, Ong LS, *et al.*: Electrocardiography of contemporary DDD pacemakers. B. Multiprogrammability, follow-up and troubleshooting. In Saksena S, Goldschlager N (eds): Electrical Therapy for Cardiac Arrhythmias. Pacing, antitachycardia devices, catheter ablation. WB Saunders, Philadelphia, 1990:265.)

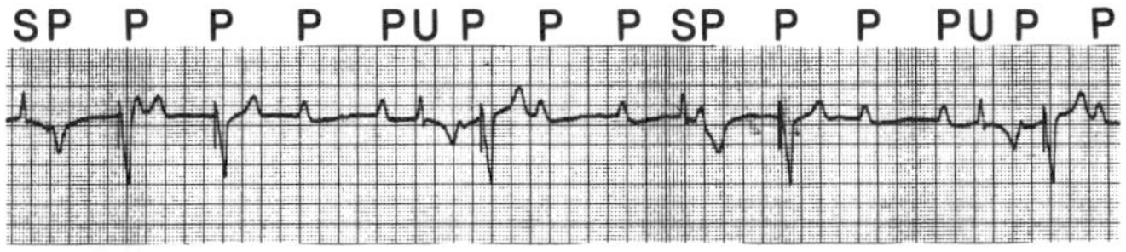

Figure 18.28. Intermittent P-wave sensing by a VVI pacemaker with a bipolar lead slightly displaced so that the proximal electrode lies in the inflow tract of the right ventricle. Although the spike-to-spike intervals vary in duration, the intervals from the onset of the sensed P wave to the next pacing stimulus are constant. (P = P wave, S = sensed QRS complex, U = unsensed QRS complex falling in the pacemaker refractory period (approximately 300 msec) generated to the preceding sensed P wave.) Undersensing of the QRS complex is secondary to oversensing of the P wave. (Reproduced with permission from Barold SS, Falkoff MD, Ong LS, *et al.*: Oversensing by single-chamber pacemakers: Mechanisms, diagnosis, and treatment. Cardiol Clin 1985;3:565.)

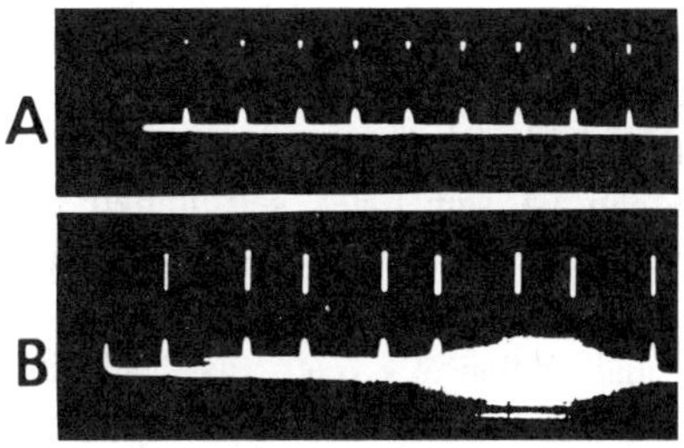

Figure 18.29. Oversensing of polarization voltage. Programmable demand pacemaker connected to an electrode lying in a saline bath. **A,** At a pulse width of 0.8 msec, the stimulation rate is 70/min without prolongation of the spike-to-spike interval. **B,** Reprogramming the pulse generator to a pulse width of 1.9 msec caused prolongation of the spike-to-spike interval resulting from intermittent sensing of the afterpotential. The pulse generator was removed from a patient who exhibited intermittent prolongation of the spike-to-spike interval (to a value equal to the sum of the automatic interval and the pacemaker refractory period) whenever the pulse width exceeded 0.6 msec. Narrowing the pulse width to 0.6 msec or less eliminated the problem in vivo. The patient continued to pace normally for several months at a narrower pulse width. The pulse generator was removed at autopsy after the patient died from noncardiac causes. (Reproduced with permission from Barold SS, Falkoff MD, Ong LS, *et al.*: Electrocardiographic diagnosis of pacemaker malfunction. In Wellens HJJ, Kulbertus HE (eds): What's New in Electrocardiography. The Hague, Martinus Nijhoff, 1981:236.)

such as ischemia or electrolyte imbalance may cause late T wave sensing. The late occurrence of T wave sensing is very rare and must be differentiated from a lead problem and pulse generator (component) failure, i.e., oversensing due to auto-interference within the pacemaker itself.

CONCEALED VENTRICULAR EXTRASYSTOLES

In 1972, Massumi, *et al.* (163) described a VVI pacemaker arrhythmia they attributed to oversensing of concealed ventricular extrasystoles (depolarization confined to the His-Purkinje system invisible on a conventional 12-lead ECG (164). Although these observations are subject to several plausible alternative interpretations, many workers believe that this phenomenon exists because remarkable pharmacologic suppression of oversensing can be achieved with antiarrhythmic drugs (165). However, oversensing of concealed ventricular extrasystoles must still be considered speculative in the absence of direct recordings from the pacing leads (159, 166).

VOLTAGES GENERATED IN THE PACING SYSTEM ITSELF INDEPENDENT OF CARDIAC ACTIVITY

Afterpotential

Delivery of the pacemaker stimulus charges the electrode-tissue interface to a large direct current potential (polarization voltage) subsequently dissipated over a relatively long period. The decay of the "afterpotential" constitutes a time change in voltage that may be sensed when the pacemaker comes out of its refractory period (Fig. 18.29). Afterpotential sensing should be suspected whenever the interval between two consecutive pacemaker stimuli lengthens to a value approximately equal to the sum of one automatic interval and the paced (delivery) refractory period of the pulse generator. Appropriate design of pacemaker circuitry has greatly minimized or even completely eliminated afterpotential sensing by the incorporation of a "fast recharge" circuit in the output stage. Despite this protection, oversensing of the afterpotential may occasionally occur when a pulse generator is programmed to a high sensitivity (or relatively short refractory period) and a high output in terms of pulse width and voltage, especially in association with an increase in the pacing rate (e.g., VVIR pacing) because the faster rate prevents full dissipation of the afterpotential (159) between pacemaker stimuli. Afterpotential oversensing can be eliminated by one of the following maneuvers: (a) prolongation of the pacemaker refractory period to contain the significant portion of the afterpotential, (b) decrease of the sensitivity (provided the QRS complex is still sensed), (c) decrease of the pulse width if capture continues, (d) avoidance of output voltage greater than the conventional 5–5.4 V.

False Signals

Abrupt and large changes in resistance within a pacing system can produce corresponding voltage changes between the anode and the cathode in the form of relatively large (false) signals (154,160,167,168). The exact diagnosis of oversensing of false signals (or voltage transients) is important to avoid the unnecessary replacement of a normally functioning pulse generator in the presence of a defective electrode system. False signals may be difficult to diagnose because they are often invisible on the standard 12-lead electrocardiogram. Such "make-break" signals may occur with intermittent derangement of a pacemaker circuit from loose connections, wire fractures with otherwise well-opposed ends, short circuits, insulation defects (159, 160,167,168), poorly designed active fixation leads (electrode chatter (169–171), or the interaction of two catheters (one active and the other one inactive) lying side by side, touching each other within the heart (172–174). Electrode chatter from a screw-in lead can be sometimes self-limited and disappear because of fibrous tissue with electrode stabilization over a period of several weeks (169).

Intermittent malfunction of a ventricular lead with oversensing constitutes the great imitator in cardiac pacing and often causes a chaotic pattern of pacing. Erratic pacemaker behavior with pauses of varying length strongly suggests defective lead system rather than pacemaker malfunction. False signals tend to occur at random and very long records will often reveal relatively long irregular and constantly changing pauses with or without spontaneous beats (Fig. 18.30). During ventricular pacing, the characteristic occurrence of false signals late in the cardiac cycle (determined by the timing of the pacemaker escape interval) permits the exclusion of P- or T-wave oversensing by simple scrutiny of the electrocardiogram. Resetting of the pacemaker (initiation of new escape intervals) from sensing false signals can mimic T wave sensing and/or afterpotential sensing. The differential diagnosis is important because T wave and/or afterpotential sensing are relatively harmless at worst causing only pacemaker bradycardia, whereas oversensing of false signals can be the earliest manifestation of a potentially catastrophic lead disruption.

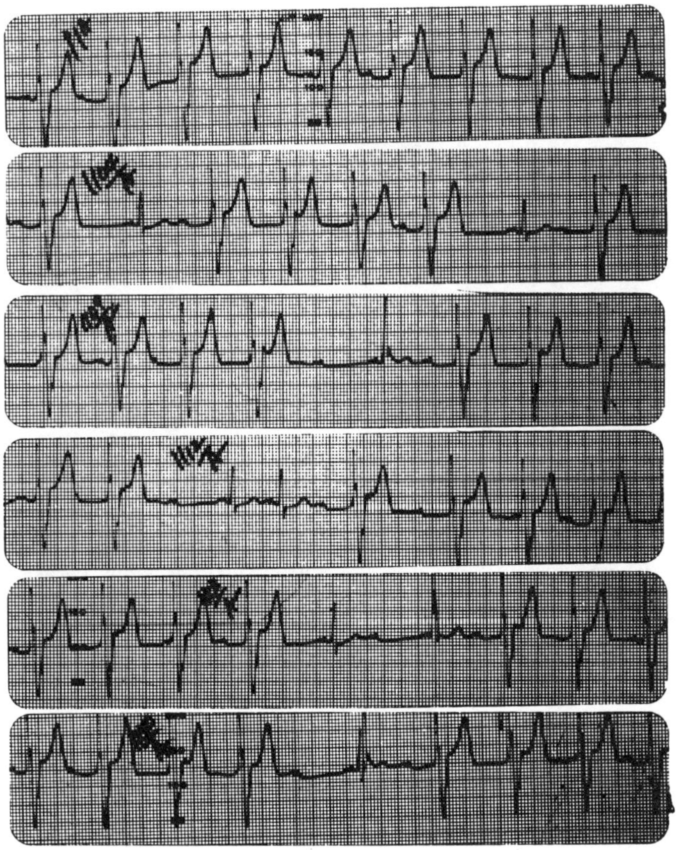

Figure 18.30. Irregular pacemaker pauses due to oversensing of false signals from a loose connection of a unipolar electrode into the pacemaker connector. (Reproduced with permission from Barold SS, Falkoff MD, Ong LS, *et al.*: Differential diagnosis of pacemaker pauses. In Barold SS (ed): Modern Cardiac Pacing. Futura Publishing Co., Mt. Kisco, NY, 1985:587.)

Testing Magnet

Conversion to asynchronous (VOO or AOO) pacing eliminates all arrhythmias related to oversensing. In the VVI mode, application of the magnet converts the irregular and constantly changing spike-to-spike intervals to a mathematically precise value that may be double, triple, or an exact multiple of the basic spike-to-spike or automatic interval (175). The demonstration of pacemaker pauses that are exact multiples of the automatic interval during asynchronous pacing (with the magnet) is diagnostic of an intermittent wire fracture (or electrode problem) and reflects the correct and undisturbed timing of a normally functioning pulse generator delivering its impulse into a transiently disrupted circuit with high impedance (175) (Fig. 18.31). When the spontaneous rhythm is faster than the present rate of the pacemaker, the absence of pacemaker stimuli conceals the occurrence of false signals. In this situation, the demonstration of mathematically precise prolongation of the spike-to-spike interval during asynchronous (AOO or VOO) pacing (as an exact multiple of the automatic interval) by means of a testing magnet may be the only diagnostic abnormality of an intermittent wire fracture.

An intermittent wire fracture can present as a pure sensing problem if its timing always allows the fractured ends to be in contact whenever the pacemaker delivers its impulse. The defective portion of the pacemaker lead may induce rhythmic recycling of a VVI pacemaker if mechanical systole consistently creates a false signal by making or breaking the circuit (168,176). Such an abnormality may be indistinguishable from T wave sensing because of its timing, regularity and conversion to normal asynchronous pacing with magnet application.

Irregularity of the Spike-to-Spike Interval Produced by Movement or Motion

Wire fractures, insulation breaks, or loose connections may produce false signals and irregular spike-to-spike intervals only in relation to certain body movements: going from the supine to sitting or standing position, pushing or applying traction on the pulse generator (and lead), deep respiration, or arm raising. Many of the body movements ordinarily associated with myopotential inhibition of unipolar pacemakers may actually unmask an occult lead problem. Thus, the pauses related to false signals may mimic oversensing of skeletal myopotentials (in unipolar pacemakers), especially if regular asynchronous (VOO or AOO) pacing occurs after application of the magnet.

Telemetry and Recording of the Intracardiac Electrogram

Telemetry permits the diagnosis of false signals noninvasively (Fig. 18.32). Lead impedance can also be determined by telemetry (high with fracture, low with insulation defect). If the diagnosis remains in doubt, the presence of false signals should

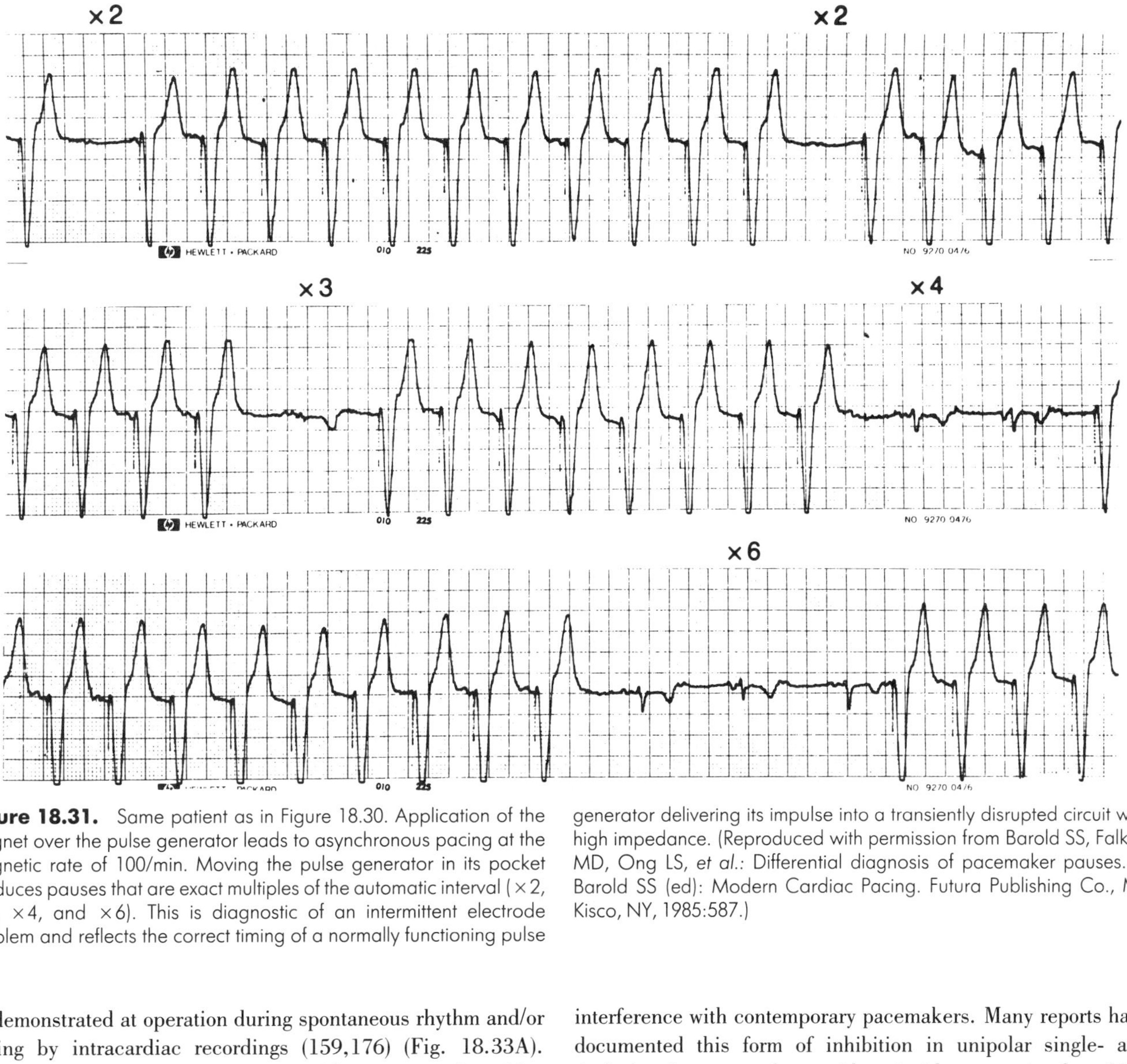

Figure 18.31. Same patient as in Figure 18.30. Application of the magnet over the pulse generator leads to asynchronous pacing at the magnetic rate of 100/min. Moving the pulse generator in its pocket produces pauses that are exact multiples of the automatic interval (×2, ×3, ×4, and ×6). This is diagnostic of an intermittent electrode problem and reflects the correct timing of a normally functioning pulse generator delivering its impulse into a transiently disrupted circuit with high impedance. (Reproduced with permission from Barold SS, Falkoff MD, Ong LS, *et al.*: Differential diagnosis of pacemaker pauses. In Barold SS (ed): Modern Cardiac Pacing. Futura Publishing Co., Mt. Kisco, NY, 1985:587.)

be demonstrated at operation during spontaneous rhythm and/or pacing by intracardiac recordings (159,176) (Fig. 18.33A). Pacemaker pauses without demonstrable corresponding false signals or other sources of interference with good intracardiac recording techniques suggest autointerference, i.e., oversensing of spurious signals generated by the pacemaker generator itself within its own internal circuity. Such autointerference may disappear upon application of the magnet, erroneously suggesting an external source of oversensing (159).

MUSCULOSKELETAL INTERFERENCE

Oversensing of myopotential interference remains by far the most common cause of pacemaker pauses and occurs almost invariably with unipolar pulse generators. Myopotential inhibition occurs rarely in bipolar systems, under special circumstances. Wirzfield, *et al.* (177) first described the inhibition of unipolar demand pulse generators by skeletal muscle potentials in 1972. Barold, *et al.* (178) recently reviewed the status of myopotential interference with contemporary pacemakers. Many reports have documented this form of inhibition in unipolar single- and dual-chamber pacemakers, with an incidence varying from 12 to 85% (178, 179) (Fig. 18.34). No unipolar pacemaker is totally immune to myopotential oversensing. The advent of advanced unipolar dual-chamber pacemakers and the need for high sensitivity to sense atrial activity have not reduced the incidence of myopotential oversensing seen with earlier generations of unipolar single-chamber pacemakers (178). As a rule, myopotential interference can be demonstrated in about 50% of patients with unipolar pulse generators by a variety of isometric exercise maneuvers, although inhibition may not be consistently reproducible. Probably only 10% of patients with demonstrable myopotential inhibition are actually symptomatic during ordinary life and require intervention such as reprogramming. Most myopotential interference originates from the deltopectoral region at the site of a unipolar pulse generator. Table 18.6 shows the various maneuvers used to bring out myopotential interference. Hyperadduction of the ipsilateral arm, reaching as far as possi-

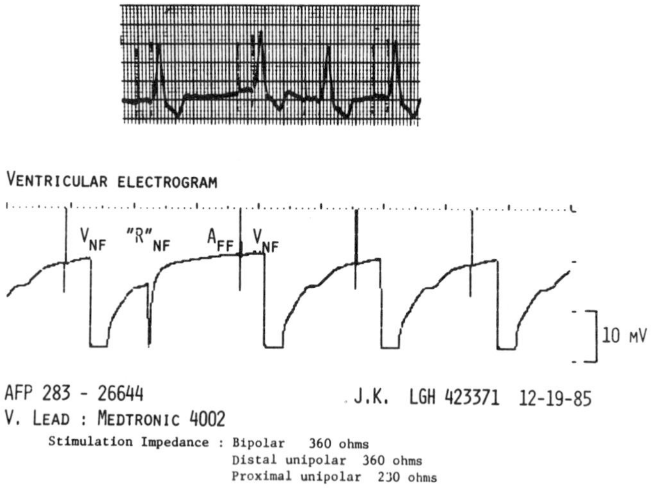

Figure 18.32. Insulation defect. Surface ECG recorded with an analog ECG machine and telemetered electrogram, A_{FF} is the far-field atrial stimulus. V_{NF} is the near-field ventricular stimulus which saturates the sense amplifier driving the telemetered recording off of the field. "R"$_{NF}$ is the near-field spurious transient which is being sensed by the pacemaker causing it to inhibit and recycle. It does not correspond to any visible event on the surface ECG nor was it associated with a repolarization phase, making it unlikely that it was a concealed ectopic beat. The invasively measured stimulation impedances are noted. (Reproduced with permission from Levine PA: Clinical manifestations of lead insulation defects. J Electrophysiol 1987;1:152.)

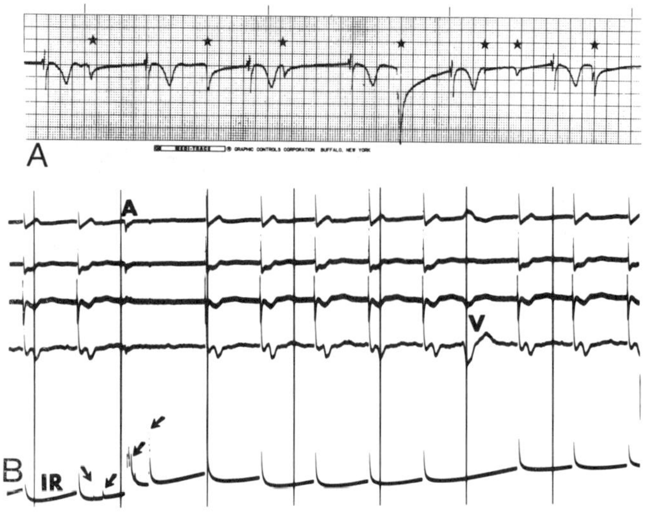

Figure 18.33. False signals demonstrated during spontaneous rhythm (rate about 40/min) by recording the unipolar ventricular (intracardiac) electrogram (1/4 standardization). There is baseline artifact (*stars*) caused by an intermittent lead fracture. Note varying morphology and amplitude of the false signals. The smaller false signals should not be misinterpreted as P waves as the latter are exceedingly small in ventricular electrograms recorded from the right ventricular apex. **B,** Diagnosis of intermittent wire fracture by intracardiac recording (IR) of the pacemaker waveform, i.e., electrogram during ventricular pacing. The four surface ECGs on **top** show prolongation of the spike-to-spike interval. There is a sudden break of lead continuity due to momentary separation of the fractured ends, with the production of false signals (*arrows*). The last arrow points to the false signal that actually initiates the last escape interval, terminating with emission of the third ventricular stimulus. **A** refers to an artifact occasionally seen during pacing on the surface ECG with intermittent unipolar lead malfunction as in a fracture. The sudden and large change of the electrical field in the heart can cause corresponding small artifacts on the surface ECG seen only in unipolar systems (Fig. 18.39). (These electrode artifacts are usually tiny, sometimes distinct only on a high-fidelity recorder when invisible on the standard ECG because of attenuation and bandwidth characteristics. Tiny deflections during bipolar pacing are almost invariably not discernible electrocardiographically.) The amplitude of the pacemaker waveform (electrogram) was considerably attenuated to allow appropriate recordings during pacing so that the false signals are much larger than those in **A** recorded during spontaneous rhythm. V = ventricular extrasystole. (Reproduced with permission from Barold SS, *et al.*: Differential diagnosis of pacemaker pauses. In Barold SS, (eds): Falkoff MD, Ong LS, *et al.*: Modern Cardiac Pacing. Futura Publishing Co., Mt. Kisco, NY, 1985:587.)

ble around the chest, coupled with pressure on the contralateral shoulder is the most sensitive test for deltopectoral myopotential interference.

Some workers claim that Holter documentation of myopotential inhibition correlates more closely than other methods with the likelihood of symptoms and demonstrable interference by a variety of maneuvers (110,180). However, others believe that most patients who display myopotential inhibition during Holter recordings show the same tendency during testing with provocative maneuvers (118). According to Gaita, *et al.* (181), Holter recordings offer few advantages over the routine provocative tests for the detection of myopotential inhibition.

Telemetry of the Intracardiac Electrogram

The capability of telemetric transmission of the intracardiac electrograms has added a new dimension to the diagnosis and treatment of myopotential oversensing (Fig. 18.35). In particular, it allows determination of the signal amplitude to guide programmability of the atrial or ventricular sensitivity to eliminate oversensing while preserving P wave and/or QRS complex sensing in AAI, VVI, and DDD pacing systems (109,112,182).

Single-Chamber Pacing

Myopotential interference may cause various combinations of oversensing and undersensing. Pacemaker pauses due to oversensing may occasionally be accompanied by periods of undersensing as a consequence of oversensing rather than pacemaker malfunction or an electrographic signal below the sensitivity of the pulse generator. Undersensing secondary to oversensing is caused by one of two mechanisms: (a) a sensed signal generates a new pacemaker refractory period. If a spontaneous signal (e.g., a QRS complex) then falls within the newly generated pacemaker refractory period, undersensing occurs (153,178); (b) repetitive signals may cause reversion of the pacemaker to its interference (noise) asynchronous mode (183). The reversion circuit depends on continuous and rapid sensing of myopotentials for the conversion to the

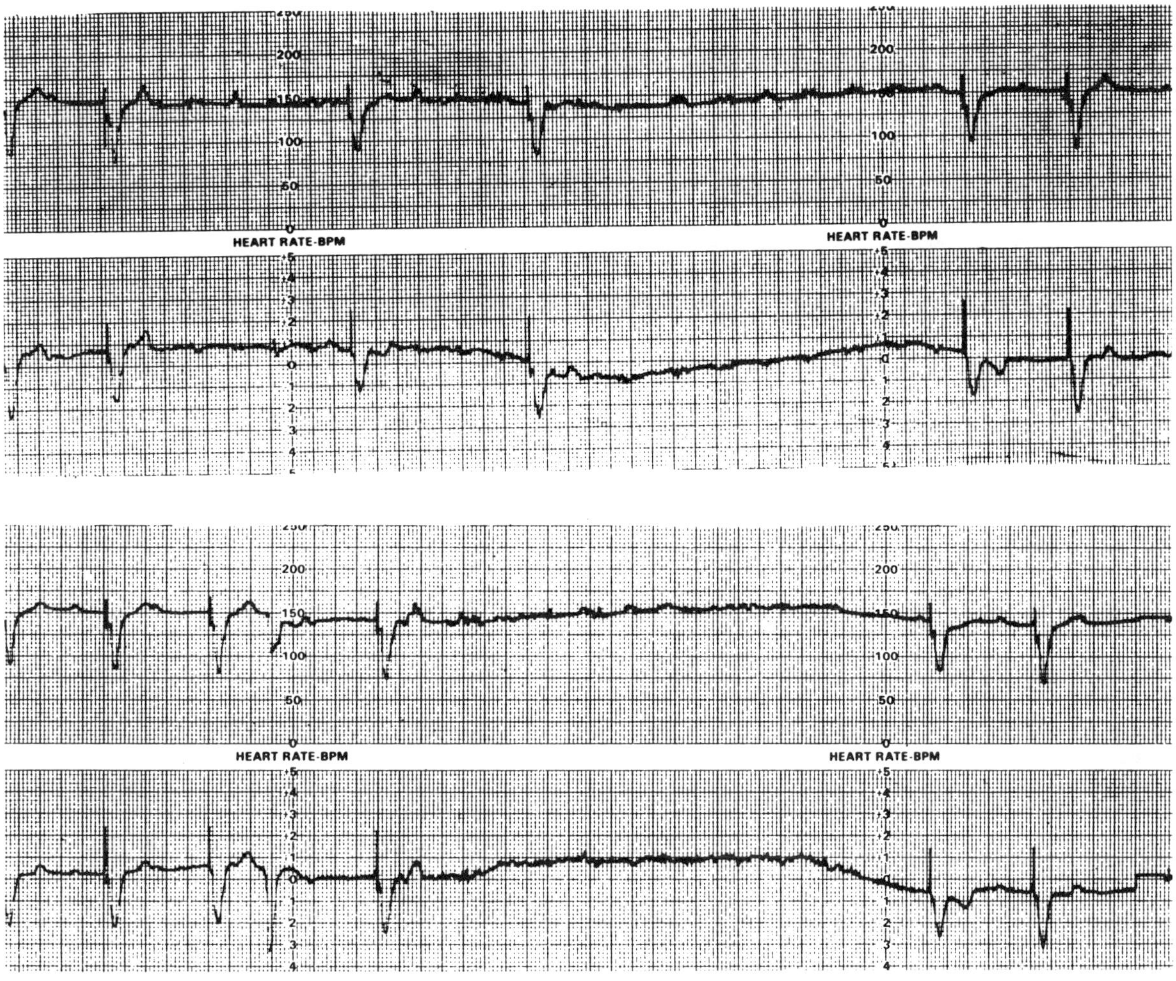

Figure 18.34. Representative tracings from a Holter recording showing marked myopotential inhibition of a unipolar pulse generator. The patient presented with near-syncope. The pauses were eliminated by reprogramming the sensitivity of the pacemaker. (Reproduced with permission from Barold SS, Falkoff MD, Ong LS, *et al.*: Differential diagnosis of pacemaker pauses. In Barold SS (ed): Modern Cardiac Pacing. Futura Publishing Co., Mt. Kisco, NY, 1985:587.)

asynchronous interference (noise) mode. The reversion circuit does not always safeguard the pulse generator from continuous inhibition. For example, if the amplitude of myopotential signals is rapidly changing, sensing may be intermittent and the sensed rate may not exceed the reversion limit. Such a situation causes inhibition rather than asynchronous pacing.

DDD Pacing

The atrial and ventricular channels of a unipolar pacemaker receive myopotential signals of identical amplitude because they arise from the same pectoral site. According to the programmed atrial and ventricular sensitivities, the following manifestations may occur (184,185):

1. Inhibition of the ventricular channel.
2. Sensing by the atrial channel with consequent triggering of a ventricular output and an increase in the pacing rate, producing a pacemaker tachycardia that may cause uncomfortable palpitations, angina, dyspnea, and hypotension if rapid ventricular pacing occurs for more than a brief period (Fig. 18.36).
3. Mixed response of alternating triggering and ventricular inhibition.
4. Reversion to interference (noise) asynchronous pacing for one or more cycles (183,184).
5. Precipitation of endless loop tachycardia by myopotential sensing by the atrial channel (186).
6. Abbreviation of the AV interval if myopotentials are sensed in the ventricular safety pacing period of a pulse generator possessing this feature (187).

Table 18.6.
Common Testing Maneuvers for Myopotential Interference

Deltopectoral muscles
Pressing palm of hand against that of observer or against wall
Pressing one hand against the other
Pushing hard against contralateral shoulder
Lifting or flexing arm against resistance
Adduction of arm against resistance
Hyperadduction reach test
Isometric handgrip
Treadmill stress test
Rectus Abdominis Muscles
Trunk lifting from or reclining backward to supine position
Lifting and holding legs 20° to the horizontal against resistance
Treadmill stress test
Diaphragm
Deep inspiration
Valsalva maneuver, straining, coughing, laughing, sneezing

Sources of Myopotentials Other than Deltopectoral Region

Pectoralis major myopotentials have been traditionally considered as the main source of pacemaker inhibition, but the rectus abdominis, diaphragm, and intercostal muscles may also contribute myopotentials capable of being sensed by pulse generators.

Rectus Abdominis

The rectus abdominis may contribute significantly to myopotential inhibition under certain circumstances (188). The rectus abdominis may be an important source of myopotential interference in about 40% of pacemakers implanted in the abdominal wall. Myopotentials from the pectoralis and rectus abdominis may act synergistically and indeed in some cases this synergy is required to provoke pacemaker inhibition irrespective of the location of the pacemaker. Thus, pulse generators implanted over the pectoral region uninfluenced by local potentials can occasionally be inhibited only by the rectus abdminis myopotentials.

Diaphragmatic Myopotentials

Oversensing of diaphragmatic myopotentials is considered rare, but well documented with normally functioning unipolar and bipolar VVI pacing systems (not necessarily related to catheter perforation) (189–192). Transient inhibition of a pacemaker by diaphragmatic myopotentials may be provoked by deep respiration and active contraction of the diaphragm during straining, Valsalva maneuver, coughing, sneezing, and laughing, especially when the pulse generator is programmed with high sensitivity (Fig. 18.37). Oversensing of diaphragmatic myopotentials

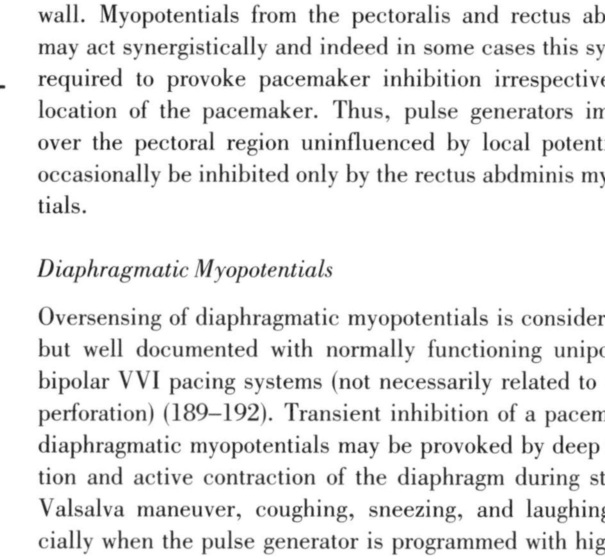

Figure 18.35. Myopotential interference recorded on the telemetered atrial electrogram in a patient with a Pacesetter 283 AFP unipolar DDD pulse generator. Note the relatively large amplitude of myopotential interference at times exceeding 2 mV. (Reproduced with permission from Barold SS, Falkoff MD, Ong LS, *et al.*: Interference in cardiac pacemakers. Endogenous sources. In El-Sherif N, Samet P (eds): Cardiac Pacing and Electrophysiology, 3rd ed. WB Saunders, Philadelphia, 1991:634.)

is an unimportant clinical problem because the pauses are relatively short and always correctable by appropriate programming of sensitivity.

Intercostal Myopotentials

I have observed myopotential triggering of unipolar DDD pulse generators with a J lead in the right atrial appendange, during deep inspiration at a very high sensitivity of the atrial channel (Fig. 18.38). In contrast, with the same or even higher sensitivity, diaphragmatic inhibition of the ventricular channel could not be demonstrated both in the DDD and VVI mode. Sensing of intercostal myopotentials by the atrial channel seems possible with both unipolar and bipolar atrial electrodes, although detection of intercostal myopotentials with bipolar systems has not yet been reported. Such intercostal myopotentials sensed by the atrial channel can be easily mistaken for other signals, such as atrial extrasystoles or myopotentials originating from the pectoral area in the case of unipolar pacemakers.

Myopotential Oversensing During Bipolar Pacing

Skeletal myopotential interference in bipolar pacing systems cannot be demonstrated under ordinary circumstances, and the geometry of the sensing electrodes makes its occurrence difficult to understand. During testing for myopotential oversensing, if the baseline of the ECG becomes grossly blurred, transient acceleration of the spontaneous rhythm with the occurrence of ventricular extrasystoles may be invisible and, if sensed, the resultant pauses may be attributed to myopotential inhibition (pseudointerference). However, myopotential sensing by a bipolar device may occur in relation to: (a) Diaphragmatic myopotentials. (b) Insulation leak of a bipolar system (193,194). An insulation leak of a pacing lead relatively close to a pulse generator may detect myopotentials and inhibit a bipolar pulse generator that has essentially been converted to a unipolar-bipolar system. (c) ? Intercostal myopotentials.

Management of Myopotential Oversensing

With multiprogrammability, there are four ways of dealing with myopotential oversensing: (a) Reduction of input sensitivity. In some pulse generators, even programming to the lowest sensitivity may not correct the problem and may also lead to undersensing of the QRS complex (or P wave in the case of AAI pacing). (b) Conversion to the triggered of VVT (AAT) mode with nominal sensitivity may allow optimal sensing of the QRS complex, but there may be periods of undesirable increase in the pacing rate (on sensing of myopotentials), and the VVT mode cannot prevent firing on the T wave. (c) Programmability from the unipolar to the bipolar mode, an option available in some pulse generators. (d) Conversion to VOO (AOO) or asynchronous mode.

Despite spectacular improvements in pacemaker technology, the incidence of myopotential interference has remained unchanged over the last 20 yr. Engineering efforts and surgical techniques have not resolved the myopotential problem during unipolar pacing. Absolute discrimination between the cardiac electrogram and skeletal muscle potentials is difficult and probably impossible in some circumstances, because the frequency spectrum of the myopotential signal overlaps that of the P wave and QRS complex. The amplitude of myopotentials may be as high as 4.5 mV. Myopotential inhibition became an important clinical problem only because of the popularity of unipolar pulse generators. In contemporary pacemaker practice, sensing and stimulating characteristics of unipolar and bipolar pacing systems are basically similar, but bipolar pulse generators provide a superior signal-to-noise ratio and better rejection of far-field interference. The previous advantages of unipolar pacing (e.g., smaller electrode size) have disappeared with the advent of multiprogrammability and smaller bipolar leads (because of changes in insulating material and introduction of coaxial conductors). Bipolar systems will probably regain their previous preeminence because of their better rejection of myopotential and other types of interference. In this way, bipolar systems permit the use of higher sensitivity settings for optimal sensing.

ABNORMAL LEAD FUNCTION

Fractures and insulation problems usually occur in the extravascular part of the lead (195,196). Extrinsic stress may cause lead damage, fracture and/or insulation at two sites: (a) at the site of the suture sleeve that anchors the lead, and (b) where the lead traverses the plane between the first rib and the clavicle on its way to the subclavian vein. Bipolar coaxial leads are particularly susceptible to the clamping effect of widening and narrowing the space between the clavicle and the first rib by arm motion, the so-called crush injury. The crush complication occurs if the point of entry into the subclavian vein is too *medial* and appears specifically related to subclavian vein access by the introducer technique (197–201). A strong ligature over the lead may also cause the same problem. Compression of the lead by a holding suture may cause the radiologic appearance of lead disruption (pseudofracture) by separating the conductor coil by the suture (202,203). A pseudofracture requires no action, but it may later become a site of insulation breakdown or fracture of the lead. With a real lead fracture, the chest x-ray can sometimes show an obvious conduction discontinuity, but the diagnostic sensitivity of x-rays is not very good in this situation.

The manifestations of an insulation break are as follows: (a) Extracardiac muscle stimulation. (b) In bipolar systems, the stimuli can increase considerably in size and the vector of the pacemaker impulse changes in direction because the pacemaker functions as a bipolar-unipolar system (distal tip electrode to proximal electrode and distal electrode to the insulation defect). These abnormalities are valid only with analog ECG recordings. (c) Loss of capture due to shunting of current away from the stimulating electrodes. Excessive current loss leads to premature battery depletion. (d) Undersensing due to signal attentuation and/or oversensing (Fig. 18.26B). Telemetry of the electro-

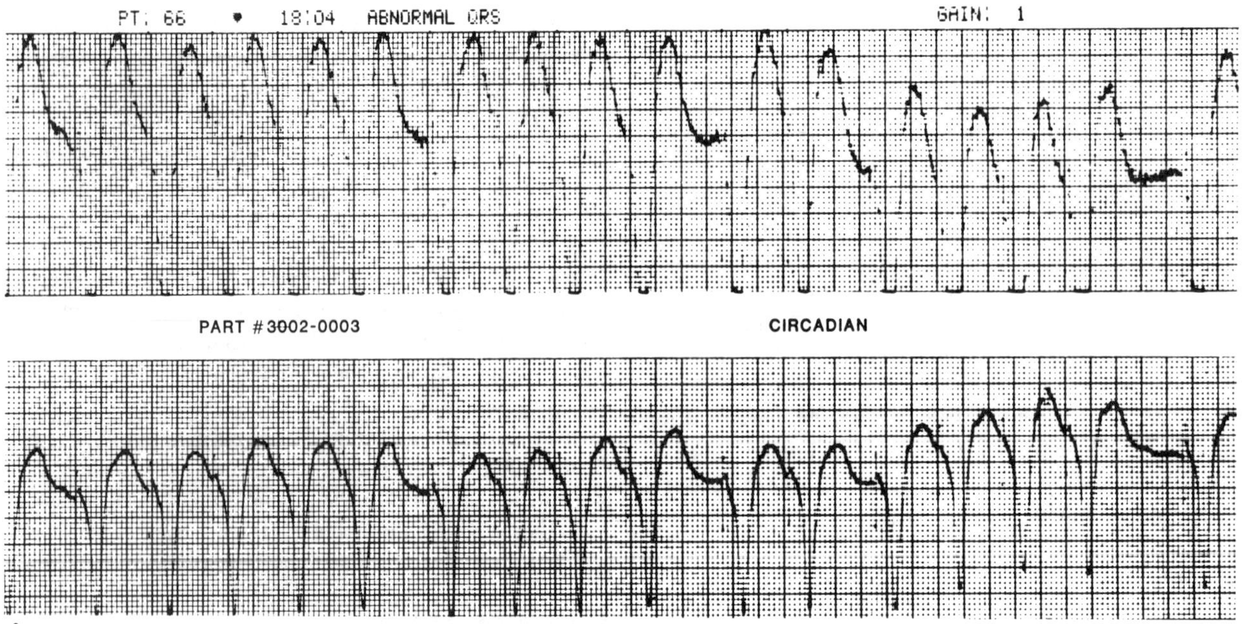

A

COSMOS DDD
LOWER RATE = 60 ppm (1000 ms)
UPPER RATE INTERVAL = 120 ppm (480 ms)
AV INTERVAL = 205 ms
PVARP = 200 ms
ATRIAL SENSITIVITY = 0.8 mV

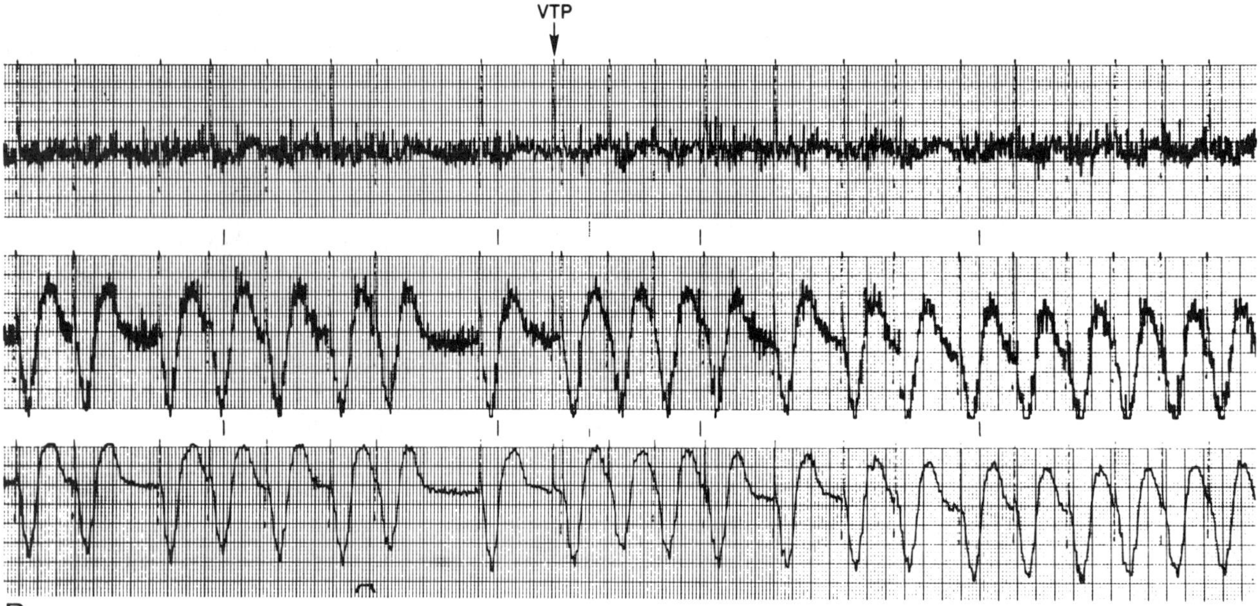

B

gram may show gradual reduction in amplitude during follow-up (111,152,205). (e) Pacemaker pauses from oversensing of false signals. Telemetry of the electrogram or event markers may reveal false signals. (f) Telemetry shows an abnormally low lead impedance (< 250 ohms).

Lead fracture is characterized by (a) no stimuli, i.e., an open circuit. (b) stimuli without capture, (c) attenuation of unipolar stimuli with or without capture (Fig. 18.39). (d) oversensing of false signals. Telemetry of electrograms or event markers may show false signals, (e) undersensing due to signal attenuation and/or oversensing (Fig. 18.26B), (f) telemetry shows an abnormally high impedance (>1000 ohms). If there is a concomitant insulation defect, the impedance may be normal or minimally elevated.

With a suspected insulation break or fracture, one should apply pressure along the course of the subcutaneous portion of the lead, extend the ipsilateral arm as high as possible, place the arm behind the back, and rotate the shoulder backward to unmask a crush injury due to clavicle-first rib compression (85).

DIFFERENTIAL DIAGNOSIS OF TACHYCARDIA DURING DDD PACING

Tachycardia during DDD pacing is a common problem, and the diagnosis is often quite simple (206). The diagnosis of tachycardia during DDD pacing is facilitated by telemetry of the atrial electrogram to identify atrial depolarization and by event markers to demonstrate how the pacemaker interprets sensed events. Carotid sinus pressure should be applied in the usual fashion for the differential diagnosis of supraventricular tachycardia. Application of the magnet (slower DOO or VOO mode) may reveal P waves. Programming the pulse generator to the VVI mode at a relatively slow rate allows analysis of atrial activity. A Wenckebach upper rate response of a DDD pacemaker suggests that the atrial rate is faster than the programmed upper rate of the pacemaker, but does not rule out sinus tachycardia, particularly if the programmed upper rate is relatively slow.

A rapid and irregular ventricular pacing rate suggests the diagnosis of atrial fibrillation or flutter (207,208). In both atrial flutter and atrial fibrillation, varying amplitude of the atrial f waves may lead to intermittent loss of atrial sensing, with the occasional delivery of atrial stimuli at the end of the atrial escape interval. Such a response coupled with periods of rapid and irregular ventricular pacing produces a chaotic pattern virtually diagnostic of underlying atrial flutter or fibrillation (Fig. 18.40). Atrial flutter or fibrillation can occasionally produce regular and rapid ventricular pacing, sometimes at the upper rate, thereby mimicking endless loop tachycardia with retrograde VA conduction. In endless loop tachycardia, application of the magnet terminates the tachycardia, while in atrial flutter or fibrillation, slower pacing in the DOO mode will reveal the regular, characteristic f waves of atrial flutter or the fibrillatory waves of atrial fibrillation, with immediate resumption of the same tachycardia on removal of the magnet. Telemetry of the atrial electrogram and/or markers facilitates the diagnosis (Figs. 18.6 and 18.41). Programming to the VVI mode at a slow rate often provides the diagnosis. The diagnosis of atrial flutter and fibrillation is one of exclusion, particularly when telemetry of the intracardiac atrial electrogram or event markers are not available.

Endless loop tachycardia related to sensing of retrograde atrial depolarization is almost always terminated upon application of the magnet (conversion to DOO or VOO mode) (209). Rarely, when endless loop tachycardia recurs after magnet removal, it can be easily terminated by chest wall stimulation to inhibit the ventricular channel of the pulse generator. The subsequent induction of a similar tachycardia by the induction of retrograde ventriculoatrial conduction substantiates the diagnosis of endless loop tachycardia. Pacemaker tachycardia triggered by myopotentials sensed by the atrial channel of a unipolar DDD pacemaker can be regular or irregular, with pacing cycles often at the upper rate interval. Myopotential triggered tachycardia may be associated with periods of myopotential inhibition (of the ventricular channel) and asynchronous pacing at the interfer-

Figure 18.36. A, Two-channel Holter recording of a patient with an Intermedics Cosmos unipolar DDD pulse generator. The programmed parameters were as follows: lower rate = 60 ppm (1000 msec), URI = 480 msec (125 ppm), AV interval = 250 msec, PVARP = 200 msec, and atrial sensitivity = 0.8 mV. There is an irregular pacemaker tachycardia. Differential diagnosis includes myopotential triggering, atrial fibrillation, and false signals from a defective atrial electrode. Reproduced with permission from Barold SS, Falkoff MD, Ong LS, *et al.*: Electrocardiography of contemporary DDD pacemakers. A. Basic concepts, upper rate response, retrograde ventriculoatrial conduction and differential diagnosis of pacemaker tachycardias. In Saksena S, Goldschlager N (eds): Electrical Therapy for Cardiac Arrhythmias, Pacing, Antitachycardia Devices, Catheter Ablation. WB Saunders, Philadelphia, 1990:225. **B,** Same patient as in **A.** The programmed parameters are identical to those indicated in **A.** Three ECG leads are recorded simultaneously. Myopotential sensing was deliberately induced by appropriate pectoral muscle exercises. Myopotential sensing by the atrial channel causes ventricular triggering at a rapid and irregular rate. Myopotential is also sensed by the ventricular channel because the interval between the seventh and eighth paced beats is approximately 1120 msec and longer than the lower rate interval (1000 msec). At the *arrow,* myopotential signals were sensed by the ventricular electrode within the ventricular safety pacing window or ventricular triggering period (VTP). This sensing causes the delivery of the ventricular stimulus at the end of the VTP, leading to abbreviation of the AV interval (110 msec). When the sensitivity of the atrial channel was decreased to 2.8 mV, P-wave sensing was still present. Consequently, atrial sensitivity was left at 2.4 mV. At this new setting, myopotential triggering could not be induced. A repeat Holter recording showed no myopotential triggering and normal sensing of P waves. (Reproduced with permission from Barold SS, Falkoff MD, Ong LS, *et al.*: Electrocardiography of contemporary DDD pacemakers. A. Basic concepts, upper rate response, retrograde ventriculoatrial conduction and differential diagnosis of pacemaker trachycardias. In Saksena S, Goldschlager N (eds): Electrical Therapy for Cardiac Arrhythmias. Pacing, Antitachycardia Devices, Catheter Ablation. WB Saunders, Philadelphia, 1990:225.)

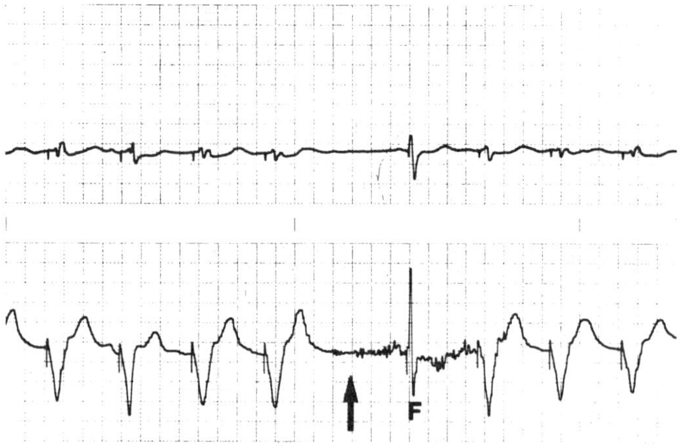

Figure 18.37. Oversensing of diaphragmatic myopotentials by *bipolar* VVI pacemaker programmed at the highest sensitivity of 0.6 mV. Two ECG leads are recorded simultaneously. The patient took a maximal inspiration at the time corresponding to the middle of the tracing. The diagnosis may be suspected in the lower strip because of interference on the baseline, but in the **upper strip** the pause in a bipolar system could be mistaken for pacemaker malfunction. After application of the magnet, no pauses were observed with deep respiration. Reprogramming the sensitivity to 0.8 mV also eliminated oversensing of diaphragmatic potentials. (Reproduced with permission from Barold SS, *et al.*: Programmable pacemakers: clinical indications, complications, and future directions. In Barold SS, Mugica J (eds): The Third Decade of Cardiac Pacing. Futura Publishing Co., Mt. Kisco, NY, 1982:37.)

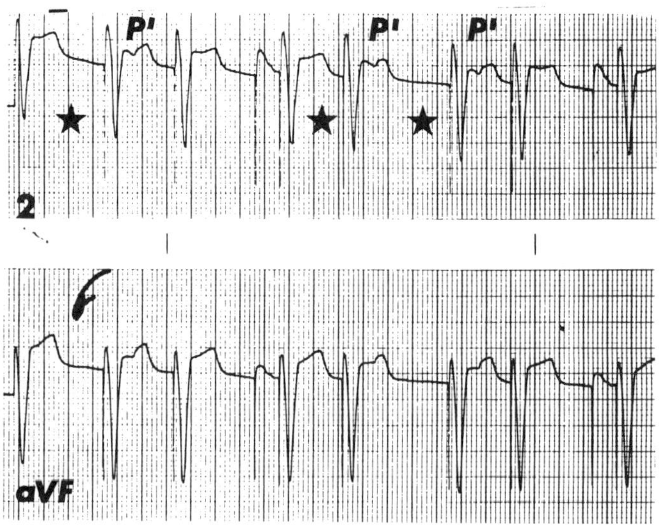

Figure 18.38. Three-lead ECG showing intercostal myopotential inhibition in a patient with a Cordis Sequicor 233F unipolar pulse generator. The parameters were as follows: lower rate = 70 beats/min (lower rate interval = 857 msec), AV delay = 200 msec, PVARP = 300 msec, ventricular refractory period = 300 msec, atrial and ventricular outputs = 6 mA at 0.6 msec, atrial sensitivity = 1.3 mV, ventricular sensitivity = 2.5 mV, upper rate interval = AV delay + PVARP = 500 msec. It appears that the atrial lead senses signals thereby triggering a ventricular output. The premature ventricular paced beat engenders retrograde VA conduction. The abnormalities were seen while the patient was basically immobile. Subsequent testing was performed during normal breathing with the patient being otherwise motionless. In this situation, myopotential interference arising from the pectoral muscles (despite lack of movement except for respiratory muscles) must be considered, but local source of myopotentials (near the unipolar plate) was ruled out because there was no myopotential inhibition of the ventricular channel in the DDD and VVI modes at 0.5, 1.3, mV and 2.5 mV sensitivity and the atrial channel exhibited no oversensing (interference) at 2.5 mV sensitivity. Oversensing by the atrial electrode was evident only at 0.5 and 1.3 mV, but not at 2.5 mV atrial sensitivity. Because both channels share the same anode, this effectively rules out well-known sources of myopotential interference such as pectoral, diaphragmatic, or rectus abdominis sites. There was no evidence of atrial lead malfunction, such as an insulation break, etc. Far-field sensing of ventricular activity by the atrial channel can be ruled out with a fairly long PVARP = 300 msec. This form of oversensing has persisted for nine years. Oversensing was accentuated with deep respiration and eliminated during held respiration. A systematic evaluation of this problem in other patients led us to consider that the atrial lead sensed myopotential interference arising from the intercostal muscles because the atrial lead in the atrial appendage lies anteriorly close to the chest-wall.

ence rate. Myopotential triggered tachycardia is easily reproducible by maneuvers that promote myopotential oversensing (Fig. 18.36B). Other types of pacemaker tachycardia are uncommon and include repetitive oversensing of atrial false signals (from a defective atrial lead—Fig. 18.42) triggering rapid ventricular pacing rate and far-field endless loop tachycardia (sensing of the tailend of the QRS complex by the atrial lead rather than the retrograde P wave).

EXOGENOUS SOURCES OF INTERFERENCE

Despite long lists of potential sources of interference, reports of clinical events from oversensing extracorporeal signals outside the hospital setting are now rare and limited to a relatively small number of environmental situations. The subject of interference from exogenous sources was recently reviewed by Barold, *et al.* (210).

Electrocautery

Electrocautery is the best known and most common form of interference in the hospital environment. Intraoperative pacemaker complications due to interference produced by electrocautery were first reported in the late 1960s and the problem has now become even more important because of different circuit designs. Unipolar and bipolar pacemakers are equally affected. Pacemaker malfunction during transurethral prostatectomy has received the most attention in the literature. However, electrocautery during any operation is a potential hazard to the pacemaker patient. With bipolar coagulation cautery, the current flow is localized across the two poles of the instrument and so far has caused no problems with pacemakers. However, bipolar electrosurgery is valuable only for small areas of coagulation, but not for cutting. Serious problems can occur during unipolar

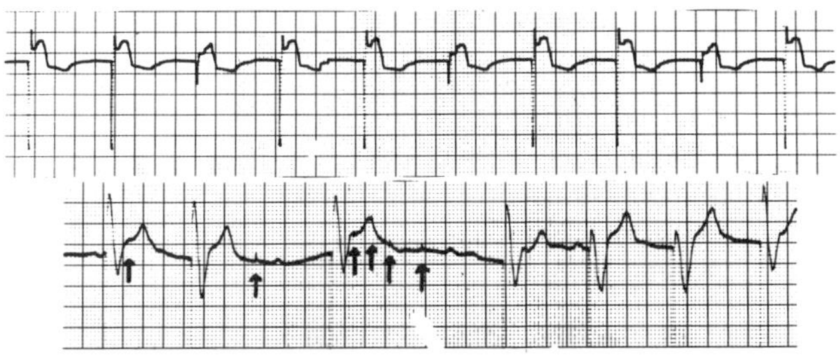

Figure 18.39. Analog ECG recordings during unipolar VVI pacing. Top: Periodic attenuation of the pacemaker spike from monitoring lead during held respiration due to a partial lead fracture. Bottom: In the same patient, there is intermittent prolongation of the spike-to-spike interval with tiny baseline artifact (*arrows*), suggestive of electrode disruption. Such false signals are rarely seen on the surface ECG. (Reproduced with permission from Barold SS, Scovil J, Ong LS, *et al.*: Periodic pacemaker spike attenuation with preservation of capture. An unusual electrocardiographic manifestation of partial pacing electrode fracture, PACE 1978;1:375.)

electrocautery (used for cutting) where electric current is not restricted to the tissue interposed between the two electrodes, but spreads out and penetrates the entire body of the patient. Obviously this stray current may be interpreted by an implanted pulse generator as a signal originating in the heart.

Electrical and thermal burns at the electrode-myocardial interface may lead to ventricular fibrillation or chronic elevation of pacing thresholds, as recorded by Shepard, *et al.* (211) who observed an increased incidence of chronic exit block in pacing systems exposed to electrocautery. There are as yet no reported cases in man of an acute increase in the pacing threshold leading to loss of capture. Chauvin *et al.* (212) observed no rise in the acute pacing threshold related to electrocautery in dogs with a transvenous right ventricular lead.

The effect of electrocautery on the pulse generator is unpredictable. Electrocautery can cause irreversible damage, random component failure, runaway behavior (213) or irreversible reduction or loss of output (214). Electrocautery can cause undesirable pacemaker programming or alteration in the random access memory (RAM). A pulse generator that picks up electrocautery artifacts can be inhibited intermittently and causes long periods of asystole, whereas the application of cautery for longer periods may revert the pulse generator temporarily to its asynchronous interference (noise) mode. The interference mode will continue until electrical interference has disappeared, whereupon the pulse generator will automatically revert to its previous mode and normal function. Inhibition from intermittent electrocautery may be prevented by conversion to the asynchronous mode with application of the magnet over the pulse generator. However, application of the magnet does not protect against ventricular fibrillation and does not prevent current pickup by the electrodes and the attendant risk of pacemaker damage.

Electrocautery may activate the reset or backup pacing circuit of a DDD pacemaker normally activated by low battery voltage (elective replacement indicator), giving rise to VOO or VVI pacing at lower rates than programmed. The reset (backup) mode which represents a normal protective response to high intensity electromagnetic interference, does not revert to the original mode and parameters when electrocautery is discontinued. Thus a DDD pulse generator converted to the reset or backup mode in the VOO or VVI mode might cause hypotension in selected patients, particularly those with the pacemaker syndrome in the VVI mode. Rate-adaptive pacemakers such as VVIR with the sensor function programmed on, may be reset to the ordinary VVI mode without rate adaptive function. Bipolar pacemakers have a lower susceptibility to reset than do unipolar ones. A reset pulse generator does not represent malfunction and can be easily reprogrammed to its previous mode.

Patients must be managed according to a careful protocol during electrocautery with pacemaker testing before and after the procedure. If unipolar cautery must be used, the ground plate should be positioned so that the current pathway does not pass through or near the pacemaker system. The unipolar or indifferent plate of the equipment should be as close as possible to the operating site and as far away as possible from the pulse generator and the pacing lead, so that the electrical pathway between the electrocautery probe and the ground plate is directed away from the pacemaker lead system. This pathway should be perpendicular to the line joining the two pacing electrodes so as to decrease transmitted interference. The unipolar probe should not be used within 15 cm of the pulse generator or lead. The electrocautery ground plate should not be located between the active electrode and the pulse generator. For transurethral resection of the prostate, the unipolar patch should be on the leg. Proper grounding of all electronic equipment used near the patient is essential. Radiofrequency catheter ablation of arrhythmias is similar to electrocautery and may cause severe disturbance of pacemaker behavior (215).

Defibrillation and Cardioversion

Defibrillation or transthoracic cardioversion involves a large amount of energy delivered to the heart during a relatively brief period. Circuitry designed to protect the pulse generator shunts energy to the lead. Contemporary pacemaker design with large-scale integrated circuits and microprocessors have made pulse generators more susceptible than in the past to this type of electrical disturbance. Unipolar systems are more susceptible to malfunction than bipolar systems. Adverse effects are related in part to burns at the myocardial-electrode interface. The following abnormalities can occur: (a) Damage to circuitry. Partial or complete destruction of the pulse generator may occur with runaway state, induction of end-of-life behavior, and reversible or irreversible alteration of the microprocessor program. (b) Acute or chronic increase in the pacing threshold, probably due to myocardial burns. Usually the threshold rise is temporary, lasting a few seconds or minutes. (c) Undersensing. Sensing

LOWER RATE = 80 ppm (750 ms)
UPPER RATE INTERVAL = 140 ppm (430 ms)
AV INTERVAL = 160 ms

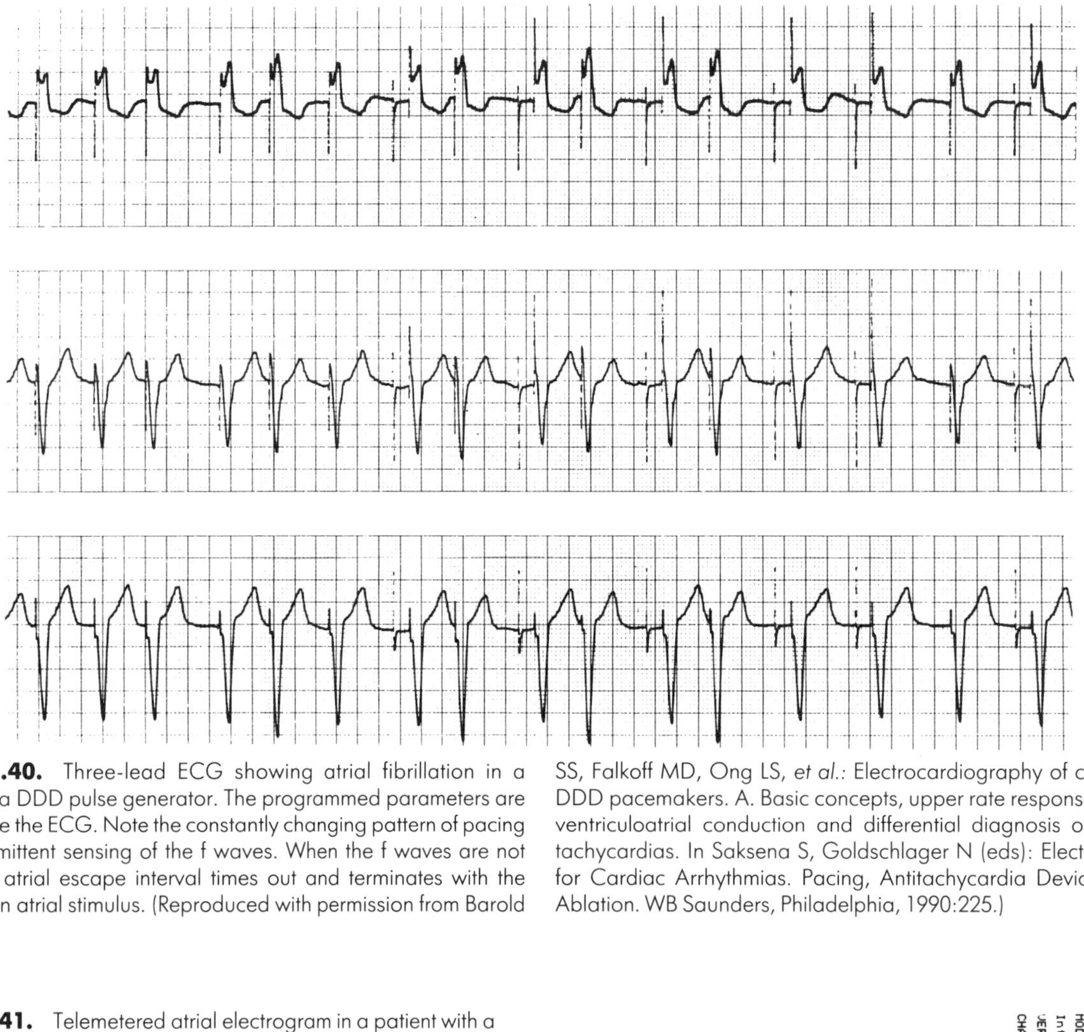

Figure 18.40. Three-lead ECG showing atrial fibrillation in a patient with a DDD pulse generator. The programmed parameters are shown above the ECG. Note the constantly changing pattern of pacing due to intermittent sensing of the f waves. When the f waves are not sensed, the atrial escape interval times out and terminates with the delivery of an atrial stimulus. (Reproduced with permission from Barold SS, Falkoff MD, Ong LS, *et al.*: Electrocardiography of contemporary DDD pacemakers. A. Basic concepts, upper rate response, retrograde ventriculoatrial conduction and differential diagnosis of pacemaker tachycardias. In Saksena S, Goldschlager N (eds): Electrical Therapy for Cardiac Arrhythmias. Pacing, Antitachycardia Devices, Catheter Ablation. WB Saunders, Philadelphia, 1990:225.)

Figure 18.41. Telemetered atrial electrogram in a patient with a Pacesetter AFP 283 DDD pulse generator programmed to the VVI mode. The atrial electrogram shows irregularly occurring f waves consistent with the presence of atrial flutter/fibrillation. (Reproduced with permission from Barold SS, Falkoff MD, Ong LS, *et al.*: Electrocardiography of contemporary DDD pacemakers. A. Basic concepts, upper rate response, retrograde ventriculoatrial conduction and differential diagnosis of pacemaker tachycardias. In Saksena S. Goldschlager N (eds): Electrical Therapy for Cardiac Arrhythmias. Pacing, Antitachycardia Devices, Catheter Ablation. WB Saunders, Philadelphia, 1990:225.)

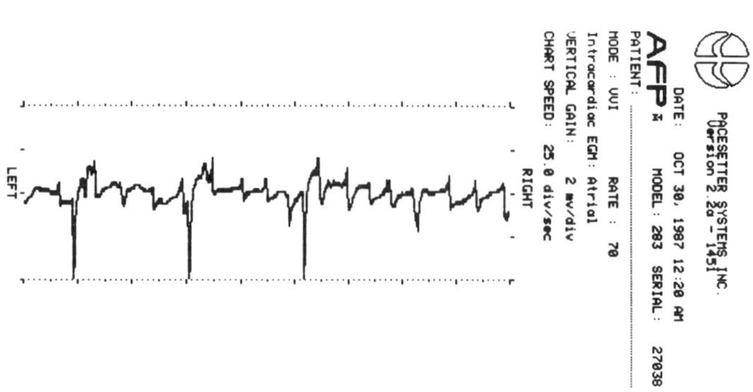

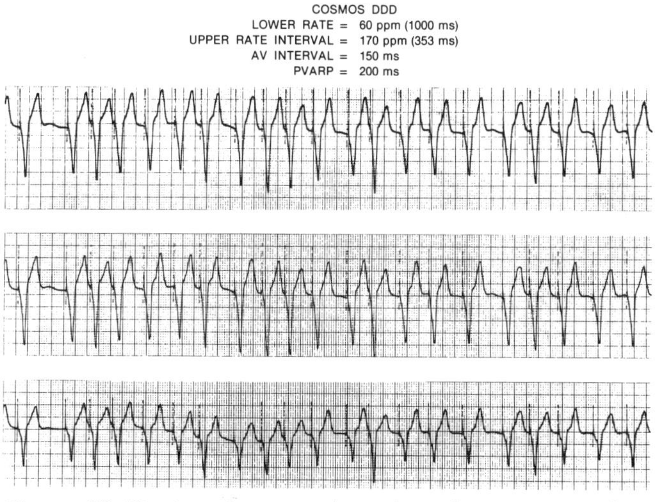

Figure 18.42. Irregular pacemaker tachycardia in a patient with an Intermedics Cosmos unipolar DDD pulse generator with a defective lead generating false signals. The defective lead produces an irregular pacemaker tachycardia which mimics atrial fibrillation. The patient demonstrated normal sinus rhythm and complete AV block in the VVI mode. Some of the paced beats appear to be followed by retrograde P waves causing notching of the ST segment and T wave. (Reproduced with permission from Barold SS, Falkoff MD, Ong LS, *et al.*: Electrocardiography of contemporary DDD pacemakers. A. Basic concepts, upper rate response, retrograde ventriculoatrial conduction and differential diagnosis of pacemaker tachycardias. In Saksena S, Goldschlager N (eds): Electrical Therapy for Cardiac Arrhythmias. Pacing, Antitachycardia Devices, Catheter Ablation. WB Saunders, Philadelphia, PA, 1990:225.)

abnormalities are usually temporary, but sometimes may last as long as 10 days. (d) Reprogramming. Programming to another mode may occur even with different parameters and reprogramming may be impossible. (e) Reset of a dual-chamber pacemaker to the VOO or VVI mode, or VVIR reset to VVI mode, as a normal response to high-level interference. The pulse generator can then be easily reprogrammed to the previous mode. Thermal and electrical burns at the electrode-myocardial interface may theoretically precipitate ventricular fibrillation, but this has not yet been clearly demonstrated in man.

Problems similar to external cardioversion/defibrillation can also occur secondary to the discharge of an implanted cardioverter/defibrillator (216) with the following manifestations: (a) temporary increase in the pacing and sensing thresholds, (b) resetting of a dual-chamber pulse generator to the VVI or VOO mode as a normal response to high-intensity electromagnetic interference. As yet, discharge of an implanted cardioverter-defibrillator has not been reported to cause irreversible pacemaker malfunction.

Guidelines for Defibrillation and Cardioversion in Pacemaker Patients

1. Use anterior-posterior paddles, if possible (their availability is not universal).
2. Do not put the paddle over the pulse generator. When using only anterior paddles, place them along a line perpendicular to the line joining the pulse generator to the tip of the ventricular pacing lead. The upward vector of the defibrillator discharge should be perpendicular to the sensing vector of the pulse generator-lead (line). In a dual-lead system in which the electrodes are roughly perpendicular to each other, give preference to the ventricular system.
3. Place the paddles at least 10 cm from the pulse generator or lead. (This may be difficult for a right pectoral implant.)
4. Use the lowest possible defibrillator energy.
5. A programmer and a transcutaneous external pacemaker should be readily available. Be prepared to increase the output of the implanted pulse generator immediately by programming.
6. Carefully monitor the patient for 24 hr. Repeated testing of threshold is important. Because of possible late malfunction, follow-up for several weeks is necessary.

Radiation

Contemporary advanced pulse generators with complementary metal oxide semiconductors (CMOS) are more sensitive to the effects of ionizing radiation, compared with the semiconductor circuits used in old pulse generator (217). Damage is variable and can be serious because it can lead to life-threatening arrhythmias. Damage to pacemaker electronics may be transient but often permanent, and depends on the type of radiation, total dose, type of device, and details of its fabrication. The deleterious effect of radiation is cumulative. Thus, the effect would be similar whether the same dose is given at one time or spread over several sessions. Given a sufficiently high cumulative absorbed dose, all pulse generators ultimately fail catastrophically. Every attempt should be made to avoid direct irradiation of a pulse generator by shielding. If this is not possible, the pulse generator should be moved to another site.

Altered function secondary to damage by radiation may produce spontaneous reprogramming in the form of a change in rate, voltage, pulse width, runaway characteristics (in one channel or both in the case of dual-chamber pacemakers), abnormal sensing, failure to reprogram, output failure, and unusual responses to application of the magnet. Because of the complexity of circuit design, the mode of failure cannot be predicted. In pulse generators tested in vitro, transient recovery of function can be followed by total failure, a response suggesting that even transient loss of function must be regarded as the precursor to permanent damage and the pacemaker should be replaced. However, during radiation therapy the pulse generator may also be influenced by electromagnetic interference from a linear accelerator; such transient malfunction is benign and does not necessitate pacemaker replacement, and it should be differentiated from more serious radiation damage.

Radiation-induced reprogramming of a pulse generator can occasionally be returned to its normal function by using a programmer, and normal pacing can continue for months without any problem. However, the pulse generator may ultimately succumb to spontaneous reprogramming representing delayed malfunction incurred during radiation (218). The pulse generator should be tested frequently during and after radiation therapy. Any unexpected behavior should be considered as pacemaker failure.

Magnetic Resonance Imaging

Despite the apparent lack of biological effects, magnetic resonance imaging (MRI) may cause important effects on pacemaker function. Radiofrequency pulsing during MRI may cause rapid pacing, inhibition, reset of DDD pulse generators, and transient reed switch malfunction. MRI is contraindicated in all patients with permanent pacemakers because serious malfunction with no output or rapid pacing may occur.

Lithotripsy

Occasionally, lithotripsy causes intermittent inhibition of VVI or DDD pulse generators or triggering of the ventricular output of DDD pulse generators by electromechanical interference. A DDD pulse generator may reach the upper rate or show irregularities in the pacing rate. Lithotripsy can induce supraventricular tachyarrhythmias that trigger the ventricular output of a DDD pulse generator with consequent increase in the ventricular pacing rate. Therefore, a DDD pulse generator should be programmed to the VVI or DOO mode during lithotripsy. Intermittent reversion to the magnet mode and rate during lithotripsy has been reported due to transient closure of the reed switch by high-energy vibration. Patients with piezoelectric activity-sensing rate-responsive pacemakers implanted in the thorax can probably undergo lithotripsy safely, provided the activity mode is deactivated. Patients with such pacemakers implanted in the abdomen should not undergo lithotripsy because of potential damage to the piezoelectric crystal.

References

1. Iliceto S, DiBiase M, Antoniolli G, *et al.*: Two-dimensional echocardiographic recognition of a pacing catheter perforation of the interventricular septum. PACE 1982;5:934.
2. Villanueva FS, Heinsimer JA, Burkman MH, *et al.*: Echocardiographic detection of perforation of the cardiac septum by a permanent pacemaker lead. Am J Cardiol 1987;59:370.
3. Gondi B, Nanda NC: Real-time, two-dimensional, echocardiographic features of pacemaker perforation. Circulation 1981;64:97.
4. Barold SS, Center S: Electrographic diagnosis of perforation of the heart by pacing catheter electrode. Am J Cardiol 1969;24:274.
5. Irwin JM, Greer GS, Lowe JE, *et al.*: Atrial lead perforation: a case report. PACE 1987;10:1378.
6. Stoney WS, Addlestone RB, Alford WC Jr, *et al.*: The incidence of venous thrombosis following long term pacing. Ann Thorac Surg 1976;22:166.
7. Seeger W, Scherer K: Asymptomatic pulmonary embolism following pacemaker implantation. PACE 1986;9:196.
8. Kinney E, Allen RP, Weidner WA, *et al.*: Recurrent pulmonary emboli secondary to right atrial thrombus around a permanent pacing catheter: a case report and review of the literature. PACE 1979;2:196.
9. Mitrovic V, Thormann J, Schlepper M, *et al.*: Thrombotic complications with pacemakers. Int J Cardiol 1983;2:363.
10. Koike R, Sasaki M, Kuroda K: Total venous obstruction. A possible complication of transvenous dual chamber pacing. Jpn Circ J 1988;52:1293.
11. Krug H, Zerbe F: Major venous thrombosis: A complication of transvenous pacemaker electrodes. Br Heart J 1980;44:158.
12. Fritz T. Richeson JF, Fitzpatrick P, *et al.*: Venous obstruction: a potential complication of transvenous pacemaker electrodes. Chest 1983;83:534.
13. Antonelli D, Turgeman Y, Kaveh Z, *et al.*: Short-term thrombosis after transvenous permanent pacemaker insertion. PACE 1989;12:280.
14. Spittell PC, Hayes DL: Venous complications after insertion of a transvenous pacemaker. Mayo Clin Proc 1992;67:258.
15. Goudevenos JA, Reid PG, Adams PC, *et al.*: Pacemaker-induced superior vena cava syndrome: Report of four cases and review of the literature. PACE 1989;12:1890.
16. Angeli SJ. Superior vena cava syndrome following pacemaker insertion post atrial septal defect repair. Am Heart J 1990;120:433.
17. Blackburn T, Dunn M. Pacemaker-induced superior vena cava syndrome. Consideration of management, Am Heart J 1988;116:893.
18. Spittell PC, Vliestra RE, Hayes DL, *et al.*: Venous obstruction due to permanent transvenous pacemaker electrodes. Treatment with percutaneous transluminal balloon venoplasty. PACE 1990;13:271.
19. Youngson GG, McKenzie RN, Nichol PM: Superior vena cava syndrome. Case report. A complication of permanent transvenous endocardial cardiac pacing requiring surgical correction. Am Heart J 1980;99:503.
20. Montgomery JH, D'Souza VJ, Dyer RB, *et al.*: Nonsurgical treatment of the superior vena cava syndrome. Am J Cardiol 1985;56:829.
21. Gray BH, Olin JW, Graor RA, *et al.*: Safety and efficacy of thrombolytic therapy for superior vena cava syndrome. Chest 1991;99:54.
22. Bradof J, Sands MJ Jr, Lakin PC: Symptomatic venous thrombosis of the upper extremity complicating permanent transvenous pacing: Reversal with streptokinase infusion. Am Heart J 1982;104:1112.
23. Murakami Y, Matsuno Y, Izumi S, *et al.*: Superior vena cava syndrome as a complication of DDD pacemaker implantation. Clin Cardiol 1990;13:298.
24. Porath A, Avnun L, Hirsch M, *et al.*: Right atrial thrombus and recurrent pulmonary embolism secondary to permanent cardiac pacing. A case report and short review of the literature. Angiology 1987;38:627.
25. Nicolosi GL, Charmet PA, Zanuttini D: Large right atrial thrombosis. Rare complication during permanent transvenous endocardial pacing. Br Heart J 1980;43:199.
26. Grunewald RA, Smith PLC, Nihoyannopoulos P, *et al.*: Right ventricular pacing wire thrombus presenting as pyrexia of unknown origin. Clin Cardiol 1989;12:106.
27. May KJ, Cardone JT, Stroebel PP, *et al.*: Streptokinase dissolution of a right atrial thrombus associated with a temporary pacemaker. Arch Intern Med 1988;148:903.
28. Mügge A, Gulba DC, Jost S, *et al.*: Dissolution of a right atrial thrombus attached to a pacemaker electrode: usefulness of recombinant tissue-type plasminogen activator. Am Heart J 1990;119:1438.
29. Ross WB, Mohiuddin SM, Pagano T, *et al.*: Malposition of a transvenous cardiac electrode associated with amaurosis fugax. PACE 1983;6:119.
30. Wohl B, Peters RW, Carliner N, *et al.*: Late unheralded pacemaker pocket infection due to Staphylococcus epidermitis: a new clinical entity. PACE 1982;5:190.
31. Wade JS, Cobbs CG: Infections in cardiac pacemakers. Curr Clin Top Infect Dis 1988;9:44.
32. Byrd CL, Schwartz SJ, Hedin NB, *et al.*: Experience with 234 pocket infections: What works? PACE 1992;15:510.
33. Bluhm G, Jolander I, Levander-Lindgren M, *et al.*: Septicaemia and endocarditis: uncommon but serious complications in connection with permanent cardiac pacing. Scand J Thorac Cardiovasc Surg 1987;16:65.

34. Choo MH, Holmes DR Jr, Gersh BJ, *et al.*: Infected epicardial pacemaker systems: partial versus total removal. J Thorac Surg 1981;8:794.
35. Choo MH, Holmes DR Jr, Gersh BJ, *et al.*: Permanent pacemaker infections: Characterization and management. Am J Cardiol 1981;48:559.
36. Enia F, LoMauro R, Meschisi F, *et al.*: Right-sided infective endocarditis with acquired tricuspid valve stenosis associated with transvenous pacemaker: a case report. PACE 1991;14:1093.
37. ElKohen M, Millaire A, Leroy O, *et al.*: Endocardites infectieuses tricuspidiennes sur sonde de stimulation permanente endocavitaire. Arch Mal Coeur 1990;83:1855.
38. Furman S: Pacemaker infection. PACE 1986;9:779.
39. Goldman BS, MacGregor DC: Management of infected pacemaker systems. Clin Prog Pacing Electrophysiol. 1984;2:220.
40. Harjula A, Järvinen A, Virtanen KS, *et al.*: Pacemaker infections—treatment with total or partial pacemaker system removal. Thorac Cardiovasc Surg 1985;33:218.
41. Hong-Barco P, O'Toole J, Gerber ML, *et al.*: Endocarditis due to six entrapped pacemaker leads and concomitant recurrent coronary arteriosclerosis. Ann Thorac Surg 1988;46:97.
42. Lewis AB, Hayes DL, Holmes DR, *et al.*: Update on infections involving permanent pacemakers: Characterization and management. J Thorac Cardiovasc Surg 1985;89:738.
43. Parry G, Goudevenos J, Jameson S, *et al.*: Complications associated with retained pacemaker leads. PACE 1991;14:1251.
44. Furman S, Behrens M, Andrews C, *et al.*: Retained pacemaker leads. J Thorac Cardiovasc Surg 1987;95:770.
45. Byrd CL, Fearnot NE, Byrd CL, *et al.*: Intravascular extraction of chronic pacing leads. The effect of physician experience. PACE 1992;15:513.
46. Fearnot NE, Smith HJ, Goode LB: Intravascular lead extraction using locking stylets, sheaths, and other techniques. PACE 1990;13:1864.
47. Byrd CL, Schwartz SJ, Hedin NB: Intravascular techniques for extraction of permanent pacemaker leads. J Thorac Cardiovasc Surg 1991;101:989.
48. Wilkoff BL, Smith HJ, Fearnot NE, *et al.*: Intravascular lead extraction: Multicenter update for 523 patients. PACE 1992;15:513.
49. Myers MR, Parsonnet P, Bernstein AD: Extraction of implanted transvenous pacing leads: A review of a persistent clinical problem. Am Heart J 1991;121:881.
50. Byrd CL, Schwartz SJ, Hedin NB, *et al.*: Intravascular lead extraction using locking stylets and sheaths. PACE 1990;13:1871.
51. Brodell BK, Castle LW, Maloney JD, *et al.*: Chronic transvenous pacemaker lead removal using a unique, sequential transvenous system. Am J Cardiol 1990;66:964.
52. Sutton K, Bourgeois I: Troubleshooting. In The Foundations of Cardiac Pacing Part 1: An Illustrated Practical Guide to Basic Pacing. Futura Publishing Co., Mt. Kisco, NY, 1991:259.
53. Byrd CL, Schwartz SJ, Gonzales M, *et al.*: Pacemaker clinic evaluations: Key to early identification of surgical problems. PACE 1986;9:1259.
54. Morgan DE, Norman R, West RO, *et al.*: Echocardiographic assessment of tricuspid regurgitation during ventricular demand pacing. Am J Cardiol 1986;58:1025.
55. Rubio PA, Al-Bassam MS: Pacemaker-lead puncture of the tricuspid valve. Successful diagnosis and treatment. Chest 1991;99:1519.
56. Fishenfeld J, Lamy Y: Laceration of the tricuspid valve by a pacemaker wire. Chest 1972;61:697.
57. Old WD, Paulsen W, Lewis SA, *et al.*: Pacemaker lead-induced tricuspid stenosis: diagnosis by Doppler echocardiography. Am Heart J 1989;117:1165.
58. Been M, Darke PG: Pacemaker twiddler: a twist in the tail? Br Med J 1988;297:1642.
59. Bayliss CE, Beanlands DS, Baird RJ: The pacemaker twiddlers syndrome. Can Med Assoc J 1968;99:371.
60. Ellis GL: Pacemaker twiddler's syndrome. A case report. Am J Emerg Med 1990;8:48.
61. Lal RB, Avery RD: Aggressive pacemaker twiddler's syndrome, dislodgement of an active fixation ventricular pacing electrode. Chest 1990;97:756.
62. Roberts JS, Wenger N: Pacemaker twiddler's syndrome. Am J Cardiol 1989;63:1013.
63. Veltri EP, Mower MM, Reid PR: Twiddler's syndrome: a new twist. PACE 1984;7:1004.
64. Anderson MH, Nathan AW: Ventricular pacing from the atrial channel of a DDD pacemaker. A consequence of pacing twiddling? PACE 1990;13:1567.
65. Mond HG: Routine testing methods. In The Cardiac Pacemaker, Function and Malfunction. Grune & Stratton, New York, 1983, p. 233.
66. Mond HG, Sloman JG: The malfunctioning pacemaker system, Part II. PACE 1981;4:168.
67. Mond HG, Sloman JG: The malfunctioning pacemaker system, Part I. PACE 1981;4:49.
68. Mond HG, Sloman JG: The malfunctioning pacemaker system, Part III. PACE 1981;4:313.
69. Broffoni T, Bonini W, Ferrari G: A new system for follow-up of patients with permanent pacemakers. PACE 1990;13:1782.
70. Steinbach KK: Pacemaker follow-up. In El-Sherif N, Samet P (eds): Cardiac Pacing and Electrophysiology, 3rd ed. WB Saunders, Philadelphia, 1991:662.
71. Schoenfeld MH: Follow-up of the pacemaker patient. In Ellenbogen KA (ed): Cardiac Pacing, Blackwell Scientific Publications. Boston, 1992:419.
72. Strathmore NJ, Mond HG: Noninvasive monitoring and testing of pacemaker function. PACE 1987;10:1359.
73. Mugica J, Henry L, Rollet M, *et al.*: The clinical utility of pacemaker follow-up visits. PACE 1986;9:1249.
74. Griffin JC, Shuenemeyer TD, Hess KR, *et al.*: Pacemaker follow-up: its rule in the detection and correction of pacemaker system malfunction. PACE 1986;9:387.
75. Furman S: Cardiac pacing and pacemakers VIII. The pacemaker follow-up clinic. Am Heart J 1977;94:795.
76. Furman S: Pacemaker follow-up. In Barold S (ed): Modern Cardiac Pacing. Futura Publishing Co., Mt. Kisco, NY, 1985:889.
77. Furman S: Pacemaker follow-up. In Furman S, Hayes DL, Holmes DR (eds): A Practice of Cardiac Pacing, 2nd ed. Futura Publishing Co., Mt. Kisco, NY 1989:511.
78. Parsonnet V, Neglia D, Bernstein AD: The frequency of pacemaker-system problems, etiologies, and corrective interventions. PACE 1992;15:510.
79. Fitzpatrick AP, Travill CM, Vardas PE, *et al.*: Recurrent symptoms after venticular pacing in unexplained syncope. PACE 1990;13:619.
80. Pavlovic SU, Kocovic D, Djordjevic M, *et al.*: The etiology of syncope in pacemaker patients. PACE 1991;14:2086.
81. Hoffman A, Jost M, Pfisterer M, *et al.*: Persisting symptoms despite permanent pacing: Incidence, causes, and follow-up. Chest 1984;85:207.
82. Dodinot B, Kubler L, Medeiros P: Syncope et malaises chez le porteur de stimulation cardiaque. Ann Cardiol Angéiol 1983;32:399.
83. Luceri RM, Hayes DL: Follow-up of DDD pacemakers. PACE 1984;7:1187.
84. Parsonnet V, Bernstein AD, Lindsay B: Pacemaker implanation complication rates: An analysis of some contributing factors. J Am Coll Cardiol 1989;13:917.
85. Levine PA: Differential diagnosis, evaluation and management of pacing system malfunction. In Ellenbogen KA (ed): Cardiac Pacing. Blackwell Scientific Publications, Boston, 1992:309.
86. Byrd CL, Schwartz SJ, Gonzales M *et al.*: DDD pacemakers maximize hemodyamic benefits and minimize complications for most patients, PACE 1988;11:1911.
87. Dreifus LS, Zinberg A, Hurzeler P, *et al.*: Ambulatory monitoring for cardiac pacemakers. Cardiovasc Clin 1988;18:83.
88. Dreifus LS, Zinberg A, Hurzeler P, *et al.*: Transtelephonic monitoring of 25,919 implanted pacemakers. PACE 1986;9:371.
89. Zinberg A: Transtelephonic follow-up. Clin Prog Pacing Electrophysiol. 1984;2:177.
90. Rubin JW, Ellison RG, Moore HV, *et al.*: Influence of telephone surveil-

lance on pacemaker patient care. J Thorac Cardiovasc Surg 1980;79: 218.

91. Furman S, Parker B, Escher DJW: Transtelephone pacemaker clinic. J Thorac Cardiovasc Surg 1971;61:827.
92. Furman S: Transtelephone pacemaker monitoring. In Chung EK (ed): Artificial Cardiac Pacing Practical Approach, 2nd ed. Williams & Wilkins, Baltimore, 1984:345.
93. Barold SS, Mugica J, Falkoff MD, *et al.*: Multiprogrammability in cardiac pacing. In Barold SS (ed): Modern Cardiac Pacing. Futura Publishing Co., Mt. Kisco, NY, 1985:377.
94. Barold SS, Falkoff MD, Ong LS, *et al.*: Electrocardiography of contemporary DDD pacemakers. B. Multiprogrammability, follow-up and troubleshooting. In Saksena S, Goldschlager N (eds): Electrical Therapy for Cardiac Arrhythmias. Pacing, Antitachycardia Devices, Catheter Ablation. WB Saunders, Philadelphia, 1990:265.
95. Barold SS, Pupillo GA, Gaidula JJ, *et al.*: Chest wall stimulation in evaluation of patients with implanted ventricular-inhibited demand pacemakers. Br Heart J 1970;32:783.
96. Barold SS: Clinical uses of chest wall stimulation in patients with DDD pulse generators. Intelligence Reports in Cardiac Pacing and Electrophysiology 1988;7:2.
97. Byrd CB, Hallberg BS, Byrd CL: Computerized pacemaker patient analysis. PACE 1990;13:1779.
98. Bernstein AD, Parsonnet V: Computer-assisted measurements in pacemaker follow-up. PACE 1986;9:392.
99. Macgregor DC, Covvey HD, Noble EJ, *et al.*: Computer-assisted reporting system for the follow-up of patients with cardiac pacemakers. PACE 1980;3:568.
100. Strathmore N, Mond H, Hunt D, *et al.*: "Pacecare"—a computerized database for pacemaker follow-up. PACE 1990;13:1787.
101. Sweesy MW, Batey RL, Forney RC: Activation times for "Emergency Back-up" Programs. PACE 1990;13:1224.
102. Castellanet MJ, Garza J, Shaner SP, *et al.*: Telemetry of programmed and measured data in pacing system evaluation and follow-up. J Electrophysiol 1987;1:360.
103. Adler S, Whistler S, Martin R: Advances in single-chamber pacemaker diagnostic data. PACE 1986;9:1141.
104. Levine PA, Venditti FJ, Podrid PJ, *et al.*: Telemetry of programmed and measured data electrograms, event markers, and event counters: Luxury or necessity? In Barold SS, Mugica J (eds): New Perspectives in Cardiac Pacing. Futura Publishing Co., Mt. Kisco, NY, 1988:187.
105. Sanders R, Martin R, Frumin H, *et al.*: Data storage and retrieval by implantable pacemakers for diagnostic purposes. PACE 1984;7:1228.
106. Levine PA, Lindenberg BS: Diagnostic data: an aid to the follow-up and assessment of the pacing system. J Electrophysiol 1987;1:396.
107. Kruse I, Markowitz T, Ryden L: Timing markers showing pacemaker behavior to aid in the follow-up of a physiologic pacemaker. PACE 1983;6:801.
108. Duffin EC Jr: The marker channel. A telemetric diagnostic aid. PACE 1984;7:1165.
109. Levine PA: The complementary role of electrogram, event marker and measured data telemetry in the assessment of pacing system function. Electrophysiol 1987;1:404.
110. Sarmiento JJ: Clinical utility of telemetered intracardiac electrograms in diagnosing a design dependent lead malfunction. PACE 1990;13:188.
111. VanBeek GJ, DenDulk K, Lindemans FW, *et al.*: Detection of insulation failure by gradual reduction in noninvasively measured electrogram amplitudes. PACE 1986;9:772.
112. Levine PA, Sholder J, Duncan JL: Clinical benefits of telemetered electrograms in assessment of DDD function. PACE 1984;7:1170.
113. Clarke M, Allen A: Use of telemetered electrograms in the assessment of normal pacemaker function. J Electrophysiol. 1987;1:388.
114. VanGelder LM, ElGamal M: Undersensing in VVI pacemakers detected by Holter monitoring. PACE 1988;11:1507.
115. Dianconi L, Ambrosini M, Serdoz R, *et al.*: Syncope in pacemaker patients. Diagnostic value of dynamic electrocardiography. In Steinbach K, Glogar D, Laszkovics, *et al.* (eds): Proceedings of VIIth World Symposium on Cardiac Pacing, Steinkopff Verlag, Darmstadt, 1983:567.
116. Famularo MA, Kennedy HL: Ambulatory electrocardiography in the assessment of pacemaker function. Am Heart J 1982;104:1086.
117. Oka Y, Ito T, Sada T, *et al.*: Ambulatory electrocardiogram obtained by Holter monitoring systems in patients with permanent demand pacemakers. Jpn Heart J 1985;26:23.
118. Janosik DL, Redd RM, Buckingham TA, *et al.*: Utility of ambulatory electrocardiography in detecting pacemaker dysfunction in the early post-implantation period. Am J Cardiol 1987;60:1030.
119. Kaul UA, Balachander J, Khalilullah M: Ambulatory monitoring in patients with implanted pacemakers. Indian Heart J 1984;36:23.
120. Hoher M, Winter UJ, Behrenbeck DW *et al.*: Pacemaker Holter ECG. Value and limitations in follow-up of pacemaker patients in cardiac pacemakers. In Behrenbeck DW, Sowton E, Fontaine G, *et al.*: (eds) Springer-Verlag, New York 1985:68.
121. Kelen GJ, Bloomfield DA, Hardage M, *et al.*: A clinical evaluation of an improved Holter monitoring technique for artificial pacemaker function. PACE 1980;3:192.
122. Tranesjo J, Fåhreus T, Nygards ME, *et al.*: Automatic detection of pacemaker pulses in ambulatory ECG recording. PACE 1982;5:120.
123. Lesh MD, Langberg JJ, Griffin JC: Pacemaker generator pseudomalfunction: an artifact of Holter monitoring. PACE 1991;14:854.
124. VanGelder LM, Bracke FALE, ElGamel MIH: Fusion or confusion on Holter recording. PACE 1991;14:760.
125. Barold SS, Falkoff MD, Ong LS, *et al.*: The abnormal pacemaker stimulus. In Barold SS (ed): Modern Cardiac Pacing. Futura Publishing Co., Mr. Kisco, NY, 1985:571.
126. Barold SS, Scovil J, Ong LS, *et al.*: Periodic pacemaker spike attenuation with preservation of capture: An unusual electrocardiographic manifestation of partial pacing electrode fracture. PACE 1978;1:375.
127. Barold SS, Falkoff MD, Ong LS, *et al.*: Normal and abnormal patterns of ventricular depolarization during cardiac pacing. In Barold SS (ed): Modern Cardiac Pacing. Futura Publishing Co., Mt. Kisco, NY; 1985:545.
128. Castellanos A Jr, Zoble R, Procacci PM, *et al.*: New sign of diagnosis of anterior myocardial infarction during right ventricular pacing. Br Heart J 1973;35:1161.
129. Barold SS, Narula OS, Javier RP, *et al.*: Significance of right bundle branch block patterns during pervenous ventricular pacing. Br Heart J 1969;31:385.
130. Klein HO, Beker B, Sareli P, *et al.*: Unusual QRS morphology associated with transvenous pacemakers. The pseudo RBBB pattern. Chest 1985;87:517.
131. Klein HO, Beker B, DiSegni E, *et al.*: The pacing electrocardiogram: How important is the QRS complex configuration? Clin Prog Electrophysiol Pacing 1986;4:112.
132. Mazzetti H, Dussaut A, Tentori C, *et al.*: Transarterial permanent pacing of the left ventricle. PACE 1990;13:588.
133. VanGelder LM, ElGamal MIH, Tielen CHJ: Changes in morphology of the paced QRS complex related to pacemaker output. PACE 1989;12:1640.
134. Kadish AH, Schmaltz S, Morady F: A comparison of QRS complexes resulting from unipolar and bipolar pacing: Implications for pace-mapping. PACE 1991;14:823.
135. Barold SS, Falkoff MD, Ong LS, *et al.*: Electrocardiographic diagnosis of myocardial infarction during ventricular pacing. Cardiol Clinics 1987;5:403.
136. Sanders R, Barold SS: Understanding elective replacement indicators and automatic parameter conversion mechanisms in DDD pacemakers. In Barold SS, Mugica J (eds): New Perspectives in Cardiac Pacing. Futura Publishing Co., Mt. Kisco, NY, 1988:203.
137. Levine PA: Magnet rates and recommended replacement time indicators of lithium pacemakers, 1986. Clin Prog Electrophysiol Pacing 1986;4:608.

138. Barold SS, Schoenfeld MH: Pacemaker elective replacement indicators. PACE 1989;12:990.
139. Barold SS, Schoenfeld MH, Falkoff MD, *et al.*: Elective replacement indicators of simple and complex pacemakers. In Barold SS, Mugica J (eds): New Perspectives in Cardiac Pacing. 2. Futura Publishing Co., Mt. Kisco, NY, 1991:493.
140. VanMechelen R, Vandekerckhove Y: Atrial capture and dual chamber pacing. PACE 1986;9:21.
141. Schüller H, Brandt J, Fåhreus T: Determination of atrial depolarization during dual chamber pacing. In Barold SS, Mugica J (eds): New Perspectives in Cardiac Pacing. Futura Publishing Co., Mt. Kisco, NY, 1988:319.
142. Barold SS, Nanda NC, Ong LS, *et al.*: Determination of successful atrial capture during unipolar dual-chamber pacing. In Barold SS (ed): Modern Cardiac Pacing, Futura Publishing Co., Mt. Kisco, NY, 1985:677.
143. Levine PA: Confirmation of atrial capture and determination of atrial capture thresholds in DDD pacing systems. Clin Prog Pacing Electrophysiol 1984;2:465.
144. Feuer JM, Florio J, Shandling AH: Alternate methods for the determination of atrial capture threshold utilizing the telemetered intracardiac electrogram. PACE 1990;13:1254.
145. VanMechelen R, Hart CT, DeBoer H: Failure to sense P waves during DDD pacing. PACE 1986;9:498.
146. Giroud D, Goy JJ: Pacemaker malfunction due to subcutaneous emphysems. Int J Cardiol 1990;26:234.
147. Hearne SF, Maloney JD: Pacemaker system failure secondary to air entrapment within the pulse generator pocket. A complication of subclavian venipuncture for lead placement. Chest 1982;82:651.
148. Mickley H, Anderson C, Nielsen LH: Runaway pacemaker: A still existing complication and therapeutic guidelines. Clin Cardiol 1989;12:412.
149. Rubenfire JJ, Laforet EG: Pacemaker runaway following intermittent output failure. PACE 1983;6:645.
150. Barold SS, Gaidula JJ: Failure of demand pacemaker from low-voltage bipolar ventricular electrograms. JAMA 1971;215:923.
151. Furman S, Hurzeler P, DeCaprio V: The ventricular endocardial electrogram and pacemaker sensing. J Thorac Cardiovasc Surg 1977;73:258.
152. Bornzin G, Stokes K: The electrode-biointerface: Sensing. In Barold SS (ed): Modern Cardiac Pacing. Futura Publishing Co., Mt. Kisco, NY, 1985:79.
153. Warnowicz MA, Goldschlager N: Apparent failure to sense (undersensing) caused by oversensing: Diagnostic use of a noninvasively obtained intracardiac electrogram. PACE 1983;6:1341.
154. Snoeck J, Decoster H, Verherstraeten M, *et al.*: Evolution of P wave characteristics after pacemaker implantation. PACE 1990;13:2091.
155. Frohlig G, Schwerdt H, Schieffer H, *et al.*: Atrial signal variations and pacemaker malsensing during exercise: A study in the time and frequency domain, J Am Coll Cardiol 1988;11:806.
156. Ross BA, Zeigler V, Zinner A, *et al.*: The effect of exercise on the atrial electrogram voltage in young patients. PACE 1991;14:2092.
157. Bricker JT, Ward KA, Zinner A *et al.*: Decrease in canine endocardial and epicardial electrogram voltage with exercise: implications for pacemaker sensing. PACE 1988;11:460.
158. Kleinert MP, Mühlenpfovdt KG, Riggert M: Necessity of exercise tests in patients with atrial programmed pacemakers. PACE 1992;15:576.
159. Barold SS, Falkoff MD, Ong LS, *et al.*: Oversensing by single-chamber pacemakers. Mechanisms, diagnosis and treatment. Cardiol Clinics 1987;3:565.
160. Barold SS, Falkoff MD, Ong LS, *et al.*: Differential diagnosis of pacemaker pauses. In Barold SS (ed): Modern Cardiac Pacing. Futura Publishing Co., Mt. Kisco, NY:587.
161. VanGelder LM, ElGamal MIH, Tielen CHJ: P wave sensing in VVI pacemakers: Useful or a problem? PACE 1988;11:1413.
162. Yokoyama M, Wada J, Barold SS: Transient early T wave sensing by implanted programmable demand pulse generator. PACE 1981;4:68.
163. Massumi RA, Mason DT, Amsterdam EA, *et al.*: Apparent malfunction of demand pacemaker caused by nonpropagated (concealed) ventricular extrasystoles. Chest 1972;61:426.
164. Rosen KM, Rahimtoola SH, Gunnar RM: Pseudo AV block secondary to premature non-propagated His bundle depolarizations. Documentations by His bundle electrocardiography. Circulation 1970;42:367.
165. Levine PA, Pirzada FA: Pacemaker oversensing. A possible example of concealed ventricular extrasystoles. PACE 1981;4:199.
166. Barold SS: Can a demand pacemaker really sense concealed ventricular extrasystoles? PACE 1981;4:226.
167. Lasseter KC, Buchanan JW, Yoshonis KF: A mechanism for "false" inhibition of demand pacemakers. Circulation 1970;42:1093.
168. Waxman MB, Berman ND, Sanz, G, *et al.*: Demand pacemaker malfunction due to abnormal sensing. Circulation 1974;50:389.
169. Chew PH, Brinker JA: Oversensing from electrode 'chatter' in a bipolar pacing lead: a case report. PACE 1990;13:808.
170. Furman S, DeCaprio V: Electrode causation of pacemaker inhibition. Chest 1977;72:117.
171. Nalos PC, Nyitray W: Benefits of intracardiac electrograms and programmable sensing polarity in preventing pacemaker inhibition due to spurious screw-in lead signals. PACE 1990;13:1101.
172. Yokoyama M, Hori M, Grechko M: Suppresion of demand mechanism by inactive myocardial electrodes. PACE 1978;1:126.
173. Waxman HL, Lazzara R, ElSherif N: Apparent malfuncton of demand pacemakers due to spurious potentials generated by contact between two endocardial electrodes. PACE 1978;1:531.
174. Widmann WC, Mangolia S, Lubow LA, *et al.*: Suppression of demand pacemakers by inactive pacemaker electrodes. Circulation 1972;45:319.
175. Coumel OP, Mugica J, Barold SS: Demand pacemaker arrhythmias caused by intermittent incomplete electrode fracture. Am J Cardiol 1975;36: 105.
176. Mugica J, Duconge R, Dubos M, *et al.*: Methods for recording intermittent contact signals in demand pacemaker arrhythmias (11 cases). PACE 1978;1:122.
177. Wirtzfeld A, Lampadius M, Ruprecht EO: Unterdruckung von demandschrittmachern durch muskelpotentiale. Dtsch Med Wochenschr 1972;97:61.
178. Barold SS, Falkoff MD, Ong LS, *et al.*: Interference in cardiac pacemakers. Endogenous sources. Myopotentials. In El-Sherif N, Samet P (eds): Cardiac Pacing and Electrophysiology, 3rd ed. WB Saunders, Philadelphia, 1991:634.
179. Watson WS: Myopotential sensing in cardiac pacemakers. In Barold SS (ed): Modern Cardiac Pacing, Futura Publishing Co., Mt. Kisco, NY, 1985:813.
180. Secemsky SI, Hauser RG, Denes P, *et al.*: Unipolar sensing abnormalities: Incidence and clinical significance of skeletal muscle interference and undersensing in 228 patients. PACE 1982;5:10.
181. Gaita F, Asteggiano R, Bocchiardo M, *et al.*: Holter monitoring and provocative maneuvers in assessment of unipolar demand pacemaker myopotential inhibition. Am Heart J 1984;107:925.
182. Halperin JL, Camunas JL, Stern EH, *et al.*: Myopotential interference with DDD pacemakers: Endocardial electrographic telemetry in the diagnosis of pacemaker-related arrhythmias. Am J Cardiol 1984;54:97.
183. Erkkila KI, Singh JB: Reversion mode activation by myopotential sensing in a ventricular inhibited demand pacemaker. PACE 1985;8:50.
184. Gabry MD, Behrens M, Andrews C, *et al.*: Comparison of myopotential interference in unipolar-bipolar programmable DDD pacemakers. PACE 1987;10:1322.
185. Zimmern SH, Clark MF, Austin WK, *et al.*: Characteristic and clinical effects of myopotential signals in a unipolar DDD pacemaker population. PACE 1986;9:1019.
186. Rozanski JJ, Blankstein RL, Lister JW: Pacer arrhythmias: myopotential triggering of pacemaker mediated tachycardia. PACE 1983;6:795.
187. Barold SS, Belott PH: Behavior of the ventricular triggering period of DDD pacemakers. PACE 1987;10:1237.

188. Gialafos J, Maillis A, Kalogeropoulos C, *et al.*: Inhibition of demand pacemakers by myopotentials. Am Heart J 1985;109:984.

189. ElGamal M, VanGelder B: Suppression of an external demand pacemaker by diaphragmatic myopotentials: A sign of electrode perforation. PACE 1979;2:191.

190. Barold SS, Ong LS, Falkoff MD, *et al.*: Inhibition of bipolar demand pacemakers by diaphragmatic myopotentials. Circulation 1977;56:679.

191. Barold SS, Falkoff MD, Ong LS, *et al.*: Diaphragmatic myopotential inhibition in multiprogrammable unipolar and bipolar pulse generators. In Steinbach K (ed): Cardiac Pacing. Proceedings of the VIIth World Symposium on Cardiac Pacing. Darmstadt, Steinkopff Verland, 1983:537.

192. Van Gelder B, ElGamal M, Bracke F, *et al.*: Are bipolar systems prone to oversensing at high sensitivity setting? PACE 1991;14:731.

193. Widlansky S, Zipes DP: Suppression of a ventricular inhibited bipolar pacemaker by skeletal muscle activity. J Electrocardiol 1974;7:371.

194. Amikam S, Prelag H, Lemer L, *et al.*: Myopotential inhibition of a bipolar pacemaker by skeletal muscle insulation defect. Br Heart J 1977;39: 1279.

195. Furman S: Troubleshooting. In Furman S, Hayes DL, Holmes DR (eds), A Practice of Cardiac Pacing, 2nd ed. Futura Publishing Co., Mt. Kisco, NY, 1989:611.

196. Alt E, Vöker R, Blömer H: Lead fracture in pacemaker patients. Thorac Cardiovasc Surg 1987;35:101.

197. Stokes K, Staffenson D, Lessar J *et al.*: A possible new complication of subclavian stick: Conductor fracture. PACE 1987;10:748.

198. Suzuki Y, Fujimori S, Sakai M, *et al.*: A case of pacemaker lead fracture associated with thoracic outlet syndrome. PACE 1988;11:326.

199. Arakawa M, Kambara K, Ito H, *et al.*: Intermittent oversensing due to internal insulation damage of temperature sensing rate responsive pacemaker lead in subclavian venipuncture method. PACE 1989;12:1312.

200. Fyke FE III: Simultaneous insulation deterioration associated with side-by-side subclavian placement of two polyurethane leads. PACE 1988;11: 1571.

201. Fink S, Jacobs DM, Miller RP, *et al.*: Anatomic evaluation of pacemaker lead compression. PACE 1992;15:510.

202. Austin SM: Pseudofracture of dual chamber pacemaker lead: Avoidance of surgical intervention. New Jersey Med 1987;84:178.

203. Witte A: Pseudo-fracture of pacemaker lead due to securing suture: a case report. PACE 1981;4:716.

204. Woscoboinik JR, Mercho N, Helguera ME, *et al.*: Diagnostic value of the chest x-ray in detection of pacemaker lead failure. PACE 1992;15: 572.

205. Levine PA: Clinical manifestations of lead insulation defects. J Electrophysiol 1987;1:144.

206. Barold SS, Falkoff MD, Ong LS, *et al.*: Electrocardiography of contemporary DDD pacemakers. A. Basic concepts, upper rate response, retrograde ventriculoatrial conduction and differential diagnosis of pacemaker tachycardias. In Saksena S, Goldschlager N (eds): Electrical Therapy for Cardiac Arrhythmias, Pacing, Antitachycardia Devices, Catheter Ablation. WB Saunders, Philadephia, 1990:225.

207. Greenspon AJ, Greenberg RM, Frankk WS: Tracking of atrial flutter by DDD pacing, another form of pacemaker mediated tachycardia. PACE 1984;7:955.

208. Levine PA, Seltzer JP: AV universal (DDD) pacing and atrial fibrillation. Clin Prog Pacing Electrophysiol 1983;1:275.

209. Barold SS, Falkoff MD, Ong LS, *et al.*: Upper rate response of DDD pacemakers. In Barold SS, Mugica J (eds): Cardiac Pacing. Futura Publishing Co., Mt. Kisco, NY, 1988:121.

210. Barold SS, Falkoff MD, Ong LS, *et al,*: Interference in cardiac pacemakers. Exogenous sources. In El-Sherif N, Samet P (eds): Cardiac Pacing and Electrophysiology, 3rd ed. WB Saunders, Philadelphia, 1991:608.

211. Shepard RV, Russo AG, Breland VC: Radiofrequency electrocoagulation hemostasis, and chronically elevated pacing threshold, in cardiopulmonary bypass procedure patients. In Meere C (ed): Proceedings of the VIth World Symposium on Cardiac Pacing, Chapter 35–2. PACESYMP, Montreal, 1979.

212. Chauvin M, Crenner F, Brehenmacher C: Does the utilization of the electrocautery affect thresholds of permanent pacing? PACE 1992;15: 574.

213. Heller LI: Surgical electrocautery and the runaway pacemaker syndrome. PACE 1990;13:1084.

214. Mangar D, Atlas GM, Kane PB: Electrocautery induced pacemaker malfunction during surgery. Can J Anaesth 1991;38:616.

215. Chin MC, Rosenqvist M, Lee MA, *et al.*: The effect of radiofrequency catheter ablation in permanent pacemakers. An experimental study. PACE 1990;13:23.

216. Calkins H, Brinker J, Veltri EP, *et al.*: Clinical interactions between pacemakers and automatic implantable cardioverter-defibrillators. J Am Coll Cardiol 1990;16:666.

217. Rodriguez F, Filimonov A, Henning A, *et al.*: Radiation-induced effects in multiprogrammable pacemaker and implantable defibrillators. PACE 1991;14:2143.

218. Jaeger M, Mirimanoff JO: La radiothérapie chez un porteur de pacemaker: une entreprise à problèmes. Stimucoeur 1990;18:96.

IV

ELECTRICAL THERAPY FOR TACHYARRHYTHMIAS

19

ELECTRICAL CARDIOVERSION AND DEFIBRILLATION

Stanley M. Bach, Jr., M.D.

Defibrillation is a term applied to the termination of rapid, uncoordinated cardiac ventricular electrical activity (ventricular fibrillation or VF). Fibrillation may be abolished by electrical or chemical means. Chemical defibrillation is accomplished by the intravascular or intracardiac injection of potassium followed by calcium. Chemical defibrillation was extensively investigated during the first three decades of the twentieth century (1). Although effective in small animals, chemical defibrillation was abandoned in favor of electrical defibrillation because of application difficulties which included ready access to equipment and peripheral vascular runoff.

Cardioversion is a term coined by Dr. Bernard Lown, who described it as a synchronized capacitor discharge for the purpose of terminating arrhythmias other than VF (2). The synchronization employed with cardioversion meant discharging the electrical pulse during the inscription of the QRS at a time when the ventricular tissue is depolarized so as to minimize the possibility of inducing VF.

The term "cardioversion" has also been applied to the termination of monomorphic ventricular tachycardia (VT). Synchronization may or may not be valuable during monomorphic VT, since there is often a complex relationship between the sensing circuit response, the sensing electrocardiogram (ECG), the partial ventricular depolarization, and the electric field produced by the shocking electrodes. Indeed, low-strength "synchronized" shocks during monomorphic VT can easily lead to VF, probably because only a portion of the ventricular myocardium is depolarized at any one time.

The use of the terms "cardioversion" and "defibrillation" in the current literature may be at variance with their original definitions. Some authors apply the term "cardioversion" to the termination of VT, usually by low-strength shocks, while reserving the term "defibrillation" for termination of VF, usually by high-strength shocks. The difficulty is that no universally accepted shock strength level separates the two. Further, the distinction between polymorphic VT and VF is not always easy to make.

NATURE OF FIBRILLATION

Ventricular fibrillation has been described as an impulse formation abnormality in which multiple ectopic foci fire asynchronously throughout the atrial or ventricular myocardium. It has also been described as an impulse conduction problem in which multiple reentry pathways are continuously changing. For established fibrillation, recent mapping studies strongly support the latter interpretation (3). However, the initiation of fibrillation is likely a local phenomenon in some area(s) of the myocardium (4).

Recent development of topology and chaos theories suggest that the behavior seen in cardiac fibrillation is not unique in nature. Colonies of light emitting marine algae may have their rhythmic bioluminescence disrupted by a properly timed stimulus (5). A water wheel, when driven at certain input flow rates, may exhibit an apparently disorganized rotational pattern (6). Even chemical systems may display this characteristic (5).

What these systems have in common is nonlinearity and feedback. *Nonlinearity* means the system input-output characteristic cannot be described by a straight line. Hence some kind of exponential function like $f(x) = x^2$ is involved. *Feedback* is a term applied to a system when a portion of its output is added or subtracted to its input to produce the output.

As a result of these characteristics, the system response is determined by the nonlinear interaction of the present system condition and input to produce the next output. Biologic systems, which have a natural period of oscillation (e.g., circadian rhythm, cardiac electrical activity) have the property of being entrainable (sychronizable) by an external stimulus. Properly applied stimuli can cause this oscillation to be reset, terminated, or to break into a complex pattern. Such patterns have been observed in a variety of experiments involving living colonies in a two-dimensional sheet (5).

Since the heart is responsible for its own blood supply, VF becomes a continuously evolving condition which was described by Wiggers as consisting of four stages (7). In the first, or undulatory stage, large areas of myocardium contract in a manner similar to premature ventricular contractions (PVCs). These contractions spread more slowly than normal conduction from the stimulation point. This stage is maintained for only a few seconds. A simultaneous surface ECG shows wide depolarization complexes.

Wiggers noted that these contractions led to subsequent patterns of contraction, probably caused by reentry, which are similar, but do not exactly repeat. If one plots the amplitude of the ECG versus its first time derivative or the current interval versus the last interval, patterns are described in what is termed "phase space." If the pattern remains confined to a finite area (volume) of this space, but never actually repeats, it is called a "strange attractor" in chaos theory. Wiggers' description is qualitatively similar to the "strange attractor in phase space" obtained from a variety of experiments involving systems other than the heart.

In the second stage, or convulsive incoordination condition, increasing contraction frequency progressively involves smaller volumes of the ventricles. It lasted 15–40 sec in Wiggers' experiments. He noted that the heart still maintained vigorous contraction during this time. The surface ECG showed diminished amplitude, higher-frequency complexes.

The third stage, or tremulous incoordination, lasts from 2 to 3 min. From his description, Wiggers indicated that even smaller areas of myocardium are contracting together. A surface ECG would presumably show fine fibrillation at this point (author's interpretation).

The final, or atonic, stage of fibrillation occurs 2–5 min after its onset. This stage is characterized by noncontractile areas of myocardium as a result of the prolonged ischemia. These noncontractile areas gradually expand to completely involve both ventricles.

Topology theory, which is the study of the properties of geometric shapes which remain unchanged when the shape is distorted, provides a theoretical basis for laboratory investigation into the origin of fibrillation. In his book, *When Time Breaks Down*, Winfree uses the topology theory to describe two different types of response, even and odd phase resetting, in externally stimulated biologic oscillators.

In odd-phase resetting, the latency, or time from the stimulus to the next natural event, decreases smoothly as the coupling interval (natural event to stimulus time) is increased. In the limiting case of odd or weak resetting, the stimulus has no effect on the timing and a plot of latency versus coupling interval is a decreasing straight line diagonal. With slightly stronger stimuli, the plot of latency against coupling interval is still decreasing and each value of latency appears an odd number of times. If the stimulus strength is further increased, a new pattern emerges. Now each value of latency appears an even number of times with no net change as the coupling interval is varied over the natural period of the biologic oscillator. Topologically, these two types of resetting are different. Odd or weak resetting results in a helix, whereas even or strong resetting presents as rings when these plots are wrapped around a cylinder.

Plotted in the three dimensions of coupling interval, stimulus strength, and latency (the time from the stimulus to the next natural event, such as depolarization), it can be shown that there is a point, known as a critical point or singularity, when the latency is undefined. The existence of this point is a result of the two different types of phase resetting. This has been demonstrated in a variety of biological systems including fruit fly reproduction and sinoatrial node (SAN) oscillation. The SAN may cease firing completely with application of a critically annihilating stimulus. When applied to a traveling wave of depolarization in ventricular myocardium, it can be shown that there are points around which rotors (rotating waves) of depolarization are generated when electric field stimulation is applied.

Frazier, *et al.* were able to demonstrate the generation and location control of these rotors in uniformly refractory canine myocardium by varying the direction of pacemaker-induced propagating wave fronts and properly timed orthogonally applied shocks. In spite of the variable rotor location, the center of the rotor (critical point) was described by a nearly constant stimulus intensity and timing (phase). The generated rotors preceded the onset of VF which was mapped by placement of an array of recording electrodes (8) (Fig. 19.1). Because of nonuniformities in stimulus strength and conduction, it can be shown that the center of the rotor generation is not a single point, but involves a U-shaped area known as a black hole (5).

In other systems as simple as water dripping from a faucet, chaotic behavior, similar to fibrillation, has been described as being confined to a finite area in phase space (6). As previously indicated, phase space plots instantaneous system variables like position and velocity along different axes. The resulting paths of the system response are confined to a small area but never repeat themselves. Recently, such patterns have been demonstrated in fibrillating human myocardium (9).

REQUIREMENTS FOR TERMINATION OF VENTRICULAR FIBRILLATION

The critical mass concept was an idea that was formulated to explain a requirement for ventricular defibrillation. It states that fibrillation must be abolished in only a certain large percentage of myocardium before it is terminated. This idea grew out of the observation that repeated dissection of myocardium would eventually render it too small to support fibrillation. These dissections were done physically or chemically with potassium chloride or were inferred from patterns of activity after electrical shocks (10–12).

More recently, mapping work by Chen, *et al.* demonstrated inability to record ventricular myocardial electrical activity for approximately 15–50 msec following an unsuccessful defibrillation shock. Further, new fibrillation wave fronts arose in areas of myocardium which had a low shock strength (electric field or potential gradient) (4). These are probably critical points or black holes around which rotating waves (rotors) of depolarization arise. Fig. 19.2A illustrates the electrical potential at various points in

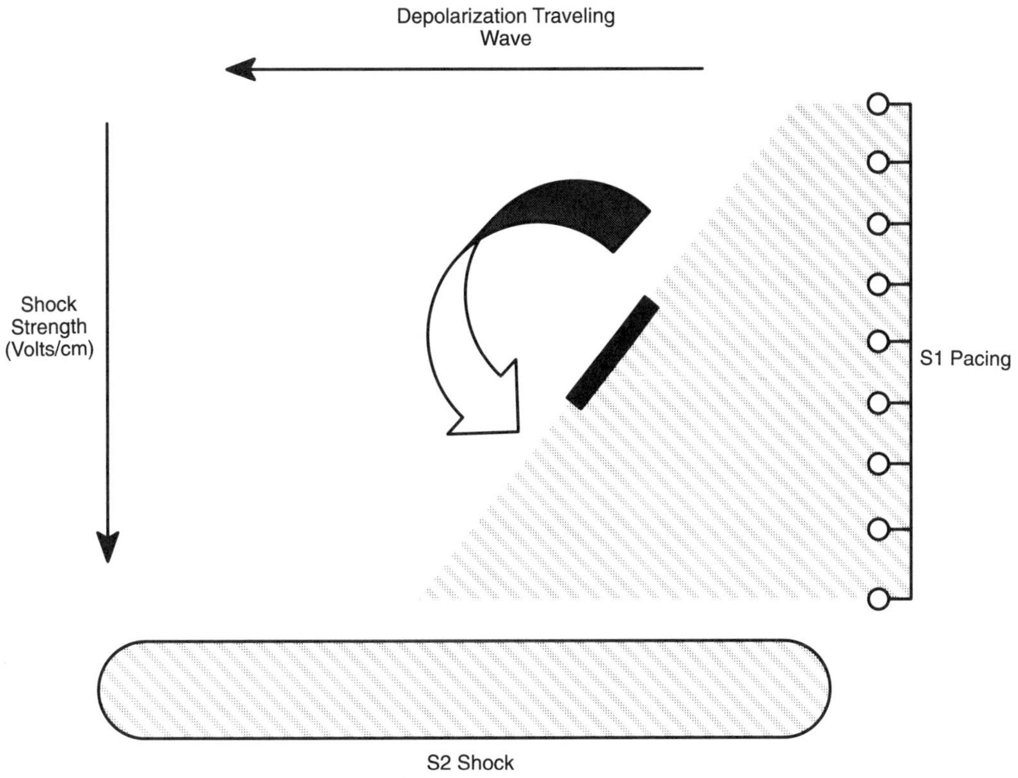

Figure 19.1. The onset of fibrillation originating in a localized area of canine myocardium. Multiple simultaneous pacing sites (S1) on the **right side** produced a planar wave of depolarization leaving a wake of varying refractoriness in the horizontal dimension. An orthogonally applied shock (S2) at the *bottom* caused a varying shock strength (potential gradient) which decreases in the vertical dimension. With proper S1–S2 coupling interval, a rotor *(rotating wave)* of depolarization around an area of functional block *(darkened bold line)* is created. This rotor progresses to fibrillation. The *cross-hatched area* is assumed to be directly excited by the shock. (Modified from Frazier DW, Wolf PD, Wharton JM, *et al.*: Stimulus-induced critical point: mechanism for electrical initiation of reentry in normal canine myocardium. J Clin Invest 1989;83:1039–1052.)

canine myocardium during an applied 1.5-V shock from right and left epicardial electrodes (usable voltages are × 100).

However, what actually stimulates tissue, and defibrillates, is the potential gradient—the spacial rate of change of potential at each point in the myocardium (Fig. 19.2B). This difference in potential at each point forces a varying current density through each area of myocardium. This varying current density results in myocardial cell stimulation depending on the gradient strength (V/cm) and timing during the cell's depolarization-repolarization cycle. During fibrillation, some cells may be completely depolarized by the shock because they have fully recovered at the time of its delivery. Other cells may be unaffected because they have just depolarized or are in an area of extremely low potential gradient. A third set of cells may have their refractory period extended by the shock, the so-called graded response (8). The ability of a particular shock waveform to prolong cellular recovery by this graded response is thought to be very important in terminating fibrillation.

As a result, during fibrillation, there may be points in the myocardium at the time of the shock which correspond to critical ones. Here the stimulus strength and timing are such that new wave fronts can arise. These new wave fronts arise both as rotors (vortices) and nonrotors.

Closely related to the requirements for defibrillation are the spatial relationships of timing and potential gradient which may give rise to fibrillation from normal rhythm. It has been demonstrated that shock strengths exist above which fibrillation will not start irrespective of the shock timing in the cardiac cycle. This strength is called the upper limit of vulnerability. It is closely related to shock strengths which are able to defibrillate. Above the upper limit of vulnerability, the singularity point, or black hole, is moved off the ventricular myocardium so that it is unlikely that induction or reinduction of fibrillation will occur (4).

Because the electric field is nonuniformly distributed throughout the myocardium (13), great efforts are being made to make it more uniform through clever electrode designs aimed toward application in implantable defibrillation.

WAVEFORMS FOR DEFIBRILLATION

Initial interest in electrical defibrillation was prompted by the early twentieth century incidence of fibrillation secondary to the introduction of 50–60 Hz alternating current (AC) power in the industrial and home environment. It also became apparent that fibrillation could accompany coronary occlusion; however, once

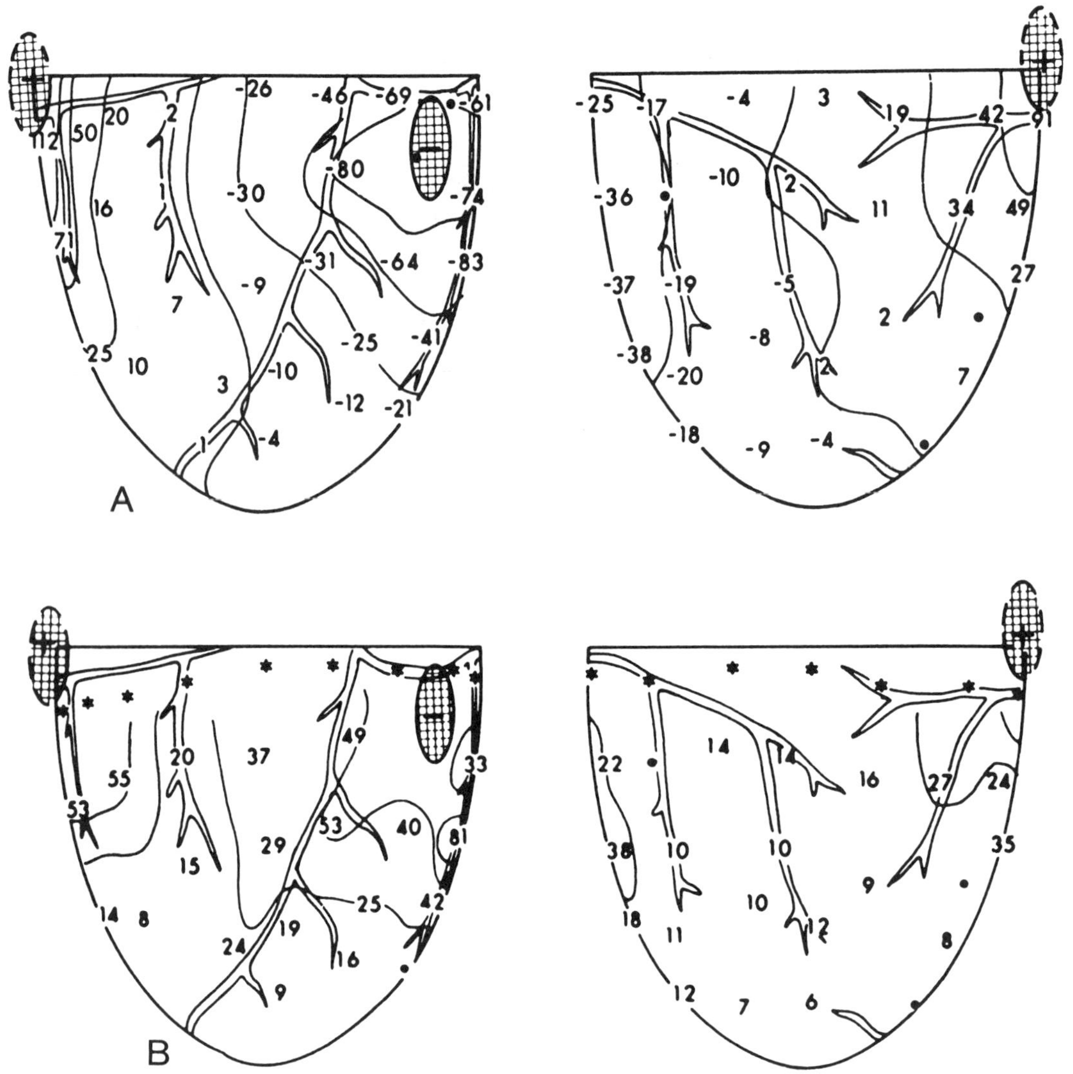

Figure 19.2. Epicardial potentials **(A)** and epicardial components of the potential gradients **(B)** for a 1.5-V shock delivered via electrodes on the bases of the left and right ventricles. **A**, The isopotential lines are more closely spaced near the two defibrillation electrodes, indicating a higher potential gradient. These measurements illustrate the highly nonuniform character of cardiac electrical stimulation from defibrillators electrodes. At voltages used for implantable defibrillators (100–750 V) the patterns are similar. This situation can lead to excessive stimulation in one portion of the myocardium and insufficient stimulation in another part. The challenge for electrode designers is to distribute the potentials and potential gradients more evenly **(B)**. **B,** High potential gradients were located around the defibrillation electrodes at the base with low gradients distant from the defibrillation electrodes at the apex. The highest gradient (55 mV/cm) was over nine times greater than the lowest gradient (6 mV/cm). Potential gradient is also the quantity that forces a current density (A/cm^2) in a given area of myocardium. (From Ideker RE, Wolf PD, Alterness C, *et al.*: Current concepts for selecting the location, size and shape of defibrillating electrodes. PACE 1991;14:232, reproduced with authors' and publisher's permission.)

it occurred, nothing could be done. Because AC power was readily available, and was often the cause of fibrillation, it was extensively studied as a method of defibrillating the heart.

The animal work of Hooker, Kouwenhoven, Langworthy, and Wiggers resulted in the first successful human electrical defibrillation by C.S. Beck in 1947. Before success, five previous failures occurred during efforts to resuscitate surgical patients by direct cardiac massage, injection of epinephrine and procaine hydrochloride, and direct cardiac application of 120 V AC electrical current (14).

The first successful use of external (transchest) AC electrical defibrillation was reported by Zoll in 1956 (15). The device consisted of a 6:1 stepup transformer with autotransformer in order to convert 120 V power to a variable voltage (up to 720 V) necessary for external conversion. The voltage was applied for 150 msec by use of a relay. The device was hazardous to the operator(s) because of the possibility of contacting the patient during the shock delivery.

The sequelae of postshock arrhythmias and respiratory arrest were not uncommon with AC defibrillation. These problems were well known because of extensive animal investigations (16). Frequencies other than 60 Hz were investigated for use in electrical defibrillation. None of them appeared to offer an advantage over the 60 Hz frequency which was readily available (15).

At the time of this first human external defibrillation, work was ongoing to investigate the use of capacitor discharge in defibrillation. Provost and Battelli first reported in 1899 that a direct current capacitor discharge could defibrillate the heart (17). Later, in 1946, Gurvich and Yuniev reported on capacitor discharge in a comparative study. Problems associated with pure capacitor discharge included a relatively large peak voltage requirement along with a propensity to produce atrioventricular (AV) block (16). In the United States, it was believed that AC defibrillation was superior to capacitor discharge. However, an AC defibrillating device could not be used with any arrhythmia other than VF since there was a high risk of inducing VF, if it were not already present.

The waveform produced by a pure capacitor discharge is shown in Fig. 19.3. It is a time-varying decrease in voltage of the form $e(t) = E^{*}\exp(-t/RC)$ where E is the maximum voltage at time zero, t is time, R is the total circuit resistance, and C is the value of the capacitor. Generation of this waveform is elementary: a step-up transformer converts 60 Hz, 120 V AC line voltage to a higher value, which is determined by the position of an autotransformer. This higher AC voltage is then converted to direct current (DC) by a rectifier device. The DC voltage is then stored on a capacitor. When delivery of the electrical charge on the capacitor is desired, a relay is closed. This connects the subject (patient or experimental animal) to the capacitor while disconnecting the charging circuit from it.

Much higher voltages than those used in AC defibrillation are required when this circuit is used. Not uncommonly, over 5000 V must be generated for external (transchest) defibrillation using capacitor discharge.

Implantable devices typically store only about one-tenth the energy of external defibrillators. They generate high voltage by use of a circuit known as a DC to DC converter which raises a battery voltage of 6 V to a voltage of approximately 100 times this value. Peleska concluded that the rapid increase at time zero of the capacitor discharge voltage causes cell damage independent of the voltage magnitude (18). Schuder has indicated that the relatively slow voltage decrease at the end of the capacitor discharge may cause refibrillation and thus render the shock ineffective, particularly for larger values of the capacitor (19).

A circuit change which addressed the problems of AC and capacitor discharge defibrillation was extensively studied by Dr. Lown at the time he investigated the cardioversion procedure

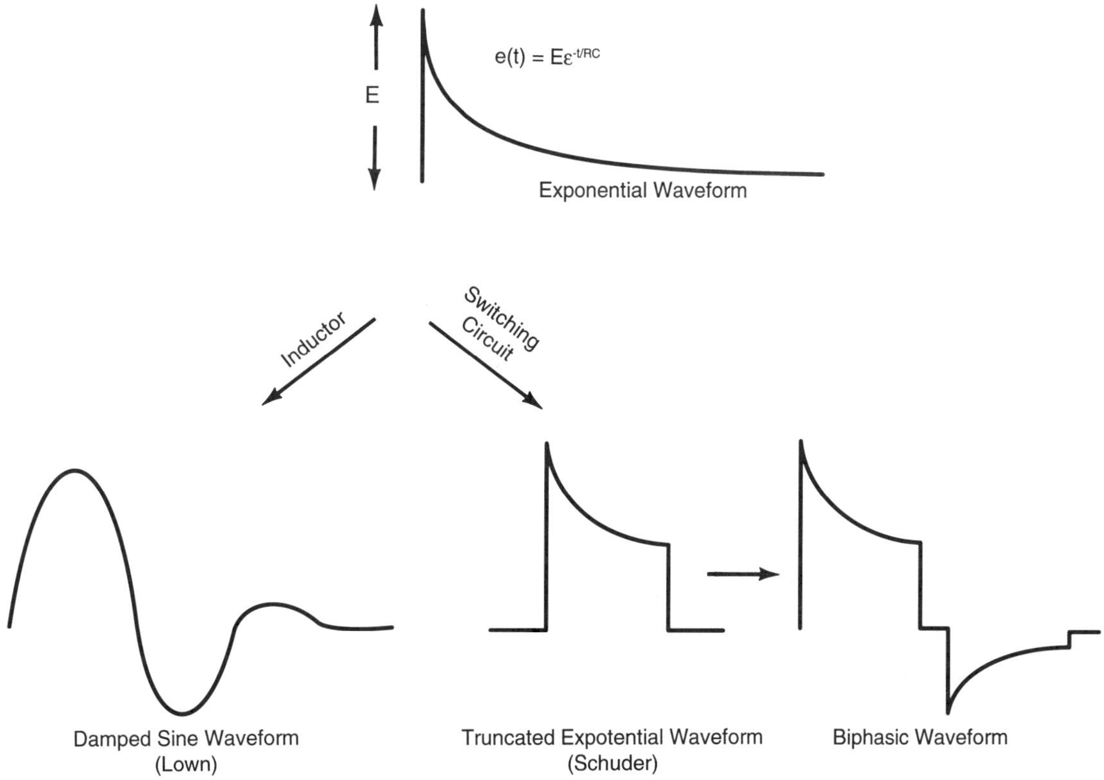

Figure 19.3. Evolution of DC defibrillation waveforms. By adding an inductor, the exponential waveform was modified into a damped sine wave. This improvement was only suitable for transchest defibrillation. Abruptly terminating the voltage decay by electronic switching produced a waveform applicable to implantable defibrillators. More elaborate electronic switching produced a biphasic waveform similar to the damped sine wave, but without the inductor.

(20). This circuit change involved the inclusion of an inductor, in series with the patient, when the capacitor was discharged. An inductor has the property of opposing a change in current, whereas a capacitor opposes a change in voltage (Fig. 19.3).

This opposition to current change greatly reduces the abruptness of current and voltage delivery. The peak current and voltage are also reduced since inductors have resistance and thus consume energy which is not delivered to the patient. The inclusion of the inductor into the capacitor circuit converts it into one which delivers a damped sine wave. That is, it is a sine wave whose amplitude decreases with each cycle.

In the case of the first use of the inductor, the sine wave usually did not provide a second positive excursion after its onset. This is due to the inductor and patient resistance. The circuit was thus somewhat "underdamped" (sinusoidal variation) with transchest electrodes which, when combined with the patient and patient-electrode resistance, resulted in a circuit resistance of 50–100 ohms. A further modification of the damped waveform occurred with the introduction of an "critically damped" (no sinusoidal variation) Edmark waveform (21). This waveform did not allow the defibrillating voltage to change polarity during the discharge.

The significance of the undershoot (polarity reversal) went unrecognized for a long time. It was extensively studied by Schuder (22,23). It is now becoming generally believed that the polarity reversal of the waveform has the ability to improve defibrillation far in excess of the slight increase in total energy it delivers. The mechanism by which this occurs is not completely understood. However, Jones and Jones have demonstrated increased ability (compared with monophasic waveforms) of long biphasic waveforms to prolong cellular repolarization (24). It has been further suggested that hyperpolarization of one end of individual cells in the first phase of the shock allows that end of the cell to be more easily depolarized during the second phase (25).

In the late 1960s, investigation of electrical waveforms that might be utilized in an implantable defibrillator was begun. Although effective, the "Lown" (underdamped sine wave) waveform was unsuitable for an implantable device for the very reason it worked: the inductor. Inductors are heavy magnetic devices which consume energy and space, both of which are at a premium in any implantable device.

Dr. John Schuder, a physicist working at the University of Missouri, developed a defibrillating circuit and waveform which were eventually incorporated into the implantable defibrillator (Fig. 19.4). As opposed to previous defibrillating devices which incorporated vacuum relays, this Schuder device accomplished electronic switching with semiconductor silicon-controlled rectifiers (SCRs). These devices have the property of remaining on until their current is reduced to a very small value. Therefore, a second switching device was utilized to short circuit the capacitor at the desired time. This caused the current that was flowing through the patient to flow through the "short circuit," turning off the "patient SCR." The waveform thus produced is known as the truncated exponential or "Schuder" waveform.

Again, the idea is a modification of the capacitor discharge. However, in this case, the capacitor is not allowed to discharge to 0 V. The voltage is abruptly removed at some point into the discharge (usually when the voltage is between 20 and 40% of its initial value). Since stored energy is proportional to the square of the voltage, the price in discarded energy was not great. Tilt is defined as "1 minus the ratio of the final voltage value to the initial voltage value." As tilt increases, it becomes more difficult to defibrillate for a given initial peak voltage or current (26).

Schuder also investigated biphasic waveforms (22,23). Biphasic waveforms reverse the polarity of the applied shock during its delivery. Although certain biphasic waveforms were known to be superior, they could not be incorporated into an implantable device until recently. Advances in the semiconductor industry produced high-voltage devices which could be easily turned on and off by low-voltage switching circuits. Such devices are known as power MOSFETs (metal oxide semiconductor field effect transistor) or IGBTs (insulated gate biopolar transistors). Various implementations using these new switching components have been incorporated into implantable cardioverter defibrillators.

The possibility of incorporating biphasic defibrillation into an implantable device has led to a variety of investigations to determine which of several conceptualized waveforms would offer the most improvement in comparison to a monophasic waveform. Tang, *et al.* determined that a second phase shorter than the first is preferable. In fact, waveforms in which the first phase is shorter than the second are inferior to monophasic waveforms (27).

Investigations into the amplitude relationship of the second phase to the first have resulted in the conclusion that the second-phase amplitude should be less than the first. This is a useful coincidence because delivery of the biphasic pulse from a single capacitor is accomplished efficiently by implantable electronics.

Single-capacitor waveforms have been reported to be superior to both two capacitor and monophasic waveforms of the same leading edge voltage and duration (28). A comparison of the improvement seen with a biphasic shock compared to a monophasic shock delivered with the same leading edge voltage is shown in Fig. 19.5. Biphasic waveforms appear to offer significant improvement in defibrillation when the electric field has a highly nonuniform distribution (as in transvenous defibrillation).

DEFIBRILLATION THRESHOLD

Prior to clinical use of implantable defibrillation, the idea of deliberately inducing ventricular fibrillation in a patient to determine whether defibrillation would be successful was almost unthinkable. Determination of defibrillation shock strength requirements in individual patients became a necessity when it slowly became known that single-shock success was not always

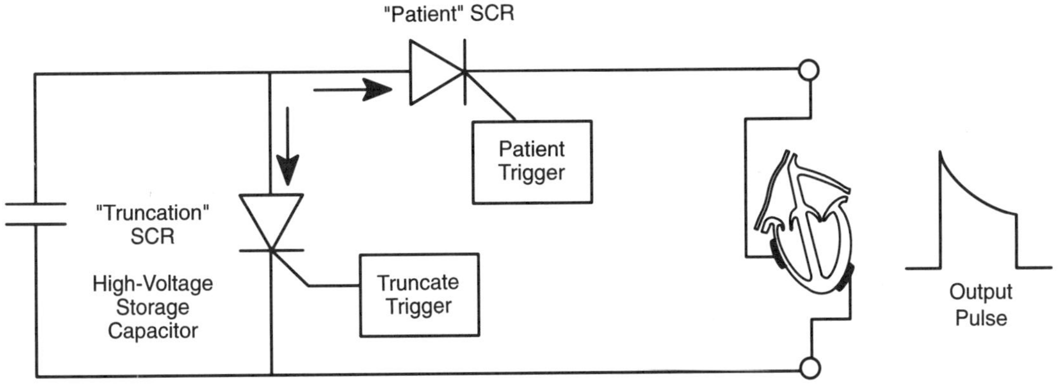

Figure 19.4. Basic Schuder circuit for generating a truncated exponential waveform. The patient SCR turns on first. At the appropriate time, the truncate SCR turns on. This removes current from the patient SCR and turns it off.

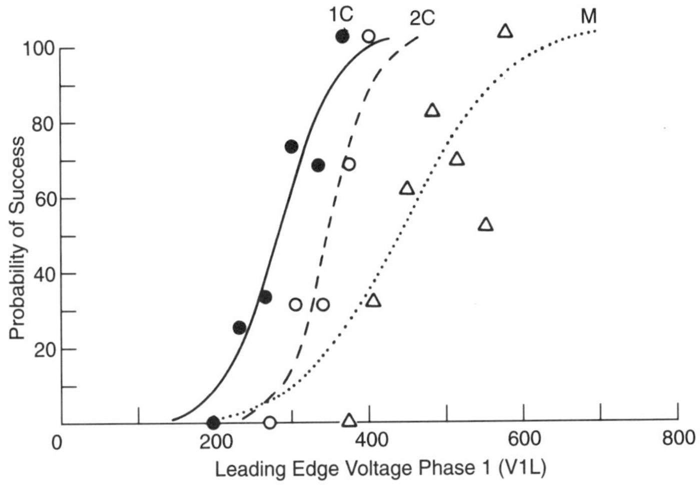

Figure 19.5. Typical sigmoid-shaped dose-response curves obtained from a defibrillator experiment. They illustrate the fact that a defibrillation "threshold" does not exist. One can arbitrarily assign a certain probability of success as the threshold. In this case, the data points were fitted to dose-response defibrillation curves with regression analysis in an experiment involving monophasic and biphasic shocks with different sized capacitors. Shown are monophasic *(triangles, dotted line)*, double-capacitor *(open circles, dashed line)*, and single-capacitor *(closed circles, solid line)* response curves in a representative dog. The voltage requirements were lowest for the single-capacitor biphasic waveform and highest for the monophasic waveform. (From Kavanagh KM, Tang ASL, Rollins DL: Monophasic, double and single capacitor Waveforms. J Am Coll Cardiol 1989;14(5):1343–1349. Reprinted with permission from the American College of Cardiology, J Am Coll Cardiol, reproduced with authors' and publisher's permission.)

reproducible and that patients differed widely in their susceptibility to VF termination.

The term "defibrillation threshold" (DFT) implies that there exists a relatively distinct boundary between shock strengths that will convert and those that will not. Such a boundary appears to exist in cardiac pacing between pulse strength that will capture and pulse strength that will not. No such boundary has been found for conversion of VF. Instead, a sigmoid-shaped dose-response curve best describes the relationship between shock strength and conversion success (Fig. 19.5). Usually shock strength is plotted in joules, peak volts, or peak current. Other variables are possible, including total electrical charge (coulombs).

At the present time, the underlying physiologic principle(s) that give rise to this characteristic are not completely understood. However, some insight can be obtained by considering the fibrillating heart as having a variety of states. At a single point in time there exists a certain geometric distribution of cells which are, at a single instant, in the transition phase of depolarization. Simultaneously, another set of cells are in the transition phase of repolarization. Lastly, a third set of cells are totally depolarized. Depending on shock strength and potential gradient (electric field) distribution, a variety of singularity points probably exists. These points are in continuous transition. A shock strength which moves these off the ventricular myocardium will probably succeed; one that does not may not succeed (4). What is still a mystery to defibrillation researchers is why some polymorphic rhythms following shocks self terminate, while others progress to sustained fibrillation.

Clinically, spontaneous polymorphic rhythms may self terminate. Electrical mapping studies indicate that often the underlying nature of these rhythms may be "figure-of-eight patterns" (29). The point is that the heart continuously varies in its ability to be converted. Smaller strength shocks terminate VF with less frequency than larger shocks and the transition between low conversion rate and near-100% conversion is not always abrupt.

Defibrillation threshold has come to mean different things depending on the context within which it is being used. To the basic researcher, it is the shock strength that gives rise to a certain stated percent success rate. To the clinician, it may be the lowest shock strength that converted fibrillation. Therefore, the term has different meaning depending on the algorithm used to obtain it. The researcher is desirous of obtaining an accurate statistical curve for the purpose of comparison to another, e.g., after pharmacologic intervention. The clinician is interested in providing a safety margin for the patient—a significant difference between the shock strength that reliably converts and the maximum output of the implantable defibrillator.

Irrespective of the algorithm, it is generally accepted that it is necessary to induce fibrillation more than one time in order to have some idea of whether the implanted lead system will reliably convert the patient. The goal is to minimize the number of inductions while retaining some confidence that the results will apply when the patient leaves the hospital.

Clinically, induction of VF is done in a variety of ways. Initially, full-wave rectified AC (120 Hz pulsed DC) was applied to an electrophysiology catheter in the right ventricle. Later, rate sensing leads of the implantable defibrillator were used. More commonly now, 60 Hz AC or pulsed DC current is applied to the device shocking leads. This provides a more uniform field distribution and more reliable induction (30). Ramp pacing from device rate sensing/pacing leads has also been used. This is especially useful when noninvasive studies are done at follow-up and the pacing commands are sent to the implantable device via telemetry. It has also been customary, both clinically and in the research environment, to consider only the first shock delivered. In the event of conversion failure, rescue shocks are not part of the formal evaluation of energy requirements. However, their effectiveness will certainly enter into any decision by the surgeon and cardiologist to revise the lead system.

DEFIBRILLATION THRESHOLD ALGORITHMS

One of the earliest published algorithms for evaluating defibrillation strength requirements assumed a relatively sharp transition between shock strengths that convert and those that do not (16). As pointed out by McDaniel, its results also depend upon whether one starts at a low shock strength, a shock strength at the theoretical 50% conversion point, or a high shock strength (31). There is a wide distribution of possible results, with the outcome biased toward the starting value.

In order to avoid these imprecise outcomes, researchers may plot a curve by delivering a certain number of shocks at each shock strength. This is usually done randomly or in balanced random order (high, then low, etc.). This can result in a large number of fibrillation-defibrillation episodes for the experimental animal. Obviously, a technique like this is clinically unacceptable.

Another experimental technique that reduces the number of shocks is called the up-down technique (32). Here, a successful shock dictates reducing the shock strength for the next trial while an unsuccessful shock dictates raising the shock strength. The benefit of this algorithm is that the trials are conducted on the most rapidly changing portion of the percent success curve. This avoids a large number of shocks at the extremes of the curve where the outcome is virtually certain.

Clinically, defibrillation requirements may be tested by starting with a large shock energy close to the maximum output of the implantable defibrillator. The logic is that if this strength doesn't convert, the lead system will have to be altered (changing defibrillating patch sizes, moving patches, etc.).

As a result of extensive canine defibrillation experiments, Lang, *et al*. recommended a concept called DFT+ or DFT++. Here, shock strengths are reduced in successive trials until a failure occurs. The lowest shock strength that converted is designated the DFT. Another one (DFT+) or two (DFT++) trials are then done at the DFT (a plus indicates successful conversion, a minus would indicate failure to convert on subsequent trial(s)). A subsequent conversion (DFT+) gives an 80% chance that the success rate is greater than 60%. Two conversions (DFT++) gives a 94% chance for the success rate to be greater than 60%. If the subsequent shock is unsuccessful on repeat trial, there is only a 40% chance that the success rate is greater than 60%. Statistically, Lang *et al*. have argued that single or two shock protocols are poor predictors of defibrillation reliability (33).

Defibrillation algorithms do not always result in simple outcomes. It is not unknown to have raised the shock strength from the lowest successful one on consecutive trials and continuously encounter unsuccessful defibrillation all the way to the maximum output. This can happen for a variety of reasons, such as a shifting electrode position on or in the heart or an air pocket under a patch electrode. In some instances, no explanation can be found. This has led some investigators to suspect that the results of trials are influenced by accumulated ischemia time.

However, some studies have not been supportive of this theory (34,35) while others have been (36). Some studies have shown a decrease in defibrillation requirements as the experiment progresses (37). The reasons for this are unknown. It is well known that the outcome of defibrillation experiments depends on the species used. Some fibrillation-defibrillation strength success curves may actually be concave downward. This means the curve has a peak, possibly at less than 100% success. At strengths greater than the peak success, the success rate decreases with increasing shock strength. This is common in the calf (22,23).

Many clinicians now prefer to do the first fibrillation-defibrillation trial at a shock strength that is half the maximum output (in joules) of the implantable device used. If successful once or twice at this energy, then the implantable device will be connected to the implanted leads and both fibrillation detection and termination are tested. The argument for this technique is that the safety margin is probably so large that the patient is likely to be converted in the ambulatory setting. There has been some evidence to suggest that even this margin underestimates the shock strength requirement for 100% defibrillation success (33).

With newer implantable devices, initial as well as subsequent shock strengths are programmable. Reducing the shock strength should then be accompanied by more extensive testing at operation or follow-up in the electrophysiology laboratory.

TRANSVENOUS ELECTRODE DESIGNS

Since the beginning of the implantable defibrillator development in the 1960s, the goal has been to make the lead implantation no more complex than that of a pacemaker. Such a lead has an electrode in the right ventricle and another in the right atrium or superior vena cava.

However, some fundamental laws of physics and physiology are working against this notion. Firstly, for a pacemaker to stimulate, it must do so only at the electrode site. The depolarization wave front then spreads over the myocardium. For defibrillation to occur, the voltage gradient in each area of the ventricular myocardium must be raised above a certain level (6 V/cm in canine experiments using a monophasic pulse (38)). This value is highly waveform dependent with some biphasic shocks having half the requirements of monophasic shocks of similar tilt (39). Field mapping studies show that wire electrodes confined to the right heart do not distribute the potential gradient as evenly as patch electrodes placed over both ventricles.

To raise the left ventricular free wall area to a high enough potential gradient, strengths that are known to cause cellular dysfunction at the electrode site may have to be used. Such strengths have the potential to reinduce fibrillation underneath the electrode (40). In essence, one may have to overdose one area of myocardium to achieve sufficient voltage gradient in another area far from the electrodes.

To overcome this limitation, and still avoid a thoracic procedure, several approaches are being explored. One approach is to increase the surface area of the right ventricular electrode. However, the design of such an electrode must take into consideration the proximity to the superior vena caval electrode and the fact that mechanical flexibility must be maintained in order to avoid right ventricular perforation. An early design approach was to separate the electrode into several sleeved sections (41,42). A second approach is to use a tightly coiled conductor with sufficiently small pitch, such as is used in pacemaker leads (43).

Concern over tricuspid valve damage limits the linear length of such an electrode. It is also desirable to have an electrode in the right atrium in order to provide a return path for current and to provide sufficient stimulation to the heart base. This also simultaneously depolarizes the atria with the shock pulse. This may be necessary because the shock could be delivered asynchronously with atrial activity and has the potential to induce atrial fibrillation if the atria are only partially stimulated.

Using a subcutaneous electrode over the left chest provides a pathway for current perpendicular to the septum and left ventricular free wall. While doing this, the return in reduced shock strength requirements is less than ideal since a significant portion of the shock energy is now dissipated in the subcutaneous tissue. In order to be useful, the area of this electrode must be large (on the order of 25 cm^2 or greater) (44). Use of a subcutaneous patch electrode as an anode and connection of an electrode in the right ventricular outflow tract and an electrode in the right ventricular apex as a common cathode has been shown to be superior to either electrode alone (45). The outflow tract electrode improves the distribution of the electric field in a location that is weak when using only the apical electrode.

Several combinations of subcutaneous and transvenous electrodes are now undergoing or have undergone clinical trial. One set of combinations is shown in Figure 19.6. Canine studies indicated that configuration 1 allowed lower defibrillation requirements than the others. However, a clinical trial showed that configuration 2 was superior (46). This was probably due to the difference in chest geometry between the canine and the human.

Another approach to this problem utilizes a right ventricular electrode, a coronary sinus electrode, and a subcutaneous electrode. Here, the coronary sinus electrode and subcutaneous electrode may or may not be connected together. This scheme also utilizes sequential shocks. The first shock is delivered between the coronary sinus electrode and the right ventricular electrode. The second shock is delivered between subcutaneous electrode and the right ventricular electrode (47).

With all of the investigation into nonthoracotomy defibrillation and the early initial success in clinical trial, it is certain that transvenous defibrillation must be the future of implantable defibrillation because of morbidity and the cost of open chest procedures. That is not to say that direct placement of epicardial patches will disappear. For the foreseeable future, patient variability in defibrillation requirements precludes this. It is still a mystery why some patients have such extremely high or low shock strength requirements.

AUTOMATIC RECOGNITION OF VENTRICULAR TACHYARRHYTHMIAS

Implantable ventricular antitachyarrhythmia devices should be capable of detecting ventricular tachycardia and fibrillation with high sensitivity while rejecting supraventricular rhythms, such as atrial fibrillation and sinus tachycardia, as "normal." Since tachyarrhythmia detection in these devices is based primarily on the interpretation of the cardiac depolarization rate, when the rate range of a patient's ventricular and supraventricular rhythms overlaps, discrimination is difficult. Electrogram morphology analysis may improve device specificity in selected patients (48,49). Other approaches to detection of ventricular tachyarrhythmias include the use of a direct physiologic sensor such as pressure or an indirect sensor such as impedance.

Atrial or ventricular rate determination is best accomplished by the placement of small, closely spaced electrodes in healthy myocardium. The electrodes should be well separated from those that deliver the shock. The signals from these electrodes are discrete depolarizations without significant repolarization activity. This greatly simplifies the electronic filtering problem. Bipolar electrodes of approximately 10 mm^2 separated by 0.5–1 cm generally provide suitable electrograms. However, bipolar electrodes are directionally sensitive. The electrograms obtained from them are dependent upon the angle between the bipole and

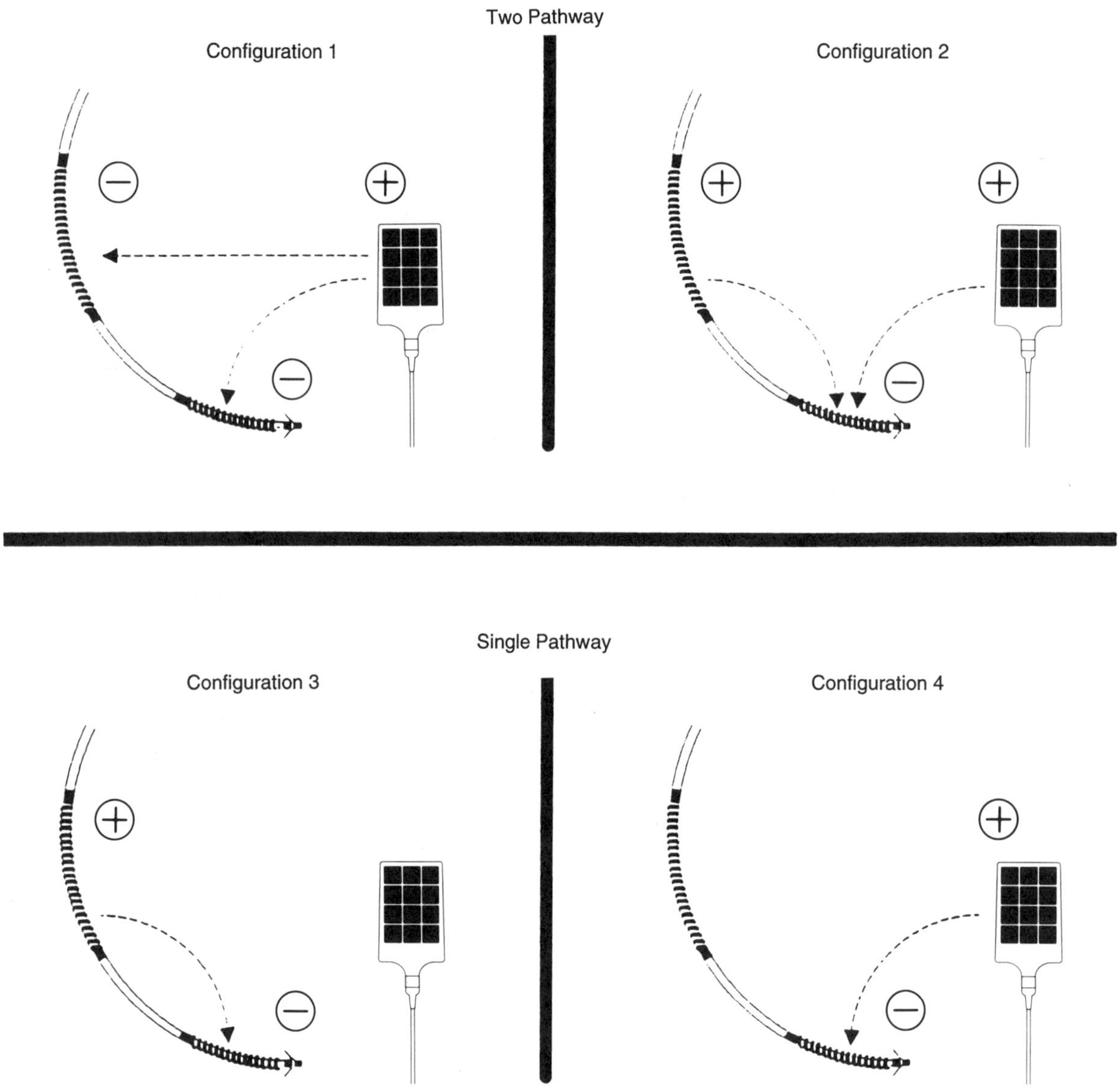

Figure 19.6. The four configurations employed in acute and chronic testing of the Endotak system for nonthoracotomy AICD implantation. Configurations 1 and 2 have dual-current paths, whereas configurations 3 and 4 have single-current paths. Based upon available clinical experience, Configuration 2 was the most favorable lead configuration tested. (From Troup PJ: Implantable cardioverters and defibrillators. Curr Prob Cardiol 1989;14:12:758, reproduced with author's and publisher's permission.)

the depolarization wave front. This depolarization wave front approaches the bipole from a variety of directions during different monomorphic tachycardias and during VF.

As a result, either an automatic sense level adjusting circuit or continuously high fixed sensitivity has been used to detect rate during normal and abnormal rhythms. High fixed sensitivity may not provide satisfactory performance because it is unable to adapt to the variability in amplitude and slew rate (signal rate of change or first derivative) which occurs during polymorphic rhythms (Fig. 19.7).

Additionally, fixed sensitivity places a burden of proof on the physician to demonstrate reliable sensing during all of a patient's rhythms. This is time consuming and, in some cases, may not be possible if spontaneously occurring rhythms are not inducible. Finally, during ventricular arrhythmias, cardiac ischemia will result in a progressive deterioration of the sensed electrogram's amplitude and slew rate. Thus, ineffective therapy may result in a signal that is less likely to be sensed by a fixed-gain amplifier compared to one controlled by some automatic level adjusting or gain control scheme which can track these changes.

Electrogram amplifiers for implantable device rate sensing have a bandpass characteristic. That is, low frequencies like 1 Hz and higher frequencies like 200 Hz are not amplified as much as frequencies near the center of the response. This characteristic is chosen to preferentially amplify depolarization signals derived from the implanted leads. For a fixed-gain amplifier of

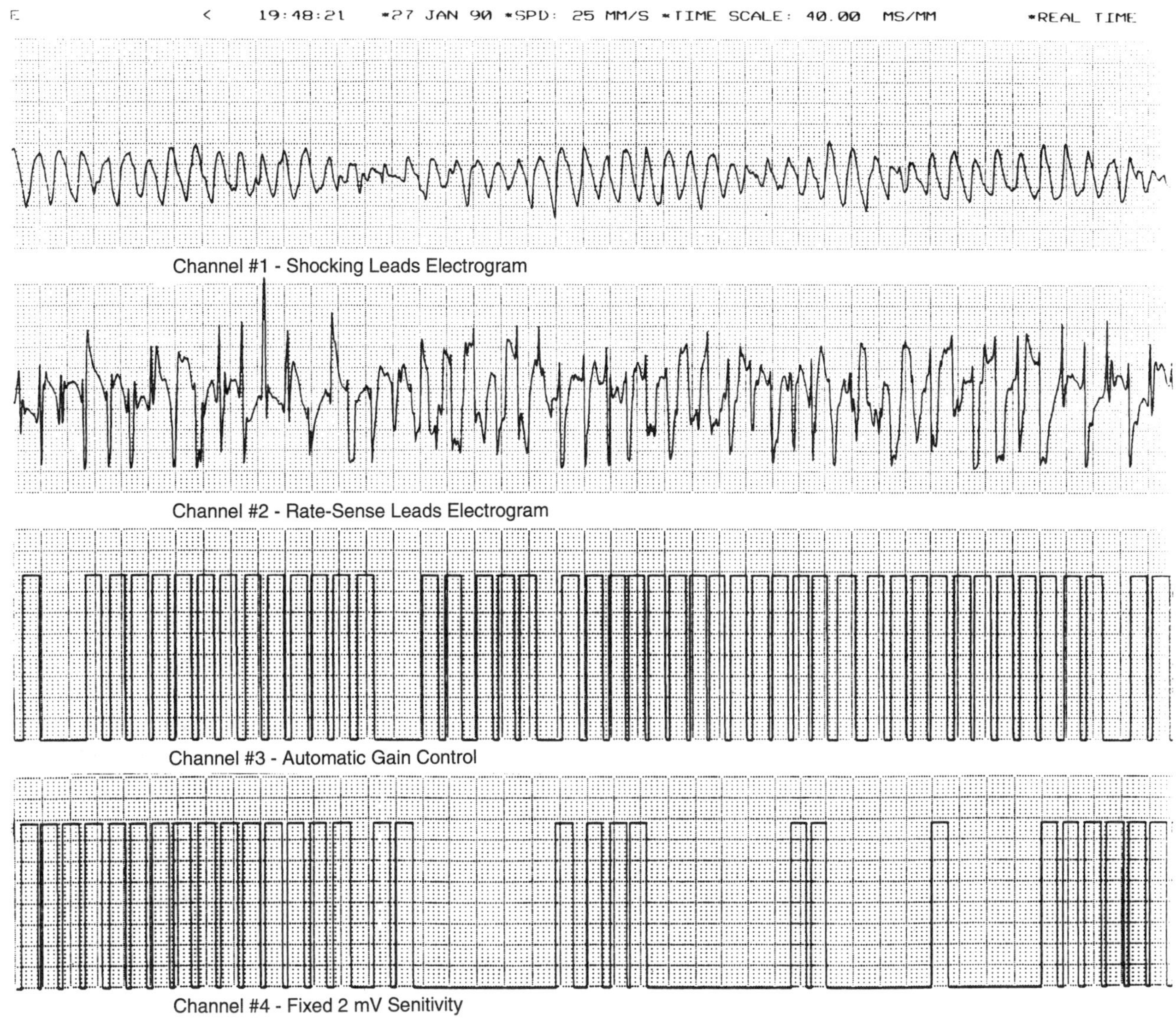

Figure 19.7. Comparison of ventricular fibrillation rate counting using automatic gain control and 2 mV fixed sensitivity. The fixed sensitivity amplifier suddenly undersenses the signal. Each sensed event is an upright pulse of 120 msec duration. (From Bach SM, Jr, Hsung JC: Implantable device algorithms for tachyarrhythmia detection/discrimination. In Proceedings of the Second International Congress on Rate Adaptive Cardiac Pacing and Implantable Defibrillators, Munich 1990, reproduced with authors' and publisher's permission.)

gain 50, a 5-mV input signal should produce a 250-mV output signal if the signal falls in the band pass (is of proper duration). For an automatic gain control amplifier set to provide a 250-mV output signal, both 1 mV and 10 mV input signals will result in the 250-mV output. In either case, the resulting output signal is compared to a fixed voltage level. When this voltage level is exceeded, a depolarization sense is declared. Automatic sensing level adjust amplifiers have a fixed gain, but vary the voltage detection level depending on the input signal magnitude.

In order to not repeatedly detect on multiple transitions, a refractory period is introduced after the first sense declaration. This refractory period (there may be more than one) may vary from several milliseconds up to several hundred milliseconds.

For tachyarrhythmia rate sensing, sensed refractory periods typically do not last more than 150 msec because of the possibility of undercounting the true rate when new depolarizations fall within this time. Theoretically, rates up to 400 beats/min may then be counted accurately. A rate just in excess of 400 beats/min would then be counted as half the signal rate. In practice this happens infrequently. These rapid rates are only seen in fibrillation in the human heart and the signals are not regular enough to allow this undercounting to occur for very long. In the adult human heart, equivalent fibrillation rates seldom exceed 400 beats/min and are often slower due to antiarrhythmic drug medication. One example of the distribution of cycle lengths detected during a polymorphic rhythm with an automatic gain control circuit is illustrated in Figure 19.8.

Onset and rate variability are two rate methods that have been

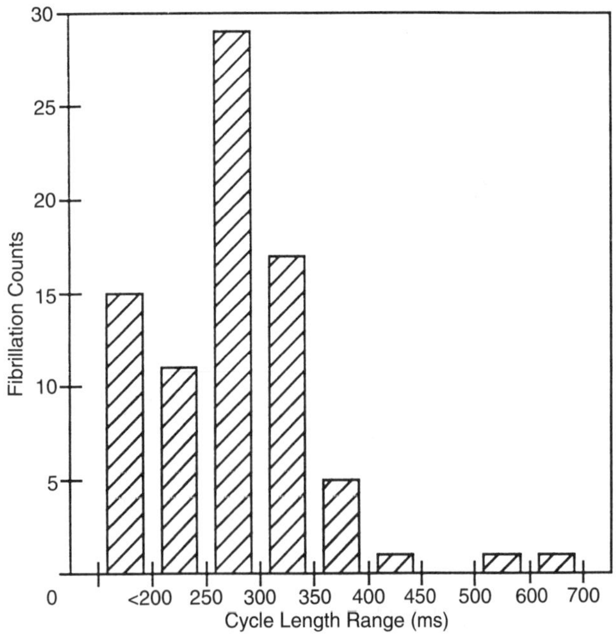

Figure 19.8. Typical frequency distribution of interval counts resulting from automatic gain control sensing of ventricular fibrillation. (From Bach Sm Jr, Hsung JC: Implantable device algorithms for tachyarrhythmia detection, discrimination. In Proceedings of the Second International Congress on Rate Adaptive Cardiac Pacing and Implantable Defibrillators, Munich 1990, reproduced with authors' and publisher's permission.)

used in implantable devices to distinguish ventricular arrhythmias from those of atrial origin. Onset is utilized to separate exercise sinus tachycardia from VT. The assumption is that VT begins abruptly whereas exercise tachycardia begins more slowly. Mercando recently reported that in the same patient there was no overlap in these cardiac rate changes (50).

Rate stability is designed to separate atrial fibrillation from monomorphic VT should the rate range of these two overlap. However, the ventricular response in atrial fibrillation may be quite regular, especially at faster rates, and ventricular tachycardia can be somewhat irregular, particularly at its onset or during nonsustained rhythms (51,52). Hence, stability may not always provide the desired diagnostic separation. One approach to stability analysis compares each cycle length to the four cycle length running average. A difference of more than a programmable number of milliseconds declares an unstable cycle length. Another approach examines the magnitude of the cycle length to cycle length changes, much as one would do when reading a surface ECG.

Morphology analysis in implantable devices is extremely simplified compared to that of cardiac care or ambulatory monitors. The main limitations are battery current drain and the computational power of the implanted microprocessor. Generally, increasing computational power translates to increased current consumption which shortens the device's battery life.

The probability density function (PDF) circuitry in the implantable cardioverter defibrillator is an analog design. It is intended to detect VF and sinusoidal-shaped (wide QRS) VT by examining the electrogram from the device shocking electrodes. This electrogram has the general character of a body surface ECG. The circuitry evaluates the fraction of time a signal spends at baseline compared to the amount of time it is changing. The entire cardiac cycle is evaluated, i.e., the depolarization and repolarization time. A signal with little isoelectric time is declared an arrhythmia. This declaration is logically ANDed with device rate criteria. That is, both the rate criteria and the PDF criteria must be met before charging of the device capacitors takes place.

Turning point morphology (TPM) is a newer microprocessor-based algorithm designed to diagnose ventricular arrhythmias via a shocking electrode electrogram. All signal rates of change are declared faster (slope) or slower (nonslope or line) than a selected value. TPM has programmable definitions of line versus slope and percent of slope necessary to declare a 2-sec segment of an electrogram as a ventricular arrhythmia. If two out of three segments are declared abnormal, the entire rhythm is declared abnormal. It is currently implemented to direct therapy to shock, bypassing antitachycardia pacing therapy. The programmable features of the algorithm are not presently available for change.

Another approach to diagnosis of arrhythmias via a morphology criterion assumes nothing about the nature of the electrogram. Instead, the algorithm learns what is normal for the patient by extracting features of the normal electrogram and then comparing those features to those of an unknown electrogram. This method of analysis is known as template matching. It has been investigated using right ventricular, 1-cm bipolar electrograms obtained during electrophysiologic study.

An example of template matching is the sequence of depolarization slopes technique (gradient pattern detection) reported by Davies, *et al.* (49). In this method, the derivative of the electrogram produces a signal whose instantaneous value is the slope (rate of change) of the original electrogram. The sequence of slopes during the depolarization of the normal electrogram is then used as a standard with which to compare an unknown electrogram (Fig. 19.9).

In implementation such practical considerations such as the necessity of obtaining a representative average normal sequence and providing usable criteria for separation of normal from abnormal must be incorporated into the algorithm.

Physiologic sensors for detection of the hemodynamic condition during ventricular tachyarrhythmias have been tested in the right ventricle and atrium (53). The difficulty, of course, is that right-sided hemodynamics do not necessarily reflect the left-sided condition. The changes in right ventricular and atrial pressure or right ventricular stroke volume (impedance technique) are small in absolute number compared to left-sided changes. This makes the measurement of these changes more critical, particularly because they are subject to alteration during normal activity. The development of a chronic pressure sensor has been plagued by moisture penetration problems while stroke volume techniques remain investigational (54).

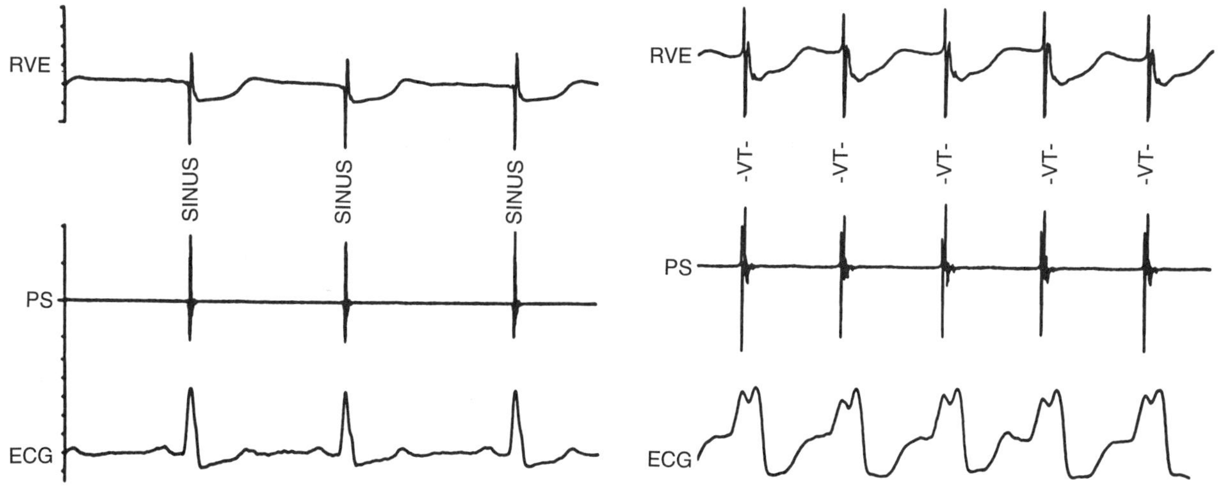

Figure 19.9. Upper panel—analogue electrogram; **middle panel**—processed signals; **lower panel**—surface ECG (CM_5); left panel— sinus rhythm; **right panel**—ventricular tachycardia. PS = processed signals; RVE = right ventricular electrogram. The alteration of electrogram morphology that occurs with the onset of ventricular tachycardia is reproduced in the processed signal allowing automatic recognition (vertical labeling). (From Davies DW, Wainwright RJ, Toley MA, *et al.*: Detection of pathological tachycardia by analysis of electrogram morphology. PACE 1986;9:200–208, reproduced with authors' and publisher's permission.)

HARDWARE ENGINEERING IN THE IMPLANTABLE CARDIOVERTER DEFIBRILLATOR PACEMAKER

To defibrillate the heart, a low voltage, on the order of 6 V, must be converted to a high voltage of about 100 times as much (600–800 V). This presents a significant challenge to the device battery, which is required to immediately supply a large current of approximately 100,000 times as much as is used in monitoring the cardiac rhythm status (1 A vs. 10 μA).

Such batteries were originally designed for military application (55) but are now being supplied by companies dedicated to their medical use (56). The electrical charge withdrawn from the battery is stored on the device output capacitor(s). These capacitors must be periodically exercised to prevent excessive deterioration of their storage ability (57). At the completion of charging, the patient-shocking electrodes are momentarily connected to the capacitor by the output switching circuits previously described. The capacitor(s) voltage polarity may be reversed midpulse (biphasic shock) or delivered sequentially over two separate pathways (47).

With the exception of the output switching, the circuitry is similar to that used in photoflash cameras. Indeed, the technology has been made available for medical application because of the commercial success of these devices. The start of capacitor charging, monitoring of the capacitor voltage, and command to deliver the pulse are controlled by dedicated circuitry or a microprocessor.

Some implantable devices have a sense amplifier connected to the shocking electrodes. The signal obtained is similar to a body surface ECG which allows the atrial depolarization (P wave) to be seen. Such a "look" at the heart may be useful to diagnose device function via telemetry if tachyarrhythmia signals are stored in the device.

Since device sense amplifiers are exposed to the high-voltage defibrillating pulse, they must be protected from damage by special circuitry. This circuitry must also allow the amplifier to quickly recover after the overload in order to immediately evaluate the patient's rhythm status. This protection circuitry should not, however, allow significant current from the shock to pass into it. This would steal useful defibrillating energy and, in the case of the rate sense/pacing leads, possibly damage the site of implantation by passing excessive current through the small surface area electrodes.

Shock protection of the device pacing output circuit is more difficult than for a pacemaker alone. Usual pacemaker overload protection allows large current to flow through the lead during a shock. Combination device (antitachycardia pacing and shock) circuitry should prevent high overload current while still allowing the pacing pulse to be delivered at the appropriate time.

Programmability is becoming increasingly complex as cardioverter-defibrillators and pacemakers blend into one unit. With this complexity comes increased data transmission speed requirements for the telemetry system. This increased speed keeps the physician informed about the implanted device's decision making during the induction and automatic conversion of tachyarrhythmias.

Combinational devices incorporate microprocessor technology or a dedicated sequencer approach. A microprocessor gets its instructions from a read-only memory (ROM), while a sequencer has its decision making process in logic gates. The microprocessor or sequencer reads the programmed parameters and saves patient history in a read-write memory (RAM). The condition of the device amplifiers and output of therapy commands are communicated through I/O (input-output) ports.

Because memory is becoming more densely packaged and

because certain kinds of memory (static RAM) consume little power when not changing, the capabilities of implantable devices are likely to continue to increase rapidly. Several device detection algorithms can be run simultaneously and the detailed event history can be stored. Event history storage and adjustment of detection parameters will become easier to use as this technology becomes more widely applied.

PACEMAKER-DEFIBRILLATOR INTERACTION

As of this writing, the most frequently implanted defibrillators do not have pacing, although many which incorporate antitachycardia pacing and bradycardia backup pacing are undergoing clinical trials. However, none of these devices are dual chamber, and thus may provide less than satisfactory pacing support for certain patients.

The major problem with simultaneous implantation of a separate pacemaker and defibrillator is one of tachyarrhythmia detection in the cardioverter-defibrillator. Canine studies conducted prior to the introduction of separate rate sensing lead defibrillators were predictive of these detection problems.

The cardioverter-defibrillator has difficulty separating pacemaker pulses from local cardiac depolarization. Since most tachyarrhythmia detection devices have an automatic sensing adjustment, the possibility exists for small fibrillation signals to be suppressed by large pacemaker spikes sensed at the cardioverter-defibrillator leads. Each pacer spike reduces the gain of the sensing circuit each time it occurs. The sensing circuit may not recover enough between pacing pulses to detect the small defibrillation depolarizations. The pacemaker continues to pace during fibrillation because its sensing circuits are fixed gain and may not detect small fibrillation depolarizations.

Separating the pacemaker electrodes and the cardioverter defibrillator rate sensing electrodes is a partial solution to this problem. It has been found that unipolar pacing does not allow this separation to take place as easily as bipolar pacing since the latter has the electric field of the pacemaker spike restricted to a smaller volume of myocardium. However, if the two sets of electrodes are widely separated, the pacemaker far field spike and local depolarization may be separated in time by more than the cardioverter defibrillator's refractory period. This can cause oversensing and lead to unwanted shocks since the defibrillator now senses the underlying heart rate at twice its true value (58). This problem may be handled by reducing the amplitude of the pacemaker output pulse.

Another problem exists when the pacemaker has capture or sensing problems. Two sets of asynchronous pulses, the pacing spikes and the local cardiac depolarization, are presented to the defibrillator. This can cause improper recycling (detection of a new arrhythmia). Pacemaker failure to capture has been documented in the early post-shock period with combined implantation of defibrillators and pacemakers (59). It is not believed to be a frequent problem. Its occurrence can be reduced by providing at least a 2-cm distance between pacing electrodes and any implanted defibrillation electrodes, because of transient conduction block in high-voltage gradient areas.

Combined use of an implantable defibrillator and separate antitachycardia pacemaker has been reported by several groups. The number of patients in each group has been small and highly selected. The patient survival statistics have been highly variable, probably as a result of the patient selection. When the devices are combined, the defibrillator rate limit is set relatively high (190–200 beats/min) as a backup to terminate high-rate arrhythmias. The pacemaker rate limit is set relatively low to terminate low rate ventricular tachycardia. In addition, burst durations are kept short. Careful attention to these details prevents the defibrillator detection circuitry from being triggered by the antitachycardia pacing (60).

The implanted defibrillator may also alter the programming of the pacemaker during delivery of the high-voltage pulse. This can have hemodynamic consequences in certain patients. It is best to attempt implantation of two separate devices in such a manner as to minimize the delivery of shock current through the pacemaker leads or case. Magnets or programmers designed for the implanted pacemaker may also affect the implanted defibrillator. Inadvertent deactivation by the magnet or false detection of an arrhythmia by the defibrillator during pacemaker reprogramming have been reported (61).

Placing the pacemaker inside the defibrillator eliminates some of the above-mentioned problems, but introduces new design challenges (62). The pacemaker output must be blanked by the pacer-defibrillator, and still recover quickly in order to sense a potential tachyarrhythmia, while avoiding the sensing of the evoked response from the pacing. These problems have been attacked by providing a separate postpacing and postsensing refractory period. How well this system will function is now under investigation in the clinical trial of several devices.

THE FUTURE OF IMPLANTABLE ANTITACHYARRHYTHMIA DEVICES

Because of the success of transvenous defibrillation, it is quite likely that the thoracotomy implantation procedure will lose its predominance within the next few years. Devices are likely to become small enough to implant in the pectoral region.

The chief obstacle to this is the development of smaller batteries and high-voltage capacitors. Detailed patient rhythm history will be displayed by device programmers in a fashion similar to that of a Holter monitor report. Finally, device specificity will improve with new detection algorithms. This will probably increase the use of these devices in patients who have been identified as being at high risk of sudden death, but as yet have not had an episode.

References

1. Wiggers CJ, Bell JR, Paine M, *et al.*: Studies of ventricular fibrillation caused by electric shock I. The revival of the heart from ventricular

fibrillation by successive use of potassium and calcium salts. Am J Physiol 1930;92:223–240.

2. Lown B, Amarasingham R, Neuman J: New method for terminating cardiac arrhythmias: Use of synchronized capacitor discharge. JAMA 1962;182:548–555.
3. Frazier DW, Krassowska W, Chen P-S, *et al.*: Transmural activations and stimulus potentials in three-dimensional anisotropic canine myocardium. Circ Res 1988;63:135–146.
4. Chen P-S, Wolf PD, Melnick SB, *et al.*: Comparison of activation during ventricular fibrillation and following unsuccessful defibrillation shocks in open chest dogs. Circ Res 1990;66:1544–1560.
5. Winfree A: When time breaks down: The three-dimensional dynamics of electrochemical waves and cardiac dynamics. Princeton University Press, Princeton, NJ, 1987:22–27,135–145,154–186.
6. Gleick J: Chaos: Making a New Science. Penguin Books, New York, 1987.
7. Wiggers CJ: The mechanism and nature of ventricular fibrillation. Am Heart J 1940;20:399–412.
8. Frazier DW, Wolf PD, Wharton JM, *et al.*: Stimulus-induced critical point. Mechanism for electrical initiation of reentry in normal canine myocardium. J Clin Invest 1989;83:1039–1052.
9. Evans SJ, Khan SS, Garfinkel A, *et al.*: Is ventricular fibrillation random or chaotic? (Abstr). Circulation 1989;80 (Suppl II):134.
10. Garry WE: The nature of fibrillary contraction of the heart and its relation to tissue mass and form. Am J Physiol 1914;33:297–414.
11. Zipes DP, Fischer J, King RM, *et al.*: Termination of ventricular fibrillation in dogs by depolarizing a critical amount of myocardium. Am J Cardiol 1975;36:37–44.
12. Mower MM, Mirowski M, Spear JF, *et al.*: Patterns of ventricular activity during catheter defibrillation. Circulation 1974;49:858–861.
13. Ideker RE, Wolf PD, Alferness C, *et al.*: Current concepts for selecting the location, size and shape of defibrillating electrodes. PACE 1991;14:227–240.
14. Beck CS, Pritchard WH, Feil HS: Ventricular fibrillation of long duration abolished by electric shock. JAMA 1947;135:985–986.
15. Zoll PM, Linenthal AJ, Gibson W, *et al.*: Termination of ventricular fibrillation in man by externally applied electric countershock. N Engl J Med 1956;254:727–732.
16. Tacker WA, Geddes LA. Electrical Defibrillation. CRC Press, Boca Raton, FL, 1980.
17. Prevost JL, Battelli F. Some effects of electric discharge on the hearts of mammals. C R Acad Sci 1899;129:1267.
18. Peleska B: Personal communication, 1984.
19. Schuder JC, Gold JH, Stoeckle H, *et al.*: Transthoracic ventricular defibrillation in the 100 kg calf with untruncated and truncated exponential stimuli. IEEE Trans Bio-Med Eng 1980;BME27-1:37–43.
20. Berkovits BV: US Patent 3236239: Defibrillator.
21. Edmark KW, Thomas GI, Jones TW: DC pulse defibrillation. J Thorac Cardiovasc Surg 1966;51:326–333.
22. Schuder JC, McDaniel WC, Stoeckle H. Transthoracic defibrillation of 100 kg calves with bidirectional truncated exponential shocks. Trans Am Soc Artif Intern Organs 1984;XXX:520–525.
23. Schuder JC, McDaniel WC, Stoeckle H. Defibrillation of 100 kg calves with asymmetrical bidirectional rectangular pulses. Cardiovas Res 1984;18:419–426.
24. Swartz JF, Jones JL, Karasik P, *et al.*: Field stimulation with symmetrical biphasic waveforms prolongs refractoriness to simulated refibrillation in human hearts (Abstr). PACE 1991;14:665.
25. Jones JL, Jones RE, Balasky G: Improved cardiac cell excitation with symmetrical biphasic defibrillator waveforms. Am J Physiol 1987;253–H1418–1424.
26. Hayes JJ, Bardy GH, Hofer B, *et al.*: A prospective evaluation of the effect of waveform tilt on defibrillation efficacy in humans (Abstr). PACE 1991;14:395.
27. Tang ASL, Yabe S, Wharton JM, *et al.*: Ventricular defibrillation using biphasic waveforms: the importance of phase duration. J Am Coll Cardiol 1989;13:207–213.
28. Kavanagh KM, Tang ASL, Rollins DL, *et al.*: A comparison of the internal defibrillation thresholds for monophasic and double and single capacitor biphasic waveforms. J Am Coll Cardiol 1989;14:1343–1349.
29. El-Sherif N, Mehra R, Gough WB, *et al.*: Ventricular activation pattern of spontaneous and induced ventricular rhythms in canine one-day-old myocardial infarction. Evidence for focal and reentrant mechanisms. Circ Res 1982;51:152–165.
30. Troup PJ: Lead system selection: Implantation and testing for automatic implantable cardioverter defibrillator. Clin Prog Electrophysiol Pacing 1986;4:260–276.
31. McDaniel WC, Schuder JC: The cardiac ventricular defibrillation threshold: Inherent limitations in its application and interpretation. Med Instrum 1987;21:170–175.
32. McDaniel WC, Schuder JC: An up-down algorithm for estimation of the cardiac ventricular defibrillation threshold. Med Instrum 1988;22:286–292.
33. Lang DJ, Swanson DK: Safety margin for defibrillation. Presented at Second International Congress on Rate Adaptive Cardiac Pacing and Implantable Defibrillators, October 10–13, 1990, Munich.
34. Tacker WA, Babbs CF, Paris RL, *et al.*: Effect of defibrillation duration on defibrillation threshold in dogs using a pervenous catheter electrode designed for use with an automatic implantable defibrillator. Med Instrum 1981;15:327–328.
35. Troup PJ, Chapman PD, Wetherbee JN, *et al.*: Do subthreshold shocks increase energy requirements for subsequent defibrillation attempts? (Abstr). Circulation 1987;76(Suppl IV):311.
36. Echt DS, Barbey JT, Black JN: Influence of ventricular defibrillation energy in dogs using bidirectional pulse discharges. PACE 1988;11:1315–1323.
37. Flaker G, Schuder JC, McDaniel W: The effect of multiple shocks on canine cardiac defibrillation. PACE 1990;13:1580–1584.
38. Zhou X, Daubert JP, Wolf PD, *et al.*: The potential gradient for defibrillation (Abstr). Circulation 1988;78:645.
39. Zhou X, Wolf PD, Rollins D, *et al.*: Potential gradient needed for defibrillation with monophasic and biphasic shocks (Abstr). PACE 1989;12:651.
40. Jones JL, Lepeschkin E, Jones RE, *et al.*: Response of cultured myocardial cells to countershock-type electric field stimulation. Am J Physiol 1978;235:H214–H222.
41. Schuder JC, Stoeckle H, West JA, *et al.*: Ventricular defibrillation in the dog with a bielectrode intravascular catheter. Arch Intern Med 1973;132:286–290.
42. Mirowski MM: US Patent 3942536: Cardioverting device having single intravascular catheter electrode system and method for its use.
43. Troup PJ: Implantable cardioverters and defibrillators. In: Current Problems in Cardiology 1989;XIV(12):673–843.
44. Nogami A, Takahashi A, Nitta J, *et al.*: Optimal size for subcutaneous plate electrode for nonthoracotomy canine defibrillation (Abstr). PACE 1991;14:718.
45. Singer I, Maldonado C, Vance F, *et al.*: Transvenous defibrillation-importance of septal recruitment (Abstr). Clin Res 1989;37(4):888.
46. Bach SM Jr, Barstad J, Moser S, *et al.*: Initial clinical experience: Endotak™ implantable transvenous defibrillator system (Abstr). J Am Coll Cardiol 1989;13:65A.
47. Bardy GH, Troutman C, Johnson G, *et al.*: Transvenous defibrillation systems: Methods of implantation and utilization success rates (Abstr). PACE 1991;14:27.
48. Callans DJ, Hook BG, Marchlinski FE: Use of bipolar recordings from patch-patch and rate sensing leads to distinguish ventricular tachycardia from supraventricular rhythms in patients with implantable cardioverter-defibrillators (Abstr). PACE 1991;14:676.
49. Davies DW, Wainwright RJ, Tooley MA, *et al.*: Detection of pathological tachycardia by analysis of electrogram morphology. PACE 1986;9:200–208.
50. Mercando AD, Gableman G, Fisher JD: Comparison of the rate of tachycar-

dia development in patients: pathologic vs. sinus tachycardias. PACE 1988;11:516.

51. Geibel A, Zehender M, Brugada P: Changes in cycle length at the onset of sustained tachycardias-importance for antitachycardia pacing. Am Heart J 1988;115:588–592.
52. Grogan EW: Role of cycle length oscillation during ventricular tachycardia in spontaneous tachycardia termination (Abstr). PACE 1990;13:507.
53. Cohen TJ, Veltri EP, Lattuca J, *et al.*: Hemodynamic responses to rapid pacing: A model for tachycardia differentiation. PACE 1988;11:1522–1528.
54. Salo R, Bach S, Lincoln W. Continuous hemodynamic monitoring during cardiac arrhythmias (Abstr). In International Symposium on Cardiac Arrhythmias, Kanazawa, Japan, 1986.
55. Horning RJ, Rhoback FW: New high rate lithium/vanadium pentoxide cell for implantable medical devices. Prog Batteries Solar Cells 1982;4:97–102.
56. Takeuchi ES, Quattrini PJ, Greatbatch W: Lithium/silver vanadium oxide batteries for implantable defibrillators. PACE 1988;11:2035–2039.
57. Aarons D, Mower M, Veltri E: Use of the elective replacement indicator in predicting time of automatic implantable cardioverter defibrillator battery depletion. PACE 1989;12:1724–1728.
58. Bach SM Jr: Technical communication: AID-B™ cardioverter defibrillator: Possible interactions with pacemakers. Intec Systems, Pittsburgh, PA, 1983.
59. Slepian M, Levine JH, Watkins L Jr., *et al.*: Automatic implantable cardioverter defibrillator/permanent pacemaker interaction: Loss of pacemaker capture following AICD discharge. PACE 1987;10:1194–1197.
60. Bonnet CA, Fogoros RN, Elson JJ, *et al.*: Long-term efficacy of an antitachycardia pacemaker and implantable defibrillator combination. PACE 1991;14:814–822.
61. Kim SG, Furman S, Matos JA, *et al.*: Automatic implantable cardioverter/defibrillator: Inadvertent discharges during permanent pacemaker magnet tests. PACE 1987;10:579–582.
62. Bach SM Jr, Hsung JC: Implantable device algorithms for detection and discrimination of tachyarrhythmia. In Alt E, Klein K, Griffin J (eds). Implantable Cardioverter Defibrillators. 1992;67–81.

20

IMPLANTABLE CARDIOVERTER DEFIBRILLATOR

Igor Singer, M.B.B.S., F.R.A.C.P., F.A.C.P., F.A.C.C., David Slater, M.D., F.A.C.C., and Morton Mower, M.D., F.A.C.P., F.A.C.C., F.C.C.P.

INTRODUCTION

The concept of an automatic implantable defibrillator, which seemed far-fetched when first proposed by Mirowski, has evolved into an effective therapeutic modality which has revolutionized treatment of patients with malignant ventricular dysrhythmias (1). The evolution from a nonprogrammable committed device capable of treating ventricular fibrillation (VF) and rapid ventricular tachycardia (VT), to a programmable, noncommitted device incorporating antitachycardia and bradycardia pacing with extensive data logging capabilities, has extended the therapeutic applications of this treatment modality (2). Viewed initially as the treatment of last resort, this therapeutic approach for therapy of VF and VT is now advocated by some as the "gold standard" against which other therapies should be compared (2).

Although not yet universally accepted taxonomy, the name implantable cardioverter defibrillator (ICD) has been seeing increasing use in recent years, both as a generic term, and as one to specifically describe the newer advanced combination devices now entering the clinical arena. A number of technical advances have occurred that make ICDs more versatile. These include: (a) improved defibrillation waveforms (4), (b) development of permanent transvenous lead systems not requiring thoracotomy for implantation of the system (5), (c) availability of antitachycardia pacing, (d) programmability of energy outputs for cardioversion and defibrillation, (e) incorporation of bradycardia pacing, and (f) extensive telemetric capabilities (6). Further, refinements are anticipated in the future with improvements in sensing, arrhythmia differentiation and classification, further reduction in device size, and improvements in transvenous defibrillation leads.

PATIENT SELECTION

Indications for ICD therapy have evolved over time due to improvements in device design, increased device programmability and wider recognition of device efficacy.

The most recent North American Society of Cardiac Pacing and Electrophysiology (NASPE) policy statement summarizes the currently accepted indications for implantation of ICD's (7).

Three separate classes of indications are recognized by this policy statement: (a) Class 1: ICD therapy is indicated, (b) Class 2: ICD therapy is a therapeutic option, but no consensus exists, and (c) Class 3: ICD therapy is not generally justified.

Class 1 Indications

Patients should be considered for ICD therapy under the following circumstances.

1. Demonstration of one or more episodes of spontaneous, sustained VT or VF and inability of electrophysiologic (EP) testing and/or Holter monitoring to predict accurately outcome of other therapies. Noninducible patients at EP study and patients with insufficient spontaneous recorded arrhythmias by Holter monitoring to render these techniques useful for subsequent analysis of therapeutic efficacy are included in this category.
2. Recurrent episodes of spontaneous sustained VT or VF despite antiarrhythmic drug therapy (guided by EP testing or noninvasive methods).
3. Episodes of spontaneous VT or VF in patients in whom antiarrhythmic therapy is limited by intolerance or noncompliance.
4. Persistent inducibility of clinically relevant sustained VT or VF at EP study on best available drug therapy or despite surgical/catheter ablation in patients with spontaneous sustained VT or VF.

Class 2 Indications

Syncope of undetermined etiology in patients with clinically relevant VT or VF induced at EP study, in whom antiarrhythmic drug therapy is limited by inefficacy, intolerance, or noncompliance.

Class 3 Indications

1. Sustained episodes of VT or VF due to reversible acute ischemia/infarction, drug toxicity, or electrolyte imbalance.
2. Recurrent syncope of undetermined etiology where sustained VT or VF cannot be induced at EP.

3. Incessant VT.
4. VF secondary to atrial fibrillation in a patient with preexcitation and antegrade conduction of the accessory pathway amenable to surgical or catheter ablation.
5. Surgical, medical, or psychiatric contraindications.

Certain trials with antiarrhythmic drug therapy have contributed to the further expansion of indications for ICDs. For example, CASCADE (Cardiac Arrest in Seattle: Conventional Versus Amiodarone Drug Evaluation) showed 17% 1-yr and 35% 3-yr incidence of recurrent cardiac arrest with amiodarone (8). The CAST study in post myocardial patients with highest ventricular ectopy showed excess mortality with encainide and flecainide and at least no significant benefit in the moricizine arm of the trial (9,10). The moricizine arm was later discontinued when it became apparent that outcome was tending toward that observed for encainide and flecainide (Cardiac Arrhythmia Suppression Trial (CAST) Oversight Committee unpublished finding).

Mortality and recurrent events are also not uncommon in patients with drug-responsive EP-guided therapy. For example, in one study (11) of 241 out-of-hospital VF survivors studied by electrophysiologic (EP) testing, 42% were noninducible, VF was induced in 16%, and sustained VT in 27%. Recurrences of sudden cardiac death ranged as high as 28% in the various groups, and those with drug-induced suppression of baseline-induced arrhythmia did not do any better than the nonsuppressible ones.

In another study (12), prognosis, predictors of survival and the prognostic value of EP study were assessed in 239 patients with sustained VT or VF in whom antiarrhythmic drug therapy was judged effective by EP study criteria. One, 2-, and 3-yr incidence of sudden death in drug responders was 17, 25, and 34% respectively. Multivariate regression analysis demonstrated that the strongest predictor of both sudden and cardiac death was a higher New York Heart Association functional class and a failure of any antiarrhythmic therapy to be identified as potentially effective by EP-guided therapy. However, even in the "drug effective" group, the incidence of sudden death was high.

These results, when contrasted with results of the largest reported series of similar patients with implanted difibrillators, which have shown sudden death rates of 2% and 5% at 1 and 3 yr (13–15) suggest that ICD therapy should be considered for the highest-risk patients.

A number of investigators feel that the use of the ICD for prophylaxis prior to cardiac arrest may be warranted in certain high-risk groups. Several large studies are underway to evaluate implantable defibrillators for prevention of sudden cardiac death, including "CABG patch" (coronary artery disease patients with positive late potentials and left ventricular (LV) ejection fraction (EF) below 0.36 who are already scheduled for bypass surgery) (16), "MADIT" (coronary artery disease patients with nonsustained ventricular tachycardia, inducible and not suppressed by procainamide, and left ventricular ejection fraction (LVEF) below 0.36, who are not suitable for bypass) (17), and "MUSTT" (asymptomatic nonsustained ventricular tachycardia, late potentials, and LVEF below 0.41) (17). Results of these studies will probably be available within the next several years. If positive, they hold promise in reducing both mortality and morbidity, as most cardiac arrest victims do not receive successful resuscitation and many that do have lasting neurologic deficits (see Chapter 6).

An interesting possible use for implantable defibrillators that has evolved over the past several years is in congestive heart failure patients awaiting cardiac transplantation. Many such patients are at high risk of dying suddenly prior to the availability of a suitable donor heart (18–20). Devices may be a useful bridge to transplantation, especially since lack of donor hearts has made for prolonged waiting time. It is expected that more rigorous studies to examine the role of defibrillator therapy in this group of patients will be launched in the near future (21).

One question regarding ICD indication, which has been subject of disputes among electrophysiologists and often presents problems in individual patients, is what to do with cardiac arrest survivor that does not have inducible arrhythmias by programmed ventricular stimulation. The results of clinical studies suggest that noninducible patients presenting with aborted sudden death are also at a high risk of recurrent cardiac arrest (11). Recently the Food and Drug Association (FDA) and Health Care Financing Administration (HCFA) have eliminated a requirement for EP inducibility in that group. They have also allowed that ICDs do not have to be considered the "last resort" therapy (22).

PREIMPLANTATION ASSESSMENT

All patients considered to be prospective candidates for an ICD should be evaluated in a clinical center that is capable of providing comprehensive therapy for ventricular dysrhythmias (23). A competent experienced team consisting of a clinical cardiac electrophysiologist, cardiovascular surgeon familiar with implantation techniques and alternative therapies for VT, anesthesiologist, and the supporting personnel, must be available. Supporting personnel include clinical arrhythmia nurse specialist, social worker, and clinical psychologist.

All prospective candidates should undergo evaluation and testing to determine their suitability for ICD or alternative therapies, and to exclude other disease processes which may influence the treatment outcome. Assessment should include history and physical examination, 12-lead electrocardiogram (ECG), chest x-ray, routine hematologic and biochemical profile, cardiac catheterization (including coronary arteriography and left ventriculography) or noninvasive assessment of left ventricular function (multigated nuclear angiography) (MUGA or two-dimensional (2D) echocardiology). Other useful information may be obtained by 24-hr Holter monitoring, exercise testing (in selected cases), or stress thallium-201 Scintigraphy.

The purpose of testing is to identify the pathophysiologic substrate, exclude concomitant disease requiring therapy, e.g., coronary or valvular disease, assess coexistent problems, e.g., ischemia, and evaluate functional and exercise capacity. Signal-averaged ECG may also be helpful for risk stratification (see Chapter 3).

Electrophysiologic study is required prior to ICD implantation. Essential information that may be obtained from an EP study includes inducibility of VT or VF, characterization of induced arrhythmias, testing of antitachycardia pacing termination techniques and pharmacologic therapy, assessment of atrioventricular (A-V) conduction, assessment of the potential for bradyarrhythmias, and exclusion of coexisting arrhythmias (e.g., supraventricular tachycardias).

Preoperative evaluation should include patient and family education about the device therapy, other available therapeutic options, psychologic evaluation of the patient, and assessment of the family support mechanisms.

THE DEVICE AND THE LEAD SYSTEM

The components of an ICD include: (a) generator (logic circuitry, capacitors, battery, connector), (b) sensing/shocking electrodes, and (c) bipolar rate-sensing electrode(s). Currently, the only approved device for clinical use in the United States is VENTAK^R (CPI, St. Paul, MN). However, a number of third- and fourth-generation devices are currently undergoing clinical trials and will soon become available for more general clinical use.

The current market-released device VENTAK^R (CPI, St. Paul, MN) weighs 293 g. Because of its relatively large size it is typically implanted in the abdominal pocket. The battery, the logic circuitry, and the capacitors are contained within a titanium casing (Fig. 20.1). Sensing/shocking electrodes are usually applied to the heart surface (intra- or extrapericardially) and are known as patch electrodes. These electrodes come in small or large sizes. A transvenous (superior vena caval) electrode is also available and may be used instead of one of the patch electrodes.

The sensing bipolar endocardial lead may be placed pervenously, in a similar fashion to a ventricular endocardial lead used for pacemakers. Alternatively an epicardial pair of electrodes may be used for rate-sensing. Currently available electrodes for VENTAK^R device(s) are shown in Figure 20.2.

The preferred electrode configuration consists of two large epicardial patches, which may be placed extra- or intrapericardially. Alternatively, a small and a large patch electrode or two small patch electrodes may be used. The choice of electrodes depends on the size of the heart and the anticipated ease of defibrillation (defibrillation threshold). In general, larger electrode surface area is likely to lower the energy requirements for defibrillation.

Another possible electrode arrangement consists of a superior vena caval (SVC) electrode and a large or a small patch electrode. Rarely, defibrillation thresholds are found to be too high with all available electrodes and an additional right or left ventricular electrode or a combination of electrodes have to be considered to increase the total surface area and improve lead geometry, thereby decreasing the defibrillation thresholds (see below).

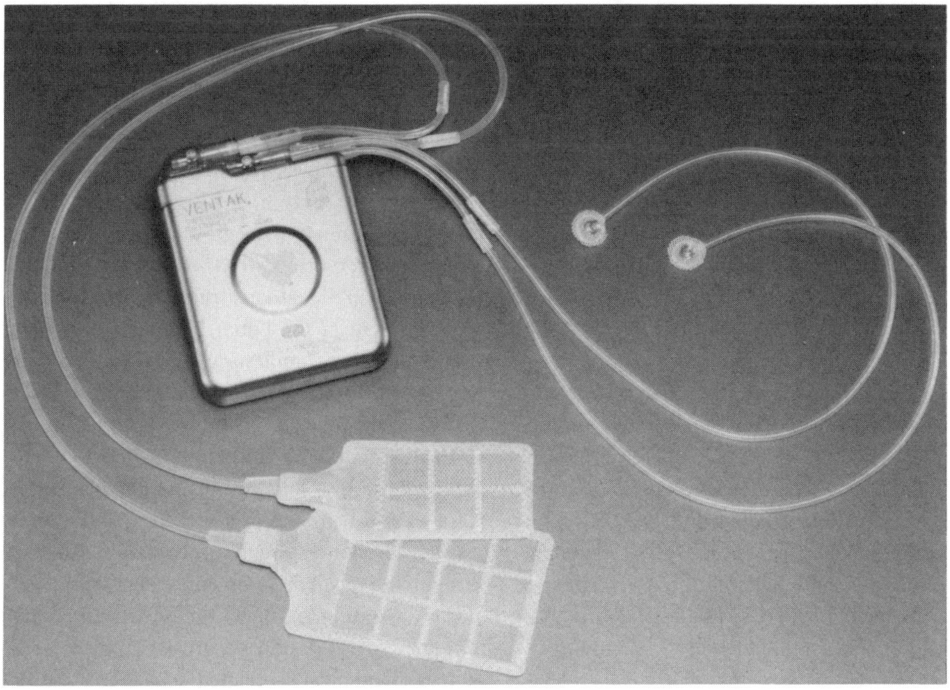

Figure 20.1. Automatic implantable cardioverter defibrillator (VENTAK^R, CPI, St. Paul, MN) attached to the defibrillation patches (large and small) and epicardial sensing leads (Courtesy of CPI, Inc., St. Paul, MN.)

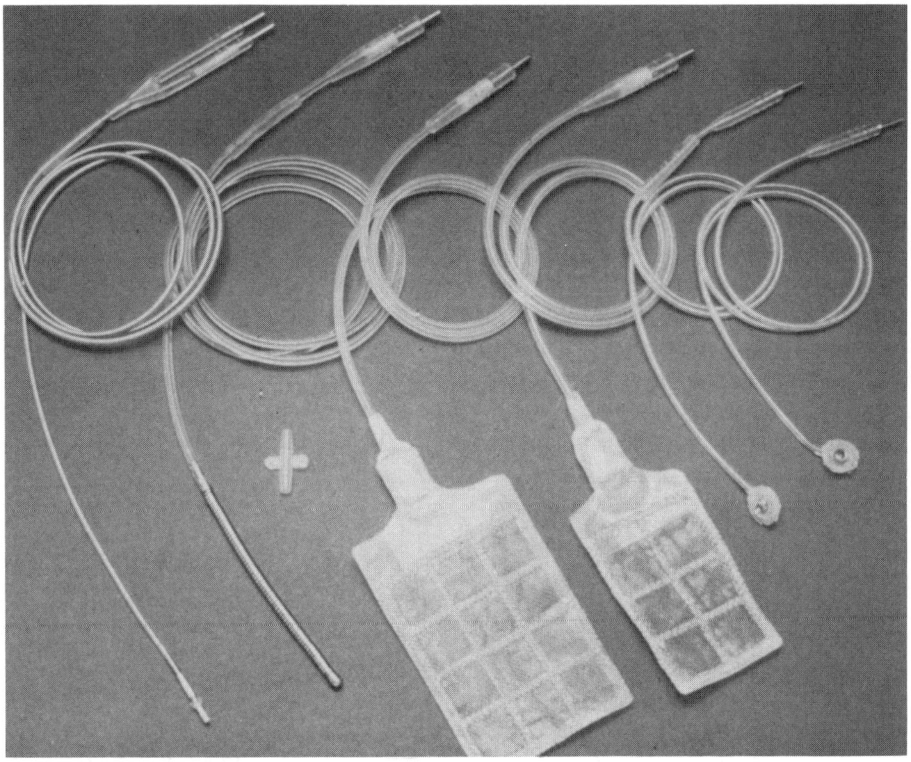

Figure 20.2. Clinically available electrodes for VENTAK^R device. From **left** to **right:** endocardial bipolar sensing lead, superior vena caval electrode, large patch lead, small patch lead, and epicardial screw-in leads. (Courtesy of CPI, Inc., St. Paul, MN.)

Another pair of electrodes is used to sense ventricular depolarization signal (electrogram). Bipolar sensing may be accomplished by either an endocardial or an epicardial pair of electrodes.

An endocardial bipolar electrode mounted on a single lead, may be positioned in the right ventricular apex. Alternatively, a pair of epicardial leads may be screwed into the left or right ventricular epicardium. Sensing must be bipolar to prevent sensing of far-field artifacts, myopotentials, and other cardiac diastolic signals (e.g., T waves or P waves). The most commonly used approach, utilizing two patch electrodes and a bipolar sensing epicardial pair of electrodes is shown in Figure 20.3.

IMPLANTATION TECHNIQUES

ICD implantation requires a close collaboration between the implanting surgeon and electrophysiologist. Surgical implantation technique depends on the need for concomitant cardiac surgery and the experience and the preference of the implanting surgeon. In general, when other cardiac surgery is required (e.g., coronary revascularization, endocardial resection, or valve surgery), median sternotomy is required (24). If an implantable defibrillator alone is contemplated, then a number of alternative techniques are available. These include lateral thoracotomy (25), subxyphoid or subcostal approaches, or a modification of these techniques.

Placement of at least one intrathoracic defibrillating patch is necessary to provide optimal defibrillation thresholds. Currently, multiple patch lead sizes are available for intrapericardial or extrapericardial placement. Patch leads may be used both for sensing and defibrillation, in an intrapericardial or an extrapericardial position. Extrapericardial patch lead placement is favored whenever possible, because of dense scarring and adhesions that can form between the patch leads and the epicardium. These adhesions may lead to pericardial restrictive physiology and make it virtually impossible for a patient to have subsequent revascularization. Occasionally, severe bleeding from erosion of coronary veins may also be encountered. Finally, in the rare instance of infection, removal of the lead system may be performed much more easily, with a lower operative risk, when the patch leads are located extrapericardially.

Placement of the patch leads requires adequate contact between the wire-conducting surface of the electrodes and the underlying myocardium or pericardium. Therefore, the patch leads should be secured to prevent motion or twisting. At least two sutures through the patch are required to ensure adequate stabilization, but four sutures (one at each corner) are preferred. Care should be taken to avoid sutures that do not ensure smooth contact. A mattress technique, placing the sutures through and through the patch allows compression of the patch while tying the suture, avoiding tearing of the underlying structures.

Larger patches provide greater surface area for defibrillation, and are generally associated with lower defibrillation thresholds (26). With concurrent cardiac procedures, one large and one

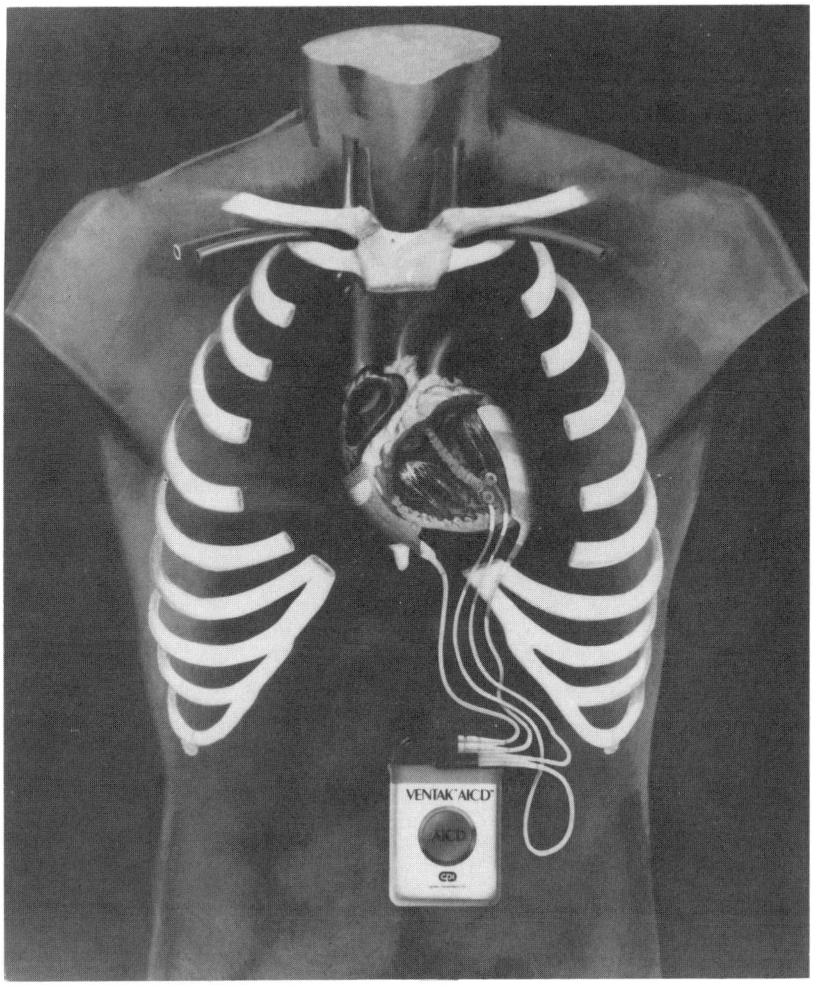

Figure 20.3. Frequently employed configuration utilizing two epicardial patch electrodes and epicardial rate sensing leads with pulse generator implanted in the subcutaneous pocket, in the left upper quadrant of abdomen. (Courtesy of CPI, Inc., St. Paul, MN.)

small patch are generally used, but in patients with small hearts, excellent results have been achieved with two small patches. The patch leads should ideally be placed in diametrically opposite positions, encompassing the largest possible transmyocardial mass and preferably, the intraventricular septum. This is not always possible, particularly in patients with previous cardiac surgery. In patients with previous cardiac surgery, placement of the patches on the left posterior or posterolateral portion of the pericardium, with a second patch placed anteriorly or on the diaphragmatic surface of the heart was found to be satisfactory. An alternative to using two patch leads is provided by the use of superior vena caval lead positioned at the junction of the superior vena cava and the right atrium, and a left ventricular patch lead.

The rate sensing lead(s) may be placed endocardially or in an epicardial position. The endocardial sensing lead is usually positioned through the left or right subclavian or cephalic vein, similar to a ventricular pacemaker lead. The lead is positioned in the apex of the right ventricle. The endocardial lead is preferred over the epicardial leads because of superior sensing characteristics and better long-term performance.

Epicardial sensing leads are positioned as close to each other as possible to provide optimal bipolar sensing. A useful technique for placement of the epicardial leads is to position one lead at a time and measure signal amplitude and pacing thresholds before placement of the second lead. With placement of the second lead, unipolar and bipolar measurements are obtained.

The pulse generator is generally placed in the left upper abdominal wall by creation of a subcutaneous or subrectus pocket. In patients with adequate adipose tissue, a subcutaneous pocket is sufficient. However, in thinner patients, a subrectus approach with division of the lateral margin of the rectus sheath, and placement of the device beneath the rectus muscle is preferred. Subcutaneous pocket can be made with a transverse, vertical, or parallel incision to the costal margin. When the device pocket is made, a meticulous hemostasis is essential, since hematoma formation significantly increases the risk of pocket infection. Leads should be carefully coiled posterior to the generator to minimize the possibility of damage to the leads subsequently at the time of generator replacement.

A variety of surgical options have been described for placement of the patch leads as well as the sutureless epicardial screw-in leads. These approaches include anterior or anterolateral thoracotomy, median sternotomy, subxiphoid, subcostal, transdiaphragmatic, and subcostal with right minithoracotomy (26–36) (Fig. 20.4). In those patients requiring additional cardiac surgical procedures, such as coronary bypass, resection of ventricular aneurysm, or valve replacement, median sternotomy used for these procedures provides excellent exposure for placement of the defibrillator lead system.

Subxiphoid Approach

The subxiphoid incision is a midline incision extending several centimeters cephalad from the xiphisternal junction, and caudally for a distance of approximately 5–6 cm. The linea alba is incised, and the xiphoid is divided or excised. With the sternum elevated, the pericardium is incised either longitudinally or transversely to expose the anterior and diaphragmatic surfaces of the heart. Patch leads can then be inserted into the pericardial space and secured to the pericardial sac. The sensing endocardial lead can be placed through the left subclavian vein, or an epicardial bipolar lead pair in the anterior or diaphragmatic surface of the right ventricle. The generator pocket is formed through a subcutaneous extension of the subxiphoid incision or by placement of a second adjacent subcostal incision, with tunneling of the leads through the abdominal wall fascia.

A major advantage of the subxiphoid incision is that it provides the least amount of surgical dissection and resultant discomfort to the patient postoperatively. Its major disadvantage is primarily related to a limited surgical exposure. In patients with previous cardiac surgery, this approach is therefore not recommended. Additionally, subxiphoid approach requires intrapericardial placement of the patch leads and limits options if defibrillation thresholds are found to be unacceptable. The use of a SVC (spring) lead and/or endocardial sensing lead requires subcutaneous tunneling from the left or right subclavian veins to the anterior abdominal wall pocket (as noted above).

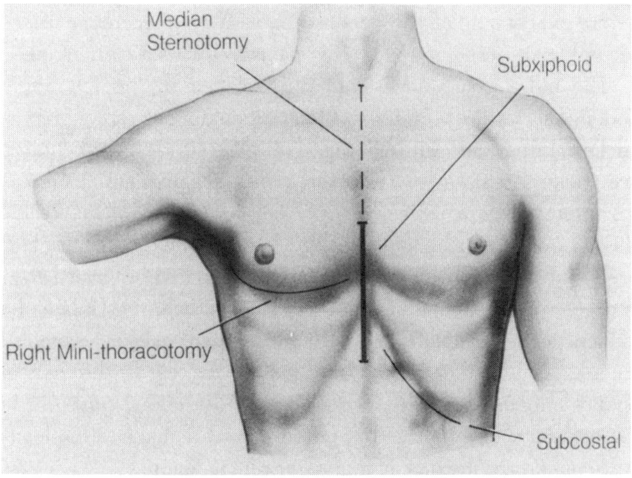

Figure 20.4. Incision sites of most commonly used surgical approaches for implantable cardioverter defibrillator.

Left Subcostal Approach

Similar to the subxiphoid approach, the subcostal incision provides greater exposure to the diaphragmatic surface of the heart and avoids the postoperative discomfort associated with a thoracotomy. Subcostal incision requires division of the left rectus muscle, which is associated with greater discomfort postoperatively than a subxiphoid incision. Placement of leads is similar to the subxiphoid approach and its advantages and disadvantages are also similar. In patients who have had previous cardiac surgery, or those patients with unacceptably high defibrillation thresholds, some authors have suggested addition of a right minithoracotomy with placement of a patch lead over the right atrium in an extrapericardial position (32). A modification of this technique, the transdiaphragmatic approach, has been described (31). The advantages and the disadvantages are virtually the same as with the subcostal approach.

Left Thoracotomy

Left thoracotomy (Fig. 20.5) provides excellent exposure to the heart. The heart is exposed through the fifth intercostal space. The technique allows placement of the leads in an intra- or extrapericardial location. It provides excellent exposure to the left ventricle with the ability to reposition leads readily if sensing or defibrillation thresholds are suboptimal. In patients who have had previous cardiac surgery, the adherence of the heart to the anterior sternum limits anterior placement of the extrapericardial patch. Adhesions within the pericardium, as well as concern

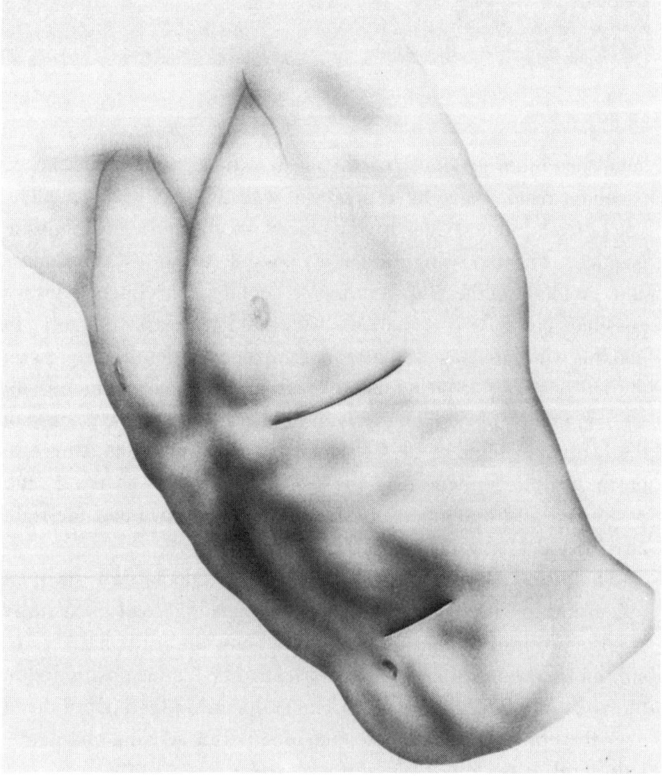

Figure 20.5. Left lateral thoracotomy approach.

for manipulation or damage to coronary bypass grafts complicates placement of intrapericardial leads. The leads are passed beneath the costal margin by placement of a curved hemostat on the costal margin, and palpation of the tip of the instrument within the pleural cavity. This avoids the risk of damage to the intra-abdominal viscera. The hemostat is then used to guide a chest tube through the space with placement of the leads inside the chest tube to protect them from injury as they are positioned in the generator pocket in the anterior abdominal wall.

The major disadvantage of the thoracotomy approach is the associated postoperative discomfort and morbidity resulting from a throacotomy incision, compared to a subxiphoid or subcostal incision.

Use of the anterior thoracotomy provides limited distraction of the ribs without injury to the anterior costal cartilages. We have, therefore, favored a more lateral approach and used a modification of the technique of muscle-sparing thoracotomy described by Bethencourt and Holmes (25,37) to eliminate the pain associated with division of the latissimus dorsi muscle (25). Through this incision, excellent exposure to the left ventricle without disruption of the costal cartilages or division of the thoracic musculature may be obtained.

Median Sternotomy

Although the median sternotomy incision provides the most optimal exposure for cardiac surgery and is advocated as the routine incision for defibrillator placement by some (38), the incision is generally not necessary for satisfactory placement of the defibrillator leads. The incision is generally well tolerated, and in many patients is associated with less discomfort than a thoracotomy. However, many patients still have significant postoperative pain and persistent discomfort related to costochondritis. Infection of a median sternotomy incision requires removal of all the defibrillator hardware and may pose a major risk to the patient in that case. This approach is generally preferred when concomitant cardiac surgery is planned.

INTRAOPERATIVE ELECTROPHYSIOLOGIC TESTING

Effectiveness of arrhythmia recognition and termination is critically dependent on adequate signal detection. It is therefore necessary to demonstrate an adequate signal amplitude and duration. In general, peak-to-peak amplitude of the rate-sensing signal should exceed 5 mV and should be less than 100 msec in duration, in the absence of an intraventricular conduction delay. The greater the amplitude and the slew rate of the signal, the greater the likelihood that the sensing will be adequate (see Chapter 13).

Pacing threshold from the sensing bipolar pair of electrodes should be routinely tested at implant. Measurements of current and lead impedance are also recommended. Testing of the unipolar pacing thresholds from the epicardial leads may also be helpful at the time of implant and to help troubleshoot possible future sensing or pacing problems (see above).

Third-generation ICDs have antitachycardia pacing capabilities and utilize rate-sensing electrodes for pacing. Therefore, adequate pacing and sensing thresholds are essential at the time of the initial implant to ensure proper device function. Lead repositioning is recommended if these basic criteria are not met.

DEFIBRILLATION THRESHOLD TESTING

To ensure that the device functions appropriately, adequate testing procedures are required at the time of device implantation. This includes testing of the minimum effective defibrillation energy, so that an effective safety margin may be programmed and to ensure that the energy output of the implanted ICD is sufficient to

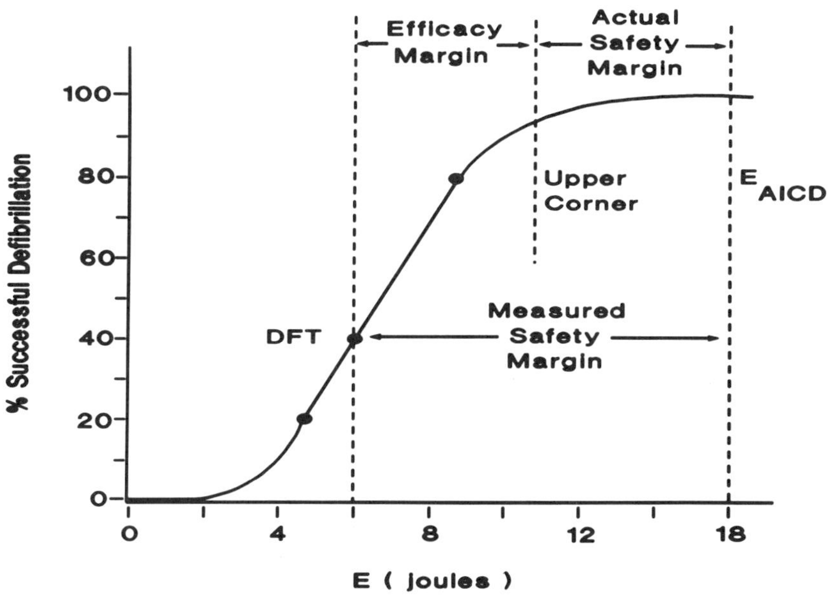

Figure 20.6. Defibrillation threshold can best be expressed by a sigmoidal probability curve relating energy to percent successful defibrillation (for discussion, see text). (Reproduced from Singer I, Lang D: Defibrillation threshold: clinical utility and therapeutic implications PACE 1992;15(6):932–949, with publisher's permission.)

defibrillate the heart. The concept of a defibrillation threshold (DFT) implies that the slope of a curve relating energy to percent success is steep, permitting a clear-cut distinction between the effective and ineffective energies, analogous to the pacing threshold. Unfortunately, no clear-cut distinction between uniformly successful and unsuccessful energies can be demonstrated (39). Defibrillation energy requirements can best be described by a dose-response curve (Fig. 20.6).

Construction of a dose-response curve is clinically impractical and may be hazardous since it requires a large number of fibrillation-defibrillation trials. Therefore, for practical purposes, most physicians adopt an abbreviated procedure to define a "safety" margin for the device. The *safety margin* may be defined as the difference in output energy of the ICD and the minimum energy requirement for consistent defibrillation. One technique that is commonly used to assess this margin is the "DFT method." A DFT is determined by using a test sequence of several fibrillation-defibrillation trials with defibrillation attempted at selected energies using an external cardioverter-defibrillator device. If the initial energy is successful, the subsequent defibrillation shock energies are decreased in successive trials until a failure is encountered. If the initial energy fails to defibrillate, subsequent energies are then incremented until a successful conversion is obtained. With this protocol, the DFT is defined as the minimum energy producing defibrillation success.

Lang and Swanson have demonstrated by using numeric modeling, that 1.5–2 times the DFT energy are needed to assure 100% defibrillation success in all patients (40,41). Safety margins for the device are measured beyond this margin of safety.

Alternative testing methods have been proposed. Church, *et al.* have proposed combining the "DFT method," i.e., stepping down to the first voltage that fails, with "incremental DFT method," i.e., stepping up to the first voltage that succeeds (42). By averaging the two DFTs, the authors obtained a threshold which is near E_{50} (energy level which is effective 50% of the time). Since the two DFT methods are distributed over opposite ends of the defibrillation curve, by using this method, one could predict 100% success in most patients at energies 1.9 times DFT.

When programming the ICD for adequate efficacy margins, one should select shock energies that also assure an energy safety margin between the defibrillation curve and the output of the device. The energy margin is needed as a buffer for proper device function, should the defibrillation curve shift to the higher energies.

One significant factor in altering the threshold for defibrillation is the duration of VF. Animal studies indicate that defibrillation energy threshold increases 30–40% with prolonged VF (30–40 sec), compared to the durations encountered for the first shock (10–15 sec) (43–46). Anecdotal human experience and preliminary human data (47–49) also suggest that prolonged durations of VF due to unsuccessful initial conversions are associated with higher defibrillation energy requirements. These studies indicate that energy thresholds after 30–40 sec of VF will increase approximately 50% compared to the thresholds for VF of 5–10 sec (47). In practice, therefore, energy safety margins should be selected so that ICD rescue shock energies are at least 50% higher than the upper end of the efficacy margin.

Historically, a measured safety margin of at least 10 J has been demonstrated to be sufficient experimentally and empirically. To minimize the potential for variability based on the arrhythmia duration, it is recommended that consistent VF duration be maintained (e.g., 10 sec) during defibrillator testing and that the time simulates the period expected during clinical ICD use. To assure proper device function, one must determine whether the measured energy margin between the DFT and the ICD is large enough to allow proper efficacy margins (whose size is determined by the testing method). If the measured margin is inadequate, the ICD should be reprogrammed or lead system revised to assure proper device function.

Efficacy and safety margins could also be assessed with an efficacy protocol which tests defibrillation success at a certain energy level one or more times. These methods differ from the DFT methods in that desired safety margin is selected before testing and is evaluated with a predetermined number of shocks. This method does not locate the defibrillation curve, but only establishes the upper boundary of its location. One advantage of this approach is that lesser number of defibrillations are required to establish the safety margin, but the disadvantage is that it limits serial comparison of DFTs over time and assessment of impact of antiarrhythmic drugs on DFTs, for example. When the testing is limited by the other clinical considerations, e.g., hemodynamic stability, this may be sufficient to determine the safety margin. Using this approach, for example three attempts at defibrillation at a prespecified energy output (3S protocol) would require $1.5 \times E_{3S}$ for 100% conversion success (41). Detailed explanation of probability calculations are beyond the scope of this manuscript and may be found elsewhere (50).

ICD TESTING

When an adequate DFT has been established by testing, an appropriate safe limit can be programmed. The programmable devices currently used are VENTAK 1550, 1555, and 1600 (St. Paul MN), but other, currently investigational devices, are anticipated for market release.

During implantable defibrillator testing, the device is usually programmed to DFT + 10 J output for the first shock and maximal output for subsequent shocks, if the anticipated dysrhythmia is VF. On the other hand, if VT is the anticipated initial dysrhythmia, based on EP testing, a low energy may be selected for the first shock (e.g., 0.5–2 J). In that case, VT cardioversion "threshold" should also be tested to ensure that the energy output is sufficient to cardiovert the VT to sinus rhythm. In the event that ventricular tachycardia does not terminate with a low-energy shock or acceleration occurs, deterioration of the rhythm to VF may ensue. Therefore, when low-energy shock is programmed as the initial device response, it is recommended that the subsequent shocks are incremented to the maximal output. The rationale for programming the maximum energy outputs for subsequent shocks is derived from the accumulated clinical and experimental experience suggesting that the ease of ventricular defibrillation declines with the duration of the fibrillation episode (44–46). On the other hand, if ventricular tachycardia is terminable by a low-energy shock, it is both reasonable and desirable to minimize the energy output of the device to lessen the patient's discomfort and to extend the battery life.

Testing in the operating room should include demonstration of VT cardioversion and ventricular defibrillation with selected programmed energies. The number of conversions and the test sequence is dictated by the clinical status of the patient on one hand, and the need to demonstrate device efficacy, with at least one successful VT cardioversion and ventricular defibrillation with the intended programming of the device, on the other hand.

With advanced (third-generation) devices which are capable of delivering antitachycardia pacing therapies, these modalities should also be tested and proven to be effective. We generally postpone testing of these modalities to a postoperative EP study. The rationale for this approach is based on the following considerations: (a) patient is awake and not under the influence of anesthesia in the electrophysiology laboratory, (b) more extensive testing is possible without consuming the operating room time, (c) antiarrhythmic therapy is often adjusted prior to testing, and (d) arrhythmias may not be inducible under general anesthesia. Principles of antitachycardia pacing and programming are further discussed in Chapter 21. Some general comments, however, can be made at this juncture.

SENSING AND ARRHYTHMIA DETECTION

Fundamental to proper functioning of the device is accurate arrhythmia detection and differentiation. Ventricular tachycardia and VF recognition in the current devices is based on two basic strategies: (a) rate and (b) morphology detection.

The first of these is easier to grasp. When a rate limit is programmed, the device will regard as tachycardia either VT or VF, or any other sustained tachycardia that is faster (has a shorter cycle length) than the programmed rate limit.

The rate detection alogorithm is more complex than that ordinarily utilized for bradycardia pacemakers. The detection algorithm must be capable of recognizing ventricular electrograms in sinus rhythm and be able to distinguish the lower-amplitude signals with a variety of slew rates and morphologies during VF, as well as the occasional complete signal dropout from VT/VF rhythms (51). The specific design feature which allows adequate signal recognition includes an automatic gain control which can amplify the signal amplitude as low as 0.1 mV and rate averaging, which keeps a cumulative record of time intervals. In some devices that lack automatic gain control, but have programmable sensitivities (e.g., Guardian^{R} ATP 4210, Telectronics, Denver, CO), the absence of automatic gain control is said to be compensated by an automatic doubling of sensitivity when VF is detected (52).

When programming the rate cutoff for the device, morphology characteristics and rate stability of VT should be considered. A rate cutoff of 10–15 beats/min below the VT rate may be sufficient for monomorphic VT. For polymorphic VTs a wider margin of programmability is required to allow adequate arrhythmia recognition (25–30 beats/min).

The second detection criterion is based on the morphology of the transcardiac electrogram and is called the probability density function (PDF). This concept was proposed initially for VF detection by Langer, *et al.* (51). PDF recognition is based on the analysis of the time spent by the transcardiac signal away from the isoelectric line. In sinus rhythm, most of the signal is at the isoelectric line. On the other hand, in sinusoidal rhythms (e.g., VF), most of the time is spent away from the baseline. It is not possible, however, for a physician to know whether a signal will satisfy the PDF criterion or not, except by programming this function and testing the arrhythmia recognition by the device of VT and VF.

This concept although of historical interest, has little practical additional value to the rate recognition criterion. Theoretically, PDF should be able to differentiate narrow QRS tachycardias (supraventricular tachycardias), from wide-complex sinusoidal VTs. However, in practice, presence of intraventricular conduction delay or bundle branch block often obscures this differentiation.

From the foregoing discussion, it should be readily apparent that using the currently available detection methodology, VT cannot be reliably distinguished from other tachyarrhythmias or even from sinus tachycardia when rate overlap occurs. With third and fourth-generation devices, which incorporate antitachycardia pacing features, additional criteria are available to help improve the specificity for VT and VF recognition. Regular (rate-stable) sustained tachycardias may be differentiated from irregular tachycardia (variable rate) by inclusion of the "rate stability" criterion. Furthermore, physiologic sinus tachycardia has a gradual onset in contradistinction to reentry tachycardias which are usually sudden in onset. Thus, an "onset delta" criterion may help differentiate physiologic (e.g., sinus tachycardia) from nonphysiologic reentry tachycardias. More accurate differentiation of VTs and supraventricular tachycardias may evolve in the future, e.g., atrial electrogram analysis, hemodynamic sensing, or signal template analysis for tachycardia detection and differentiation.

POSTOPERATIVE TESTING AND FOLLOW-UP

Deactivation of ICD for the first few days postoperatively to avoid inappropriate shocks triggered by atrial fibrillation with a rapid ventricular response should be balanced against the risk of leaving the patient relatively unprotected from VT or VF, with the possibility of decreased efficacy of external defibrillation consequent on the "shielding" effect of the patch leads (53). One way to solve this seeming dilemma is to program the device temporarily to a higher rate cutoff (e.g., 195–200 beats/min) in the immediate postoperative period.

Prior to hospital discharge, EP testing is advisable to demonstrate efficacy of the ICD (54). Predischarge ICD testing is strongly recommended when intraoperative testing determines that the DFT safety margin approximate(s) the maximum output of the device (output of the device is less than DFT plus 10 J) (55) or a change in antiarrhythmic therapy is made which has a potential to increase the DFTs or alter the rate of the VT. When antitachycardia pacing therapy is used to terminate VT, postoperative testing of VT termination is mandatory.

Patient education predischarge is recommended to increase patient compliance and to allay anxieties of the patient and family about the life-threatening aspects of the disease and possible anxieties surrounding the device function.

Follow-up

Follow-up of patients postoperatively should address the following goals: (a) assessment of the drug efficacy and the appropriateness of therapy, (b) assessment of ICD battery, capacitor, and lead system integrity, and (c) assessment of associated medical and possible psychosocial problems. When antiarrhythmic therapy is altered, subsequent EP assessment may be required to assess the adequacy of therapy and the appropriateness of the programmed parameters. More extensive discussion of this important subject may be found in Chapter 21.

DRUG-DEVICE INTERACTIONS

Effects of Antiarrhythmic Drugs on Defibrillation Thresholds

Concurrent antiarrhythmic drug therapy is frequently used with ICDs to suppress frequent episodes of VT or to slow the tachycardia rate. Antiarrhythmic therapy may also be required for therapy of supraventricular arrhythmias. Potential interactions that may occur between antiarrhythmic drugs and ICDs are listed in Table 20.1.

Some antiarrhythmic drugs may alter the DFTs significantly (56). Although limited human data are available about the effects of antiarrhythmic drugs on DFTs, the known effects are listed in Table 20.2

In general, Class IC agents (flecainide and encainide) increase the DFTs (57,58). Class IB agents (lidocaine and mexiletene) also tend to increase the DFTs (59,60).

Type IA drugs (quinidine and procainamide) have no significant effects on DFTs in therapeutic concentrations (61–64). Similarly, bretylium (a Type III antiarrhythmic) does not have a significant effect on DFTs.

Amiodarone, a Class III agent, has a more complex effect on defibrillation. When administered acutely (intravenously), it decreases the DFTs (65,66). However, when administered chronically, it elevates the DFTs (65–69). This apparent bimodal effect may be due to its metabolite, desethylamiodarone, or it may be a concentration-dependent effect, since tissue levels of amiodarone increase progressively with time and chronicity of administration (70,71).

Cathecolamines facilitate defibrillation (72). Similar effects are also observed in response to aminophylline (73). The beneficial effect of cathecolamines are important clinically, since their administration facilitates defibrillation during cardiopulmonary resuscitation (see Chapters 25 and 26).

The effects of antiarrhythmic drugs should be carefully considered at the time of ICD implant, or when alteration in antiarrhythmic therapy is contemplated.

Effects of Antiarrhythmic Drugs on Arrhythmia Recognition by ICD

Antiarrhythmic drugs may have other clinically significant effects that can potentially impact on the arrhythmia recognition by the ICD. Antiarrhythmic drugs may increase latency, cause PR prolongation or QRS widening, or prolong QT interval. This may result in double counting if diastolic signals are oversensed. Alterations in QRS morphology or intraventricular conduction delay may result in morphology indistinguishable from VT during supraventricular tachycardia or atrial fibrillation. Probability density function criteria may be met. If the rate then exceeds the minimum programmed rate for the device, an inappropriate shock may result.

A potentially beneficial effect of antiarrhythmic drugs besides complete suppression of arrhythmia, is to convert a previously sustained ventricular tachycardia to a nonsustained rhythm. In committed ICDs (VENTAK[R] 1550 or 1600), this may result in an inappropriate shock if the VT is sensed but spontaneously terminates prior to the shock administration. This problem may be in part overcome by a programmable delay function

Table 20.1.
Possible Effects of Antiarrhythmic Drugs that May Affect ICD Function

1. Alteration in DFT
2. Change in QRS morphology resulting in satisfaction of PDF criteria
3. Alteration in ventricular tachycardia cycle length
4. Change from sustained to nonsustained ventricular tachycardia, resulting in inappropriate shocks during nonsustained ventricular tachycardia in committed devices
5. Alteration in postshock excitability
6. Increase in pacing thresholds
7. Increase in latency, PR interval, or alteration in conduction velocity leading to double counting

Table 20.2.
Effect of Antiarrhythmic Drugs on Defibrillation Threshold

Increase	No Change	Decrease
Encainide	MODE	Amiodarone (acute)
ODE	Quinidine	
Flecainide	Procainamide	Clofilium
Recainam	Bretylium	Isoproterenol
Lidocaine		Sotalol
Mexiletene		NAPA
Amiodarone (chronic)		

Abbreviations: MODE, 3-methoxy, NAPA = *N*-acetyl procainamide; *O*-desethyl encainide; ODE, *O*-desmethylencainide.

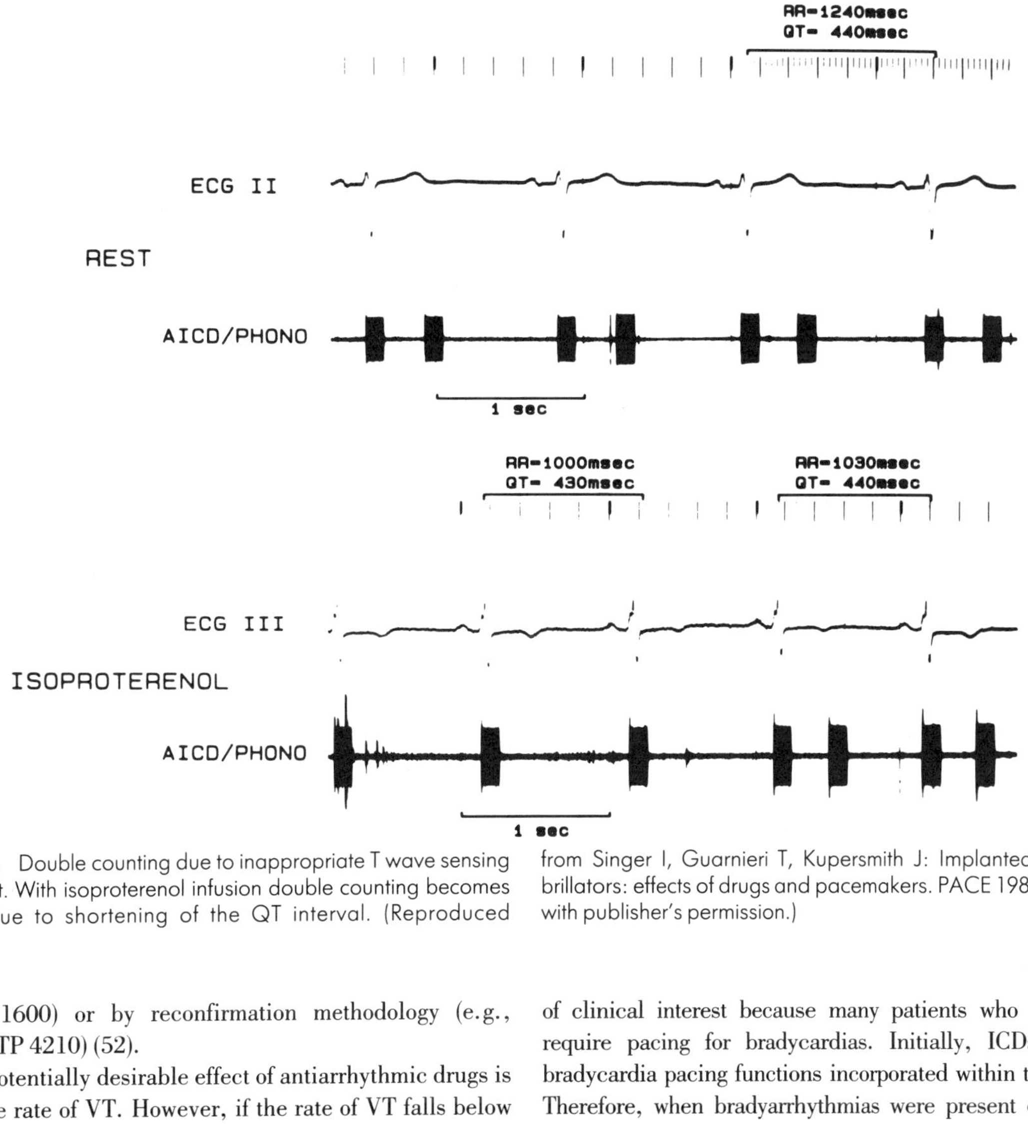

Figure 20.7. Double counting due to inappropriate T wave sensing is noted at rest. With isoproterenol infusion double counting becomes intermittent due to shortening of the QT interval. (Reproduced from Singer I, Guarnieri T, Kupersmith J: Implanted automatic defibrillators: effects of drugs and pacemakers. PACE 1988;11:2250–2252, with publisher's permission.)

(VENTAK^{R} 1600) or by reconfirmation methodology (e.g., Guardian^{R} ATP 4210) (52).

Another potentially desirable effect of antiarrhythmic drugs is slowing of the rate of VT. However, if the rate of VT falls below the programmed rate cutoff for the device, VT may not be treated by the device. This problem may be overcome by the use of tiered therapy in third-generation devices and reprogramming of the device when therapy is altered significantly. Reprogramming of the device requires repeated EP testing to demonstrate device efficacy and function. Altered latency and increased conduction delay may have an effect on the device sensing. Thus, double counting is possible if T waves are sensed inappropriately, resulting in inappropriate discharges (Fig. 20.7).

Antiarrhythmic drugs may affect postshock tissue excitability leading to prolonged pauses postdefibrillation, requiring pacing support. They may also elevate pacing thresholds postshock, resulting in pacemaker capture failure postdefibrillation.

INTERACTIONS OF ICDs WITH PACEMAKERS

Potential interactions between pacemakers and ICDs are listed in Table 20.3.

The interactions between implanted pacemakers and ICDs are of clinical interest because many patients who have ICDs also require pacing for bradycardias. Initially, ICDs did not have bradycardia pacing functions incorporated within the same device. Therefore, when bradyarrhythmias were present or resulted from concomitant antiarrhythmic drug therapy, pacemakers had to be implanted as well. This situation has been partially remedied in the second-generation devices (Guardian^{R} 4202 and 4203) and the third-generation devices (Guardian^{R} ATP, PRx^{R}, PCD^{R}, Res-Q^{R}, and Cadence^{R}) although even in these devices pacing can only be accomplished in VVI mode at present, which may be inappropriate for those patients who have limited cardiac reserve and require A-V synchrony to maintain adequate cardiac output.

Potential interactions may be one of the following: (a) effect of defibrillation shock on the pacemaker lead system, (b) effect of defibrillation shock on the pacing thresholds acutely, (c) sensing problems related to the pacemaker signals, and (d) interactions between an ICD and an antitachycardia pacemaker.

Anecdotal evidence exists documenting pacemaker damage post-external defibrillation. Pacemaker reprogramming by an internal or external defibrillation shock has also been documented (74–78). Internal defibrillator discharge has not been documented to produce permanent pacemaker damage, however. Current pacemakers have protective circuits incorporated which shunt the excessive energy during defibrillation away from the internal electrodes of the pulse generator.

Levine has described transient loss of capture, sensing or both and chronic threshold rise following external cardioversion or defibrillation (79). Similar rise in thresholds was reported by Slepian, *et al.* following internal cardioversion defibrillation by automatic implantable cardioverter-defibrillator (AICD) (80).

Possible sensing problems may also arise due to ICD detection of pacemaker stimulus artefacts. Double counting may occur if the device senses both the pacemaker stimulus and the native QRS (Fig. 20.8). On the other hand, during VF, if the sensing amplifier detects stimulus artefact and "locks on" the stimulus, it may not be able to detect VF, with potentially disastrous consequences. This is especially true for unipolar pacemakers. Therefore, unipolar pacemakers are contraindicated in patients with implanted ICDs (81).

Effect of internal shock on pacemaker capture threshold is another important consideration, since postshock transient asystole is not uncommon. Guarnieri, *et al.* have demonstrated a transient increase in pacing threshold post–ICD shock (82). Duration of capture loss was related to current amplitude of the pacemaker and was independent of the pacing site (endocardial or epicardial). Time to capture was significantly prolonged due to Type IC drug flecainide.

When pacing and defibrillation function is built into the same electrode, it is important to consider a possibility that internal defibrillation shock may alter postshock pacing threshold. Yee, *et al.* have demonstrated serial changes in QRS amplitude and stimulation threshold after catheter internal shock using the pig as the animal model for transvenous defibrillation (83). On the other hand, Winkle, *et al.* have not observed such changes using the CPI tripolar transvenous catheter (ENDOTAK^R, CPI, St. Paul, MN), suggesting that the design feature of the catheter itself may influence postdefibrillation threshold alteration, and that the specific design features of the catheter may also be important (84).

Sensing problems may occur in the presence of pacemaker signals which may lead to inappropriate discharges by the ICD if double or triple counting occurs. The following interaction may occur between pacemakers and ICDs: (a) detection inhibition, (b) double counting, and (c) countershock-induced loss of sensing by the pacemaker resulting in asynchronous pacing (81).

Detection inhibition may occur with either temporary or permanent ventricular or atrial pacemakers. For example, if a patient with a pacemaker develops VT or VF, the pacemaker may not sense the QRS signal appropriately and will thus continue to pace. If the resulting pacemaker artifacts are sensed by the ICD detection circuitry, then the ICD may "lock on" the pacemaker signal and "ignore" the VT. Thus, VF detection may be inhibited with potentially disastrous consequences.

Cohen, *et al.* have reported seeing pacing during VF in 24 episodes in seven patients. In three patients, all with unipolar pacemakers, the inappropriate sensing caused ICD inhibition

Table 20.3.
Possible Pacemaker and ICD Interactions

Pacemaker–ICD interactions
VF nondetection due to sensed pacemaker stimuli
Double, triple, and multiple counting resulting in inappropriate shocks
ICD–pacemaker interactions
Pacemaker reprogramming by the defibrillation discharge
Sensing/capture failure postdefibrillation
ATP–ICD interactions
Arrhythmia acceleration by ATP resulting in VF
ATP triggering ICD discharge when ATP pacemaker and ICD are combined

Abbreviations: ATP = antitachycardia pacemaker

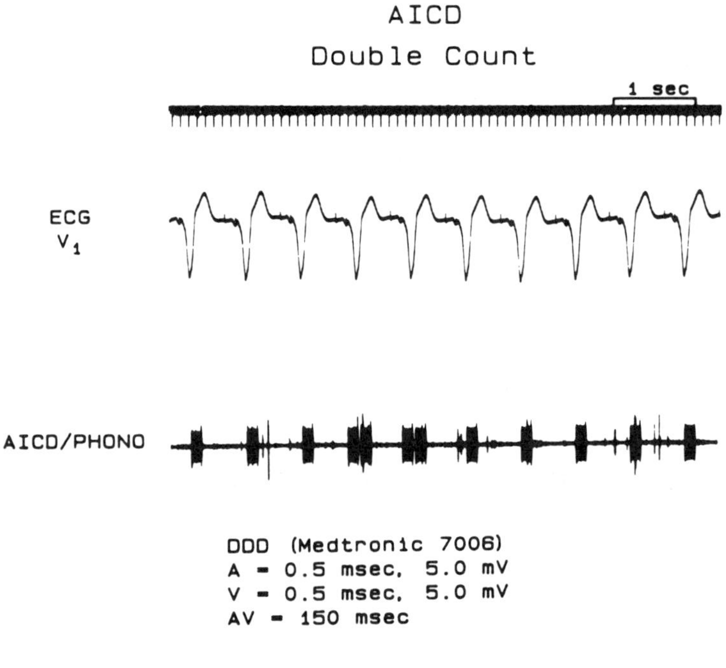

Figure 20.8. Double counting due to intermittent sensing of pacemaker and QRS electrograms. (Reproduced from Singer I, Guarnieri T, Kupersmith J: Implanted automatic defibrillators: effects of drugs and pacemakers. PACE 1988;11:2250–2262, with publisher's permission.)

during VF (85). Therefore, unipolar pacemakers should **never** be used in conjunction with an ICD.

Double counting may occur in patients with a ventricular pacemaker if intraventricular conduction delay which results in sufficient artifact-to-QRS signal separation to exceed ICD refractory period. Under these circumstances, both signals will be interpreted as QRS depolarizations and double counting may result, leading to inappropriate shocks.

Failure of the pacemaker to sense ventricular or atrial depolarization may also lead to inappropriate discharges of the ICD, due to multiple counting of pacemaker artifacts and QRS signal and asynchronous pacing resulting from the sensing failure.

Diastolic T-wave sensing may also occur and result in double counting (86). Antiarrhythmic drugs that slow the sinus rate, prolong the QT interval, and distort the ST segment are particularly prone to predispose to double counting due to inappropriate T-wave sensing.

ANTITACHYCARDIA DEVICES COMBINED WITH ICDs (see also Chapter 21)

Antitachycardia pacemakers may be used to interrupt VT by causing temporary refractoriness in one of the tachycardia circuit pathways. This may be accomplished by appropriately timed single, double, triple, or multiple extrastimuli. Multiple extrastimuli and bursts are more effective by "peeling back" refractoriness and permitting earlier entry of extrastimuli in the excitable gap (see also Chapter 2). Pacing techniques are generally more effective for slower and hemodynamically better tolerated monomorphic VTs and generally ineffective for polymorphic VTs or VF. Because antitachycardia pacing may result in VT acceleration or VF, antitachycardia pacing should never be used alone in the ventricle without an implanted ICD. Newer, third-generation devices incorporate antitachycardia pacing as part of a tiered therapeutic response, using the less "aggressive" strategies for slow VT termination (e.g., antitachycardia pacing), cardioversion/defibrillation for VT, and defibrillation for VF.

Interaction between antitachycardia pacemakers and ICDs may occur if two devices are used separately (87, 88). For example, VT may be accelerated by antitachycardia pacing (ATP) triggering ICD defibrillation. ICD defibrillation may result in conversion of VF to VT, resulting in antitachycardia pacing activation or asystole, leading to pacing. Antitachycardia pacing if it falls within the sensing window of a committed device may inappropriately trigger defibrillation by the ICD. A comprehensive treatment strategy is emerging with third-generation devices which combines features of antitachycardia pacemakers and defibrillators and is capable of dealing specifically with a wide variety of tachyarrhythmias and bradyarrhythmias.

CLINICAL RESULTS

A substantial body of clinical data has been collected documenting efficacy of implantable defibrillator therapy. In addition, there were observations in monitored patients of automatic termination of malignant arrhythmias via the devices. In some patients these were bystanders' observation of dizziness or collapse being reversed after a diffuse muscular contraction or other evidence of an internal discharge (89,90).

Over the years, the therapy has evolved from a "last resort" effort to one that is part of the initial thinking of physician caring for sudden death survivor and others with comparable ventricular arrhythmia. This change in approach is based on substantial differences in sudden death survival curves between patients with implanted defibrillators and historical controls in patients previously treated in other ways.

In the earliest published study (89), 1 yr sudden death rate (defined as deaths without a clear other cause) for the first 52 implantations was 8.5%, total deaths 22.9%. This is a 52% decrease from an estimated mortality for this group. Figure 20.9 shows actual mortality for the two early models of the device, "orig model" of the automatic implantable defibrillator (AID) which was specifically designed to sense ventricular fibrillation only, and the AICD. This is compared to a hypothetical "expected" mortality. With the more recent devices (the integrated circuit models available since 1986 have been considered more reliable) as well as with the extended arrhythmia indications, survival in later studies has been greater (90–92).

Currently, there are no prospective randomized studies comparing the survival of ICD-treated patients with a comparable group of patients treated by EP-guided drug therapy. Some insight may be gained by comparing survival statistics of AICD-treated patients with similar patients treated by antiarrhythmic drugs, from other studies. Figure 20.10 shows data from Winkle, *et al.* (13) showing considerably less sudden and total deaths in the AICD group versus antiarrhythmic drug nonresponders (12, 92).

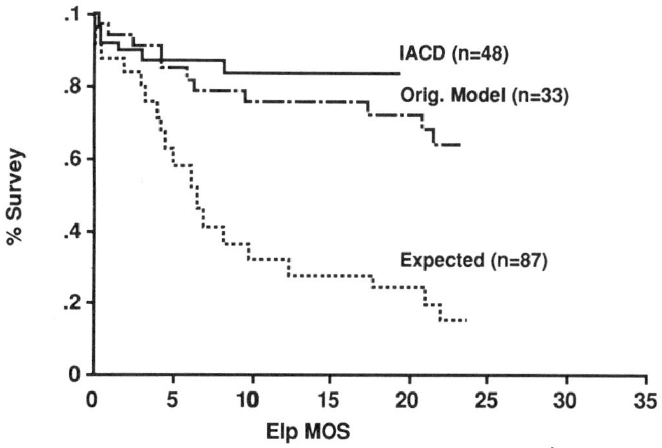

Figure 20.9. Survival curves for initial 87 patients implanted in Baltimore. The first 33 patients received the original model AID (automatic implantable defibrillator). Patients who underwent replacement of that device with the more advanced IACD (implantable automatic cardioverter defibrillator) were withdrawn alive from the first group and reentered into the second group. A hypothetical mortality curve was constructed assuming episodes of symptomatic arrhythmia would have resulted in death had the defibrillator not been implanted. Note the improvement in mortality with the devices, and the improved units performing even better than the original one.

Some investigators have compared survival statistics of the AICD-treated group with an earlier, similar group of patients in whom EP-guided drug therapy was used. Data from Massachusetts General Hospital comparing patients who had AICDs implanted from 1983 to 1988 with an earlier group of similar arrhythmia patients, from 1978 to 1983 was as follows: for the earlier group, mean ejection fraction was 43%, 77% had arrhythmias responsive to drugs, and 1- and 5-yr cardiac deaths were 15 and 37%, respectively. In the later AICD group, mean ejection fraction was 31%, only 15% were drug responders, but cardiac death rate was much less at 4 and 16% at 1 and 5 years (93).

The largest database on ICDs now available has been compiled by Cardiac Pacemakers, Inc., manufacturers of the first device available. Sudden death mortality has been extremely low. For example, Table 20.4 shows that sudden death survival for all devices at 1 yr was 98.9% and for earlier models at 1 yr was 97.5% (Table 20.5). Total survival for all causes of cardiac deaths were 96.9 and 91.6% at 1 and 5 yr, respectively (Table 20.4). Tables 20.6 and 20.7 show clinical information and concomitant therapy, respectively, in this group of patients. One issue with this type of data is possible underreporting of deaths to a manufacturing company. However, mortality in this database seems generally comparable to that in the studies described above.

All of the above data show an impressive reduction in mortality following ICD implantation. This has led to widespread acceptance of this therapy for treatment of patients with aborted sudden death (Fig. 20.11) and VT refractory to therapy. However, none of the data are from a randomized study and this fact has created controversy among investigators. While many investigators feel that the reduction in sudden death post-ICD implantation is so striking as to make a randomized trial unnecessary, others disagree (94,95). The critics of AICD data cite possible bias in studies with historical controls in selection of patients, improvements in other types of care over the later time periods, etc. Although their objections appear to be overstated, randomized trials comparing ICDs with amiodarone therapy are underway in various countries as well as those examining new prophylactic indications for ICDs (See Indications) which will perhaps help clarify this controversy.

COMPLICATIONS OF ICD THERAPY

Reliability of the devices, as opposed to patient survival, relates to engineering factors such as random component failures. From this standpoint, the present generators seem reliable. Table 20.8 shows data on the longevity of the devices independent of how

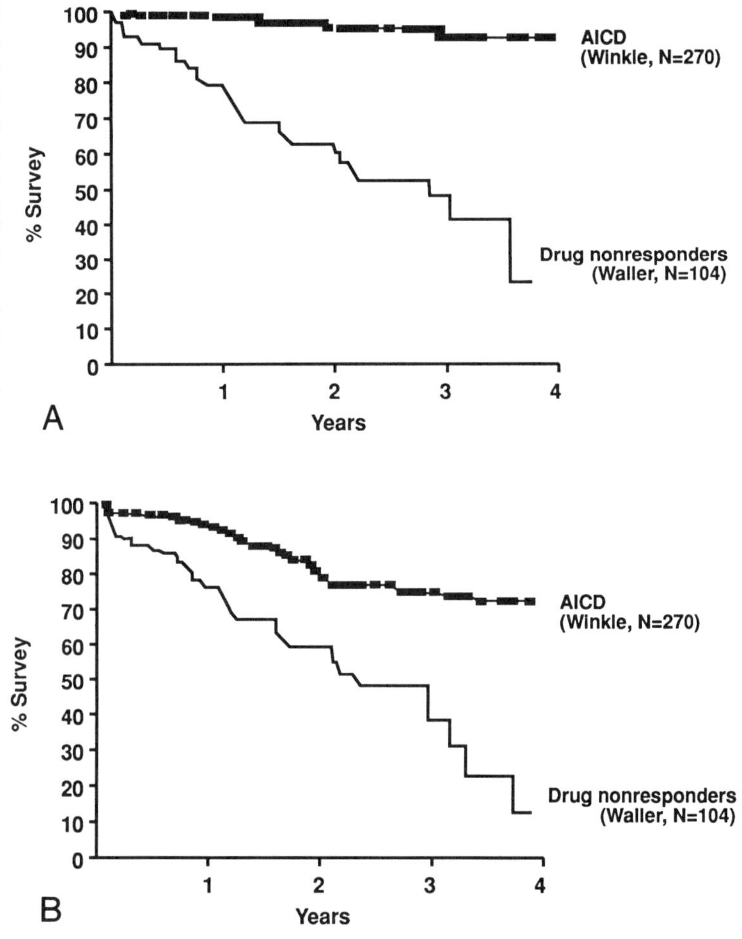

Figure 20.10. Freedom from sudden cardiac death (**A**) and freedom from total death (**B**) in one large single center study compared to similar groups treated with drug therapy. The AICD has a beneficial effect for drug nonresponders, raising them to the level of survival enjoyed by drug responders. AICD data are replotted from Winkle R, Mead H, Ruder M, *et al.*: Long-term outcome with the automatic implantable cardioverter-defibrillator. J Am Coll Cardiol 1989;13:1353–1361; and drug data from Swerdlow CD, Winkle RA, Mason JW: Determinants of survival in patients with ventricular tachyarrhythmias. N Engl J Med 1983;24:1436–1442; and Walter T, Kay HR, Spielman SR, *et al.*: Reduction in sudden death and total mortality by antitachycardia therapy evaluated by electrophysiologic drug testing: criteria of efficacy in patients with sustained ventricular tachyarrhythmia. J Am Coll Cardiol 1987;10:83–89. Reproduced with permission from the authors and publisher.)

Table 20.4.
Actuarial Survival Free of Events in the Overall AICD Implant Cohort[a]

	1 yr	2 yr	3 yr	4 yr	5 yr
Sudden cardiac death	98.9	98.3	98.0	97.4	97.0
Nonsudden cardiac death	98.0	97.0	96.0	95.4	94.5
Total cardiac death	96.9	95.2	94.0	93.0	91.6
Death from all causes	94.3	91.6	89.2	87.0	84.5
Sample size	11,723	6,770	3,481	1,450	671

[a]Data analysis through August 15, 1991.

Table 20.5.
Survival Free from Sudden Death Rates for Newer Devices After Market Release Compared to Earlier Ones Through August 15, 1991[a]

	1 yr	2 yr	3 yr	4 yr	5 yr
AID B/BR	97.5	95.9	94.7	94.0	94.0
sample size	1,110	684	363	211	103
VENTAK[R]	98.4	97.7	97.5	97.4	
sample size	5,937	4,977	1,398	191	
VENTAK[R] P	99.4	99.4			
sample size	963	282			
VENTAK[R] 1550	99.5	99.4			
sample size	5,612	740			

[a]AID B/BR corresponds to the early AICD. The VENTAK is the integrated circuit version AICD. Ventak 1550 and Ventak-P are partially and fully programmable units, respectively.

Table 20.6.
Age Distribution and Primary Clinical Diagnosis for Overall Cohort through August 15, 1991

	Number	Percent
Patient Age		
<25	217	1.2
25–44	1,398	7.7
45–64	8,602	47.4
65+	7,936	43.7
Not Reported	817	
Average age = 61.5 years	Std dev = 11.6	
Age range = 7.7–91.4 years		
Primary Clinical Diagnosis		
Coronary Artery Disease	11,315	74.2
Nonischemic Cardiomyopathy	1,609	10.5
Other: Long Q-T, Valvular Primary Electrical, Congenital	2,330	15.3
Not Reported	3,814	

Table 20.7.
Concomitant Therapy for Overall Cohort through August 15, 1991

	Number	Percent
Pharmacologic Therapy	11,399	46.8
Antiarrhythmics (AA)	6,995	61.4
Beta Blockers (BB)	1,035	9.1
AA + BB	531	4.6
Other	2,838	25.0
Surgical Therapy	4,889	30.0
CABG	3,334	68.2
Mapping, resection, ablation, etc.	176	3.6
Combination	539	11.0
Other	840	17.2

the patients do and absent normal battery depletion. The units are seen to have steadily improved.

The pulse generators have been relatively large, to date, and the major complication of implantation, which is in part related to this fact, has been infection. Table 20.9 lists the incidence of this and other complications through October 15, 1988 compiled by CPI. The incidence of complications associated with defibrillator therapy is undoubtedly related to the relative experience, the surgical volume, and the population mix in a given clinical center. It is also dependent on physician preference for a particular type of therapy, economic constraints restricting the use of ICD therapy, differences in definition of what constitutes a complication, and differences in study designs. There is no doubt that complications are more common in the highest risk patients. With respect to the data shown in Table 20.9, it should be noted that the incidence of complications is likely to be underreported in series compiled by a manufacturer, as it is obtained indirectly.

Perioperative mortality may in part be related to the implant technique. There is evidence that even in centers reporting relatively higher mortality from thoracotomy insertion (96), use of a transvenous system (Endotak[R], CPI, St. Paul, MN) is associated with an extremely low perioperative mortality (97). Perioperative mortality in experienced centers is reported to be 1.5–3% (13,14).

Incidence of lead-related complications in the experienced

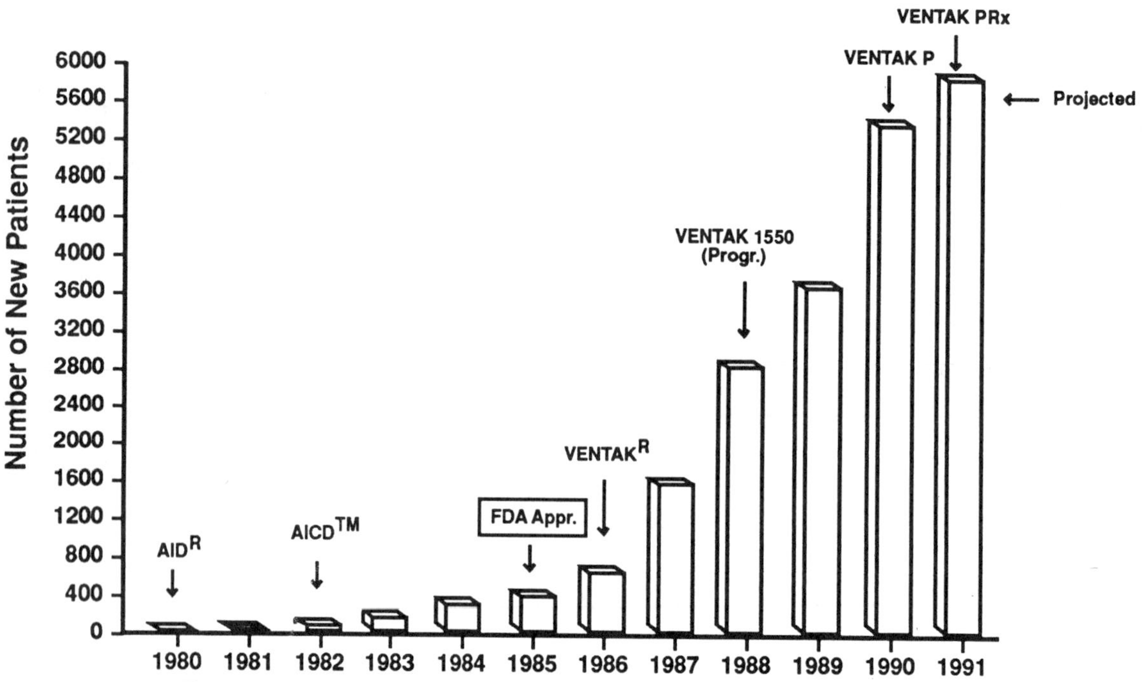

Figure 20.11. Growth in use of implantable defibrillators since first implant in 1980.

Table 20.8.
Longevity of Devices Themselves, A Measure of Freedom from Events Such as Random Component Failure, Is Independent of How the Patients Do[a]

	6 mo	12 mo	18 mo	24 mo	30 mo
AID B/BR	96.8	88.8	83.3	81.5	81.1
sample size	1709	1419	1080	524	169
VENTAK[R]	99.4	98.9	98.3	98.1	97.3
sample size	6325	6032	5696	4955	2965
VENTAK[R] P	99.5	99.1	98.8		
sample size	1490	956	521		
VENTAK[R] 1550	99.6	99.2	98.9	98.8	
sample size	8747	5542	2638	721	

[a]This is a measure of device reliability. Normal battery depletion does not appear.

centers has been low. These were primarily associated with the SVC lead. In one of the largest reported series (13), 10% of patients with SVC lead had complications, including lead migration or lead fracture. Patch lead complications were uncommon, reported in 2% of patients, including patch cracking and patch fracture. Fractures associated with the sensing leads are also relatively uncommon (1%). Infection was reported in 1% of patients, with the most common organism being *Staphylococcus aureus*.

Other reported complications include device discharges due to nonsustained VT (in the current generation of committed devices) or inappropriate therapy for supraventricular tachycardias. The true incidence of undesirable discharges cannot be determined with certainty, since current devices have no data logging capabilities. This issue may be clarified and probably largely eliminated with the use of third-generation noncommitted devices (see below).

Although the absolute incidence of infections is low, when it occurs, it is devastating and uniformly demands explanation of the hardware. Aside from infection, pulse generator complications include erosion or extrusion (0.7%) and pulse generator migration (0.2%) (13). Careful surgical technique can prevent most generator-related complications. Pocket effusion is relatively common and usually insignificant, since most resorb spontaneously.

Endocardial lead displacement may occur. Loss of sensing or capture may occur acutely or chronically. This may result in inappropriate shocks (due to oversensing) or failure to deliver therapy (due to undersensing). Lead repositioning is required in that event. Endocardial lead fracture is relatively uncommon.

Lead migration was a problem encountered early on with the superior vena caval lead due to inadequate lead fixation. Since this lead is used less frequently now, with the majority of patients having patch leads implanted, this complication is now seen less frequently. This may change in the future, however, with the use of endocardial defibrillation electrodes.

Acute pericarditis and pleuritis associated with patch leads is seen relatively frequently. The true incidence of these complications is most likely underreported in the registry. These complications rarely lead to serious sequelae, but occasionally, significant pericardial or pleural effusion may accumulate, requiring fluid removal by paracenthesis.

Adverse psychologic reactions to ICDs have been reported in some patients, but this issue has not been studied systematically. In our experience, severe psychologic reactions are rare,

Table 20.9.
Incidence of Most Common Complications Through October 15, 1988 reported to CPI[a]

Infection	1.3
Erosion/extrusion	0.7
Pulse generator migration	0.2
Pocket effusion/fluid accumulation	0.4
Pacemaker interaction	0.2
Lead dislodgment/migration	0.4
Lead fracture	0.7
Pericardial effusion	0.1
Psychologic reactions	0.1
Elevated chronic DFT	0.5
Nondetection (due to PDF)	0.1
Multiple counting	2.0
Pulse misdirection during magnet test	0.8

[a]One of the most important of these is infection, although low in absolute incidence, devastating when present, and usually demanding removal of all hardware.

but continuing support is desirable for the patient, the spouse, and the immediate family.

NEWER TECHNOLOGIES

The implantable defibrillator has evolved from a committed device, capable only of treating VF to a programmable noncommitted device, i.e., one that can change if the arrhythmia changes or is terminated, and is capable of antitachycardia and bradycardia pacing with a tiered, hierarchical approach to VT therapy.

Antitachycardia Pacing

The original device conceived by Mirowski and Mower has undergone important transformation. As the implantable defibrillator concept became widely recognized and appreciated, limitations of such therapy became clear as well. First, it was recognized that the initiating rhythm prior to VF was in most cases VT and that lower energies are as efficacious as higher energies for therapy of VT. Second, it was recognized that for most slow, monomorphic and stable VTs antitachycardia pacing is effective and that in most cases, higher-energy shock (30 J) was not required to terminate the VT (98,99). Therefore, addition of antitachycardia pacing capability was considered advantageous since the ability to terminate VT with antitachycardia pacing alone could conserve battery life and eliminate unpleasant shocks.

Although efficacious in most instances, antitachycardia pacing is ineffective for rapid or polymorphic VT and in some cases is known to accelerate the tachycardia and cause deterioration of the rhythm to VF. It may also result in a prolonged episode of hypotension due to repeated attempts at antitachycardia pacing. Because of these considerations, a concept of tiered therapy was advanced where different "zones" of tachycardia could be managed by more or less "aggressive" therapy consisting of antitachycardia pacing for slow VT, low-energy cardioversion for faster VT, and higher-energy defibrillation for VF (Fig. 20.12).

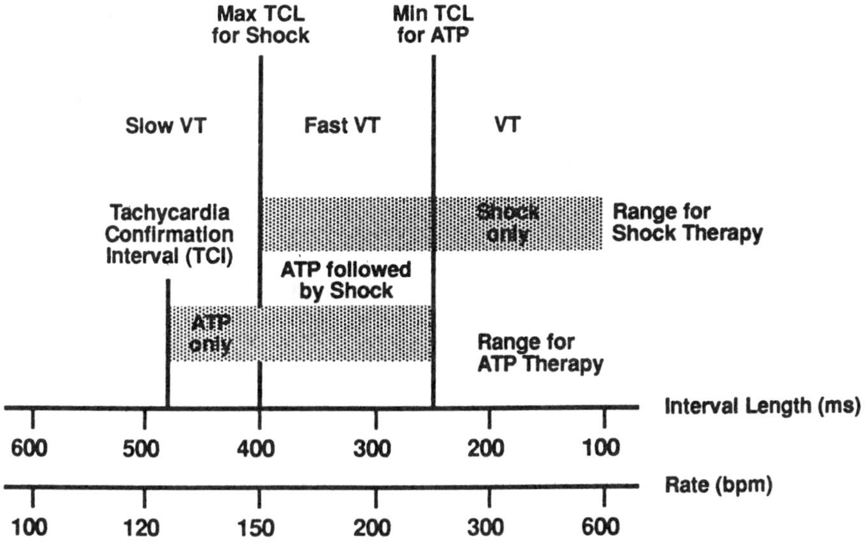

Figure 20.12. Tiered therapy concept implemented for Guardian[R] ATP 4210 (Telectronics, Inc.) with therapy "zones": for *slow* VT—only ATP therapy is administered; for *fast* VT—ATP therapy is followed by shock; for *very fast* VT and VF only high-energy shock is administered. (Reproduced from Singer I, Austin E, Nash W, *et al.*: The initial clinical experience with an implantable cardioverter defibrillator/antitachycardia pacemaker. PACE 1991;14: 1119–1128, with permission.)

09:16 AM 16SEP90

0 seconds
Tachy detection
TCL 330ms (181PPM)
0 seconds
Sense History (ms)
310 290 300
330 385 365
340 345 295
360
Detection

2 seconds
Sense History (ms)
330 290 330
350 330 365
Confirmation

2 seconds
Tachy still present
TCL 340ms (177PPM)
PASAR-0 therapy
II = 270ms
CI = 270ms
10 pulses delvrd

5 seconds
Sense History (ms)
360 405 260
360 260 370
Reversion

7 seconds
Reversion

09:15 AM 16SEP90

0 seconds
Tachy detection
TCL 345ms (175PPM)
0 seconds
Sense History (ms)
280 340 360
270 470 425
350 410 295
260 350 405
305 330 405
360 315 310

Detection
1 seconds
Sense History (ms)
385 330 275
260 365
Reversion
1 seconds
Reversion

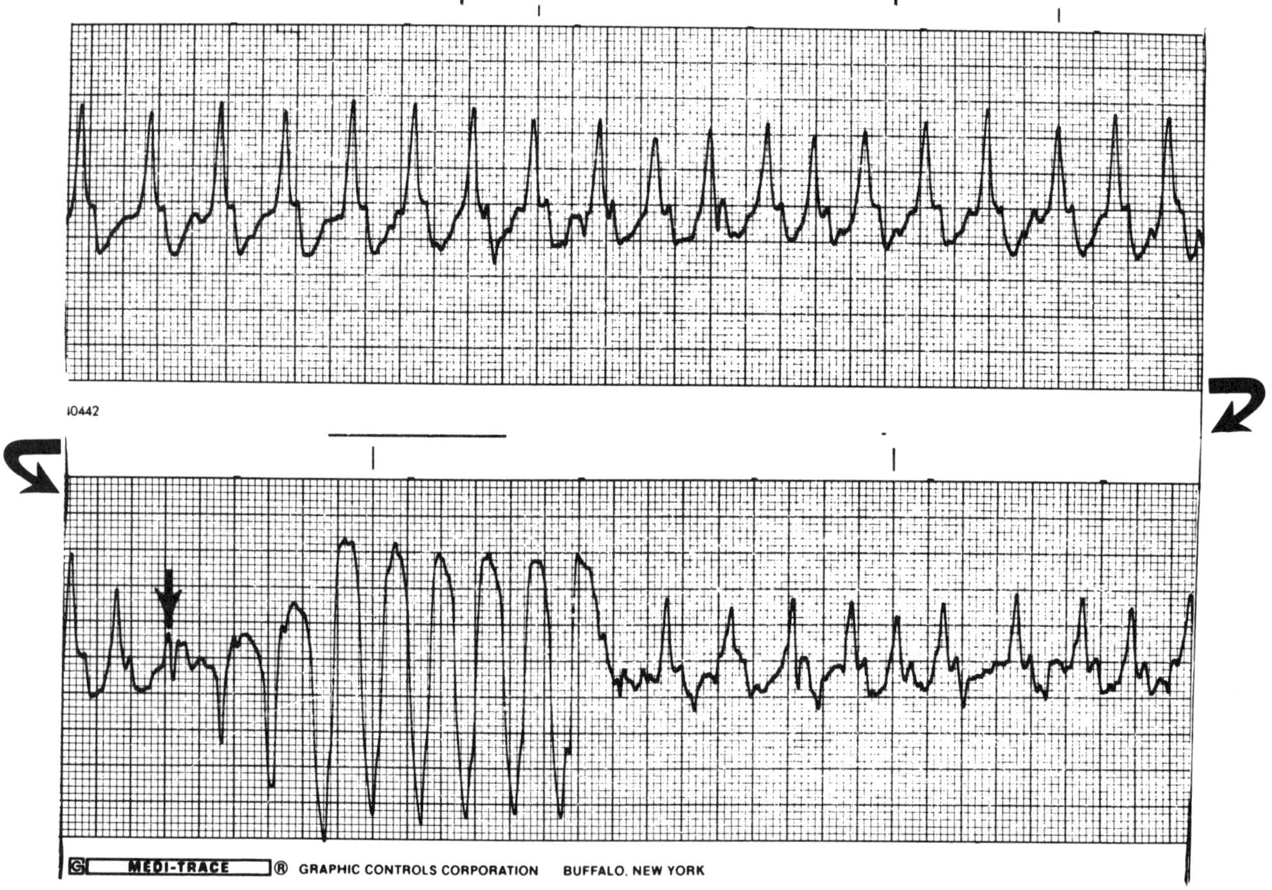

While this concept is attractive conceptually, a number of technical problems have to be overcome to enable this approach to be implemented optimally. These include but are not limited to the following considerations: (a) accurate arrhythmia detection and differentiation (this is currently not possible in all cases since many supraventricular tachycardias overlap in their rates with VTs), (b) ability to accurately classify hemodynamically stable from unstable VTs, (c) implementation of the most effective but least aggressive therapy immediately, and (d) prevention of inappropriate therapy, i.e., shocks, etc. for non-sustained, self-terminating tachycardias.

Accurate arrhythmia classification depends on precise differentiation of supraventricular from ventricular dysrhythmias. Since all currently available devices have only a ventricular-sensing electrode, the available options for tachycardia recognition are limited and include rate, suddenness of onset, and rate stability (in some devices). Though able to differentiate paroxysmal regular tachycardias from nonparoxysmal tachycardias, these criteria are limited in their specificity and may decrease sensitivity for detection (Fig. 20.13). For further discussion of these concepts, see Chapter 21.

To enhance arrhythmia differentiation, further advances are required. To this end, atrial sensing with A-V electrogram relationship analysis is being developed. Alternative approaches such as template matching, a technique where normal QRS complexes during sinus rhythm are compared to VT complexes, are also being considered.

Bradycardia Pacing

Significant number of patients with implanted ICDs may require bradycardia pacing. It has been estimated that up to 20% of patients may require concommitant pacing or pacing after the shock delivery (56,100,101). Initially, in patients requiring pacing, pacemakers were implanted in addition to the implanted ICDs. This was disadvantageous in several respects: (a) additional procedure and device was required and (b) potential for device-pacemaker interactions was present (see above). To avoid these problems, all third- and some second-generation devices (e.g., Guardian^R 4202 and 4203) incorporate bradycardia pacing capabilities. Currently available devices do not provide dual-chamber pacing. Patients who need dual-chamber pacing for optional hemodynamics may still require concommitant pacemaker implantation presently.

Diagnostic Capabilities

Early devices provided no diagnostic information regarding the arrhythmias initiating the device therapy. The only information that could be retrieved was the number of shocks and the device capacitor charge times. The lack of diagnostic capabilities limited the interpretation of the shock validity, i.e., whether a defibrillation shock was appropriate or inappropriate. This information could only be gleaned from the patient's history and fortuitous ECG or Holter recordings. Since palpitations and presyncope may occur with hemodynamically destabilizing supraventricular arrhythmias, inferences regarding appropriateness of device therapy were at best educated guesses.

With programmability, the need for stored electrogram data retrieval has become even more important. Some investigational, third-generation devices incorporate electrogram data storage (Guardian ATP^R and Cadence^R) and provide documentation of RR intervals (Fig. 20.13), cycle length of arrhythmias detected, detection zone satisfied and the therapy delivered, impedance during the shock delivery, and the date and the time of the event. Real-time ventricular electrograms may be stored. These are particularly valuable in the diagnosis of rate-sensing lead fracture or lead connection electronic noise which may mimic real arrhythmia detection and result in inappropriate therapy (Fig. 20.14).

Hemodynamic Sensing

Hemodynamic sensing has been proposed as an alternative to accurately classify stable arrhythmias, potentially amenable to antitachycardia pacing from unstable tachycardias requiring prompt termination. A variety of sensors have been proposed including the pressure sensor (dP/dt), detection of the right ventricular volume (dV/dt), pace depolarization integral (PDI) sensing, measurement of Doppler derived cardiac output, and other possible approaches. While the concept of hemodynamic sensing is attractive, addition of hemodynamic sensors would vastly complicate the lead design and further complicate the detection and therapy delivery algorithm. Stability of the signal over time and accurate signal to noise detection present formidable engineering challenges. It also remains to be proven that the added complexity of devices incorporating such hemodynamic feedback mechanisms would prove to be superior to the simpler devices where rate alone is used to differentiate arrhythmias.

With respect to nonsustained arrhythmias, various strategies have been proposed, are currently either in clinical use, or are under clinical investigation in the investigational third generation devices. These include programmable shock delay (Ventak P^R, CPI, St. Paul, MN) and reconfirmation methodology (e.g., Guardian ATP^R 4210, Telectronics, Englewood, CO) (52). Although successful in most cases, these strategies are imperfect and may delay definitive therapy occasionally. Nevertheless, noncommitted devices are superior to committed devices and help prevent unnecessary therapy for nonsustained VT (Fig. 20.15). The available

Figure 20.13. Lack of specificity for VT detection: **A,** telemetry printout from a patient with implanted Guardian^R ATP 4210 (Telectronics, Inc.). Telemetry demonstrates two episodes of tachycardia meeting detection criteria, the first resulting in ATP therapy with apparent reversion, and the second terminating spontaneously. Note that RR intervals vary considerably (280–470 msec) suggesting atrial fibrillation. **B,** Real-time recording demonstrates atrial fibrillation with intraventricular conduction delay, resulting in inappropriate ATP therapy (*arrow*). **Top** and **bottom strips** are continuous.

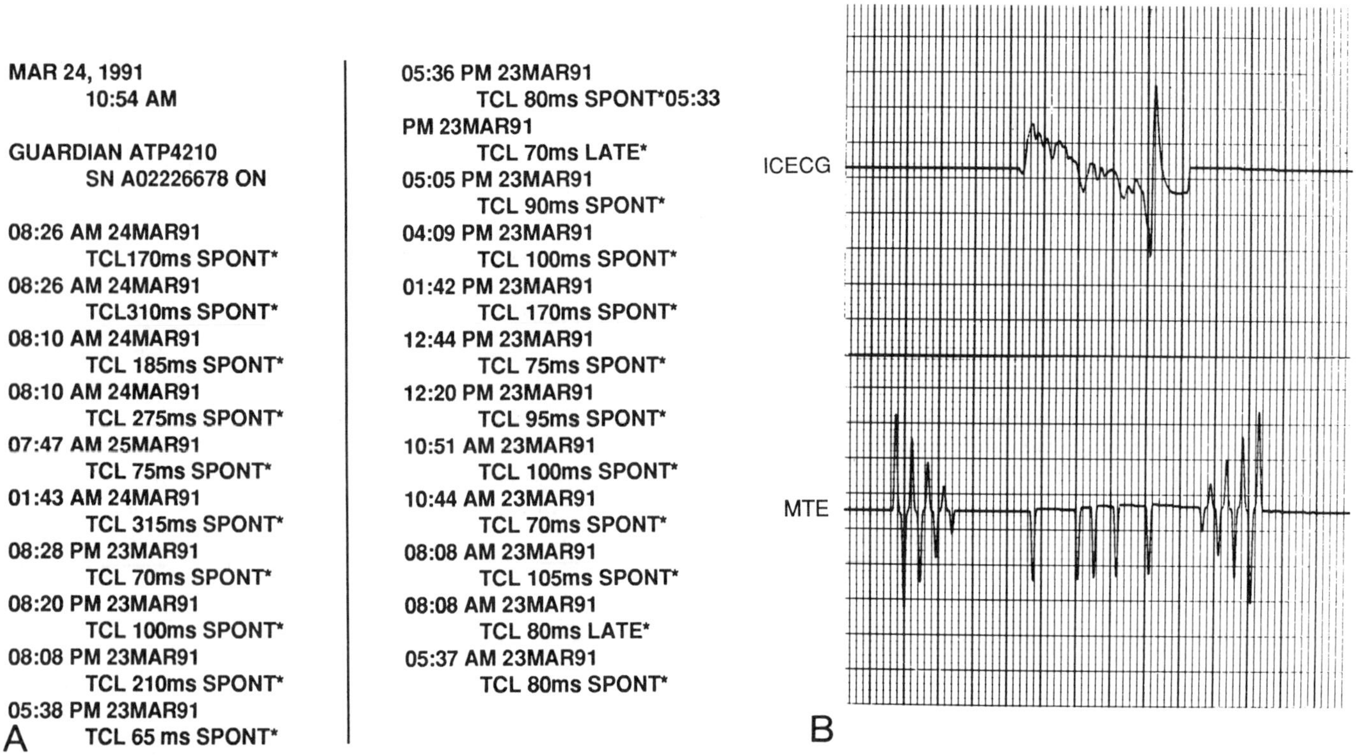

Figure 20.14. Lead fracture detection on telemetry readout and confirmed by intracardiac electrogram "snapshots". **A,** Multiple apparently spontaneously terminating tachyarrhythmias, with several episodes less than 100 msec are detected, suggesting oversensing and a possible lead problem. **B,** Intracardiac electrogram (ICECG) and main timing event log (MTE) of a 1-sec "snapshot" demonstrates multiple signals due to lead fracture.

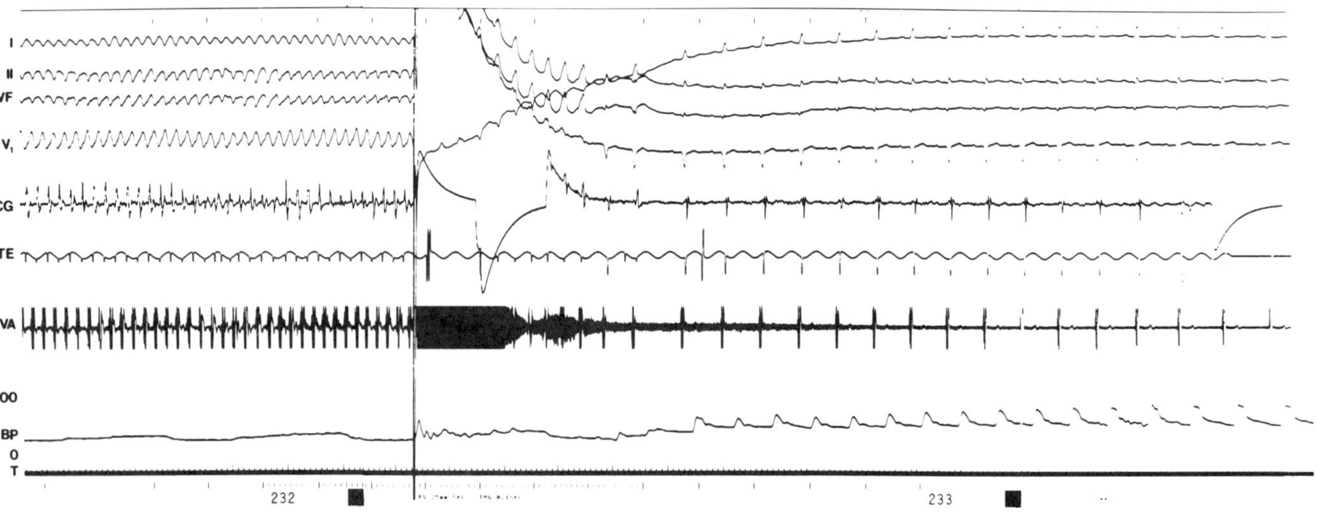

Figure 20.15. Advantage of reconfirmation prior to therapy delivery. Patient with implanted Guardian[R] ATP 4210 device (Telectronics, Inc.). From **top** to **bottom:** surface leads I, II, aVF, V_1, intracardiac electrogram (ICECG), main timing events (MTE), right ventricular apex electrogram (RVA), and blood pressure (BP). Note VF with appropriate detection and delivery of shock, followed by nonsustained VT, with appropriate redetection (*sinusoidal line* on MTE channel indicates therapy mode for the device). The device starts recharging but after detection of sinus rhythm, no therapy is delivered (termination of the sinusoidal line).

Table 20.10.
Technologies Available in Investigational, Third-Generation Devices

Company Device	CPI PRX[R]	Telectronics Guardian ATP[R]	Medtronic PCD[R]	Ventritex Cadence[R]	Intermedics RES-Q[R]	Siemens Siecure[R]
Programmability	+[a]	+	+	+	+	+
Rate	+	+	+	+	+	+
Energy	+	+	+	+	+	+
Antitachycardia pacing	+	+	+	+	+	+
Bradycardia pacing	+	+	+	+	+	+
Tiered therapy	+	+	+	+	+	+
Committed	No	No	No(VT) Yes(VF)	No	Yes	Yes
Stored electrograms	–[b]	+	–	+	–	—[c]
Noninvasive EPS	+	+	+	+	+	+

Adapted from Winkle RA: State of the art of the AICD. PACE 1991;14:961–966.
[a](+) Available.
[b](–) Not available.
[c]Presently unknown.
Abbreviations: EPS, electrophysiologic study.

programmable options in currently investigational devices, which are likely to be market released in the next several years, are summarized in Table 20.10.

NONTHORACOTOMY ICD SYSTEMS

ICD therapy in the past was limited to patients able to undergo thoracotomy. Morbidity and mortality as well as the cost of implementation may be reduced by nonthoracotomy systems. To this end, development of nonthoracotomy lead systems, downsizing of pulse generators, and application of alternative defibrillation waveforms is being considered.

An important area of advancement in ICD technology is development of endocardial lead systems which can be implanted transvenously, thus obviating thoracotomy in most instances. The first of these systems tested was Endotak[R] (CPI, St. Paul, MN) (97). This lead system is used in conjunction with a subcutaneous electrode placed in the left axillary region (Fig. 20.16). Although successful in achieving adequate defibrillation thresholds in about two-thirds of implanted patients, the system uses a relatively large endocardial lead (11F) (Fig. 20.17). In the initial implementation of this lead, lead fracture was encountered, causing short-circuiting within the lead and inappropriate shocks (97). The lead was redesigned, and at present clinical trials are continuing to establish the long-term safety and stability of this lead.

Alternative lead designs have been proposed which utilize smaller electrodes. One such system is Accufix DF[R] lead system (Telectronics, Englewood, CO) (102) (Fig. 20.18). Braided technology (see Chapter 13) is used for defibrillation electrode design, with pacing and sensing electrode located at the tip of the lead. This lead has also been adapted for atrial use. By providing atrial anchoring (Fig. 20.18B), it is used as superior vena caval defibrillation lead, in a two-lead arrangement (atrial–right ventricular apex), with a subcutaneous patch electrode.

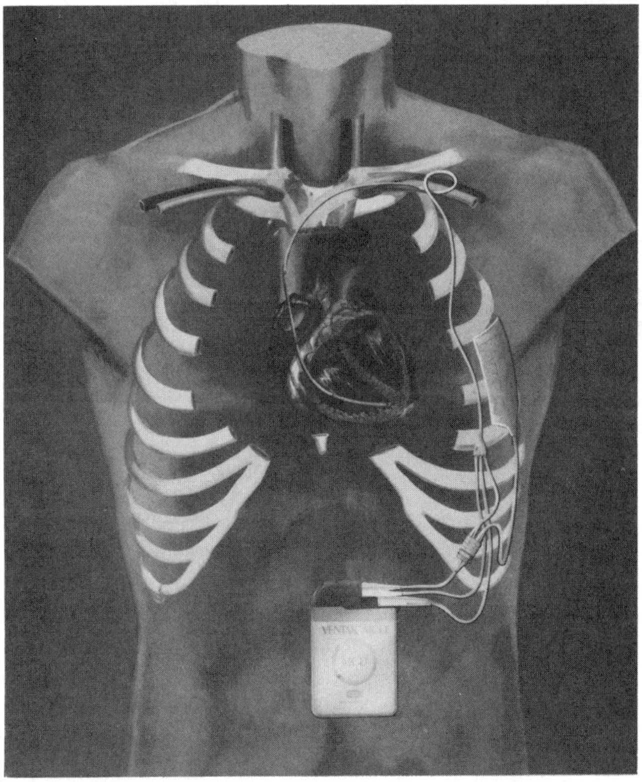

Figure 20.16. Endocardial defibrillation lead of Endotak[R] shown, with a subcutaneous patch electrode as it is usually implanted. (Courtesy of CPI, St. Paul, MN.)

Other endocardial leads are undergoing clinical trials. Several different lead configurations have been proposed, including the coronary sinus lead used in conjunction with the right ventricular apical lead and a subcutaneous patch electrode (103), and right ventricular outflow and right ventricular apex cathode to subcutaneous patch lead (anode) configuration (104). Introduction of more efficacious endocardial lead designs and

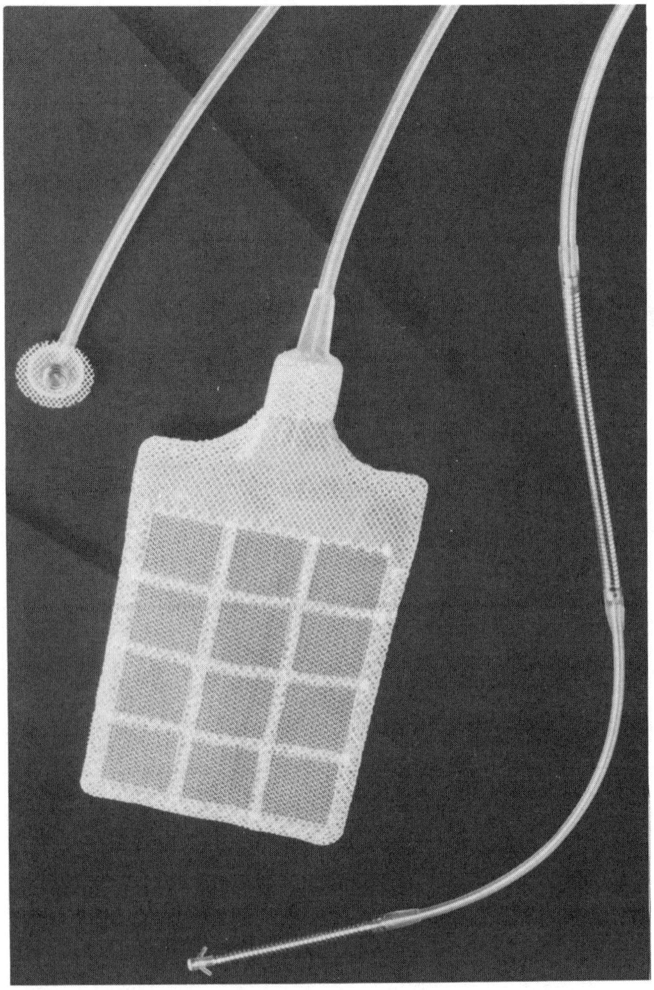

Figure 20.17. Endotak[R] defibrillation lead shown with a patch electrode. (Courtesy of CPI, St. Paul, MN.)

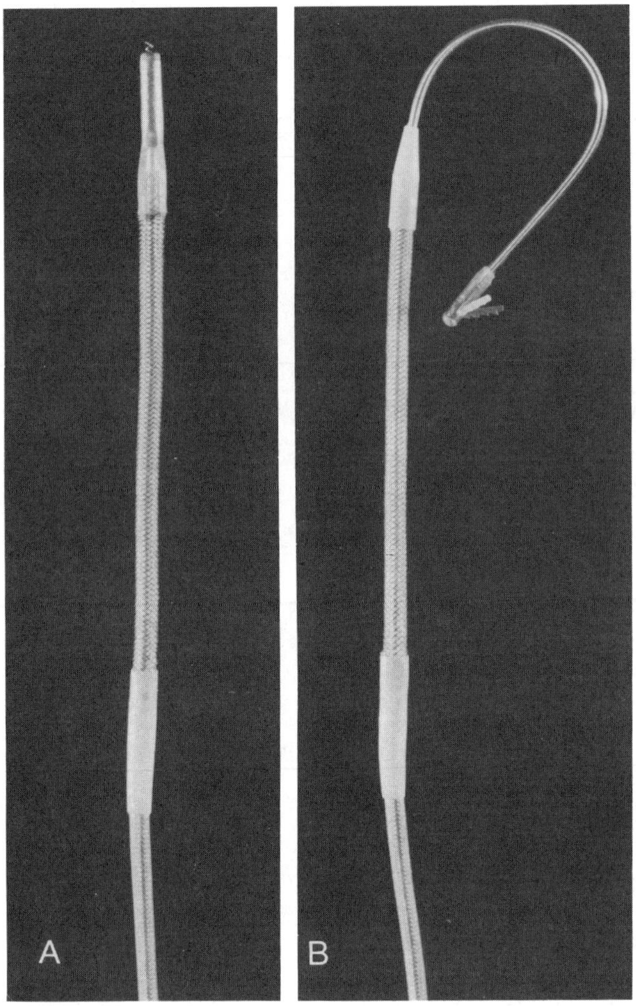

Figure 20.18. Accufix DF[R] lead system. Note the braided defibrillation coil and distal pacing electrode with extendable, active fixation screw, ventricular (**A**), and SVC lead (**B**), with passive atrial anchoring mechanism. (Courtesy of Telectronics, Englewood, CO.)

configurations will obviate the need for a thoracotomy in the majority of patients, thereby decreasing the cost, morbidity and mortality associated with ICD implantation.

Other technological advances such as downsizing of capacitors and batteries and improvements in energy delivery, by improving the energy waveform lead designs and geometry, are likely to result in downsizing of the pulse generators, thereby enabling pectoral implants similar to the current techniques for pacemaker implantation.

More efficient energy waveforms have been described recently. For example, it has been demonstrated that biphasic shocks, where the initial pulse duration is equal to or greater than the duration of the second negative pulse, are superior to monophasic waveforms (105). It is likely that all future ICD designs will incorporate biphasic as well as monophasic shocks. Other concepts have been tried including sequential shocks, triphasic waveforms, and others. To date, clinical advantage of these waveforms has not been demonstrated.

IMPACT OF CURRENT RANDOMIZED TRIALS ON ICD THERAPY

ICD therapy has been demonstrated to be effective for VT and VF and in preventing sudden death due to these causes (see above).

Impressive results have accumulated demonstrating overall efficacy of ICD therapy for prevention of sudden cardiac death. However, no prospective data are available comparing this treatment strategy to other available treatment strategies. Reliable data on the overall impact of ICD therapy on survival, as opposed to freedom from sudden cardiac death due to VT/VF, will likely emerge from the randomized clinical trials. Several randomized trials are currently in progress. If these trials demonstrate superiority of ICD therapy to antiarrhythmic drug therapy in a prospective fashion, and demonstrate improvement in survival over and above its benefit in preventing sudden cardiac deaths, it is possible that indications for ICD therapy will be further extended. Other related issues, such as the role of EP testing, value of adjunctive surgical therapy, and device cost effectiveness should also be addressed in future studies.

SUMMARY

Progress in the first decade of ICD therapy has been truly remarkable. Availability of new technologies may further broaden the applicability of this therapy to new subsets of patients thus far not considered for ICD therapy. Results of ongoing clinical trials examining the role of prophylactic device therapy, if the device is proven superior, may further advance ICD therapy for patients at risk of sudden cardiac death but who have not yet had an aborted cardiac episode due to VT or VF.

References

1. Akhtar M, Garan H, Lehmann M, *et al.*: Sudden cardiac death: management of high-risk patients. Ann Intern Med 1991;114:499–512.
2. Lehmann MH, Steinman RT, Schuger CD, *et al.*: Editorial: The automatic implantable cardioverter defibrillator as antiarrhythmic treatment modality of choice for survivors of cardiac arrest unrelated to acute myocardial infarction. Am J Cardiol 1988;62:803–805.
3. Nabih MA, Jackson K, Steinusan RT, *et al.*: Relationship between presenting ventricular tachyarrhythmias and terminal (sudden death) arrhythmias: implications for implantable cardioverter-defibrillator (ICD) therapy (Abstr). PACE 1991;14:679.
4. Winkle RA, Mead RH, Ruder MA, *et al.*: Improved low energy defibrillation efficacy in man with the use of a biphasic truncated exponential waveform. Am Heart J 1989;117:122–127.
5. Saksena S, Parsonnet V: Implantation of a cardioverter/defibrillator without thoracotomy using a triple electrode system. JAMA 1988;259:69–72.
6. Winkle RA, Fain ES, Mead RH, *et al.*: Clinical feasibility of an automatic combined antitachycardia device (Abstr). Circulation 1988;(Suppl II)78:II–220.
7. Lehmann MH, Saksena S: Implantable Cardioverter Defibrillators in Cardiovascular Practice: Report of the Policy Conference of the North American Society of Pacing and Electrophysiology. PACE 1991;14:969–979.
8. Greene L, Bardy G, CASCADE Investigators: Cardiac arrest in Seattle: conventional versus amiodarone drug evaluation (the CASCADE Study). Am J Cardiol 1991;67:578–584.
9. Echt D, Liebson P, Mitchell B, *et al.*: Mortality and mobidity in patients receiving encainide, flecainide or placebo. N Engl J Med 1991;324(12): 781–788.
10. Advisory letter to physicians. Dow Chemical Co., 1991.
11. Poole J, Mathison T, Kudenchuk P, *et al.*: Longterm outcome in patients who survived out of hospital ventricular fibrillation and undergo electrophysiology studies. J Am Coll Cardiol 1990;16:657–665.
12. Swerdlow CD, Winkle RA, Mason JW: Determinants of survival in patients with ventricular tachyarrhythmias. N Engl J Med 1983;24:1436–1442.
13. Winkle R, Mead H, Ruder M, *et al.*: Long-term outcome with the automatic implantable cardioverter-defibrillator. J Am Coll Cardiol 1989;13:1353–1361.
14. Kelly P, Cannom D, Garan H, *et al.*: The automatic implantable cardioverter defibrillator. Efficacy, complications, and survival in patients with malignant ventricular arrhythmias. J Am Coll Cardiol 1988;11:1278–1286.
15. Tchou P, Kadric N, Anderson J: *et al.*: Automatic implantable cardioverter defibrillators and survival of patients with left ventricular dysfunction and malignant ventricular arrhythmias. Ann Intern Med 1988;109:529–534.
16. Bigger JT: A discussion of the CABG patch trial. CPI AICD ADVANCES, First Quarter, 1991.
17. Moss AJ: MUSTT and MADIT trials examine role of antiarrhythmic therapy in nonsustained VT patients. CPI AICD ADVANCES, Fourth Quarter, 1990.
18. Mullins PA, Scott JP, Dunning JJ, *et al.*: Cardiac transplant waiting lists, donor shortage and retransplantation and implications for using donor hearts. Am J Cardiol 1991;68:408–409.
19. Troester J, Klein H, Haverich A, *et al.*: Incidence of sudden cardiac death in patients considered too well for transplant. PACE 1991;14(II):679.
20. Stevenson LW, Bolling SF: Improving survival of patients awaiting transplant. CPI AICD ADVANCES, Third Quarter, 1990.
21. Lehmann M, for the DEFIBRILLAT Study Group: Actuarial risk of sudden death while awaiting cardiac transplantation in patients with atherosclerotic heart disease. Am J Cardiol 1991;68:545–546.
22. Congressional Record. HCFA Guidelines for AICD reimbursement. 1991
23. Singer I, Kupersmith J: AICD Therapy: Patient Selection. Primary Cardiol 1990;16(5):27–37.
24. Singer I, Kupersmith J: AICD Therapy: implantation techniques and clinical results. Primary Cardiol 1990;16(6):37–49.
25. Slater D, Singer I, Stavens C, *et al.*: Lateral thoracotomy for automatic defibrillator. Arch Surg 1991;126:778–781.
26. Troup PS, Chapman PD, Olinger GN, Kleinman LH, *et al.*: The implanted defibrillator: relation of defibrillator lead configuration and clinical variances to fibrillation on threshold. J Am Coll Cardiol 1985;6:1315–1321.
27. Brodman R, Fisher JD, Furman S, *et al.*: Implantation of automatic cardioverter-defibrillators via median sternotomy. PACE 1984;7:1363–1369.
28. Lawrie GM, Griffin JC, Wyndham CRC: Epicardial implantation of the automatic implantable defibrillator by left subcostal thoracotomy. PACE 1984;7:1370–1374.
29. Shapira N, Cohen AI, Wish M, *et al.*: Transdiaphragmatic implantation of the automatic implantable cardioverter defibrillator. Ann Thorac Surg 1989;48:371–375.
30. Cannom DS, Winkle RA: Implantation of the automatic implantable cardioverter defibrillator (AICD): practical aspects. PACE 1986;9:793–808.
31. Lawrie GM, Kanshik RR, Pacifico A: Right minithoracotomy: an adjunct to left subcostal automatic implantable cardioverter defibrillator implantation. Ann Thorac Surg 1989;47:780–781.
32. Winkle RA, Stinson EB, Echt DS, *et al.*: Practical aspects of automatic cardioverter/defibrillator implantation. Am Heart J 1984;108:1335–1346.
33. Watkins L, Guarnieri T, Griffith L, *et al.*: Implantation of the automatic implantable cardioverter defibrillator. J Cardiac Surg 1988;3:1–7.
34. Thurer RJ, Luceri RM, Bolooki H. Automatic implantable cardioverter defibrillator: techniques of implantation and results. Ann Thorac Surg 1986;42:143–147.
35. Watkins L, Mirowski M, Mower MM, *et al.*: Implantation of the automatic defibrillator: the subxiphoid approach. Ann Thorac Surg 1982;34:515–520.
36. Watkins L, Mower MM, Reid PR, *et al.*: Surgical techniques for implanting the automatic implantable defibrillator. PACE 1984;7:1357–1362.
37. Bethencourt DM, Holmes EC: Muscle sparing posterolateral thoracotomy. Ann Thorac Surg 1988;45:337–339.
38. Blakeman BM, Wilkes D, Pifarre R: Median sternotomy for implantable cardioverter/defibrillator. Arch Surg 1989;124:1065–1066.
39. Dixon EG, Tang ASL, Wolf PD, *et al.*: Improved defibrillation thresholds with large contoured epicardial electrodes and biphasic waveforms. Circulation 1987;76:1176–1184.
40. McDaniel WC, Schuder JC: The cardiac ventricular defibrillation threshold—inherent limitations in its application and interpretation. Med Instrum 1987;21:170–176.
41. Lang DJ, Swanson DK: Safety margin for defibrillation. 1990, Presented at Second International Congress on Rate Adaptive Cardiac Pacing and Implantable Defibrillators, October 10–13, Munich.
42. Church T, Martinson M, Kallok M, *et al.*: A model to evaluate alternative methods of defibrillation threshold determination. PACE 1988;11:200–285.
43. Echt DS, Barbey JT, Black NJ: Influence of ventricular fibrillation duration

on defibrillation energy in dogs using bidirectional pulse discharges. PACE 1988;11:1315–1323.

44. Fujimura C, Jones DL, Klein GJ: Effects of time to defibrillation and subthreshold preshocks on defibrillation success in pigs. PACE 1989;12:358–365.
45. Jones JL, Swartz JF, Jones RE, *et al.*: Increasing fibrillation duration enhances relative asymmetrical biphasic versus monophasic defibrillator waveform efficacy. Circ Res 1990;67:376–384.
46. Bardy GH, Stewart RS, Ivey TD, *et al.*: Potential risk of low energy cardioversion attempts by implantable cardioverters (Abstr). J Am Coll Cardiol 1987;9:168.
47. Bardy GH, Ivey TD, Allen M, *et al.*: A prospective, randomized evaluation of effect of ventricular fibrillation duration on defibrillation thresholds in humans. J Am Coll Cardiol 1989;13:1362–1366.
48. Bardy GH, Ivey TD, Johnson G, *et al.*: Prospective evaluation of initially ineffective defibrillation pulses on subsequent defibrillation success during ventricular fibrillation in survivors of cardiac arrest. Am J Cardiol 1988;62:718–722.
49. Deeb GM, Griffith BP, Thompson ME, *et al.*: Lead systems for internal ventricular fibrillation. Circulation 1981;64:242–245.
50. Singer I, Lang D: Defibrillation threshold: clinical utility and therapeutic implications. PACE 1992;15(6):932–949.
51. Langer A, Heilman MS, Mower MM, *et al.*: Considerations in the development of the automatic implantable defibrillator. Med Intrum 1976;10:163–167.
52. Singer I, Austin E, Nash W, *et al.*: The initial clinical experience with an implantable cardioverter defibrillator/antitachycardia pacemaker. PACE 1991;14:1119–1128.
53. Lerman BB, Deale OC: Effect of epicardial patch electrodes on transthoracic defibrillation. Circulation 1990;81:1409–1414.
54. Schamp DJ, Langberg JJ, Lesh MD, *et al.*: Post-implant/pre-discharge automatic implantable defibrillator testing: Is it mandatory? (Abstr). PACE 1990;13:510.
55. Marchlinski FE, Flores B, Miller JM, *et al.*: Relation of the intraoperative defibrillation threshold to successful postoperative defibrillation with an automatic implantable cardioverter defibrillator. Am J Cardiol 1988;62:393–398.
56. Singer I, Guarnieri T, Kupersmith J: Implanted automatic defibrillators: effects of drugs and pacemakers. PACE 1988;11:2250–2262.
57. Fain ES, Dorian P, Davy JM, *et al.*: Effects of encainide and its metabolites on energy requirements for defibrillation. Circulation 1986;73:1334–1341.
58. Reiffel JA, Coromilas J, Zimmerman JM, *et al.*: Drug-device interactions: Clinical considerations. PACE 1985;8:369–373.
59. Dorian P, Fain ES, Davy JM, *et al.*: Lidocaine causes a reversible, concentration-dependent increase in defibrillation energy requirements. J Am Coll Cardiol 1986;8:327–332.
60. Marinchak RA, Friehling TD, Line RA, *et al.*: Effect of antiarrhythmic drugs on defibrillation threshold: Case report of an adverse effect of Mexiletene and review of the literature. PACE 1988;11:7–12.
61. Dorian P, Fain ES, Davy JM, *et al.*: Effect of qunidine and bretylium on defibrillation energy requirements. Am Heart J 1986;112:19–25.
62. Deeb GM, Hardesty RL, Griffith BP, *et al.*: The effects of cardiovascular drugs on the defibrillation threshold and the pathological effects on the heart using an automatic implantable defibrillator. Ann Thoracic Surg 1983;35:361–366.
63. Woolfolk DI, Chaffee WR, Cohen W, *et al.*: The effect of quinidine on electrical energy required for ventricular defibrillation. Am Heart J 1966;72:659–663.
64. Koo CC, Allen JD, Pantridge JF: Lack of effect of bretylium tosylate on electrical ventricular defibrillation in a controlled study. Cardiovasc Res 1984;18:762–767.
65. Fain ES, Lee JT, Winkle RA: Effects of acute intravenous and chronic oral amiodarone on defibrillation energy requirements. Am Heart J 1987;114:8–17.
66. Kentsch M, Kunze KP, Bleifeld W: Effect of intravenous amiodarone on ventricular fibrillation during out-of-hospital cardiac arrest (Abstr). J Am Coll Cardiol 1986;7:82.
67. Fogoros RN: Amiodarone-induced refractoriness to cardioversion. Ann Intern Med 1984;100:699.
68. Guarnieri T, Levine JH, Veltri EP: Success of chronic defibrillation and the role of antiarrhythmic drugs with the automatic implantable cardioverter/defibrillator. Am J Cardiol 1987;60:1061–1064.
69. Haberman RJ, Veltri EP, Mower MM: The effect of amiodarone on defibrillation threshold. J Electrophysiol 1988;2(5):415–423.
70. Holt DW, Tucker GT, Jackson PR, *et al.*: Amiodarone pharmacokinetics. Am Heart J 1983;106:840–847.
71. Barbieri E, Conti F, Zampieri P, *et al.*: Amiodarone and desethylamiodarone distribution in the atrium and adipose tissue of patients undergoing short and long-term treatment with amiodarone. J Am Coll Cardiol 1986;8:210–215.
72. Ruffy R, Schechtman K, Moaje E, *et al.*: B-adrenergic modulation of direct defibrillation energy in anesthetized dog heart. Am J Physiol 1985;248(17):H674–H677.
73. Ruffy R, Monje E, Schechtman K: Facilitation of cardiac defibrillation by aminophylline in the conscious, closed-chest dog. J Electrophysiol 1988;2(6):450–454.
74. Aylward P, Blood R, Tonkin A: Complications of defibrillation with permanent pacemaker in situ. PACE 1979;2:462–465.
75. Gould L, Patel S, Gomes GI, *et al.*: Pacemaker failure following external defibrillation. PACE 1981;4:575–577.
76. Giedwoyn JO: Pacemaker failure following external defibrillation. Circulation 1971;44:293–299.
77. Palac RT, Hwang MH, Klodnycky ML, *et al.*: Delayed pulse generator malfunction after D.C. Countershock. PACE 1981;4:163–167.
78. Das G, Eaton J: Pacemaker malfunction following transthoracic countershock. PACE 1981;4:487–490.
79. Levine PA, Barold SS, Fletcher RD, *et al.*: Adverse acute and chronic effects of electrical defibrillation and cardioversion on implanted unipolar cardiac pacing systems. J Am Coll Cardiol 1983;6:1413–1422.
80. Slepian M, Levine JH, Watkins L, *et al.*: The automatic implantable cardioverter defibrillator-permanent pacemaker interaction: Loss of pacemaker capture following AICD discharge. PACE 1987;10:1194–1197.
81. Bach JM: AID-B cardioverter-defibrillator: possible interactions with pacemakers. Intec. Systems Technical Communication 1983, Document 1650095.
82. Guarnieri T, Datorre SD, Bondke H, *et al.*: Increased pacing threshold after an automatic defibrillator shock in dogs: Effects of Class I and Class II antiarrhythmic drugs. PACE 1988;11:1324–1330.
83. Yee R, Jones DL, Jarvis E, *et al.*: Changes in pacing threshold and R wave amplitude after transvenous catheter countershock. J Am Coll Cardiol 1984;4:543–549.
84. Winkle RA, Bach SM, Mead HR, *et al.*: Comparison of defibrillation efficacy in humans using a new catheter and superior vena caval spring-left ventricular patch electrodes. J Am Coll Cardiol 1988;11:365–370.
85. Cohen AI, Wish MW, Fletcher RD, *et al.*: The use and interaction of permanent pacemakers and the automatic implantable cardioverter defibrillator. PACE 1988;11:704–711.
86. Singer I, DeBorde R, Veltri EP, *et al.*: The automatic implantable cardioverter defibrillator: T wave sensing in the newest generation. PACE 1988;11:1584–1591.
87. Luderitz R, Gerckens U, Manz M: Automatic implantable cardioverter/defibrillator (AICD) and antitachycardia pacemaker (Tachylog): combined use in ventricular tachyarrhythmias. PACE 1986;9:1356–1360.
88. Manz M, Gerckens U, Funke HD, *et al.*: Combination of antitachycardia pacemaker and automatic implantable cardioverter/defibrillator for ventricular tachycardia. PACE 1986;9:676–684.
89. Mirowski M, Reid PR, Mower MM, *et al.*: Successful conversion of out-of-hospital life-threatening ventricular tachyarrhythmias with the implanted automatic defibrillator. Am Heart J 1981;103:147–148.

90. Mirowski M, Reid PR, Mower MM, *et al.*: Automatic Implantable Cardioverter-Defibrillator: clinical results. PACE 1984;7:1345–1350.
91. Mirowski M, Reid PR, Winkle RA, *et al.*: Mortality in patients with implanted defibrillators. Ann Intern Med 1983;98:585–588.
92. Waller T, Kay HR, Spielman SR, *et al.*: Reduction in sudden death and total mortality by antitachycardia therapy evaluated by electrophysiologic drug testing: criteria of efficacy in patients with sustained ventricular tachyarrhythmia. J Am Coll Cardiol 1987;10:83–89.
93. Tordjman-Fuchs T, Garan H, McGovern B, *et al.*: Out of hospital cardiac arrest: improved long-term outcome in patients with automatic implantable cardioverter defibrillator (AICD). Circulation 1989;80(II):121.
94. Furman S: AICD Benefit. PACE 1989;12:399–400.
95. Fogoros RN: The implantable defibrillator backlash. Am J Cardiol 1991;67:1424–1427.
96. Pinski SL, Sgarbossa EB, Maloney JD, *et al.*: Survival in patients declining implantable cardioverter-defibrillators. Am J Cardiol 1991;68;(8):800–801.
97. Endotak clinical database. CPI, for PMA filing with FDA, 1991.
98. Fisher JD, Kim SG, Mercando AD: Electrical devices for treatment of arrhythmias (Suppl). Am J Cardiol 1988;61:45A–57A.
99. Rosenthal ME, Josephson ME: Current status of antitachycardia devices. Circulation 1990;82:1879–1890.
100. Saksena S, Lindsay DD, Parsonnet V: Development for future implantable cardioverters and defibrillators. PACE 1987;10:1342–1356.
101. Calkins H, Brinker J, Vetri EF, *et al.*: Clinical interactions between pacemakers and automatic implantable cardioverter-defibrillators. J Am Coll Cardiol 1990;16:666–673.
102. Singer I, Maldonado C, Scott C, *et al.*: Permanent Accufix DF[R] and BEDL[R] electrodes for transvenous defibrillator in the canine model. In: Antonioli GE, Aubert AE, Ector M (eds): Proceedings of the Second International Symposium on Pacing Leads. Ferrara, 1991. Elsevier Science Publishers, 1991:309–316.
103. Bardy GH, Allen MD, Mehra, *et al.*: Transvenous defibrillation in humans via the coronary sinus. Circulation 1990;81(4):1252–1259.
104. Singer I, Maldonado C, Vance F, *et al.*: Defibrillation efficacy using two low profile endocardial electrodes. Am J Med Sci 1991;302(2):82–88.
105. Chapman PD, Vetter JW, Scuzia JJ, *et al.*: Comparison of monophasic with dual capacitor biphasic waveforms for nonthoracotomy canine internal defibrillation. J Am Coll Cardiol 1989;14(1):242–245.
106. Winkle RA: State of the art of the AICD. PACE 1991;14:961–966.

21

ANTITACHYCARDIA PACEMAKERS

Igor Singer, M.B.B.S., F.R.A.C.P., F.A.C.P., F.A.C.C.

ELECTROPHYSIOLOGIC MECHANISMS

Tachycardias most suitable for antitachycardia pacing techniques have reentry as their underlying mechanism. Reentry usually requires two physiologically distinct conduction pathways with differing electrophysiologic (EP) properties. The reentry circuit may be either anatomically (1) or functionally determined (2). Reentry requires that two pathways are connected proximally and distally. Unidirectional block is required in one pathway and a slow conduction in the other to provide the condition for reentry to occur (Fig. 21.1). Presence of antegrade unidirectional block in one pathway forces the impulse to travel in the alternate pathway. If the conduction velocity and the refractory periods of the two pathways are such that by the time the impulse returns it is capable of conducting again in retrograde direction, reentry will result. A delicate balance of conduction and refractoriness is required to perpetuate the tachycardia.

The excitation wave front propagates leaving behind it tissue which is temporarily refractory to further conduction. The duration of the refractoriness depends on the effective and the functional refractory periods of tissues comprising the reentry loop. The difference in the time required for the impulse to recirculate in the reentry loop and the duration of refractoriness constitutes the excitable component of the circuit, the so-called excitable gap. Partial or complete abolition of the excitable gap by electrical stimulation interrupts the propagation of the excitation wave front and terminates the reentry tachycardia. Also, an impulse may enter the reentrant circuit during the excitable gap and entrain the arrhythmia; following cessation of such stimulation the tachycardia may terminate.

Factors that influence the ability of external impulse(s) to terminate reentrant tachycardias are: (a) tachycardia cycle length (rate), (b) refractory periods of components of the reentry circuit and the tissue between the pacing site and the reentry circuit, (c) distance between the pacing site and the reentry circuit, and (d) conduction velocity of the tissue between the pacing site and the reentry circuit (3) (see Chapter 2).

Antitachycardia pacing techniques are designed to alter the property of the excitable tissue (myocardial cells) transiently, by depolarizing the cardiac tissue at a critical moment, thereby altering the tissue refractoriness, so that the recirculating impulse conduction is blocked and reentry tachycardia terminated.

Value of antitachycardia pacing techniques for termination of reentrant tachycardias in the clinical setting is well documented (4–11). Clinical tachycardias in which antitachycardia pacing techniques are useful, for either acute therapy or chronic management, are listed in Table 21.1.

ANTITACHYCARDIA PACING TECHNIQUES

A variety of techniques are available for antitachycardia pacing therapy. They are listed in Table 21.2.

Underdrive Pacing

Slow competitive asynchronous pacing at a rate less than the tachycardia rate is referred to as underdrive pacing. By pacing asynchronously, provided that the pacing rate is not an exact multiple of the tachycardia rate, progressive scanning of the cardiac cycle may find the excitable gap of the tachycardia circuit and terminate the tachycardia. This technique may be implemented with implanted pacemakers (atrial or ventricular) which pace asynchronously when a magnet is applied over the pacemaker. Dual-chamber pacemakers may also be effective in this regard (10,11).

Stimuli should be delivered in the atrium for supraventricular tachycardia and to the ventricle for ventricular tachycardia (VT). For reciprocating tachycardias of Wolff-Parkinson-White (WPW) syndrome, stimuli may be delivered in either chamber, since both atria and ventricles are necessary components of the reentry circuit.

Interruption of a reentry tachycardia by a single extrastimulus, on which this technique relies, is the least effective method for termination of reentry tachycardia. Its efficacy requires a large excitable gap and a relatively close proximity of the pacing stimulus to the tachycardia circuit. It is estimated that approximately 50% of slow tachycardias (rates <150 beats/min) may be

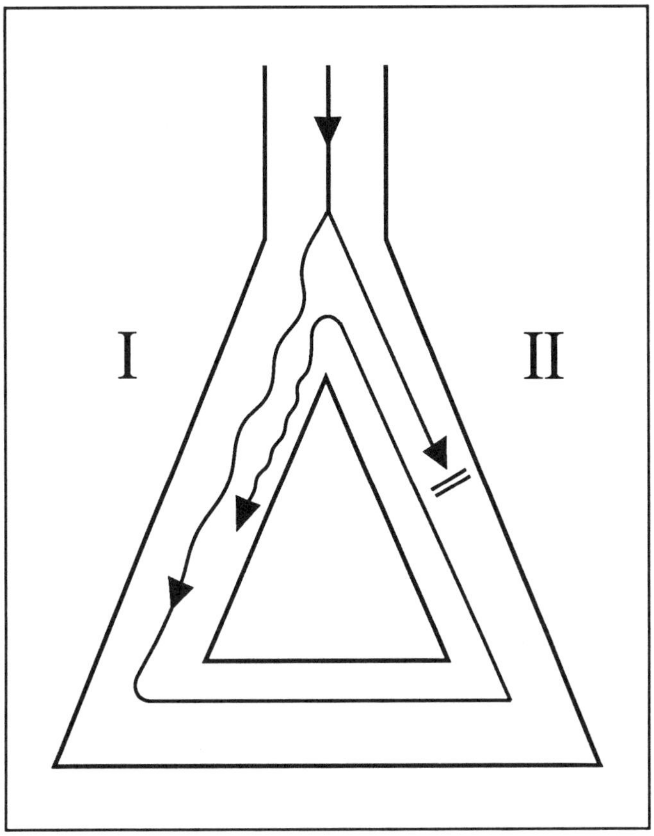

Figure 21.1. A schematic representation of a reentry loop. The prerequisites for reentry are two anatomically and/or physiologically separate conduction pathways connected proximally and distally. Pathway I has a shorter refractory period, but slower conduction velocity than pathway II, enabling the impulse to conduct slowly in antegrade direction in pathway I. Pathway II has a substantially longer refractory period than pathway I, but faster conduction velocity. As the impulse enters both pathways, it is blocked antegradely in pathway II but is conducted slowly in pathway I. By the time the impulse returns, pathway II has recovered sufficiently to conduct the impulse in retrograde direction and reentry tachycardia may be initiated (see text). Adapted from Fogoros RN. "Electrophysiologic Testing," Fig 2.6, p 19, Blackwell Scientific Publications, 1990, Cambridge, Mass., with permission.

converted by a single extrastimulus method, though it is also the least likely of the available antitachycardia pacing techniques to accelerate the tachycardia (0.5%) (12).

Overdrive Pacing

Overdrive pacing is implemented by pacing the heart at rates above the tachycardia rate. The rationale for this approach is based on the concept of "peeling back of the refractoriness," where the refractoriness of the intervening tissue between the stimulus site and the excitable gap of the tachycardia is shortened by the preceding extrastimulus to allow easier delivery of the subsequent extrastimuli into the excitable gap of the tachycardia circuit. This method of pacing is effective for rapid tachycardias (>160 beats/min) and may be used to treat atrial flutter, AV nodal reentry tachycardia, atrioventricular (A-V) reciprocating tachycardia, and VT.

Although more effective than single extrastimulus technique for terminating tachycardia, burst pacing is also more likely to cause acceleration of tachycardia. For this reason, antitachycardia pacing should never be employed as a "stand-alone" therapy for VT without a backup implantable cardioverter-defibrillator (ICD). A variety of strategies are available for overdrive pacing. These are discussed below.

Table 21.1.
Tachycardias Amenable to Antitachycardia Pacing

Atrioventricular reciprocating tachycardia
AV nodal reentry tachycardia
Atrial flutter
Ventricular tachycardia

Abbreviations: AV = atrioventricular.

Table 21.2.
Antitachycardia Pacing Techniques

Underdrive pacing
Overdrive pacing
Ramp pacing
Burst pacing
Autodecremental burst pacing
Shifting burst
Scanning burst
Scanning burst with ramp pacing
Centrifugal scans
Adaptive pacing with delays in number of extrastimuli
Ultrarapid train stimulation
Programmed stimulation
Single extrastimulus
Double, triple, and multiple extrastimuli

Ramp Pacing

Ramp pacing refers to a method of pacing where burst pacing is delivered with gradual acceleration (ramp up) or deceleration (ramp down) if rates are in excess of the tachycardia rate (13–16). The sequence of pacing may be altered within the ramp to alternately decelerate and then accelerate, or in a reverse sequence. It is also possible to combine features of ramp pacing and scanning by altering the timing of the first stimulus within the ramp.

Burst Pacing

Burst pacing delivers multiple extrastimuli with the same coupling interval (Fig. 21.2, top panel). On subsequent attempts, coupling intervals are equally reduced within the burst sequence (17). Burst pacing may also be combined with independently timed extrastimuli at the end of the burst sequence. This technique is more likely to cause tachycardia acceleration (12).

Autodecremental (Adaptive) Burst Pacing

In this mode of pacing, the burst cycle length is a preset percentage of the tachycardia cycle length (Fig. 21.2, bottom panel).

Shifting Bursts

With this technique, the timing of the first and the subsequent extrastimuli are decremented on successive attempts (14).

Scanning Burst with Ramp Pacing

In this mode of pacing, the timing of the first stimulus of the ramp changes. The ramp may be either decremental or incremental.

Centrifugal Scans

Centrifugal scans employ alternatively shortening and lengthening of extrastimulus coupling intervals. Single or multiple extrastimuli may be employed (20) (Fig. 21.3).

Adaptive Pacing with Changes in the Number of Extrastimuli

In this technique, the timing of the first extrastimulus is selected as a percentage of the tachycardia cycle length. If the tachycardia persists, a second and subsequently multiple stimuli are added at a percentage of the cycle length (21) (Fig. 21.4).

Ultrarapid Train Stimulation

A short burst of pacing is delivered at a rapid rate (3000–6000/min) in the refractory period and timed to produce a single capture with the shortest possible coupling interval. Although effective, this technique may produce acceleration and fibrillation (22).

Programmed Extrastimulation

Programmed extrastimulation is used extensively in the electrophysiology laboratory to terminate reentrant tachycardias. This technique utilizes single, double, triple, or multiple extrastimuli which are delivered with predetermined timing within the tachycardia cycle (Fig. 21.5). Multiple extrastimuli are superior to single extrastimulus techniques because of "peeling of refractoriness" by preceding extrastimuli (see above). The memory of the coupling intervals that are effective in termination of the tachycardia are features of some devices.

TACHYCARDIA SENSING

Automatic antitachycardia pacemakers and third-generation ICDs, which combine features of antitachycardia pacemakers and cardioverters/defibrillators (see Chapter 20), utilize a variety of detection algorithms. These include rate (19,23), suddenness of onset (24,25), rate stability (25), and probability density function (26) (for VF detection). None of these criteria provide an absolute differentiation of physiologic from pathologic tachycar-

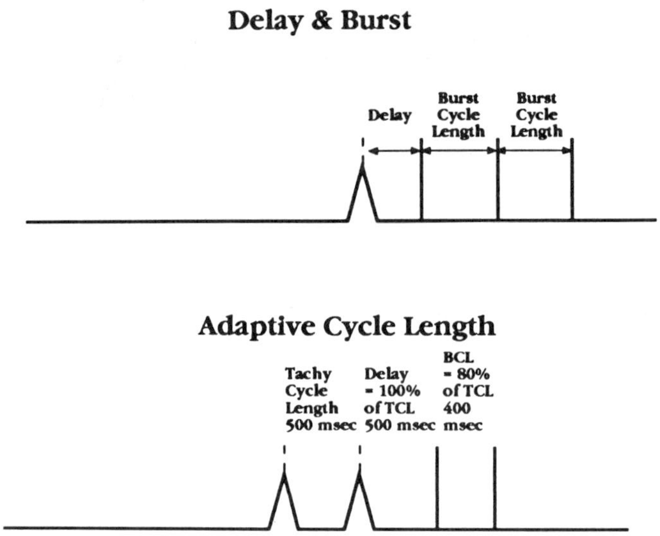

Figure 21.2. Schematic illustration of autodecremental burst pacing.

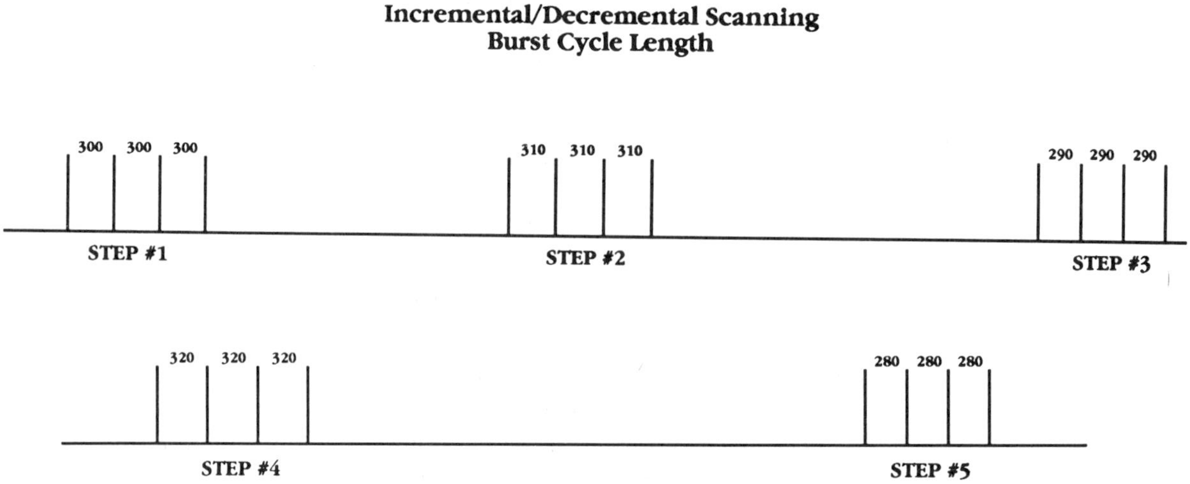

Figure 21.3. An illustration of centrifugal scanning technique.

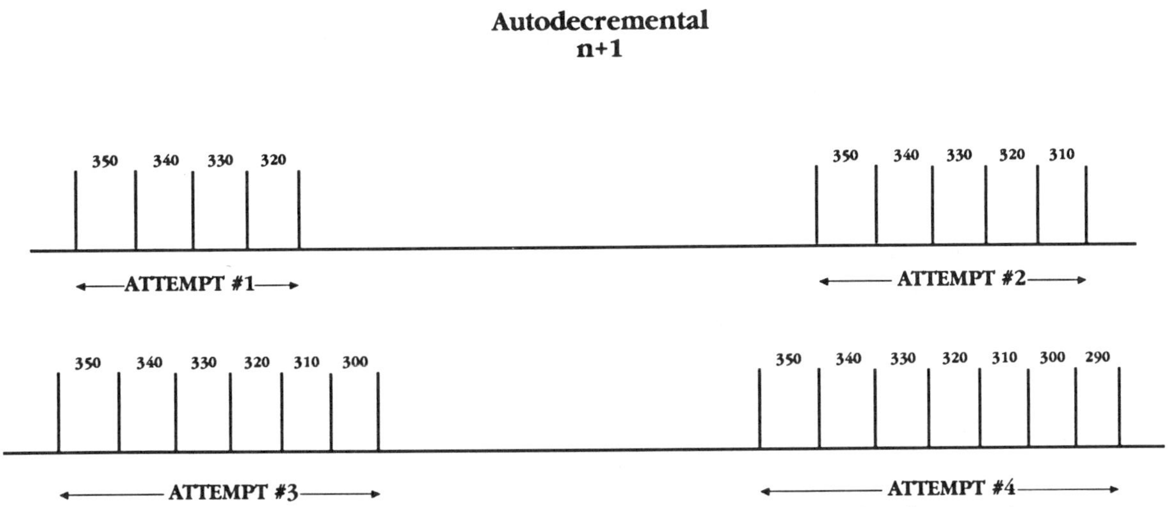

Figure 21.4. Schematic illustration of adaptive pacing with changes in number of extrastimuli.

dias. Overlaps in rate, tachycardia stability, slew rate, morphology, and signal amplitude between physiologic (sinus) tachycardia and pathologic tachycardias exist, making differentiation of sinus from pathologic tachycardias difficult at times (27–30).

Heart Rate

Heart rate measurement is the simplest method to detect tachycardia. Unfortunately, it lacks specificity, since physiologic and pathologic tachycardias often overlap (19,23). To improve the specificity, other criteria have been proposed and are often useful to further separate physiologic from pathologic tachycardias.

Suddenness of Onset

Physiologic tachycardia that occurs during exercise or emotional arousal is characterized by gradual onset. In contrast, pathologic tachycardias, especially of reentrant type, have an abrupt onset. However, a substantial overlap exists which may render this criterion of limited utility as well. Commercial devices with rate acceleration detection algorithm are available (24,25).

Rate Stability

Rate stability may be used to differentiate irregular from regular tachycardias (25). Measurement of RR intervals during tachycardia may separate atrial fibrillation from VT. Although this criterion is generally useful, it should be noted that some VTs also exhibit considerable rate variability (e.g., polymorphic VT). Careful programming is therefore required to differentiate pathologic from physiologic tachycardias.

Morphologic Differentiation

A number of techniques have been proposed to separate sinus rhythm from pathologic rhythms. These include probability density function (26), frequency content analysis (31), area under the electrogram curve (32), and intrinsic deflection timing (31). Each of these techniques attempts to separate sinus rhythm from pathologic rhythms by analyzing the morphologic characteristics of the electrogram. Detailed discussion of each of these techniques is beyond the scope of this manuscript and may be found elsewhere in the literature (26,31,32).

Activation Sequence Analysis

Analysis of A-V relationships during tachycardia may provide further clues to the tachycardia origin. Using an analysis of A-V relationships, Arzbacher, *et al.* were able to classify tachycardias accurately in 95% of cases (33). Clearly, this algorithm is also imperfect, since 1:1 V-A relationship may also exist during VT, AV node reentry tachycardia, or A-V reciprocating tachycardia.

Physiologic Correlates of Tachycardia

During tachycardia, blood pressure, stroke volume, intracardiac wall tension, and cardiac output change. During prolonged tachycardia, oxygen extraction by the tissues increases and oxygen saturation of mixed venous blood decreases. Alteration in these physiologic variables may be used to provide hemodynamic correlates of tachycardia. Although not specific for any given tachycardia, measurement of physiologic variables that characterize the hemodynamic consequences of tachycardia may be incorporated into automatic response algorithms, to enable the device to respond more or less aggressively, depending on the physiologic consequences of tachycardia. Ongoing research will determine the usefulness of such sensors as dP/dt, dV/dt, paced depolarization integral (PDI), oxygen sensor, and others.

PATIENT EVALUATION

All patients who are considered potential candidates for an implantable device must undergo EP studies to evaluate: (a) the

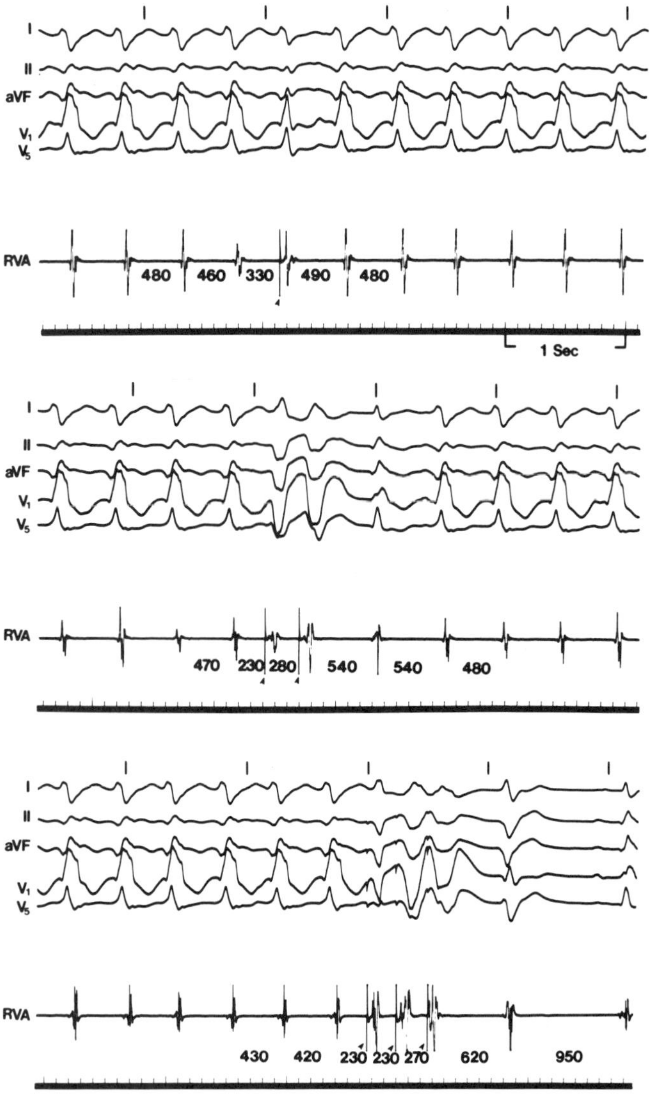

Figure 21.5. Programmed extrastimulation. From **top** to **bottom:** each panel is labeled identically: surface leads I, II, aVF, V_1, and V_5, and right ventricular electrogram (RVA). Single, double and triple extrastimuli are introduced in an attempt to terminate ventricular tachycardia (VT). Extrastimuli are marked with *arrowheads.* Note that single and double extrastimuli fail to terminate VT (**top** and **middle** panels) but triple extrastimuli are effective in terminating the VT.

mechanism of the tachycardia, (b) rate and stability of the tachycardia, (c) the most effective consistent sequence for its termination, (d) the most effective site of stimulation to terminate the tachycardia, and (e) adequate detection and termination of the arrhythmia by the device.

The following are the recommendations for EP studies in patients considered for implantable devices based on the American College of Cardiology/American Heart Association (ACC/AHA) task force report (34): Class I (general agreement exists): (a) all patients who are candidates for implantation of an electrical device, (b) patients in whom an electrical device is already implanted, but in whom changes in antiarrhythmic drug therapy are contemplated, which may influence the functioning of the device; Class II (electrophysiologic studies are frequently performed, but no general consensus exists): patients with implantable antitachycardia device, to confirm acceptable device function during follow-up; Class III (electrophysiologic study not indicated): patients who are not considered candidates for an implantable device.

Table 21.3.
Proposed Evaluation of a Prospective Patient Considered for Antitachycardia Device[a]

Clinical evaluation
History and physical examination
Noninvasive evaluation
12-lead ECG
Holter monitoring
Event recorder
Exercise testing
Signal-averaged ECG (VT)
Left ventricular function—2D echo, MUGA
Invasive evaluation
Coronary arteriography
Left ventriculography
Electrophysiologic study

[a]See also Chapters 3 and 4.
Abbreviations: MUGA = multigated nuclear cineangiography; 2D echo = two-dimensional echocardiography.

Evaluation of patients for antitachycardia device therapy is similar to evaluation of patients selected for pharmacologic or ablative therapy. Suggested evaluation is summarized in Table 21.3. Clinical noninvasive assessment of patients presenting with arrhythmias is discussed in Chapter 3 and invasive EP studies in Chapter 4. Special comments regarding specific goals of EP evaluation for patients considered for antitachycardia pacing therapy are addressed here.

Electrophysiologic Study

The role of EP study is to define the nature of the arrhythmia, determine its mechanism, and to select and test specific antitachycardia pacing modalities. At the time of the device implantation, an intraoperative study is conducted to demonstrate effective functioning of the device. Finally, a postoperative EP study (prior to patient discharge) is advisable to assess the device function.

Evaluation of Antitachycardia Pacing Therapy for Supraventricular Tachycardia

A number of alternative strategies for therapy of supraventricular tachycardias are available and include pharmacologic, ablative, and surgical options. Antitachycardia pacing therapy may be selected for patients who are either unresponsive or intolerant to pharmacologic therapy, or are unwilling to undergo catheter ablative or surgical therapy. Since the advent of catheter ablation for therapy or WPW syndrome and AV nodal reentry tachycardia, the indications for antitachycardia pacing for su-

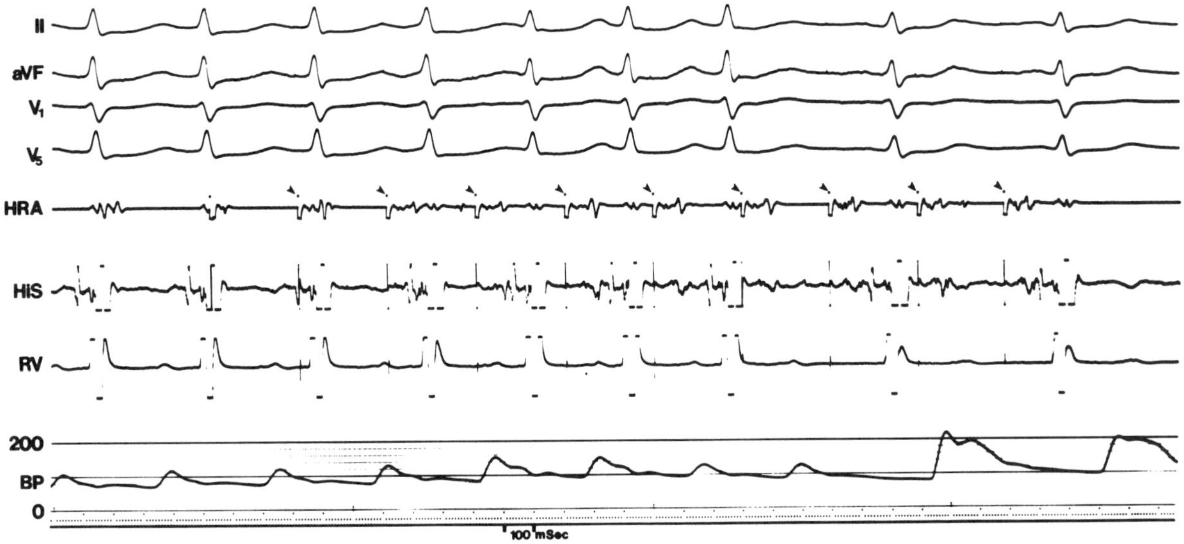

Figure 21.6. Termination of AV nodal reentry tachycardia by burst extrastimuli (arrowheads). From **top** to **bottom:** surface leads II, aVF, V_1 and V_5, intracardiac electrograms—high right atrium (HRA), His bundle (HiS) and right ventricular apex (RV), blood pressure (BP), and time line.

praventricular tachycardias have narrowed further. However, relative simplicity of antitachycardia pacing therapy and its effectiveness makes this option attractive for some patients (Fig. 21.6).

Specific questions to be addressed by EP study prior to the device implant are the following: (a) What is the mechanism of the tachycardia? (b) Is there a single or are there multiple tachycardias? (c) What is the reproducibility of tachycardia termination? (d) What is the most optimal sequence of stimulation for tachycardia termination? (e) What is the risk of acceleration with the chosen termination sequence? (f) What is the role of the antiarrhythmic therapy for tachycardia slowing and termination? During testing, tachycardia should be induced multiple times and the device's ability to terminate the tachycardia documented.

Evaluation of Antitachycardia Pacing Therapy for Ventricular Tachycardia

Antitachycardia devices for therapy of VT as "stand-alone" devices have no role in therapy of ventricular tachycardia because of the risk of acceleration and deterioration of VT to VF (Fig. 21.7). Antitachycardia pacing therapy was initially employed in combination with ICD therapy for therapy of ventricular tachycardias. With the development of advanced cardioverters/defibrillators, which incorporate antitachycardia pacing therapy, it is now feasible to utilize antitachycardia pacing techniques for therapy of stable monomorphic VTs.

Further discussion of implantation techniques and testing of ICDs may be found in Chapter 20. Programming of third-generation devices that incorporate antitachycardia pacing strategies require thorough preoperative, operative and postoperative testing to insure that the sensing is adequate, that the detection criteria are appropriate and that the sequenced therapy is effective. Recommended sequencing of therapy for therapy of VT is summarized in Table 21.4.

RESULTS

The long-term results of therapy with antitachycardia pacing for supraventricular tachycardias reported in the literature by different investigators are difficult to compare due to a small number of patients in some series, and a variety of devices employed in others. The results of the largest series of patients are listed in Table 21.5 (35–42). In most series, the majority of patients had favorable results with antitachycardia pacing, although the follow-up period varied considerably in the reported series. Most investigators used concurrent antiarrhythmic therapy. Fisher, *et al.* (39) reported efficacy rates of 93% at 1 yr and 78% at 5 yr.

The results of antitachycardia pacing for ventricular tachycardia are listed in Table 21.6 (39–43). Relatively large numbers of deaths have been reported due to VT/VF in some series (39,40,41,44). This is undoubtedly due to VT acceleration and deterioration to VF. Hence, antitachycardia pacing should not be employed alone in the ventricle without an implanted ICD or as a part of an ICD device. Advantages of antitachycardia pacing therapy in combination with, or as a part of an ICD device however, are obvious. Majority of slow monomorphic VTs may be terminated by antitachycardia pacing, obviating the use of an electrical shock, and thus enhancing patient's comfort. Battery longevity may be improved since the energy requirements for pacing are many orders of magnitude smaller than that required for defibrillation. Combination of antitachycardia pacing therapy for VT with cardioversion/defibrillation introduces new complexities on the other hand, which include: (a) imperfect specificity of arrhythmia recognition, (b) tachycardia acceleration, and (c) a possible delay of "definitive" therapy for VT/VF (see Fig. 21.7).

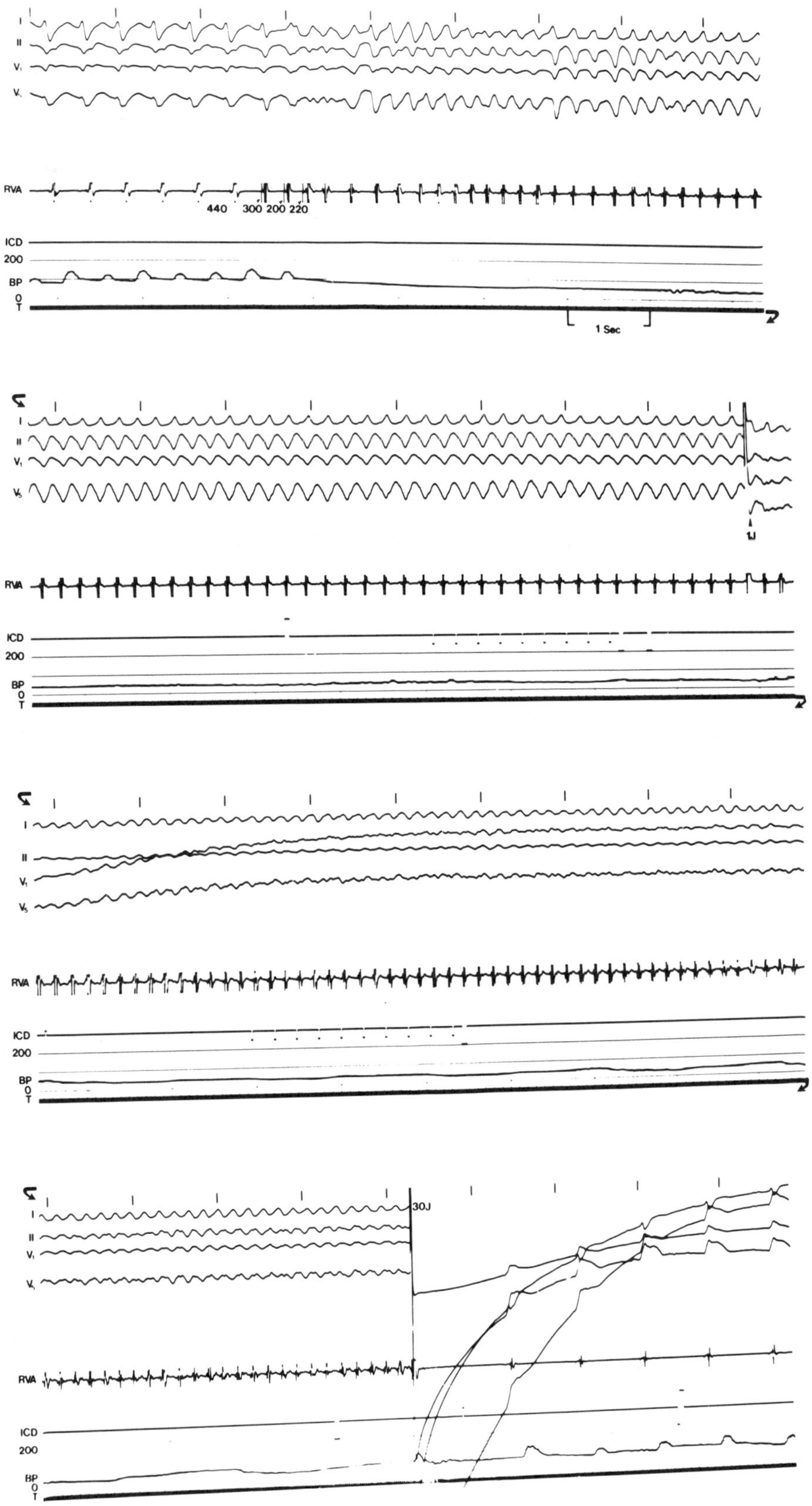

Figure 21.7. Ventricular tachycardia acceleration by antitachycardia pacing and failure of low energy cardioversion, requiring high energy output by ICD for defibrillation. Panels **1** through **4** (**top** and **bottom**) are a continuous recording. Each panel is identically labeled: surface leads I, II, V_1, and V_5, intracardiac electrogram (RVA), internal cardioverter defibrillator (ICD—Ventak[R] P), blood pressure (BP), and time lines (T). **Note:** monomorphic VT (C.L. 440 msec) acceleration when triple extrastimuli are delivered, to ventricular flutter. Low-energy cardioversion is delivered (1 J), resulting in ventricular fibrillation (VF). Ventricular fibrillation is again appropriately detected by the device which subsequently delivers a second shock at 30 j, converting VF to sinus rhythm.

FOLLOW-UP OF PATIENTS WITH IMPLANTED ANTITACHYCARDIA DEVICES

The need for careful follow-up of all patients with antitachycardia devices cannot be overemphasized. The frequency of follow-up varies depending on the type of device being followed. The goals of follow-up are: (a) assessment of device efficacy, (b) assessment of the system (generator and lead/s) integrity, (c) evaluation of concomitant problems not directly related to the device, and (d) collation of the data for clinical research.

Since the information is highly focused, these patients should be seen in a dedicated clinic or in an office staffed by experienced personnel. A separate database is recommended, since clinical charts are often displaced or unavailable at the time of the patient follow-up visit. A computerized database has obvious advantages, including the ease of information retrieval and data collation.

All patients with implanted antitachycardia devices for therapy of supraventricular tachycardias should be seen within 1 mo of implantation and then at three monthly intervals for up to a year, and six monthly intervals thereafter. The schedule for implanted devices in the ventricle depends on the type of device implanted and the need for capacitor reformation of ICD, when antitachycardia pacemakers are combined with ICDs. Ventak^R (CPI, St. Paul, MN) series of devices require two monthly follow-ups until a significant rise in charge time is detected, then at 1 monthly intervals until ERI is reached. Patients should also be seen with first out-of-hospital ICD discharge or if frequent or atypical circumstances surround the ICD discharge.

Transtelephonic monitoring may become available in future devices. Patients with third generation ICD devices that do not require external capacitor reformation (e.g., Guardian^R ATP 4210) may need to be seen less frequently.

Assessment at each follow-up visit should include the following: (a) careful history and physical examination, (b) 12-lead electrocardiogram (ECG), (c) noninvasive telemetry of diagnostic data, (d) testing of sensing and pacing thresholds, lead impedance, and battery status, (e) for ICDs: charge times and capacitor reformation times and examination of log counters to examine for intervening shocks, antitachycardia, or bradyarrhythmia pacing. Elective replacement indicator (ERI) criteria should be checked against the latest manufacturer's recommendations.

Table 21.4.
Selection of Treatment Strategies Based on Ventricular Tachycardia Characteristics

Based on tachycardia rate and morphology
Slow MVT—ATP followed by low-energy cardioversion and defibrillation
Rapid MVT—defibrillation
Based on hemodynamic stability
Stable—ATP followed by low-energy cardioversion and defibrillation
Unstable—defibrillation

Abbreviations: ATP = antitachycardia pacing; MVT = monomorphic ventricular tachycardia.

TROUBLESHOOTING

The tools available for troubleshooting are clinical history and examination, 12-lead ECG, examination of diagnostic data

Table 21.5.[a]
Results for Device Therapy of SVT

Investigator	No. Patients	Pacer Type	Duration of Follow-up (mos)	Antiarrhythmic Therapy (No. Patients)	Results: Good	Results: Unsatisfactory
Bertholet (35)	13	PASAR^R 4151 (Telectronics) SPO 500 (Medtronic)	5–30	5	10	3
Spurrell (19)	21	PASAR^R 4151 and 4171	2–40	8	16	—[b]
Zipes (36)	21	SYMBIOS^R 7008 (Medtronic)	NA	NA	21	—
Sowton (20)	16	TACHYLOG^R (Siemens-Elema)	5–19	3	14	—[c]
Den Dulk (37)	12	SPO 510 (Medtronic)	3–26	8	12	—
Peters (38)	10	5998 (Medtronic)	24–60	4	7	3
Fisher (39)	16	Miscellaneous	6–177	All	16	—
Griffin (40) (multicenter)	91	CYBERTACH^R (Intermedics)	>21	NA	82%	18%[d]
Rothman (41) (multicenter)	16	ORTHOCOR^R (Cordis)	1–40	NA	88%	—
Kahn (42) (multicenter)	12	5998 (Medtronic)	15–36	8	10	—[e]

[a]Table lists only series of 10 patients or more.
[b]Two sudden deaths, three deactivated (patients underwent surgical therapy).
[c]Two patients underwent surgical resection of accessory pathway for Wolff-Parkinson-White syndrome.
[d]Eight units explanted due to inadequate sensing.
[e]One explant, one patient died of CVA, 2 patients died of chronic pericarditis.
Abbreviations: CVA = cerebrovascular accident; NA = not available; SVA = supraventricular tachycardia.

Table 21.6.
Antitachycardia Devices for Therapy of Ventricular Tachycardia

Investigator	No. of Patients	Pacemaker Model	Concurrent Antiarrhythmic Therapy	Duration of Follow-up (mos)	Results (%) Good	Results (%) Unsatisfactory
Herre (43)	28	5998 (Medtronic)	18	1–25	9[b]	1
Fisher (39)	20	Miscellaneous	All	2–92	18[c]	2
Saksena (44)	11	ORTHOCOR[R] (Cordis)	All	NA	3	
Rothman (41) (multicenter)	53	ORTHOCOR[R] (Cordis)	NA	1–41	84%[d]	
Griffin (40) (multicenter)	52	CYBERTACH[R] (InterMedics)	NA	12	58%[e]	

[a]Table lists only series of 10 or more patients.
[b]No spontaneous VT in 19 patients, one sudden death.
[c]One explanted at 1 mo, four disarmed at 1 mo, four sudden deaths.
[d]Six sudden deaths, three documented due to VT/VF.
[e]14 nontachycardia-related deaths, 4 sudden deaths.
Abbreviations: NA = not available.

stored in the device, event recorders or Holter recordings, and at times EP testing and ultimately, intraoperative lead recordings may be required. With sound-emitting ICDs (Ventak[R] series), phonocardiograms (or "beepograms," as they are called) may be useful to diagnose sensing of diastolic events (e.g., T waves) or multiple sensing associated with lead connector problems or lead fractures (see Chapter 20). If lead malposition is suspected, chest x-ray or fluoroscopy may be helpful in confirming the clinical suspicion. Occasionally, prolonged observation on a telemetry unit is required to diagnose a particular problem. Graphic display of telemetered electrograms from the device's stored memory of arrhythmic events is possible with newer devices as well as a printout of log counters to help critically evaluate RR intervals, noise events, and therapies applied. A thorough knowledge and familiarity with intricacies of various devices is required of the follow-up team.

DEVICE PROGRAMMING

In general, output and sensitivity values are chosen to provide a sufficient safety margin. Detection criteria should be tailored to the tachycardias treated. The first and the simplest of the detection criteria is rate. Rate criterion should be ideally selected so that the detection rate cutoff is below the rate of a stable tachycardia (10–15 beats/min) or (15–25 beats/min) for irregular, polymorphous tachycardias. Rate criterion should, however, be chosen to be higher than the maximum rate of physiologic (sinus) tachycardia. If that is not possible, additional criteria may be used to differentiate physiologic from nonphysiologic tachycardias. These include rate stability and sudden onset criteria. These additional criteria may be sufficient to differentiate atrial fibrillation from reentry tachycardias.

Additional criteria, such as sustained high rate, should be incorporated as a "fail safe" mechanism to permit activation of antitachycardia pacing therapy if a tachycardia persists longer than a prespecified period. More sophisticated criteria are likely to be developed in the future, including analysis of A-V electrogram relationships, template recognition and possibly, hemodynamic sensing (see above).

For ventricular use, antitachycardia therapy needs to be "fine-tuned" and thoroughly tested in the electrophysiologic laboratory (Fig. 21.8), since failure to prescribe an effective therapy may result in frequent or inappropriate ICD discharges. During follow-up, such historical information as near-loss or loss of consciousness, number of defibrillations, and frequency of antitachycardia pacing should be carefully elicited and corroborated by the telemetered data.

COMPLICATIONS OF ANTITACHYCARDIA PACING THERAPY

The reader is also directed to Chapter 20 for discussion of possible complications associated with ICD therapy. Complications related to the lead and the pulse generators may arise with antitachycardia pacemakers similar to the pacemakers designed for bradyarrhythmia therapy. Specific to antitachycardia pacemakers are: (a) problems of inappropriate tachycardia detection, (b) tachycardia acceleration due to antitachycardia pacing therapy and (c) alterations in effectiveness of antitachycardia pacing over time, which may be related to disease progression, alterations in antiarrhythmic therapy, changes in autonomic tone, or drug-device interactions.

Problems with Tachycardia Detection

For most devices, differentiation of physiologic from pathologic tachycardias is imperfect. When rates overlap, rate alone is insufficient to differentiate sinus tachycardia from atrial fibrillation, for example. As a result of inaccurate differentiation, pacemaker-induced tachycardia may result (45–47). Characteristics of tachycardia, including rate, mode of onset, regularity, and changes with adrenergic tone and body position, should be carefully considered. It is important to consider heart rate response to exercise, and posture. If substantial overlap exists between physiologic heart rate responses and tachyarrhythmias,

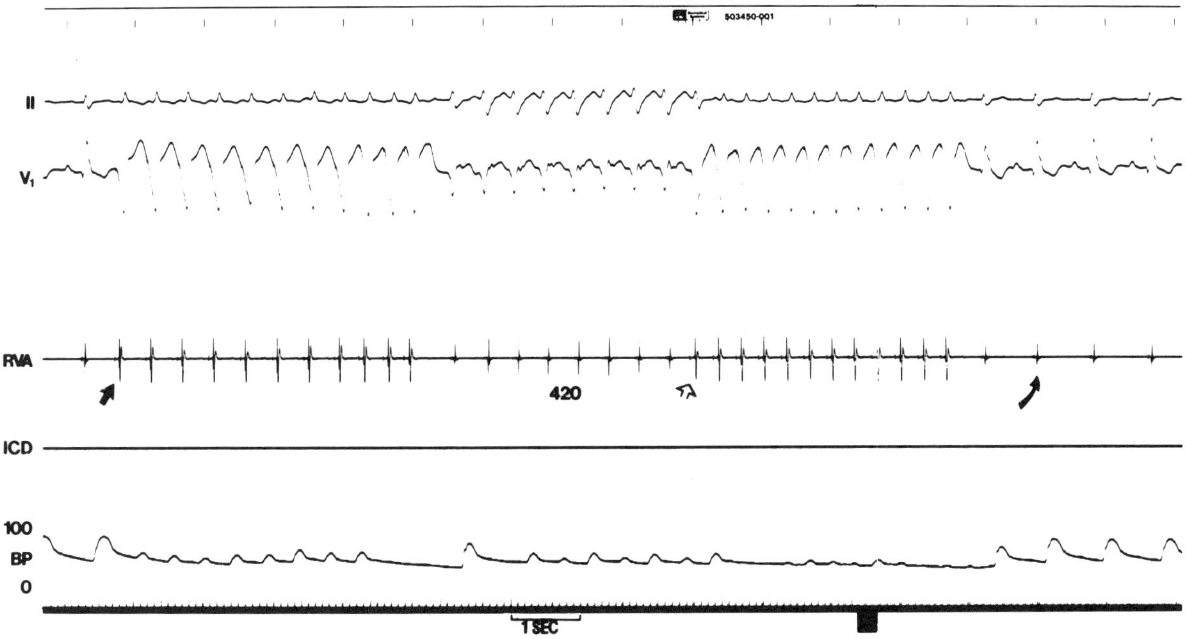

Figure 21.8. Device testing. Testing of possible interaction of antitachycardia device (Intertach II, Intermedics, Angleton, TX) and ICD (Ventak[R] P (CPI, St. Paul, MN). Ventricular tachycardia is induced using the antitachycardia pacemaker (*solid arrow*). The rhythm is appropriately detected and terminated by a burst of 12 extrastimuli (*open arrow*) followed by the return of sinus rhythm (*curved solid arrow*). From **top** to **bottom:** surface leads II, V_1, right ventricular apex (RVA), ICD channel, blood pressure (BP), and time lines (T).

additional detection criteria should be considered, i.e., "high rate," "sudden onset," and "rate stability."

Adequate sensing of intracardiac electrograms during sinus rhythm and during tachycardia should be insured at the time of implant and during the predischarge EP study. Inappropriate sensing (undersensing) may lead to asynchronous pacing or signal nondetection during VF (Fig. 21.9). Careful intraoperative testing with documentation of signal amplitude and slew rates during sinus rhythm and during tachycardia induction is therefore essential. Oversensing, on the other hand, may lead to false-positive tachycardia detection during sinus rhythm with inappropriate antitachycardia therapy or defibrillation (45).

Alterations in antiarrhythmic drug therapy may also cause previously effective therapy to become ineffective, due to alterations in tachycardia cycle length or tissue refractoriness. Therefore, when alterations in therapy are considered, device-antiarrhythmic drug interactions should be considered. Changes in programming may require both an alteration of arrhythmia detection criteria and antitachycardia pacing therapy.

Tachycardia Acceleration

When antitachycardia pacing therapy is delivered in the atrium, the most commonly induced arrhythmia during therapy is atrial fibrillation (47,48). Patients with WPW syndrome are at the greatest risk, particularly if A-V accessory pathways are capable of conducting very rapidly (have short antegrade refractory periods). During atrial fibrillation the rhythm may deteriorate to VF under such circumstances (49). Therefore, antitachycardia therapy is not recommended in WPW syndrome patients with short antegrade functional refractory period of the accessory pathways, nor with documented history of atrial fibrillation or cardiac arrest.

Acceleration of VT is potentially even more hazardous (Fig. 21.7). Ventricular tachycardia and VF are well-documented complications of the antitachycardia pacing therapy in the ventricle (45,49–51). Therefore, we do not recommend implantation of an antitachycardia device in the ventricle under *any* circumstances without a backup ICD or as a part of an ICD system. The value of antitachycardia pacing therapy is dependent on careful patient selection.

Alterations in Effectiveness of Therapy over Time

In an individual patient, effectiveness of antitachycardia pacing may change over time (48,51). This is due to the diurnal as well as the day to day variability in tachycardia reproducibility and stability, effects of autonomic tone, posture, electrolyte status, serum levels of antiarrhythmic drugs, progression of disease, ischemia, or other less-well defined factors.

Newer antitachycardia devices have adaptive features which deliver antitachycardia pacing therapy at intervals calculated as a percentage of tachycardia cycle lengths, or have a memory of prior termination, which may facilitate finding the most appropriate termination sequence rapidly (52,53). Careful retesting

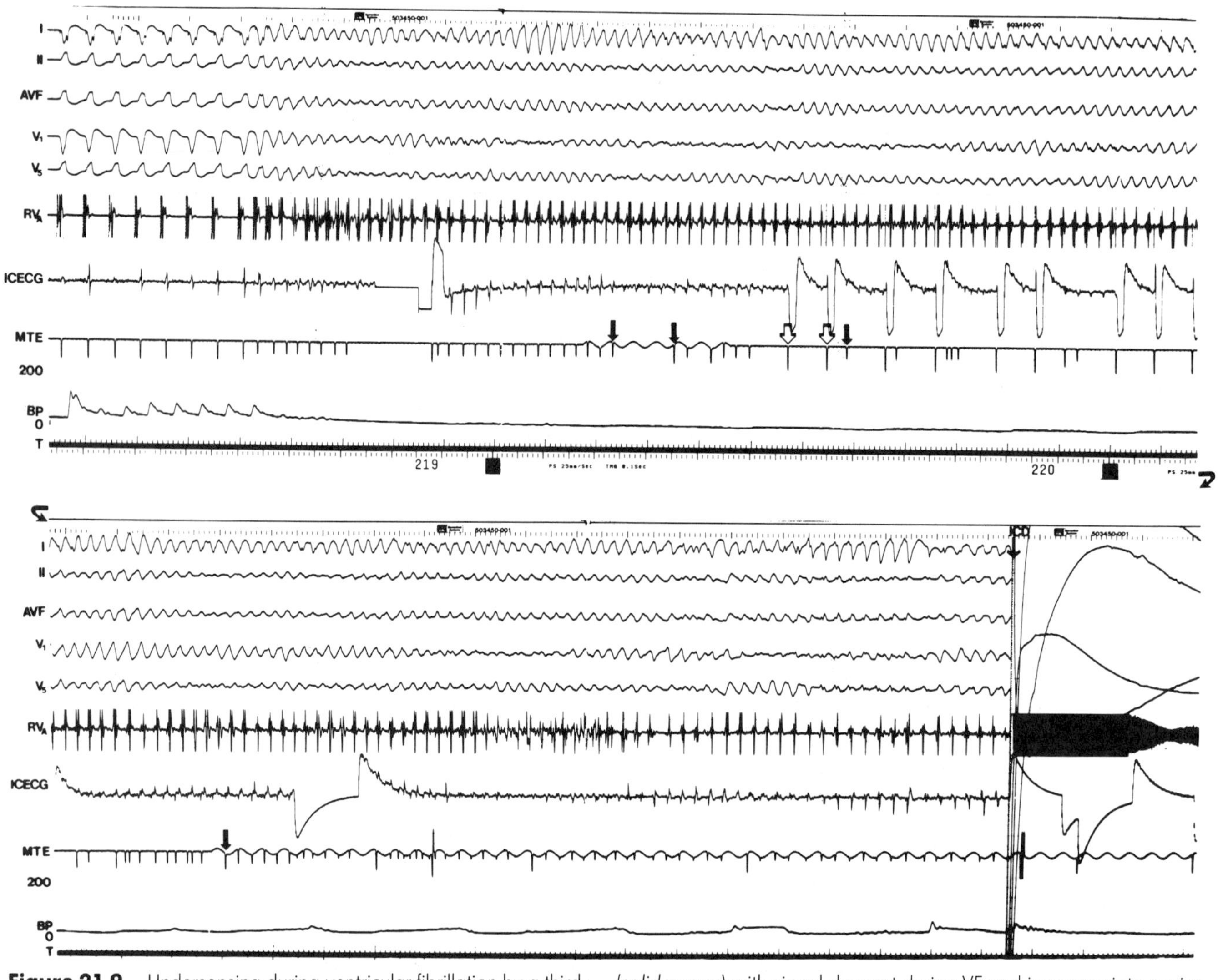

Figure 21.9. Undersensing during ventricular fibrillation by a third-generation programmable defibrillator (Guardian[R] ATP 4210), with fixed gain control. From **top** to **bottom:** Surface leads I, II, AVF, V_1 and V_5, intracardiac signal from the right ventricular apex (RV_A), intracardiac electrogram (ICECG), main timing event channel (MTE), blood pressure (BP), time lines (T). Note intermittent undersensing (*solid arrows*) with signal dropout during VF and inappropriate pacing during VF (open arrows). Ventricular fibrillation is eventually redetected with appropriate ICD shock and return of normal sinus rhythm. Programmed sensitivity is 1mV which is halved when VF is detected. *Top* and *bottom tracings* are continuous.

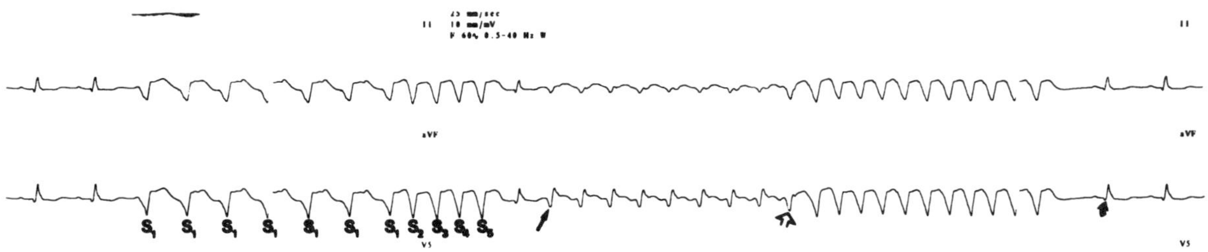

Figure 21.10. Noninvasive testing of antitachycardia device. Patient with Intratach[R]II device (in combination with ICD) is tested using the pacemaker for VT induction. Noninvasive induction of VT with a six-beat drive (S_1), followed by four extrastimuli (S_2, S_3, S_4, S_5) (*solid arrow*). Ventricular tachycardia is promptly detected by the antitachycardia device (*open arrow*) and terminated (*wide solid arrow*).

may be required to reprogram antitachycardia devices when previously effective therapy becomes less effective or ineffective (Fig. 21.10).

CONCLUSION

Antitachycardia devices are effective for therapy of supraventricular and ventricular tachycardias of reentry type. Thorough knowledge and training are necessary for the personnel involved in evaluation, implantation, and follow-up of patients with antitachycardia devices. Implantation and follow-up of such patients may be best suited for specialized EP centers with well-trained staff and a capability of providing alternative therapies for arrhythmias.

References

1. Mines GR: On dynamic equilibrium in the heart. J Physiol 1913;46:349–383.
2. Allessie MA, Bonke FIM, Schopman FJG: Circus movement in rabbit atrial muscle as a mechanism of tachycardia. III. The "leading circle" concept. Circ Res 1977;41:9–18.
3. Wellens HJJ, den Dulk K, Brugada P: Pacemaker management of cardiac arrhythmias. In Dreifus LS, Brest AN (eds): Pacemaker Therapy. Philadelphia, FA Davis, 1983:165–175.
4. Griffin JC, Mason JW, Calfee RV: Clinical use of an implantable automatic tachycardia-termination pacemaker. Am Heart J 1980;100:1093–1096.
5. Spurrell RAJ, Nathan AW, Bexton RS, *et al.*: Implantable automatic scanning pacemaker for termination of SVT. Am J Cardiol 1982;49:753–760.
6. Sowton E: Clinical results with tachylog antitachycardia pacemaker. PACE 1984;1313–1317.
7. Barold SS, Falkoff MD, Ong LS, *et al.*: New pacing techniques for the treatment of tachycardias. The golden age of cardiac pacing. In Barold SS, Mugica JM (eds): The Third Decade of Cardiac Pacing. Futura Publishing Co., Mt. Kisco NY 1982:309–332.
8. Den Dulk K, Bertholet M, Brugada P, *et al.*: A versatile pacemaker system for termination of tachycardias. Am J Cardiol 1983;52:731–738.
9. Den Dulk K, Bertholet M, Brugada P, *et al.*: Clinical experience with implantable devices for control of tachyarrhythmias. PACE 1984;7:548–556.
10. Fisher JD, Kim SG, Mercando AD: Electrical devices for treatment of arrhythmias. Am J Cardiol 1988;61:45A–57A.
11. Medina-Ravell V, Maduro C, Portillo B, *et al.*: Follow-up of twenty-five patients with implantable antitachycardia DVI, MN pulse generators (Abstr). PACE 1983;6:145.
12. Castellanos A, Waxman HL, Moleiro F, *et al.*: Preliminary studies with an implantable multimodal A-V pacemaker for reciprocating AV tachycardias. PACE 1980;3:257–265.
13. Escher DJW, Furman S: Emergency treatment of cardiac arrhythmias: emphasis on use of electrical pacing. JAMA 1970;214:1028–2034.
14. Furman S: Therapeutic uses of atrial pacing. Am Heart J 1973;86:835–840.
15. Charos GS, Haffajee CI, Gold RL, *et al.*: A theoretically and practically more effective method for interruption of ventricular tachycardia: self-adapting autodecremental overdrive pacing. Circulation 1986;73:309–315.
16. Den Dulk K, Kersschot IE, Brugada P, *et al.*: Is there a universal antitachycardia mode? Am J Cardiol 1986;57:950–955.
17. Spurrel RAJ, Nathan AW, Camm AJ: Clinical experience with implantable scanning tachycardia reversion pacemakers. PACE 1984;7:1296–1300.
18. Jantzer JH, Hoffman RM: Acceleration of ventricular tachycardia by rapid overdrive pacing combined with extrastimuli. PACE 1984;7:922–924.
19. Spurrel RAJ, Nathan AW, Camm AJ: Clinical experience with implantable scanning tachycardia reversion pacemakers. PACE 1984;7:1296–1300.
20. Sowton E: Clinical results with the tachylog antitachycardia pacemaker. PACE 1984;7:1313–1317.
21. Den Dulk K, Kersschot IE, Brugada P, *et al.*: Is there a universal antitachycardia mode? Am J Cardiol 1986;57:950–955.
22. Fisher JD, Ostrow E, Kim SG, *et al.*: Ultrarapid single-capture train stimulation for termination of ventricular tachycardia. Am J Cardiol 1983;51:1334–1338.
23. Fisher JD, Johnston DR, Furman S, *et al.*: Long-term stability of antitachycardia devices (Abstr). Clin Res 1986;34:298.
24. Griffin JC, Mason JW, Calfee RV: Clinical use an implantable automatic tachycardia-termination pacemaker. Am Heart J 1980;100:1093–1096.
25. Pless BD, Sweeney MB: Discrimination of supraventricular tachycardia from sinus tachycardia of overlapping cycle length. PACE 1984;7:1318–1324.
26. Mirowski M: The automatic implantable cardioverter-defibrillator: an overview. J Am Coll Cardiol 1985;6:461–466.
27. Davies DW, Wainwright RJ, Tooley MA, *et al.*: Detection of pathological tachycardia by analysis of electrogram morphology. PACE 1986;9:200–208.
28. Fisher JD, Kim SG, Furman S, *et al.*: Role of implantable pacemakers in control of recurrent ventricular tachycardia. Am J Cardiol 1982;49:194–206.
29. Fisher JD, Goldstein M, Ostrow E, *et al.*: Maximal rate of tachycardia development: Sinus tachycardia with sudden exercise vs. spontaneous ventricular tachycardia. PACE 1983;6:221–228.
30. Furman S, Fisher JD, Pannizzo F: Necessity of signal processing in tachycardia detection. In Barold S., Mugica J (eds): The Third Decade of Cardiac Pacing. Futura Publishing Co., New York, 1982.
31. Davies DW, Wainwright RJ, Tooley MA, *et al.*: Endocardial electrogram analysis for the automatic recognition of ventricular tachycardia (Abstr). Circulation 1985;72(Suppl II):III–474.
32. Langberg JD, Griffin JC: Arrhythmic identification using the morphology of the endocardial electrogram (Abstr). Circulation 1985;(Suppl III):III–474.
33. Arzbacher R, Burp T, Jenkins J, *et al.*: Automatic tachycardia recognition. PACE 1984;7:541–547.

34. Zipes DP, Akhtar M, Denes P, *et al*.: Guidelines for clinical intracardiac electrophysiologic studies. A report of the American College of Cardiology/American Heart Association Task Force on Assessment of Diagnostic and Therapeutic Cardiovascular Procedures (Subcommittee to Assess Clinical Intracardiac Electrophysiologic Studies). J Am Coll Cardiol 1989; 14(7):1827–1842.
35. Bertholet M, Demoulin JC, Wefejle A, *et al*.: Programmable extrastimulus pacing for long-term management of supraventricular and ventricular tachycardias: Clinical experience in 16 patients. Am Heart J 1985;110:582–589.
36. Zipes DP, Prystowsky EN, Miles WM, *et al*.: Initial experience with Symbios model 7008 pacemaker. PACE 1984;7:1301–1305.
37. Den Dulk K, Bertholet M, Brugada P, *et al*.: Clinical experience with implantable devices for control of tachyarrhythmias. PACE 1984;7:548–556.
38. Peters RW, Scheinman MM, Morady F, *et al*.: Long-term management of recurrent paroxysmal tachycardia by cardiac burst pacing. PACE 1985;8:35–44.
39. Fisher JD, Johnston DR, Furman S, *et al*.: Long-term efficacy of antitachycardia pacing for supraventricular and ventricular tachycardia. Am J Cardiol 1987;60:1311–1316.
40. Griffin JC, Sweeney M: The management of paroxysmal tachycardia using the Cybertach-60. PACE 1984;7:1291–1295.
41. Rothman MT, Keefe JM: Clinical results with Omni-Orthocor[R], an implantable antitachycardia pacing system. PACE 1984;7:1306–1312.
42. Kahn A, Morris JJ, Citron P: Patient-initiated rapid atrial pacing to manage supraventricular tachycardia. Am J Cardiol 1976;38:200–204.
43. Herre JM, Griffin JC, Nielsen AP, *et al*.: Permanent triggered antitachycardia pacemakers in the management of recurrent sustained ventricular tachycardia. J Am Coll Cardiol 1985;6:206–212.
44. Saksena S, Pantopoulous D, Parsonnet V, *et al*.: Usefulness of an implantable antitachycardia pacemaker system for supraventricular or ventricular tachycardia. Am J Cardiol 1986;58:70–74.
45. Echt DS: Potential hazards of implanted devices for the electrical control of tachyarrhythmias. PACE 1984;7:580–587.
46. Fahraeus T, Lassuik C, Sonthag C: Tachycardias initiated by automatic antitachycardia pacemakers. PACE 1984;7:1049–1054.
47. Lerman BB, Waxman HL, Buxton AE, *et al*.: Tachyarrhythmias associated with programmable automatic atrial antitachycardia pacemakers. Am Heart J 1983;106:1029–1035.
48. Spurrell RAJ, Nathan AW, Bexton RS, *et al*.: Implantable automatic scanning pacemaker for termination of supraventricular tachycardia. Am J Cardiol 1982;49:753–760.
49. Spurrell RAJ, Nathan AW, Camm AJ: Clinical experience with implantable scanning tachycardia reversion pacemakers. PACE 1984;7:1296–1300.
50. Jentzer JH, Hoffman RM: Acceleration of ventricular tachycardia by rapid overdrive pacing combined with extrastimuli. PACE 1984;7:922–924.
51. Falkoff MD, Barold SS, Goodfriend MA, *et al*.: Long-term management of ventricular tachycardia by implantable automatic burst tachycardia-terminating pacemakers. PACE 1986;9:885–895.

V

ABLATIVE THERAPY: SURGERY AND CATHETER ABLATION CARDIOPULMONARY RESUSCITATION

22

OPERATIVE TREATMENT OF SUPRAVENTRICULAR TACHYCARDIA

Andrea Natale, M.D., Gerard M. Guiraudon, M.D., F.R.C.S.(C), F.A.C.C., Raymond Yee, M.D., F.R.C.P.(C), F.A.C.C., and George J. Klein, M.D., F.R.C.P.(C), F.A.C.C.

INTRODUCTION

Operative treatment of supraventricular tachycardia is dependent on understanding the mechanism of tachycardia sufficiently to allow a procedure directed at a portion of the arrhythmia substrate critical to perpetuation of tachycardia. This is identified by electrophysiologic techniques. Operative therapy of supraventricular tachycardia has become highly sophisticated and successful following the elucidation of the mechanism of the supraventricular tachycardias by electrophysiological techniques (1–3). In addition, operative ablation is directed at atrial tissue and is consequently generally not associated with left ventricular dysfunction (1–3). More recently, the lessons learned from operative therapy have been applied to catheter ablation, a procedure in which the identified substrate is destroyed by applying energy (usually radiofrequency) to the end of a catheter (4–7). Although catheter ablative therapy has rapidly become the primary nonpharmacologic treatment for the supraventricular tachycardias, operative therapy will continue to have a role in those tachycardias where ablation is not feasible or in individuals in whom ablation is technically difficult. In addition, patients may require concomitant cardiac surgery during which it is most convenient to deal with the associated arrhythmia under direct visualization of the heart. Virtually all recurrent supraventricular tachycardias are amenable to operative therapy including atrial-ventricular (A-V) reentry, atrial ventricular (AV) node reentry, atrial flutter, atrial fibrillation, and atrial tachycardia.

GENERAL PRINCIPLES

Regardless of the tachycardia, the general approach to the patient considered for operative surgery is uniform and includes the following:

Complete Medical Assessment

This is necessary to evaluate a potential primary cause of the arrhythmia (e.g., hyperthyroidism, pulmonary embolism) and to define cardiac anatomy even when no primary cause is found. The latter allows elucidation of concomitant abnormalities that must be either corrected or at least considered in the operative plan including cardiac anomalies and other structural abnormalities.

Preoperative Electrophysiologic Assessment

The major goal of the preoperative assessment is to reproduce the observed arrhythmia and other potential arrhythmias and to determine their mechanism. Anatomic localization of the area destined for ablation (accessory pathway, atrial focus) is then carried out in considerable detail and an obligatory part of the reentrant circuit is identified and localized in the case of atrial reentrant tachycardia. A multicatheter study is generally required with electrode catheters in the high right atrium, His bundle region, right ventricle, and coronary sinus (8). Other catheters may be required for localization depending on the mechanism of arrhythmia, e.g., a left atrial catheter for left atrial tachycardias. The electrophysiology study should ideally be definitive and informative enough to proceed with surgery even in the event that intraoperative mapping is not possible by virtue of failure to induce the offending arrhythmia intraoperatively or temporary obtundation of the arrhythmia mechanism.

Intraoperative Mapping Studies

A clear idea of the arrhythmia mechanism and a detailed operative plan should be available prior to intraoperative mapping. A major purpose of intraoperative mapping is to verify the preoperative findings and provide increased resolution of anatomic localization with exposure of the heart. Activation sequence mapping is the pivotal tool. In most cases, a hand-held probe is moved sequentially in the area of interest during a stable rhythm with the data reconstructed at the end of the procedure to provide the activation sequence (9). Mapping systems are also available in which the area of interest is covered with multiple electrodes which can record data necessary to reproduce the activation sequence from a single cycle (10). The latter systems can be computerized to provide activation times from local electrodes and isochronal maps on line. The hand-held probe method is perfectly adequate in the Wolff-Parkinson-White (WPW) syndrome (2) but computerized mapping systems can be helpful in more complex arrhythmias such as atrial tachycardias, especially where a stable sustained arrhythmia is not available.

Wolff-Parkinson-White Syndrome

The first successful operative ablation of an accessory pathway was reported by Cobb, et al. at Duke University (11) in 1968 and this is widely acknowledged to be the beginning of the era of modern arrhythmia surgery. Surgery directed at accessory pathways evolved rapidly and became the model for operative treatment of all arrhythmias. WPW syndrome is perhaps the best understood of all the paroxysmal rhythm disorders and lends itself most ideally to an ablation procedure. The critical arrhythmia substrate in WPW syndrome is, in the great majority of cases, the accessory atrioventricular (AV) pathway, a small muscular strand traversing the AV annulus. Elimination of this pathway in a small and discrete area of the AV ring eliminates all arrhythmias associated with WPW syndrome. The electrocardiogram provides a useful first approximation to the site of the accessory pathway in the presence of overt preexcitation (12). The arrhythmias observed are invariably reproducible at the electrophysiologic study, the most common of which is orthodromic atrioventricular reciprocating tachycardia (13). Electrophysiologic assessment focuses on localization of the accessory pathway, the elucidation of unsuspected multiple accessory pathways and the diagnosis of other potential tachycardias such as AV node reentry not suspected clinically. The atrial insertion of the accessory pathway is best identified by atrial activation sequence mapping along the AV annulus during orthodromic reciprocating tachycardia, namely, by the site of earliest atrial activation during this arrhythmia. Accessory pathway potentials may also be observed at or in close proximity to this site (14). Localization by these techniques is sufficient to proceed with arrhythmia surgery. Localization of the ventricular insertion of the accessory pathway can also be performed by endocardial ventricular mapping at the AV ring under the mitral and tricuspid annuli (15). This is technically more difficult (especially in the right ventricular) and is most useful for catheter ablative therapy by this approach. Electrophysiologic mapping in WPW syndrome is reliable in localizing the accessory pathway to one of four surgical areas, namely, anteroseptal, posteroseptal, right lateral, and left lateral. The intraoperative mapping can be brief and focused. The most useful steps in intraoperative mapping include mapping of the epicardial ventricular aspect of the AV ring during preexcitation to determine the ventricular insertion site of the accessory pathway and mapping of the atrial aspect of the AV ring during reciprocating tachycardia to determine the atrial insertion (16) (Fig. 22.1). Although the atrial and ventricular insertions of the accessory pathway may not align "exactly" (17) they are generally within 10–20 mm and well within the limit of the surgical area to be ablated for any particular pathway location. Two operative approaches have been described. In the endocardial approach, the involved atrium is opened under cardiopulmonary bypass and the pathway approached by endocardial incision along the AV ring in the area of interest (18) (Fig. 22.2A). In the epicardial approach, the pathway is approached by epicardial dissection through the AV fat pad in the area of interest (19) (Fig. 22.2B). The latter does not require cardiopulmonary bypass or cardioplegia and allows the procedure to proceed simultaneously with continuous mapping on the normothermic beating heart. Although there are theoretical advantages to either procedure, both can be highly successful and the technique of choice is largely a matter of operator preference.

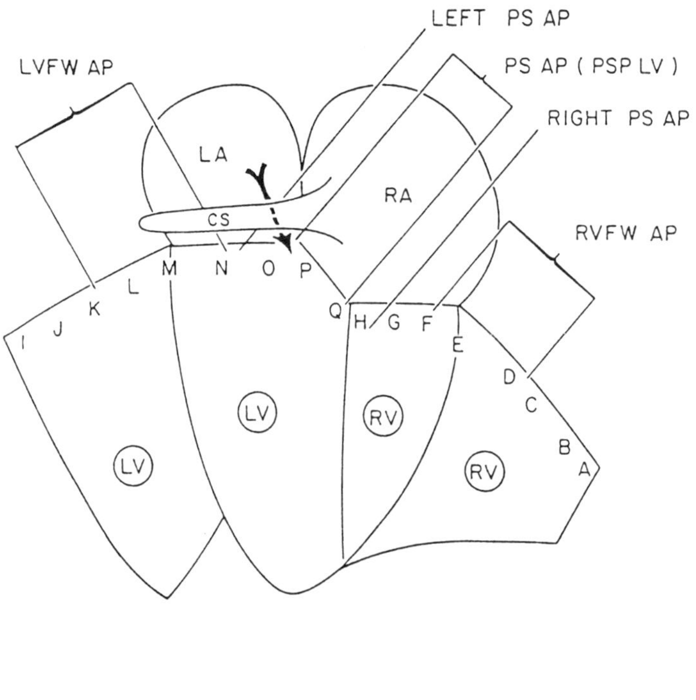

Figure 22.1. Operative classification of accessory pathway location. The heart is displayed as if it were cut along the anterior interventricular groove and flattened. The right ventricle (RV) is labeled from A to H. The left ventricle (LV) is labeled from I to Q. (AP = accessory pathway; CS = coronary sinus; LA = left atrium; LVFW = left ventricular free wall; RA = right atrium; RVFW = right ventricular free wall. (From Klein GJ, Guiraudon GM, Sharma AD, *et al.*: Surgical treatment of tachycardias: indications and electrophysiological assessment. In Yu P, Goodwin F (eds): Progress in Cardiology. Lea & Febiger, Philadelphia, 1986:139–153, reproduced with permission.)

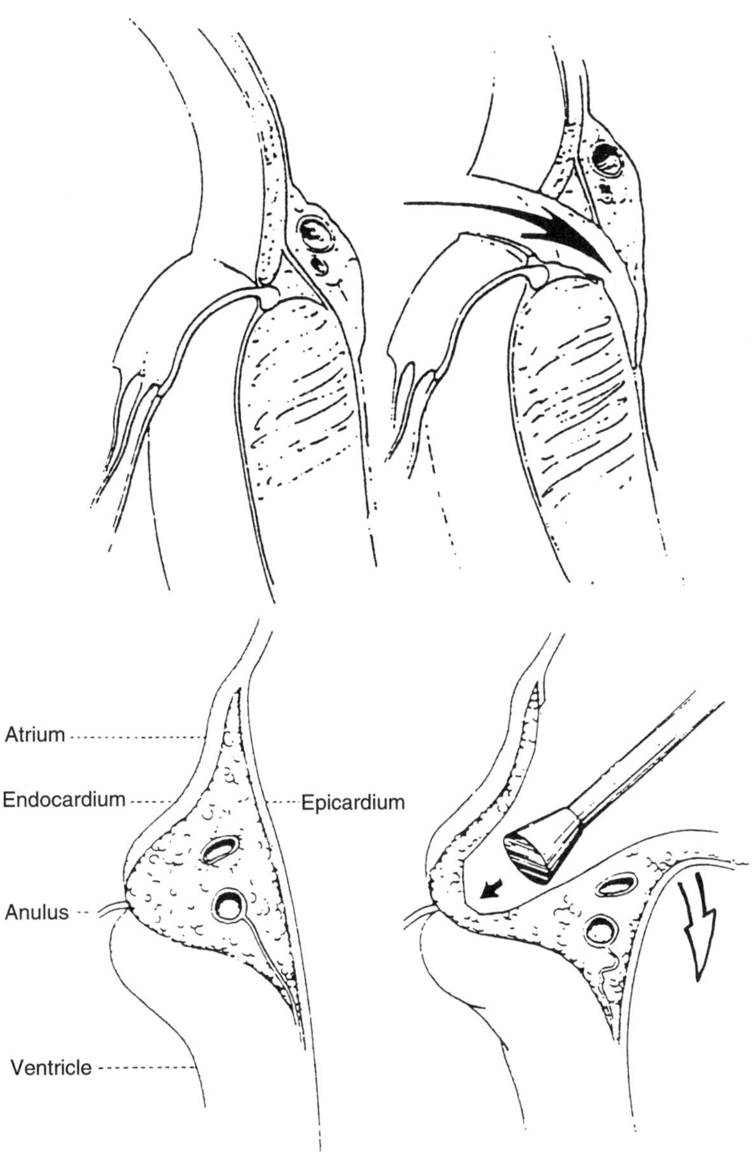

Figure 22.2. Operative technique for accessory pathway ablation. **Top,** The endocardial technique for accessory pathway interruption. A supranular incision from the endocardial surface of the atrium allows access to the atrioventricular fat pad. (From Klein GJ, Guiraudon GM, Perkins DG, *et al.*: Surgical correction of the Wolff-Parkinson-White syndrome in the closed heart using cryosurgery: A simplified approach. J Am Coll Cardiol 1984;3:405–409.) **Bottom,** The epicardial approach to accessory pathway ablation. The fat pad and vascular contents are dissected away and the cryoprobe is applied to this region. (From Klein GJ, Guiraudon GM, Perkins DG, *et al.*: Surgical correction of the Wolff-Parkinson-White syndrome in the closed heart using cryosurgery: A simplified approach. J Am Coll Cardiol 1984;3:405–409, reproduced with permission.)

Operative therapy of accessory pathways has been highly successful with success rates in the range of 98% and mortality and morbidity in the range of 1% reported by experienced centers (18–20). Catheter ablation has largely supplanted operative therapy for primary therapy of WPW syndrome (4,6,7) but operative therapy is still useful where ablative therapy has not been successful or where concomitant cardiac surgery is required. In some instances, operative therapy may be preferable to prolonged radiation exposure sometimes associated with catheter ablation.

Atrioventricular Node Reentry Tachycardia

There has been abundant evidence of at least two functionally distinct pathways involved in AV node reentry (21) but the anatomic correlates of these pathways have not been clearly identified. Surgery was initially not attempted for this arrhythmia because of the view that the reentrant pathways were entirely intranodal. The fortuitous operative cure of AV node reentry after a failed attempt at AV node ablation described by Pritchett, et al. (22) clearly demonstrated that operative cure was feasible without resorting to AV nodal block. There is now mounting evidence that at least part of the required reentrant circuit is extranodal providing the current rationale for both catheter and operative ablative approaches (5,7,22–26). The role of preoperative electrophysiologic testing in suspected AV node reentrant tachycardia is quite different than for WPW syndrome. Electrophysiologic testing is essentially done to verify the diagnosis and exclude other causes of supraventricular tachycardia. A detailed intraoperative mapping is considerably less useful. When catheter mapping is performed, retrograde atrial activation mapping during AV node reentry tachycardia is the most feasible. Generally, this will identify the retrograde limb as coming from the anterior portion of the AV node or the AV node proper (great majority of cases, especially the "common" type of AV node reentry tachycardia) or, alternatively, retrograde activation will occur first in the region of the coronary sinus orifice posteriorly (much less frequent, often with the "uncommon" type of AV node reentry tachycardia). Potentials possibly representing extranodal pathways have been described and the identification of these may eventually prove to be useful in delineating the circuit (27).

The success of surgery is not dependent on intraoperative mapping for several reasons. First, the region is small and the resolution of mapping by conventional techniques is generally not sufficient to be anatomically explicit. Multichannel recording with specially constructed fine electrodes in a small dense array may eventually become more informative (28–29). Second, contusion to the AV node region intraoperatively may render induction of tachycardia difficult. Finally, the available operative approaches generally do not depend a great deal on the results of mapping. The first successful prospective operative cure of AV node reentry tachycardia was described in a case report by Marquez-Montes (26). However, the first systematic series demonstrating operative cure of AV node reentry tachycardia was described by Ross, et al. (30). The surgery essentially involved perinodal dissection with the dissection more focused anteriorly where retrograde conduction demonstrated the anterior portion of the AV node to be early, and posteriorly, near the coronary sinus orifice, where this was demonstrated to be the site of retrograde activation (Fig. 22.3). Guiraudon described an entirely anatomically oriented dissection which did not utilize the results of mapping (31) (Fig. 22.4). This approach aimed to dissect the AV node free from all its atrial attachments save the deep atrial attachments. Finally, Cox, et al. described a cryosurgical technique where a series of cryolesions encircled the AV node in a fence-like fashion aiming to disrupt perinodal imputs (32) (Fig. 22.5). All three operative approaches have proved highly successful with success in the range of 90% or greater and an incidence of AV block in the range of 5% or less (31–33). The technique of Cox appears to be technically simpler and less operator dependent (34) although this may be a value judgment.

The success of all of these operative approaches while maintaining "normal" AV node conduction to a greater or lesser degree clearly demonstrated the requirement of the perinodal region for AV node reentry and paved the way for cure of this arrhythmia by catheter techniques. The latter have supplanted surgery as primary nonpharmacological therapy for AV node reentry tachycardia (5,7,35–36). Currently, operative therapy may be recommended in those instances where catheter ablation has failed or is technically not feasible or for a patient undergoing concomitant cardiac surgery.

Atrial Tachycardia

The atrial tachycardias are a heterogeneous group of tachycardias where the arrhythmia mechanism is entirely within the

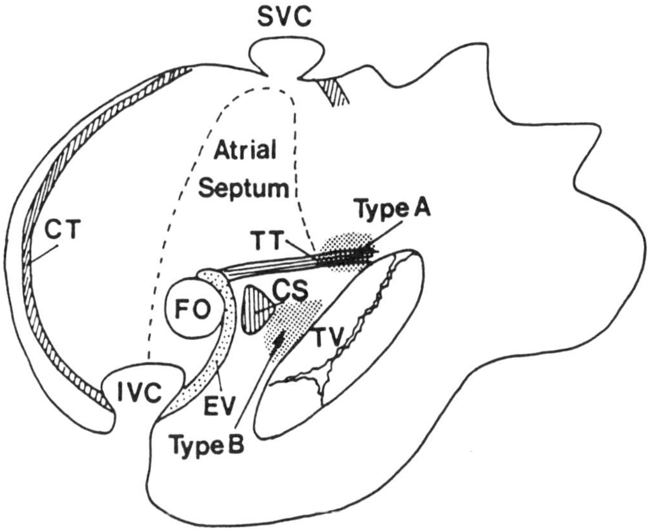

Figure 22.3. Location of earliest retrograde activation during AV nodal reentry tachycardia. In type A, earliest activation is anteromedial to the AV node, whereas in type B it is posterior to the AV node in the vicinity of the coronary sinus os. CS = coronary sinus; CT = crista terminalis; EV = eustachian valve; FO = foramen ovale; IVC = inferior vena cava; SVC = superior vena cava; TT = tendon of Todaro. (From Brugada P, Wellens HJJ, (eds): Cardiac Arrhythmias: Where to Go from Here? Futura Publishing Co., Mt. Kisco, NY, 1987:591–603, reproduced with permission.)

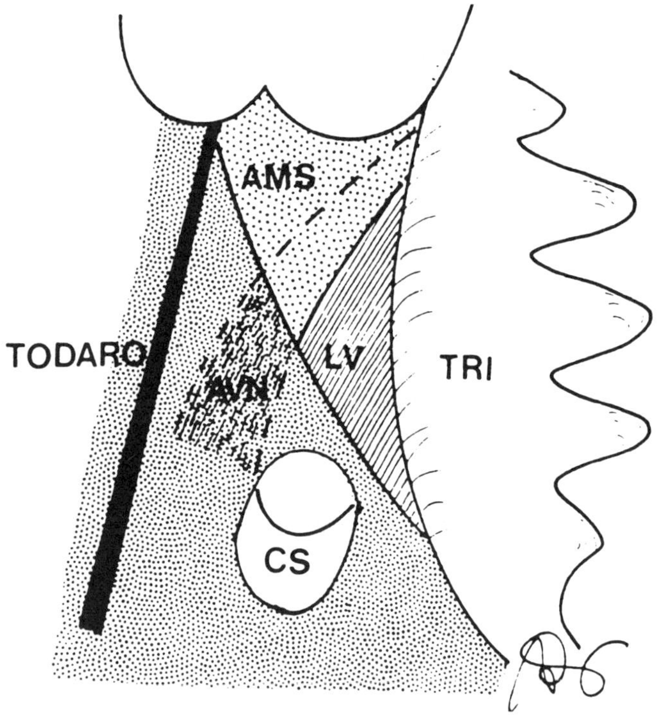

Figure 22.4. Landmarks used for anatomically guided AV nodal dissection. Atrial membranous septum (AMS), os of the coronary sinus (CS), left ventricle (LV), tendon of Todaro (TODARO), and tricuspid valve (TRI) are shown. The atrioventricular node (AVN) is situated underneath the septal atrial wall at the apex of the triangle of Koch. (From Fujimura O, Guiraudon GM, Yee R, *et al.*: Operative therapy of Atrioventricular node reentry: results of an anatomically guided procedure. Am J Coll Cardiol 1989;64:1327–1332, reproduced with permission.)

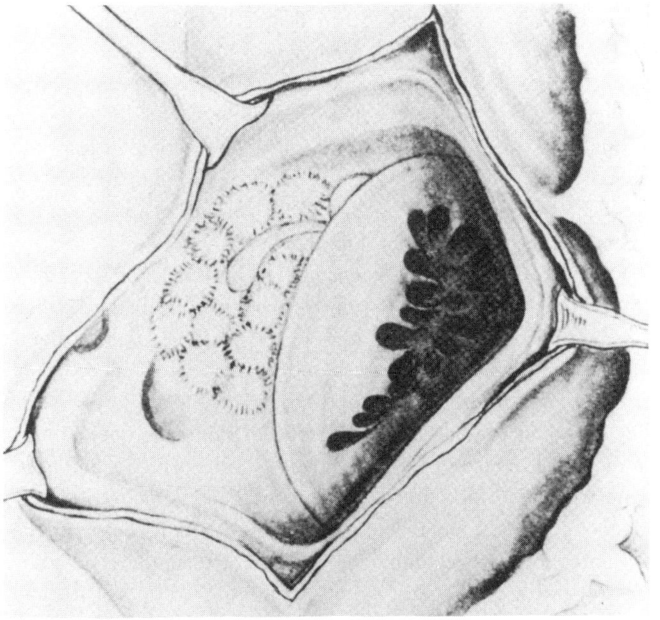

Figure 22.5. Encircling perinodal cryoablation. The cryoprobe is placed sequentially around the AV node and within the triangle of Koch. At each site, the tissue is cooled to −60°C for 2 min or until temporary heart block occurs. (From Ferguson TB, Cox JL: Surgical therapy for patients with supraventricular tachycardia. In Scheinman MM, (ed): Cardiol Clin 1990;8(3):535–555, reproduced with permission.)

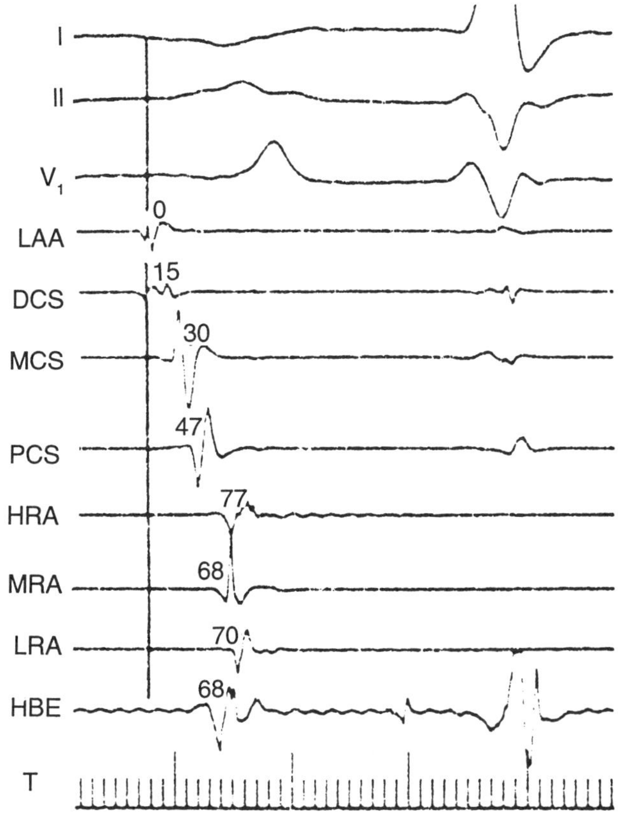

Figure 22.6. Endocardial mapping of the atria during atrial tachycardia. Activation recorded from the catheters is related to the onset of the P wave on the surface electrocardiogram (ECG). The earliest atrial activity is recorded in the left atrial appendage. I, II, V_1 are surface ECG leads; DCS = distal coronary sinus; HBE = His bundle region; HRA = high right atrium; LAA = left atrial appendage; LRA = low right atrium; MDC = mid-coronary sinus; MRA = mid-right atrium; PCS is proximal coronary sinus. (From Platia EV (ed): Management of Cardiac Arrythmias:the Nonpharmacologic Approach. JB Lippincott, Philadelphia, 1987:304–339, reproduced with permission.)

atrium and does not depend on the AV node or ventricle as part of the mechanism. They are readily distinguished clinically from the junctional tachycardias (AV node reentry, atrial ventricular reentry) by their response to adenosine or vagotonic maneuvers. The atrial tachycardias will demonstrate atrial-ventricular (A-V) block in the face of these maneuvers but the atrial tachycardia will continue unchanged in spite of this. The mechanisms of atrial tachycardia are heterogeneous but, broadly speaking, are either due to reentry in the atrium or abnormal impulse formation. They are much less frequent than the junctional tachycardias, accounting for up to 10% of cases in infancy and childhood and up to 3% in adults (37–39). They are frequently resistant to medical therapy and dilated cardiomyopathy may result in instances where the tachycardia is incessant (40). Approximately two-thirds of atrial tachycardias are localized in the right atrium with most of the remainder in the left atrium (41). Atrial reentry is more probable when the arrhythmia occurs in the setting of previous atrial surgery for congenital heart disease.

The role of electrophysiologic testing depends on the clinical presentation. If the tachycardia is incessant, the major aim of testing is atrial mapping with multiple catheters to delineate the "site of origin" as well as possible. Another important goal is to establish the mechanism or at least determine if the arrhythmia can be terminated and is inducible by programmed stimulation with or without autonomic facilitation. When the tachycardia is intermittent, the first goal of electrophysiologic testing is to determine if the arrhythmia can be reliably induced by programmed stimulation. If so, the "site of origin" is determined by careful and detailed endocardial atrial mapping (Fig. 22.6). Radiographic documentation of catheter position at the "site of origin" facilitates subsequent anatomic localization intraoperatively. It may help the surgeon to be present during the atrial mapping procedure to visualize the catheter positions fluoroscopically. The electrophysiologic study is of minimal use if the tachycardia is not inducible. Under these circumstances, it may be reasonable to bring the patient back to the laboratory during tachycardia at a subsequent time for the purposes of mapping. It is tenuous to take the patient to the operating room without good preoperative localization of the tachycardia.

Even when the arrhythmia is reproducibly induced in the laboratory, it may not be inducible under intraoperative conditions. If the arrhythmia is inducible intraoperatively, a detailed activation sequence map is the most useful procedure for delineating the "site of origin" and areas of critical conduction delay. This enables a more focused operation directed at a critical part of the arrhythmia mechanism regardless of the ablative techniques favored by the surgeon (excision, cryosurgery, laser) (42–46). If the surgery can only be guided by the results of preoperative mapping, the operative intervention should be more generous to provide a greater margin of safety. A more gross procedure be it excision, cryosurgery or laser surgery is then carried out (47–49). Isolation procedures have also been described which electrically exclude the desired atrial section (generally a large part or all of one atrium) by creating a fibrous scar around this region to "trap" electrical activity therein (41,50). It is difficult to evaluate the results of surgery since the patients and arrhythmia mechanisms reported have been eclectic and the patient numbers reported relatively few. Nonetheless, it would appear that greater than 90% success can be obtained in well-selected cases with mortality in the range of 1–5% (41). Failure is usually related to inability to map the arrhythmia with sufficient resolution or the reoccurrence of arrhythmia at alternate sites possibly due to diffuse atrial disease (1,16,38).

Atrial Flutter

Atrial flutter is an atrial tachycardia characterized by its rapid rate (approximately 300 cycles/min) and characteristic "flutter wave" morphology. Generally, the "common" type of flutter is associated with negative P waves in the inferior electrocardiographic leads and the "uncommon" type is associated with positive waves in the same leads. Atrial flutter has now been clearly shown to be due to atrial reentry and the common type in particular has been well documented to involve macroreentry in the right atrium associated with an anatomic "obstacle" (51–57). In this type, activation during flutter moves cephalad from the coronary sinus region, around the fossa ovalis, and returns via the crista terminalis caudad around the inferior vena cava to the region of the coronary sinus (Fig. 22.7).

Operative therapy may be considered in drug refractory cases when pure flutter is consistently observed clinically. When concomitant atrial fibrillation is observed in a given patient, operative therapies directed at flutter alone will generally not suffice. The purpose of electrophysiologic testing is to verify the diagnosis and provide an endocardial activation sequence map for the arrhythmia and identify zones of slow conduction felt to be critical in the circuit. Intraoperative mapping is focused mainly on activation sequence mapping of the atrium. This can be facilitated by multichannel recording and computerized interpretation although single-point mapping is quite satisfactory when the arrhythmia is sustained and reproducible. "Ice mapping" can be useful to identify sites considered to be essential components of the circuit. If tachycardia persists during cooling of a given region to −10°Centigrade it is clearly not an integral part of the circuit whereas reproducible termination of tachycardia by this maneuver implies the opposite. Multiple operative approaches are feasible for this large right atrial reentrant circuit including transection of the fossa ovalis and the two adjacent regions (58) or cryoablation of the zone of slow conduction in the region of the coronary sinus (16,53). The latter technique at-

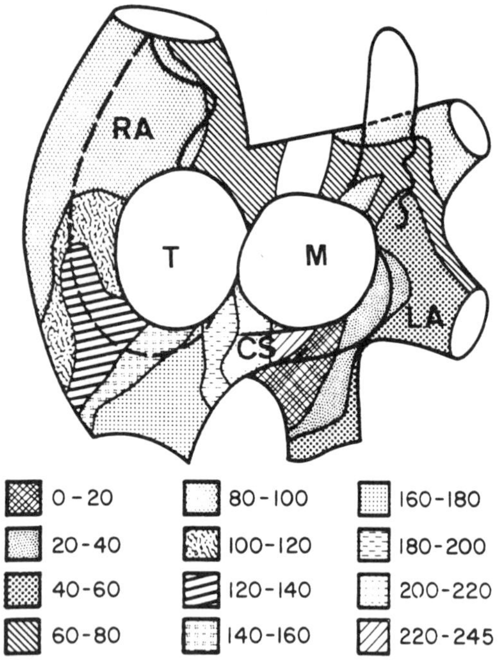

Figure 22.7. Epicardial mapping during the "common" type of atrial flutter. The atria are viewed from below as if they were "lifted" off the ventricles. Zones of equal activation time are indicated by different hatching. Earliest activation is recorded in the area close to the coronary sinus os and proceeds counterclockwise around the right atrium to return to its origin. The left atrium is activated passively. CS = coronary sinus; LA = left atrium; M = mitral valve; RA = right atrium; T = tricuspid valve. (From Guiraudon GM, Klein GJ, Sharma AD, *et al.*: Surgery for atrial flutter, atrial fibrillation and atrial tachycardia. In Zipes DP, Jalife J (eds): Cardiac Electrophysiology: from Cell to Bedside. WB Saunders, Philadelphia, 1990:915–921, reproduced with permission.)

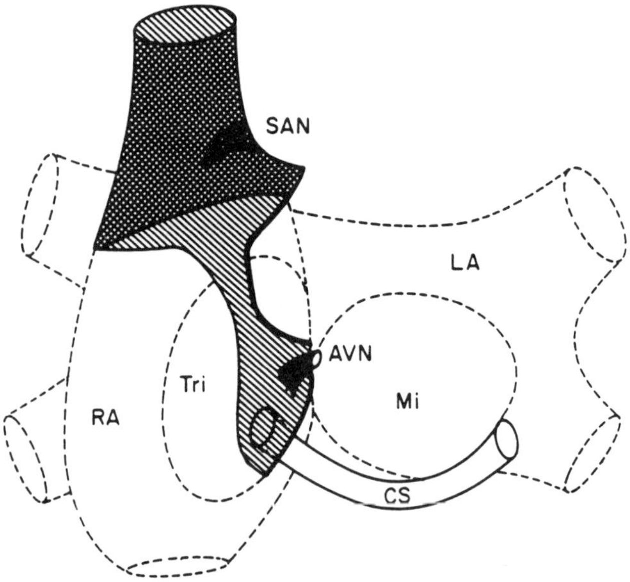

Figure 22.8. Schematic representation of the "corridor" that includes the sinus node and the AV node. AVN = AV node; CS = coronary sinus; LA = left atrium; Mi = mitral annulus; RA = right atrium; SAN = sinus node; Tri = tricuspid annulus. (From Guiraudon GM, Klein GJ, Sharma AD, *et al.*: Surgery for atrial flutter, atrial fibrillation, and atrial tachycardia. In Zipes DP, Jalife J (eds): Cardiac Electrophysiology: from Cell to Bedside. WB Saunders, Philadelphia, 1990;915–921, reproduced with permission.)

tempts to interrupt the circuit by cryoablating the region bounded by the coronary sinus orifice, the posterior inferior tricuspid annulus and the inferior vena cava. The latter is possible using cryoablation on the normothermic beating heart. Indications for surgery in atrial flutter are uncommon since the majority of patients do not have this tachycardia as a single isolated rhythm disorder. Most frequently, it is associated with atrial fibrillation and often occurs in the setting of diffuse atrial disease. In addition, it may be possible to deal with this arrhythmia using catheter ablative techniques (59). In well-selected cases, the operative approach should be highly successful with minimal morbidity (1,16,53).

Atrial Fibrillation

Atrial fibrillation is perhaps the most prevalent supraventricular tachycardia present in 0.4% of the general population and in 4–10% of people over 60 yr of age (60–62). Current evidence suggests that the mechanism involves multiple reentrant wavelets circulating over the atria seeking nonrefractory tissue (63). Experimentally, it has been shown that fibrillation can only be maintained when the tissue mass exceeds a critical volume, compatible with a view that fibrillation is maintained by multiple reentrant circuits "without an anatomic obstacle" (64). Unlike the other supraventricular tachycardias, it has not been possible to identify a discrete site critical to the perpetuation of atrial fibrillation and consequently approaches to operative therapy have been more obtuse. The role of electrophysiologic testing in preoperative evaluation is limited. It is more useful in the assessment of sinus node function and AV node conduction under baseline conditions since the presence of severe sinus node or AV node dysfunction might be associated with pacemaker requirement which would blunt the potential benefit of the surgery. In addition, electrophysiologic testing may be useful in uncovering "primary" rhythm disorder such as AV reentry or AV node reentry which in some cases may be the real trigger mechanism for atrial fibrillation. Otherwise, current approaches to operative therapy are not dependent on the results of electrophysiologic testing.

The initial attempt at operative therapy of atrial fibrillation was described by Williams, et al. (65). They hypothesized that the left atrium was responsible for atrial fibrillation in patients with mitral valve disease and suggested that operative electrical "isolation" of the left atrium would prevent manifest atrial fibrillation. This approach was not further developed by these authors, possibly because the approach would not be applicable to the majority of patients with atrial fibrillation who do not have mitral valve disease. An alternate approach was described by Guiraudon, an operation that has become to be known as the "corridor operation" (16). In this procedure, a strip of atrial tissue including the sinus node and the AV node is electrically excluded from the remainder of the atria using dissection and cryosurgery (Fig. 22.8). Thus, sinus node function is left intact and in control of the heart. The impulse travels down the "corridor" to the ventricle and atrial fibrillation is much less likely in this small "island" of atrial tissue. Reasonable success with this procedure has been reported by both Guiraudon, et al. (66) and by others (67). The procedure has the potential to maintain normal chronotropic function of the heart in the absence of intrinsic sinus node dysfunction. This appears to be the

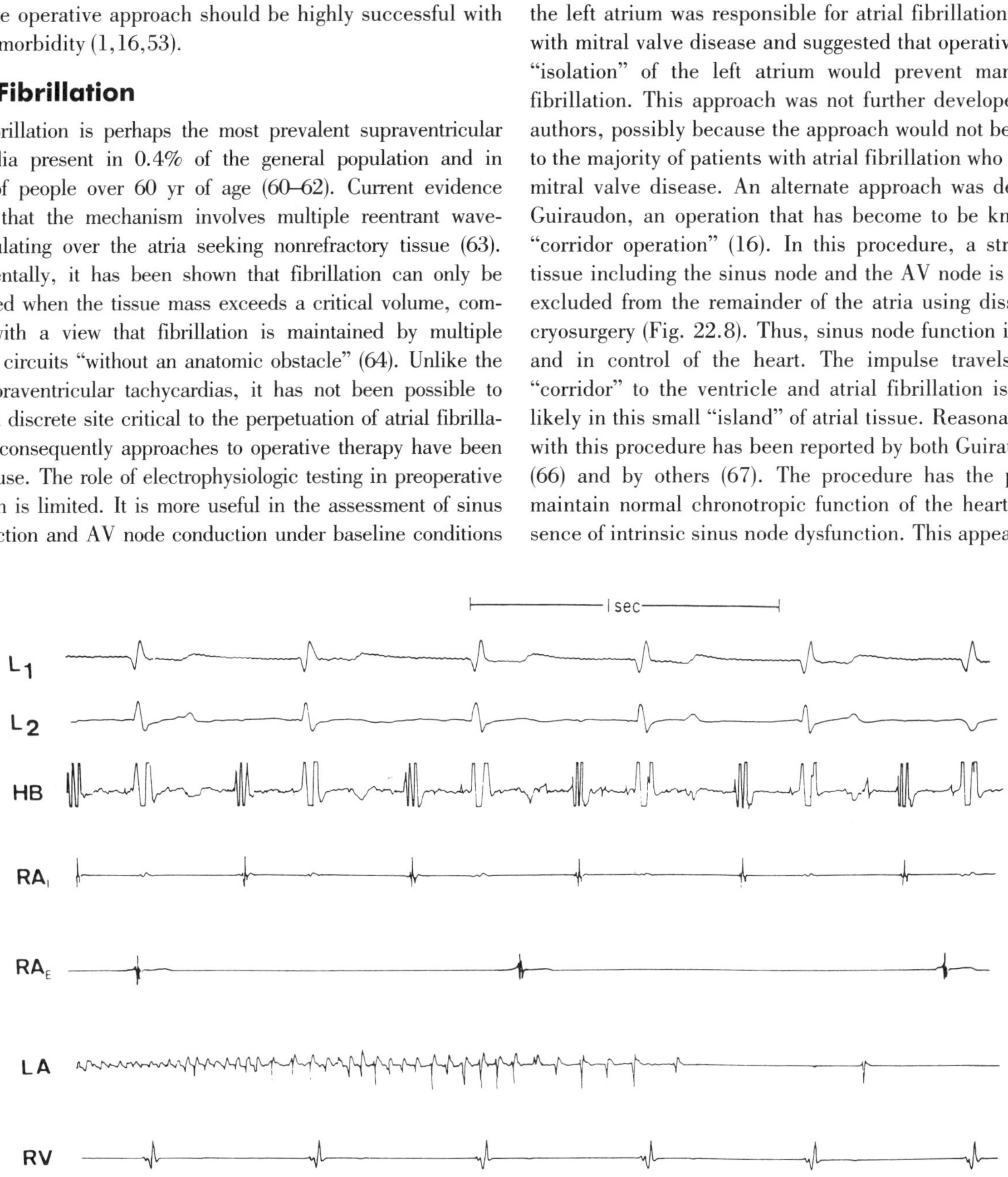

Figure 22.9. Recording during postoperative electrophysiologic study showing sinus rhythm in the corridor (RAI), an independent atrial rhythm in the excluded right atrium (RAE), and atrial fibrillation in the excluded left atrium (LA). L_1, L_2 = surface leads I, II; HB = His bundle electrogram; RV = right ventricular electrogram. (From Guiraudon GM, Klein GJ, Sharma AD, *et al.*: Surgery for atrial flutter, atrial fibrillation, and atrial tachycardia. In Zipes DP, Jalife J (eds): Cardiac Electrophysiology: from Cell to Bedside. WB Saunders, Philadelphia, 1990:915–921, reproduced with permission.)

major benefit of this surgery. Atrial contractility is not maintained and one or more of the excluded portions may continue to fibrillate resulting in a continued need for anticoagulation (Fig. 22.9). Cox, et al. have described an alternate approach which they term the "maze" procedure (68). This procedure is apparently based on the rationale that the multiple wavelets required for continuous reentry can be disrupted by forcing the sinus node impulse through a circumscribed pathway created by incision and suturing (69). The sinus impulses are "herded" through this maze to the AV node. The initial report of this procedure is promising but the results are preliminary (70). It has the theoretical advantages of maintaining contractile function and obviating the need for anticoagulation but this remains to be verified by long-term follow-up. It is clear that an ideal operation similar to ablation of an accessory pathway for WPW is currently not available. The difficulties include failure to identify a discrete focus causing tachycardia, the high prevalence of this arrhythmia in the elderly, and the frequent presence of diffuse atrial disease in this patient population. Current practice favors AV node ablation with pacemaker implantation as the nonpharmacologic therapy of choice for refractory atrial fibrillation, reserving the operative approaches for the few patients in whom the possibility of therapy without pacemaker implantation is critically important.

SUMMARY

The past two decades have witnessed great advances in our understanding of supraventricular tachycardias and the development of excellent approaches for cure of many of the supraventricular tachycardias. Indeed, this important milestone paved the way for the emergence of the newer catheter ablative therapies. Operative therapy will continue to play a smaller but important role in the management of the supraventricular tachycardias in the foreseeable future.

References

1. Guiraudon GM, Klein GJ, Sharma AD, *et al.*: Surgical alternatives for supraventricular tachycardias. Am J Cardiol 1989;64:92J–96J.
2. Klein GJ, Guiraudon GM, Sharma AD, *et al.*: Surgery for tachycardia: indications and electrophysiological assessment. Circulation 1987;75 (suppl III):III 186-9.
3. Gallagher JJ, Selle JG, Svenson RH, *et al.*: Surgical treatment of arrhythmias. Am J Cardiol 1988;61:27A–44A.
4. Jackman WM, Wang X, Friday KJ, *et al.*: Catheter ablation of accessory atrioventricular pathways (Wolff-Parkinson-White Syndrome) by radiofrequency current. N Engl J Medl 1991;324:1605–1611.
5. Epstein LM, Scheinman MM, Langberg JJ, *et al.*: Percutaneous catheter modification of the atrioventricular node. A potential cure for atrioventricular nodal tachycardia. Circulation 1989;80:757–68.
6. Kuck KH, Schluter M, Geiger M, *et al.*: Radiofrequency current catheter ablation of accessory atrioventricular pathways. Lancet 1991;337:1557–1561.
7. Calkins H, Sousa J, El-Atassi R, *et al.*: Diagnosis and cure of the Wolff-Parkinson-White syndrome or paroxysmal supraventricular tachycardia during a single electrophysiologic test. N Engl J Med 1991;324:1612–1618.
8. Leitch J, Klein GJ, Yee R, *et al.*: Invasive electrophysiologic evaluation of patients with supraventricular tachycardia. Cardiol Clin 1990;8:465–477.
9. Gallagher JJ, Kasell JH, Cox JL, *et al.*: Techniques of intraoperative electrophysiologic mapping. Am J Cardiol 1982;49:221–240.
10. Smith WM, Wharton JM, Blanchard SM, *et al.*: Direct cardiac mapping. In: Zipes DP, Jalifé J (eds): Cardiac electrophysiology: from cell to bedside. WB Saunders, Philadelphia, 1990;:849–858.
11. Cobb FR, Blumenschein SD, Sealy WC, *et al.*: Successful surgical interruption of the bundle of kent in a patient with Wolff-Parkinson-White syndrome. Circulation 1968;38:1018–1029.
12. Milstein S, Sharma AD, Guiraudon GM, *et al.*: An algorithm for the electrocardiographic localization of accessory pathway in the Wolff-Parkinson-White syndrome. PACE 1987;10:555–563.
13. Prystowsky EN: Diagnosis and management of the preexcitation syndrome. Curr Prob Cardiol 1988;13:230–310.
14. Jackman WM, Kuck KH, Friday KJ, *et al.*: Catheter recordings of accessory atrioventricular pathway activation. In Zipes DP, Jalife J (eds): Cardiac Electrophysiology: from Cell to Bedside. Philadelphia, WB Saunders, 1990:941–502.
15. Szabo TS, Klein GJ, Guiraudon GM, *et al.*: Localization of accessory pathways in the Wolff-Parkinson-White syndrome. PACE 1989;12:1691–1705.
16. Guiraudon GM, Klein GJ, Sharma AD, *et al.*: Surgery for atrial flutter, atrial fibrillation and, atrial tachycardia. In Zipes DP, Jalife J (eds): Cardiac Electrophysiology: from Cell to Bedside. WB Saunders, Philadelphia, 1990:915–920.
17. Jackman WM, Friday KJ, Yeung-Lai-Wah JA, *et al.*: New catheter technique for recording left-free accessory atrioventricular pathway activation: identification of pathway fiber orientation. Conclusion 1988;78:598–611.
18. Ferguson TB, Cox JL: Surgical treatment for the Wolff-Parkinson-White syndrome: the endocardial approach. In Zipes DP, Jalife J (eds): Cardiac Electrophysiology: from Cell to Bedside. WB Saunders, Philadelphia, 1990:897–906.
19. Guiraudon GM, Klein GJ, Sharma AD, *et al.*: Surgery for the Wolff-Parkinson-White syndrome: the epicardial approach. In Zipes DP, Jalife J (eds): Cardiac Electrophysiology: from Cell to Bedside. WB Saunders, Philadelphia, 1990:907–914.
20. Guiraudon GM, Klein GJ, Yee R, *et al.*: Surgery for Wolff-Parkinson-White syndrome using the epicardial approach. Experience with 490 patients. Circulation 1990;82 (Suppl III):III-473.
21. Denes P, Wu D, Dhingra R, *et al.*: Demonstration of dual A-V nodal pathways in patients with paroxysmal supraventricular tachycardia. Circulation 1973;48:549.
22. Pritchett ELC, Anderson RW, Benditt DG, *et al.*: Reentry within the atrioventricular node: surgical cure with preservation of atrioventricular conduction. Circulation 1979;60:440–446.
23. Iinuma H, Dreifus LS, Mazgalev T, *et al.*: Role of the perinodal region in atrioventricular nodal reentry: evidence in an isolated rabbit heart preparation. J Am Coll Cardiol 1983;2:465–473.
24. Kerr CR, Benson DW, Gallagher JJ: Role of specialized conducting fibers in the genesis of "AV nodal" re-entry tachycardia. PACE 1983;6:171–184.
25. Mazgalev T, Dreifus LS, Bianchi J, *et al.*: The mechanism of AV junctional reentry: role of the atrio-nodal junction. Anat Rec 1981;201:179–188.
26. Marquez-Montes J, Rufilanehas JJ, Estene JJ, *et al.*: Paroxysmal nodal reentrant tachycardia, surgical cure with preservation of atrioventricular conduction. Chest 1983;4:690–694.
27. Roman CA, Wang X, Friday FJ, *et al.*: Catheter technique for selective ablation of slow pathway in AV nodal reentrant tachycardia. PACE 1990;13:498.
28. Prystowsky EN, Irwin JM, Wharton JM, *et al.*: Intraoperative endocardial mapping of atrial septal activation sequences during atrioventricular reentry. Circulation 1988;78 (Suppl II):II-44.
29. Chang BC, Schuessler RB, Stone CM, *et al.*: Computerized activation

sequence mapping of the human atrial septum. Ann Thorac Surg 1990;49:231–241.

30. Ross DL, Johnson DC, Denniss AR, *et al.*: Curative surgery for atrioventricular junctional ("AV nodal") reentrant tachycardia. J Am Coll Cardiol 1985;6:1383–1392.
31. Guiraudon GM, Klein GJ, Sharma AD, *et al.*: Skeletonization of the atrioventricular node. Surgical alternative for AV nodal reentrant tachycardia: experience with 32 patients. Ann Thorac Surg 1990;49:565–572.
32. Cox JL, Ferguson TB, Lindsay BD, *et al.*: Perinodal cryosurgery for atrioventricular node reentry tachycardia in 23 patients. J Thorac Cardiovasc Surg 1990;99:440–450.
33. Johnson DC, Ross DL, Uther JB: The surgical cure of atrioventricular junctional reentrant tachycardia. In Zipes DP, Jalife J, (eds): Cardiac Electrophysiology: from Cell to Bedside. WB Saunders, Philadelphia, 1990:921–923.
34. Santarelli P, Alessandrini F, Montenero AS, *et al.*: Surgical therapy for supraventricular tachycardias. In D'Alessandro LC (ed): Heart Surgery 1991. Rome, CESI, 1991:145–158.
35. Hassaguerre M, Warin JF, Lemetayer P, *et al.*: Closed-chest ablation of retrograde conduction in patients with atrioventricular nodal reentrant tachycardia. N Engl J Med 1989;320:426–433.
36. Lee MA, Morady F, Kadish A, *et al.*: Catheter modification of the atrioventricular junction with radiofrequency energy for control of atrioventricular nodal reentry tachycardia. Circulation 1991;83:827–835.
37. Wu D, Denes P, Amat-y-Leon F, *et al.*: Clinical, electrocardiographic and electrophysiologic observations in patients with paroxysmal supraventricular tachycardia. Am J Cardiol 1978;41:1045–1051.
38. Guiraudon GM, Klein GJ, Sharma AD, *et al.*: Surgical treatment of supraventricular tachycardia. A five-year experience. PACE 1986;9:1376–1380.
39. Mehta AV, Sanchez GR, Sacks EJ, *et al.*: Ectopic automatic atrial tachycardia in children: clinical characteristics, management and follow-up. J Am Coll Cardiol 1988;11:379–385.
40. Packer DL, Bardy GH, Worley SJ, *et al.*: Tachycardia-induced cardiomyopathy: a reversible form of left ventricular dysfunction. Am J Cardiol 1986;57:563–570.
41. Lowe JE, Hendry PJ, Packer DL, *et al.*: Surgical management of chronic ectopic atrial tachycardia. Semi Thorac Cardiovasc Surg 1989;1:58–66.
42. Gillette PC, Wampler DG, Garson A Jr, *et al.*: Treatment of atrial automatic tachycardia by ablation procedures. J Am Coll Cardiol 1985;6:405–409.
43. Ott DA, Gillette PC, Garson A Jr, *et al.*: Surgical management of refractory supraventricular tachycardia in infants and children. J Am Coll Cardiol 1985;5:124–129.
44. Anderson BP, Stinson EB, Mason JW: Surgical exclusion of focal paroxysmal atrial tachycardia. Am J Cardiol 1982;49:869–874.
45. Josephson ME, Spear JF, Harken AH, *et al.*: Surgical excision of automatic atrial tachycardia. anatomic and electrophysiologic correlates. Am Heart J 1982;104:1076–1085.
46. Iwa T, Ichihashi T, Hashizume Y, *et al.*: Successful surgical treatment of left atrial tachycardia. Am Heart J 1985;109:160.
47. Hendry PJ, Packer DL, Anstadt MP, *et al.*: Surgical treatment of automatic atrial tachycardias. Ann Thorac Surg 1990;49:253–260.
48. Seals AA, Lawrie GM, Magro S, *et al.*: Surgical treatment of right atrial focal tachycardia in adults. J Am Coll Cardiol 1988;11:1111–1117.
49. Chang JP, Chang CH, Yeh SJ, *et al.*: Surgical cure of automatic atrial tachycardia by partial left atrial isolation. Ann Thorac Surg 1990;49:466–468.
50. Harada A, D'Agostino HJ, Schuesser RB, *et al.*: Right atrial isolation: a new surgical treatment for supraventricular tachycardia. J Thorac Cardiovasc Surg 1988;95:643–650.
51. Wells JL, MacLean WAH, James TN, *et al.*: Characterization of atrial flutter. Studies in man after open heart surgery using fixed atrial electrodes. Circulation 1979;60:665–673.
52. Waldo AL: Some observations concerning atrial flutter in man. PACE 1983;6:1181–1189.
53. Klein GJ, Guiraudon GM, Sharma AD, *et al.*: Demonstration of macroreentry and feasibility of operative therapy in the common type of atrial flutter. Am J Cardiol 1986;57:587–591.
54. Waldo AL: Atrial flutter. New directions in management and mechanism. Circulation 1990;81:1142–1143.
55. Feld GK: Activation patterns in canine atrial flutter. Circulation 1990;82 (Suppl II):III:56.
56. Chang BC, Schuessler RB, Stone CM, *et al.*: Computerized mapping of the atrial septum in patients with atrial flutter. Circulation 1989;80 (Suppl II):II-221.
57. Feld GK: Activation pattern during induction and entrainment of canine atrial flutter. Circulation 1990;82 (Suppl III):III-318.
58. Guiraudon GM, Klein GJ, Sharma AD, *et al.*: Use of old and new anatomic, electrophysiologic, and technical knowledge to develop operative approaches to tachycardia. In Brugada P, Wellens HJJ (eds): Cardiac Arrhythmias: Where to Go from Here? Futura Publishing Co., Mt. Kisco, NY, 1987;639–652.
59. Saoudi N, Atallah G, Kirkorian G, *et al.*: Catheter ablation of the atrial myocardium in human type I atrial flutter. Circulation 1990;81:762–771.
60. Kannel WB, Abbott RD, Savage DD, *et al.*: Epidemiologic features of chronic atrial fibrillation. The Framingham Study. N Engl J Med 1982;306:1018–1022.
61. Treseder AS, Sastry BS, Thomas TP, *et al.*: Atrial fibrillation and stroke in elderly hospitalized patients. Age Aging 1986;15:89–92.
62. Martin A, Benbow LJ, Butrous GS, *et al.*: Five year follow-up of 101 elderly subjects by means of long-term ambulatory cardiac monitoring. Eur Heart J 1984;5:592–596.
63. Moe GK: On the multiple wavelet hypothesis of atrial fibrillation. Arch Int Pharmacodyn 1962;140:183–188.
64. Allessie MA, Lammers WJEP, Bonke FIM, *et al.*: Experimental evaluation of Moe's multiple wavelet hypothesis of atrial fibrillation. In Zipes DP, Jalife J (eds): Cardiac Electrophysiology and Arrhythmias. Grune & Stratton, Orlando, FL, 1985:265–275.
65. Williams JM, Ungerleider RM, Lofland GK, *et al.*: Left atrial isolation: a new technique for the treatment of supraventricular arrhythmias. J Thorac Cardiovasc Surg 1980;80:373–380.
66. Leitch JW, Klein GJ, Yee R, *et al.*: Sinus node-atrioventricular node isolation: long-term results with the "corridor" operation for atrial fibrillation. J Am Coll Cardiol 1991;17:970–975.
67. DeFauw JJ, van Hemel NM, Vermuelen FE, *et al.*: Short-term results of the "corridor operation" for drug-refractory paroxysmal atrial fibrillation. Circulation 1988;78(Suppl):II-43.
68. Cox JL, Schuessler RB, Cain ME, *et al.*: Surgery for atrial fibrillation. Semin Thorac Cardiovasc Surg 1989;1:67–73.
69. Cox JL, Canavan TE, Schuessler RB, *et al.*: The surgical treatment of atrial fibrillation: II. Intraoperative electrophysiologic mapping and description of the electrophysiologic basis of atrial flutter and atrial fibrillation. J Thorac Cardiovasc Surg 1991;101:406–426.
70. Cox JL, Schuessler RB, D'Agostino HJ, *et al.*: The surgical treatment of atrial fibrillation. III Development of a definitive surgical procedure. J Thorac Cardiovasc Surg 1991;101:569–583.

23

SURGICAL MANAGEMENT OF VENTRICULAR TACHYCARDIA

Andrea Natale, M.D., Gerard M. Guiraudon, M.D., F.R.C.S.(C), F.A.C.C., Raymond Yee, M.D., F.R.C.P.(C), F.A.C.C., and George J. Klein, M.D., F.R.C.P.(C), F.A.C.C.

INTRODUCTION

Despite significant advances in our understanding and pharmacologic management of sustained ventricular tachycardia (VT), this potentially lethal arrhythmia continues to pose a major challenge (1–5). Surgical approaches continue to represent an important mode of therapy for drug refractory VT even with the development of implantable antitachycardia devices such as the implantable cardioverter defibrillator (6–9). While catheter ablative techniques are being actively pursued, their application to VT management remains experimental and surgical ablation of VT remains the principal curative therapy option available (10,11). This review focuses on the surgical approach to the management of patients with refractory VT.

PATIENT SELECTION AND PREOPERATIVE ASSESSMENT

The selection of suitable candidates for operative ablation of VT impacts on the surgical results. Arrhythmia surgery is considered for the patient in whom the VT is a primary arrhythmia and not secondary to some reversible cause such as myocardial ischemia or electrolyte imbalance. Patients are traditionally referred after one or more antiarrhythmic agents, given in adequate doses to achieve therapeutic blood concentrations, have failed to suppress spontaneous or inducible VT (12). The underlying etiology in the majority of these patients is ischemic heart disease due to coronary atherosclerosis with previous myocardial infarction while the remainder consists of a heterogeneous group including dilated or hypertrophic cardiomyopathy, valvular heart disease, isolated right ventricular (RV) dysplasia, repaired congenital heart disease, neoplasm, or previous cardiac trauma (13). Rarely patients may have no identifiable structural heart disease and the refractory VT represents a primary electrical disturbance.

Objective assessment of potential surgical candidates is directed toward defining (a) the anatomic substrate for the VT and functional status of the ventricles and coronary circulation and (b) the electrophysiologic (EP) substrate of the VT and correlation with the anatomic disease by careful mapping. Following a careful history and physical examination, the 12-lead electrocardiogram (ECG) of normal sinus rhythm and during spontaneous VT provides critical information such as infarct location, number of morphologic types of VT, and their putative sites of origin and rate (14). Note should be made of the hemodynamic state of the patient during the various VT types (monomorphic or polymorphic) since these impact on the ability to map the VT. Graded treadmill exercise testing may reveal the role of acute ischemia in triggering VT episodes although the induction of sustained monomorphic VT by exercise testing is uncommon (15). Noninvasive tests such as two-dimensional echocardiography and radionuclide angiography provide relevant quantitative information on cardiac structure and function and may be helpful for early identification of the patient with extremely poor LV function who would be an extremely poor surgical candidate for ablative surgery without resorting to cardiac catheterization. Two-dimensional echocardiography and radionuclide wall motion studies may also provide initial evidence of myocardial disease predominating in the right ventricle (16,17). The majority of patients undergo contrast left ventriculography and selective coronary arteriography to identify (a) the extent and location of the myocardial infarct scar or left ventricular (LV) aneurysm, (b) the functional status of noninfarcted myocardium and, (c) the extent and severity of coronary atherosclerosis that might require concomitant revascularization during ablative surgery. Contrast right ventriculography is vital in patients with VT originating from the right ventricle myocardium such as in arrhythmogenic right ventricular dysplasia or repaired tetralogy of Fallot (18). In selected patients, myocardial biopsy must also be considered to rule out a subclinical acute myocarditis since, in this case, the spontaneous remission of VT may occur or LV function may deteriorate in the postoperative period (19,20).

Refractoriness to antiarrhythmic drugs may occasionally be determined by ambulatory monitoring in hospital if VT episodes are frequent (5,21,22) but usually this is established by electrophysiology study–guided drug testing when VT is infrequent and hemodynamically unstable (1,23,24). Invasive electrophysiologic studies verify that the VT is reproducibly inducible by programmed stimulation and permit (a) serial drug testing (25–33) and (b) in the event of drug refractoriness, a preoperative endocardial map using multipolar electrode catheters (34,35). The types of VT induced in the laboratory must be carefully compared with spontaneous VT episodes. The presence of multiple VT morphology types may represent different exit points and conduction patterns for a common reentrant circuit or might reflect discreetly separate "foci" (36). Endocardial catheter mapping is vital prior to surgery because (a) it provides preliminary information to correlate the site of VT origin with the sites of anatomic lesions and (b) it may constitute the only information available to the surgeon regarding the VT site(s) of origin if VT is not inducible intraoperatively. One or more electrode catheters systematically moved to various endocardial locations during the VT provide a map of the VT endocardial activation pattern. The site of the earliest recorded ventricular electrogram activity (preferably preceding onset of the QRS complex during VT) represents the site of VT origin (Fig. 23.1). If VT is not inducible by programmed stimulation or is poorly tolerated, pacing from multiple endocardial sites and comparing the "pace map" QRS morphology on a 12-lead ECG with that obtained during the clinical VT may provide important clues as to the likely site of origin (35,37). Similarly, endocardial catheter mapping during sinus rhythm may reveal areas of slow conduction critical to a reentrant mechanism for VT as manifested in low-amplitude fragmented diastolic potentials and in some cases continuous electrical activity (38–41). It may be difficult to perform a complete VT endocardial map of the patient with multiple VT morphologies.

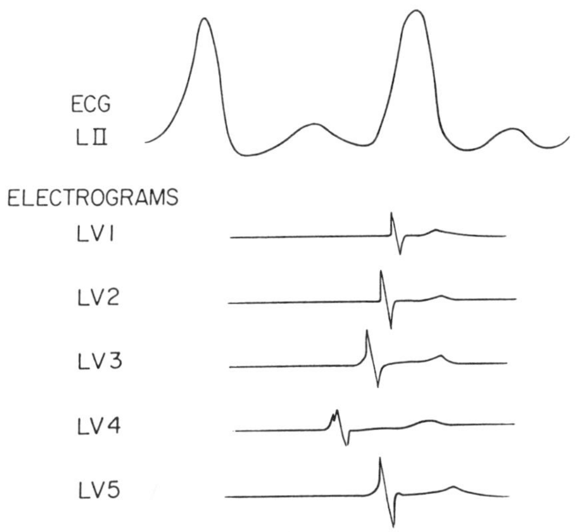

Figure 23.1. Schematic diagram of endocardial catheter mapping of ventricular activation during ventricular tachycardia. The electrogram recorded at the earliest activation point (LV4) precedes the QRS on the surface ECG. LII = surface ECG lead II; LV1, LV2, LV3, LV4, LV5 are left ventricle bipolar electrograms recorded at different sites. (From Tyagi S, Sharma AD, Giraudon GM, *et al.*: Intraoperative cardiac mapping of preexcitation syndromes and ventricular tachycardia. J Electrophysiol 1989;3:47–64, reproduced with permission.)

All data from noninvasive and invasive tests are then assimilated to create a profile of the patient. The ideal candidate for ablative surgical procedure is a patient who (a) has discrete anatomic lesion in the right or left ventricle such as an LV aneurysm but in whom the remaining myocardium is normal so that myocardial contractility of the remaining myocardium is excellent with an ejection fraction > 35–40%; (b) has absence of any other disease such as coronary artery stenosis requiring revascularization or valvular heart disease requiring a prosthetic replacement; (c) in a patient with a single VT type; and (d) in a patient with excellent general medical health. Unfortunately, this type of patient is encountered infrequently. All too often, the typical patient is an older male with a large aneurysmal scar with global hypokinesis, perhaps associated with papillary muscle dysfunction and multiple documented VT morphologic types, some of which might be associated with hemodynamic instability and require cardioversion. Some patients may have only polymorphic VT inducible at EP study that degenerates rapidly to VF. The spectrum of patients is diverse but it is clear that the mortality and success rate associated with VT surgery is related to ventricular function (ejection fraction less than 20%), ability to adequately map the arrhythmia, and presence of multiple sites of origin (42–44). The efficacy of VT surgery is highest with sustained monomorphic VT that can clearly be mapped to a discrete site and is worst for polymorphic or pleomorphic VT or if only ventricular fibrillation (VT) is inducible at surgery. In these cases other options should probably be considered.

SURGICAL APPROACHES

The operative techniques developed over the past several decades have paralleled advances in the understanding of the mechanism and pathophysiologic processes underlying VT of various etiologies. They have evolved from blind and aggressive approaches aimed at resecting the entire structural lesion presumed to be the originating site of the ventricular arrhythmia toward more focused surgery guided by multielectrode computerized mapping systems and directed at the specific zones within diseased myocardium proven to be the site of origin.

Prior to 1978 the most common method employed by surgical centers was an aneurysmectomy and coronary artery revascularization, if necessary (45–47). The success rate reported by various surgical centers ranged from 30–50%. The perioperative mortality associated with aneurysmectomy with revascularization ranged from 20–40% (45–47). This variability likely reflected differences in patient selection, specific surgical techniques, and level of surgical experience.

Insights gained from mapping of the VT led to a recognition that the transitional zone (border zone) between diseased and normal myocardium often gave rise to VT (36,48–50). Recognizing this, Guiraudon, *et al.* introduced the encircling endocardial ventriculotomy (EEV) wherein a transmural incision was made along the entire circumference of the border zone of the infarct scar (51) thereby disrupting the reentrant circuit or isolating the reentrant circuit from the normal myocardium (exit block) (Fig. 23.2). The major concern with this technique was a potential detrimental effect on global ventricular function in these patients (52–54), many of whom had borderline ventricular function preoperatively. Nonetheless, efficacy of the surgical technique was superior to that of simple aneurysmectomy, with mortality of approximately 13% (55). Neither the EEV nor aneurysmectomy required precise localization by mapping and both methods depended on the presence of an obvious discrete scar. The encircling endocardial cryoablation technique (56) and the "partial" encircling endocardial ventriculotomy (57,58) were a slight modification of the EEV method but used cryoablative technology or a map-guided ventriculotomy to try to reduce the impact of surgery on normal myocardium. The results of these techniques have been encouraging with mortality rate of 6% reported by Guiraudon (56) and of 7.6% using the partial ventriculotomy (58).

In 1979, Harken and Josephson introduced the method of subendocardial resection of arrhythmogenic scar tissue (59,60). The technique could be applied diffusely to all evident scars (61–64) or in a limited manner to peel or remove the scar tissue following careful VT mapping (65–76) (Fig. 23.3). Results from different centers with this technique have shown impressive long-term results in affecting a cure with an acceptable mortality rate of approximately 10–15% (59–76). Cryoablation has been combined with subendocardial resection to approach certain areas difficult to approach with the scalpel (papillary muscle, interventricular septum) to avert concomitant prosthetic implant (67,72,76,78,79) because cryoablation disrupts excitable tissue while leaving the supportive connective tissue intact (77). Cryoablation has also been successfully used as the sole surgical technique whenever a distinct scar was not present or to reduce the size of myocardial damage (80–82). However, cryoablation of a large mass of tissue may prolong the time of the procedure (13,81).

Several centers are investigating the application of laser technology to photoablate the arrhythmogenic substrate (72,83,84). Laser coagulation, while sharing some of the advantages of cryoablation, provides additional benefits in that a more rapid ablation can be achieved and it can be performed on the normothermic beating heart (83,84). Whether the replacement of the surgeon's scalpel or cryoprobe by the laser probe or other more expensive technologies will incrementally improve mortality and success rates, is uncertain.

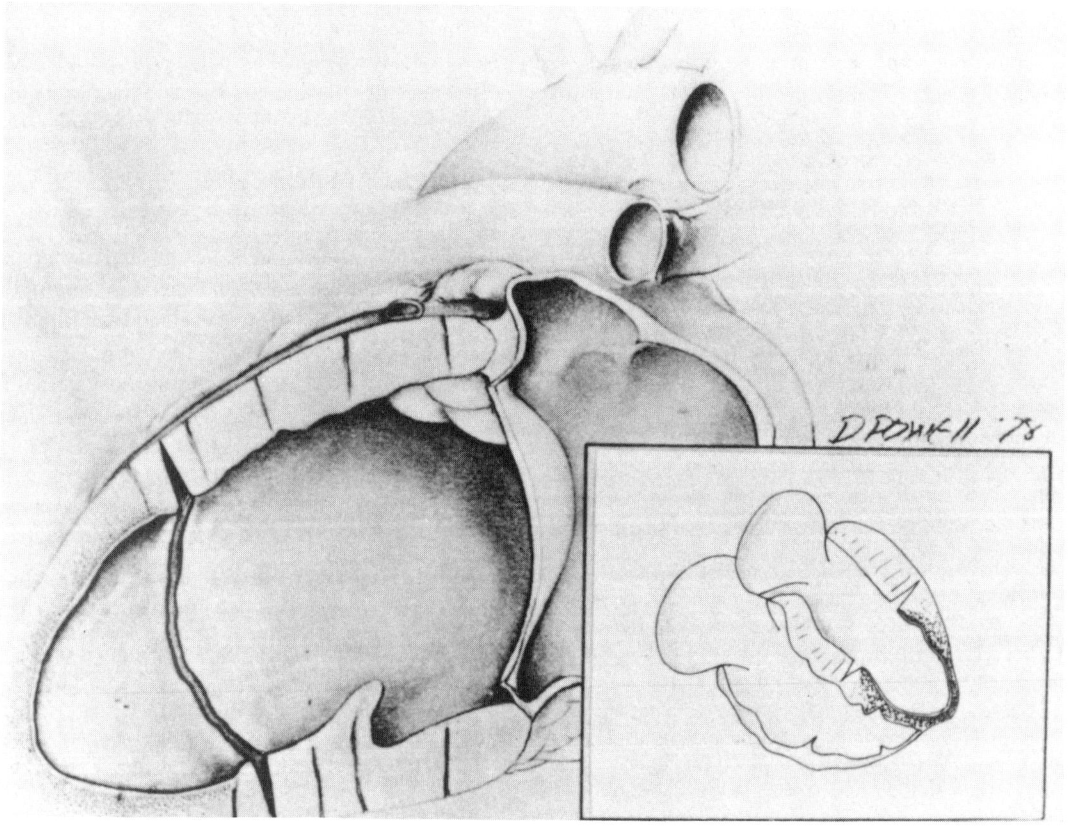

Figure 23.2. Encircling endocardial ventriculotomy. An incision completely isolates the diseased tissue from the viable myocardium. The depth of the ventriculotomy is demonstrated in the **inset.** (From Guirandon GM, Fontaine G, Frank R, *et al.*: Encircling endocardial ventriculotomy: a new surgical treatment for life threatening ventricular tachycardias resistant to medical treatment. Ann Thorac Surg 1978;26:438–444, reproduced with permission.)

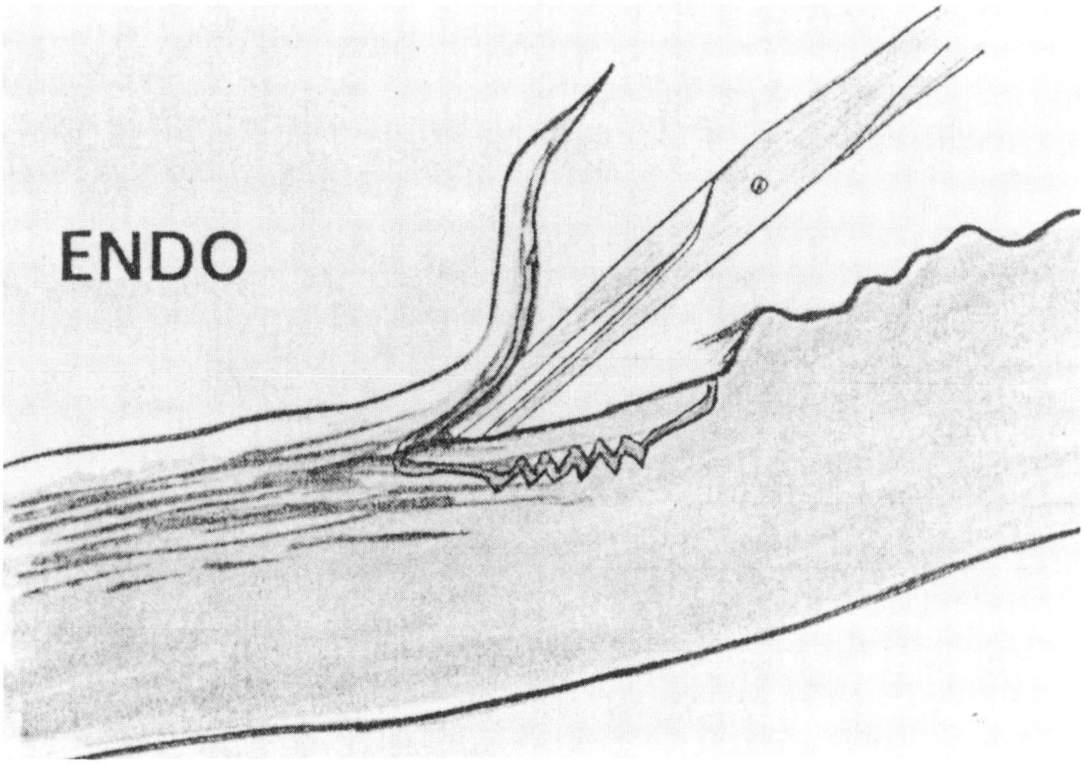

Figure 23.3. Subendocardial resection of the ventricular tachycardia substrate. After a plane of dissection is identified between the scar and the normal myocardium a scissors is used for the resection. ENDO is the endocardial surface. (From Fontaine G, Giraudon GM, Frank R, *et al.*: Surgical treatment of chronic ventricular tachycardia. In Levy S, Scheinman M (eds): Cardiac Arrhythmias. From Diagnosis to Therapy. Futura Publishing Company, Mt. Kisco, NY, 1984:479–495, reproduced with permission.)

Whether one particular surgical approach is clearly superior to any other is difficult to answer because (a) most reports from centers with extensive VT surgery experience involve a relatively small number of patients, and (b) the potential for selection bias undoubtedly exists between centers (Table 23.1). Table 23.1 lists many of the reports published by various centers detailing the surgical methods employed, study size and results. Currently there are no prospective randomized trials comparing two or more of the surgical approaches. Regardless of the specific technique used, the objective is now to disrupt the arrhythmogenic tissue with a minimum of damage to adjacent healthy myocardium.

VENTRICULAR TACHYCARDIA UNRELATED TO ISCHEMIC HEART DISEASE

The majority of patients who require surgery for VTs have ischemic heart disease. However, a significant proportion of these arrhythmias are associated with other etiologies, especially in younger patients. In an international surgical registry of 665 patients, 10% had no coronary disease (13).

Arrhythmogenic RV dysplasia historically served as a model for testing some of the principles of VT surgery. This is a condition in which the ventricular myocardium is replaced by fibrous-fatty infiltration. Although initially described as involving the right ventricle exclusively (85,86), it has been demonstrated that the process may progress to affect the left ventricle (87). In their initial experience, Guiraudon, *et al.* performed a map-guided local ventriculotomy or a resection at the site of VT origin or where delayed or fractionated electrograms were recorded (88). However, the high incidence of long-term relapses (50%) led them to design a more extensive RV disconnection procedure. The RV free wall was dissected from its septal and left ventricular attachments thereby confining the tachycardia to the right chamber (89) (Fig. 23.4). The rate of success in preventing VT recurrence was good but deterioration of LV function have been reported late after this procedure (90). This may in part be attributable to natural progression of the disease and may be avoided through a careful selection of patients (91,92). The total disconnection should be attempted when the disease only involves the right ventricle and when the arrhythmia is demonstrated to originate from the right ventricle alone. Patients with extensive or progressive involvement of both ventricles should be considered for alternative treatment modalities such as the implantable cardioverter-defibrillator or cardiac transplantation if LV function is severely depressed. Ventricular tachycardia associated with other cardiac abnormalities has also been treated successfully by operative approaches. Among these, the nonischemic dilated cardiomyopathy and the idiopathic form of VT represent the most common conditions (13,92). Excellent results have been reported in carefully selected patients with these disorders when intraoperative mapping of VT was adequate (92). Indeed, because visible and well-demarcated endocardial scars are often not present, accurate intraoperative mapping is critical in guiding surgical ablation.

Ventricular tachycardia has also been observed in postoperative tetralogy of Fallot and valvular heart disease. In the former situation, the VT typically originates from the RV outflow tract where previous surgery was directed at the obstruction and a surgical cure is possible in patients with drug-unresponsive VT (92–95). In cases of VT secondary to valvular heart disease, correction of the valve abnormality with improvement of hemodynamic function may resolve the arrhythmia without the need for

Table 23.1.
Results of Surgery for Ventricular Tachycardia

Series	No.	Operative Technique(s)	Mortality Rate (%)	Postoperative Inducibility (%)
Moran (63)	65	DSER	12	9
Hargrove (68)	289	SER + cryo	15	33
Brodman (43)	22	SER	14	NR
Ivey (43)	11	SER	9	20
Swerdlow (115)	98	Multiple	17	32
Garan (65)	36	SER	17	33
Krafchek (76)	39	SER + cryo	10	3
Hammon (43)	32	Multiple	12	NR
Balooki (45)	18	Multiple	16	25
Saksena (83)	24	SER	0	33
Vigano (13)	36	SER	8	NR
Kron (70)	70	SER	13	13
Ostermeyer (58)	93	PEEV	5	19
Selle (84)	15	Laser	13	0
Yee (71)	62	Multiple	8	NR
McGiffin (43)	123	Multiple	21	38
Manolis (72)	30	Multiple	10	30
Guiraudon (55)	30	EEV	13	6
Zee-Cheng (62)	46	Multiple	7	37
Landymore (64)	26	DSER	12	4
Guiraudon (56)	16	EE cryo	6	6
Saksena (83)	5	Laser	0	20
Caceres (81)	39	Cryo + SER	5	24
Pagé (82)	33	Cryo	6	13
Cox (43)	65	SER + cryo	14	2
Willems (13)	64	Multiple	18	NR

Abbreviations: cryo = cryoablation; DSER = diffuse subendocardial resection; EE cryo = encircling endocardial cryoablation; EEV = encircling endocardial ventriculotomy; multiple = more than two different techniques; NR = not reported; PEEV = partial encircling endocardial ventriculotomy; SER = subendocardial resection.

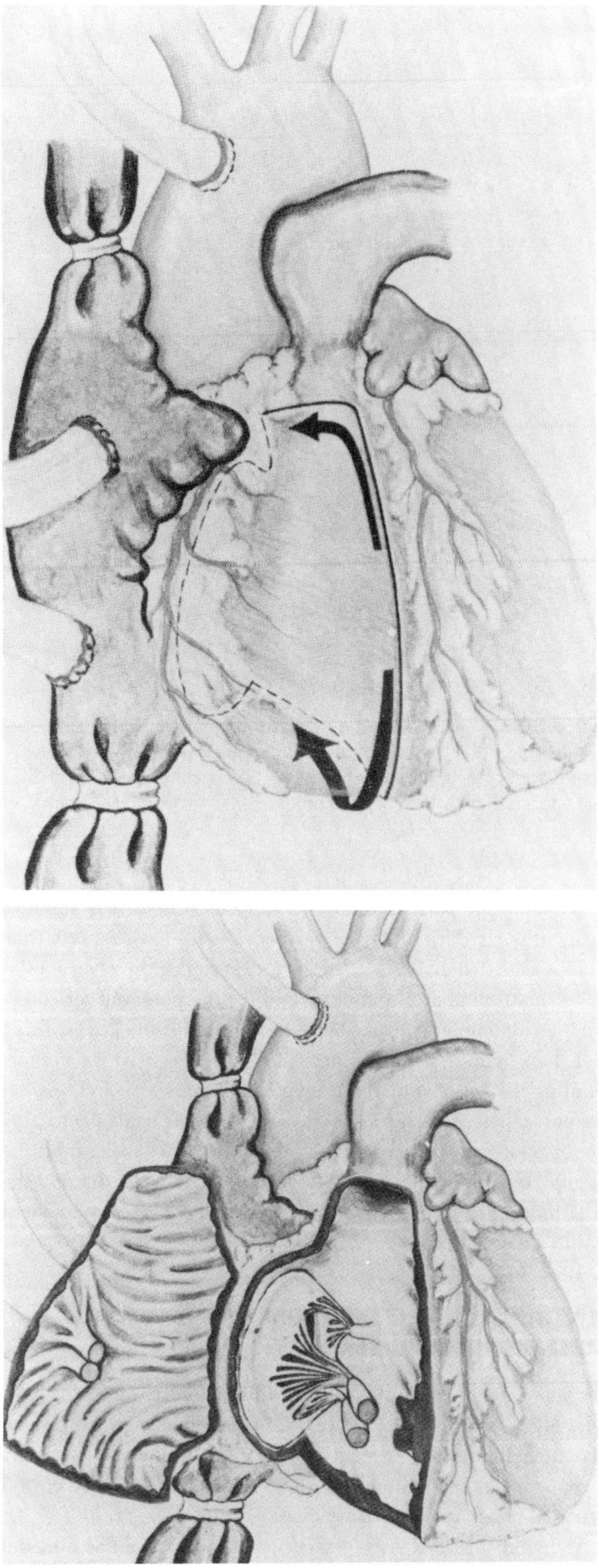

Figure 23.4. Total right ventricular disconnection. **Upper panel:** the arrows indicate the direction of the incision. **Lower panel:** the right ventricle free wall is disconnected from its attachment and the anterior papillary muscle. (From Guiraudon GM, Klein GJ, Gulamhusein SS, *et al.*: Total disconnection of the right free wall. Surgical treatment of right ventricular tachycardia associated with right ventricular dysplasia. Circulation 1983;67:463–470, reproduced with permission.)

arrhythmia surgery (92,96,97) but electrophysiology studies should be performed after valve surgery. Where the left ventricle is severely compromised and persists postoperatively despite good prosthetic valve function, concomitant automatic cardioverter-defibrillator implantation may be considered. Rarely, VT may be associated with a cardiac tumor (98,99) or with idiopathic LV aneurysm (85). The presence of a discrete lesion with healthy residual myocardium make many of these patients good candidates for ablative surgery.

Role of intraoperative cardiac mapping

Advances in intraoperative cardiac mapping technology have contributed importantly to our understanding of the genesis of VT and have served as a catalyst to improve surgical approaches and certainly allowed a more precise definition of the arrhythmogenic area. Following their introduction by Fontaine, *et al*. in 1974 (100), cardiac mapping systems were custom designed by individual centers and commercially available computerized signal acquisition and analysis cardiac mapping systems have only recently become available. Historically, the simplest available mapping system consisted of a single hand-held probe which could be manipulated over the epicardial or endocardial surface to map individual sites (Fig. 23.5) (101–103). Analog signals were recorded on paper or magnetic tape to be played back later for visual analysis. Such systems were sufficient for mapping a limited number of sites such as the atrioventricular annulus during accessory pathway ablation for the Wolff-Parkinson-White syndrome. Later on a multielectrode band array was developed for simultaneous acquisition of signals from multiple sites (101–103). However, such simple systems were difficult to apply to more complex VT surgery. Without computer on-line analysis, manual analysis of incoming signals was tedious, time consuming and difficult to perform in 30–40% of patients. Such systems utilizing limited numbers of electrodes mandated that the patient have sustained, easily inducible, monomorphic VT that was hemodynamically stable to allow complete mapping of the epicardial or endocardial surface (101–105).

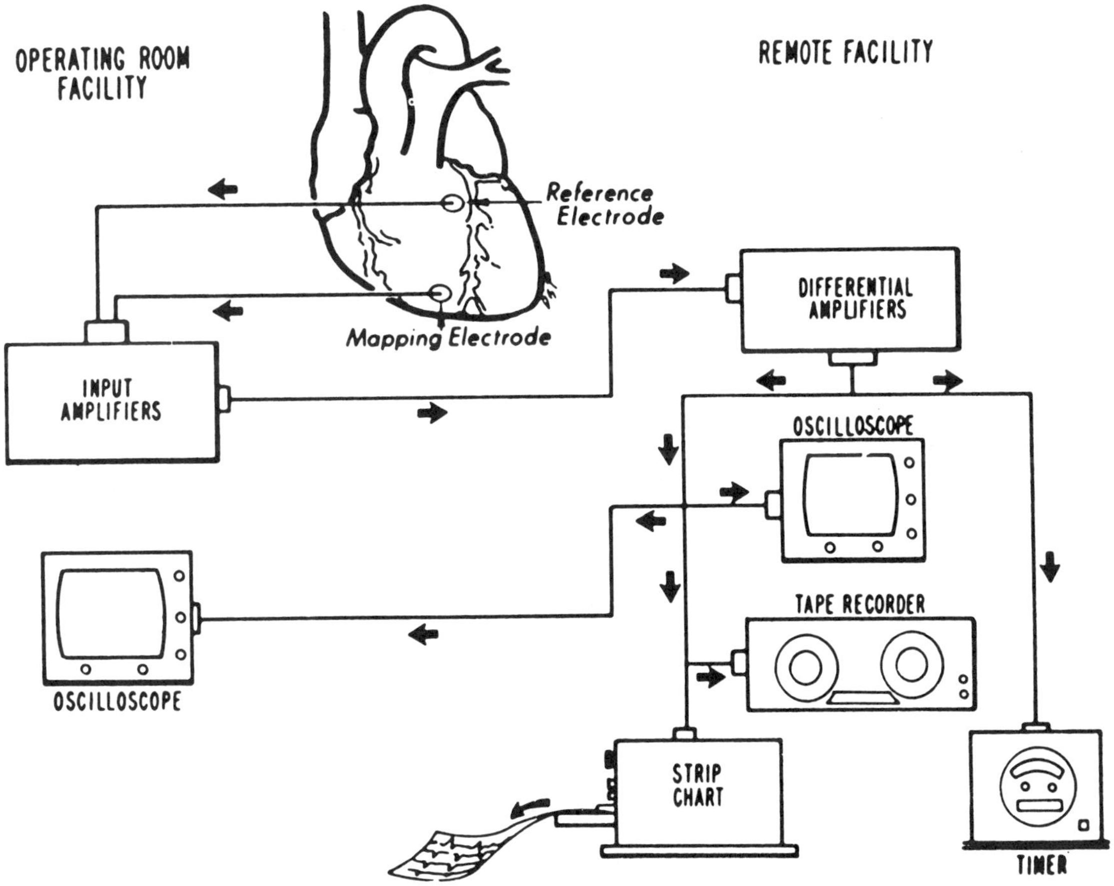

Figure 23.5. Schematic representation of the system originally used for single point intraoperative mapping. The system used a fixed reference electrode and a roving bipolar electrode. Activation times recorded from the roving electrode were compared with the activation at the fixed electrode, and the activation sequence obtained shown according to a predetermined grid. The data were sent from differential amplifiers to a digital timer which displays the signals simultaneously in two distinct oscilloscopes in the operating room and in a remote facility. Data could also be stored on a magnetic tape and retrieved to be printed when necessary. (From Gallagher JJ, Kasell J, Sealy WB, *et al*.: Epicardial mapping in the Wolff Parkinson White syndrome. Circulation 1978;57:854–866, reproduced with permission.)

The introduction of multielectrode systems using sock and balloon mounted array developed to map the entire epicardial or endocardial surface simultaneously was an important advance in surgical management (Fig. 23.6). It was then possible to map a particular VT episode using several beats of VT and a map could be generated within an acceptable period of time (106,107). In the mid-1980s, Downar introduced a custom designed computerized mapping system which provided on-line continuous display of the epicardial activation pattern using a sock electrode array simultaneous with the endocardial activation pattern mapped using a balloon-mounted electrode array introduced through an atriotomy (108–111). Placing the balloon array through the mitral or aortic valve obviated a ventriculotomy which may prevent induction of tachycardia in up to 40% of patients (111). While mapping of the epicardial activation pattern may be sufficient in many patients with VT (Fig. 23.7), it is clear that in a certain proportion of patients, the earliest site of epicardial breakthrough may be distant from the reentrant circuit (112). The ventricular wall is a three-dimensional structure and microreentrant circuits may exist at any level between the endocardial and epicardial surfaces. It has been suggested that up to 81–90% of VTs may demonstrate earliest activation on the endocardial surface (69,82,83,112). While this may be true, it remains to be seen whether endocardial activation mapping will yield an improved rate of success.

Finally, there remains some divergence of opinion regarding the necessity and value of cardiac mapping to guide VT surgery (113). A recent retrospective analysis of surgical series suggests that postoperative noninducibility is directly related to the completeness of tachycardia mapping (Fig. 23.8) (68,114) while more localized, map-guided surgical procedures are associated with lower mortality (13,75,115). The patient with a single discrete well-demarcated scar or aneurysm resulting from acute myocardial infarction who has only one VT morphology and an otherwise healthy ventricle is the optimal but infrequent patient. In this situation, cardiac mapping at the time of surgery, while helpful, likely is not critical to achieving success. On the other hand, the patient who presents with a dilated cardiomyopathy suffering from multiple VT types, some of which may be associated with hemodynamic instability, constitutes a major challenge to the surgeon. Complete ablation of VT may not be possible even after careful and complete cardiac mapping. Between the two extremes lies a spectrum of patients and one can only say that the presence of a computerized cardiac mapping system would allow any surgical service the flexibility required to handle a broad range of patients suffering from ventricular tachycardia.

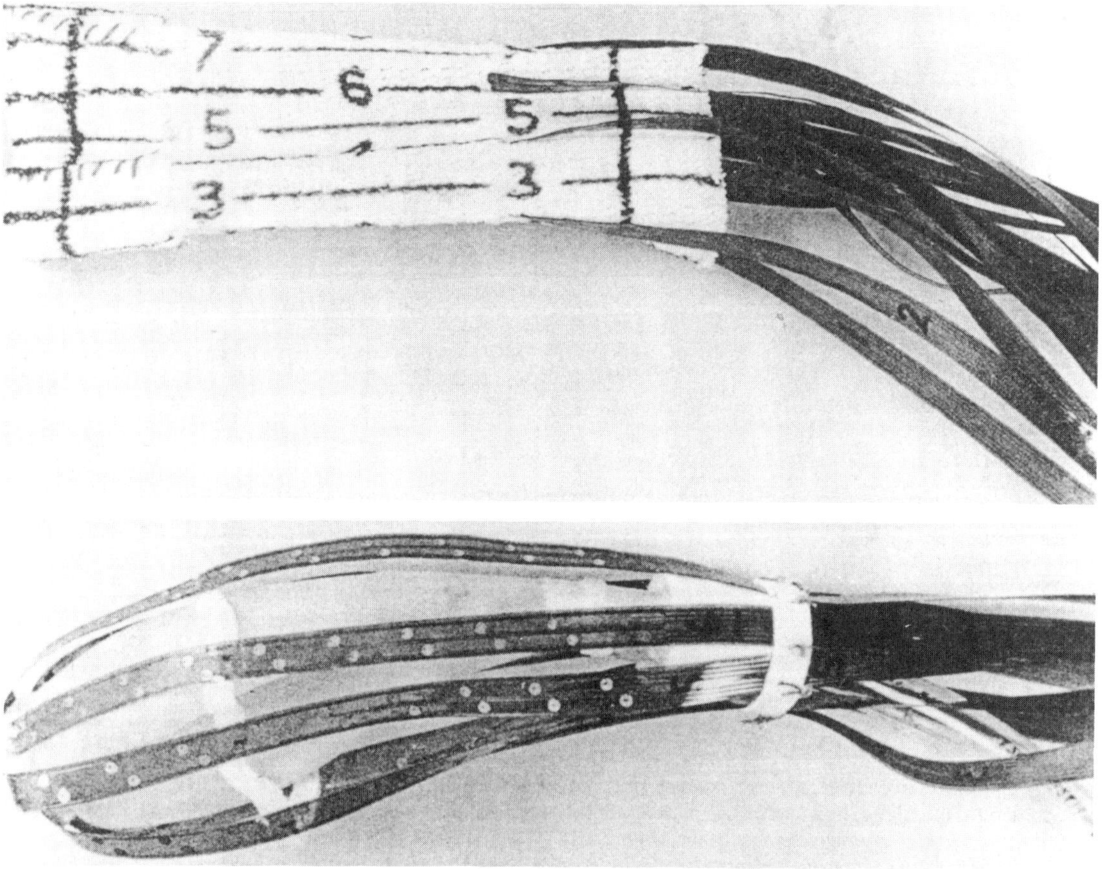

Figure 23.6. Upper panel: Sock electrode array used for epicardial mapping. Several bipolar electrode pairs are mounted on each strip. **Lower panel:** balloon electrode array used for endocardial mapping. The balloon is mounted on a semi-rigid support and is inflated only after insertion in the ventricle. Each strip consists of multiple electrode pairs. (From Lawrie GM, *et al.*: Ann Surg 1989;209:716–727, reproduced with permission.)

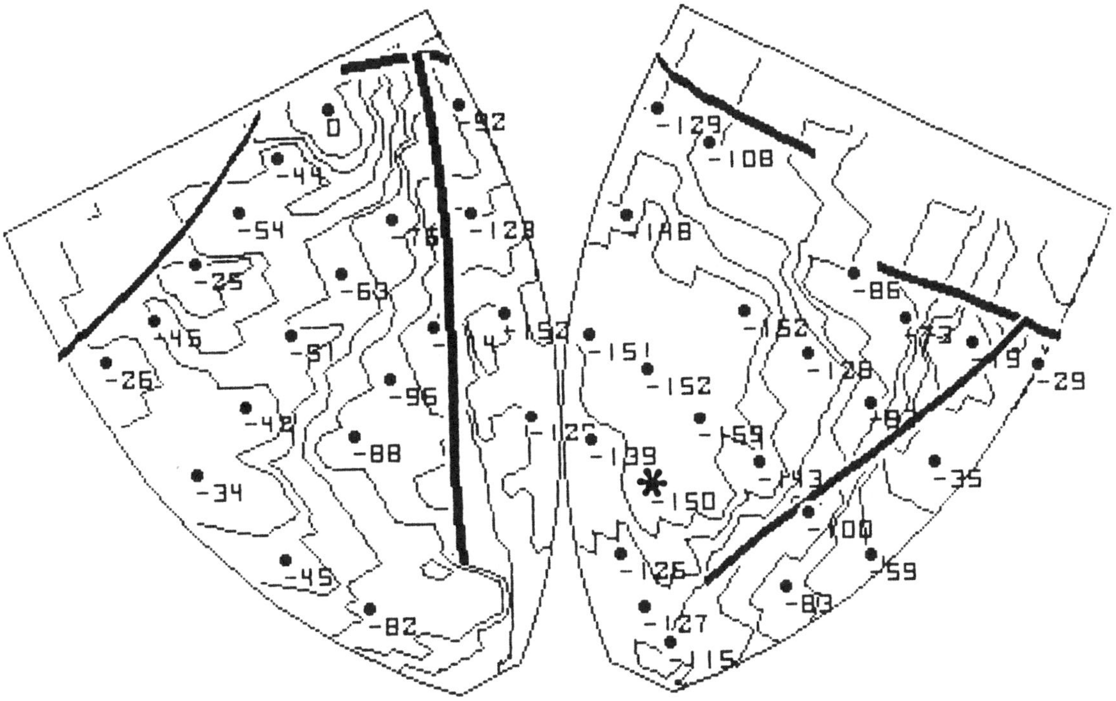

Figure 23.7. Epicardial activation sequence obtained using a sock array connected to the computerized mapping system. In the diagram the heart is cut along the posterior interventricular sulcus and unfolded for display. The **left side** of the diagram shows the right ventricle and part of the left ventricle divided by the left anterior descendant coronary artery. The **right side** of the diagram shows the left ventricle and part of the right ventricle divided by the left posterior descendant coronary artery. The *asterisk* indicates the earliest activation point near the left ventricle apex.

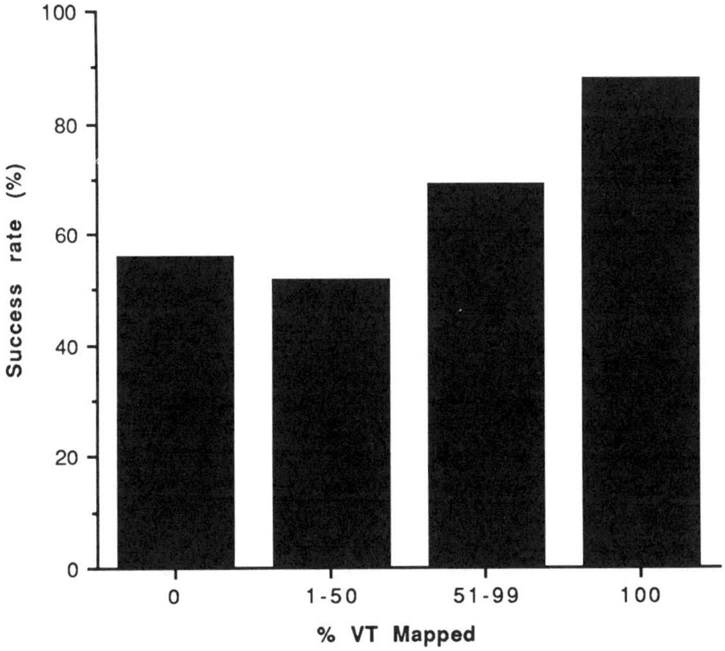

Figure 23.8. Comparison between completeness of ventricular tachycardia mapping in the operating room, expressed as percentage, and success rate of surgical therapy. Success rate increases considerably from less than 60% to approximately 90% when the completeness of the mapping approaches 100%. (Readapted by Hargrove WC, Miller JM: Risk stratification and management of patients with recurrent ventricular tachycardia and other malignant ventricular arrhythmias. Circulation 1989;79(Supp I):178–181, reproduced with permission.)

CONCLUSIONS

The development of surgical ablative techniques for life-threatening ventricular tachyarrhythmia has been an ongoing evolutionary process. At present, the optimal surgical approach should incorporate a careful selection of patients, complete intraoperative mapping and a relatively wide surgical ablation of the arrhythmogenic tissue. In the future, more sophisticated mapping systems and greater experience with new surgical procedures may yield a higher success rate and lower mortality. At the same time, developments in other treatment modalities such as catheter ablation (10,11,116), drug therapy and implantable antitachycardia devices (117) will challenge the current role of surgery in the management of VT.

References

1. Wellens H, Brugada P, Stevenson W: Programmed electrical stimulation of the heart in patients with life-threatening ventricular arrhythmias. What is the significance of induced arrhythmias and what is the correct stimulation protocol? Circulation 1985;72:1–7.
2. Panidis I, Morganroth J: Sudden death in hospitalized patients: cardiac rhythm disturbances detected by ambulatory electrocardiographic monitoring. J Am Coll Cardiol 1983;2:798–805.
3. Denniss AR, Richards DA, Cody DV, *et al.*: Prognostic significance of ventricular tachycardia and fibrillation induced at programmed stimulation and delayed potentials detected on the signal-averaged electrocardiograms of survivors of acute myocardial infarction. Circulation 1986;74:731–745.
4. Marchlinski FE, Waxman HL, Buxton AE, *et al.*: Sustained ventricular tachyarrhythmias during the early postinfarction period: electrophysiologic findings and prognosis for survival. J Am Coll Cardiol 1983;2:240–250.
5. Mitchell LB, Duff HJ, Manyari DE, *et al.*: A randomized clinical trial of the noninvasive and invasive approaches to drug therapy of ventricular tachycardia. N Engl J Med 1987;317:1681–1687.
6. Mirowski M: The automatic implantable cardioverter-defibrillator. An overview. J Am Coll Cardiol 1985;6:461–466.
7. Winkle RA, Mead RH, Ruder MA, *et al.*: Long-term outcome with the automatic implantable cardioverter-defibrillator. J Am Coll Cardiol 1989; 13:1353–1361.
8. Kelly PA, Cannom DS, Garan H, *et al.*: The automatic implantable cardioverter-defibrillator: efficacy, complications and survival in patients with malignant ventricular arrhythmias. J Am Coll Cardiol 1988;11:1278–1286.
9. Marchlinksi FE, Flores BT, Buxton AE, *et al.*: The automatic implantable cardioverter-defibrillator: efficacy, complications, and device failures. Ann Intern Med 1986;104:481–488.
10. Morady F, Scheinman MM, DiCarlo LA, *et al.*: Catheter ablation of ventricular tachycardia with intracardiac shocks: results in 33 patients. Circulation 1987;75:1037–1049.
11. Belhassen B, Miller HI, Geller E, *et al.*: Transcatheter electrical shock ablation of ventricular tachycardia. J Am Coll Cardiol 1986;7:1347–1355.
12. Wellens HJJ, Bar FWHM, Vanagt EJDM, *et al.*: Medical treatment of ventricular tachycardia: considerations in the selection of patients for surgical treatment. Am J Cardiol 1982;49:186–193.
13. Borgreffe M, Podczeck A, Ostermeyer J, *et al.*: Long-term results of electrophysiologically guided antitachycardia surgery in ventricular tachyarrhythmias. A collaborative report on 665 patients. In G. Breithart, M. Borgreffe, Zipes DP (eds): Non pharmacological therapy of tachyarrhythmias. Mt. Kisco, NY, Futura Publishing Co. 1987:109–132.
14. Miller JM, Marchlinski FE, Buxton AE, *et al.*: Relationship between the 12-lead electrocardiogram during ventricular tachycardia and endocardial site of origin in patients with coronary artery disease. Circulation 1986; 77(4):759–766.
15. Woelfel A, Foster JR, Simpson RJ, *et al.*: Reproducibility and treatment of exercise-induced ventricular tachycardia. Am J Cardiol 1984;53:751–56.
16. Gaffney FA, Nicod P, Lin JC, *et al.*: Noninvasive recognition of the parchment right ventricle (Uhl' anomaly, arrhythmogenic right ventricular dysplasia) syndrome. Clin Cardiol 1983;6:235–242.
17. Manyari DE, Duff HJ, Kostuk WJ, *et al.*: Usefulness of noninvasive studies for diagnosis of right ventricular dysplasia. Am J Cardiol 1986;57:1147.
18. Robertson JH, Bardy GH, German LD, *et al.*: Comparison of two dimensional echocardiographic and angiographic findings in arrhythmogenic right ventricular dysplasia. Am J Cardiol 1985;55:1506–1508.
19. Strain JE, Grose RM, Factor SM, *et al.*: Results of endomyocardial biopsy in patients with spontaneous ventricular tachycardia but without apparent structural heart disease. Circulation 1983;68:1171–1181.
20. Faitelson L, Pacifico A, Weilbacher D, *et al.*: Endomyocardial biopsy in patients with malignant ventricular arrhythmias without coronary artery disease. Circulation 1988;78(Suppl 2):240.
21. Kim AG: The management of patients with life-threatening tachyarrhythmias: programmed stimulation or Holter monitoring (either or both?). Circulation 1987;76:1 5.
22. Swerdlow CD, Peterson J: Prospective comparison of Holter montoring and electrophysiologic study in patients with coronary artery disease and sustained ventricular tachyarrhythmias. Am J Cardiol 1985;56:577–585.
23. Buxton AE, Waxman HL, Marchlinski FE, *et al.*: Role of triple extrastimuli during electrophysiologic study of patients with documented sustained ventricular tachyarrhythmias. Circulation 1984;69:532–540.
24. Wilber DJ, Garan H, Finkelstein D, *et al.*: Out-of-hospital cardiac arrest. Use of electrophysiologic testing in the prediction of long term outcome. N Engl J Med 1986;318:19–24.
25. Horowitz LN: Intracardiac electrophysiologic studies for drug selection in ventricular tachycardia. Circulation 1987;75(Suppl III):III-134-6.
26. Graboys T: Long-term survival of patients with malignant ventricular arrhythmia treated with antiarrhythmic drugs. Am J Cardiol 1982;50:437–443.
27. Reddy CP, Chen TJ, Guillory WR: Electrophysiologic studies in selection of antiarrhythmic agents: use with ventricular tachycardia. PACE 1986;9:756–763.
28. Rae AP, Greenspan AM, Spielman SR, *et al.*: Antiarrhythmic drug efficacy for ventricular tachyarrhythmias associated with coronary artery disease as assessed by electrophysiologic studies. Am J Cardiol 1985;55:1994–1999.
29. Waller TJ, Kay HR, Spielman SR, *et al.*: Reduction in sudden death and total mortality by antiarrhythmic therapy evaluated by electrophysiologic drug testing: criteria of efficacy in patients with sustained ventricular tachyarrhythmia. J Am Coll Cardiol 1987;10:1083–1089.
30. Garan H, Stavens CS, McGovern B, *et al.*: Reproducibility of ventricular tachycardia suppression by antiarrhythmic drug therapy during serial electrophysiologic testing in coronary artery disease. Am J Cardiol 1986; 58:977–980.
31. Oseran DS, Gang E, Rosenthal ME, *et al.*: Electropharmacologic testing in sustained ventricular tachycardia associated with coronary heart disease: value of the response to intravenous procainamide in predicting the response to oral procainamide and oral quinidine treatment. Am J Cardiol 1985;56:883–886.
32. Waxman HL, Buxton AE, Sadowski LM, *et al.*: The response in procainamide during electrophysiologic study for sustained ventricular tachyarrhythmias predicts the response to other medication. Circulation 1982;67:30–37.
33. Kuchar DL, Rottman J, Berger E, *et al.*: Prediction of successful suppression of sustained ventricular tachyarrhythmias by serial drug testing from data derived at the initial electrophysiologic study. J Am Coll Cardiol 1988;12:982–988.
34. Josephson ME, Horowitz LN, Spielman SR, *et al.*: The role of catheter mapping in the preoperative evaluation of ventricular tachycardia. Am J Cardiol 1982;49:207–220.
35. Waxman HL, Josephson ME: Ventricular activation during ventricular

endocardial pacing: I. Electrocardiographic patterns related to the site of pacing. Am J Cardiol 1982;50:1–10.

36. Josephson ME, Gottlieb CD: Ventricular tachycardia associated with coronary artery disease. In Zipes DP, Jalife J (eds): Cardiac Electrophysiology: from Cell to Bedside. WB Saunders, Philadelphia, 1990:571–580.
37. Marchlinski FE: Ventricular tachycardia: clinical presentation, course, and therapy. In Zipes DP, Jalife J (eds): Cardiac Electrophysiology: from Cell to Bedside. WB Saunders, Philadelphia, 1990:756–777.
38. Josephson ME, Horowitz LN, Farshidi A: Continuous electrical activity: a mechanism of recurrent ventricular tachycardia. Circulation 1978;57:659–666.
39. Josephson ME, Wit AL: Fractioned electrical activity and continuous electrical activity: fact or artifact? Circulation 1984;70:529–532.
40. Cassidy DM, Vassallo JA, Buxton AE, *et al.*: The value of catheter mapping during sinus rhythm to localize site of origin of ventricular tachycardia. Circulation 1984;63:1103.
41. Klein H, Karp RB, Kouchoukos NT, *et al.*: Intraoperative electrophysiologic mapping of the ventricle during sinus rhythm in patients with a previous myocardial infarction: Identification of the electrophysiologic substrate of ventricular arrhythmias. Circulation 1982,66:847–853.
42. Miller JM, Gottlieb CD, Hargrove WE, *et al.*: Factors influencing operative mortality in surgery for ventricular tachycardia. Circulation 1988;78:II-44.
43. Cox LJ: Patient selection criteria and results of surgery for refractory ischemic ventricular tachycardia. Circulation 1989;79(Suppl I):163-I-177.
44. Lawrie GM, Wyndham CRC: Importance of preoperative variables in predicting operative mortality in direct surgery for drug resistent ventricular tachycardia (Abstr). J Am Coll Cardiol 1988;11:113.
45. Balooki H, Palatiano GM, Zaman L, *et al.*: Surgical management of postmyocardial infarction ventricular tachyarrhythmia by myocardial debulking, septal isolation, and myocardial revascularization. J Thorac Cardiovasc Surg 1986;92:716–725.
46. Brawley R, Magovern G, Gott V, *et al.*: Left ventricular aneurysmectomy: factors influencing post-operative results. J Thorac Cardiovasc Surg 1983;85:712–717.
47. Couch OA: Cardiac aneurysm with ventricular tachycardia and subsequent excision of aneurysm. Circulation 1959;20:251–253.
48. Scherlang BJ, el-Sherif N, Hope R, *et al.*: Characterization and localization of ventricular arrhythmias resulting from myocardial ischemia and infarction. Circ Res 1974;35:372–383.
49. Horowitz LN, Josephson ME, Harken AN: Epicardial and endocardial activation during sustained ventricular tachycardia in man. Circulation 1980;61:1227.
50. de Bakker JMT, Janse MJ, van Capelle FJL, *et al.*: Endocardial mapping by simultaneous recording of endocardial electrograms during cardiac surgery for ventricular aneurysm. J Am Coll Cardiol 1983;19:947.
51. Guiraudon GM, Fontaine G, Frank R, *et al.*: Encircling endocardial ventriculotomy. A new surgical treatment for life-threatening ventricular tachycardias resistant to medical treatment following myocardial infarction. Ann Thorac Surg 1978;26:438–444.
52. Ungerleider RM, Holman WL, Stanley TE III, *et al.*: Encircling endocardial ventriculotomy for refractory ischemic ventricular tachycardia. II. Effects on regional myocardial blood flow. J Thorac Cardiovasc Surg 1982;83:850–856.
53. Ungerleider RM, Holman WL, Calcagno D, *et al.*: Encircling endocardial ventriculotomy for refractory ischemic ventricular tachycardia. II. Effects on regional left ventricular function. J Thorac Cardiovasc Surg 1982;83:857–864.
54. Cox JL, Gallagher JJ, Ungerleider RM, *et al.*: Encircling endocardial ventriculotomy for refractory ischemic ventricular tachycardia. IV. Clinical indication, surgical technique, mechanism of action, and results. J Thorac Cardiovasc Surg 1982;83:865–872.
55. Guiraudon GM, Klein GJ, Sharma AD, *et al.*: Use of old and new anatomic, electrophysiologic, and technical knowledge to develop operative approaches to tachycardia. In Brugada P, Wellens HJJ (eds): Cardiac Arrhythmias: Where to Go from Here? Mount Kisco, NY, Futura Publishing Co., 1987:639–652.
56. Guiraudon GM, Klein GJ, Jones DL, *et al.*: Encircling endocardial cryoablation for ventricular arrhythmia after myocardial infarction: further experience (Abstr). Circulation 1985;72(Suppl 3):322.
57. Ostermeyer J, Breithardt G, Borgreffe M, *et al.*: Surgical treatment of ventricular tachycardias: complete versus partial encircling endocardial ventriculotomy. J Thorac Cardiovasc Surg 1984;87:517–525.
58. Ostermeyer J, Borgreffe M, Breithardt, *et al.*: Direct operations for the management of life-threatening ischemic ventricular tachycardia. J Thorac Surg 1987;94:848–865.
59. Harken AH, Josephson ME, Horowitz LN: Surgical endocardial resection for the treatment of malignant ventricular tachycardia. Ann Surg 1979;190–456.
60. Josephson ME, Harken AH, Horowitz LN: Endocardial excision. A new surgical technique for the treatment of recurrent ventricular tachycardia. Circulation 1979;60:1430–1439.
61. Landymore R, Kinley CE, Gardner M: Encircling endocardial resection with complete removal of endocardial scar without intraoperative mapping for the ablation of drug-resistant ventricular tachycardias. J Thorac Cardiovasc Surg 1985;89:18–24.
62. Zee-Cheng CS, Kouchoukos NT, Connors JP, *et al.*: Treatment of life-threatening ventricular arrhythmias with nonguided surgery supported by electrophysiologic testing and drug therapy. J Am Coll Cardiol 1989;13: 153–162.
63. Moran JM, Kehoe RF, Loeb JM, *et al.*: Extended endocardial resection for the treatment of ventricular tachycardia and ventricular fibrillation. Ann Thorac Surg 1982;43:538–562.
64. Landymore RW, Gardner MA, McIntyre AJ, *et al.*: Surgical intervention for drug-resistant ventricular tachycardia. J Am Coll Cardiol 1990;16:37–41.
65. Garan H, Nguyen K, McGovern B, *et al.*: Perioperative and long-term results after electrophysiologically directed ventricular surgery for recurrent ventricular tachycardia. J Am Coll Cardiol 1986;8:201–209.
66. Hargrove WC III: Surgery for ventricular tachycardia associated with ischemic heart disease. In Zipes DP, Jalife J (eds): Cardiac Electrophysiology: from Cell to Bedside. WB Saunders, Philadelphia, 1990:924–925.
67. Hargrove WC III: Surgery for ischemic ventricular tachycardia. Operative techniques and long-term results. Seminars in Thoracic and Cardiovascular Surgery 1989;1:83–87.
68. Hargrove WC, Miller JM: Risk stratification and management of patients with recurrent ventricular tachycardia and other malignant ventricular arrhythmias. Circulation 1989;79(Suppl I):178–181.
69. Downar E, Harris L, Michelborough LL, *et al.*: Endocardial mapping of ventricular tachycardia in the intact human ventricle. Evidence for a reentrant mechanism. J Am Coll Cardiol 1988;11:783–791.
70. Kron IL, Lerman BB, Nolan SP, *et al.*: Sequential endocardial resection for the surgical treatment of refractory ventricular tachycardia. J Thorac Cardiovasc Surg 1987;94:843–847.
71. Yee ES, Schienman MM, Griffin JC, *et al.*: Surgical options for treating ventricular tachyarrhythmia and sudden death. J Thorac Cardiovasc Surg 1987;94:866–873.
72. Manolis AS, Rastegar H, Payne D, *et al.*: Surgical therapy for drug-refractory ventricular tachycardia: results with mapping-guided subendocardial resection. J Am Coll Cardiol 1989;14:199–208.
73. Bourke JP, Hilton CJ, McComb J, *et al.*: Surgery for control of recurrent life-threatening ventricular tachyarrhythmias within 2 months of myocardial infarction. J Am Coll Cardiol 1990;16:42–48.
74. Haines DE, Lerman BB, Kron IL, *et al.*: Surgical ablation of ventricular tachycardia with sequential map-guided subendocardial resection: electrophysiologic assessment and long-term follow-up. Circulation 1988;77:131–141.
75. Harken AH, Horowitz LN, Josephson ME: Comparison of standard aneurysmectomy with directed endocardial resection for the treatment of recur-

rent sustained ventricular tachycardia. J Thorac Cardiovasc Surg 1980;80:527–534.

76. Krafchek J, Lawrie GM, Roberts R, *et al.*: Surgical ablation of ventricular tachycardia: improved results with a map-directed regional approach. Circulation 1986;73:1239–1247.

77. Klein GJ, Harrison L, Ideker RF, *et al.*: Reaction of the myocardium to cryosurgery: electrophysiologic and arrhythmogenic potential. Circulation 1970;59:364–372. Mt. Kisco, NY: Futura Publishing Co., 1987;109–132.

78. Krafchek J, Lawrie GM, Wyndham CRC: Cryoablation of arrhythmias from the interventricular septum: initial experience with a biventricular approach. J Thorac Cardiovasc Surg 1986;91:419–427.

79. Guiraudon GM, Jones DL, Klein GJ, *et al.*: Feasibility of cryoablation of the posterior papillary muscle in the dog (Abstr). J Am Coll Cardiol 1986;7(Suppl A):236A.

80. Caceres J, Werner P, Jazayeri M, *et al.*: Efficacy of cryosurgery alone for refractory monomorphic sustained ventricular tachycardia due to inferior wall infarction. J Am Coll Cardiol 1988;11:1254—1259.

81. Caceres J, Akhtar M, Werner P, *et al.*: Cryoablation of refractory sustained ventricular tachycardia due to coronary artery disease. Am J Cardiol 1989;63:296–300.

82. Pagé PL, Cardinal R, Shenasa M, *et al.*: Surgical treatment of ventricular tachycardia. Regional cryoablation guided by computerized epicardial and endocardial mapping. Circulation 1989;80(Suppl I):124-I-134.

83. Saksena S, Hussain MS, Gielchinsky I, *et al.*: Intraoperative mapping-guided argon laser ablation of malignant ventricular tachycardia. Am J Cardiol 1987;59:78–83.

84. Selle JG, Svenson RH, Sealy WC, *et al.*: Successful clinical laser ablation of ventricular tachycardia: a promising new therapeutic method. Ann Thorac Surg 1986;42:380–384.

85. Guiraudon GM, Klein GJ, Sharma AD, *et al.*: Surgical treatment of ventricular arrhythmia in the absence of coronary artery disease. In Iwa T, Fontaine G (eds): Cardiac Arrhythmias: Recent Progress in Investigation and Management. New York:Elsevier Science Publisher, 1988;265–269.

86. Guiraudon GM, Klein GJ, Sharma AD, *et al.*: Surgical therapy for arrhythmogenic right ventricular adiposis. Eur Heart J 1989;10(Suppl D):82–83.

87. Manyari De, Klein GJ, Gulamshusein S, *et al.*: Arrhythmogenic right ventricular dysplasia: a generalized cardiomyopathy? Circulation 1983;68: 251–257.

88. Guiraudon GM, Fontaine G, Frank R, *et al.*: Surgical treatment of ventricular tachycardia guided by ventricular mapping in 23 patients without coronary artery disease. Ann Thorac Surg 1981;32:439–450.

89. Guiraudon GM, Klein GJ, Gulamhusein SS, *et al.*: Total disconnection of the right free wall. Surgical treatment of right ventricular tachycardia associated with right ventricular dysplasia. Circulation 1983;67:463–470.

90. Cox JL, Bardy GH, Damiano RJ, *et al.*: Right ventricular isolation procedures for nonischemic ventricular tachycardia. J Thorac Cardiovasc Surg 1985;90:212.

91. Jones DL, Guiraudon GM, Klein GJ: Total disconnection of the right ventricular free wall: physiological consequences in the dog. Am Heart J 1984;107:1169–1177.

92. Lawrie GM, Pacifico A, Kaushik R: Results of direct surgical ablation of ventricular tachycardia not due to ischemic heart disease: Ann Surg 1989;6:716–725.

93. Garson A Jr, Randall DC, Gillette PC, *et al.*: Prevention of sudden death after repair of Tetralogy of Fallot: treatment of ventricular arrhythmias. J Am Coll Cardiol 1985;6:221—227.

94. Garson A Jr, Porter CJ, Gillette PC, *et al.*: Induction of ventricular tachycardia during electrophysiologic study after repair of Tetralogy of Fallot. J Am Coll Cardiol 1983;1:1493–1502.

95. Harken AH, Horowitz LN, Josephson ME: Surgical correction of recurrent sustained ventricular tachycardia following complete repair of Tetralogy of Fallot. J Thorac Cardiovasc Surg 1980;80:779–781.

96. von Olshausen K, Amann E, Hoffman M, *et al.*: Ventricular arrhythmias before and late after valve replacement. Am J Cardiol 1984;54:142–146.

97. Gradman AH, Harbison MA, Berger HJ, *et al.*: Ventricular arrhythmias late after aortic valve replacement and their relation to left ventricular performance. Am J Cardiol 1981;48:824–831.

98. Strauss R, Merliss R: Primary tumors of the heart. Arch Pathol 1945;39:74–78.

99. Reece IJ, Cooley DA, Frazier OH, *et al.*: Cardiac tumors: clinical spectrum and prognosis of lesion other than classical benign myxoma in 20 patients. J Thorac Cardiovasc Surg 1984;88:439–446.

100. Fontaine G, Guiraudon G, Frank R, *et al.*: La cartographie epicardique et le traitement chirurgical por simple ventriculotomie de certaines tachycardies ventriculaires rebelles par reentree. Arch Mal Coeur 1975;68:113–124.

101. Gallagher JJ, Kasell JH, Cox JL, *et al.*: Techniques of intraoperative electrophysiologic mapping. Am J Cardiol 1982;49:221–240.

102. Tyagi S, Sharma AD, Guiraudon GM, *et al.*: Intraoperative cardiac mapping of preexcitation syndromes and ventricular tachycardia. J Electrophysiol 1989;3:47–64.

103. Cox JL: The evolution of intraoperative mapping techniques in cardiac arrhythmia surgery. Semin Thorac Cardiovasc Surg 1989;1:11–20.

104. Ideker RE, Smith WM, Wallace AG, *et al.*: A computerized method for the rapid display of ventricular activation during the intraoperative study of arrhythmias. Circulation 1979;59:449–458.

105. Smith WM, Ideker RE, Kinicki RE, *et al.*: A computer system for the intraoperative mapping of ventricular arrhythmias. Comput Biomed Res 1980;13:61.

106. Mickleborough LL: Surgery for ventricular tachycardia: intraoperative mapping techniques. Semin Thorac Cardiovasc Surg 1989;1:74–82.

107. Smith WM, Wharton JM, Blanchard SM, *et al.*: Direct Cardiac Mapping. In Zipes DP, Jalife J (eds): Cardiac Electrophysiology: from Cell to Bedside. WB Saunders, Philadelphia, 1990:849–858.

108. Downar E, Parson ID, Mickleborough LL, *et al.*: On-line epicardial mapping of intraoperative ventricular arrhythmias. Initial clinical experience. J Am Coll Cardiol 1984;4:703–714.

109. Mickleborough LL, Harris L, Downar E, *et al.*: A new intraoperative approach for endocardial mapping of ventricular tachycardia. J Thorac Cardiovasc Surg 1988;95:271–280.

110. Mickleborough L, Chen T, Gray G: Experience with simultaneous RV and LV endocardial mapping during surgery for ventricular tachycardia (VT). PACE 1991;14(Abstr II):646.

111. Mickleborough LL, Usui A, Downar E, *et al.*: Transatrial balloon technique for activation mapping during operations for recurrent ventricular tachycardia. J Thorac Cardiovasc Surg 1990;99:227–233.

112. Spielman SR, Michelson EI, Horowitz LN, *et al.*: The limitations of epicardial mapping as a guide to the surgical therapy of ventricular tachycardia. Circulation 1978;57:566.

113. Josephson ME, Horowitz LN, Spielman SR, *et al.*: Comparison of endocardial catheter mapping with intraoperative mapping of ventricular tachycardias. Circulation 1980;61:395.

114. Cox JL: Ventricular tachycardia surgery: a review of the first decade and a suggested contemporary approach. Semin Thorac Cardiovasc Surg 1989;1:97–103.

115. Swerdlow CD, Mason JW, Stintson EB, *et al.*: Results of operations for ventricular tachycardia in 105 patients. J Thorac Cardiovasc Surg 1986; 92:105–113.

116. Fontaine G, Frank R, Tonet J, *et al.*: Fulguration of chronic ventricular tachycardia: results of forty-seven consecutive cases with follow-up ranging from 11 to 65 months. In Zipes DP, Jalife J (eds): Cardiac Electrophysiology: from Cell to Bedside. WB Saunders, Philadelphia, 1990:979–985.

117. Hammon JW: The role of the automatic implantable cardioverter-defibrillator in the treatment of ventricular tachycardia. Semin Thorac Cardiovasc Surg 1989;1:88–96.

24

CATHETER ABLATION FOR ARRHYTHMIAS

Andrea Natale, M.D., George J. Klein, M.D., F.R.C.P.(C), F.A.C.C.,
Raymond Yee, M.D., F.R.C.P.(C), F.A.C.C., and Mark Wathen, M.D.

Inadvertent production of atrioventricular (AV) block after cardioversion during electrophysiologic testing (1) suggested the feasibility of ablation of the AV node by energy delivery through a catheter. Atrioventricular node ablation using direct current (DC) high-energy shock through an electrode catheter was initially demonstrated in animals by Gonzales, *et al.* (2) and subsequently in patients by Scheinman, *et al.* (3) and Gallagher (4). This technique involved delivering shock through a standard electrode catheter interfaced with a standard cardiac defibrillator. Catheter ablation has evolved considerably since these early reports and has become standard therapy for many arrhythmias.

ENERGY SOURCES AND TECHNICAL ASPECTS

The original ablation system utilized a standard defibrillator delivering a DC high-energy shock through an electrode catheter at the target site. Multiple physical events occur which contribute to the mechanism of tissue injury with this method (5,6). There is an early phase of energy transfer characterized by resistive heating at the catheter-tissue interface lasting 1–2 msec (7). Vaporization of blood in contact with the catheter generates small quantities of gas which insulate the electrode from blood. This is associated with impedance rise and peak voltage of several thousand volts (8). Sparks are generated with increases in temperature up to 1700°C and pressures greater than 38 atm observed (9). Although barotrauma and arcing have been considered important mechanisms of injury, the high electrical field generated during energy discharge may also be important (10,11). Excessive tissue destruction leading to complications with this technique have been attributed to arcing and barotrauma (12–15). Both changes in the shape and polarity of the discharge (16,17) and changes in the geometry of the electrode (18) were attempted to minimize these effects. Rowland, *et al.* (19) suggested that reducing the duration of the shock waveform to 10 msec using lower energies with a brief time-constant capacitative discharge limits gas formation and provides adequate ablation with fewer complications.

Radiofrequency energy is currently the most widely used energy source for ablation. This energy is generated over a frequency range of 300 KHz–2 MHz and is very similar to that used in standard cautery or coagulation units. In contrast to DC shock, radiofrequency energy is relatively painless, does not result in barotrauma, and produces small, discrete lesions (20). D'Arsonval was the first to demonstrate that radiofrequency current can be passed through humans without untoward effects (21). Clark reported the potential usefulness of radiofrequency energy to cut and coagulate living tissue in 1911 (22) and this technique was established in medicine after the work of Cushing and Bovie in 1928 (23). The feasibility of producing radiofrequency lesions through a catheter was appreciated in 1979 by Geddes, *et al.* who inadvertently shunted radiofrequency current through a pacing electrode (24).

Tissue damage with radiofrequency energy results from resistive energy transfer which generates heat at the electrode-tissue interface (25). Temperature at the catheter tip rises rapidly in the first 5 secs. Temperatures greater than 50°C are required to permanently injure tissue whereas temperatures exceeding 120°C result in carbonization and uncontrolled tissue disruption (20,26,27). Whether a radiofrequency unit cuts or coagulates depends on waveform and power output (20). The high-voltage, continuous, unmodulated sinusoidal current results in rapid temperature rise to the boiling point which produces vapor bubbles at the catheter. This leads to impedance rise associated with gas ionization and sparking. Continuous sparking provides the cutting ability of such units (28). Superficial coagulation of tissue is achieved by a damped, modulated current which consists of bursts of energy repeated at regular intervals. The pause between bursts prevents excessive temperature rise and arcing (28). Catheter ablation utilizes similar but unmodulated waveform and lower energy levels. Impedance is closely monitored during clinical ablation since sudden impedance rise is associated with arcing and potentially excessive tissue destruction

(29). This impedance rise is usually related to coagulum at the tip of the catheter (20). The size of the radiofrequency lesion depends on power, pulse duration and contact pressure at the tissue-electrode interface (30). A setting of 5 watts for at least 5 secs is required for some tissue damage. A lesion rapidly increases in size during the first 5 secs and reaches its maximum size within 30 to 40 secs (31). The size of a lesion is dependent upon the size of the ablating electrode with a 4-mm length shown to be optimal for a given fixed current (32,33).

It has been suggested that monitoring of temperature at the tip of the ablation catheter is the best guide to ablation as tissue injury results mainly by heat production (34). Rise in temperature reflects delivery of electrical energy to the myocardium and correlates better with lesion size than power setting (35). Maintaining temperature below the boiling point also prevents impedance rise and coagulum formation (36). Positioning of the catheter at the target site is another critical consideration in achieving a successful ablation. The development of tip-deflectable catheters has greatly facilitated catheter positioning at the desired site. Undoubtedly, further evolution in catheters allowing multidirectional deflection or region specific design will further simplify ablation procedures (37–39).

The widespread use of catheter ablation for rhythm problems in all age groups has raised concern about the long-term effects of radiation exposure required by the procedure. Calkins, *et al.* (40) evaluated the amount of radiation received by patients and physicians during ablation sessions. They estimated that a fluoroscopy time in the order of 44 min provided a risk of malignancy or genetic defect comparable to that after coronary angioplasty and recommended that individual physicians not perform more than 15 ablations per month. Undoubtedly, further refinements in ablation techniques will reduce the time of ablation sessions and advances in fluoroscopy technology will further minimize radiation exposure. Catheter ablation has become front-line therapy for patients with problematic supraventricular tachycardia associated with Wolff-Parkinson-White syndrome or AV nodal reentry. It is also proving increasingly useful in some patients with atrial flutter, ectopic atrial tachycardia, and ventricular tachycardia.

PREEXCITATION SYNDROMES

An overwhelming majority of preexcitation syndromes are related to an accessory A-V pathway, a muscular strand providing abnormal continuity between the atria and ventricles at the AV rings. This pathway is amenable to destruction by a discrete lesion with cure of tachycardia. The ablation catheter is guided to the area of interest under fluoroscopic control with the optimal site established by electrogram morphology recorded at the catheter tip. Early experience using DC shock energy was disappointing with low success rates and potentially disastrous complications occurring during energy delivery into the coronary sinus (12–15). Excellent success was achieved by utilizing endocardial shocks near the AV ring and avoiding high-energy shocks within the coronary sinus although the technique was still burdened by a small incidence of serious complications including cardiac tamponade, late ventricular fibrillation, and inadvertent AV block (41–43). More recently, Lemery and coworkers used low-energy, short-pulse techniques and achieved excellent results but not entirely free from potentially serious complications (44).

The radiofrequency technique has virtually supplanted the DC shock technique for accessory pathway ablation. Borggrefe, *et al.* (45) first described successful ablation of an accessory pathway using this technique in 1987. Subsequently, excellent results have been reported in larger numbers of patients using this technique with success rates in excess of 90% and a nonfatal complication rate in the range of up to 4% (46–51). However, complications have included myocardial infarction, myocardial perforation, aortic valve perforation and systemic embolus. Success rates with left lateral accessory pathways approach 100% with somewhat lesser success at other locations.

Localization of the accessory pathway is achieved by standard electrophysiologic techniques (52). Because of the relatively small size of the ablative lesion, precise mapping and stable catheter positioning are required. The ablation catheter may be advanced to the atrioventricular ring underneath the mitral or tricuspid leaflets (ventricular approach) or over the leaflets (atrial approach). Localization can be achieved by mapping during atrial rhythm (anterograde mapping) or during ventricular rhythm or reciprocating tachycardia (retrograde mapping). The appearance of a "ring" electrogram displaying prominent atrial and ventricular deflections indicates proximity to the atrioventricular border. Criteria for accessory pathway localization during anterograde mapping include: (a) the presence of accessory pathway potential, (b) a satisfactory "ring electrogram" as described above, (c) earliest ventricular activity on the local electrogram with ventricular activation occurring prior to the onset of the delta wave on the surface electrocardiogram (ECG) (Fig. 24.1).

The criteria during retrograde mapping include: (a) presence of accessory pathway potential, (b) recording of a ring electrogram, (c) site of earliest recorded atrial activation (shortest ventriculoatrial interval) (Fig. 24.2).

A transseptal approach to the left atrium is useful for ablation of left-sided accessory pathways from the atrial side and is a reasonable alternative to ablation under the mitral valve leaflets via a retrograde aortic approach (53). The anteroseptal pathway can be approached from either the atrial side or the ventricular side (i.e., underneath the tricuspid leaflet). These pathways are near the His bundle and the ideal electrogram at this site includes a prominent accessory pathway potential with a smaller, more far field His potential (48–51). Right-sided accessory pathways may be technically difficult. A subvalvular approach is complicated by right ventricular trabeculation and catheter stability may be a problem with the atrial approach. Finally, posteroseptal pathways can be challenging and require very careful mapping and a versatile approach. These pathways

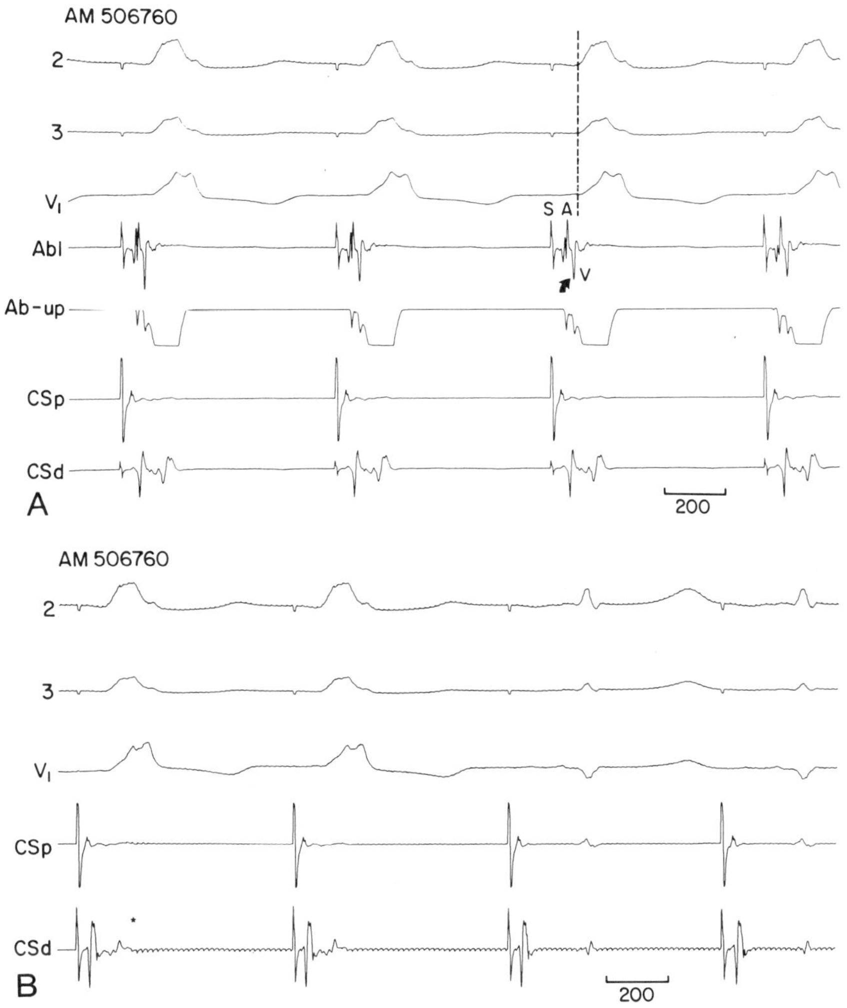

Figure 24.1. Radiofrequency ablation in a patient with a left-sided accessory pathway. **A,** Endocardial recording from the ablation catheter at the successful site shows that the intrinsic deflection of the ventricular electrogram (V) precedes the onset of the delta wave indicating close proximity to the accessory pathway. The *arrow* indicates a potential possibly arising from the accessory pathway. **B,** Radiofrequency ablation at the same site resulted in normalization of the QRS within two beats. 2, 3, V1 are electrocardiographic leads: A = atrial electrogram; Abl = bipolar recording from the ablation catheter; AB-up = unipolar recording from the ablation catheter; CSd = distal coronary sinus; CSp = proximal coronary sinus; SA = stimulus artifact. The onset of radiofrequency ablation is indicated by an *asterisk*.

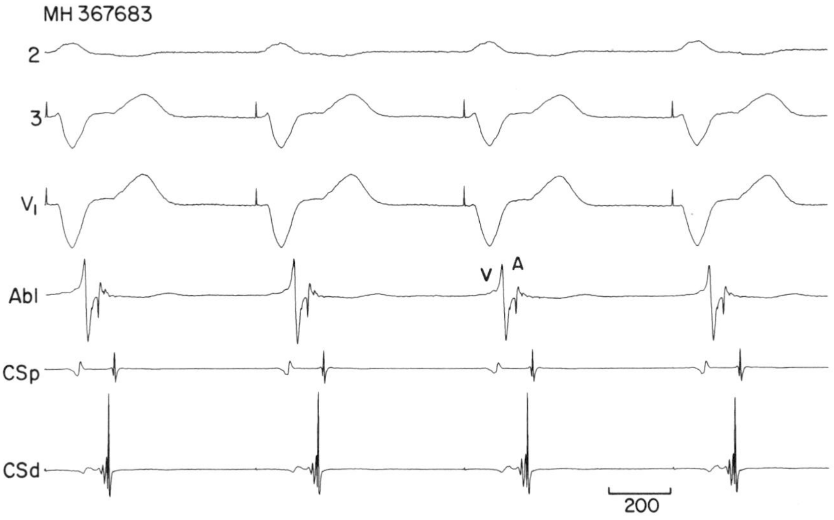

Figure 24.2. Endocardial mapping in a patient with a left-sided accessory pathway at a successful site during ventricular pacing. Recording from the ablation catheter (Abl) showed a short VA interval with no isoelectric line between the ventricular (V) and the atrial (A) electrogram. Abbreviations as in Figure 24.1.

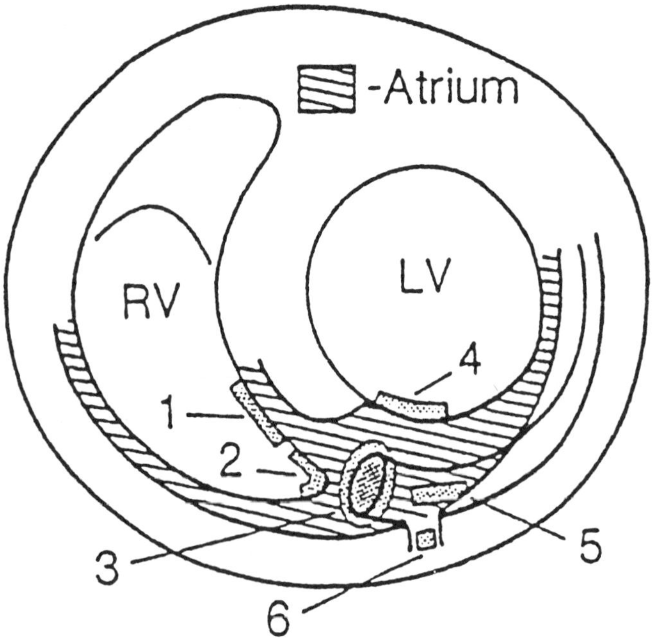

Figure 24.3. Diagram showing possible successful ablation sites of posteroseptal accessory pathways. 1 and 2 are at the right posteroseptal region, 3 is at the ostium of the coronary sinus, 4 is in the left ventricle, 5 is inside the coronary sinus, 6 is inside the middle cardiac vein. LV = left ventricle; RV = right ventricle (From Wang X; Jackman WM, McClelland J, *et al.*: PACE 1992;15-II:533, reproduced with permission.)

may be ablated near the orifice of the coronary sinus on the right atrial side, within the coronary sinus, within the cardiac venous system, or from the left side, depending on the results of mapping (52,54,55) (Fig. 24.3). Catheter ablation is currently considered to be reasonably primary therapy for problematic Wolff-Parkinson-White syndrome. Operative therapy is useful in cases where catheter ablation has failed or where the patient is undergoing concomitant cardiac surgery.

ATRIOVENTRICULAR NODE REENTRANT TACHYCARDIA

The tachycardia circuit in AV node reentry was initially considered to be confined entirely to the AV node and not amenable to any ablative therapy without incurring an AV block. Pritchett, *et al.* (56) initially reported cure of AV node reentrant tachycardia with preservation of AV node conduction in a patient after a failed attempt at AV node ablation. This proved the feasibility of ablative cure of AV node reentry without producing AV block. Several successful operative approaches were then described which had in common cryosurgery or dissection in the perinodal region (57,58). Catheter ablation was then applied to AV node reentry in an attempt to achieve a similar result. The initial goals of catheter ablation were similar to those described for operative therapy, namely mapping earliest retrograde atrial activation during tachycardia (57) or creating lesions in the periphery of the AV node that would result in "modification" of the AV node, preserving the AV node conduction and eliminating the ability to sustain AV node reentrance (59–61). Initial results using the DC shock technique (62,63) were reasonably successful but were limited by inconsistency, the occurrence of inadvertent total AV block and other potential adverse effects related to the DC shock technique.

The introduction of radiofrequency ablation for AV nodal reentry has resulted in more consistent cure of AV node reentry with fewer adverse effects. Two basic approaches have been described. The "anterior" or "fast pathway" approach selects a site posterior and inferior to the usual His recording site. The electrogram at this site shows a large atrial deflection and a relatively much smaller and slurred His deflection. Total AV block can be readily achieved at this site but modification results with a more conservative ablation and careful monitoring of the PR interval. Current between 300 and 500 mA is applied while closely observing the AH interval. The end point is prolongation of the AH interval and current is immediately discontinued after this is achieved. Rapid junctional tachycardia is also an indication for cessation of current with this technique as it may herald complete AV block. Excellent results with success rates greater than 80% can be expected. Inadvertent AV block ranging from 2 to 20% has been reported (64–66). Electrophysiologic testing after this approach suggests ablation of the "fast pathway" with residual prolongation of the PR interval and loss of retrograde conduction. The latter is not a constant finding, suggesting that the anterograde fast pathway and the retrograde fast pathway are not necessarily the same anatomical entities.

Recently, Jackman, *et al.* (67) suggested that the slow pathway is a distinct anatomic entity that can be ablated. A potential can be recorded, usually between the orifice of the coronary sinus and the tricuspid valve ring ("base" of Koch's triangle) which may represent activation of the "slow" pathway. This potential has been a useful marker for successful slow pathway ablation in the hands of these investigators. Other investigators (66,68) have used anatomically guided radiofrequency ablations in a similar region (near the orifice of the coronary sinus at the base of Koch's triangle) and have reported excellent results without recording these potentials. In our institution, we use a stepwise anatomically guided approach which involves a series of radiofrequency lesions starting in the vicinity of the coronary sinus (Fig. 24.4). The first lesion is placed at the rim of the tricuspid ring in the area of interest at a site where a relatively small atrial and large ventricular electrogram is recorded. The catheter is progressively pulled back with the atrial electrogram becoming relatively larger. Successful slow pathway ablation is invariably heralded by a junctional tachycardia and the endpoint for successful ablation is elimination of the slow pathway and all AV nodal echoes (Fig. 24.5). If the initial site is unsuccessful, progressive lesions are repeated at higher levels approaching the AV node. Electrophysiologic testing after the slow pathway approach shows loss of slow pathway conduction and preservation of anterograde fast and retrograde fast pathway conduction. The initial results are encouraging with an incidence of inadver-

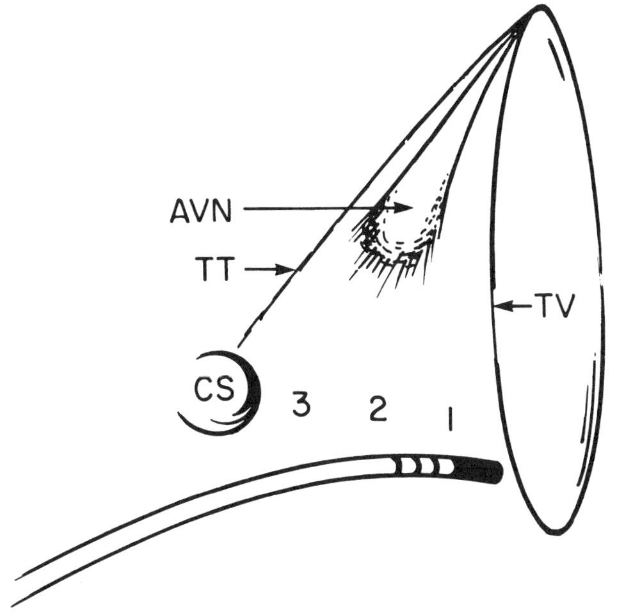

Figure 24.4. Schematic representation of the region of Koch's triangle from the right anterior oblique view. To ablate the fast pathway, the catheter is placed near the anterior aspect of the AV node (AVN). Anatomically guided ablation of the slow pathway consists of radiofrequency applications starting caudally at the coronary sinus ostium (CS) and moving progressively toward the AV node. Each "run" of lesions includes ablation from a site closer to the ventricle (1) toward the atrium (2) and (3). TT = tendon of Todaro; TV = tricuspid valve.

tent AV block in the range of 1% (66–68). Although further long-term follow-up is required to assess potential adverse effects including late AV block, it seems likely that this technique will become the standard of therapy in the future.

ATRIAL TACHYCARDIAS

Atrial tachycardias have been defined as tachycardias originating in atrial tissue, and include focal atrial tachycardia ("ectopic" atrial tachycardia), atrial flutter, and atrial fibrillation. The technique of catheter ablation is most amenable to a tachycardia in which the focus of tachycardia or a critical part of a tachycardia circuit is localized to a relatively small area but can be identified and ablated. Curative catheter ablation is therefore feasible for focal atrial tachycardia and atrial flutter.

Focal atrial tachycardia may result from abnormal automaticity, triggered activity or atrial reentry. Ablation is generally directed to the site of earliest atrial activation during focal tachycardia (Fig. 24.6), and preferably directed at the site of critical conduction delay for atrial reentrant tachycardias. The technical problems with ablating atrial tachycardia can be formidable. The tachycardia may not be reproducibly inducible to allow detailed mapping. Catheter manipulation in the complex, three-dimensional structure of the atria may be difficult. Finally, there may be multiple foci of atrial tachycardia. Perhaps for these reasons, experience with ablation in the atrial tachycardias has been slower to emerge. Early experience with DC shock

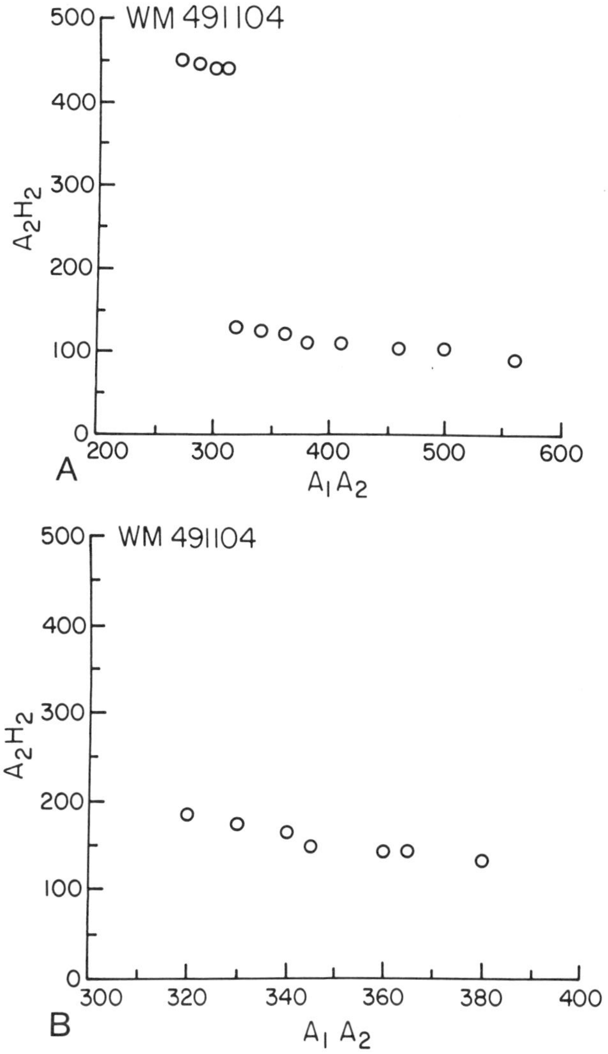

Figure 24.5. AV node function curve before and after slow pathway ablation in a patient with AV node reentry tachycardia. **A,** Before ablation progressively premature atrial extrastimulus showed the presence of dual AV node pathways. **B,** Radiofrequency ablation in the Koch's triangle area results in elimination of the slow pathway physiology and the postablation atrioventricular conduction is maintained by the fast pathway only. A_1A_2 = interval between the last pacing beat of the drive and atrial extrastimulus; A_2H_2 = atrio-Hisian interval observed during atrial extrastimulus testing.

(69,70) and radiofrequency (71,72) techniques are nonetheless encouraging and there is little doubt that this will become the nonpharmacologic therapy of choice for the atrial tachycardias as experience is gained.

ATRIAL FLUTTER

Atrial flutter is generally classified as "common" or typical atrial flutter (Type 1) or "uncommon" flutter (Type II). Common flutter is characterized by atrial flutter cycle length of approximately 200–250 msec and initially negative flutter waves in the inferior electrocardiographic leads. Uncommon flutter is faster and has the opposite flutter wave morphology. Common flutter has been the most widely studied and is better understood. It is due to right atrial macro-reentry with the wavefront circulating in a caudal-cranial direction on the anterior right atrium and septum and the reverse direction in the lateral and posterior atrium (73). The site of critical conduction delay in the circuit is the narrow isthmus of tissue in the vicinity of the orifice of the inferior vena cava, the tricuspid valve ring and the orifice of the coronary sinus (74,75), and this has been the "target" for operative (76) and catheter ablation. Experience has been gained with both the DC shock technique (77,78) and the radiofrequency technique (79,80). The electrophysiology laboratory at University Hospital, London, Canada, currently uses an anatomically guided technique in the critical regions described and utilizes termination of atrial flutter (Fig. 24.7) as an indication of proximity to a critical area of the circuit. Although the use of catheter ablation for atrial flutter will expand, it must be remembered that most patients with this arrhythmia have associated heart disease and atrial pathology which will certainly predispose many patients to concomitant atrial fibrillation.

ATRIAL FIBRILLATION

The mechanism of atrial fibrillation is currently thought to be multiple wavelet reentry (81) and the rationale for a focal ablative procedure is not present. Ablation of the AV node with implantation of a rate-responsive pacemaker has nonetheless emerged as a useful technique in patients with refractory atrial fibrillation. The catheter is guided to the AV node region using anatomic landmarks and electrogram morphology, with the ideal site usually being that recording a relatively large atrial deflection and a smaller but distinct His deflection. The DC shock technique was originally used and was highly successful but was associated with potentially serious complications including myocardial infarction, cardiac perforation, cardiac tamponade, and late sudden death (82). The radiofrequency technique has sup-

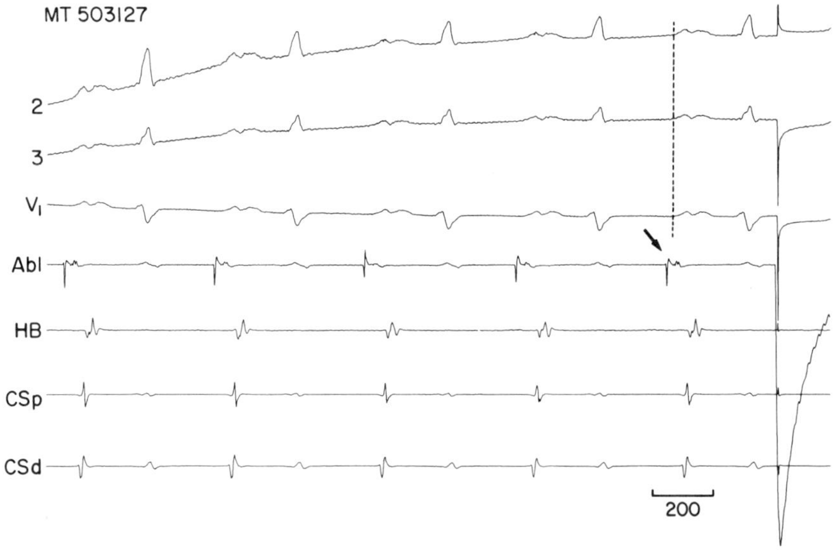

Figure 24.6. Radiofrequency ablation in a patient with incessant atrial tachycardia and tachycardia-induced cardiomyopathy. Tachycardia originated in the left atrium and recording from the ablation catheter *(arrow)* at the successful site showed an atrial electrogram preceding the onset of the P wave by 30 msec. Abbreviations as in Figure 24.1. HB = His bundle.

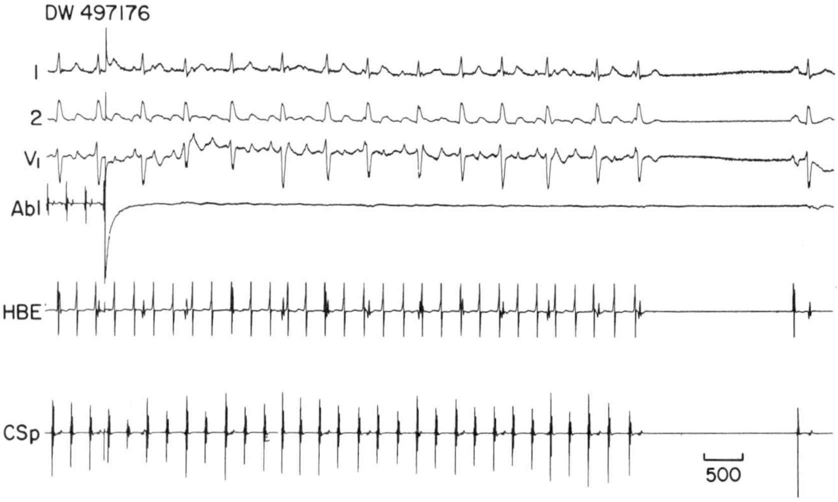

Figure 24.7. Radiofrequency ablation in a patient with "common" atrial flutter. Anatomically guided radiofrequency ablation in the posterior inferior region of the right atrium resulted in acute termination and permanent interruption of atrial flutter. Abbreviations as in Figure 24.1.

planted the DC shock technique and is successful in greater than 90% of patients with few adverse affects (82–86). For technically difficult cases, a left-sided approach through the aortic valve can be utilized (87). The His bundle is recorded on the ventricular septum immediately below the aortic valve cusp. Successful AV node ablation is heralded by rapid accelerated junctional rhythm followed by a narrow QRS junctional escape rhythm.

VENTRICULAR TACHYCARDIA WITHOUT STRUCTURAL HEART DISEASE

Ventricular tachycardia in the absence of structural heart disease is generally not associated with mortality but can be problematic in drug refractory patients. The mechanism for tachycardia in the context is probably not homogeneous but most of such tachycardias originate in a focal area of ventricle and are associated with normal intramyocardial conduction and normal ventricular electrograms (88). The focal origin of these tachycardias in this context make them amenable to catheter ablation techniques. The "target" for ablation is earliest recorded ventricular activity at least at the onset of the QRS on the surface ECG (Fig. 24.8) with pace mapping serving as an ancillary localizing technique. The most common type of idiopathic ventricular tachycardia was described as early as 1922 by Gallaverdin (89). It is characterized by left bundle branch block, inferior axis QRS morphology and is frequently aggravated by exercise. The site of "origin" is in the right ventricular outflow tract, frequently at the junction of the right ventricular free wall and septum in that region. Ablation using DC shock (90) and later radiofrequency energy (91,92) has demonstrated success rates greater than 80%. Another less common type of ventricular tachycardia in patients with normal ventricles was initially observed by Blanchot in 1973 (93) and further characterized by Belhassen in 1981 (94). This tachycardia has a typical QRS morphology with right bundle branch block and left axis deviation. The tachycardia is usually verapamil responsive. The "site of origin" of tachycardia is in the inferoposterior septal region of the left ventricle (Fig. 24.9). Early experience with ablation of this type of tachycardia is encouraging (91,92,95).

VENTRICULAR TACHYCARDIA DUE TO BUNDLE BRANCH REENTRY

Tachycardia due to reentry in the bundle branches has been observed in up to 6% of patients referred for ventricular tachycardia and is usually seen in the presence of dilated cardiomyopathy (96,97). The circuit generally involves antegrade conduction over the right bundle branch with retrograde conduction over the left bundle branch system (98). The right bundle branch is easily localized and is generally a relatively simple target for catheter ablation using DC (99–101) or preferably radiofrequency energy (96,102). However, patients with this type of tachycardia generally have significant myocardial dysfunction and ventricular tachycardias due to other mechanisms frequently coexist (96).

VENTRICULAR TACHYCARDIA WITH STRUCTURAL HEART DISEASE

Ventricular tachycardia in the presence of structural heart disease, generally ischemic heart disease, is associated with logistic complexities that make endocardial catheter ablation a more formidable challenge. These include the following difficulties: (a) intramural clot or fibrosis may overlay the arrhythmogenic zone; (b) the zone of critical conduction delay (site of origin of tachycardia) may be intramyocardial or epicardial; (c) the critical arrhythmogenic zone to be ablated may be extensive; (d) interpretation of electrograms indicating the zone of critical

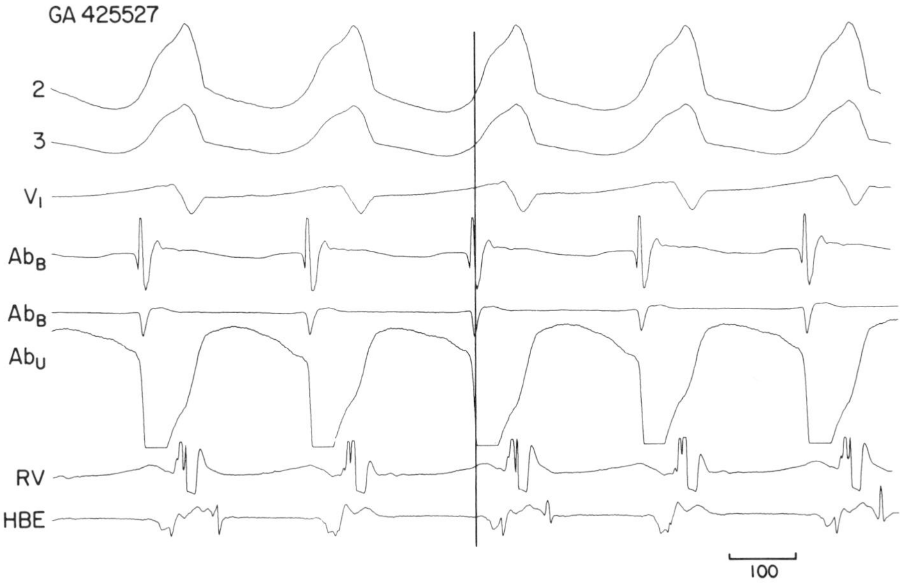

Figure 24.8. Endocardial mapping at the successful site in a patient with right ventricular (*RV*) outflow tract ventricular tachycardia. Recording from the ablation catheter shows the ventricular electrogram coincident with the onset of the QRS. Abbreviations as in Figure 24.1. HBE = His bundle electrogram.

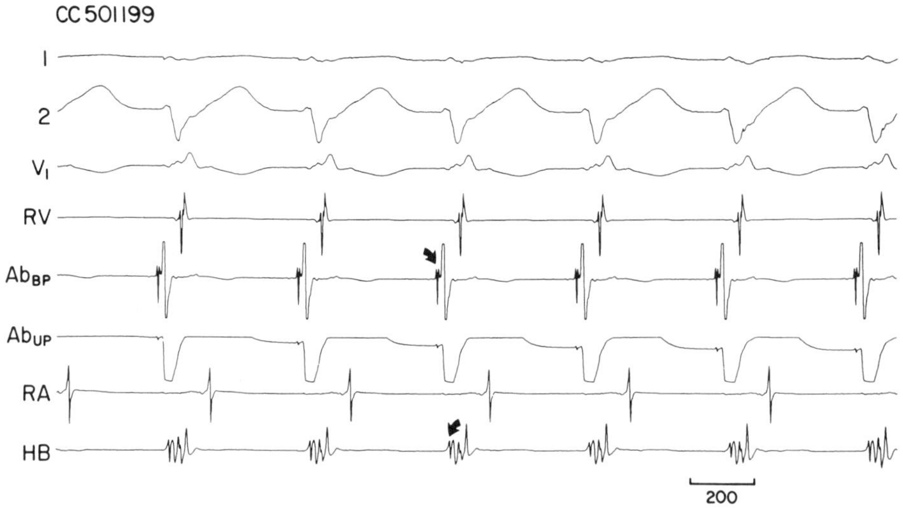

Figure 24.9. Intracardiac recordings at a successful site in a patient with no structural heart disease and ventricular tachycardia originating in the left ventricle. At the successful site the ventricular electrogram precedes the onset of the QRS. The QRS is preceded by a large potential *(upper arrow)* at this site. The *bottom arrow* indicates His bundle electrogram. Abbreviations as in Figure 24.1. Ab_{BP} = Ablation catheter bipolar recording.

conduction delay may be very complex even if this zone is accessible to the catheter.

Nonetheless, progress in ablation of ventricular tachycardia has been made since the first attempt by Hartzler, *et al.* (103). Patients undergoing catheter ablation for ventricular tachycardia generally have monomorphic ventricular tachycardia, have failed drug therapy, and are not candidates for operative ablation or defibrillator implantation. A major challenge is identifying a target for ablation. In contrast to patients with normal hearts, identification of earliest ventricular activation just prior to the onset of the QRS on the surface ECG may be inadequate and attention has been focused on identifying the zone of critical conduction delay (104,105). This has been achieved by locating mid-diastolic potentials necessary for tachycardia perpetuation (106,107) or by locating sites at which pacing can accelerate tachycardia without altering the QRS morphology and with a long stimulus to QRS interval (concealed entrainment) (108). Initial results utilizing either DC shock or radiofrequency with efficacy in the range of 15–50% have been reported (104,105,109,110). In addition, a significant incidence of serious complications including new tachycardias, incessant ventricular tachycardia, electromechanical dissociation, and cardiogenic shock have been reported.

CONCLUSIONS

Since initial pioneering attempts, catheter ablation has greatly evolved and is currently accepted as initial therapy in Wolff-Parkinson-White syndrome and other supraventricular rhythm disorders. Ablation of ventricular tachycardia associated with structural heart disease is the current frontier. Novel catheter design and newer energy sources will ultimately expand the horizon of this procedure to most arrhythmias.

References

1. Vedel J, Frank R, Fontaine G, *et al.*: Bloc auriculo-ventriculaire intra-hisien definitif induit au coeurs d'une exploration endoventriculaire droite. Arch Mal Coeur 1985;72:107–112.
2. Gonzalez R, Scheinman M, Margaretten W, *et al.*: Closed-chest electrode-catheter technique for His bundle ablation in dogs. Am J Physiol 1982;241:H283–H287.
3. Scheinman MM, Morady F, Hess DS, *et al.*: Catheter-induced ablation of the atrioventricular junction to control refractory supraventricular arrhythmia. JAMA 1982;248:851–855.
4. Gallagher JJ, Svenson RH, Kasell JH, *et al.*: Catheter technique for closed-chest ablation of the atrioventricular conduction system. N Engl J Med 1982;306:194–200.
5. Bardy GH, Coltorti F, Ivey TD, *et al.*: Some factors affecting bubble formation with catheter-mediated defibrillator pulses. Circulation 1986;73:525–538.
6. Holt PM, Boyd EGCA: Hematologic effects of the high-energy endocardial ablation technique. Circulation 1986;73:1029.
7. Fontaine G, Volmen W, Nienaltowska E, *et al.*: Approach to the physics of fulguration. In Fontaine G, Scheinman MM (eds): Ablation in Cardiac Arrhythmias. Mt. Kisco, NY, Futura 1987:101–116.
8. Holt PM, Boyd EGCA: Physical and experimental aspects of ablation with direct-current shocks. In Saksena S, Goldschlager N (eds): Electrical therapy for cardiac arrhythmia. Philadelphia, WB Saunders, 1990:619–626.
9. Holt PM, Boyd EGCA: Biolectric effects of high energy, electrical discharges. In Scheinman MM (ed): Catheter Ablation of Cardiac Arrhythmia. Dordrecht, Martinus Nijhoff, 1988:1–36.
10. Levine JH, Spear JF, Weisman HF, *et al.*: The cellular electrophysiologic changes induced by high-energy electrical ablation in canine myocardium. Circulation 1986;73:818–829.
11. Jones JL, Proskauer CC, Paull WK, *et al.*: Ultrastructural injury to check myocardial cells in vitro following "electrick countershock." Circ Res 1980;46:387–394.
12. Fisher JD, Broadman R, Kim SG, *et al.*: Attempted nonsurgical electrical ablation of accessory pathways via the coronary sinus in the Wolff-Parkinson-White syndrome. J Am Coll Cardiol 1984;4:685.
13. Bardy GH, Ivey TD, Coltorti F, *et al.*: Developments, complications and limitations of catheter-mediated electrical ablation for posterior accessory atrioventricular pathways. Am J Cardiol 1988;61:309–316.
14. Morady F, Scheinman MM, Winston SA, *et al.*: Efficacy and safety of transcatheter ablation of posteroseptal accessory pathways. Circulation 1985;72:170–177.
15. Ruder MA, Mead RH, Gaudian V, *et al.*: Transvenous catheter ablation of extranodal accessory pathways. J Am Coll Cardiol 1988;11:1245–1253.
16. Coltorti F, Rackson MM, Hanson K, *et al.*: Current waveform modulation to avoid plasma arcing and barotrauma with catheter mediated electric discharges (Abstr). Circulation 1985;72(Suppl III):III-474.

17. Boyd EG, Holt PM: Haematologic effects of the ablation technique: a comparison between anodal and cathodal delivery (Abstr). J Am Coll Cardiol 1986;7:131A.
18. Cunningham D, Rowland E, Rickards A: A new nonarcing electrode for catheter ablation. Design and trial performance. (Abstr). Circulation 1987;76(Suppl IV):IV-405.
19. Rowland E, Cunningham D, Ahsan A, *et al.*: Transvenous ablation of atrioventricular conduction with a low energy power source. Br Heart J 1989;62:361–366.
20. Borggrefe M, Haverkamp W, Budde TH, *et al.*: Radiofrequency ablation. In Zipes DP, Jalife J (eds): Cardiac Electrophysiology. From Cell to Bedside. Philadelphia: WB Saunders, 1990:997–1004.
21. d'Arsonval A. Action physiologique des courants alternatifs à grand frequence. Arch Physiol Norm Pathol 1983;5:401.
22. Clark W. Oscillatory desiccation in the treatment of accessible malignant growths and minor surgical conditions. J Adv Ther 1911;29:169–172.
23. Cushing H. Bovie WT. Electro-surgery as an aid to the removal of intracranial tumors. Surg Gynecol Obstet 1928;47:751–758.
24. Geddes LA, Tacker WA, Cabler PQ. A new electrical hazard associated with the electrocautery. Med Instr 1975;9:112–116.
25. Haines D, Watson D, Halperin C. Characteristics of heat transfer and determination of temperature gradient and viability threshold during radiofrequency fulguration of isolated perfused canine right ventricle (Abstr). Circulation 1987;76:IV-1109.
26. Haines D, Verow A. Observation on electrode-tissue interface temperature and effect on electrical impedance during radiofrequency ablation of ventricular myocardium. Circulation 1990;82;82:1034–1038.
27. Huang SKS: Radiofrequency catheter ablation of cardiac arrhythmias: appraisal of an evolving therapeutic modality. Am Heart J 1989;118:1317–1323.
28. Haverkamp W, Hindricks G, Gulker H, *et al.*: Coagulation of ventricular myocardium using radiofrequency alternating current: biophysical aspects and experimental findings. PACE 1989;12-II:187–194.
29. Ring ME, Huang SKS, Gorman G, *et al.*: Determinants of impedance rise during catheter ablation of bovine myocardium with radiofrequency energy. PACE 1989;12:1502–1513.
30. Hoyt RH, Huang SK, Marcus FI, *et al.*: Factors influencing trans-catheter radiofrequency ablation of the myocardium. J Appl Cardiol 1986;1:469–474.
31. Pecson RD, Roth DA, Mark VH. Experimental temperature control of radiofrequency brain lesion size. J Neurosurg 1969;30:703–710.
32. Langberg J, Lee M, Chin M, *et al.*: Radiofrequency catheter ablation. The effect of electrode size on lesion volume in vitro. PACE 1990;13:1242–1248.
33. Blouin LT, Marcus FI. The effect of electrode design on the efficiency of delivery of radiofrequency energy to cardiac tissue in vitro. PACE 1989;12-II:136–143.
34. Haverkamp W, Hindricks G, Rissel U, *et al.*: Determinanten der endokardialen Hochfrequenz-Katheterablation. Herzsschrittmacher 1987;7:63–70.
35. Haverkamp W, Hindricks G, Rissel U, *et al.*: Temperature-guided radiofrequency coagulation of myocardial tissue (Abstr). J Am Coll Cardiol 1989;13:169A.
36. Haines D: Impedance rise during radiofrequency ablation is due to sudden boiling at the catheter tip and is prevented by tip temperature monitoring (Abstr). Circulation 1988;78:II-156.
37. Avitall B, Hare J, Lessila C, *et al.*: New generation of catheter for mapping and ablation: a rotating tip and lateral defectable catheters (Abstr). Circulation 1991;84:II-24.
38. Avitall B, Dhala A, Hare J, *et al.*: Ablation of left side accessory pathways: criteria for catheter design (Abstr). PACE 1992;15-II:581.
39. Wittkampf F, Wever E, Hauer R: Improved catheter shape for radiofrequency ablation of left sided posteroseptal and posterior accessory pathways (Abstr). PACE 1992;15-II:582.
40. Calkins H, Niklason L, Sousa J, *et al.*: Radiation exposure during radiofrequency catheter ablation of accessory atrioventricular connections. Circulation 1991;84:2376–2382.
41. Morady F, Scheinman MM, William HK, *et al.*: Long-term results of catheter ablation of a posteroseptal accessory atrioventricular connection in 48 patients. Circulation 1989;79:1160–1170.
42. Haissaguerre M, Warin JF, Le Metayer P, *et al.*: Catheter ablation of Mahaim fibers with preservation of atrioventricular nodal conduction. Circulation 1990;82:418–427.
43. Warin J, Haissaguerre M, D'ivernoi C, *et al.*: Catheter ablation of accessory pathways. Technique and results in 248 patients. PACE 1990;13:1609–1614.
44. Lemery R, Talajic M, Roy D, Coutu B, *et al.*: Success, safety, and late electrophysiological outcome of low-energy direct-current ablation in patients with the Wolff-Parkinson-White syndrome. Circulation 1992;85:957–962.
45. Borggrefe M, Budde T, Podceck A, *et al.*: High frequency alternating current ablation of accessory pathway in humans. J Am Coll Cardiol 1987;10:576–582.
46. Calkins H, Sousa J, El-atassi R, *et al.*: Diagnosis and cure of the Wolff-Parkinson-White syndrome or paroxysmal supraventricular tachycardia during a single electrophysiologic test. N Engl J Med 1991;324:1612–1618.
47. Jackman WM, Wang X, Friday KJ, *et al.*: Catheter ablation of accessory atrioventricular pathways (Wolff-Parkinson-White syndrome) by radiofrequency current. N Engl J Med 1991;324:1601–1611.
48. Calkins H, Langberg J, Sousa J, *et al.*: Radiofrequency catheter ablation of accessory atrioventricular connection in 250 patients. Circulation 1992;85:1337–1346.
49. Leather RA, Leitch JW, Klein GJ, *et al.*: Radiofrequency catheter ablation of accessory pathways: a learning experience. Am J Cardiol 1991;68:1651–1655.
50. Macdonald D, O'Connor BK, Serwer GA, *et al.*: Use of radiofrequency current to ablate accessory connection in children. Circulation 1991;84:2318–2324.
51. Schluter M, Geiger M, Siebel J, *et al.*: Catheter ablation using radiofrequency current to cure symptomatic patients with tachyarrhythmias related to an accessory atrioventricular pathway. Circulation 1991;84:1644–1661.
52. Calkins H, Kim YN, Schmaltz S, *et al.*: Electrogram criteria for identification of appropriate target sites for radiofrequency catheter ablation of accessory atrioventricular connections. Circulation 1992;85:565–573.
53. Natale A, Klein GJ, Yee R, *et al.*: Radiofrequency ablation of left lateral accessory pathway: transseptal vs. retrograde aortic approach (Abstr). PACE 1992;15-II:518.
54. Wang X, Jackman WM, McClelland J, *et al.*: Sites of successful radiofrequency ablation of posteroseptal accessory pathways (Abstr). PACE 1992;15-II:535.
55. Oren J, McClelland J, Beckman K, *et al.*: Epicardial posteroseptal accessory pathways requiring ablation from the middle cardiac vein (Abstr). PACE 1992;15-II:535.
56. Pritchett LC, Anderson RR, Benditt DG, *et al.*: Reentry within the atrioventricular node: surgical cure with preservation of the atrioventricular conduction. Circulation 1979;60:440–446.
57. Ross DL, Johnson DC, Denniss AR, *et al.*: Curative surgery for atrioventricular junctional ("AV nodal") reentrant tachycardia. J Am Coll Cardiol 1985;6:1383–1392.
58. Fujimura O, Guiraudon GM, Yee R, *et al.*: Operative therapy of atrioventricular node reentry and results of anatomically guided procedure. Am J Cardiol 1989;64:1327–1332.
59. Marcus FI, Blouin LT, Bharati S, *et al.*: Production of chronic first degree atrioventricular block in dogs using closed-chest electrode catheter with radiofrequency energy. J Electrophysiol 1988;2:315–326.
60. Lopez Merino V, Sanchis J, Chorro FJ, *et al.*: Induction of partial alteration in atrioventricular conduction in dogs by percutaneous emission of high frequency currents. Am Heart J 1988;115:1214–1221.

61. Huang SKS, Chenarides J, Gasdia G. Chronic incomplete atrioventricular block induced by radiofrequency catheter ablation. Circulation 1989;80: 951–961.
62. Haissaguerre M, Warin JF, Lemetayer P, *et al.*: Closed-chest ablation of retrograde conduction in patients with atrioventricular nodal reentrant tachycardia. N Engl J Med 1989;320:426–433.
63. Epstein L, Scheinman M, Langberg J, *et al.*: Percutaneous catheter modification of the atrioventricular node. Circulation 1989;80:757–768.
64. Lee MA, Morady F, Kadish A, *et al.*: Catheter modification of the atrioventricular junction with radiofrequency energy for control of atrioventricular nodal reentry tachycardia. Circulation 1991;83:827–835.
65. Sanjuan R, Morell S, Garcia Civera R, *et al.*: Transvenous ablation with high frequency energy for atrioventricular junctional (AV nodal) reentrant tachycardia. PACE 1989;12:1631–1639.
66. Jazayeri MR, Hempe SL, Sra JS, *et al.*: Selective transcatheter ablation of the fast and slow pathways using radiofrequency energy in patients with atrioventricular nodal reentrant tachycardia. Circulation 1992;85:1318–1328.
67. Roman CA, Wang X, Friday KJ, *et al.*: Catheter technique for selective ablation of slow pathway in AV nodal reentrant tachycardia (Abstr). PACE 1990;13:498.
68. Key GN, Epstein AE, Daily SM, *et al.*: Selective radiofrequency ablation of the slow pathway for the treatment of atrioventricular nodal reentrant tachycardia. Circulation 1992;85:1675–1688.
69. Silka MJ, Gillette PC, Garson A, *et al.*: Transvenous catheter ablation of a right atrial automatic ectopic tachycardia. J Am Coll Cardiol 1985;5:999–1001.
70. Gillette PC, Wampler DG, Garson A, *et al.*: Treatment of atrial automatic tachycardia by ablation procedures. J Am Coll Cardiol 1985;6:405–409.
71. Tracy CM, Swartz JF, Hoops HG, *et al.*: Radiofrequency catheter ablation of ectopic atrial tachycardia using activation pace mapping (Abstr). J Am Coll Cardiol 1982;19:185A.
72. Ehlert FA, Goldberger J, Deal BJ, *et al.*: Radiofrequency current catheter ablation for drug refractory automatic supraventricular tachycardia (Abstr). PACE 1992;15-II:549.
73. Touboul P, Saoudi N, Atallah G, *et al.*: Electrophysiologic basis of catheter ablation in atrial flutter. Am J Cardiol 1989;64:79J–82J.
74. Klein GJ, Guiraudon GM, Sharma AD, *et al.*: Demonstration of macroreentry and feasibility of operative therapy in the common type of atrial flutter. Am J Cardiol 1986;57:587–591.
75. Cosio FG, Arribas F, Barbero JM, *et al.*: Validation of double-spike electrograms as markers of conduction delay or block in atrial flutter. Am J Cardiol 1988;61:775–780.
76. Cosio FG, Arribas F, Palacios J, *et al.*: Fragmented electrogram and continuous electrical activity in atrial flutter. Am J Cardiol 1986;57:1309–1314.
77. Saoudi A, Atallah G, Kirkorian G, *et al.*: Catheter ablation of the atrial myocardium in human type I atrial flutter. Circulation 1990;81:762–771.
78. Saoudi N, Mouton-Schleiffer D, Letac B: Direct catheter ablation of atrial flutter. Lancet 1987;5:568–69.
79. Feld G, Chen PS, Fleck P, *et al.*: Radiofrequency catheter ablation of type 1 atrial flutter in humans (Abstr). PACE 1992;15-II:584.
80. Numain SO, Linker NJ, Debbas NMG, *et al.*: Successful catheter ablation of atrial flutter substrate using low energy DC shocks (Abstr). J Am Coll Cardiol 1991;17:367A.
81. Moe GK, Abildskov JA: Atrial fibrillation as a self-sustaining arrhythmia independent of focal discharge. Am Heart J 1959;58:59–70.
82. Scheinman MM. Catheter ablation for cardiac arrhythmias, personnel, and facilities. PACE 1992;15:715–721.
83. Jackman WM, Wang X, Friday KJ, *et al.*: Catheter ablation of atrioventricular junction using radiofrequency current in 17 patients. Circulation 1991;83:1562–1576.
84. Yeung-Lai-Wah JA, Alison J, Lonergan L, *et al.*: High success rate of atrioventricular node ablation with radiofrequency energy. J Am Coll Cardiol 1991;18:1753–1758.
85. Langberg JJ, Chin MC, Rosenqvist M, *et al.*: Catheter ablation of the atrioventricular junction with radiofrequency energy. 1989;80:1527–1535.
86. Langberg JJ, Chin MC, Schamp DJ, *et al.*: Ablation of the atrioventricular junction with radiofrequency energy using a new electrode catheter. Am J Cardiol 1991;67:142–147.
87. Sousa J, El-Atassi R, Rosenheck S, *et al.*: Radiofrequency catheter ablation of the atrioventricular junction from the left ventricle. Circulation 1991;84:567–571.
88. Marchlinski FE: Ventricular tachycardia: clinical presentation, course, and therapy. In Zipes DP, Jalife J (eds): Cardiac Electrophysiology. From Cell to Bedside. WB Saunders, Philadelphia, 1990:756–777.
89. Gallavardin L. Extrasystolie ventriculaire à paroxysmes tachycardiques prolongés. Arch Mal Coeur 1922;15:298–306.
90. Morady F, Kadish AH, DiCarlo L, *et al.*: Long-term results of catheter ablation of idiopathic right ventricular tachycardia. Circulation 1990; 82:2093–2099.
91. Calkins H, Langberg J, El-Atassi R, *et al.*: Catheter ablation of idiopathic ventricular tachycardia using radiofrequency energy (Abstr). PACE 1992;15-II:584.
92. Klein LS, Shih HT, Hackett FK, *et al.*: Radiofrequency catheter ablation of ventricular tachycardia in patients without structural heart disease. Circulation 1992;85:1666–1674.
93. Blanchot P, Warin JF: Un nouveau cas de tachycardie ventriculaire par reentrée. Arch Mal Coeur 1973;66:915–923.
94. Belhassen B, Rotmensch HH, Laniado S: Response of recurrent sustained ventricular tachycardia to verapamil. Br Heart J 1981;46:679–682.
95. Ruffy R, Kim SS, Lal R: Paroxysmal fascicular tachycardia: electrophysiologic characteristics and treatment by catheter ablation. J Am Coll Cardiol 1985;5:1008–1014.
96. Cohen TJ, Chien WW, Lurie KG, *et al.*: Radiofrequency catheter ablation for treatment of bundle branch ventricular tachycardia: results and long-term follow-up. J Am Coll Cardiol 1991;18:1767–1773.
97. Caceres J, Jazayeri M, McKinnie J, *et al.*: Sustained bundle branch reentry as a mechanism of clinical tachycardia. Circulation 1989;79:256–270.
98. Akhtar M, Damato AN, Batsford WP, *et al.*: Demonstration of reentry in His-Purkinje system in man. Circulation 1974;50:1150–1159.
99. Touboul P, Kirkorian G, Atallah G, *et al.*: Bundle branch reentrant tachycardia treated by electrical ablation of the right bundle branch. J Am Coll Cardiol 1986;7:1404–1409.
100. Tchou P, Jazayeri M, Denker S, *et al.*: Transcatheter electrical ablation of right bundle branch: a method of treating macroreentrant ventricular tachycardia attributed to bundle branch reentry. Circulation 1988;78:246–257.
101. Volkmann H, Kunhnert H, Dannberg G, *et al.*: Bundle branch reentrant tachycardia treated by transvenous catheter ablation of the right bundle branch. PACE 1989;12:258–261.
102. Langberg JJ, Desai J, Dullet N, *et al.*: Treatment of macroreentrant ventricular tachycardia with radiofrequency ablation of the right bundle branch. Am J Cardiol 1989;63:1010–1013.
103. Hartzler GO: Electrode catheter ablation of refractory ventricular tachycardia. J Am Coll Cardiol 1983;2:1107–1113.
104. Morady F, Scheinman MM, Di Carlo LA, *et al.*: Catheter ablation of ventricular tachycardia with intracardiac shocks: results in 33 patients. Circulation 1987;75:1037–1049.
105. Belhassen B, Miller HI, Geller E, *et al.*: Transcatheter electrical shock ablation of ventricular tachycardia. J Am Coll Cardiol 1986;7:1347–1355.
106. Morady F, Frank R, Kou WH, *et al.*: Identification and catheter ablation of a zone of slow conduction in the reentrant circuit of ventricular tachycardia in humans. J Am Coll Cardiol 1988;11:775–782.

107. Fitzgerald DM, Friday KJ, Yeung JA, *et al.*: Electrogram patterns predicting successful catheter ablation of ventricular tachycardia. Circulation 1988;77:806–814.
108. Morady F, Kadish A, Rosenheck S, *et al.*: Concealed entrainment as a guide for catheter ablation of ventricular tachycardia in patients with prior myocardial infarction. J Am Coll Cardiol 1991;17:678–689.
109. Evans GT, Scheinman MM: Catheter ablation for control of ventricular tachycardia: a report of the percutaneous cardiac mapping and ablation registry. PACE 1986;9-II:1391–1395.
110. Scheinman MM, Laks MM, DiMarco J, *et al.*: Current role of catheter ablative procedures in patients with cardiac arrhythmias. Circulation 1991;83:2146–2153.

25

CARDIOPULMONARY RESUSCITATION

Alan D. Guerci, M.D., F.A.C.C.

Cardiopulmonary resuscitation (CPR) consists of a series of measures designed to deliver oxygenated blood to the heart and brain until effective cardiac activity is restored. This chapter will review basic life support, i.e., airway management and chest compression, and advanced cardiac life support, therapies that are intended to terminate specific arrhythmias.

MECHANISMS OF BLOOD FLOW DURING CHEST COMPRESSION

Kouwenhoven, Jude, and Knickerbocker, the developers of the currently accepted technique of chest compression, assumed but never proved that blood flows as a result of direct compression of the heart between the sternum and vertebral column (1). This assumption has since been challenged by a series of observations which suggest that blood flow during chest compression is a consequence of fluctuations in intrathoracic pressure. In this scheme, elevated intrathoracic pressure is transmitted efficiently to extrathoracic large arteries, but retrograde venous flow is prevented by venous valves in the internal jugular veins and the extremities (2–6). As a result of this differential transmission of intrathoracic pressure to the periphery, arteriovenous pressure gradients are established and blood flow ensues.

The intrathoracic pressure hypothesis derives most of its support from three observations. First, patients in ventricular fibrillation can maintain consciousness for up to 40 sec by rapid and vigorous coughing. Coughing increases intrathoracic pressure without compressing the heart between the sternum and vertebral column. Second, during sternal compression or cough, pressure changes are similar in a variety of locations in the thorax: right atrium, pulmonary artery, left ventricle, aorta, esophagus, and lateral pleural space. Third, ascending aortic pressure increases before blood flows during chest compression (7,8). This inversion of the usual physiologic sequence of flow induced changes in pressure is consistent with the intrathoracic pressure hypothesis in that intrathoracic pressure increases first and then literally drives blood out of the thorax.

Echocardiographic studies have provided support for both the direct compression and intrathoracic pressure hypotheses, and it is not known which mechanism is predominant in any one patient. Two observations of overriding importance have been derived from the many studies which have attempted to identify the mechanism of blood flow during chest compression. First, the direct compression and intrathoracic pressure hypotheses are not mutually exclusive. Both are critically dependent on vigorous chest compression. Up to the point at which sternal compression causes extensive chest wall trauma, cardiac output is proportional to compression force. Second, cardiac output during external chest compression is extremely low, probably only 5–10% of normal. Although forceful chest compression may in some cases generate sufficient cerebral perfusion sufficient to prevent brain damage, myocardial perfusion is probably never sufficient to prevent a rapid and relentless downward spiral of ischemia and acidosis. This fact should be borne in mind when considering the timing and priority of other treatments of arrest victims. Above all, chest compression should never interfere with defibrillation.

BASIC LIFE SUPPORT

The American Heart Association recommends that ventilation be initiated before chest compression. This sequence (airway, breathing, chest compression) is essential in prolonged arrest situations, in which the circulation of unoxygenated blood would provide minimal, if any, benefit, but may not be necessary if endotracheal intubation is expected within a minute or two. Ventilatory requirements during chest compression are proportional to pulmonary blood flow (cardiac output) and, therefore, may be very small. As long as the patient has not been hypoventilating prior to the arrest, brief periods of chest compression may be beneficial even without ventilation. The drawback to this approach is that the patient's prearrest ventilatory status may be unknown.

If defibrillation is unsuccessful, or if a defibrillator is not immediately available, ventilation and chest compression should be started. Respiratory arrest is usually obvious. When in doubt, the rescuer can evaluate the adequacy of the arrest victim's ventilatory efforts by looking, listening, or feeling for air flow. This is done by placing one ear next to the victim's nose, listening and feeling for air flow while watching the chest wall.

If air flow is absent or inadequate, the neck should be extended in order to raise the base of the tongue away from the oropharynx. This may be accomplished by pushing the forehead back with one hand while pulling the chin with the other. This maneuver is particularly important in cases of upper airway obstruction, which may be caused by the tongue and which may be evidenced by ventilatory efforts (diaphragmatic descent, intercostal retractions, etc.) with minimal or no air flow. In cases of suspected cervical spine injury, this movement should be restricted as much as possible to extension of the mandible.

Once the airway has been repositioned, two deep breaths should be delivered to the victim. Resistance to airflow should be interpreted as evidence of airway obstruction and should stimulate efforts to reposition the airway. If repositioning the airway fails to facilitate air flow, it is assumed that the problem lies at the level of the larynx or trachea.

The Heimlich maneuver must be modified in unconscious arrest victims. The heel of one hand is placed inferior to the xiphoid, the second hand is placed over the first, and both are driven cephalad and posteriorly. If this modified Heimlich maneuver fails, it may be supplemented by chest compressions or back blows. The chest compressions are the same as those delivered during CPR. Back blows are administered by rolling the arrest victim on the side and applying one or two forceful blows to the mid-thoracic spine. Since back blows are intended only to dislodge foreign material, they should be followed either by the modified Heimlich maneuver or by sternal compression. These actions will raise intrathoracic pressure and, at least in theory, propel foreign material into the oropharynx, where it can be removed by inserting two fingers into the victim's mouth and sweeping laterally across the oropharynx.

Once the airway obstruction is relieved, the rescuer should deliver two deep breaths at approximately 10-sec intervals. Fifteen chest compressions, performed at a rate of 80–100/min, should be applied in the interval between ventilations.

Chest compression should be as vigorous as the patient's thorax can withstand because cardiac output during CPR is directly proportional to sternal displacement. The rapidity of the compression stroke and the maintenance of the compression stroke for 50% of each cycle of chest compression and release both appear to be important (6,8,9). At the currently recommended compression rate of 80–100/min, compression duration of 50% tends to occur naturally.

TREATMENT OF ARRHYTHMIAS

Blind Defibrillation

Several observations support a policy of immediate, "blind" defibrillation in unmonitored arrest victims. First, a high percentage of arrests are due to ventricular tachycardia and ventricular fibrillation. For practical purposes, defibrillation is the only effective treatment of these patients. Second, it is extremely unlikely that defibrillation will convert asystole or a bradyarrhythmia into ventricular fibrillation. Since brady-asystolic arrests are nearly always fatal, the induction of ventricular fibrillation would be expected to have little effect on outcome. Finally, since defibrillation is performed repeatedly in the course of cardiac arrest, ventricular fibrillation induced by defibrillation would be quickly converted back to the original rhythm.

The American Heart Association recommends that defibrillation be performed at 200, 300 and 400 J. Provided that at least 200 J are delivered, the energy level of defibrillation is probably less important than the speed with which defibrillation is applied. In cases of unmonitored arrest or monitored ventricular fibrillation, nothing should be allowed to delay defibrillation by more than 15 or 30 sec. This includes CPR, airway management, insertion of intravenous lines, or attempts to establish electrocardiographic monitoring.

General Approach

It is useful to approach arrhythmias causing cardiac arrest on the basis of the rate of ventricular activation. Treatment of tachyarrhythmias is aimed at the restoration of organized electrical activity and subsequent evaluation of the patient's hemodynamic status. This means that defibrillation is the treatment of first choice, and it should be understood that drug treatment of tachyarrhythmias causing cardiac arrest is intended to promote the likelihood of defibrillation when initial defibrillatory discharges have failed. Treatment of asystole and severe bradyarrhythmias is designed to increase heart rate into the physiologic range, at which time judgments can be made about manipulation of inotropic state. Finally, if the heart rate is within the physiologic range and the patient remains pulseless or profoundly hypotensive, attention should be directed to extramyocardial causes of arrest, such as hypovolemia, tension pneumothorax, or pericardial tamponade.

Epinephrine is the mainstay of drug therapy for cardiac arrest. In high doses, epinephrine causes intense peripheral vasoconstriction, maximizes coronary and cerebral perfusion for any level of chest compression, and promotes resuscitation from experimental asystolic and fibrillatory arrest (10–13). Thus, epinephrine should be given to any patient requiring chest compression to support his or her circulation.

The dose of epinephrine used clinically, one mg every five minutes, is taken directly from experiments involving 10- to 12-kg dogs. It is now known that this dose does not induce a full vasopressor response in humans (14). This has stimulated a controversy over the proper dosing of epinephrine during CPR. Proponents of "high-dose" epinephrine, usually defined as around 10 mg at 5-min intervals, advocate its use on the grounds that the 1-mg dose was selected arbitrarily, that higher doses are known to raise coronary perfusion pressure, and that restoration of spontaneous circulation is related to coronary perfusion pressure. Opponents point out that the heart is more resistant to ischemia than the brain and raise the possibility that high-dose epinephrine may promote the resuscitation of patients who have already sustained severe ischemic brain damage.

Randomized clinical trials will soon characterize the effects of high-dose epinephrine in out-of-hospital arrest but may fail to define its role for inpatient arrests. It seems appropriate to make a distinction between these two patient populations on the basis of time to treatment. Time to treatment is usually long in out-of-hospital arrest, by which time brain damage may have already occurred. In contrast, the early administration of high-dose epinephrine is likely to promote cerebral preservation as well as coronary perfusion.

Until the results of these trials are available, several comments appear to be in order. First, 1 mg of epinephrine should be retained as the initial dose whenever it can be given in the first few minutes of cardiac arrest, because the 1-mg dose often works and higher doses may be dangerous if the patient is resuscitated after only a brief period of arrest. Second, if 1 mg fails to promote resuscitation early in arrest, it is unlikely to do so later, when progressive ischemia and acidosis further depress catecholamine responsiveness. Finally, based on current knowledge, fear that high-doses of epinephrine given late in cardiac arrest will lead to the resuscitation of someone in whom severe brain damage is already established is really another way of saying that severe brain damage is already established. Under such circumstances, resuscitative efforts should be discontinued.

Ventricular Tachyarrhythmias

Ventricular fibrillation and hypotensive ventricular tachycardia rarely respond to drug therapy alone and nearly always respond to a 200-J countershock. Consequently, direct current (DC) countershock is the treatment of choice. It should be applied as quickly as possible and, if unsuccessful, whenever drug therapy is thought to have changed the metabolic or pharmacologic milieu. In practice, countershock is usually repeated 2–4 min after each round of drug treatment.

Drug therapy for ventricular tachyarrhythmias causing cardiac arrest is aimed at maximizing coronary perfusion with epinephrine and promoting defibrillation with antiarrhythmics. Lidocaine is the drug of first choice, but the low cardiac output of CPR necessitates modification of the usual infusion regimen. An initial bolus of 1 mg/kg is followed by 0.5 mg/kg every 8 min up to a total dose of 3 mg/kg. Because hepatic blood flow and, therefore, lidocaine metabolism are negligible during CPR, this regimen provides therapeutic serum levels throughout the arrest.

Lidocaine levels are therapeutic within a few minutes of the first dose with this regimen. If lidocaine does not lead quickly to successful defibrillation, it is reasonable to add a second antiarrhythmic, usually bretylium. There are two justifications for this approach. First, if lidocaine does not by itself promote resuscitation early in the course of an arrest, it is unlikely that it will do so later, when the patient's heart is more ischemic and more acidotic. Second, the onset of action of bretylium is slow. To be most effective, it should be given early. The dose is 5–10 mg/kg, which may be repeated at 10-min intervals up to a total of 25 mg/kg.

Due to the vasodilatory and negative inotropic properties of procainamide solutions, procainamide can be given at a rate of only 20 mg/min. Since the usual intravenous loading dose is 1 g, 50 min would be required to fully load a patient with procainamide. This is obviously unsatisfactory during cardiac arrest.

Amiodarone, 300–500 mg IV at 5- to 10-min intervals, appears to be remarkably effective in refractory ventricular fibrillation and ventricular tachycardia. It is also not yet approved by the Food and Drug Administration for intravenous use.

Propranolol, 0.1 mg/kg IV over 5 min, may be effective when acute myocardial ischemia is thought to have caused the arrest.

Magnesium sulfate given in a 2-g intravenous bolus, may also be effective in patients with ventricular tachyarrhythmias, particularly torsades de pointes (15). Its mechanism is uncertain but may be related to inhibition of calcium entry during ventricular depolarization.

Ventricular tachyarrhythmias may be caused by temporary transvenous pacing wires or by catheter tips which have migrated into the right ventricle. Catheters and pacing wires should be withdrawn to the vena cava if there is any doubt about their position in patients with refractory ventricular tachyarrhythmias.

Asystole

The first goal in the treatment of asystolic arrest is the generation of organized electrical activity. Once this is accomplished, contractile state may be evaluated by palpating pulses and measuring blood pressure.

In high doses, epinephrine probably saturates β_1-receptors and is an extremely powerful positive chronotrope. Because of this property and the peripheral vasoconstrictive effect of high doses of epinephrine, which maximizes coronary perfusion, epinephrine is the drug of choice in asystole. Isoproterenol is no longer recommended because it reduces aortic pressure and may actually abolish coronary perfusion.

Atropine, 1 mg IV at 5- to 10-min intervals up to a total of 2 mg, is also recommended for asystolic arrest. In patients refractory to epinephrine, atropine is rarely if ever successful in restoring cardiac activity. Its administration in this setting is also probably harmless.

If ventricular pacing is to be effective, it should be initiated early in asystolic arrest.

Severe Bradyarrhythmias

Severe bradyarrhythmias, a category which includes slow, pulseless idioventricular rhythms, are treated with epinephrine and vigorous ventilation. The goals of therapy are to increase heart rate and inotropic state. Temporary pacing may be helpful in cases of severe bradycardia with a pulse.

Electromechanical Dissociation

Electromechanical dissociation is characterized by pulselessness or profound hypotension despite a relatively normal heart rate. It is usually the result of end-stage heart disease, sepsis, or overwhelming metabolic derangements. Under these conditions, electromechanical dissociation is almost always fatal. Electromechanical dissociation may also result from hypovolemia, hypoxemia, tension pneumothorax, or pericardial tamponade. Thus, the appropriate treatment of electromechanical dissociation involves the administration of epinephrine and fluids while these causes are being investigated.

MISCELLANEOUS ISSUES IN DRUG THERAPY

Sodium Bicarbonate

Although severe acidosis depresses contractility, the administration of sodium bicarbonate or other alkalinizing agents has not influenced outcome from carefully controlled experimental models of cardiac arrest (16–19). This failure is probably a consequence of low levels of coronary blood flow during CPR and a resulting inability to deliver enough alkalinizing agent to the (metabolically active) myocardium (19). The use of bicarbonate is therefore permitted but not encouraged for arrest victims with metabolic acidosis. Hyperventilation is the preferred treatment.

Calcium

Calcium gluconate and calcium carbonate are moderately potent but short-acting positive inotropes. They do not effect long-term outcome from routine cases of electromechanical dissociation. However, calcium salts may be lifesaving in patients with overdose of calcium channel blockers or severe hyperkalemia. In the latter case, calcium partially antagonizes the membrane effects of potassium.

Route of Drug Administration

The route of drug administration during cardiac arrest is a serious issue. Peak concentration of flow indicators in femoral arterial blood occurs within 1 or 2 min of subclavian or internal jugular venous injection, but not until 5–10 min after peripheral venous injection. If drugs must be given into peripheral veins, they should probably be flushed in with 20 to 30 ml of normal saline or 5% dextrose in water.

OPEN CHEST MASSAGE

Cardiac output is nearly normal during open chest massage and it is likely that many patients who would otherwise die can be revived with this technique (20,21). The disadvantages of open chest massage include the morbidity of emergency thoracotomy and the very real possibility of resuscitating the heart of a patient who has already sustained severe brain damage. This being the case, it seems appropriate to reserve open chest massage for previously healthy arrest victims in whom it is reasonable to presume that the cerebral cortex is still alive. This includes young patients with hypothermic arrest or young patients with witnessed arrest for whom CPR was started promptly but who have failed to respond to initial resuscitative measures.

IS RESUSCITATION WORTHWHILE?

Approximately half of inpatient arrest victims are resuscitated, and about one-third of these (15% overall) survive to hospital discharge. One study reported that 80% of patients surviving to hospital discharge were alive 6 mo later, and that memory was intact in 75% of these patients (22). Outcomes from out-of-hospital arrest vary according to time to provision of CPR, initial rhythm, and time to first attempt to defibrillation. In Seattle, bystander initiation of CPR increased survival to hospital discharge from 21 to 43% and reduced the incidence of gross neurologic deficits from 55 to 4% (23). When paramedics were authorized to defibrillate patients at the scene, as opposed to waiting until arrival in the hospital emergency department, long-term survival increased from 4 to 19% (24). Indeed, the culmination of the massive commitment to basic and advanced cardiac life support in Seattle has been stunning. For witnessed arrests due to ventricular fibrillation with bystander initiation of CPR and arrival of paramedics within 4 min, survival to hospital discharge approaches 70% (25). Seventy-five percent of these survivors were able to return to work, and 49% were alive 4 yr later (26).

Deciding when to terminate resuscitative efforts is often difficult. Patient comorbidity, heart rhythm, and response to treatment all provide guidance on the utility of continuing CPR. The probability of survival is directly proportional to the patient's prearrest life expectancy. Extramyocardial causes of electromechanical dissociation, ventricular tachycardia, and ventricular fibrillation usually respond to therapy. Patients with asystole, pulseless idioventricular rhythms, myocardiogenic electromechanical dissociation, and asystole alternating with ventricular fibrillation seldom respond to therapy; survival to hospital discharge is even more unusual.

Finally, it is extremely difficult to resuscitate normothermic, normovolemic patients who remain in full arrest after 15–20 min of continuous CPR and advanced cardiac life support, and survival with intact neurologic function after more than 30 min of uninterrupted cardiac arrest is truly rare. Thus, it may be appropriate to terminate resuscitative efforts after as little as 10 min in some cases, but to continue for 20 or even 30 min in others.

References

1. Kouwenhoven WB, Jude JR, Knickerbocker GG: Closed-chest cardiac massage. JAMA 1960;73:1064–1067.
2. Rudikoff MT, Maughan WL, Effron M, *et al.*: Mechanisms of blood flow during cardiopulmonary resuscitation. Circulation 1980;61:258–265.

3. Criley JM, Blaufuss AH, Kissel GL: Cough-induced cardiac compression. JAMA 1976;236:1246–1250.
4. Chandra N, Guerci A, Weisfeldt ML, *et al.*: Contrasts between intrathoracic pressures during external chest compression and cardiac massage. Crit Care Med 1981;9:789–792.
5. Niemann JT, Roseborough JR, Hausknecht M, *et al.*: Pressure synchronized cineangiography during experimental cardiopulmonary resuscitation. Circulation 1981;64:985–991.
6. Halperin H, Tsitlik JE, Guerci AD, *et al.*: Determinants of blood flow to vital organs during cardiopulmonary resuscitation in dogs. Circulation 1986;73:539–550.
7. Guerci AD, Halperin HR, Beyar R, *et al.*: Aortic diameter and pressure flow sequence identify mechanism of blood flow during external chest compression in dogs. J Am Coll Cardiol 1989;14:790–798.
8. Maier GW, Tyson GS, Olsen CO, *et al.*: The physiology of external cardiac massage: high impulse cardiopulmonary resuscitation. Circulation 1984;70:86–101.
9. Taylor GJ, Tucker WM, Greene HL, *et al.*: Importance of prolonged compression during cardiopulmonary resuscitation. N Engl J Med 1977;296:1515–1517.
10. Michael JR, Guerci AD, Koehler RC, *et al.*: Mechanisms by which epinephrine augments cerebral and myocardial perfusion during cardiopulmonary resuscitation in dogs. Circulation 1984;69:822–835.
11. Pearson JW, Redding JS: Influence of peripheral vascular tone on cardiac resuscitation. Anesth Analg 1965;44:746–750.
12. Redding JS, Pearson JW: Resuscitation from ventricular fibrillation. Drug therapy. JAMA 1968;203:93–98.
13. Otto CW, Yaleaitis RW, Blitt CD: Mechanism of action of epinephrine in resuscitation from asphyxial arrest. Crit Care Med 1981;9:321–326.
14. Gonzalez ER, Ornato JP, Garnett AR, *et al.*: Dose dependent vasopressor response to epinephrine during CPR in humans. Ann Emerg Med 1989;18:920–926.
15. Tzivoni D, Banai S, Schuger C, *et al.*: Treatment of torsade de pointes with magnesium sulfate. Circulation 1988;77:392–397.
16. Guerci AD, Chandra N, Johnson E, *et al.*: Failure of sodium bicarbonate to improve resuscitation from ventricular fibrillation in dogs. Circulation 1986;74(Suppl IV):IV-75–IV-79.
17. von Planta M, Gudipati C, Weil MH, *et al.*: Effects of tromethamine and sodium bicarbonate buffers during cardiac resuscitation. J Clin Pharmacol 1988;28:594–599.
18. Gazmuri RJ, von Planta M, Weil MH, *et al.*: Cardiac effects of carbon dioxide-consuming and carbon dioxide-generating buffers during cardiopulmonary resuscitation. J Am Coll Cardiol 1990;15:482–490.
19. Kette F, Weil MH, von Planta M, Gazmuri RJ, Rackow EC. Buffer agents do not reverse intramyocardial acidosis during cardiac resuscitation. Circulation 1990;81:1660–1666.
20. Del Guercio LR, Feins NR, Cohn JD, *et al.*: Comparison of blood flow during external and internal cardiac massage in man. Circulation 1965;31 (Suppl I):I-171-I-180.
21. Kern KB, Sanders AB, Badylak SF, *et al.*: Long term survival with open chest cardiac massage after closed chest compression in a canine preparation. Circulation 1987;75:498–503.
22. Bedell SE, Delbanes TL, Cook EF, *et al.*: Survival after cardiopulmonary resuscitation. N Engl J Med 1983;309:569–576.
23. Thompson RG, Hallstrom AP, Cobb LA: Bystander initiated cardiopulmonary resuscitation in the management of ventricular fibrillation. Ann Intern Med 1979;90:737–740.
24. Eisenberg MS, Copass MK, Hallstrom AP, *et al.*: Treatment of out-of-hospital cardiac arrest by emergency medical technicians. N Engl J Med 1980;302:1379–1385.
25. Eisenberg M, Hallstrom A, Bergner L: The ACLS score. Predicting survival from out-of-hospital cardiac arrest. JAMA 1981;246:50–52.
26. DeBard ML: Cardiopulmonary resuscitation. Analysis of six year's experience and review of the literature. Ann Emerg Med 1981;10:408–415.

26

APPROACH TO RESUSCITATION IN THE ELECTROPHYSIOLOGY LABORATORY

Igor Singer, M.B.B.S., F.R.A.C.P., F.A.C.P., F.A.C.C.

Electrophysiologic (EP) studies are associated with minimal mortality and morbidity in experienced centers (1,2), despite the fact that many patients who are referred for EP studies have serious, advanced cardiac dysfunction and many have significant coronary artery disease. Even in young, healthy patients, life-threatening arrhythmias are induced at times to study their mechanisms and evaluate therapeutic options. The safety of EP studies may be enhanced by : (a) continuous monitoring of intra-arterial blood pressure during EP studies (see Chapter 4), (6) immediate availability of defibrillation (by the use of R_2 pads or equivalent), a backup defibrillator in case the first malfunctions, and availability of experienced staff and anesthesia backup support. As interventional techniques, such as catheter ablation, become more widely used for therapy of supraventricular and ventricular tachycardias (VTs), the risk associated with invasive electrophysiologic studies may increase.

Arrhythmias which may result in cardiac arrest include: (a) ventricular fibrillation (VF), (b) VT, (c) atrial fibrillation with rapid antegrade conduction via the accessory tract in Wolff-Parkinson-White (WPW) syndrome, and (d) asystole or extreme bradycardias associated with sick sinus syndrome or complete heart block without an adequate ventricular escape rhythm. Other complications, related to the cardiac catheterization technique per se, may lead to, precipitate or complicate arrhythmia management or result in hemodynamic compromise. These include: (a) profound vasovagal syncope, (b) pericardial tamponade due to catheter perforation of the ventricle or atrium, (c) pneumothorax and (d) acute myocardial ischemia or infarction precipitated by spontaneous or induced tachycardias.

VENTRICULAR FIBRILLATION

Therapy for VF is prompt defibrillation. The defibrillation shock should be administered in asynchronous mode, with the initial energy of 300–360 J (in adults). Although lower energies (e.g., 200 joules) may be effective, the author does not recommend routinely trying lower energies, since delaying an effective shock increases the defibrillation threshold, and if VF is allowed to persist beyond 20–30 sec, later shocks may be less effective (3–7).

Correct placement of R_2 defibrillation pads (R_2 Corp., Skokie, IL) or equivalent, is of paramount importance. It has been shown that lead geometry as well as the surface area of the defibrillation electrodes are important determinants of defibrillation efficacy. Poor lead geometry or inadequate tissue contact may result in unsuccessful defibrillation (8). In general, anteroposterior positioning of the electrodes is optimal (Figs. 26.1 and 26.2). It is imperative that the electrophysiologist personally checks the positioning of the electrodes and connections prior to the EP study. A backup defibrillator should always be on the standby, in the event that the first defibrillator malfunctions (Fig. 26.2).

If the first defibrillation shock is ineffective, the energy should be incremented to the maximum available energy on the second and subsequent shocks. Position of the defibrillation electrodes must be checked quickly and if suboptimal, electrodes should be repositioned prior to the administration of subsequent shocks.

Defibrillation is almost always effective. Factors that may interfere with successful defibrillation include: (a) inadequate energy, (b) inadequate defibrillation electrode positioning, (c) large tissue impedance, (e.g., in obese patients) (9), (d) increase in defibrillation thresholds due to antiarrhythmic drugs, especially type IC (10,11), Type IB (12,13), and amiodarone (chronic administration (14,16), see Chapter 20), and (e) severe electrolyte disturbance, acidosis or ongoing myocardial ischemia.

Administration of epinephrine intravenously has been shown to decrease the defibrillation thresholds (17,18), whereas administration of lidocaine has been demonstrated to increase the defibrillation thresholds in experimental animals (12). In refractory VF, the author would advise rapid intravenous administra-

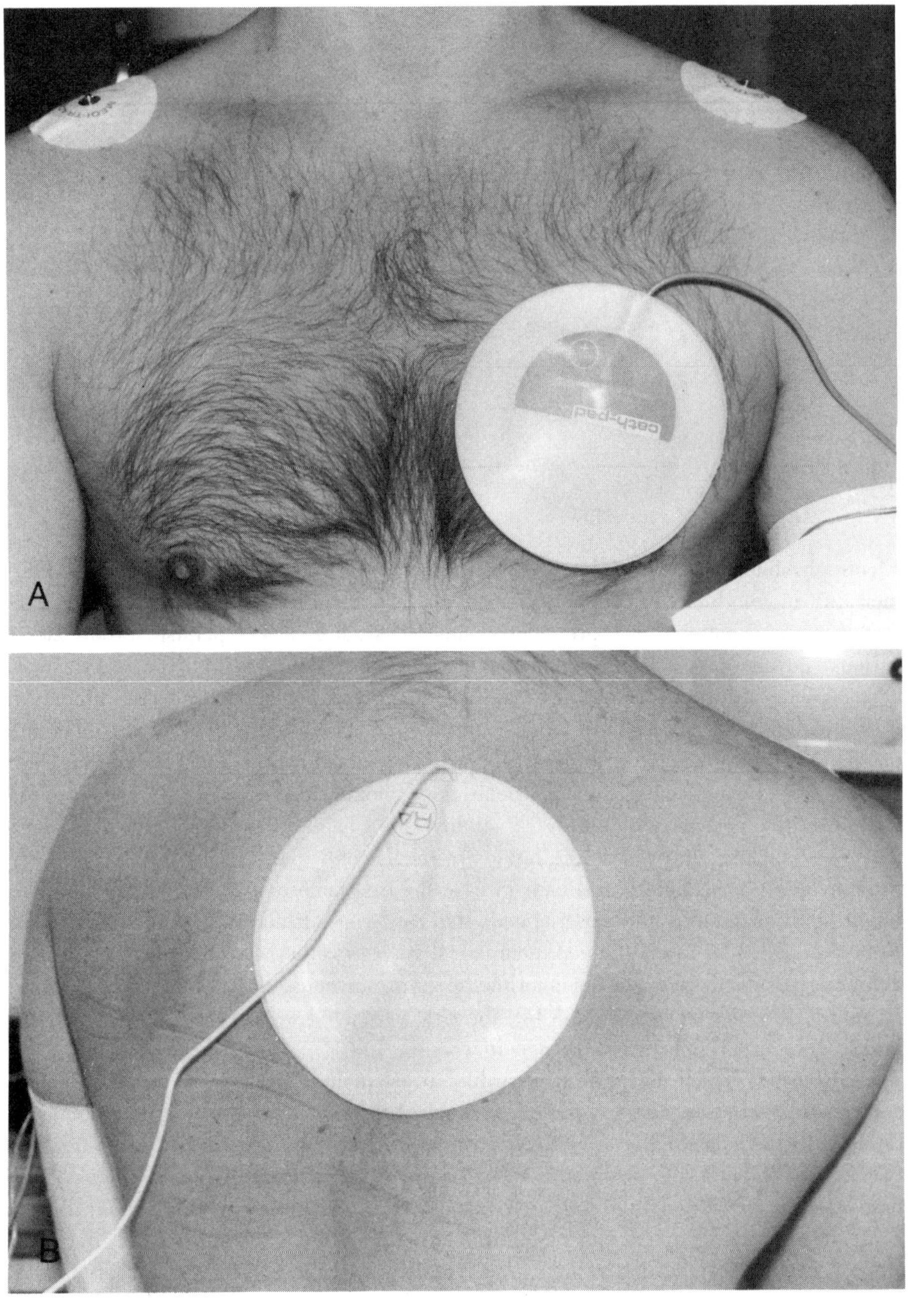

Figure 26.1. Positioning of R_2 defibrillation pads on the chest **(A)** anterior and **(B)** posterior.

tion of epinephrine (1 mg every 5 min) via the central line (femoral or subclavian), initiation of cardiopulmonary resuscitation (CPR) and after 15–20 sec of cardiac compression, repeat defibrillation. Epinephrine is beneficial during resuscitation by causing peripheral vasoconstriction, thereby maximizing coronary and cerebral perfusion, as well as by lowering the defibrillation thresholds (18–20). In the author's experience, in the rare case where VF does not respond promptly to defibrillation, epinephrine facilitates subsequent defibrillation (personal observation).

The role of lidocaine in VF is controversial. Although the standard CPR protocol (see Chapter 25) recommends the use of lidocaine during CPR, Type IB drugs have been shown to increase defibrillation thresholds in experimental animals (12). In recurrent VF secondary to long-QT syndrome, or due to ischemia, lidocaine may be helpful.

Amiodarone 300–500 mg IV at 5 to 10 min intervals has also been shown to be effective in "chemical" defibrillation (21). This drug is currently not approved by the Food and Drug Administration (FDA) for this indication, but may be available to some investigators under specific investigational protocols.

Sedation of the patient is appropriate when VF is expected (e.g., during implantable cardioverter/defibrillator (ICD) testing) or after defibrillation to allay the anxiety and induce amne-

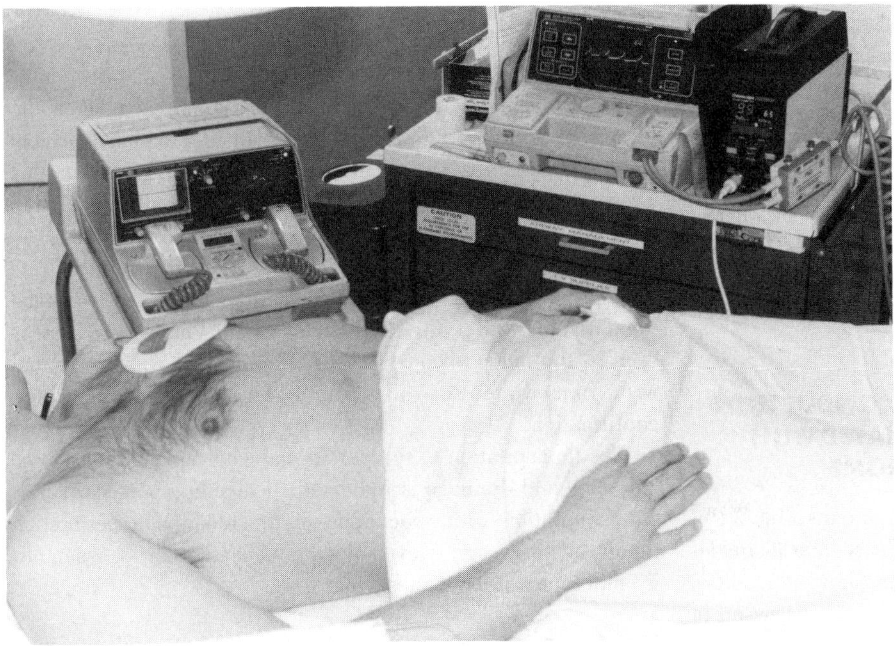

Figure 26.2. Defibrillation pads are connected on line to the defibrillator **(right)**. A back up defibrillator **(left)** is available in case of defibrillator malfunction.

sia for the event. We generally use the short-acting drug midazolam hydrochloride (Versed) 1–5 mg IV. This may be combined with intravenous morphine sulfate (2–4 mg IV) or Demerol (25 mg IV) for added analgesic effect. Respiratory depression or confusion may be undesirable side effects and patients should be carefully monitored during the drug administration.

VENTRICULAR TACHYCARDIA

Induction of VT is common in the electrophysiology laboratory and is in fact an endpoint for programmed ventricular stimulation (see Chapters 4 and 8). Methods for induction and termination of VT are discussed in Chapters 2, 4, and 8. In most cases, if VT is monomorphic, blood pressure stable and tissue perfusion adequate, antitachycardia pacing, programmed ventricular stimulation or overdrive (burst) pacing are usually successful in terminating VT. However, when VT is rapid (cycle length <250 msec), polymorphic or associated with significant hypotension and systemic hypoperfusion, immediate cardioversion is required. Although energies of 100 J or less are often effective for VT termination, we routinely start with 200 J, since a theoretical advantage of using less energy is outweighed by the need to restore stable rhythm and adequate perfusion rapidly. Discomfort to the patient is not significantly reduced with lesser energies (e.g., a 100-J shock may be as unpleasant to the patient as a 200-J shock). Caveats with respect to sedation are the same as for VF.

Ventricular tachycardia may deteriorate to VF with antitachycardia pacing. The frequency with which this occurs depends on the aggressivity of the pacing protocol (it is more likely to occur with multiple extrastimuli, rapid ventricular pacing, and decremental protocols—see also Chapter 21).

Occasionally, VT does not terminate with programmed ventricular stimulation, antitachycardia pacing, or cardioversion. This situation is occasionally encountered due to proarrhythmic effects of the antiarrhythmic drugs. Horowitz, *et al.* reported a 3% incidence of severe proarrhythmic responses due to antiarrhythmic therapy in 397 patients undergoing EP studies for ventricular tachyarrhythmias (2).

In this setting, VT may result in significant hypotension and may lead to intractable heart failure and death. In this situation, supportive measures consisting of volume expansion to maintain preload and pressors (dobutamine or dopamine) in judicious doses may be required. Rarely, we have resorted to catheter ablation in this situation.

A special emergency is presented by incessant ventricular tachycardia refractory to antiarrhythmic therapy with steadily deteriorating hemodynamic picture. In this situation, the author recommends consideration of catheter ablation guided by endocardial mapping. Surgical intervention, using intraoperative endocardial mapping and subendocardial resection, cryoablation, or laser-assisted endocardial fulguration is another alternative in patients who are otherwise operative candidates. Intraaortic balloon pump or percutaneous cardiopulmonary bypass may be useful in this situation to support the patient during catheter ablation and mapping.

The role of antiarrhythmic drug therapy for VT is discussed in Chapters 4, 8, 10, and 11. Antiarrhythmic drugs are rarely used in the EP laboratory to terminate ventricular tachycardia. This is so, because administration of antiarrhythmic drugs alters the "baseline state" and interferes with subsequent EP testing. Furthermore, most reentrant arrhythmias are either amenable to overdrive (burst) pacing or may be terminated by cardioversion. When the baseline programmed ventricular stimulation protocol is completed, antiarrhythmic drugs are routinely tested for therapy of VT in a sequential manner. Usually Type IA drugs (procainamide or quinidine) are tested first, followed by Type IB drugs (lidocaine or mexiletene) or Type III drugs (amiodarone) on subsequent studies. Infusions of antiarrhythmic drugs are appropriate if VT recurs spontaneously after electrical cardioversion or if it cannot be readily terminated by burst pacing and the patient becomes hemodynamically unstable. This situation may arise if the mechanism of VT is not reentry, e.g., it is due to abnormal automaticity, or is enhanced by ischemia or catecholamine stimulation (anxiety, stress or β-adrenergic drug administration).

ATRIAL FIBRILLATION WITH RAPID CONDUCTION VIA THE ACCESSORY TRACT ASSOCIATED WITH WOLFF-PARKINSON-WHITE SYNDROME

Rapid conduction via the accessory tract in patients with WPW syndrome may result in hemodynamic collapse due to inadequate ventricular filling (due to shortened diastole) and result in ventricular fibrillation. This subject is extensively discussed in Chapter 9.

Hemodynamic collapse due to extremely rapid ventricular rates or VF is treated by prompt cardioversion/defibrillation. Recurrence of atrial fibrillation immediately after cardioversion, with subsequent deterioration to VF, is uncommon. If it occurs, however, infusion of intravenous procainamide (15–20 mg/kg body/weight) with a maintenance dose of 20–50 μg/kg/min may be followed by a repeat attempt at cardioversion. Often atrial fibrillation will terminate spontaneously with procainamide infusion, rendering repeat cardioversion unnecessary.

Asystole

Asystole is rare in the electrophysiology laboratory. It is precluded by the ready availability of ventricular, atrial, and atrioventricular synchronous pacing. With right atrial and ventricular pacing catheters, pacing may be initiated within seconds of the onset of asystole or extreme sinus bradycardia.

Patients with chronotropic incompetence, severe sinus node disease or patients with vasovagal syncope may have profound bradycardias associated with hypotension. The therapy for bradyarrhythmias is pacing, which is readily available in the electrophysiology laboratory. In patients with vasovagal syncope, administration of atropine 1–1.5 mg IV is necessary since the vasodepressor component of syncope does not respond to pacing alone. Rapid volume expansion with 0.9% normal saline may also be required.

OTHER CAUSES OF HEMODYNAMIC COLLAPSE IN THE ELECTROPHYSIOLOGY LABORATORY

Other complications arising from the cardiac catheterization may cause, contribute to, or initiate hemodynamic deterioration, exacerbate hypotension, and cause death. These complications must be diagnosed promptly and treated expeditiously.

Pericardial Tamponade

Catheter placement for EP studies is rarely complicated by perforation of the cardiac chambers or pericardial tamponade. Most ventricular perforations do not result in tamponade except when the patient is anticoagulated. However, atrial perforation almost always leads to tamponade, since the atrial tissue is thin and relatively inelastic. Tamponade is usually heralded by substernal chest pain, anxiety, and increased respiratory rate and is followed by tachycardia, hypotension, and engorged jugular veins with positive Kussmaul's sign. Pulsus paradoxus is seen in the more advanced cases. Rapid diagnosis is essential with immediate two-dimensional (2D) echocardiographic confirmation.

Needle aspiration of the pericardial sack under fluoroscopic guidance and drainage is indicated. If bleeding persists, surgical exploration with evacuation of the blood and perforation repair is necessary. Reversal of anticoagulation is essential. Prompt intervention is lifesaving.

Pneumothorax

Placement of subclavian or internal jugular sheaths and catheters may be complicated by pneumothorax. This is also a possible complication of permanent pacemaker implantation, when subclavian vein puncture is used for lead placement.

Pneumothorax may be small and unrecognized. Therefore, whenever the central veins are cannulated during EP study or pacemaker placement, it is a good clinical practice to obtain chest x-ray after the procedure, to exclude that possibility. A large pneumothorax, particularly a tension pneumothorax, may result in hemodynamic collapse. Signs of pneumothorax are usually cough (due to pleural irritation), followed by dyspnea and hypotension (tension pneumothorax), deteriorating arterial saturation, tachypnea, anxiety, and eventually confusion and restlessness secondary to hypoxemia and cerebral hypoperfusion.

Diagnosis is confirmed by fluoroscopy. The collapsed lung is readily apparent ipsilateral to the needle puncture. If tension pneumothorax is present, it is a true emergency which should be handled by an immediate chest tube insertion or if not immediately available, needle decompression of the pleural space (16-gauge needle). Hypotension and hypoxemia may trigger VT or VF. Therefore, prompt intervention is mandatory.

Acute Ischemia or Myocardial Infarction

Patients with severe coronary artery disease may develop ischemia during the course of an EP study due to pacing, sympathetic stimulation, or induced tachycardias, which increase oxygen utilization and impair coronary perfusion.

The approach to therapy is the same as conventionally employed and includes: (a) termination of the precipitating cause, e.g., tachycardia, (b) reversal of ischemia with intravenous or sublingual nitroglycerin, beta-blocking drugs, and other supportive measures. Ischemia is usually readily reversible and self-limiting. In our experience, ischemia is rarely a consequence of EP studies in appropriately selected patients.

CONCLUSION

Despite the invasive nature of EP studies, adverse and fatal complications are extremely uncommon. In laboratories where the experience is extensive, low complication rates have been reported (1,2). It should be emphasized that the safety of EP studies is enhanced by adequate patient assessment and preparation, adequate supportive measures, availability of trained electrophysiology personnel, and meticulous quality control.

References

1. Horowitz LN: Safety of electrophysiologic studies. Circulation (Suppl) 1986;73:28.
2. Horowitz LN, Kay HR, Kutalek SP, *et al.*: Risks and complications of clinical electrophysiologic studies: a prospective analysis of 1,000 consecutive patients. J Am Coll Cardiol 1987;9:1261–1268.
3. Echt DS, Barbey JT, Black NJ: Influence of ventricular fibrillation duration on defibrillation energy in dogs using bidirectional pulse discharges. PACE 1988;11:1315–1323.
4. Fujimura C, Jones DL, Klein GJ: Effects of time to defibrillation and subthreshold preshocks on defibrillation success in pigs. PACE 1989;12:358–365.
5. Jones JL, Swartz JF, Jones RE, *et al.*: Increasing fibrillation duration enhances relative asymmetrical biphasic versus monophasic defibrillator waveform efficacy. Circ Res 1990;67:376–384.
6. Bardy GH, Ivey TD, Allen M, *et al.*: A prospective, randomized evaluation of effect of ventricular fibrillation duration on defibrillation thresholds in humans. J Am Coll Cardiol 1989;13:1362–1366.
7. Bardy GH, Ivey TD, Johnson G, *et al.*: Prospective evaluation of initially ineffective defibrillation pulses on subsequent defibrillation success during ventricular fibrillation in survivors of cardiac arrest. Am J Cardiol 1988;62:718–722.
8. Lerman BB, Deale OC: Effects of epicardial patch electrodes on transthoracic defibrillation. Circulation 1990;81:1409–1414.
9. Singer I, Lang D: Defibrillation threshold: clinical utility and therapeutic implications. PACE 1992;15:932–949.
10. Fain ES, Dorian P, Davy JM, *et al.*: Effects of encainide and its metabolites on energy requirements for defibrillation. Circulation 1986;73:1334–1341.
11. Reiffel JA, Coromilas J, Zimmerman JM, *et al.*: Drug-device interactions: clinical considerations. PACE 1985;8:369–373.
12. Dorian P, Fain ES, Davy JM, *et al.*: Lidocaine causes a reversible, concentration-dependent increase in defibrillation energy requirements. J Am Coll Cardiol 1986;8:327–332.
13. Marinchak RA, Friehling TD, Line RA, *et al.*: Effect of antiarrhythmic drugs on defibrillation threshold: case report of an adverse effect of Mexiletene and review of the literature. PACE 1988;11:7–12.
14. Fogoros RN: Amiodarone-induced refractoriness to cardioversion. Ann Intern Med 1984;100:699.
15. Guarnieri T, Levine JH, Veltri EP: Success of chronic defibrillation and the role of antiarrhythmic drugs with the automatic implantable cardioverter/defibrillator. Am J Cardiol 1987;60:1061–1064.
16. Haberman RJ, Veltri EP, Mower MM: The effect of amiodarone on defibrillation threshold. J Electrophysiol 1988;2(5)415–423.
17. Ruffy R, Schechtuan K, Moaje E, *et al.*: β-adrenergic modulation of direct defibrillation energy in anesthetized dog heart. Am J Physiol 1985;248(17):H674–H677.
18. Ruffy R, Monje E, Schechtman K: Facilitation of cardiac defibrillation by aminophylline in the conscious, closed-chest dog. J Electrophysiol 1988;2(6)450–454.
19. Michael JR, Guerci AD, Koehler RC, *et al.*: Mechanisms by which epinephrine augments cerebral and myocardial perfusion during cardiopulmonary resuscitation in dogs. Circulation 1984;69:822–835.
20. Otto CW, Yaleaitis RW, Blitt CD: Mechanism of action of epinephrine in resuscitation from asphyxial arrest. Crit Care Med 1981;9:321–326.
21. Kentsch M, Kunze KP Bleifeld W: Effect of intravenous amiodarone on ventricular fibrillation during out-of-hospital cardiac arrest (Abstract). J Am Coll Cardiol 1986;7:82.

INDEX

Page numbers in *italics* denote figures; those followed by "t" denote tables.